Fourth Edition

IRVING GLICKMAN, B.S., D.M.D., F.A.C.D., F.I.C.D.

Late Professor and Chairman of the Department of Periodontology and
Research Professor of Oral Pathology, Tufts University School of
Dental Medicine; Chief of Periodontology Service, New England Medical
Center Hospitals; Consultant in Periodontology, Forsyth Dental
Center, Boston, Massachusetts; Consultant to the Armed Forces Institute
of Pathology, Washington, D.C.

ILLUSTRATED WITH 942 FIGURES

Clinical
Periodontology

PREVENTION, DIAGNOSIS AND TREATMENT OF
PERIODONTAL DISEASE IN THE
PRACTICE OF GENERAL DENTISTRY

W. B. SAUNDERS COMPANY · PHILADELPHIA · LONDON · TORONTO

W. B. Saunders Company: West Washington Square
Philadelphia, PA 19105

1 St. Anne's Road
Eastbourne, East Sussex BN21 3UN, England

1 Goldthorne Avenue
Toronto, Ontario M8Z 5T9, Canada

Listed here is the latest translated edition of this book, together with the
language of the translation and the publisher.
French (4th Edition)—Julian Prelat, Paris, France
Italian (2nd Edition)—Editrice Scientifica, Milan, Italy
Spanish (3rd Edition)—Editorial Mundi, Buenos Aires, Argentina
Spanish (4th Edition)—NEISA, Mexico City, Mexico

Clinical Periodontology   ISBN 0-7216-4137-7

Print No.   9   8   7

To my wife,
Violeta
and to my children, Alan and Denise

Preface
to the Fourth Edition

There have been many important advances in periodontics since the third edition of this book. The emphasis has shifted dramatically to prevention; the goals of treatment have been expanded to include the reconstruction of tissues destroyed by disease, while at the same time there has been a revival of the simpler treatment procedures. The role of dental plaque in the etiology of periodontal disease has been extensively documented, and scientists are busily seeking plaque and calculus preventives. Increased awareness of the importance of occlusion in the preservation of periodontal health has added a challenging new dimension to periodontal practice.

Most important of all, a new aura of social responsibility pervades the periodontal field. The already overwhelming backlog of untreated periodontal disease continues to grow more rapidly than it can be coped with. Every effort is being made to alert the public to its stake in the periodontal problem, and to develop universally applicable simple preventive measures and broaden the manpower base capable of providing effective treatment.

This edition reflects these changes and others yet to come. It contains an entirely new section on Preventive Periodontics; new chapters on Dental Plaque, Acquired Pellicle and Calculus; and on Microorganisms in the Etiology of Gingival and Periodontal Disease. The chapters on Occlusion and Occlusal Adjustment have been rewritten, drawing upon the author's electronic telemetric studies of the functioning dentition. There is a new expanded chapter on Muco-gingival and Reconstructive Surgery, extensively illustrated to demonstrate how each procedure is performed. The Treatment of Infrabony Pockets has been re-written to include the newest clinical developments using bone and marrow im-plants. All other chapters have been brought up to date and carefully annotated with the most recent clinical and laboratory research developments.

I have drawn upon international and diversified sources to continue the use-fulness and preserve the objectivity of this book. A revision of this magnitude is impossible without colleagues and friends who give generously of their time and material. The assistance of the following of my colleagues is acknowledged with appreciation: Kenneth Berman, Sol Bernick, Edward Cohen, Milton Dines, Samuel Dreizen, Neville Gilmore, Abraham Haddad, Mark Hirsh, Claude Ibbott, Shail Kuba, William Less, Mayer Liebman, Max Listgarten, Noshir Mehta, Abraham Nizel, Benjamin Patur, Stanley Ross, Max Schmidt, Knut Selvig, Samuel Turesky and Michael Weissman.

I am indebted to Jerome B. Smulow, who collaborated with me in the development of many of the concepts presented in this book; to Lydia C. Pitzi and Ann Marie Previti for their untiring secretarial assistance; to Rachel Hill, who prepared the microscopic material; to Leo Goodman and Harry W. Maskell for their excellent photography; and to Robert H. Ullrich, Jr., medical artist, for his skillfully executed, explicit illustrations.

Special appreciation goes to Janice El Qudsi for organizing the illustrations and checking the accuracy of the references; and to my friends at the W. B. Saunders Company for the expertise with which they prepared this beautiful edition.

IRVING GLICKMAN
Boston, Massachusetts

Preface
to the First Edition

This is a textbook for practitioners of general dentistry and students preparing to be general practitioners. It was the author's desire to create an analytical text, fostered by a critical objectivity. An effort has been made to differentiate between fact and unsubstantiated hypothesis. This constitutes a challenge, especially when it means parting with tradition. However, difficult though it may be, it is sometimes necessary to guard against the hampering influence of habit which tends to nudge us along the well travelled pathways of thought.

This book is predicated on the premise that the periodontal care of the American public is primarily the concern of the practitioner of general dentistry. The establishment of periodontia as a specialty should be a stimulus for improved periodontal care by the general practitioner. The existence of a group of dentists who desire to limit their practices or specialize in periodontia cannot be hailed as a sign that the obligation of the general practitioner in regard to periodontal problems is diminished. If anything, the opposite is true. The existence of individuals with a primary interest in cardiology who limit their practices accordingly has not meant that medical schools have diminished their teaching of the anatomy and physiology of the heart and the diagnosis and management of cardiac dysfunction—or that practitioners of general medicine have discarded their stethoscopes.

The need for training the general practitioner so that he can fulfill his responsibility to provide periodontal care for all his patients has stimulated a reorientation in the philosophy of dental education and intensification in the teaching of periodontology at both the undergraduate and postgraduate levels. The general practitioner should know enough to handle most periodontal problems which confront him. The availability of a well-trained group of specialists for unusual problems should serve to supplement the dental care available to our population. The establishment of periodontia as a specialty and continued improvement in the ability of the general practitioner to cope with periodontal problems are interdependent movements—mutually dependent upon each other for continued stimulation and progress.

Much information is available regarding the nature of periodontal disease and its treatment. Many problems are as yet unsolved. The existing status of knowledge does not warrant an attitude of complacency. On the other hand, a sizable accumulation of knowledge has resulted from the industry of clinicians and research workers. A considerable portion of this information is applicable in the practice of dentistry. It is the purpose of this textbook to present existing knowledge regarding periodontal problems in such a manner that it can be incorporated in the practice of general dentistry. It was planned with the following objectives in mind:

> The application of basic principles of periodontology in the prevention, diagnosis and treatment of periodontal disease.

> An appreciation of the extent to which the initiation of periodontal disease and tooth loss from pathological destruction of the periodontal tissues can be prevented.

> An evaluation of the interrelation of local and systemic factors in the causation of periodontal disease.

> An appreciation of the effect of treatment procedures upon the tissue changes underlying clinical disease.

> The presentation of treatment techniques that can be performed with the degree of skill possessed by every qualified practitioner of general dentistry.

> An explanation of the application of various treatment techniques to specific clinical periodontal problems.

> The clarification of the interrelation of clinical periodontal procedures with the other aspects of general dentistry.

It has been the experience of the author that the type of preparation which dental students and dentists engaged in graduate and postgraduate training find most useful in the clinical management of periodontal problems is an understanding of clinical phenomena in terms of underlying tissue changes. All clinical periodontal problems are basically gross expressions of microscopic tissue changes. The microscopic changes underlying clinical periodontal disease are essentially manifestations of the composite effects of disease-causing factors. The effectiveness of treatment procedures is reflected in terms of microscopic tissue changes. It is understandable why the interpretation of clinical phenomena in terms of tissue changes is of such practical value in the periodontal field. Crystallization of the clinical management of periodontal problems in terms of microscopic tissue changes is therefore the keynote of this book.

Terminology in the periodontal field is still in a somewhat unsettled state. Conscientious efforts are in progress to clarify this situation. Disagreement over terminology tends to divert attention from more basic considerations. Emphasis is therefore placed upon the explanation of the nature of various conditions, rather than upon the terms by which they are designated. Recommendations of the Terminology Committee of the American Academy of Periodontology which appeared in the Journal of Periodontology in nineteen hundred and fifty are presented and indicated in italics.

IRVING GLICKMAN

Boston, Massachusetts

Contents

PART IV.   CLASSIFICATION OF GINGIVAL AND
                    PERIODONTAL DISEASE

*Section Three.   The Prevention of Gingival and
                          Periodontal Disease*

*Section Four.   The Treatment of Gingival and
                        Periodontal Disease*

PART I.   DIAGNOSIS; DETERMINATION OF THE PROGNOSIS;
                  THE TREATMENT PLAN

Introduction

THE HISTORICAL BACKGROUND OF PERIODONTOLOGY*

THE PAST

Periodontal disease is a major problem in modern dental practice. Paleopathological studies indicate that man has been subject to periodontal disease since prehistoric times, and our earliest historical records reveal an awareness of periodontal disease and the need for treating it.

Periodontal disease was the commonest of all diseases of which there was evidence in the embalmed bodies of the **Egyptians** of 4000 years ago.[6] Much of the present-day knowledge of Egyptian medicine comes from the Ebers and Edwin Smith Surgical Papyri.[1] The Ebers papyrus contains many references to gingival disease and prescriptions for strengthening the teeth, and also makes mention of specialists in the care of the teeth.

Oral hygiene was practiced by the **Sumerians** of 3000 B.C., and elaborately decorated **golden toothpicks** found in the excavations at Ur in Mesopotamia suggest an interest in cleanliness of the mouth.[7] The **Babylonians** and **Assyrians** following the earlier Sumerian civilization apparently suffered from periodontal conditions, and a clay tablet of the period tells of treatment by gingival massage combined with various herbal medications. Medicinal mouthwashes were also used, and Jastrow[4] refers to a tablet where six different drugs are suggested for the treatment of "sickness of the mouth," presumably periodontal disease.

In the oldest known **Chinese** medical work, written about 2500 B.C. by **Hwang-Fi,** oral disease is divided into three types, as follows: (1) Fong Ya or inflammatory condi-

tions. (2) Ya Kon or diseases of the soft investing tissues of the teeth. (3) Chong Ya or dental caries.[7] Gingival inflammations, periodontal abscesses and gingival ulcerations are described in accurate detail. One gingival condition is described as follows: "The gingivae are pale or violet red, hard and lumpy, sometimes bleeding; the toothache is continuous." Herbal remedies, "Zn-hine-tong," are mentioned for the treatment of these conditions. The Chinese were among the earliest people to use the "chew stick" as a **toothpick and toothbrush** to clean the teeth and massage the gingival tissues.

The importance of oral hygiene was recognized by the early **Hebrews.** Many pathologic conditions of the teeth and their surrounding structures are described in the Talmudic writings. Vestiges of the **Phoenician civilization** include a specimen of **wire splinting** apparently constructed to stabilize teeth loosened by chronic destructive periodontal disease.

Among the ancient **Greeks, Hippocrates of Cos (460–335 B.C.)** was the father of modern medicine, the first to institute a systematic examination of the patient's pulse, temperature, respiration, excreta, sputum, and pains. He discussed the function and eruption of the teeth and also the etiology of periodontal disease. He believed that inflammation of the gums could be produced by accumulations of pituita or calculus with gingival hemorrhage occurring in cases of persistent disease. He described different varieties of splenic

---

*Periodontology is the *science and study of the periodontium and periodontal disease.*

maladies, to one of which he assigned the following symptoms: "The belly becomes swollen, the spleen enlarged and hard, the patient suffers from acute pain. The gums are detached from the teeth and smell bad."[7]

The **Etruscans**, much before 735 B.C., were adept in the art of constructing artificial dentures, but there is no evidence of their awareness of the existence of periodontal disease or its treatment.

Among the **Romans, Aulus Cornelius Celsus (first century A.D.)** referred to diseases which affect the soft parts of the mouth and their treatment as follows: "If the gums separate from the teeth, it is beneficial to chew unripe pears and apples and keep their juices in the mouth." He described looseness of the teeth caused by the weakness of their roots or by flaccidity of the gums and noted that in these cases it is necessary to touch the gums lightly with a red hot iron and then smear them with honey. The Romans were very interested in oral hygiene. Celsus believed that stains on the teeth should first be removed and the teeth then rubbed with a **dentifrice**. The use of the **toothbrush** is mentioned in the writings of many of the Roman poets. Gingival massage was an integral part of oral hygiene. **Paul of Aegina** during the seventh century differentiated between epulis, a fleshy excrescence of gums in the neighborhood of a tooth, and parulis, which he described as an abscess of the gums. He wrote that tartar incrustations must be removed either with scrapers or a small file, and that the teeth should be carefully cleansed after the last meal of the day.

Rhazes (850–923), an Arabian of the Middle Ages, recommended opium, oil of roses, and honey in the treatment of periodontal disease. To strengthen loosened teeth he recommended **astringent mouth washes and dentifrice powders**. He described a procedure of scarification of the gingiva, and strong counterirritants in the treatment of disease of the gums. A voluminous writer, he has seven chapters in his "Al-Fakkir" on the teeth. They are entitled, *The Teeth, Teeth on Edge, Decay of the Teeth, Looseness of the Gums, Suppuration of the Gums, Pyorrhea* and *Bleeding Gums, and Halitosis.* **Avicenna (980–1037)** discussed the filing of elongated teeth and reported that "in order to have loosened teeth become firm again, one must avoid using same in mastication." He wrote extensively on diseases of the gingiva such as ulcers, suppuration, recession and fissures.

Albucasis (936–1013) stressed the care and treatment of the supporting structures. He recognized an interrelation between tartar and disease of the gums. Albucasis referred to the treatment of periodontal disease as follows:[3] **"Sometimes on the surface of the teeth, both inside and outside, as well as under the gums, are deposited rough scales, of ugly appearance, and black, green or yellow in colour; thus corruption is communicated to the gums, and so the teeth are in the process of time denuded. It is necessary for thee to lay the patient's head upon thy lap and to scrape the teeth and molars, on which are observed either true incrustations, or something similar to sand, and this until nothing more remains of such substance, and until also the dirty colour of the teeth disappears, be it black or green, or yellowish, or of any other colour. If a first scraping is sufficient, so much the better; if not, thou shalt repeat it on the following day, or even on the third or fourth day, until the desired purpose is obtained. Thou must know however, that the teeth need scrapers of various shapes and figures, on account of the very nature of this operation. In fact the scalpel with which the teeth must be scraped on the inside, is unlike that with which thou shalt scrape the outside; and that with which thou shalt scrape the interstices between the teeth shall likewise have another shape. Therefore thou must have all this series of scalpels ready if so it pleases God."**

A set of instruments was designed by Albucasis for scaling the teeth. These instruments were crude but their role in the heritage of the modern periodontal instrumentarium is quite apparent.

In the fifteenth century, **Valescus of Montpellier (1382–1417)** stated that in order to treat disease of the gums tartar must be removed little by little either with iron instruments or with dentifrices. In the fourteenth and fifteenth centuries reference is also made to white wine, roasted salt and aromatic substances as adjuncts in periodontal therapy.

Bartholomeus Eustachius, in a book published in **Venice (1563),** explained the firmness of teeth in the jaws as follows: "There exists besides a very strong ligament, principally attached to the roots by which these latter are tightly connected with the alveoli." The gums also contribute to their firmness, and here he compares it to the joining of the skin to the finger nails.

With the beginning of the eighteenth century dentistry developed the early signs of scientific curiosity which were the precursors of present-day research disciplines. **Pierre Fauchard (1678–1761)**, the father of modern dentistry, in the first and second editions of his epochal treatise *"Le Chirurgien Dentiste"* discussed many aspects of the subject of periodontology. He described chronic periodontal disease as a "kind of scurvy" which attacked the gums, the alveoli and the teeth. The clinical acuity of the observation of Fauchard is shown by his statement, **"Not only are the gums affected by it (periodontal disease) which are livid, swollen, and inflamed, but those which do not show these symptoms as yet are not immune from this affliction. It is recognized by a yellowish almost white pus and by a little glutinous material which is emitted from the gums when a rather heavy pressure is applied by the finger."*** Fauchard believed that internal remedies were not effective in treating periodontal disease. He recommended careful scaling of the teeth to remove the calculus deposits, and he developed many instruments for this purpose; dentifrices, mouthwashes and splinting of loose teeth were included in his therapeutic procedures.

John Hunter, the eighteenth century English physiologist and surgeon, published two books on dentistry in which he discussed diseases of the alveolar process which he believed to be the site of suppurative periodontal disease. The nineteenth century brought new names and developments to the periodontal field, such as **Kunstmann** and his surgical measures for the treatment of periodontal disease, and **Robiscek** and the "flap operation." **John M. Riggs,** the first of many North American contributors, was credited by his contemporaries with "originating and first publicly describing a new treatment for the cure of . . . absorption of the alveolar process . . . thereby saving and restoring to firmness the loosened teeth." His treatment consisted of **subgingival curettage.** He described periodontal disease in detail, and chronic

destructive disease of the supporting tissues was for many years called "Riggs' disease."[5]

With the beginning of the twentieth century there developed a prolific group of clinicians and scientists throughout the world with a major interest in the periodontal field. Their names and contributions are documented throughout the pages of this book. Dentists and members of allied fields are now organized in societies devoted to further knowledge in periodontology, and worldwide interchange of ideas regarding periodontal problems is fostered by journals and international meetings.

PRESENT-DAY PERIODONTICS IN THE PRACTICE OF DENTISTRY

Before undertaking a detailed study of periodontal disease, it is important to have a proper perspective regarding the role of periodontics* in the practice of dentistry.

Periodontal disease is the major cause of tooth loss in adults, and for many years periodontics was thought of as a conglomeration of treatment techniques for the purpose of trying to save teeth suffering from advanced disease.

It gradually became apparent that the periodontal disease which caused the tooth loss in adults was the terminal stage of processes which started, but were untreated, in youth. Attention shifted to early treatment because it is simpler, produces more predictable results and spares the patient unnecessary loss of tooth-supporting tissues.

Today the emphasis is upon preventing periodontal disease, because most periodontal disease is preventable. No longer confirmed within the limitations of an autonomous branch of dentistry, periodontics has become a philosophy underlying all dental practice.

Every dental procedure is performed with concern for its effect upon the periodontium, and effective chairside measures for preventing periodontal disease are part of the total dental care of all patients. In addition, educational programs are being developed to alert the public to the impor-

---

*Darby, quoted in Weinberger.[7]

*Periodontics is the branch of dentistry that deals with the science and treatment of periodontal diseases. Synonym: periodontia.

tance of periodontal disease and to motivate them to take advantage of available methods of preventing it. **The priority of periodontics in the practice of dentistry has shifted from repairing damage done by preventable disease to keeping healthy mouths healthy.**[2]

REFERENCES

1. Castiglione, A.: History of Medicine. 2nd ed. New York, Alfred A. Knopf, 1941.

2. Glickman, I.: Preventive Periodontics — A Blueprint for the Periodontal Health of the American Public. J. Periodont., 38:361, 1967.

3. Guerini, V.: History of Dentistry. Philadelphia, Lea & Febiger, 1909.

4. Jastrow, N.: The Medicine of the Babylonians and Assyrians. Proc. Soc. Med., London, 7:109, 1914.

5. Merritt, A. H.: The Historical Background of Periodontology. J. Periodont., 10:7, 1939.

6. Ruffer, M. A.: Studies in the Palaeopathology of Egypt. Chicago, University of Chicago Press, 1921.

7. Weinberger, B. W.: An Introduction to the History of Dentistry. St. Louis, C. V. Mosby, 1948.

Section One • The Tissues of the Periodontium

The periodontium is the investing and supporting tissues of the tooth, and consists of the *periodontal ligament,* the *gingiva, cementum* and *alveolar bone.* The cementum is considered a part of the periodontium because, with the bone, it serves as the support for the fibers of the periodontal ligament. The periodontium is subject to morphologic and functional variations as well as changes with age. This section deals with the normal features of the tissues of the periodontium, knowledge of which is necessary for an understanding of periodontal disease.

Chapter 1

THE GINGIVA

The *oral mucosa* consists of the following three zones: the gingiva and the covering of the hard palate, termed the masticatory mucosa; the dorsum of the tongue, covered by specialized mucosa; and the remainder of the oral mucous membrane. The *gingiva* is that part of the oral mucous membrane that covers the alveolar processes of the jaws and surrounds the necks of the teeth.

NORMAL CLINICAL FEATURES

The gingiva is divided into the marginal, attached and interdental areas.

The marginal gingiva (unattached gingiva)

The marginal gingiva is the unattached gingiva surrounding the teeth in collar-like fashion (Fig. 1–1) and demarcated from the adjacent attached gingiva by a shallow linear depression, the *free gingival groove.*[1] Usually slightly more than a millimeter wide, it forms the soft tissue wall of the gingival sulcus. It may be separated from the tooth surface with a blunt probe.

THE GINGIVAL SULCUS. The gingival sulcus is the shallow groove around the tooth bounded by the surface of the tooth and the epithelium lining the free margin of the gingiva. It is a V-shaped depression and barely permits the entrance of a thin blunt probe. The average depth of the normal sulcus has been reported as 1.8 mm., with a variation of from 0 to 6 mm.;[108] 2 mm.;[14] 1.5 mm.;[160] and 0.69 mm.[47] (Gottlieb considered the "ideal" sulcus depth to be zero.[52, 55])

The attached gingiva

The attached gingiva is continuous with the marginal gingiva. It is firm, resilient and tightly bound to the underlying cementum and alveolar bone. The facial aspect of the attached gingiva extends to the relatively loose and movable alveolar mucosa from

7

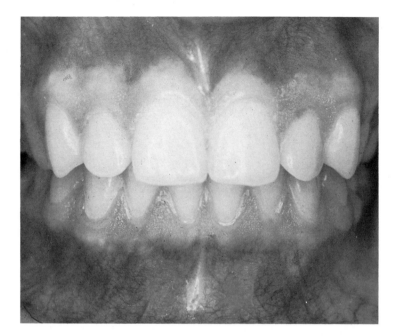

Figure 1–1 Normal Gingiva in Young Adult. Note the demarcation (mucogingival line) between the attached gingiva and darker alveolar mucosa.

which it is demarcated by the mucogingival line (*mucogingival junction*) (Fig. 1–1). The width of the attached gingiva on the facial aspect in different areas of the mouth varies from less than 1 mm. to 9 mm.[13] On the lingual aspect of the mandible, the attached gingiva terminates at the junction with the mucous membrane lining the sublingual sulcus in the floor of the mouth. The palatal surface of the attached gingiva in the maxilla blends imperceptibly with the equally firm, resilient palatal mucosa. The terms *cemental gingiva* and *alveolar gingiva* are sometimes used to designate the different portions of the attached gingiva according to their areas of attachment.

The interdental gingiva

The interdental gingiva occupies the *gingival embrasure*, which is the interproximal space beneath the area of tooth contact. It consists of two papillae, one facial, and one lingual, and the *col*.[23] The latter is a valley-like depression which connects the papillae and conforms to the shape of the interproximal contact area (Figs. 1–2 and 1–3).

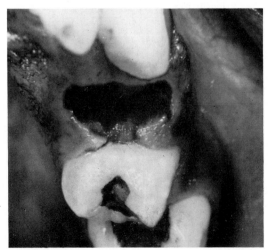

Figure 1–2 Site of extraction showing the facial and palatal interdental papillae and the intervening col.

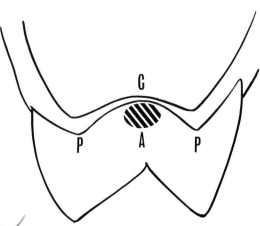

Figure 1–3 Interdental papillae (P), col (C) and relationship to contact area (A) on mesial surface.

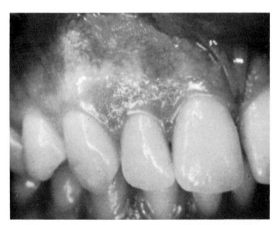

Figure 1–4 Interdental Papillae with Central Portion Formed by Attached Gingiva. The shape of the papillae varies according to the dimension of the gingival embrasure.

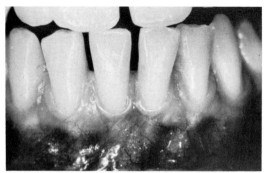

Figure 1–5 Absence of interdental papillae and col where proximal tooth contact is missing.

Each interdental papilla is pyramidal; the outer surface is tapered toward the interproximal contact area, and the mesial and distal surfaces are slightly concave. The lateral borders and tip of the interdental papillae are formed by a continuation of the marginal gingiva from the adjacent teeth. The intervening portion consists of attached gingiva (Fig. 1–4).

In the absence of proximal tooth contact, the gingiva is firmly bound over the interdental bone and forms a smooth rounded surface without interdental papillae or a col (Fig. 1–5).

NORMAL MICROSCOPIC FEATURES

The Marginal Gingiva (Unattached Gingiva)

The marginal gingiva consists of a central core of connective tissue covered by strati-fied squamous epithelium (Fig. 1–6). The epithelium on the crest and outer surface of the marginal gingiva is keratinized, parakeratinized or both, contains prominent **rete pegs**, and is continuous with the epithelium of the attached gingiva. The epithelium along the inner surface is devoid of rete pegs, is neither keratinized nor parakeratinized, and forms the lining of the gingival sulcus.

The gingival fibers

The connective tissue of the marginal gingiva is densely collagenous, containing a prominent system of **collagen fiber bundles** called the gingival fibers. The gingival fibers have the following functions: to brace the marginal gingiva firmly against the tooth; to provide the rigidity necessary to withstand the forces of mastication without being deflected away from the tooth surface; and to unite the free marginal gingiva with the cementum of the root and the adjacent attached gingiva. The gingival fibers are arranged in three groups: gingivodental, circular and transseptal.[3, 44]

GINGIVODENTAL GROUP. These are the fibers of the facial, lingual and interproximal surfaces. They are embedded in the cementum just beneath the epithelium at the base of the gingival sulcus. On the facial and lingual surfaces they project from the cementum in fan-like conformation toward the

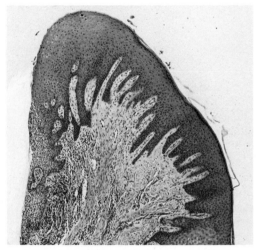

Figure 1–6 Section of Clinically Normal Gingiva, showing inflammation which is almost always present near the base of the sulcus. Keratinized strands are visible on the outer surface.

crest and outer surface of the marginal gingiva and terminate short of the epithelium (Figs. 1–7 and 1–8). They also extend external to the periosteum of the facial and lingual alveolar bone and terminate in the attached gingiva or blend with the periosteum of the bone. Interproximally, the gingivodental fibers extend toward the crest of the interdental gingiva (Fig. 1–6).

CIRCULAR GROUP. These fibers course through the connective tissue of the marginal and interdental gingiva and encircle the tooth in ring-like fashion.

TRANSSEPTAL GROUP. Located interproximally, the transseptal fibers form

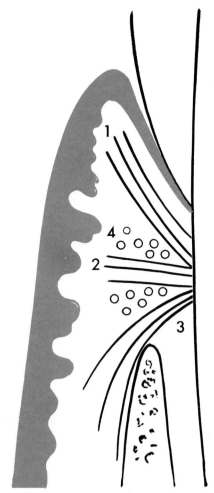

Figure 1–8 Diagrammatic Illustration of the Gingivodental Fibers extending from the cementum (1) to the crest of the gingiva (2) to the outer surface and (3) external to the periosteum of the labial plate. Circular fibers (4) are shown in cross section.

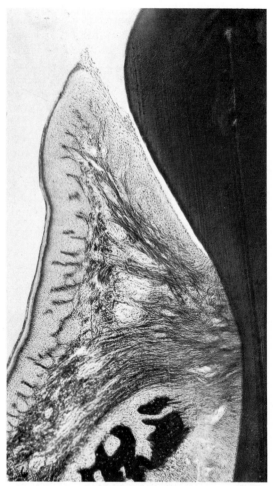

Figure 1–7 Faciolingual Section of Marginal Gingiva, showing gingival fibers extending from the cementum to the crest of the gingiva, to the outer gingival surface and external to the periosteum of the bone. Circular fibers are shown in cross section between the other groups. (Courtesy of Dr. Sol Bernick.)

horizontal bundles that extend between the cementum of approximating teeth into which they are embedded. They lie in the area between the epithelium at the base of the gingival sulcus and the crest of the interdental bone and are sometimes classified with the principal fibers of the periodontal ligament.

In clinically normal gingiva, small foci of plasma cells and lymphocytes are almost always found in the connective tissue near the base of the sulcus. They represent a chronic inflammatory response to irritation from constantly present bacteria and their products in the sulcus area.

Mast cells

Mast cells, which are distributed throughout the body, are numerous in the connective tissue of the oral mucosa and the gingiva.[157] They contain a variety of **biologically active substances** such as histamine, proteolytic-esterolytic enzymes, "slow-reacting substance" and lipolecithins which may be involved in the development and progress of gingival inflammation, and heparin which is a factor in bone resorption. Other products such as serotonin, unsaturated fatty acids and β-glucuronidase appear to be less important, whereas the function of mast cell ascorbic acid and phosphatase is not clear.[165]

Although some disagree,[125] it is the consensus that mast cells are increased in chronic gingival inflammation, except in areas of dense leukocytic infiltration and ulceration.[124, 164] The active chemicals are liberated by degranulation of the mast cells, possibly by enzyme products of bacterial dental plaque, or by a local antigen-anti-body reaction. By stimulating the inflammatory response, mast cell chemicals may increase local resistance to injurious agents.

The Gingival Sulcus, Sulcus Epithelium and Epithelial Attachment

The marginal gingiva forms the soft tissue wall of the gingival sulcus, and is joined to the tooth at the base of the sulcus by the epithelial attachment (Fig. 1–9). The sulcus is lined with thin, nonkeratinized stratified squamous epithelium without rete pegs. It extends from the coronal limit of the epithelial attachment at the base of the sulcus to the crest of the gingival margin. The sulcus epithelium is extremely important, because it acts as a **semipermeable membrane** through which injurious bacterial products pass into the gingiva and tissue fluid from the gingiva seeps into the sulcus.[140]

The **epithelial attachment** consists of a collar-like band of stratified squamous epi-

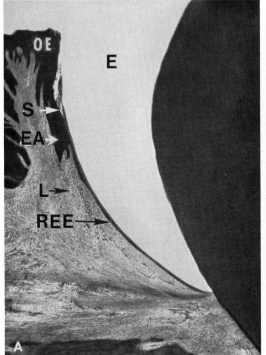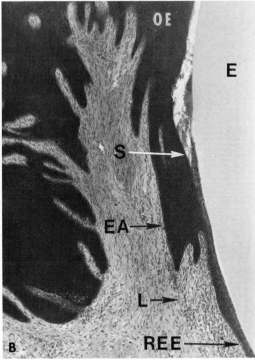

Figure 1–9 Gingival Sulcus. *A,* Gingival sulcus (S) on the enamel (E) at the junction of the epithelial attachment (EA) with the tooth surface. Note the oral epithelium (OE), the reduced enamel epithelium (REE) and the leukocytic infiltration (L) (monkey). *B,* Detailed section showing the sulcus (S) being formed by separation of the epithelial attachment (EA) from the enamel (E). Note that the epithelial attachment proliferates along the tooth, replacing the reduced enamel epithelium (REE). Remnants of the reduced enamel epithelium are in the gingival sulcus. Leukocytic infiltration (L) usually present in clinically normal gingiva is shown beneath the base of the sulcus.

thelium. It is three to four layers thick in early life, but the number of layers increases to 10 or even 20 with age; its length ranges from 0.25 to 1.35 mm. The length and level at which the epithelium is attached depend upon the stage of tooth eruption and differ on individual tooth surfaces.

The epithelial attachment is attached to the enamel by a **basal lamina (basement membrane)**[82] comparable to that which attaches epithelium to tissue elsewhere in the body. The basal lamina consists of a **lamina densa** (adjacent to the enamel) and a **lamina lucida** to which **hemidesmosomes** are attached (Figs. 1–10 and 1–11). The hemidesmosomes are enlargements on the inner leaflet of the epithelial cells called attachment plaques. The cell membrane consists of an inner and outer leaflet separated by a clear zone. Organic strands from the enamel extend into the lamina densa.[134] As it moves along the tooth, epithelium attaches to **afibrillar cementum** on the crown (Figs. 1–10 and 1–11) and to **root cementum** in a similar manner. An extramembranous **sticky**

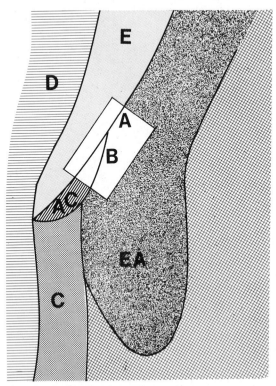

Figure 1–10 Dentogingival Junction, showing EA, epithelial attachment; E, enamel; D, dentin; C, cementum; AC, afibrillar cementum. Electron micrographs of areas A and B in the inset are shown in Figure 1–11.

coating elaborated by the epithelial cells, consisting of proline and/or hydroxyproline and neutral mucopolysaccharide,[145] also **binds the epithelial attachment to the tooth.**

The epithelial attachment to the tooth is reinforced by the gingival fibers, which brace the marginal gingiva against the tooth surface. For this reason the epithelial attachment and the gingival fibers are considered a functional unit, referred to as the *dentogingival junction.*

Development of the Epithelial Attachment and Gingival Sulcus

Gottlieb's initial description of the origin of the epithelial attachment was based upon observations made with the light microscope. Additional information has evolved from subsequently developed research techniques such as histochemistry, radioautography[41] and electron microscopy.[65, 118, 130] To understand the development of the epithelial attachment and its relationship to the teeth, it is best to start with the unerupted tooth.

After enamel formation is complete, the enamel is covered with reduced enamel epithelium and is attached to the tooth by a basal lamina containing hemidesmosomes of the ameloblast cell wall.[83, 135] When the tooth penetrates the oral mucosa, the stratum intermedium of the reduced enamel epithelium unites with the oral epithelium to form what Gottlieb termed the *epithelial attachment*[53, 56] and described as organically attached to the enamel. As the tooth erupts, the **united epithelium proliferates along the crown,** displacing the ameloblasts, which form the inner layer of the reduced enamel epithelium (Fig. 1–12). The epithelial attachment forms a proliferating collar around the tooth which is attached to the enamel in the same manner as the ameloblasts it displaced.

The epithelial attachment is a constantly **self-renewing structure** with mitotic activity occurring in all cell layers.[93] The regenerating epithelial cells move toward the tooth surface and along it in a coronal direction to the gingival sulcus, where they are shed[9] (Fig. 1–12). The proliferating cells provide a continuous and sliding attachment to the tooth surface. Although the epithelial attachment is biologically bonded to the tooth surface by the hemidesmosomes

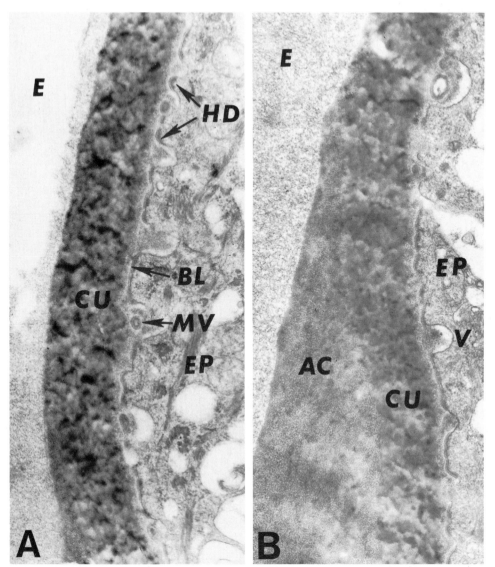

Figure 1–11   Electron Micrograph of Epithelial Attachment and Dental Cuticle (Secondary Dental Cuticle of Gottlieb).
Sections taken from areas A and B in inset in Figure 1–10. *A,* Dental cuticle (CU) on enamel (E), with basal lamina (BL) and hemidesmosomes (HD) of the epithelial attachment (EP) attached to the cuticle. Also shown are the microvilli of the epithelial cell wall (MV). *B,* Dental cuticle (CU) on afibrillar cementum (AC) and enamel (E). The cells of the epithelial attachment (EP) are attached to the cuticle by a basal lamina and hemidesmosomes. Also shown is a secretory vacuole (V) containing material similar to that of the basal lamina. (From Dr. Max A. Listgarten.[82])

and basement lamina, the strength of the attachment has not been measured.

The *gingival sulcus* is formed at the junction of the epithelial attachment and the enamel when the tooth erupts into the oral cavity. At that time the epithelial attachment forms a broad band from the tip of the crown to the cemento-enamel junction. As the tooth erupts, the most coronal portion of the epithelial attachment progressively separates from the enamel and deposits a cuticle from its surface onto the tooth (the

secondary cuticle). The shallow V-shaped space between the cuticle on the tooth and the surface of the epithelial attachment from which it separated becomes the **gingival sulcus.** Its base is located at the most coronal level at which the epithelium is attached to the tooth (Fig. 1–13).

Gottlieb's concept of the formation of the gingival sulcus and the epithelial attachment has been challenged in several respects. Weski,[160] Gross,[60] and Wodehouse[163] contend that the gingival sulcus is formed by a split in the epithelial attachment (intra-epithelial split) rather than by separation from the tooth. Becks[10] and Skillen[126] maintain that the reduced enamel epithelium degenerates and disappears when the gingival sulcus is formed and that it does not persist as an epithelial attachment.

Waerhaug[152,153] claims that the epithelial attachment is not *attached* to the enamel but is in close apposition with it, and therefore should be called the *epithelial cuff*.

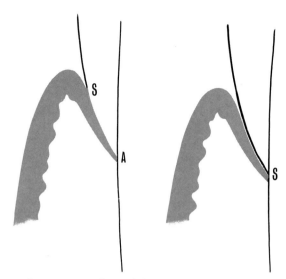

Figure 1–13 *Left,* **Gottlieb's Concept** of broad epithelial attachment and shallow gingival sulcus (S). The base of the sulcus is at the most superficial level of the attached epithelium. *Right,* **Waerhaug's Concept** of a broad non-attached epithelial cuff with a deep gingival sulcus (S) with its base at the most apical level of the epithelium.

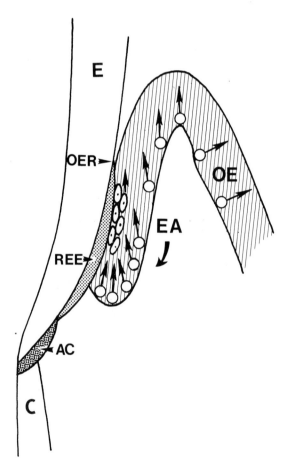

Figure 1–12 Epithelial Attachment Migrates on the Tooth. The epithelial attachment (EA), formed by the joining of the oral epithelium and the stellate reticulum of the reduced enamel epithelium (OER), proliferates along the enamel (E) in the direction of the single arrow, replacing the remaining ameloblastic layer of the reduced enamel epithelium (REE). Afibrillar cementum, sometimes formed on enamel after degeneration and shrinkage of the reduced enamel epithelium, is shown at AC. It is often covered by root cementum (C). The straight arrows indicate the coronal movement of the regenerating epithelial cells, which multiply more rapidly in the epithelial attachment than in the outer oral epithelium (OE). (From Dr. Max A. Listgarten.[81])

According to this opinion, the bottom of the sulcus is at the deepest point of the epithelial cuff rather than at its most superficial level (Fig. 1–13). However, other investigators[8,82,88,143,151] have reaffirmed the concept that the epithelial attachment is attached to the tooth, and one of them (Orban[106]) suggested the term *attached epithelial cuff* as preferable to epithelial attachment.

Gingival Fluid (Crevicular Fluid)

The gingival sulcus contains a fluid which seeps into it from the gingival connective tissue through the thin sulcular wall.[17,89] The gingival fluid (1) cleanses material from the sulcus; (2) contains sticky plasma proteins which may improve adhesion of the epithelial attachment to the tooth; (3) possesses antimicrobial properties; and (4) may exert antibody activity in defense of the gingiva. It may also serve as a medium for bacterial growth and contribute to the formation of dental plaque and calculus.

Gingival fluid occurs in minute amounts in the sulci of normal gingiva,[12,156] suggesting that it is a physiologic filtration product from the blood vessels, modified as it seeps through the sulcus epithelium. However, it is the prevalent opinion that **gingival fluid is an inflammatory exudate.**[85] Its presence in normal sulci is considered an artefact caused by increased permeability of capillaries damaged when the fluid is collected by inserting filter paper strips to the base of the sulcus instead of confining them to the crest of the gingival margin.[35] The question of whether gingival fluid is a product of normal gingiva is complicated by the fact that, **with few exceptions,**[104] **gingiva which appears normal clinically invariably exhibits inflammation when examined microscopically.**

The *amount of gingival fluid* increases with inflammation,[104] sometimes proportional to its severity.[34, 107] Gingival fluid is also increased by chewing coarse foods, by toothbrushing and massage, by ovulation[75] and by hormonal contraceptives.[78] Progesterone and estrogen increase the permeability of gingival vessels and the flow of gingival fluid in animals with and without gingivitis.[76, 77, 79]

The *composition of gingival fluid* is similar to blood serum except in the proportions of some of its components. Thus far reported as included in gingival fluid are electrolytes (K^+, Na^+, Ca^{++}), amino acids, plasma proteins, fibrolytic factors, gamma G globulin, gamma A globulin, gamma M globulin (immunoglobulins), albumin and lysozyme, fibrinogen and acid phosphatase.[15, 16, 29, 136] In gingival fluid from nearly normal gingiva the level of sodium is below that of serum, calcium approximately equals the serum level and potassium is more than three times higher. In inflamed gingiva the sodium content of gingival fluid equals the serum level, and calcium and phosphorus are more than three times higher;[68] the potassium : sodium ratio is elevated and the acid phosphatase content is increased.[10] Also contained in gingival fluid are microorganisms, desquamated epithelial cells and leukocytes (polymorphonuclears, lymphocytes and monocytes), which migrate through the sulcal epithelium.[33, 37, 127] Bacteria and leukocytes are increased in inflammation.

The Attached Gingiva

The attached gingiva is continuous with the marginal gingiva and consists of stratified squamous epithelium and an underlying connective tissue stroma. The epithelium is differentiated into (1) a cuboidal basal layer, (2) a spinous layer comprised of polygonal cells, (3) a multi-layered granular component consisting of flattened cells with prominent basophilic keratohyaline granules in the cytoplasm and shrunken hyperchromic nucleus, and (4) a cornified layer that may be keratinized, parakeratinized or both.

The gingival epithelium is similar to epidermis in that it shows a distinct sex difference. In the female, a large Feulgen-positive particle has been found adjacent to the nuclear membrane in 75 per cent of the cases; in the male, a similar but smaller particle is present in 1 to 2 per cent of the cells.[91]

Electron microscopy reveals that the cells of the gingival epithelium are connected to each other by structures along the cell periphery called *desmosomes.*[84] Each desmosome consists of two dense *attachment plaques* approximately 150 Å thick, formed by thickening of the cell membranes, separated by an *intervening space* of 300 to 350 Å (Fig. 1–14). Between the attachment plaques there is a *lamellated structure*, consisting of four layers of low electron density separated by three darker osmophilic layers (two lateral dense lines and a central line called the intercellular contact layer) approximately 75Å apart. The space between the cells is filled with a granular and fibrillar "cement" substance, and cytoplasmic projections of the cell wall resembling *microvilli* extend into the intercellular space. *Tonofibrils* radiate in brush-like fashion from the attachment plaques into the cytoplasm of the cells (Fig. 1–14).

In the stratum corneum of highly keratinized gingiva (palate) the **desmosomes are modified.** The cell membranes are thickened and separated by a three-layered structure (a central thick, dark osmophilic band between two narrow, less dense lines).

Less frequently observed forms of epithelial cell connections are[141] *tight junctions* (zonula occludens), areas where the outer membranes of adjoining cells are fused; and *intermediate junctions* (zonula adherens), areas in which the cell membranes are parallel and separated by a 200 to 300 Å wide space filled with amorphous material.

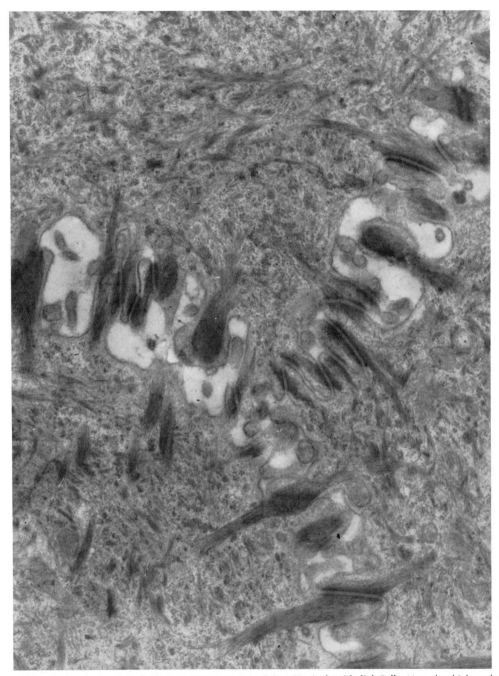

Figure 1–14 Electron Micrograph Showing Desmosomes Joining Gingival Epithelial Cells. Note the thickened attachment plaque in adjoining cell membranes and the spaces between them which form each desmosome. Brush-like tonofibrils project from the desmosomes into the cytoplasm. Magnification × 2600. (Courtesy of Dr. Max A. Listgarten.)

The Basal Lamina (Basement Membrane)

The epithelium is joined to the underlying connective tissue by a basal lamina 300 to 400 Å thick, which lies approximately 400 Å beneath the basal epithelial layer.[71,119,133] The basal lamina consists of lamina lucida and lamina densa. Hemidesmosomes of the basal epithelial cells abut on and extend into the lamina lucida.

The basal lamina is synthesized by the basal epithelial cells and consists of a **polysaccharide-protein complex and embedded collagen and reticulin fibers.**[102] *Anchoring fibrils* extend from the underlying connective tissue into the basal lamina, some of which penetrate through the lamina densa and lamina lucida to the membrane of the basal epithelial cells.[137] The basement lamina is permeable to fluids but acts as a barrier to particulate matter.

The Lamina Propria

The connective tissue of the gingiva is known as the lamina propria. It is densely collagenous with few elastic fibers. Argyrophilic reticulin fibers ramify between the collagen fibers and are continuous with reticulin in the blood vessel walls.[94] The lamina propria consists of two layers: (1) a papillary layer subjacent to the epithelium which consists of papillary projections between the epithelial rete pegs, and (2) a reticular layer contiguous with the periosteum of the alveolar bone.

Blood Supply, Lymphatics and Nerves

There are *three sources of blood supply to the gingiva* (Fig. 1–15): (1) *Supraperiosteal arterioles* along the facial and lingual surfaces of the alveolar bone, from which capillaries extend along the sulcus epithelium and between the rete pegs of the external gingival surface.[36,69] Occasional branches of the arterioles **pass through the alveolar bone to the periodontal ligament,** or run over the crest of the alveolar bone. (2) *Vessels of the periodontal ligament,* which extend into the gingiva and anastomose with capillaries in the sulcus area. (3) *Arterioles, which emerge from the crest of the interdental septa*[42] and extend parallel to the crest of the bone to anastomose with vessels of the periodontal ligament,

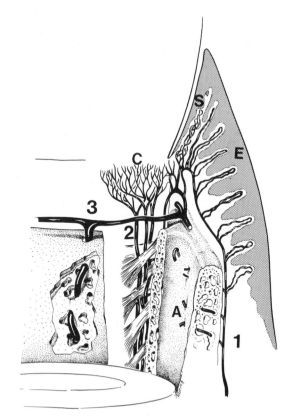

Figure 1–15 Periodontal Blood Supply. Diagrammatic representation of the three sources of blood supply to the gingiva as follows: (1) Supraperiosteal arterioles along the facial and lingual bone surfaces supply capillaries along the gingival sulcus (S) and external surface (E). Supraperiosteal branches also enter and pass through the bone to reach the periodontal ligament as alveolar penetrating vessels (A). (2) Longitudinal vessels of the periodontal ligament supply the col (C) and anastomose with capillaries in the sulcus area (S). (3) Arterioles penetrate the crest of the interdental septa and run along the crest of the bone to anastomose with vessels of the periodontal ligament and capillaries of the sulcus area (S) and with other vessels along the crest of the bone.

with capillaries in the gingival crevicular areas, and with vessels which run over the alveolar crest.

Beneath the epithelium on the outer gingival surface, capillaries extend into the papillary connective tissue between the epithelial rete pegs in the form of terminal hairpin loops with efferent and afferent branches,[62,67] spirals and varices (Fig. 1–16). The loops are sometimes linked by cross communications,[43] and there are also flattened capillaries which serve as reserve vessels when the circulation is increased in response to irritation.[49] Along the sulcus epithelium, capillaries are arranged in a flat anastomosing plexus which extends

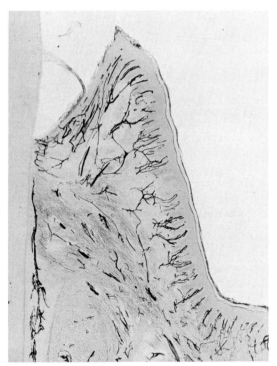

Figure 1–16   Blood Supply and Peripheral Circulation of the Gingiva. Tissues perfused with India ink. Note the capillary plexus parallel to the sulcus, and the capillary loops in the outer papillary layer. Note also the supraperiosteal vessels external to the bone which supply the gingiva and a periodontal ligament vessel anastomosing with the sulcus plexus. (Courtesy of Dr. Sol Bernick.)

parallel to the enamel from the base of the sulcus to the gingival margin.[21] In the col area there is a mixed pattern of anastomosing capillaries and loops.

The *lymphatic drainage* of the gingiva begins in the lymphatics of the connective tissue papillae. It progresses into the collecting network external to the periosteum of the alveolar process and then to the regional lymph nodes (particularly the submaxillary group).[123] In addition, lymphatics just beneath the epithelial attachment extend into the periodontal ligament and accompany the blood vessels.

Gingival innervation is derived from fibers arising from nerves in the peridontal ligament and from the labial, buccal and palatal nerves.[11] The following nerve structures are present in the connective tissue: a meshwork of *terminal argyrophilic* fibers, some of which extend into the epithelium; *Meissner-type tactile corpuscles; Krause-type end bulbs,* which are temperature receptors; and *encapsulated spindles.*[71]

The Interdental Gingiva and the Col

As the proximal tooth surfaces contact in the course of eruption, the oral mucosa between the teeth is separated into the facial

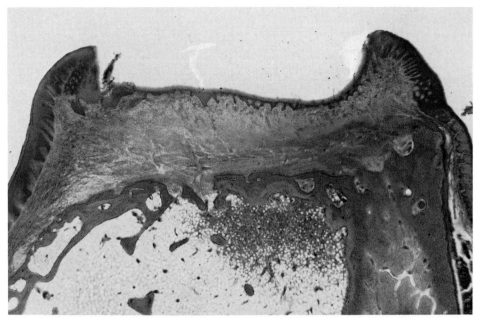

Figure 1–17   Faciolingual Section (Monkey) Showing Col Between the Facial and Lingual Interdental Papillae. The col is covered with stratified squamous epithelium.

and lingual interdental papillae joined by the col.[23] Each interdental papilla consists of a central core of densely collagenous connective tissue covered by stratified squamous epithelium. There are *oxytalan* fibers in the connective tissue of the col[70] as well as in other areas of the gingiva.[45]

At the time of eruption and for a period thereafter, the col is covered by *reduced enamel epithelium* derived from the approximating teeth. This is gradually undermined and replaced by *stratified squamous epithelium* from the adjacent interdental papillae (Fig. 1–17). It has been suggested that during the period that the col is covered by reduced enamel epithelium it is *highly susceptible to injury and disease* because the protection provided by this type of epithelium is inadequate.[95]

CORRELATION OF THE NORMAL CLINICAL AND MICROSCOPIC FEATURES

To understand the normal clinical features of the gingiva, one must be able to interpret them in terms of the microscopic structures they represent.

Color

The color of the attached and marginal gingiva is generally described as coral pink, and is produced by the vascular supply, the thickness and degree of keratinization of the epithelium and the presence of pigment-containing cells. The color varies in different persons and appears to be correlated with the cutaneous pigmentation. It is lighter in blond individuals with a fair complexion than in swarthy brunettes.

The attached gingiva is demarcated from the adjacent alveolar mucosa on the buccal aspect by a clearly defined mucogingival line. The alveolar mucosa is red, smooth and shiny rather than pink and stippled. Comparison of the microscopic structure of the attached gingiva and alveolar mucosa affords an explanation for the difference in appearance. The epithelium of the alveolar mucosa is thinner, nonkeratinized, and contains no rete pegs (Fig. 1–18). The connective tissue of the alveolar mucosa is loosely arranged and the blood vessels are more numerous.

PHYSIOLOGIC PIGMENTATION (MELANIN). Melanin, a non-hemoglobin–derived brown pigment is responsible for the normal pigmentation of the skin, gingiva and remainder of the oral mucous membrane. It is present in all individuals, often not in sufficient quantities to be detected clinically, but is absent or severely diminished in albinism. Melanin pigmentation in the oral cavity is prominent in Negroes (Fig. 1–19) and in some Arabs, Ceylonese,

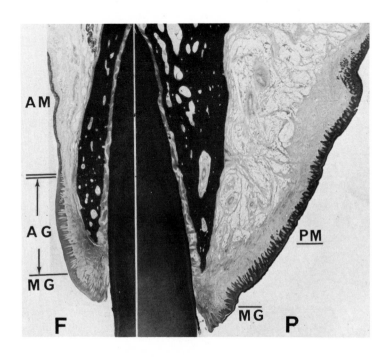

Figure 1–18 Oral Mucosa, Facial and Palatal Surfaces. *F,* Facial surface showing the marginal gingiva (MG), attached gingiva (AG) and alveolar mucosa (AM). The double line (=) marks the mucogingival junction. Note the differences in the epithelium and connective tissue in the attached gingiva and alveolar mucosa. *P,* Palatal surface showing the marginal gingiva (MG) and thick keratinized palatal mucosa (PM).

Chinese, East Indians, Filipinos, Greeks, Gypsies, Italians, Japanese, Javanese, Peruvians, Puerto Ricans, Rumanians and Syrians.

Melanin is formed by dendritic *melanocytes* in the basal and spinous layers of the gingival epithelium (Fig. 1–20). It is synthesized in *organelles* within the cells called *premelanosomes* or *melanosomes*.[25, 117, 131] These contain tyrosinase, which hydroxylates tyrosine to dihydroxyphenylalanine (dopa), which in turn is progressively converted to melanin. Melanin granules are phagocytosed by and contained within other cells of the epithelium and connective tissue called *melanophages* or *melanophores*.

According to Dummett,[32] the distribution of oral pigmentation in the Negro is as follows: gingiva, 60 per cent; hard palate, 61 per cent; mucous membrane, 22 per cent; and tongue, 15 per cent. Gingival pigmentation occurs as a diffuse, deep purplish discoloration or as irregularly shaped brown and light brown patches. It may appear in the gingiva as early as three hours after birth, and often is the only evidence of pigmentation.

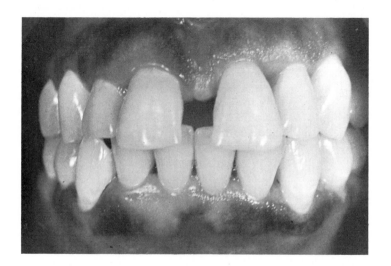

Figure 1–19 Physiologic melanotic pigmentation of the gingiva.

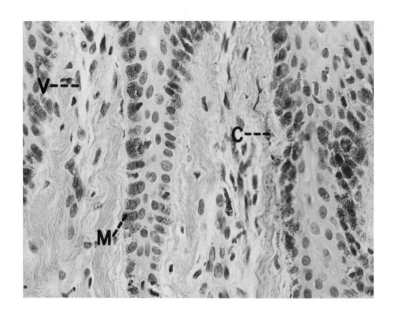

Figure 1–20 Pigmented Gingiva, showing melanocytes (M) in the basal epithelial layer and melanophores (C) in the connective tissue. Also shown is a capillary (V) in the papillary connective tissue.

Size

The size of the gingiva corresponds to the sum total of the bulk of cellular and intercellular elements and their vascular supply. Alteration in size is a common feature of gingival disease.

Contour

The contour or shape of the gingiva varies considerably, and depends upon the shape of the teeth and their alignment in the arch, the location and size of the area of proximal contact, and the dimensions of the facial and lingual gingival embrasures. The marginal gingiva envelops the teeth in collar-like fashion, and follows an escalloped outline on the facial and lingual surfaces. It forms a straight line along teeth with relatively flat surfaces. On teeth with pronounced mesiodistal convexity (e.g., maxillary canines), or in labial version, the normal arcuate contour is accentuated and the gingiva is located further apically. On teeth in lingual version the gingiva is horizontal and thickened (Fig. 1–21).

The *shape* of the _interdental gingiva_ is governed by the contour of the proximal tooth surfaces, the location and shape of the contact area, and the dimensions of the gingival embrasures. When the proximal surfaces of the crowns are relatively flat

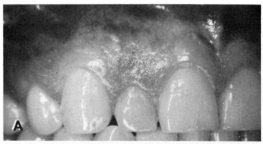
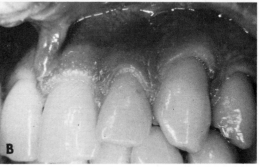

Figure 1–22 Shape of interdental gingival papillae correlated with shape of teeth and embrasures. *A,* Broad interdental papillae; *B,* narrow interdental papillae.

faciolingually, the roots are close together, the interdental bone is thin mesiodistally, and the gingival embrasures and interdental gingiva are narrow mesiodistally. Conversely, with proximal surfaces that flare away from the area of contact, the mesiodistal diameter of the interdental gingiva is broad (Fig. 1–22). The height of the interdental gingiva varies with the location of the proximal contact.

Consistency

The gingiva is firm and resilient and, with the exception of the movable free margin, tightly bound to the underlying bone. The collagenous nature of the lamina propria and its contiguity with the mucoperiosteum of the alveolar bone determines the firm consistency of the attached gingiva. The gingival fibers contribute to the firmness of the gingival margin.

Surface texture

The gingiva presents a minutely lobulated surface like an orange peel, and is referred to as being _stippled_. Stippling is

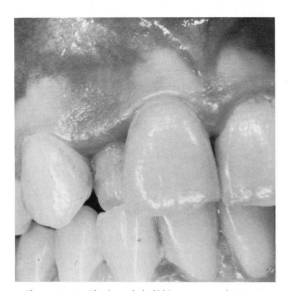

Figure 1–21 Thickened shelf-like contour of gingiva on tooth in lingual version aggravated by local irritation.

best viewed by drying the gingiva (Fig. 1–23). The attached gingiva is stippled; the gingival margin is not. The central portion of the interdental papillae is usually stippled, but the margin borders are smooth. The pattern and extent of stippling vary from person to person, and in different areas of the same mouth.[58,114] It is less prominent on lingual than on facial surfaces, and may be absent in some patients.

Stippling varies with age. It is absent in infancy, appears in some children at about five years of age, increases until adulthood, and frequently begins to disappear in old age.

Microscopically, stippling is produced by alternate rounded protuberances and depressions in the gingival surface. The papillary layer of the connective tissue projects into the elevations, and both the elevated and depressed areas are covered by stratified squamous epithelium (Fig. 1–24). The degree of keratinization and the prominence of stippling appear to be related.

Stippling is a form of adaptive specialization or reinforcement for function. It is a feature of healthy gingiva, and **reduction or loss of stippling is a common sign of gingival disease.** When the gingiva is restored to health following treatment, the stippled appearance returns.

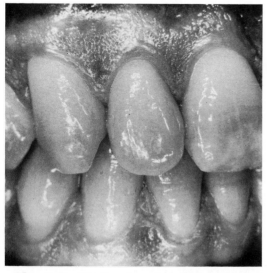

Figure 1–23 **Stippling** of attached gingiva and central portions of interdental papillae. The gingival margin is smooth.

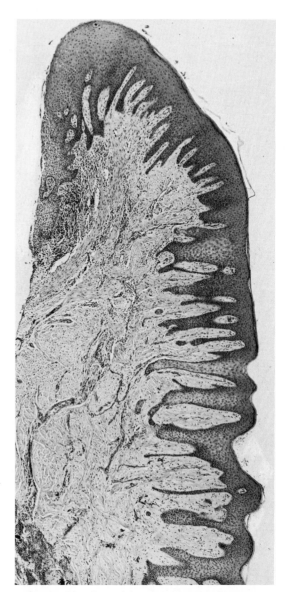

Figure 1–24 Gingival biopsy of patient shown in Figure 1–23, demonstrating alternate elevation and depressions in the attached gingiva responsible for stippled appearance.

Keratinization

The epithelium covering the outer surface of the marginal gingiva and the attached gingiva is keratinized or parakeratinized or presents varied combinations of both conditions.[116] The surface layer is shed in thin strands and replaced by cells from the underlying granular layer. Keratinization is considered to be a protective adaptation to function which in-

creases when the gingiva is stimulated by toothbrushing.

Keratinization of the oral mucosa varies in different areas in the following order: palate (most keratinized), gingiva, tongue and cheek (least keratinized).[98] The degree of gingival keratinization is not necessarily correlated with the different phases of the menstrual cycle,[66, 99] and diminishes with age and the onset of menopause.[109]

Renewal of gingival epithelium

The oral epithelium undergoes continuous renewal. Its thickness is maintained by a balance between new cell formation in the basal and spinous layers and the shedding of old cells at the surface. The *mitotic activity* exhibits a 24-hour periodicity, with highest and lowest rates occurring in the morning and evening respectively.[147] The mitotic rate is higher in nonkeratinized gingival epithelium than in keratinized areas, and is increased in gingivitis, without significant sex differences. Opinions differ as to whether the mitotic rate is increased[87, 96] or decreased[6] with age.

The mitotic rate in experimental animals varies in different areas of the oral epithelium in the following descending order: buccal mucosa, hard palate, sulcus epithelium, epithelial attachment, outer surface of the marginal gingiva and attached gingiva.[2, 61, 86, 147] The following have been reported as the turnover times for different areas of the oral epithelium in experimental animals: palate, tongue, and cheek, 5 to 6 days; gingiva, 10 to 12 days, with the same or more time required with age; and epithelial attachment, 1 to 6 days.[9, 128]

Position

The position of the gingiva refers to the level at which the **gingival margin is attached to the tooth.** When the tooth erupts into the oral cavity, the epithelial attachment is at the tip of the crown; as eruption progresses, it moves in the direction of the root. As the apical portion of the epithelial attachment proliferates along the enamel, the coronal portion separates from the tooth. Coordinated with this migration the gingival margin undergoes atrophy and "**follows the epithelial attachment,**" thereby preserving the physiologic depth of the sulcus. Without accompanying atrophy of the gingival margin, proliferation and detachment of the epithelial attachment would result in a deepened gingival sulcus or a pathological periodontal pocket.

Continuous tooth eruption

According to the *concept of continuous eruption* (Gottlieb[57]), eruption does not cease when teeth meet their functional antagonists, but continues throughout life. It consists of an *active* and *passive* phase. *Active eruption* is the movement of the teeth in the direction of the occlusal plane, whereas *passive eruption* is the exposure of the teeth by separation of the epithelial attachment from the enamel and migration onto the cementum.

Inherent in the concept is the distinction between the *anatomic crown* (the portion of the tooth covered by enamel) and the *anatomic root* (the portion of the tooth covered by cementum), and the *clinical crown* and *clinical root*. The clinical crown is the part of the tooth that has been denuded of epithelium and projects into the oral cavity; the clinical root is that portion of the tooth covered by periodontal tissues.

When the teeth reach their functional antagonists, the gingival sulcus and epithelial attachment are still on the enamel,[105] and the clinical crown is approximately two thirds of the anatomic crown.

Active and passive eruption proceed together, and under ideal conditions are synchronized as follows:

ACTIVE ERUPTION. Active eruption is coordinated with attrition. The teeth erupt to compensate for tooth substance worn away by attrition. Attrition reduces the clinical crown and prevents it from becoming disproportionately long in relation to the clinical root, thus avoiding excessive leverage on the periodontal tissues. Ideally, the rate of active eruption keeps pace with tooth wear, preserving the *vertical dimension* of the dentition.

As the teeth erupt, cementum is deposited at the apices and furcations of the roots, and bone is formed along the fundus of the alveolus and at the crest of the alveolar bone. In this way part of the *tooth substance lost by attrition is replaced by*

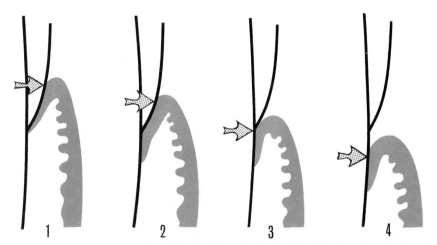

Figure 1–25 Diagrammatic Representation of the Four Stages in Passive Eruption According to Gottlieb.[57]
1, Base of the gingival sulcus (arrow) and the epithelial attachment are on the enamel. 2, Base of the gingival sulcus (arrow) is on the enamel and part of the epithelial attachment is on the root. 3, Base of the gingival sulcus (arrow) is at the cemento-enamel line, and the entire epithelial attachment is on the root. 4, Base of the gingival sulcus (arrow) and the epithelial attachment are on the root.

lengthening of the root, and socket depth is maintained to support the root.

PASSIVE ERUPTION. Passive eruption, which accompanies and is coordinated with active eruption, is divided into four stages (Fig. 1–25).

Stage One. The teeth reach the line of occlusion. The epithelial attachment and base of the gingival sulcus are on the enamel.

Stage Two. The epithelial attachment proliferates so that part is on the cementum and part on the enamel. The base of the sulcus is still on the enamel.

Stage Three. The entire epithelial attachment is on the cementum, and the base of the sulcus is at the cemento-enamel junction. As the epithelial attachment proliferates from the crown onto the root, it remains no longer at the cemento-enamel junction than at any other area of the tooth.

Stage Four. The epithelial attachment has proliferated further on the cementum. The base of the sulcus is on the cementum, a portion of which is exposed.

Proliferation of the epithelial attachment onto the root is accompanied by degeneration of gingival and periodontal ligament fibers and their detachment from the tooth. The cause of this degeneration is not understood. Some consider it a physiologic change to create space for the epithelium; others suggest that the proliferating epithelium causes the fiber degeneration.

As noted above, apposition of bone accompanies active eruption, but it is also correlated with the rate of passive eruption. The distance between the apical end of the epithelial attachment and the crest of the alveolus remains constant throughout continuous tooth eruption (1.07 mm.).[47]

Gingival recession (gingival atrophy)

According to the concept of continuous eruption, the gingival sulcus may be located on the crown, cemento-enamel junction or root, depending upon the age of the patient and the stage of eruption. **Exposure of the root by the apical migration of the gingiva is called gingival recession,** or atrophy. Some root exposure is considered normal with age and is referred to as *physiologic recession;* excessive exposure is termed *pathologic recession* (see Chap. 8). The distinction is one of degree. Investigators who do not accept the concept of continuous eruption maintain that the cemento-enamel junction is the normal location of the gingiva and that any exposure of the root is pathological.[161, 162]

Cuticular structures on the tooth

The term cuticle is used to describe a strand-like acellular structure with a homogeneous matrix, sometimes enclosed within clearly demarcated linear borders.

The following cuticular structures have been described on the teeth:

1. *Acquired pellicle (acquired cuticle).* This is an acquired rather than anatomical structure deposited on the tooth surface by the saliva as a *thin acellular translucent adherent film.* (For additional information regarding the acquired pellicle, see Chap. 22).

2. *Primary cuticle (enamel cuticle, Nasmyth's membrane).* Originally described by Nasmyth[103] and subsequently by Gottlieb, this cuticle is present *on the enamel* of the unerupted tooth. It is considered to be the final product of degenerating ameloblasts after completion of enamel formation. It is calcified and slightly more resistant to acids and alkalis than is the enamel. After eruption the cuticle tends to be worn off in areas exposed to the abrasive effect of foods. It persists at the gingival third of the enamel, particularly interproximally, less frequently on the occlusal surface of the posterior teeth in the developmental grooves. Initially colorless, it becomes stained by adherent food debris and bacteria. The green stain on children's teeth is produced in this manner.

Electron microscopy reveals that the structure designated as "primary cuticle" consists of **ameloblasts of the reduced enamel epithelium attached to the enamel by a basal lamina (basement lamina).**[81, 83, 135] This consists of a lamina densa (adjacent to the enamel) and a lamina lucida to which hemidesmosomes of the ameloblasts are attached.

3. *Secondary cuticle (cuticula dentis, transposed crevicular cuticle).*[52] This cuticle occurs upon both the enamel (theoretically external to the enamel cuticle, with which it combines) and on the cementum, but not on all teeth. It is deposited by the epithelial attachment as it migrates along the tooth and separates from crown and root (Fig. 1–26). It is not present on cementum to which the periodontal ligament is attached. It was originally described as keratinized,[52] but this observation has not been supported by subsequent histochemical studies.[158, 159]

Electron microscopy reveals a coarsely granular structure (0.5 micron) adherent to the enamel and cementum in the location of the secondary cuticle.[82] The epithelial attachment is attached to it by a basal lamina (0.1 micron) (Figs. 1–10 and 1–11). **The**

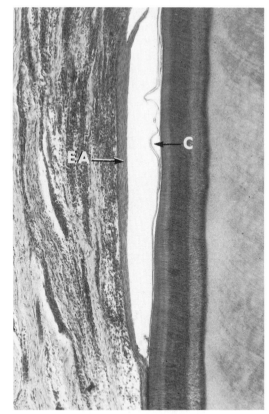

Figure 1–26 Formation of Secondary Cuticle (C) by Separation Away From Epithelial Attachment (EA).

secondary cuticle appears to be a nonkeratinized product of the epithelial attachment cells, possibly contributed to by gingival fluid and saliva.[81] Others describe it as a pathologic product of inflamed gingiva,[97] or a pathologic conglutinate of erythrocytes.[64]

The cuticular covering on the enamel may be more resistant to caries than that on the cementum. This impression is based upon the observation that caries which starts at the cemento-enamel junction of exposed teeth often spreads to adjacent cementum and underlying dentin, without involving the contiguous enamel surface.

HISTOCHEMICAL ASPECTS OF NORMAL GINGIVA

Histochemical techniques provide useful information regarding the chemical components and enzyme systems of normal gingiva. In addition to adding to our understanding of physiologic processes in the gingiva, this information provides **guidelines for interpreting the changes which occur in gingival disease.**

The connective tissue of normal gingiva contains a PAS-positive (periodic acid–Schiff stain) *heteropolysaccharide intercellular ground substance*[40] that is also present in the walls of the blood vessels and between the cells of the epithelium.[122] A thin PAS-positive basement membrane demarcates the connective tissue from the epithelium (Fig. 1–27). Electron microscopy reveals this to be a band of reticulin on the connective tissue side of the lamina densa of the basal lamina, rather than the basal lamina itself which is not involved in the PAS reaction.[138]

PAS-negative acid mucopolysaccharides, hyaluronic acid and *chondroitin sulfate A, C and B*[121,144] demonstrated between the epithelial cells are considered by some[142] to be intercellular cementing substances and by others[50] to be stained portions of the intercellular attachment apparatus. *Neutral mucopolysaccharides* also occur intercellularly in the epithelium.

Glycogen, which is PAS-positive, is distributed throughout the intercellular substance of the connective tissue and in the smooth muscle of the arterioles.[150] In the epithelium, glycogen occurs intracellularly, in concentrations inversely related to the degree of keratinization. Some consider it a normal component of epithelium;[120,155,160] others find it only in acanthosis, usually associated with inflammation.[31] *Phosphorylase activity* generally occurs in the epithelium where glycogen is located.[113]

RNA is found in large quantities in the basal cells of normal gingival epithelium, decreasing toward the superficial layers, and in lowest concentration in the crevicular epithelium.[74] *DNA*, normally present in the nucleus of all gingival cells, is increased in gingival hyperplasia. The DNA and RNA activity of the epithelium at the gingival margin and epithelial attachment is greater than in the remaining oral mucosa.[59]

Sulfhydryls and *disulfides* are normal components of the gingival epithelium and connective tissue.[148] In the keratinization process sulfhydryls are oxidized to disulfides and both are significant in a wide range of biologic activities such as enzymatic and antibody reactions, cell growth and division, and cell permeability and detoxification. Sulfhydryls and disulfides are present throughout the gingival epithelium; the former is increased in keratinized and parakeratinized layers,[148] and the latter in the surface keratinized cells.[92] In the connective tissue, sulfhydryls and disulfides

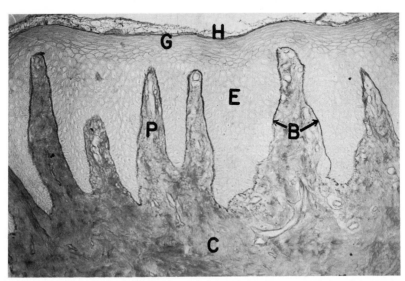

Figure 1–27 Normal Human Gingiva Stained with the Periodic Acid-Schiff (P.A.S.) Histochemical Method. The basement membrane (B) is seen between the epithelium (E) and underlying connective tissue (C). In the epithelium there is glycoprotein material between the cells and in the cell membrane of the superficial hornified (H) and underlying granular layers (G). The connective tissue presents a diffuse amorphous ground substance and interspersed streakings of collagen fibers. The blood vessel walls stand out clearly in the papillary projections of the connective tissue (P).

occur intercellularly and in the fibroblasts and endothelial cells. The *phospholipid* and *cholesterol* content of the gingiva is comparable to that of skin,[63] and lipids have been demonstrated in keratohyaline granules in the epithelium.[28]

Enzymes

Alkaline phosphatase is present in the endothelial cells, in the capillary walls and possibly in the fibers of the connective tissue. It has been described in keratinized and parakeratinized surface layers,[24] but some doubt that it occurs in epithelium.[20]

Acid phosphatase, found in the epithelium in greatest concentration in the surface and prickle cell layers,[154] is related to keratinization.[22] It is not present in the epithelial attachment or sulcus lining. *Disphospho- and triphosphopyridine nucleotide reductases,* present in all epithelial cells except keratin and parakeratin, in desmosomes, tonofibrils and nucleoli, suggest an oxidative metabolic pathway for the formation of the keratin precursor substance and keratin.[39] In tissue culture mucopolysaccharides and acid phosphatase are present in epithelial and fibroblast-like gingival cells, but the amount of alkaline phosphatase is negligible.[129]

Acetylcholinesterase and nonspecific *cholinesterase* are present in gingival connective tissue.[5] *Endogenous reducing enzymes, succinic dehydrogenase, glucose-6-phosphate dehydrogenase, lactic dehydrogenase,[38] beta-D-glucuronidase, beta-glucosidase, beta-galactosidase[80]* and *aminopeptidase[101, 112]* have been observed in gingiva. *Esterase[80]* occurs in the basal and granular layers of the epithelium and in the connective tissue near periodontal pockets.[20]

Collagenase is produced in epithelium and connective tissue of normal gingiva as well as in the periodontal ligament and alveolar bone.[46] *Cytochrome oxidase* activity occurs in the sulcal and attachment epithelium, in the basal layers of marginal and attached gingiva and in the connective tissue.[111] *5-Nucleotidase* occurs in the blood vessels and surface epithelial cells of keratinized gingiva and only in the blood vessels of nonkeratinized and parakeratinized gingiva.[27] *Lysosomes* have been demonstrated in exfoliated cells of the epithelial attachment.[73]

The *oxygen consumption of normal gingiva* (QO_2 1.6 ± 0.37) is comparable to that of skin (QO_2 1.48 ± 0.48).[51] The respiratory activity of the epithelium is approximately three times greater than that of the connective tissue,[100] and the sulcal epithelium is approximately twice that of whole gingiva.[72]

REFERENCES

1. Ainamo, J., and Loe, H.: Anatomical Characteristics of Gingiva. A Clinical and Microscopic Study of the Free and Attached Gingiva. J. Periodont., 37:5, 1966.
2. Anderson, G. S., and Stern, I.: The Proliferation and Migration of the Attachment Epithelium on the Cemental Surface of the Rat Incisor. Periodontics, 4:115, 1966.
3. Arnim, S. S., and Hagerman, D. A.: The Connective Tissue Fibers of the Marginal Gingiva. J.A.D.A., 47:271, 1953.
4. Avery, J. K., and Rapp, R.: Pain Conduction in Human Dental Tissues. Dent. Clin. North America, July 1959, p. 489.
5. Avery, J. K., and Rapp, R.: Presence of Acetylcholinesterase in Human Gingiva. J. Periodont., 30:152, 1959.
6. Barakat, N. J., Toto, P. D., and Choukas, N. C.: Aging and Cell Renewal of Oral Epithelium. J. Periodont.-Periodontics, 40:599, 1969.
7. Bass, C. C.: A Demonstrable Line in Extracted Teeth Indicating the Location of the Outer Border of the Epithelial Attachment. J. D. Res., 25:401, 1946.
8. Baume, J. L.: The Structure of the Epithelial Attachment Revealed by Phase Contrast Microscopy. J. Periodont., 24:99, 1953.
9. Beagrie, G. S., and Skougard, M. R.: Observations in the Life Cycle of the Gingival Epithelial Cells of Mice as Revealed by Autoradiography. Acta Odont. Scandinav., 20:15, 1962.
10. Becks, H.: Normal and Pathologic Pocket Formation. J.A.D.A., 16:2167, 1929.
11. Bernick, S.: Innervation of the Teeth and Periodontium. Dent. Clin. North America, July 1959, p. 503.
12. Björn, H. L., Koch, G., and Lindhe, H.: Evaluation of Gingival Fluid Measurements. Odont. Revy, 16:300, 1965.
13. Bowers, G. M.: A Study of the Width of the Attached Gingiva. J. Periodont., 34:201, 1963.
14. Box, H. K.: Treatment of the Periodontal Pocket. Toronto, The University of Toronto Press, 1928.
15. Brandtzaeg, P.: Immunochemical Comparison of Proteins in Human Gingival Pocket Fluid, Serum and Saliva. Arch. Oral Biol., 10:795, 1965.
16. Brandtzaeg, P., and Mann, W.: A Comparative Study of the Lysozyme Activity of Human Gingival Pocket Fluid. Acta Odont. Scandinav., 22: 441, 1964.
17. Brill, N., and Björn, H.: Passage of Tissue Fluid into Human Gingival Pockets. Acta Odont. Scandinav., 17:11, 1959.
18. Burnett, G. M., Gouge, S., and Toye, A. E.: Lyso-

zyme Content of Human Gingiva and Various Rat Tissues. J. Periodont., 30:148, 1959.

19. Cabrini, R. L., and Carranza, F. A., Jr.: Histochemical Distribution of Acid Phosphatase in Human Gingiva, J. Periodont., 29:34, 1958.

20. Cabrini, R. L., and Carranza, F. A., Jr.: Histochemistry of Periodontal Tissues. A Review of the Literature. Internat. D. J., 16:466, 1966.

21. Carranza, F. A., et al.: A Study of Periodontal Vascularization in Different Laboratory Animals. J. Periodont. Res., 1:120, 1966.

22. Carranza, F. A., Jr., and Cabrini, R. L.: Histochemical Distribution of Acid Phosphatase in Healing Wounds. Science, 135:672, 1962.

23. Cohen, B.: Morphological Factors in the Pathogenesis of Periodontal Disease. Brit. D. J., 107:31, 1959.

24. Cohen, L.: Alkaline Phosphatase Activity in Human Gingival Epithelium. Periodontics, 6:23, 1968.

25. Cohen, L.: ATPase and Dopa Oxidase Activity in Human Gingival Epithelium. Arch. Oral Biol., 12:1241, 1967.

26. Cohen, L.: Keratinization of the Gingivae. D. Practit., 18:134, 1967.

27. Cohen, L.: Presence of 5-Nucleotidase in Human Gingiva. J. D. Res., 46:757, 1967.

28. Cohen, L.: Presence of Lipids in Keratohyaline Granules of Human Gingiva. J. D. Res., 46:630, 1967.

29. Cowley, G. C.: Fluorescence Studies of Crevicular Fluid. J. D. Res., 45:655, 1966.

30. Cruz Ortis, F.: Proteolytic Action in Normal and Pathologic Gingival Tissues and in the Granulation Tissue of Periodontal Pockets. Santiago, University of Chile Press, 1946.

31. Dewar, M. R.: Observations on the Composition and Metabolism of Normal and Inflamed Gingivae. J. Periodont., 26:29, 1955.

32. Dummett, C. O.: Physiologic Pigmentation of the Oral and Cutaneous Tissues in the Negro. J. D. Res., 25:422, 1946.

33. Egelberg, J.: Cellular Elements in Gingival Pocket Fluid. Acta Odont. Scandinav., 21:283, 1963.

34. Egelberg, J.: Gingival Exudate Measurements for Evaluation of Inflammatory Changes of the Gingivae. Odont. Revy, 15:381, 1964.

35. Egelberg, J.: Permeability of the Dento-gingival Vessels. II. Clinically Healthy Gingivae. J. Periodont. Res., 1:276, 1966.

36. Egelberg, J.: The Topography and Permeability of Blood Vessels at the Dento-gingival Junction in Dogs. J. Periodont. Res., 2:Suppl. 1, 1967.

37. Egelberg, J., and Attstrom, R.: Presence of Leukocytes within Crevices of Healthy and Inflamed Gingiva and Their Immigration from the Blood. J. Periodont. Res., Suppl., 4:23, 1969.

38. Eichel, B.: Oxidation Enzymes of Gingiva. Ann. New York Acad. Sc., 85:479, 1960.

39. Eichel, B., Shahrik, H. A., and Lisanti, V. F.: Cytochemical Demonstration and Metabolic Significance of Reduced Diphospho-Pyridinenucleotide and Triphospho-Pyridinenucleotide Reductases in Human Gingiva. J. D. Res., 43:92, 1964.

40. Engel, M. B.: Water-soluble Mucoproteins of the Gingiva. J. D. Res., 32:779, 1953.

41. Engler, W. O., Ramfjord, S. P., and Hiniker, J. J.: Development of Epithelial Attachment and Gin-

42. Folke, L. E. A., and Stallard, R. E.: Periodontal Microcirculation as Revealed by Plastic Microspheres. J. Periodont. Res., 2:53, 1967.

43. Forsslund, G.: Structure and Function of Capillary System in the Gingiva in Man. Development of Stereophotogrammetric Method and Its Application for Study of the Subepithelial Blood Vessels in Vivo. Acta Odont. Scandinav., 17:9, Suppl. 26, 1959.

44. Frohlich, E.: Veränderungen im Gefüge des Zahnfleischbindegewebes bei den entzündlichen marginalen Zahnbetterkrankungen. Deutsche Zahnärzt. Zeitschr., 7:477, 1952.

45. Fullmer, H. M.: Critique of Normal Connective Tissue of the Periodontium and Some Alterations with Periodontal Disease. J. D. Res., 41 (Suppl. 1): 223, 1962.

46. Fullmer, H. M., et al.: The Origin of Collagenase in Periodontal Tissues of Man. J. D. Res., 48:636, 1969.

47. Gargiulo, A. W., Wentz, F. M., and Orban, B.: Dimensions and Relations of the Dentogingival Junction in Humans. J. Periodont., 32:261, 1961.

48. Glickman, I., and Bibby, B. G.: The Existence of Cuticular Structures on Human Teeth. J. D. Res., 22:91, 1943.

49. Glickman, I., and Johannessen, L.: Biomicroscopic (Slit-Lamp) Evaluation of the Normal Gingiva of the Albino Rat. J.A.D.A., 41:521, 1950.

50. Glickman, I., and Smulow, J. B.: Histopathology and Histochemistry of Chronic Desquamative Gingivitis. Oral Surg., 21:325, 1966.

51. Glickman, I., Turesky, S., and Hill, R.: Determination of Oxygen Consumption in Normal and Inflamed Human Gingiva Using the Warburg Manometric Technic. J. D. Res., 28:83, 1949.

52. Gottlieb, B.: Aetiologie und Prophylaxe der Zahnkaries. Ztschr. f. Stomatol., 19:129, 1921.

53. Gottlieb, B.: Der Epithelansatz am Zahne. Deutsch. Monatschr. f. Zahnhk., 39:142, 1921.

54. Gottlieb, B.: Tissue Changes in Pyorrhea. Trans. 7th Int. Dent. Congress, 1:421, 1926.

55. Gottlieb, B.: What is a Normal Pocket? J.A.D.A., 13:1747, 1926.

56. Gottlieb, B.: Zur Biologie des Epithelansatzes und des Alveolarrandes. Deutsch. Zahnärztl. Wchnschr., 25:434, 1922.

57. Gottlieb, B., and Orban, B.: Active and Passive Eruption of the Teeth, J. D. Res., 13:214, 1933.

58. Greene, A. H.: A Study of the Characteristics of Stippling and Its Relation to Gingival Health. J. Periodont., 33:176, 1962.

59. Greulich, R. C.: Epithelial DNA and RNA Synthetic Activities of the Gingival Margin. J. D. Res., 40:682, 1961.

60. Gross, H.: Zur Genese der vertieften Zahnfleischtasche Paradentium, 3:69, 1930.

61. Hansen, E. R.: Mitotic Activity of the Gingival Epithelium in Colchicinized Rats. Odont. T., 74:229, 1966.

62. Hansson, B. O., Lindhe, J., and Branemark, P. I.: Microvascular Topography and Function in Clinically Healthy and Chronically Inflamed Dentogingival Tissues—A Vital Microscopic Study in Dogs. Periodontics, 6:265, 1968.

63. Hodge, H. C.: Gingival Tissue Lipids. J. Biol. Chem., 101:55, 1933.

64. Hodson, J.: The Distribution, Structure, Origin, and Nature of the Dental Cuticle of Gottlieb. Periodontics, 5:295, 1967.

65. Ito, H., Enomoto, S., and Kobayashi, K.: Electron Microscopic Study of the Human Epithelial Attachment. Bull. Tokyo Med. Dent. Univ., 14:267, 1967.

66. Iusem, R.: A Cytological Study of the Cornification of the Oral Mucosa in Women. Oral Surg., Oral Med. & Oral Path., 3:1516, 1950.

67. Karring, T., and Löe, H.: Blood Supply of the Periodontium. J. Periodont. Res., 2:74, 1967.

68. Kaslick, R. S., et al.: Quantitative Analysis of Sodium, Potassium and Calcium in Gingival Fluid from Gingiva in Varying Degrees of Inflammation. J. Periodont., 41:93, 1970.

69. Kindlova, M.: The Blood Supply of the Marginal Periodontium in Macacus Rhesus. Arch. Oral Biol., 10:869, 1965.

70. Kohl, J., and Zander, H. A.: Fibres Conjunctive Oxytalan dans le Tissue Gingival Interdentaire. Paradontol., 16:23, 1962.

71. Kurahashi, Y., and Takuma, S.: Electronmicroscopy of Human Gingival Epithelium. Bull. Tokyo D. Col., 3:29, 1962.

72. Lainson, P. A., and Fisher, A. K.: Endogenous Oxygen Consumption Rates of Bovine Attached Gingiva. J. Periodont. Res., 3:132, 1968.

73. Lange, D., and Camelleri, G. E.: Cytochemical Demonstration of Lysosomes in the Exfoliated Epithelial Cells of the Gingival Cuff. J. D. Res., 46:625, 1967.

74. Leng, A., et al.: Determination of the Nucleic Acids in Normal and Pathologic Gingiva. Rev. Dental de Chile, 45:809, 1955.

75. Lindhe, J., and Attström, R.: Gingival Exudation During the Menstrual Cycle. J. Periodont. Res., 2:194, 1967.

76. Lindhe, J., Attström, R., and Björn, A. L.: Influence of Sex Hormones on Gingival Exudation in Dogs with Chronic Gingivitis. J. Periodont. Res., 3:279, 1968.

77. Lindhe, J., Attström, R., and Björn, A. L.: Influence of Sex Hormones on Gingival Exudation in Gingivitis-Free Female Dogs. J. Periodont. Res., 3:273, 1968.

78. Lindhe, J., and Björn, A. L.: Influences of Hormonal Contraceptives on the Gingiva of Women. J. Periodont. Res., 2:1, 1967.

79. Lindhe, J., and Brånemark, P. I.: Changes in Vascular Proliferation after Local Application of Sex Hormones. J. Periodont. Res., 2:266, 1967.

80. Lisanti, V. F.: Hydrolytic Enzymes in Periodontal Disease. Ann. New York Acad. Sc., 85:461, 1960.

81. Listgarten, M. A.: Changing Concepts About the Dento-epithelial Junction. J. Canad. D. Assn., 36:70, 1970.

82. Listgarten, M. A.: Electron Microscopic Study of the Gingivo-dental Junction of Man. Am. J. Anat., 119:147, 1966.

83. Listgarten, M. A.: Phase Contrast and Electron Microscopic Study of the Junction between Reduced Enamel Epithelium and Enamel in Unerupted Human Teeth. Arch. Oral Biol., 11:999, 1966.

84. Listgarten, M. A.: The Ultrastructure of Human Gingival Epithelium. Am. J. Anat., 114:49, 1964.

85. Löe, H., and Holm-Pedersen, P.: Absence and Presence of Fluid from Normal and Inflamed Gingivae. Periodontics, 3:171, 1965.

86. Löe, H., and Karring, T.: A Quantitative Analysis of the Epithelium-Connective Tissue Interface in Relation to Assessments of the Mitotic Index. J. D. Res., 48:634, 1969.

87. Löe, H., and Karring, T.: Mitotic Activity and Renewal Time of the Gingival Epithelium of Young and Old Rats. J. Periodont. Res., Suppl., 4:18, 1969.

88. Macapanpan, L. C.: Union of the Enamel and Gingival Epithelium. J. Periodont., 25:243, 1954.

89. Mandel, J. I., and Weinstein, E.: The Fluid of the Gingival Sulcus. Periodontics, 2:147, 1964.

90. Manhold, J. H., and Volpe, A. P.: Effect of Inflammation in the Absence of Proliferation on the Oxygen Consumption of Gingival Tissue. J. D. Res., 42:103, 1963.

91. Marwah, A. S., and Weinmann, J. P.: A Sex Difference in Epithelial Cells of Human Gingiva. J. Periodont., 26:11, 1955.

92. McHugh, W. D.: Keratinization of Gingival Epithelium in Laboratory Animals. J. Periodont., 35:338, 1964.

93. McHugh, W. D., and Zander, H. A.: Cell Division in the Periodontium of Developing and Erupted Teeth. D. Practit., 15:451, 1965.

94. Melcher, A. H.: Gingival Reticulin: Identification and Role in Histogenesis of Collagen Fibers. J. D. Res., 45:426, 1966.

95. Melcher, A. H.: Pathogenesis of Chronic Gingivitis. II. The Effect of Inflammatory Changes in the Corium on the Overlying Epithelium. D. Practit. & D. Record, 13:50, 1962.

96. Meyer, J., Marwah, A. S., and Weinmann, J. P.: Mitotic Rate of Gingival Epithelium in Two Age Groups. J. Invest. Derm., 27:237, 1956.

97. Meyer, W.: Controversial Questions Regarding the Histology of the Enamel Cuticle. Vierteljhschr. f. Zahnheilk., 46:42, 1930.

98. Miller, S. C., Soberman, A., and Stahl, S.: A Study of the Cornification of the Oral Mucosa of Young Male Adults. J. D. Res., 30:4, 1951.

99. Montgomery, P. W.: A Study of Exfoliative Cytology of Normal Human Oral Mucosa. J. D. Res., 30:12, 1951.

100. Morgan, R. E., and Wingo, W. J.: The Oxygen Consumption of Gingival Crevicular Epithelium. Oral Surg., 22:257, 1966.

101. Mori, M., and Kishiro, A.: Histochemical Observation of Aminopeptidase Activity in the Normal and Inflamed Oral Epithelium. J. Osaka Univ. D. Sch., 1:39, 1961.

102. Moss, M. L.: Phylogeny and Comparative Anatomy of Oral Ectodermal-Ectomesenchymal Inductive Interactions. J. D. Res., 48:732, 1969.

103. Nasmyth, A.: On the Structure, Physiology, and Pathology of the Persistent Capsular Investments and Pulp of the Tooth. Medico-Chirurgical Transactions of the Royal Medical & Chirurgical Society of London, 22:310, 1839.

104. Oliver, R. C., Holm-Pedersen, P., and Löe, H.: The Correlation between Clinical Scoring, Exudate Measurements and Microscopic Evaluation of Inflammation in the Gingiva. J. Periodont.-Periodontics, 40:201, 1969.

105. Orban, B., and Kohler, J.: The Physiologic Gingival Sulcus. Ztschr. f. Stomatol., 22:353, 1924.

106. Orban, B., et al.: The Epithelial Attachment (The Attached Epithelial Cuff). J. Periodont., 27:167, 1956.

107. Orban, J. E., and Stallard, R. E.: Gingival Crevicular Fluid: A Reliable Predictor of Gingival Health? J. Periodont.-Periodontics, 40:231, 1969.

108. Ostrom, C. A., Skillen, W. G., and Fosdick, L. S.: Chemical Studies in Periodontal Disease VIII. Gingival Glycogen Concentration in Experimental Occlusal Trauma, J. D. Res., 29:55, 1950.

109. Papic, M., and Glickman, I.: Keratinization of the Human Gingiva in the Menstrual Cycle and Menopause. Oral Surg., Oral Med. & Oral Path., 3:504, 1950.

110. Pelzer, R. H.: A Method for Plasma Phosphatase Determination for the Differentiation of Alveolar Crest Bone Types in Periodontal Disease. J. D. Res., 19:73, 1940.

111. Person, P., Felton, J., and Fine, A.: Biochemical and Histochemical Studies of Aerobic Oxidative Metabolism of Oral Tissues. III. Specific Metabolic Activities of Enzymatically Separated Gingival Epithelium and Connective Tissue Components. J. D. Res., 44:91, 1965.

112. Quintarelli, G.: Histochemistry of the Gingiva III. The Distribution of Aminopeptidase in Normal and Inflammatory Conditions. Arch. Oral Biol., 2:271, 1960.

113. Quintarelli, G., and Cheraskin, E.: Histochemistry of the Gingiva VI. Distribution and Localization of Phosphorylase. J. Periodont., 32:339, 1961.

114. Rosenberg, H., and Massler, M. J.: Gingival Stippling in Young Adult Males. J. Periodont., 38:473, 1967.

115. San Martín Sánchez, A.: Spectrographic Analysis of the Normal and Pyorrhetic Mucosa. Santiago, University of Chile Press, 1946.

116. Schilli, W.: The Most Superficial Zone of the Stratum Corneum of the Gingiva. Oral Surg., 25:896, 1968.

117. Schroeder, H. E.: Melanin Containing Organelles in Cells of the Human Gingiva. J. Periodont. Res., 4:1, 1969.

118. Schroeder, H. E.: Ultrastructure of the Junctional Epithelium and Human Gingiva. Helv. Odont. Acta, 13:65, 1969.

119. Schroeder, H. E., and Theilade, J.: Electron Microscopy of Normal Human Gingival Epithelium. J. Periodont. Res., 1:95, 1966.

120. Schultz-Haudt, S. D., and From, S.: Dynamics of Periodontal Tissues. I. The Epithelium. Odont. Tskr., 69:431, 1961.

121. Schultz-Haudt, S. D., From, S. H. J., and Nordbo, H.: Histochemical Staining Properties of Isolated Polysaccharide Components of Human Gingiva. Arch. Oral Biol., 9:17, 1964.

122. Schultz-Haudt, S. D., Paus, S., and Assev, S.: Periodic Acid–Schiff Reactive Components of Human Gingiva, J. D. Res., 40:141, 1961.

123. Schweitzer, G.: Lymph Vessels of the Gingiva and Teeth. Arch. f. Mik. Anat. und Ent., 69:807, 1907.

124. Shapiro, S., Ulmansky, M., and Scheuer, M.: Mast Cell Population in Gingiva Affected by Chronic Destructive Periodontal Disease. J. Periodont.-Periodontics, 40:276, 1969.

125. Shelton, L., and Hall, W.: Human Gingival Mast Cells. J. Periodont. Res., 3:214, 1968.

126. Skillen, W. G.: The Morphology of the Gingivae of the Rat Molar. J.A.D.A., 17:645, 1930.

127. Skougaard, M. R., Bay, I., and Klinkhamer, J. M.: Correlation between Gingivitis and Orogranulocytic Migratory Rate. J. Res., 48:716, 1969.

128. Skougaard, M. R., and Beagrie, G. S.: The Renewal of Gingival Epithelium in Marmosets (Callithrix jacchus) as Determined Through Autoradiography with Thymidine-H_3. Acta Odont. Scandinav., 20:467, 1962.

129. Smulow, J. B., and Glickman, I.: In Vitro Cultural and Histochemical Characteristics of Human Oral Mucosa. Arch. Oral Biol., 11:1143, 1966.

130. Soni, N. N., Silberkweit, M., and Hayes, R. L.: Pattern of Mitotic Activity and Cell Densities in Human Gingival Epithelium. J. Periodont., 36:15, 1965.

131. Squier, C. A., and Waterhouse, L. P.: The Ultrastructure of the Melanocyte in Human Gingival Epithelium. J. D. Res., 46:112, 1967.

132. Stallard, R. E., Diab, M. A., and Zander, H. A.: The Attaching Substance between Enamel and Epithelium – A Product of the Epithelial Cells. J. Periodont., 36:40, 1965.

133. Stern, I. B.: Electronmicroscopic Observations of Oral Epithelium. I. Basal Cells and the Basement Membrane. Periodontics, 3:224, 1965.

134. Stern, I. B.: Further Electron Microscopic Observations of the Epithelial Attachment. Internat. Ass. Dent. Res. Abstr., 45th General Meeting, 1967, p. 118.

135. Stern, I. B.: The Fine Structure of the Ameloblast – Enamel Junction in Rat Incisors, Epithelial Attachment and Cuticular Membrane. 5th Internat. Congress for Electron Micros., 2:6, 1966.

136. Sueda, T., and Cimasoni, G.: The Origins of Acid Phosphatase in Human Gingival Fluid. Arch. Oral Biol., 13:553, 1968.

137. Susi, F.: Histochemical Autoradiographic and Electron Microscopic Studies of Keratinization in Oral Mucosa. Ph.D. Thesis, Tufts University, 1967.

138. Swift, J. A., and Saxton, C. A.: The Ultrastructural Location of the Periodate-Schiff Reactive Basement Membrane of the Dermoepidermal Junctions of Human Scalp and Monkey Gingiva. J. Ultrastruct. Res., 17:23, 1967.

139. Talbot, E.: Histopathology of the Jaws and Apical Dental Tissues: The So-Called Nasmyth's Membrane. D. Cosmos, 1920.

140. Thilander, H.: Permeability of the Gingival Pocket Epithelium. Internat. Dent. J., 14:416, 1964.

141. Thilander, H., and Bloom, G. D.: Cell Contacts in Oral Epithelia. J. Periodont. Res., 3:96, 1968.

142. Thonard, J. C., and Scherp, H. W.: Histochemical Demonstration of Acid Mucopolysaccharides in Human Gingival Epithelial Intercellular Spaces. Arch. Oral Biol., 7:125, 1962.

143. Toller, J. R.: The Organic Continuity of the Dentine, the Enamel and the Epithelial Attachment in Dogs. Brit. D. J., 67:443, 1939.

144. Toto, P. D., and Grundel, E. R.: Acid Mucopolysaccharides in the Oral Epithelium. J. D. Res., 45:211, 1966.

145. Toto, P. D., and Sicher, H. J.: Mucopolysaccharides in the Epithelial Attachment. J. D. Res., *44*:451, 1965.

146. Trott, J. R.: An Investigation into the Glycogen Content of the Gingivae. D. Practit., 7:234, 1957.

147. Trott, J. R., and Gorenstein, S. L.: Mitotic Rates in the Oral and Gingival Epithelium of the Rat. Arch. Oral Biol., 8:425, 1963.

148. Turesky, S., Crowley, J., and Glickman, I.: A Histochemical Study of Protein-Bound Sulfhydryl and Disulfide Groups in Normal and Inflamed Human Gingiva. J. D. Res., *36*:225, 1957.

149. Turesky, S., Glickman, I., and Fisher, B.: The Effect of Physiologic and Pathologic Processes Upon Certain Histochemically Detectable Substances in the Gingiva. J. Periodont., 30:116, 1959.

150. Turesky, S., Glickman, I., and Litwin, T.: A Histochemical Evaluation of Normal and Inflamed Human Gingivae. J. D. Res., 30:792, 1951.

151. Ussing, M. J.: The Development of the Epithelial Attachment. Acta Odont. Scandinav., *13*:123, 1956.

152. Waerhaug, J.: Current Views on the Epithelial Cuff. Periodontics, 4:278, 1966.

153. Waerhaug, J.: The Gingival Pocket. Odont. Tskr. 60. Suppl. 1, 1952, Oslo.

154. Waterhouse, J. P.: The Gingival Part of the Human Periodontium. Its Ultrastructure and the Distribution in It of Acid Phosphatase in Relation to Cell Attachment and the Lysosome Concept. D. Practit., *15*:409, 1965.

155. Weinmann, J. P., et al.: Occurrence and Role of Glycogen in the Epithelium of the Alveolar Mucosa and of the Attached Gingiva. Am. J. Anat., *104*:381, 1959.

156. Weinstein, E., Mandel, I. D., Salkind, A., Oshrain, H. I., and Pappas, G. D.: Studies of Gingival Fluid. Periodontics, 5:161, 1967.

157. Weinstock, A., and Albright, J. T.: The Fine Structure of Mast Cell in Normal Human Gingiva. J. Ultrastruct. Res., *17*:245, 1967.

158. Wertheimer, F. W.: A Histologic Comparison of Apical Cuticles, Secondary Dental Cuticles and Hyaline Bodies. J. Peridont., *37*:5, 1966.

159. Wertheimer, F. W., and Fullmer, H. M.: Morphologic and Histochemical Observations on the Human Dental Cuticle. J. Periodont., 33:29, 1962.

160. Weski, O.: Die chronischen marginalen Entzündungen des Alveolar-fortsatzes mit besonderer Berücksichtigung der Alveolarpyorrhoe. Vierteljahrschr. f. Zahnheilk., 38:1, 1922.

161. Wilkinson, F. C.: A Patho-histological Study of the Tissue of Tooth Attachment. D. Record, *55*: 105, 1935.

162. Williams, C. H. M.: Present Status of Knowledge Regarding the Etiology of Periodontal Disease. Oral Surg., Oral Med. & Oral Path., 2:729, 1949.

163. Wodehouse, W. B.: The Gingival Trough—Its Early Development. Australian J. D., *33*:139, 1929.

164. Zachrisson, B. U.: Mast Cells of the Human Gingiva. IV. Experimental Gingivitis. J. Periodont. Res., *4*:46, 1969.

165. Zachrisson, B. U., and Schulz-Haudt, S. D.: Biologically Active Substances of the Mast Cell. J. Periodont. Res., 2:21, 1967.

166. Zander, H. A.: The Distribution of Phosphatase in Gingival Tissue. J. D. Res., *20*:347, 1941.

THE PERIODONTAL LIGAMENT

The periodontal ligament is the connective tissue structure that surrounds the root and connects it with the bone. It is continuous with the connective tissue of the gingiva and communicates with the marrow spaces through vascular channels in the bone.

NORMAL MICROSCOPIC FEATURES

Principal fibers

The most important elements of the periodontal ligament are the principal fibers, which are collagenous, arranged in bundles, and follow a wavy course (Figs. 2–1 and 2–2). Terminal portions of the principal fibers that insert into cementum and bone are termed Sharpey's fibers.

PRINCIPAL FIBER GROUPS OF THE PERIODONTAL LIGAMENT. The principal fibers are arranged in the following groups: transseptal, alveolar crest, horizontal, oblique and apical (Figs. 2–3 and 2–4).

Transseptal Group. These fibers extend interproximally over the alveolar crest and are embedded in the cementum of adjacent teeth (Fig. 2–5). The transseptal fibers are a remarkably constant finding. They are reconstructed even after destruction of the alveolar bone has occurred in periodontal disease.

Alveolar Crest Group. These fibers extend obliquely from the cementum just beneath the epithelial attachment to the alveolar crest. Their function is to counterbalance the coronal thrust of the more apical fibers, thus helping to retain the tooth within its socket and resist lateral tooth movements.

Horizontal Group. These fibers extend at right angles to the long axis of the tooth from the cementum to the alveolar bone. Their function is similar to those of the alveolar crest.

Oblique Group. These fibers, the largest group in the periodontal ligament, extend from the cementum in a coronal direction obliquely to the bone. They bear the brunt of vertical masticatory stresses and transform them into tension on the alveolar bone.

Apical Group. The apical group of fibers radiate from the cementum to the bone at the fundus of the socket. They do not occur on incompletely formed roots.

Other fibers

Other well-formed fiber bundles interdigitate at right angles or splay around and between regularly arranged fiber bundles.

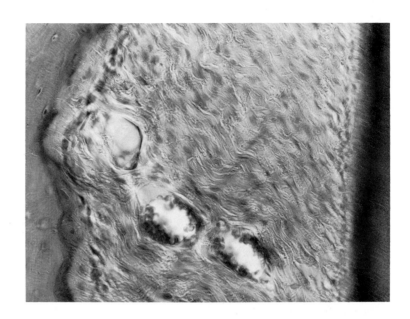

Figure 2-1 Principal Fibers on the Periodontal Ligament Follow a Wavy Course. The formative function of the periodontal ligament is illustrated by the newly formed osteoid and osteoblasts along a previously resorbed bone surface (*left*) and the cementoid and cementoblasts (*right*). Note the fibers embedded in the forming calcified tissues.

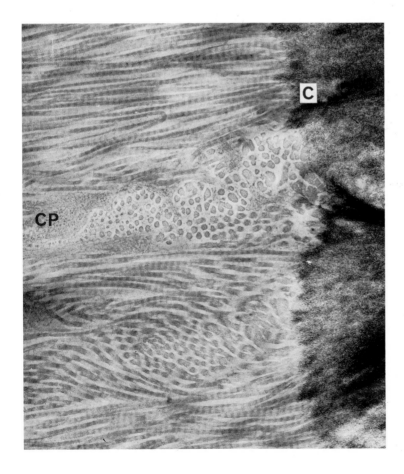

Figure 2-2 Electron Micrograph of Periodontal Fiber Attachment to Cementum. The periodontal fibers consist of bundles of parallel fibrils which insert into the cementum (C) at varying angles. The fibrils have a periodic cross banding typical of collagen. CP, cellular process. Magnification × 30,000. (Courtesy of Dr. Knut A. Selvig.)

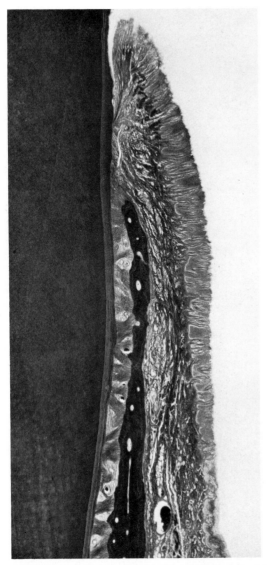

Figure 2-3 Principal Fiber Bundles of the Periodontal Ligament on the facial surface of a mandibular premolar (Silver stain).

Less regularly arranged *collagen fibers* are found in the interstitial connective tissue between the principal fiber groups which contains the blood vessels, lymphatics and nerves. Other fibers of the periodontal ligament are the *elastic fibers,*[45] which are relatively few, and oxytalan[19, 23] (acid-resistant) fibers, which are distributed mainly around the blood vessels and embedded in cementum in the cervical third of the root. Their function is not understood.

THE INTERMEDIATE PLEXUS. The principal fiber bundles consist of individual fibers which form a continuous anastomosing network between tooth and bone.[11] It has been suggested that instead of being continuous the individual fibers consist of two separate parts spliced together midway between cementum and bone in a zone called the *intermediate plexus.* The plexus has been reported in the periodontal ligament of continuously growing incisors of animals,[27, 32, 40] but not in the posterior teeth;[51] and in actively erupting human teeth, but not after they reach occlusal contact. Rearrangement of the fiber ends in the plexus is supposed to accommodate tooth eruption, without necessitating the embedding of new fibers into tooth and bone.[32] There are doubts regarding the existence of such a plexus;[6, 46] some consider it a microscopic artefact,[20] whereas others find no evidence of it when collagen fiber formation is traced with radioactive proline.[15]

Cellular elements

The cellular elements of the periodontal ligament are fibroblasts, endothelial cells, cementoblasts, osteoblasts, osteoclasts, tissue macrophages and strands of epithelial cells, termed the "epithelial rests of Malassez" or "resting epithelial cells."[49]

The *epithelial rests* form a latticework in the periodontal ligament and appear as either isolated clusters of cells or interlacing strands, depending on the plane in which the microscopic section is cut. Continuity with the epithelial attachment in experimental animals has been suggested.[24] They are considered to be remnants of the Hertwig root sheath, which disintegrates during root development when cementum is formed on the dentin surface, but this concept has been questioned.[17]

Epithelial rests are distributed throughout the periodontal ligament of most teeth, close to the cementum, and are most numerous in the apical[39] and cervical areas.[50] They diminish in number with age[41] by degenerating and disappearing or undergoing calcification to become cementicles. They are surrounded by a PAS-positive, argyrophilic, fibrillar, sometimes hyaline capsule from which they are separated by a distinct basement lamina or membrane. Epithelial rests proliferate when stimulated[44, 47] and participate in the formation of periapical cysts and lateral root cysts or deepen peri-

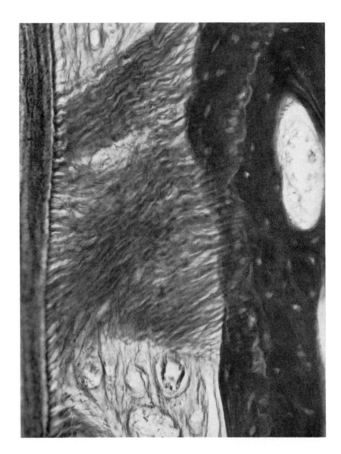

Figure 2–4 Detailed view of Figure 2–3 showing continuous collagen fibers embedded in the cementum (*left*) and bone (*right*) (silver stain). Note the Sharpey's fibers within the bone.

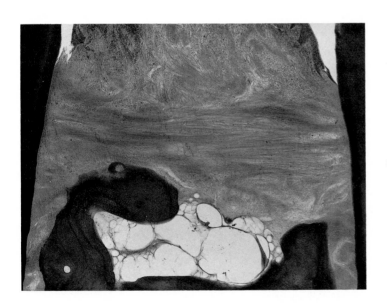

Figure 2–5 Transseptal Fibers at the crest of the interdental bone.

odontal pockets by fusing with proliferating gingival epithelium.

The periodontal ligament may also contain calcified masses called cementicles (see Chap. 3) which are adherent to, or detached from, the root surfaces.

Vascular supply

The blood supply is derived from the *inferior* and *superior alveolar arteries* and reaches the periodontal ligament from three sources: *apical vessels, penetrating vessels from the alveolar bone,* and *anastomosing vessels from the gingiva.*[12] The apical vessels enter the periodontal ligament at the apical region and extend to the gingiva, giving off lateral branches in the direction of the cementum and bone. The vessels within the periodontal ligament are connected in a net-like plexus which receives its principal supply from alveolar perforating arteries and small vessels which penetrate through channels in the alveolar bone[18] (Figs. 2–6 and 2–7). The blood

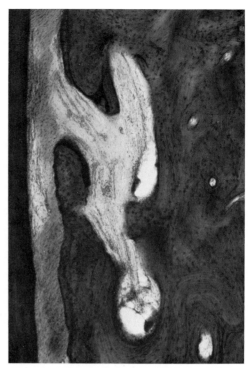

Figure 2–7 Small Vessels in Channel connecting the periodontal ligament and alveolar bone.

supply from this source increases from the incisors to molars; is greatest in the gingival third of single-rooted teeth, less in the apical third and least in the middle; is equal in the apical and middle thirds of multirooted teeth; is slightly greater on the mesial and distal surfaces than on the facial and lingual; and is greater on the mesial surfaces of mandibular molars than on the distal.[8] The vascular supply from the gingiva is derived from branches of deep vessels in the lamina propria. The venous drainage of the periodontal ligament accompanies the arterial supply.

Lymphatics

Lymphatics supplement the venous drainage system. Those draining the region just beneath the epithelial attachment pass into the periodontal ligament and accompany the blood vessels into the periapical region.[9] From there they pass through the alveolar bone to the inferior dental canal in the mandible, or the infraorbital canal in the maxilla, and to the submaxillary group of lymph nodes.

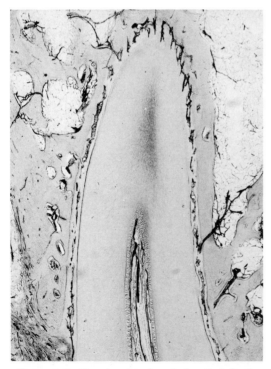

Figure 2–6 Vascular Supply of the Periodontium (monkey perfused with India ink). Note the longitudinal vessels in the periodontal ligament and alveolar perforating arteries in channels between the bone marrow and periodontal ligament. (Courtesy of Dr. Sol Bernick.)

Innervation

The periodontal ligament is abundantly supplied with sensory nerve fibers capable of transmitting *tactile, pressure* and *pain* sensations by the trigeminal pathways.[2, 5] Nerve bundles pass into the periodontal ligament from the periapical area and through channels from the alveolar bone. The nerve bundles follow the course of the blood vessels and divide into single myelinized fibers, which ultimately lose their myelin sheath and terminate either as free nerve endings or elongate spindle-like structures. The latter are *proprioceptive receptors* that account for the sense of localization when the tooth is touched.

Development of the periodontal ligament

The periodontal ligament develops from the *dental sac,* a circular layer of fibrous connective tissue surrounding the tooth bud. As the developing tooth erupts, the loose connective tissue of the sac differentiates into three layers: an outer layer adjacent to the bone, an inner layer along the cementum, and an intermediate layer of unorganized fibers.[35] The principal fiber bundles are derived from the intermediate layer and are thickened and arranged according to functional requirements when the tooth reaches occlusal contact.[31]

FUNCTIONS OF THE PERIODONTAL LIGAMENT

The functions of the periodontal ligament are *physical, formative, nutritional* and *sensory.*

Physical function

The physical functions of the periodontal ligament entail the following:[33] transmission of occlusal forces to the bone; attachment of the teeth to the bone; maintenance of the gingival tissues in their proper relationship to the teeth; resistance to the impact of occlusal forces (shock absorption); and provision of a "soft tissue casing" to protect the vessels and nerves from injury by mechanical forces.

RESISTANCE TO THE IMPACT OF OCCLUSAL FORCES (SHOCK ABSORPTION). According to Parfitt[36] the initial responsibility for resisting occlusal forces rests in four systems of the periodontal ligament rather than in the principal fibers. The fibers serve a secondary role of restraining the tooth against lateral movement and preventing deformity of the periodontal ligament under compressive force. The four systems that initially resist occlusal forces are (1) the *vascular system,* which acts as a shock absorber and takes up strains of sudden occlusal forces; (2) the *hydrodynamic system,* consisting of tissue fluid and fluid which passes through small vessel walls[7] and is squeezed into the surrounding areas through foramina in the alveoli to resist axial forces; (3) the *pitch system,* which is probably closely related to the hydrodynamic system and controls the pitch or level of the tooth in the socket, and (4) the *resilient system,* which causes the tooth to spring back into position when the occlusal forces are removed. These systems are phenomena of the blood vessels and the ground substance–collagen complex of the periodontal ligament.

TRANSMISSION OF OCCLUSAL FORCES TO THE BONE. The arrangement of the principal fibers is similar to a suspension bridge or a hammock. When an axial force is applied to a tooth, there is a tendency toward displacement of the root into the alveolus. The oblique fibers alter their wavy untensed pattern, assume their full length, and sustain the major part of the axial force.

When a horizontal or tipping force is applied, there are **two characteristic phases** of tooth movement: the first is **within the confines of the periodontal ligament,** and the second produces a **displacement of the facial and lingual bony plates.**[16] The tooth rotates about an axis which may change as the force is increased. The apical portion of the root moves in a direction opposite to the coronal portion. In areas of tension the principal fiber bundles are taut rather than wavy. In areas of pressure the fibers are compressed, the tooth is displaced and there is a corresponding distortion of bone in the direction of root movement.[37]

In single-rooted teeth the axis of rotation is located slightly apical to the middle third of the root (Fig. 2–8). The root apex[33] and

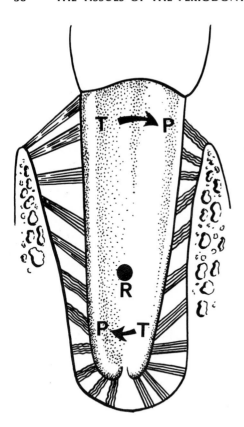

Figure 2–8 Distribution of Faciolingual Forces (arrows) around the axis of rotation (R) in a mandibular premolar. The periodontal ligament fibers are compressed in areas of pressure (P) and taut in areas of tension (T).

the coronal half of the clinical root have been suggested as other locations of the axis of rotation. The periodontal ligament, shaped like a hourglass, is narrowest in the region of the axis of rotation[14, 30] (Table 2–1). In multirooted teeth the axis of rotation is located in the bone between the roots.

In compliance with the physiologic mesial migration of the teeth (see page 39), the periodontal ligament on the mesial root surface is thinner than on the distal surface (Figs. 2–9 and 2–10).

OCCLUSAL FUNCTION AND THE STRUCTURE OF THE PERIODONTAL LIGAMENT. **Just as the tooth depends upon the periodontal ligament to support it during function, so does the periodontal ligament depend upon stimulation provided by occlusal function to preserve its structure.** Within physiologic limits the periodontal ligament can accommodate increased function by an increase in width, a thickening of the fiber bundles and an increase in diameter and number of Sharpey's fibers (Table

TABLE 2–1 THICKNESS OF PERIODONTAL MEMBRANE OF 172 TEETH FROM FIFTEEN HUMAN JAWS (COOLIDGE[14])

	Average of Alveolar Crest	Average of Midroot	Average of Apex	Average of Tooth
Ages 11–16				
83 teeth from 4 jaws	0.23	*0.17*	0.24	0.21
Ages 32–50				
36 teeth from 5 jaws	0.20	*0.14*	0.19	0.18
Ages 51–67				
35 teeth from 5 jaws	0.17	*0.12*	0.16	0.15
Age 25 (1 case)				
18 teeth from 1 jaw	0.16	*0.09*	0.15	0.13

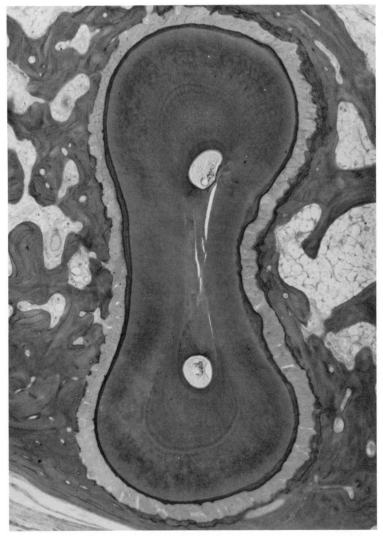

Figure 2–9 Physiologic Mesial Migration. Horizontal section through molar root. The periodontal ligament is thinner on the side toward which the tooth is migrating (mesial surface, *left*) than on the distal surface (*right*). The distal fibers are taut.

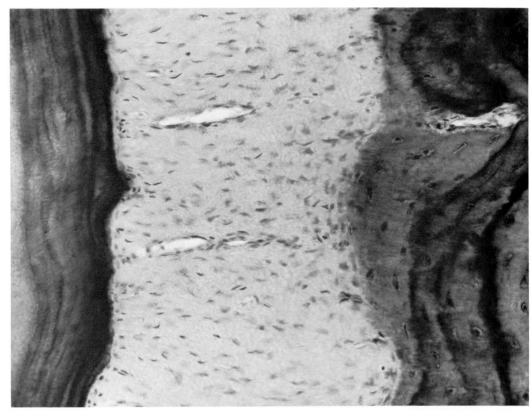

Figure 2–10 Detailed View of Figure 2–9; distal surface, showing cementum, periodontal ligament and bone. The tooth is migrating mesially (toward the cleft). Note the osteoblasts in the periodontal ligament and new bone formation (*right*).

TABLE 2–2 COMPARISON OF PERIODONTAL WIDTH OF FUNCTIONING AND FUNCTIONLESS TEETH IN A MALE AGED 38 (KRONFELD[30])

	Heavy Function Left Upper 2nd Bicuspid	Light Function Left Lower 1st Bicuspid	Functionless Left Upper 3rd Molar
Average width of periodontal space at entrance of alveolus	0.35 mm.	0.14 mm.	0.10 mm.
Average width of periodontal space at middle of alveolus	0.28 mm.	0.10 mm.	0.06 mm.
Average width of periodontal space at fundus of alveolus	0.30 mm.	0.12 mm.	0.06 mm.

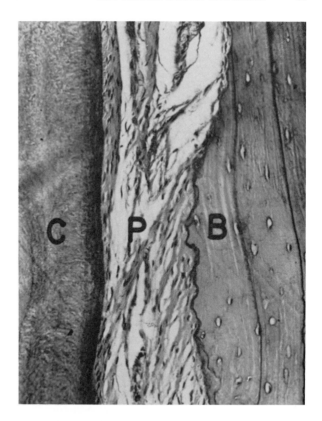

Figure 2–11 Atrophic Periodontal Ligament (P) of Tooth Devoid of Function. Note the lacunar resorption of the alveolar bone (B). Cementum (C).

2–2). Occlusal forces which exceed what the periodontal ligament can withstand produce injury called *trauma from occlusion* (see Chap. 24).

When function is diminished or absent, the periodontal ligament atrophies. It is thinned, and the fibers are reduced in number and density, become disoriented,[1] and ultimately are arranged parallel to the root surface (Fig. 2–11). In addition, the cementum is unaffected[13] or thickened, and the distance from the cemento-enamel junction to the alveolar crest is increased.[38]

Periodontal disease alters the functional demands upon the periodontal ligament

Destruction of the periodontal ligament and alveolar bone by periodontal disease disrupts the balance between the periodontium and occlusal forces. When supporting tissues are reduced by disease, the burden upon the tissue which remains is increased. Occlusal forces which were beneficial to the intact periodontal ligament may become injurious.

Formative function

The periodontal ligament serves as the periosteum for cementum and bone. Cells of the periodontal ligament participate in the formation and resorption of these tissues which occur in physiologic tooth movement, in the accommodation of the periodontium to occlusal forces and in the repair of injuries. Variations in cellular enzyme activity (certain dehydrogenases[20] and nonspecific esterase[22]) are correlated with the remodeling process. In areas of bone formation, osteoblasts, fibroblasts and cementoblasts stain intensely for nonspecific alkaline phosphatase, glucose-6-phosphatase and thiamine pyrophosphate.[21] In areas of bone resorption osteoclasts, fibroblasts, osteocytes and cementocytes stain for nonspecific acid phosphatase. Cartilage formation in the periodontal ligament is unusual and represents a metaplastic phenomenon in the repair of the periodontal ligament following injury.[3]

Like all structures of the periodontium, the periodontal ligament is constantly undergoing remodeling. Old cells and fibers are broken down and replaced by new ones, and mitotic activity can be observed in the fibroblasts and endothelial cells.[34] Fibroblasts form the collagen fibers and also develop into osteoblasts and cementoblasts. The rate of formation and differentiation of fibroblasts affects the rate of formation of collagen cementum and bone. Collagen formation increases with the rate of eruption.[42]

Radioautographic studies with radioactive thymidine, proline and glycine indicate a high rate of collagen metabolism in the periodontal ligament. Formation of new fibroblasts and collagen is most active adjacent to the bone and in the middle of the ligament and least active on the cementum side.[15, 43] Collagen turnover is greatest at the crest and apex.[10] There is also rapid turnover of sulfated mucopolysaccharides in the cells and amorphous ground substance of the periodontal ligament.[4]

Nutritional and sensory functions

The periodontal ligament supplies nutrients to the cementum, bone and gingiva by way of the blood vessels and provides lymphatic drainage. The innervation of the periodontal ligament provides *proprioceptive* and *tactile sensitivity*,[29, 48] which detects and localizes external forces acting upon the individual teeth and serves an important role in the neuromuscular mechanism controlling the masticatory musculature (see Chap. 52).

REFERENCES

1. Anneroth, G., and Ericsson, S. G.: An Experimental Histological Study of Monkey Teeth Without Antagonist. Odont. Revy, 18:345, 1967.
2. Avery, J. K., and Rapp, R.: Pain Conduction in Human Dental Tissues. Dent. Clin. North America, July 1959, p. 489.
3. Bauer, W. H.: Effect of a Faulty Constructed Partial Denture on a Tooth and Its Supporting Tissue, with Special Reference to Formation of Fibrocartilage in the Periodontal Membrane as a Result of Disturbed Healing Caused by Abnormal Stresses. Am. J. Orthodont. & Oral Surg., 27:640, 1941.
4. Baumhammers, A., and Stallard, R.: S35-Sulfate Utilization and Turnover by Connective Tissues of the Periodontium. J. Periodont. Res., 3:187, 1968.
5. Bernick, S.: Innervation of the Teeth and Periodontium. Dent. Clin. North America, July 1959, p. 503.
6. Bevelander, G., and Nakara, H.: The Fine Structure of the Human Periodontal Ligament. Anat. Rec., 162:313, 1968.
7. Bien, S. M.: Hydrodynamic Damping of Tooth Movement. J. D. Res., 45:907, 1966.
8. Birn, H.: The Vascular Supply of the Periodontal Membrane. J. Periodont. Res., 1:51, 1966.
9. Box, K. F.: Evidence of Lymphatics in the Periodontium. J. Canad. D. Assn., 15:8, 1949.
10. Carneiro, J., and Fava de Moraes, F.: Radioautographic Visualization of Collagen Metabolism in the Periodontal Tissues of the Mouse. Arch. Oral Biol., 10:833, 1965.
11. Ciancio, S. C., Neiders, M. E., and Hazen, S. P.: The Principal Fibers of the Periodontal Ligament. Periodontics, 5:76, 1967.
12. Cohen, L.: Further Studies into the Vascular Architecture of the Mandible. J. D. Res., 39:936, 1960.
13. Cohn, S. A.: Disuse Atrophy of the Periodontium in Mice. Arch. Oral Biol., 10:909, 1965.
14. Collidge, E. D.: The Thickness of the Human Periodontal Membrane. J.A.D.A., 24:1260, 1937.
15. Crumley, P. J.: Collagen Formation in the Normal and Stressed Periodontium. J. Am. Soc. Periodont., 2:53, 1964.
16. Davies, R., and Picton, D. C. A.: Dimensional Changes in the Periodontal Membrane of Monkey's Teeth with Horizontal Thrusts. J. D. Res., 46:114, 1967.
17. Diab, M. A., and Stallard, R. E.: A Study of the Relationship Between Epithelial Root Sheath and Root Development. Periodontics, 3:10, 1965.
18. Folke, L. E. A., and Stallard, R. E.: Periodontal Microcirculation as Revealed by Plastic Microspheres. J. Periodont. Res., 2:53, 1967.
19. Fullmer, H. M.: A Critique of Normal Connective Tissues of the Periodontium and Some Alterations with Periodontal Disease. J. D. Res., 41 (Suppl. to No. 1):223, 1962.
20. Gibson, W., and Fullmer, H.: Histochemistry of the Periodontal Ligament. I. The Dehydrogenases. Periodontics, 4:63, 1966.
21. Gibson, W., and Fullmer, H.: Histochemistry of the Periodontal Ligament: II. The Phosphatases. Periodontics, 5:226, 1967.
22. Gibson, W., and Fullmer, H.: Histochemistry of the Periodontal Ligament. III. The Esterases. Periodontics, 6:71, 1968.
23. Goggins, J. F.: The Distribution of Oxytalan Connective Tissue Fibers in Periodontal Ligaments of Deciduous Teeth. Periodontics, 4:182, 1966.
24. Grant, D., and Bernick, S.: A Possible Continuity between Epithelial Rests and Epithelial Attachment in Miniature Swine. J. Periodontics, 40:87, 1969.
25. Griffin, J. C.: Fine Structure of the Synthetizing Periodontal Fibroblasts and the Maturation of Periodontal Collagen. J. D. Res., 46:1311, 1967.
26. Grupe, H. E., Ten Cate, A. R., and Zander, H. A.: A Histochemical and Radiobiological Study of In Vitro and In Vivo Human Epithelial Cell Rest Proliferation. Arch. Oral Biol., 12:1321, 1967.
27. Hindle, M. C.: Quantitative Differences in Periodontal Membrane Fibers. J. D. Res., 43:953, 1964.
28. Inoue, M., and Akiyoshi, M.: Histologic Investigation on Sharpey's Fibers in Cementum of Teeth in Abnormal Function, J. D. Res., 41:503, 1962.
29. Kizior, J. E., Cuozzo, J. W., and Bowman, D. C.: Functional and Histologic Assessment of the Sensory Innervation of the Periodontal Ligament of the Cat. J. D. Res., 47:59, 1968.

30. Kronfeld, R.: Histologic Study of the Influence of Function on the Human Periodontal Membrane. J.A.D.A., 18:1242, 1931.

31. Levy, B. M., and Bernick, S.: Studies on the Biology of the Periodontium of Marmosets: II. Development and Organization of the Periodontal Ligament of Deciduous Teeth in Marmosets (*Callithrix Jacchus*) J. D. Res., 47:27, 1968.

32. Melcher, A. H.: Remodelling of the Periodontal Ligament During Eruption of the Rat Incisor. Arch. Oral Biol., 12:1649, 1967.

33. Muhlmann, H. R.: The Determination of Tooth Rotation Centers. Oral Surg., Oral Med. & Oral Path., 7:392, 1954.

34. Muhlmann, H. R., Zander, H. A., and Halberg, F.: Mitotic Activity in the Periodontal Tissues of the Rat Molar. J. D. Res., 33:459, 1954.

35. Orban, B.: Embryology and Histogenesis. Fortschr. d. Zahnheilk., 3:749, 1927.

36. Parfitt, G. H.: The Physical Analysis of Tooth Supporting Structures. In: The Mechanism of Tooth Support. Bristol, J. Wright and Sons, Ltd., 1967, p. 154.

37. Picton, D. C. S., and Davies, W. I. R.: Dimensional Changes in the Periodontal Membrane of Monkeys (*Macaca Irus*) Due to Horizontal Thrusts Applied to the Tooth. Arch. Oral Biol., 12:1635, 1967.

38. Pihlstrom, B. L., and Ramfjord, S. P.: The Effect of Non-Function on the Periodontium of Rhesus Monkeys. I.A.D.R. Abstr., 48th General Meeting, 1970, p. 201.

39. Reeve, C. M., and Wentz, F. J.: The Prevalence, Morphology and Distribution of Epithelial Rests in the Human Periodontal Ligament. Oral Surg., Oral Med. & Oral Path., 15:785, 1962.

40. Sicher, H.: The Axial Movement of Continuously Growing Teeth. J. D. Res., 21:201, 1942.

41. Simpson, H. E.: The Degeneration of the Rests of Malassez with Age as Observed by the Apoxestic Technique. J. Periodont., 36:288, 1965.

42. Stallard, R. E.: The Effect of Occlusal Alterations on Collagen Formation Within the Periodontal Ligament. Periodontics, 2:49, 1964.

43. Stallard, R. E.: The Utilization of H_3-Proline by the Connective Tissues of the Periodontium. J. Am. Soc. Periodont., 1:185, 1963.

44. Ten Cate, A. R.: The Histochemical Demonstration of Specific Oxidative Enzymes and Glycogen in the Epithelial Cell of Malassez. Arch. Oral Biol., 10:207, 1965.

45. Thomas, N. G.: Elastic Fibers in Periodontal Membrane and Pulp. J. D. Res., 7:325, 1927.

46. Troth, J. R.: The Development of the Periodontal Attachment in the Rat. Acta Anat., 51:313, 1962.

47. Trowbridge, H. O., and Shibata, F.: Mitotic Activity in Epithelial Roots of Malassez. Periodontics, 5:109, 1967.

48. Tryde, G., Frydenberg, O., and Brill, N.: An Assessment of the Tactile Sensibility in Human Teeth. An Evaluation of a Quantitative Method. Acta Odont. Scandinav., 20:233, 1962.

49. Valderhaug, J. P., and Nylen, M. U.: Function of Epithelial Rests as Suggested by their Ultrastructure. J. Periodont. Res., 1:69, 1966.

50. Valderhaug, J. P., and Zander, H.: Relationship of "Epithelial Rests of Malassez" to Other Periodontal Structures. Periodontics, 5:254, 1967.

51. Zwarych, P. D., and Quigley, M. B.: The Intermediate Plexus of the Periodontal Ligament: History and Further Observations. J. D. Res., 44:383, 1965.

Chapter 3

THE CEMENTUM

NORMAL MICROSCOPIC FEATURES

Cementum is the calcified mesenchymal tissue that forms the outer covering of the anatomic root. It may exert a far more critical role in the development of periodontal disease than has thus far been demonstrated.

There are two types of cementum: *acellular* (primary) and *cellular* (secondary). Both consist of a calcified interfibrillar matrix and collagen fibrils. The cellular type contains cementocytes in individual spaces (lacunae) which communicate with each other through a system of anastomosing canaliculi. There are two types of collagen fibers (a fiber consists of a bundle of submicroscopic fibrils): Sharpey's fibers, the embedded portion of principal fibers of the periodontal ligament[37, 48] which are formed by the fibroblasts, and a second group of fibers presumably produced by the cementoblasts,[45] which also form the glycoprotein interfibrillar ground substance.

Acellular and cellular cementum are arranged in *lamellae* separated by incremental lines parallel to the long axis of the root. They represent rest periods in cementum formation and are more mineralized than the adjacent cementum.[54] Sharpey's fibers make up most of the structure of *acellular cementum*, which has a principal role in supporting the tooth. Most of the fibers are inserted at approximately right angles into the root surface and penetrate deep into the cementum (Fig. 3–1), but others enter from several different directions.[9] Their size, number and distribution increase with function.[21] Sharpey's fibers are completely calcified with the mineral crystals parallel to the fibrils as they are in dentin and bone, except in a 10 to 50 micron wide zone near the cementodentinal junction where they are partly calcified. Acellular cementum also contains other collagen fibrils which are calcified and irregularly arranged or parallel to the surface. (For a comprehensive presentation of the electron microscopy of cementum, see the monograph by K. A. Selvig).[44]

Cellular cementum is less calcified than the acellular type.[22] Sharpey's fibers occupy a lesser portion of cellular cementum and are separated by other fibers which are either parallel to the root surface or arranged at random (Fig. 3–2). Some of Sharpey's fibers are completely calcified, others are partially calcified, and in some there is a central uncalcified core surrounded by a calcified border.[45]

The distribution of acellular and cellular cementum varies. The coronal half of the root is usually covered by the acellular type, and cellular cementum is more common in the apical half. With age the greatest increase in cementum is of the cellular type in the apical half of the root and in the furcation areas.

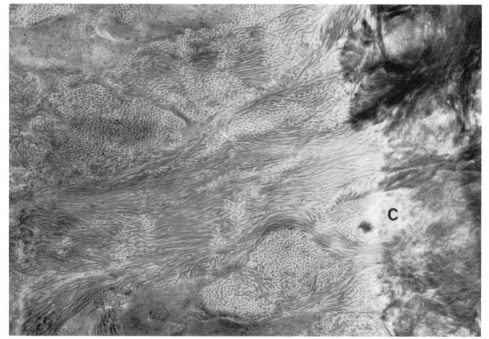

Figure 3–1   Electron Micrograph of the Surface of Acellular Cementum. Bundles of densely packed collagen fibrils are inserted into the cementum (C) more or less at right angles to its surface. × 10,000. (From Dr. Knut A. Selvig.[44])

Figure 3–2   Electron Micrograph of the Surface of Cellular Cementum. The cementum matrix contains irregularly arranged bundles of fibrils (C). Calcification foci are present in the precementum within a 5-micron wide zone at the surface of the cementum. × 10,000. (From Dr. Knut A. Selvig.[44])

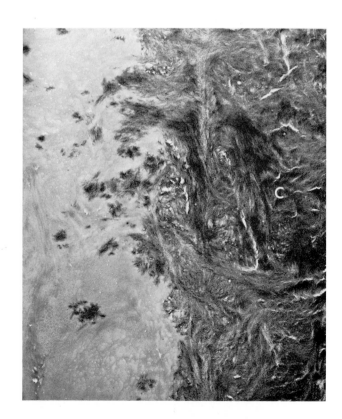

Intermediate cementum is an ill-defined zone of the cementodentinal junction which contains cellular remnants of Hertwig's sheath embedded in calcified ground substance.[12]

The *inorganic content* of cementum (hydroxyapatite, $Ca_{10}(PO4)_6(OH)_2$) is 46 per cent, which is less than that of bone (70.9 per cent), enamel (95.5 per cent) or dentin (69.3 per cent). The calcium and magnesium-phosphorus ratio is higher in apical than in cervical areas.[46] Opinions differ as to whether the microhardness increases[31] or decreases with age,[52] and no relationship has been established between aging and the mineral content of cementum.

Histochemical studies indicate that the *matrix of cementum* contains a *carbohydrate-protein complex*, with a protein component which contains *arginine and tyrosine. Neutral and acid mucopolysaccharides* are present in the matrix and cytoplasm of some cementoblasts. The lining of the lacunae, the incremental lines and the precementum are rich in *acid mucopolysaccharides, possibly chondroitin sulfate B.*[40] Precementum stains metachromatically,[18] and the ground substance of acellular and cellular cementum is orthochromatic.

The cemento-enamel junction

The cementum at and immediately subjacent to the cemento-enamel junction is of particular clinical importance in root scaling procedures.[36] Three types of relationships involving the cementum may exist at the cemento-enamel junction.[32] Cementum *overlaps the enamel* in about 60 to 65 per cent of the cases (Fig. 3–3). In about 30 per cent, there is an *edge-to-edge butt joint*, and in 5 to 10 per cent, the *cementum and enamel fail to meet.* In the latter instance gingival recession may be accompanied by an accentuated sensitivity because the dentin is exposed.

A layer of *granular afibrillar cementum* sometimes extends a short distance on the enamel at the cemento-enamel junction. It contains acid mucopolysaccharides and nonfibrillar collagen, in contrast with root cementum which is rich in collagen fibers. It has been hypothesized that this material is deposited on the enamel by connective tissue following degeneration and shrinkage of the reduced enamel epithelium.[29] The afibrillar cementum may be partially covered by root cementum. Cementum occurs on the enamel in swine, covering more of the surface than in humans, and over the entire enamel of bovine teeth.[14, 42]

In periodontal disease, the cementum adjacent to the enamel usually undergoes disintegration. The enamel then forms an overhanging ledge that may be confused with calculus when the tooth is scaled (Fig. 3–4).

The thickness of cementum on the coronal half of the root varies from 16 to 60 microns, or about the thickness of a hair. It attains its greatest thickness of up to 150 to 200 microns in the apical third, and also in the bifurcation and trifurcation areas.[34] Between the ages of 11 and 70 the average thickness of the cementum increases threefold, with the greatest increase in the apical region. Average thicknesses of 95 microns at age 20 and 215 microns at age 60 have been reported.[55]

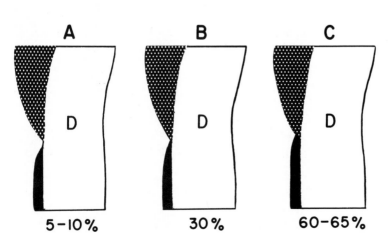

Figure 3–3 Statistical Representation of Normal Variations in Tooth Morphology at the Cemento-Enamel Junction. *A,* Space between enamel and cementum with dentin exposed (D). *B,* End-to-end relationship of enamel and cementum. *C,* Cementum overlapping the enamel. (After Hopewell-Smith.)

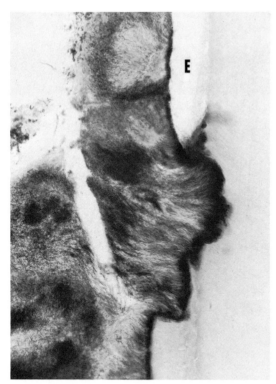

Figure 3–4 Cemento-Enamel Junction. Disintegration of cementum and dentin leaves overhanging ledge of enamel (E). The area is covered with calculus.

In very young animals, both cellular and acellular cementum are very permeable and permit the diffusion of dyes from the pulp canal and from the external root surface. In cellular cementum the canaliculi in some areas are contiguous with the dentinal tubuli. Devitalized teeth take up about one tenth as much radioactive phosphorus (P[32]) through the cementum as vital teeth.[53]

With age, the permeability of cementum diminishes.[10] There is also a relative diminution in the contribution of the pulp to the nutrition of the tooth, which increases the importance of the periodontal ligament as a pathway for metabolic exchange.[51] In the very aged, the phosphate exchange in the tooth by way of the periodontal ligament and cementum increases to 50 per cent of the total.[50]

CEMENTOGENESIS

Cementum formation starts with the mineralization of a meshwork of irregularly arranged collagen fibrils sparsely distributed in an interfibrillar ground substance or matrix (Fig. 3–5).[42, 43] It increases in thickness by the addition of ground substance and the progressive mineralization of collagen fibrils of the periodontal ligament (Fig. 3–6). Hydroxyapatite crystals are deposited first within and on the surface of the fibers and then in the ground substance. Periodontal ligament fibers being incorporated into the cementum at approximately right angles to the surface (Sharpey's fibers) appear under the electron microscope as a series of mineralized spurs from which a fiber projects into the periodontal ligament.

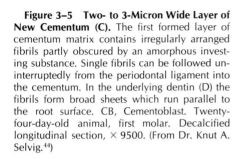

Figure 3–5 Two- to 3-Micron Wide Layer of New Cementum (C). The first formed layer of cementum matrix contains irregularly arranged fibrils partly obscured by an amorphous investing substance. Single fibrils can be followed uninterruptedly from the periodontal ligament into the cementum. In the underlying dentin (D) the fibrils form broad sheets which run parallel to the root surface. CB, Cementoblast. Twenty-four-day-old animal, first molar. Decalcified longitudinal section, × 9500. (From Dr. Knut A. Selvig.[44])

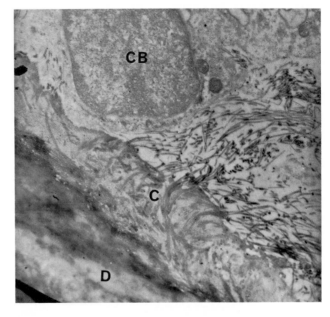

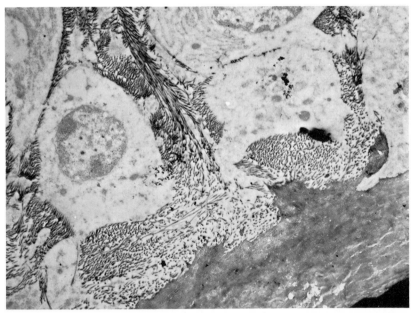

Figure 3–6   Root Surface at Some Distance From the Apex. More advanced stage of development of attachment apparatus. Cross-sectioned bundles of collagen fibrils are seen near the cementum surface. Decalcified, × 6000. (From Dr. Knut A. Selvig.[44])

Cementoblasts, initially separated from the cementum by uncalcified collagen fibrils, are enclosed within it by the mineralization process. Cementum formation is a continuous process which proceeds at a varying rate.

CONTINUOUS DEPOSITION OF CEMENTUM

Cementum deposition continues after the teeth have erupted into contact with their functional antagonists and throughout life. This is part of the over-all process of continuous tooth eruption. The teeth erupt in an effort to keep pace with tooth substance lost by occlusal and incisal wear. As they erupt, less of the root remains in the socket, weakening the support of the teeth. This is compensated for by continuous deposition of cementum on the root surface, in greatest amounts in the apices and furcation areas,[26] plus the formation of bone at the crest of the alveolus. The combined effect is to lengthen the root and deepen the socket. The physiologic width of the periodontal ligament is preserved by continuous deposition of cementum, and bone formation along the inner socket wall as the tooth continues to erupt.

An uncalcified surface layer of precementum, part of the process of continuous cementum deposition, is considered by Gottlieb[15] to be the natural barrier to excessive apical migration of the epithelial attachment. Impaired cementum formation ("cementopathia") was thought to be a cause of pathologic periodontal pocket formation because it reduced the restraint on epithelial migration.

FUNCTION AND CEMENTUM FORMATION

No clear-cut correlation has been established between occlusal function and cementum deposition.[25] From the findings of well-developed cementum on the roots of teeth in dermoid cysts, and from the presence of thicker cementum on embedded teeth than on teeth in function,[17] it has been inferred that function is not necessary for cementum formation. Cementum is thinner in areas of injury caused by excessive occlusal forces,[4] but thickening of cementum may also occur in these areas.

HYPERCEMENTOSIS

The term *hypercementosis* (cementum hyperplasia) refers to a prominent thickening of the cementum. It may be localized to one tooth or may affect the entire dentition. Because of considerable physiologic variation in the thickness of cementum among different teeth of the same person and among teeth of different persons, it is sometimes difficult to distinguish between hypercementosis and physiologic thickening of cementum.

Hypercementosis occurs as a generalized thickening of the cementum, with nodular enlargement of the apical third of the root. It also appears in the form of spike-like excrescences (cemental spikes) created by either the coalescence of cementicles that adhere to the root[17] or the calcification of periodontal fibers at the sites of insertion into the cementum.[27]

The etiology of hypercementosis varies and is not completely understood. The spike-like type of hypercementosis generally results from excessive tension from orthodontic appliances or occlusal forces. The generalized type occurs in a variety of circumstances. In teeth without antagonists, it is interpreted as an effort to keep pace with excessive tooth eruption. In teeth subject to low-grade periapical irritation arising from pulp disease, it is considered as compensation for the destroyed fibrous attach-

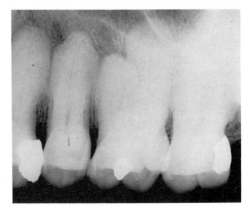
Figure 3–7   Hypercementosis in Paget's Disease.

ment to the tooth. The cementum is deposited adjacent to the inflamed periapical tissue. Hypercementosis of the entire dentition may be hereditary,[56] and also occurs in Paget's disease[39] (Fig. 3–7). Localized hypercementosis occurs at the insertion of the transseptal fibers in experimental lathyrism.[13] Cementum formation is diminished in hypophosphatasia.[3]

CEMENTICLES

Cementicles are globular masses of cementum arranged in concentric lamellae that lie free in the periodontal ligament or adhere to the root surface (Fig. 3–8). Cementicles may develop from calcified epi-

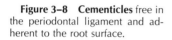
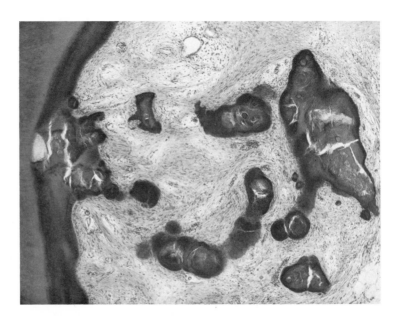
Figure 3–8   Cementicles free in the periodontal ligament and adherent to the root surface.

thelial rests, around small spicules of cementum or alveolar bone traumatically displaced into the periodontal ligament, from calcified Sharpey's fibers, and from calcified thrombosed vessels within the periodontal ligament.[30]

CEMENTOMA

Cementomas are masses of cementum generally situated apical to the teeth to which they may or may not be attached. They are considered as either odontogenic neoplasms or developmental malformations. Cementomas occur more frequently in females than in males, more often in the mandible than in the maxilla,[7] and may occur singly or multiply.[41] Usually harmless, they are generally discovered upon radiographic examination. In some cases they produce deformity of jaw contour.

The microscopic structure of the cementoma varies with regard to the proportions of connective tissue and cementum. The cementum may be arranged either as numerous coalescent cementicles or as an irregular mesh-work of trabeculae separated by fibrous connective tissue.[15]

The surface of the cementoma is generally formed by a layer of newly formed incompletely calcified cementoid lined by cementoblasts and surrounded by a connective tissue capsule. With continued deposition of cementum, the proportion of connective tissue within the lesion is reduced.

The radiographic appearance of the cementoma varies, depending upon the proportion of calcified cementum and fibrous connective tissue in the lesion. When composed principally of cementum, the lesion appears as a discrete, circumscribed, dense, radiopaque mass within which isolated radiolucent markings may be seen.

CEMENTUM RESORPTION AND REPAIR

The cementum of erupted as well as unerupted teeth is subject to resorption. The resorptive changes may be of microscopic proportions or sufficiently extensive to present a radiographically detectable alteration in the root contour. Cementum resorption is extremely common. In a microscopic study of 261 teeth it occurred in 236 (90.5

per cent).[20] The average number of resorption areas per tooth was 3.5. Of the 922 areas of resorption, 708 (76.8 per cent) were located in the apical third of the root, 177 (19.2 per cent) in the middle third, and 37 (4.0 per cent) in the gingival third of the root. Seventy per cent of all resorption areas were confined to the cementum without involving the dentin.

Cementum resorption may be due to local or systemic causes or may occur without the etiology being apparent (idiopathic) (Fig. 3–9). Among the local conditions under which it occurs are trauma from occlusion[35] (Fig. 3–10), orthodontic movement,[19, 24, 33, 38] pressure from malaligned erupting teeth, cysts and tumors,[25] teeth without functional antagonists, embedded teeth, replanted and transplanted teeth,[1] periapical disease and periodontal disease. Peculiar susceptibility of the cervical area to resorption has been attributed to the absence of either uncalcified precementum or reduced enamel epithelium.[47] Among the systemic conditions suspected as predisposing to or inducing cemental resorption are debilitating infections such as tuberculosis and pneumonia;[16] deficiencies of calcium,[23] vitamin D[6] and vitamin A;[11] hypothyroidism,[5] hereditary fibrous osteodystrophy,[49] and Paget's disease.[39]

Cementum resorption appears microscopically as bay-like concavities in the root surface. Multinucleated giant cells and large mononuclear macrophages are generally found adjacent to cementum undergoing active resorption (Fig. 3–11). Several sites of resorption may coalesce to form a large area of destruction. The resorptive process may extend into the underlying dentin and even into the pulp, but it is usually painless.

Cementum resorption is not necessarily continuous and may alternate with periods of repair and the deposition of new cementum. The newly formed cementum is demarcated from the root by a deeply staining irregular line, termed a reversal line, which designates the border of the previous resorption (Fig. 3–12). Embedded fibers of the periodontal ligament reestablish a functional relationship in the new cementum. Cementum repair requires the presence of viable connective tissue. If epithelium proliferates into an area of resorption, repair will not take place. Cementum repair can occur in devitalized as well as vital teeth.

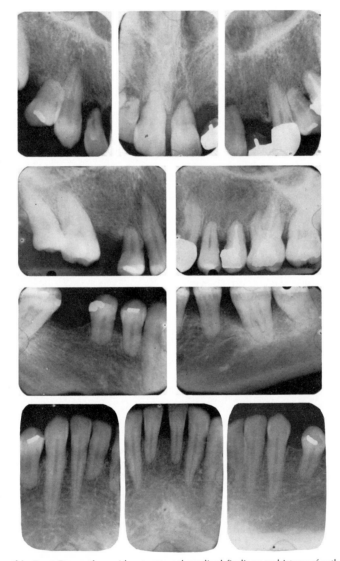

Figure 3–9 **Idiopathic Root Resorption** without unusual medical findings or history of orthodontic treatment.

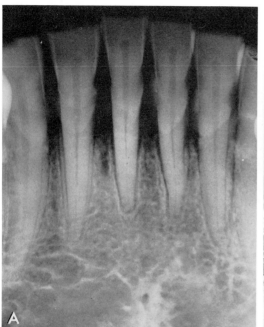

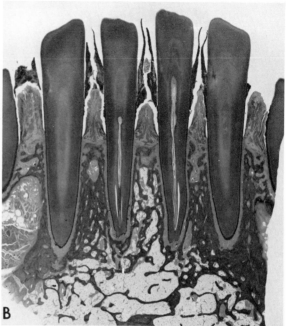

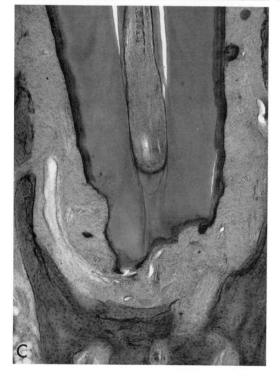

Figure 3–10 Cemental Resorption Associated With Excessive Occlusal Forces. *A,* Mandibular anterior teeth. Note the thickening of the periodontal ligament space and lamina dura with blunting of the apices of the central incisors. *B,* Survey section of the mandibular anterior teeth. *C,* Left central incisor shortened by resorption of cementum and dentin. Note partial repair of the eroded areas.

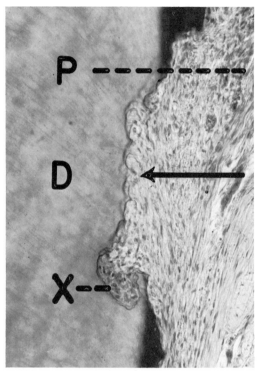

Figure 3–11   Resorption of Cementum and Dentin (D). A multinuclear osteoclast is seen at (X), inflammatory infiltration of the periodontal ligament (P). The direction of resorption is indicated by the arrow.

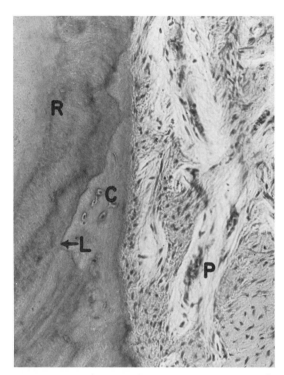

Figure 3–12   Section Showing Repair of Previously Resorbed Root. The defect is filled in with cellular cementum (C), which is separated from the older cementum (R) by an irregular indented line (L), which indicates the preexistent outline of the resorbed root. Periodontal ligament (P).

Fusion of the cementum and alveolar bone with obliteration of the periodontal ligament is termed *ankylosis*. Ankylosis invariably occurs in teeth with cemental resorption, suggesting that it may represent a form of abnormal repair. Ankylosis may also develop following chronic periapical inflammation, tooth replantation, occlusal trauma, and around embedded teeth.

INJURIES TO CEMENTUM

Fracture

When a tooth is subjected to a severe external force, such as a blow or biting on a hard object, fracture of the root (Fig. 3–13) or "tearing" of the cementum may occur. Complete horizontal or oblique fractures may be followed by repair, which includes the deposition of calcified tissues and the embedding of new periodontal fibers. Several factors influence the likelihood of such repair. Exposure of the site of fracture to the oral cavity with subsequent infection will interfere with repair. Even in unexposed fractures, the deposition of calcified tissue is reduced upon *proximity of the fracture to the oral cavity*.[8] The distance between the fractured root ends and the inherent reparative capacity of the individual also influence repair of complete horizontal or oblique root fractures.

Cemental tear

Detachment of a fragment of cementum from the root surface is known as a *cemental tear*. The separation of cementum may be complete, with displacement of a fragment into the periodontal ligament, or it may be incomplete, with the cementum fragment remaining partially attached to the root (Figs. 3–14 and 3–15).

Cementum fragments displaced into the periodontal ligament may undergo a variety of changes. New cementum may be deposited at the periphery, and periodontal fibers may be-

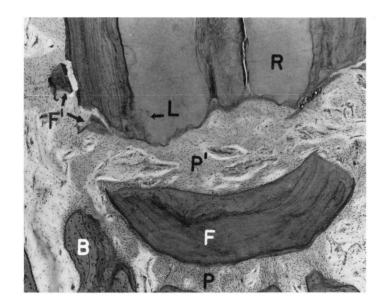

Figure 3–13 Root Repair After Traumatic Fracture. Detached fragments of cementum are shown at F'. The apical section of cementum (F) is separated from the remainder of the root (R) by dense connective tissue (P') and attached to the bone (B) by the periodontal ligament (P).

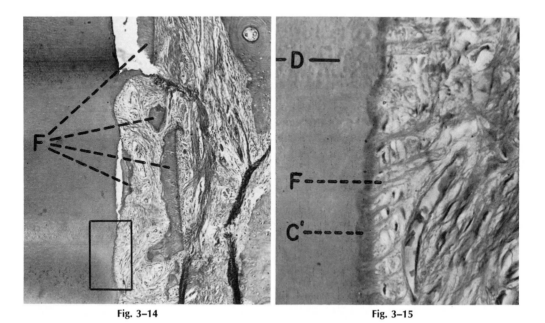

Fig. 3–14   Fig. 3–15

Figure 3–14   Traumatic "Cemental Tear" with fragments of cementum (F) free in the periodontal ligament.

Figure 3–15   High-power section of area within rectangle in Figure 3–14. New cementum (C') is shown along dentin (D). Periodontal fibers (F) are embedded in the new cementum.

come embedded in it, so as to establish a functional relationship between the tooth on one aspect and alveolar bone on the other. The detached cementum may be reunited to the root surface by new cementum. Detached cementum fragments may be completely resorbed or may undergo partial resorption followed by addition of new cementum and embedding of collagen fibers.

REFERENCES

1. Agnew, R. G., and Fong, C. C.: Histologic Studies on Experimental Transplantation of Teeth. Oral Surg., Oral Med. & Oral Path., 9:18, 1956.
2. Albright, J. T., and Flanagan, J. B.: Electronmicroscopy of Cementum. I.A.D.R. Abstracts of the 40th Meeting, 1962, p. 77.
3. Baer, P., Brown, N., and Hamner, J. E.: Hypophosphatasia. J. Am. Soc. Periodont., 2:209, 1964.
4. Balbe, R., Carranza, R., and Erausquin, R.: The Periodontal Structures in Case Number 8. Revista Odontológica. Buenos Aires, July, 1938.
5. Becks, H.: Root Resorptions and Their Relation to Pathologic Bone Formation, Internat. J. Orthodont. & Oral Surg., 22:445, 1936.
6. Becks, H., and Weber, M.: The Influence of Diet on the Bone System with Special Reference to the Alveolar Process and the Labyrinthine Capsule. J.A.D.A., 18:197, 1931.
7. Bernier, J. L., and Thompson, H. C.: The Histogenesis of the Cementoma. Am. J. Orthodont., 32:543, 1946.
8. Bevelander, G.: Tissue Reactions in Experimental Tooth Fracture. J. D. Res., 21:481, 1942.
9. Bevelander, G., and Nakahara, H.: The Fine Structure of the Human Periodontal Ligament. Anat. Rec., 162:313, 1968.
10. Blayney, J. R., Wasserman, F., Groetzinger, G., and DeWitt, T. G.: Further Studies in Mineral Metabolism of Human Teeth by the Use of Radioactive Isotopes. J. D. Res., 29:559, 1941.
11. Burn, C. G., Orten, A. I., and Smith, A. H.: Changes in the Structure of the Developing Tooth in Rats Maintained on a Diet Deficient in Vitamin A. Yale J. Biol. & Med., 13:817, 1940–1.
12. El Mostehy, M. R., and Stallard, R. E.: Intermediate Cementum. J. Periodont. Res., 3:24, 1968.
13. Gardner, A. F.: Alterations in Mesenchymal and Ectodermal Tissues During Experimental Lathyrism. Apposition and Calcification of Cementum. Paradontol., 20:111, 1966.
14. Glimcher, M., Friberg, U., and Levine, P.: The Identification and Characterization of a Calcified Layer of Coronal Cementum in Erupted Bovine Teeth. J. Ultrastruct. Res., 10:76, 1964.
15. Gottlieb, B.: Biology of the Cementum. J. Periodont., 17:7, 1942.
16. Gottlieb, B.: Tissue Changes in Pyorrhea. J.A.D.A., 14:2178, 1927.
17. Gottlieb, B., and Orban, B.: Biology and Pathology of the Tooth and Its Supporting Mechanism. Trans. by M. Diamond, New York, The Macmillan Co., 1938, p. 70.
18. Haim, G.: Histochemische Untersuchungen des Zementgewebes. Deutsche Zahnärtz. Zeitschr., 16:71, 1962.
19. Hemley, S.: The Incidence of Root Resorption of Vital Permanent Teeth. J. D. Res., 20:133, 1941.
20. Henry, J. L., and Weinmann, J. P.: The Pattern of Resorption and Repair of Human Cementum. J.A.D.A., 42:271, 1951.
21. Inoue, M., and Akiyoshi, M.: Histological Investigation on Sharpey's Fibers in Cementum of Teeth in Abnormal Function. J. D. Res., 41:503, 1962.
22. Ishikawa, J., Yamamoto, H., Ito, K., and Masuda, M.: Microradiographic Study of Cementum and Alveolar Bone. J. D. Res., 43:936, 1964.
23. Jones, M. R., and Simonton, F. V.: Mineral Metabolism in Relation to Alveolar Atrophy in Dogs. J.A.D.A., 15:881, 1928.
24. Ketcham, A. H.: A Progress Report of an Investigation of Apical Root Resorption of Permanent Teeth. Internat. J. Orthodont., 15:310, 1929.
25. Kronfeld, R.: Biology of the Cementum. J.A.D.A., 25:1451, 1938.
26. Kronfeld, R.: Cement Hyperplasia in Non-Functioning Teeth (Die Zementhyperplasien und Nicht-Functionierenden Zähne). Ztschr. f. Stomatol., 25:1218, 1927.
27. Kronfeld, R.: Cementum and Sharpey's Fibers. Ztschr. f. Stomatol., 26:714, 1928.
28. Listgarten, M. A.: A Light and Electron Microscopic Study of Coronal Cementogenesis. Arch. Oral Biol., 13:93, 1968.
29. Listgarten, M. A.: Changing Concepts about the Dento-epithelial Junction. J. Canad. D. Assn., 36:70, 1970.
30. Mikola, O. J., and Bauer, W. H.: Cementicles and Fragments of Cementum in the Periodontal Membrane. Oral Surg., Oral Med. & Oral Path., 2:1063, 1949.
31. Nihei, I.: A Study of the Hardness of Human Teeth. J. Osaka Univ. Dent. Soc., 4:1, 1959.
32. Noyes, F. B., Schour, I., and Noyes, H. J.: A Textbook of Dental Histology and Embryology. 5th ed. Philadelphia, Lea & Febiger, 1938, p. 113.
33. Oppenheim, A.: Human Tissue Response to Orthodontic Intervention of Short and Long Duration. Am. J. Orthodont. & Oral Surg., 28:263, 1942.
34. Orban, B.: Oral Histology and Embryology. 2nd ed. St. Louis, C. V. Mosby Co., 1944, p. 161.
35. Orban, B.: Tissue Changes in Traumatic Occlusion. J.A.D.A., 15:2090, 1928.
36. Riffle, A. B.: Cemento-Enamel Junction. J. Periodont., 23:41, 1952.
37. Romaniuk, K.: Some Observations of the Fine Structure of Human Cementum. J. D. Res., 46:152, 1967.
38. Rudolph, C. E.: An Evaluation of Root Resorption Occurring during Orthodontic Therapy. J. D. Res., 19:367, 1940.
39. Rushton, M. A.: Dental Tissues in Osteitis Deformans. Guy's Hosp. Rpt., 88:163, 1938.
40. Sasso, W.: Histochemical Study of Human Dental Cementum. Rev. Fac. Odont., 4:189, 1966.
41. Scannell, J. M.: Cementoma. Oral Surg., Oral Med. & Oral Path., 2:1169, 1949.
42. Selvig, K. A.: An Ultrastructural Study of Cementum Formation. Acta Odont. Scandinav., 22:105, 1964.
43. Selvig, K. A.: Electron Microscopy of Hertwig's Epithelial Sheath and of Early Dentin and Ce-

mentum Formation in the Mouse Incisor. Acta Odont. Scandinav., *21*:175, 1963.

44. Selvig, K. A.: Studies on the Genesis, Composition and Fine Structure of Cementum. Bergen-Oslo-Tromsö, Universitetsforlaget, 1967.

45. Selvig, K.: The Fine Structure of Human Cementum. Acta Odont. Scandinav., *23*:423, 1965.

46. Selvig, K. A., and Selvig, S. K.: Mineral Content of Human and Seal Cementum. J. D. Res., *41*:624, 1962.

47. Southam, J.: Clinical and Histological Aspects of Peripheral Cervical Resorption. J. Periodont., *38*:534, 1967.

48. Stern, I.B.: An Electron-Microscopic Study of the Cementum, Sharpey's Fibrils and Periodontal Ligament in the Rat Incisor. Am. J. Anat., *115*:377, 1964.

49. Thoma, K. H., Sosman, M. C., and Bennett, G. A.: An Unusual Case of Hereditary Fibrous Osteodystrophy (Fragilitas Ossium) with Replacement of Dentine by Osteocementum. Am. J. Orthodont. & Oral Surg., *29*:1 (Oral Surg), 1943.

50. Volker, J. F.: The Phosphate Metabolism of the Erupted Tooth as Indicated by Studies Utilizing the Radioactive Isotope. Tufts Outlook, *16*:3, 1942.

51. Volker, J. F., Gilda, J. E., and Ginn, J. T.: Radiophosphorus Metabolism of Pulpless Teeth. J. D. Res., *21*:322, 1942.

52. Warren, E. B., et al.: Effects of Periodontal Disease and of Calculus Solvents on Microhardness of Cementum. J. Periodont., *35*:505, 1964.

53. Wasserman, F., Blayney, J. R., Groetzinger, G., and DeWitt, T. G.: Studies on the Different Pathways of Exchange of Minerals in Teeth with the Aid of Radioactive Phosphorus. J. D. Res., *20*:389, 1941.

54. Yamamoto, H., et al.: Microradiographic and Histopathological Study of the Cementum. Bull. Tokyo D. Univ., *9*:141, 1962.

55. Zander, H. A., and Hurzeler, B.: Continuous Cementum Apposition. J. D. Res., *37*:1035, 1958.

56. Zemsky, J. L.: Hypercementosis and Heredity: An Introduction and Plan of Investigation. D. Items Int., *53*:355, 1931.

Chapter 4

THE ALVEOLAR BONE

NORMAL MICROSCOPIC FEATURES

The *alveolar process* is the bone which forms and supports the tooth sockets (alveoli). It consists of the inner socket wall of thin compact bone called the *alveolar bone proper (cribriform plate)*, the *supporting alveolar bone* which consists of cancellous trabeculae and the facial and lingual plates of compact bone. The interdental septum consists of cancellous supporting bone enclosed within a compact border (Fig. 4–1).

The alveolar process is divisible into separate areas on an anatomic basis, *but it functions as a unit. All parts are interrelated in the support of the teeth.* Occlusal forces which are transmitted from the periodontal ligament to the inner wall of the alveolus are supported by the cancellous trabeculae, which in turn are buttressed by the labial and lingual cortical plates. Designation of the entire alveolar process as alveolar bone is more consistent with its functional unity.

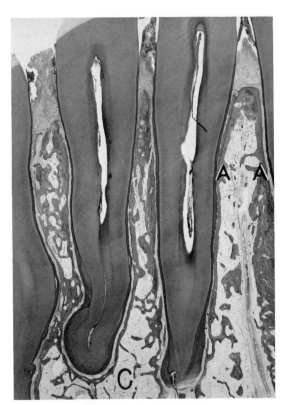

Figure 4–1 Mesiodistal Section Through Mandibular Canine and Premolars Showing Interdental Bony Septa. The dense bony plates (A) in relation to the teeth are separated by cancellous bony structure (C). Note the vertical blood vessels in the interdental septum at the right.

Cells and intercellular matrix

Alveolar bone consists of a calcified matrix with osteocytes enclosed within spaces called lacunae. The osteocytes extend into minute canals (canaliculi), which radiate from the lacunae. The canaliculi form an anastomosing system through the intercellular matrix of the bone, which brings oxygen and nutrients to the osteocytes and removes metabolic waste products.

Bone is composed principally of the minerals calcium and phosphate, along with hydroxyl, carbonates and citrate and trace amounts of other ions such as Na, Mg and F. The mineral salts are arranged in hydroxyapatite crystals of ultramicroscopic size. The spaces between the crystals are filled with organic matrix, with a predominance of collagen, plus water, solids not included in the crystalline structure and small quantities of mucopolysaccharides, principally chondroitin sulfate.[14, 17]

In the cancellous trabeculae the matrix is arranged in lamellae demarcated from each other by prominent cement lines. Occasionally, there are regularly arranged Haversian systems in the cancellous trabeculae. The compact alveolar bone consists of closely arranged lamellae and Haversian systems.

The socket wall

The principal fibers of the periodontal ligament which anchor the tooth in the socket are embedded for a considerable distance into the alveolar bone where they are referred to as *Sharpey's fibers*. Some Sharpey's fibers are completely calcified, but most contain an uncalcified central core within a calcified outer layer.[7, 22] The socket wall consists of dense lamellated bone, some of which is arranged in Haversian systems and *"bundle bone."* Bundle bone is the term given to bone adjacent to the periodontal ligament because of its content of Sharpey's fibers[24] (Fig. 4–2). It is arranged in layers with intervening appositional lines, parallel to the root (Fig. 4–3). Bundle bone is not unique to the jaws; it occurs throughout the skeletal system where ligaments and muscles are attached. Bundle bone is gradually resorbed on the side of the marrow spaces and replaced by lamellated bone.

The *cancellous portion of the alveolar bone* consists of trabeculae which enclose irregularly shaped marrow spaces lined with a layer of thin, flattened endosteal

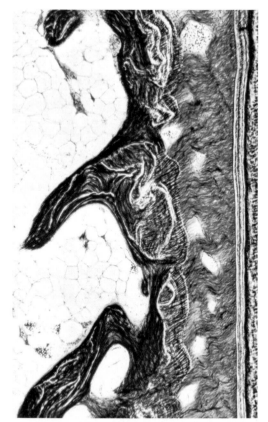

Figure 4–2 Deep Penetration of Sharpey's Fibers Into Bundle Bone on the Distal Surface of Tooth. Compare with the dense bone lining marrow spaces that replaced pre-existent bundle bone as tooth migrated mesially (to the right). (Courtesy of Dr. Sol Bernick.)

cells. There is wide variation in the trabecular pattern of the cancellous bone,[18] which is affected by occlusal forces. The matrix of the cancellous trabeculae consists of irregularly arranged lamellae separated by deeply staining incremental and resorption lines indicative of previous bone activity, with an occasional Haversian system.

Vascular supply, lymphatics and nerves

The bony wall of the tooth socket appears radiographically as a thin, radiopaque line, termed the *lamina dura*. However, it is perforated by numerous channels containing blood, lymph vessels and nerves, which link the periodontal ligament with the cancellous portion of the alveolar bone (Fig. 4–4). The vascular supply of the bone is derived from blood vessels in the peri-

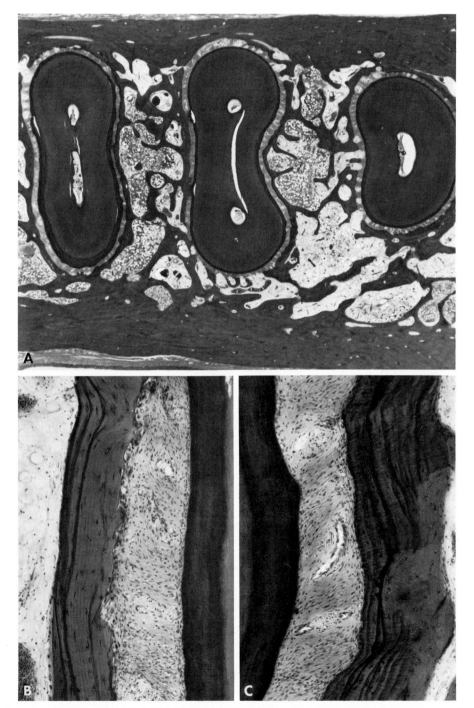

Figure 4–3   Bundle Bone Associated With Physiologic Mesial Migration of the Teeth. *A,* Horizontal section through molar roots in the process of mesial migration (mesial, *left;* distal, *right*). *B,* Mesial root surface showing osteoclasis of bone. *C,* Distal root surface showing bundle bone which has been partially replaced with dense bone on the marrow side.

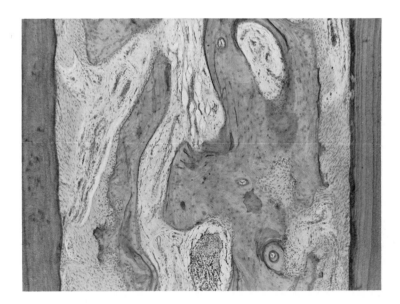

Figure 4–4 Interdental Bone showing vessel channel connecting the marrow spaces with the periodontal ligament.

odontal ligament and in the marrow spaces, and also from small branches of peripheral vessels that penetrate the cortical plates.

The interdental septum

The interdental septum consists of cancellous bone bordered by the socket walls of approximating teeth and the facial and lingual cortical plates (Fig. 4–5).

The mesiodistal angulation of the crest of the interdental septum parallels a line drawn between the cemento-enamel junction of the approximating teeth. The average distance between the crest of the alveolar bone and the cemento-enamel junction in the mandibular anterior region of young adults varies between 0.96 mm. and 1.22 mm.[11] With age, the distance between the bone and the cemento-enamel junction increases throughout the mouth (1.88 mm. to 2.81 mm.).[8]

The marrow

In the embryo and newborn, the cavities of all the bones are occupied by red hematopoietic marrow. The red marrow gradually undergoes a physiologic change to the fatty or yellow inactive type of marrow. In the adult, the marrow of the jaw is normally of the latter type, and red marrow is found only in the ribs, sternum, vertebrae, skull and humerus. However, foci of red bone marrow are occasionally seen in the jaws, often accompanied by resorption of bone trabeculae.[3] Common locations are the maxillary tuberosity (Fig. 4–6) and the maxillary and mandibular molar and premolar areas, which may be visible radiographically as zones of radiolucence. It has been suggested that they may be (1) remnants of the original marrow that has not undergone physiologic change to the fatty state, (2) localized manifestations of a generalized increase in red blood cell formation or of systemic disease such as tuberculosis,[4] or (3) the response to local injury or dental infection.

Bone is the calcium reservoir of the body, and the alveolar bone participates in the maintenance of the body calcium balance. *Calcium is constantly being deposited and withdrawn from the alveolar bone to provide for the needs of other tissues and to maintain the calcium level of the blood.* The calcium in the cancellous trabeculae is more readily available than that in compact bone. Conversely, easily mobilizable calcium is deposited in the trabeculae rather than the cortex of adult bone.

So persistent is the effort to maintain a normal calcium level in the blood, that even in cases of skeletal osteoporosis the blood calcium may be normal. In experimental animals the rate of metabolism of alveolar bone is more rapid than that of the diaphysis of the femur and slower than the metaphysis or "growth zone."[20]

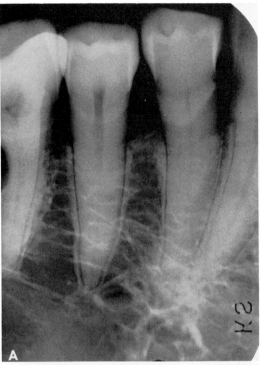
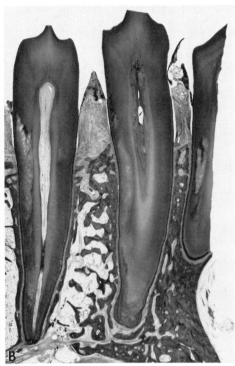
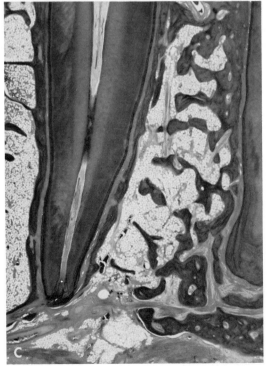

Figure 4–5 Interdental Septa. *A,* Mandibular premolar area. Note the prominent lamina dura. *B,* Interdental septa between the canine (*right*) and premolars. In the latter the central cancellous portion is bordered by dense bony plates of the socket wall. (This forms the lamina dura around the teeth in the radiograph.) *C,* Interdental septum between the premolars, showing central cancellous bone and dense plate around the teeth.

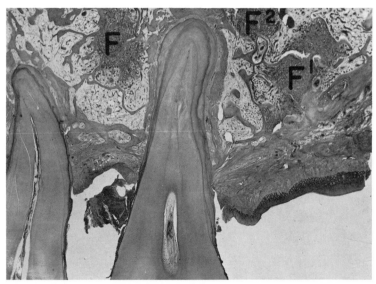

Figure 4–6 Mesiodistal section in the molar area of the maxilla of a 59-year-old male, showing foci of hematopoiesis in the marrow (F, F¹, F²).

THE EXTERNAL CONTOUR OF ALVEOLAR BONE

The bone contour normally conforms to the prominence of the roots, with intervening vertical depressions which taper toward the margin (Fig. 4–7).

The height and thickness of the facial and lingual bony plates are affected by the alignment of the teeth and angulation of the root to the bone and by occlusal forces. On teeth in labial version, the margin of the labial bone is located farther apically than on teeth in proper alignment. The bone margin is thinned to a knife edge and presents an accentuated arc in the direction of

the apex (Fig. 4–8). On teeth in lingual version, the facial bony plate is thicker than normal. The margin is blunt and rounded, and horizontal rather than arcuate. The effect of the *root to bone angulation* upon the height of alveolar bone is most noticeable on the palatal roots of maxillary molars. *The bone margin is located farther apically on the roots, which form relatively acute angles with the palatal bone.*[12] The cervical portion of the alveolar plate is sometimes considerably thickened on the facial surface, apparently as reinforcement against occlusal forces (Fig. 4–9).

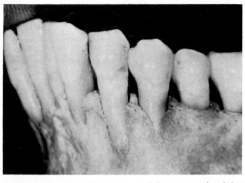

Figure 4–8 Apical location of bone on the labially placed mandibular canine and first premolars. Compare with higher level and thicker margin of the bone on the second premolar.

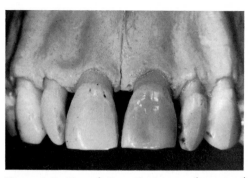

Figure 4–7 Normal Bone Contour conforms to the prominence of the roots.

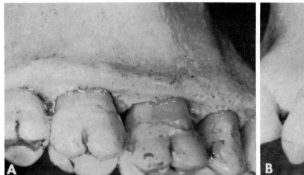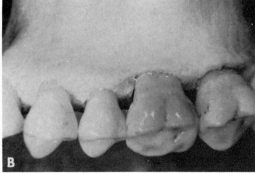

Figure 4–9 Variation in the cervical portion of the buccal alveolar plate. *Left,* Shelf-like conformation. *Right,* Comparatively thin buccal plate.

Fenestrations and dehiscences

Isolated areas in which the root is denuded of bone and the root surface is covered only by periosteum and overlying gingiva are termed *fenestrations* if the marginal bone is intact, and *dehiscences* if the denuded areas extend to the margin (Fig. 4–10). Such defects occur on approximately 20 per cent of the teeth; they occur more often on the facial bone than on the lingual, are more commonly on anterior teeth than on posterior teeth, and are frequently bilateral. There is microscopic evidence of lacunar resorption at the margins. The cause is not clear, but trauma from occlusion is suspected.[23] Prominent root contours, malposition and labial protrusion of the root combined with a thin bony plate are predisposing factors.[6] Fenestration and dehiscences are important, because they may complicate the outcome of mucogingival surgery (see Chap. 46).

THE LABILITY OF ALVEOLAR BONE

In contrast to its apparent rigidity, alveolar bone is the least stable of the periodontal tissues; its structure is in a constant state of flux.[16] The physiologic lability of alveolar bone is maintained by a sensitive balance between bone formation and bone resorption, regulated by local and systemic influences (Fig. 4–11). Bone is resorbed in areas of pressure and formed in areas of tension. The cellular activity which affects the height, contour and density of alveolar bone is manifested in three areas: (1) *adjacent to the periodontal ligament,* (2) *in relation to the periosteum of the facial and lingual plates,* and (3) *along the endosteal surface of the marrow spaces.*

Figure 4–10 **Dehiscence** on the canine and **Fenestration** of the first premolar.

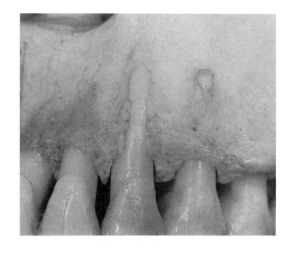

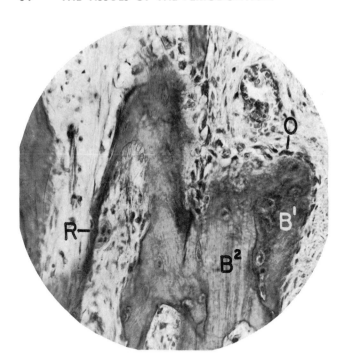

Figure 4–11 Bone Formation and Bone Resorption in Close Proximity in Alveolar Bone. Osteoblasts (O) at the periphery of new bone (B¹) formed on older lamellated bone (B²) at site of previous resorption, indicated by irregular reversal line. Note osteoclast (R) along adjacent partially resorbed trabecula.

Mesial migration of the teeth and reconstruction of alveolar bone

With time and wear the proximal contact areas of the teeth are flattened and the teeth tend to move mesially. This is referred to as *physiologic mesial migration,* a gradual process with intermittent periods of activity, rest and repair. By age 40, it effects a reduction of 0.5 cm. in the length of the dental arch from the midline to the third molars.[2] **Alveolar bone is reconstructed in compliance with the physiologic mesial migration of the teeth.** Bone resorption is increased in areas of pressure along the mesial surfaces of the teeth, and new layers of bundle bone are formed in areas of tension on the distal surfaces (Figs. 4–3 and 4–12).

Occlusal forces and alveolar bone

There are two aspects to the relationship between occlusal forces and alveolar bone. **The bone exists for the purpose of supporting teeth during function,** and, in common with the remainder of the skeletal system, **depends upon the stimulation it receives from function for the preservation of its structure.** There is therefore a constant and sensitive balance between occlusal forces and the structure of alveolar bone.[15]

Alveolar bone undergoes constant remodeling in response to occlusal forces (Fig. 4–13). Osteoclasts and osteoblasts redistribute bone substance to meet new functional demands most efficiently. Bone is removed from where it is no longer needed and added where new needs arise.

When an occlusal force is applied to a tooth either through a food bolus or by contact with opposing teeth, several things happen, depending upon the direction, intensity and duration of the force. The tooth is displaced against the resilient periodontal ligament, in which it creates areas of tension and compression. The facial and lingual walls of the socket bend in the direction of the force.[19] When the force is released, the tooth, ligament and bone spring back to their original positions.

The socket wall reflects the responsiveness of alveolar bone to occlusal forces. Osteoblasts and newly formed osteoid line the socket in areas of tension; osteoclasts and lacunar resorption occur in areas of pressure.

The number, density and alignment of cancellous trabeculae are also influenced by occlusal forces. Experimental systems

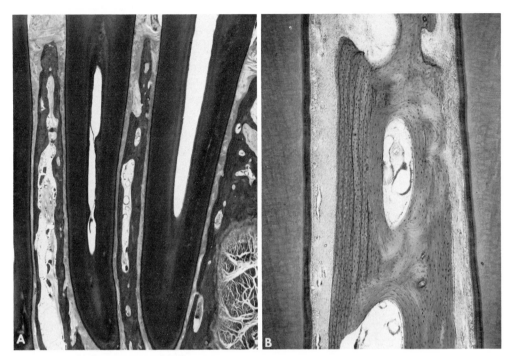

Figure 4–12 **Bone Response to Physiologic Mesial Migration.** *A,* Interdental septa between the canine (*left*) and first and second premolars. *B,* Interdental septum between the first and second premolars, showing bundle bone on the distal of the first premolar (*left*) and resorption on the mesial of the second (*right*).

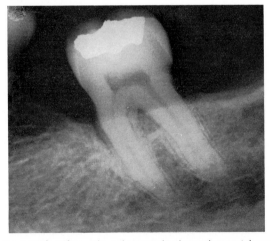

Figure 4–13 **Bone Trabeculae** realigned perpendicular to the mesial root of tilted molar.

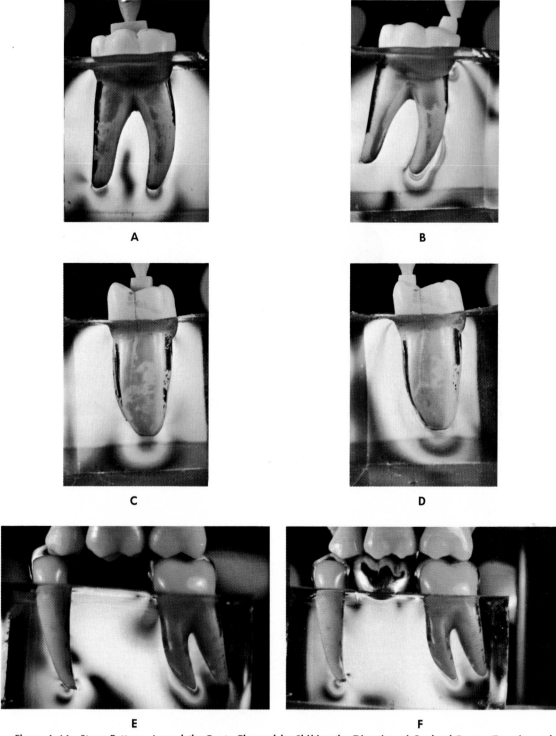

Figure 4–14 Stress Patterns Around the Roots Changed by Shifting the Direction of Occlusal Forces (Experimental Model Using Photoelastic Analysis). *A,* Buccal view of ivorine molar subjected to an **axial force.** The colored fringes indicate that the internal stresses are at the root apices. *B,* Buccal view of ivorine molar subjected to a **mesial tilting force.** The color fringes indicate that the internal stresses are along the mesial surface and at the apex of the mesial root. *C,* Ivorine molar subjected to **axial force** viewed from the mesial proximal surface. The colored fringes indicate that the stresses are concentrated at the apex. *D,* Ivorine molar subjected to **lingual tilting force** viewed from the mesial proximal surface. The colored fringes indicate that the internal stresses are along the lingual surface and at the apex. *E,* **Stress patterns around the roots of teeth adjacent to an edentulous space.** Note particularly the stress fringes in the mesial cervical region of the molar. *F,* **Changes in stress patterns produced by inserting a fixed bridge.** Note the disappearance of the fringes in the cervical region of the molar (compare with *E.)*

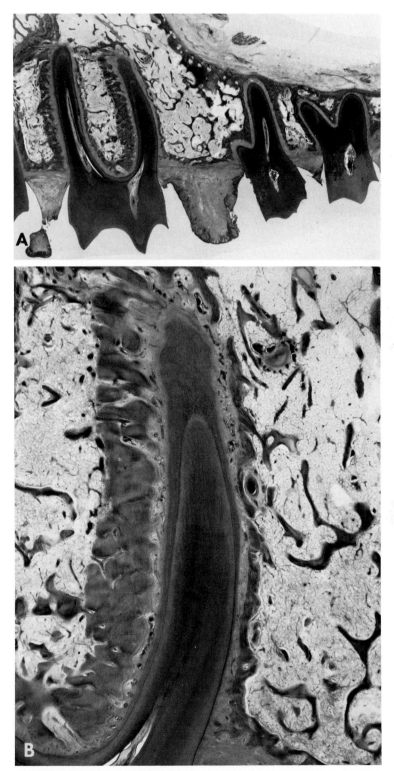

Figure 4–15   Bone Response to Increased Occlusal Forces. *A,* Mesiodistal section through maxillary molar and premolars subjected to increased occlusal forces. *B,* Mesiobuccal root of the second molar, showing thickening of bone along the distal surface in response to increased tension and thinning of the bone on the mesial aspect caused by increased pressure.

utilizing photoelastic analysis indicate alterations in stress patterns in the periodontium created by changes in the direction and intensity of occlusal forces[9] (Fig. 4–14). The bone trabeculae are aligned in the path of the tensile and compressive stresses so as to provide maximum resistance to the occlusal force with a minimum of bone substance (Fig. 4–15).[21] Forces which exceed the adaptive capacity of the bone produce injury called trauma from occlusion (see Chap. 24).

When occlusal forces are increased, the cancellous trabeculae are increased in number and thickness, and bone may be added to the external surface of the labial and lingual plates (Fig. 4–9). When occlusal forces are reduced, bone is resorbed, bone height is diminished, and the number and thickness of the trabeculae are reduced.[5,13] This is termed *disuse or afunctional atrophy.* Although occlusal forces are extremely important in determining the internal architecture and external contour of alveolar bone, other factors such as local physiochemical conditions, vascular anatomy and the individual systemic condition are also involved.[1]

REFERENCES

1. Anderson, B. G., Smith, A. H., Arnim, S. S., and Orten, A. V.: Changes in Molar Teeth and Their Supporting Structures in Rats Following Extraction of the Upper Right First and Second Molars. Yale J. Biol. & Med., 9:189, 1936.
2. Black, G. V.: Pathology of the Hard Tissues of the Teeth. Oral Diagnosis. 8th ed. Woodstock, Ill., Medico-Dental Publishing Co., 1948, p. 389.
3. Box, H. K.: Bone Resorption in Red Marrow Hyperplasia in Human Jaws. Bull. 21, Canadian D. Res. Found., 1936.
4. Cahn, L. R.: Red Marrow in the Jaws. J.A.D.A., 27:1056, 1940.
5. Cohn, S. A.: Disuse Atrophy of the Periodontium in Mice. Arch. Oral Biol., 10:909, 1965.
6. Elliot, J. R., and Bomers, G. M.: Alveolar Dehiscence and Fenestration. Periodontics, 1:245, 1963.
7. Frank, R., Lindemann, G., and Vedrine, J.: Structure sub-microscopique de l'os alvéolaire des maxillaires à l'état normal. Rev. Franç. Odonto-stomat., 5:1507, 1958.
8. Garguilo, A. W., Wentz, F. M., and Orban, B.: Dimensions and Relations of the Dentogingival Junction in Humans. J. Periodont., 32:216, 1961.
9. Glickman, I., Roeber, F. W., Brion, M., and Pameijer, J. H. N.: Photoelastic Analysis of Internal Stresses in the Periodontium Created by Occlusal Forces. J. Periodont.-Periodontics, 41:30, 1970.
10. Glickman, I., and Wood, H.: Bone Histology in Periodontal Disease. J. D. Res., 21:35, 1942.
11. Herulf, G.: On det marginala alveolarbenet hos ungdom i studieåldernenröntgenstudie. Svensk Tandkläkare-Tidsskrift., 43:42, 1950.
12. Hirschfeld, I.: A Study of Skulls in the American History in Relation to Periodontal Disease. J. D. Res., 5:241, 1923.
13. Kellner, E.: Histologic Findings on Teeth Without Antagonists. Ztschr. f. Stomatol., 26:271, 1928.
14. Loe, H.: Bone Tissue Formation. A Morphological and Histochemical Study. Acta Odont. Scandinav., 17:311, 1959.
15. MacMillan, H. W.: A Consideration of the Structure of the Alveolar Process, with Special Reference to the Principle Underlying Its Surgery and Regeneration. J. D. Res., 6:251, 1924–6.
16. Manson, J. D.: Age Changes in Bone Activity in the Mandible. Proc. First European Bone and Tooth Symposium. Oxford, Pergamon Press, 1964, pp. 343–349.
17. McLean, F. C., and Urist, M. R.: Bone. 2nd ed. Chicago, University of Chicago Press, 1961, p. 38.
18. Parfitt, G. J.: An Investigation of the Normal Variations in Alveolar Bone Trabeculation. Oral Surg., Oral Med. & Oral Path., 15:1453, 1962.
19. Picton, D. A.: On the Part Played by the Socket in Tooth Support. Arch. Oral Biol., 10:945, 1965.
20. Rogers, H. J., and Weidman, S. M.: Metabolism of Alveolar Bone. Brit. D. J., 90:7, 1951.
21. Sepel, C. M.: Trajectories of Jaws. Acta Odont. Scandinav., 8:81, 191, 1948.
22. Selvig, K. A.: The Fine Structure of Human Cementum. Acta Odont. Scandinav., 23:423, 1965.
23. Stahl, S. S., Cantor, M., and Zwig, E.: Fenestrations of the Labial Alveolar Plate in Human Skulls. Periodontol., 1:99, 1963.
24. Stein, G., and Weinmann, J. P.: The Physiologic Movement of the Teeth. Ztschr. f. Stomatol., 23:733, 1925.

Chapter 5

AGING AND THE PERIODONTIUM

Disease of the periodontium occurs in childhood, adolescence and early adulthood, but the prevalence of periodontal disease and the tissue destruction and tooth loss it causes increase with age. Many tissue changes occur with aging, some of which may affect the disease experience of the periodontium. *It is sometimes difficult to draw a sharp line between physiologic aging and the cumulative effects of disease.*

Aging is a slowing down of natural function, a disintegration of the balanced control and organization that characterize the young.[30] It is a process of physiologic and morphologic disintegration, as distinguished from infancy and adolescence, which are processes of integration and coordination. Aging is described in detail in texts devoted to the subject.[6] Some general age changes and alterations in the periodontium will be considered here.

GENERAL EFFECTS OF AGING

Aging is manifested to a different degree and in a different manner in various tissues and organs, but it includes general changes[39, 42, 43] such as tissue desiccation, reduced elasticity, diminished reparative capacity, altered cell permeability, and increased calcium content in the cells of many organs.[27]

In the skin, the dermis and epidermis are thinned, keratinization is diminished,[21] the blood supply is decreased, and there is degeneration of the nerve endings. Patchy peripheral anesthesia, indicative of central nervous system deterioration, is common in senility. Tissue elasticity is reduced with aging,[23] and there is degeneration of the elastic tissue fibers of the corium. The atrophic skin changes are less marked in females, and may be reversed in local areas by application of estrogen.

Bone undergoes osteoporosis with aging.[10] The bone is rarefied, trabeculae are reduced in number, the cortical plates are thinned, vascularity is reduced, lacunar resorption is more prominent, and susceptibility to fracture is increased. Generalized osteoporosis occurs in aged females more commonly than in males, and has been associated with sex hormone dysfunction.[22] With age, water content of bone is reduced, the mineral crystals are increased in size, and collagen fibrils are thickened.[19]

AGE CHANGES IN THE PERIODONTIUM

Gingiva and other areas of the oral mucosa

In the gingiva the following changes have been identified with aging: recession, diminished keratinization both in males[42] and females,[33] stippling reduced[17] or unchanged,[35] decreased connective tissue cellularity, increased intercellular substances,[47] and reduced oxygen consumption, a measure of metabolic activity.[46] In menopausal patients the gingiva is less keratinized than in patients of comparable age with active menstrual cycles.

Changes in other areas of the oral mucosa include atrophy of the epithelium and connective tissue with loss of elasticity;[37] decrease in protein-bound hexoses and mucoproteins,[7] which may reduce resilience and increase susceptibility to trauma;[12] increase in mast cells; atrophy of the papillae of the tongue, with the filiform papillae more severely affected; decrease in the number of taste buds in the circumvallate papillae;[6] nodular varicose enlargement of veins on the ventral surface of the tongue; and increase in the sebaceous glands in the lip and cheek.

Periodontal ligament

In the periodontal ligament, increase in elastic fibers;[18] decrease in vascularity, mitotic activity,[44] fibroplasia,[20, 28] collagen fibers and mucopolysaccharides,[34, 40, 45] increase in arteriosclerotic changes;[16] and both an increase[24] and a decrease[9] in width have been described in aging. The decreased width may result from encroachment upon the ligament by continuous deposition of cementum and bone.[26]

Alveolar bone

In addition to reduction in height[14] (senile atrophy), changes occur in alveolar bone with aging that are similar to changes in the remainder of the skeletal system. These include osteoporosis,[2, 22] decreased vascularity, and a reduction in metabolism and healing capacity.[43] Resorption activity is increased,[29] bone formation is decreased[15, 41] and bone porosity may result. Ability of the alveolar bone to withstand occlusal forces is diminished after the age of 30.[11]

Tooth-periodontium relationships

The most obvious change in the teeth with aging is a loss of tooth substance caused by attrition. Occlusal wear reduces cusp height and inclination (Fig. 5–1), with a resultant increase in the food table area and loss of sluiceways. The degree of attrition is influenced by the musculature, consistency of the food, tooth hardness, occupational factors and habits such as bruxism and clenching.[25, 36]

The rate of attrition is coordinated with other age changes such as continuous tooth eruption and gingival recession (Fig. 5–2). Reduction in bone height which occurs with aging is not necessarily related to occlusal wear.[3] In those cases in which bone support is reduced, the clinical crown tends to become disproportionately long and creates excessive leverage upon the bone. **By reducing the clinical crowns, attrition preserves the balance between the teeth and their bony support.**

Wear of teeth also occurs on the proximal surfaces, accompanied by mesial migration of the teeth.[32] Proximal wear reduces the anteroposterior length of the dental arch by approximately 0.5 cm. by age 40.[48] Anteroposterior narrowing from proximal wear is greater in teeth that taper toward the cervical such as the incisors.[48] Progressive attrition and proximal wear result in a reduced maxillary-mandibular overjet in the molar area and an edge-to-edge bite anteriorly.

Other effects of aging

Regressive changes in the salivary glands with retention cyst formation and associated xerostomia have been identified with

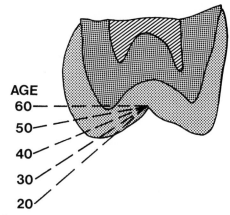

Figure 5–1 Diminution in Cuspal Inclination with increasing age.

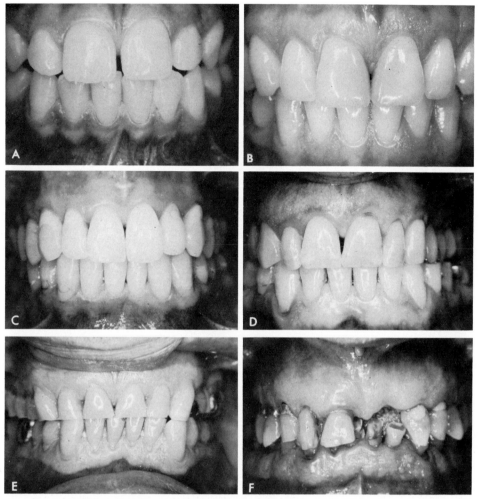

Figure 5–2 Tooth-Periodontium Relationships at Different Ages. *A,* Age 12. The gingiva is located on the enamel and the clinical crown is shorter than the anatomic crown. *B,* Age 25. The gingiva is attached close to the cemento-enamel junction. *C,* Age 30. Gingiva at cemento-enamel junction, with slight signs of recession. *D,* Age 50. Slight occlusal wear and slight recession. *E,* Age 72. Moderate attrition and slight to moderate recession. *F,* Age 73. Marked attrition with reduction in the height of the clinical crowns.

aging.[37] Decrease in salivary flow and in the amount of ptyalin have been described as the causes of inadequate lubrication of food during mastication and poor starch digestion. Fatty degeneration of the parotid gland occurs in aged experimental animals.[1]

Masticatory efficiency

Slight atrophy of the buccal musculature has been described as a physiologic feature of aging.[13] However, reduction in masticatory efficiency in aged individuals is more likely to be the result of unreplaced missing teeth, loose teeth, poorly fitting dentures, or an unwillingness to wear dentures. Re-duced masticatory efficiency leads to poor chewing habits and the possibility of associated digestive disturbances. Aged persons select carbohydrates and foods requiring less chewing effort when masticatory efficiency is impaired.

Avitaminosis is common in aged persons, but the extent to which it results from impaired masticatory efficiency has not been established. The vitamin requirement of older persons may be increased because of their dietary habits. Long-standing calcium deficiency has been considered a causative factor in senile osteoporosis.[22] The advisability of increased calcium intake in aged individuals is doubtful, but a diet high in

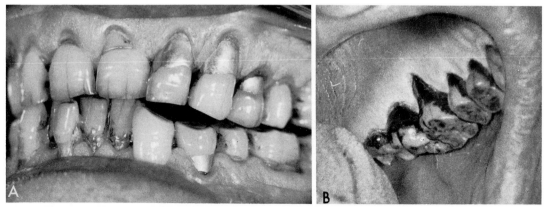

Figure 5–3 *A,* **Attrition of the Teeth** and gingival recession in a 65-year-old male. Note the elliptical contour of the tooth wear associated with pipe smoking. *B,* Lingual view showing accentuated recession on the first molar.

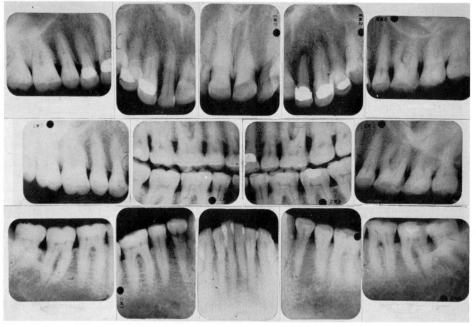

Figure 5–4 Radiographs of the patient shown in Figure 5–3. Aside from a few localized areas of bone loss there is little evidence of reduced bone height considered to be a physiologic feature of aging.

protein and vitamins and comparatively low in carbohydrates and fat may be beneficial.

AGING AND THE CUMULATIVE EFFECTS OF ORAL DISEASE

With time, chronic disease can produce many oral changes, and it is difficult to determine how much physiologic aging contributes to the total picture. Some contend that gingival recession, attrition and reduction in bone height in the aged result more from disease and factors in the oral environment than from physiologic aging.[4] Although gingival recession, attrition and bone loss commonly occur with age, they are not present in all patients, and vary considerably in the same age group. An aged individual with marked attrition may present relatively little alveolar bone loss (Figs. 5–3 and 5–4). Marked attrition may also be produced in young and middle-aged adults by bruxing and clenching habits (Figs. 5–5 and 5–6).

Increased alveolar bone loss in the aged has been related to less efficient oral hygiene.[38] Bone loss, pathologic migration of the teeth and loss of vertical dimension in the aged may be the results of periodontal disease and failure to replace missing teeth.

Leukoplakia of the oral mucosa and staining of the teeth are common in aged individuals who are inveterate smokers. Wearing artificial dentures for years without rebasing, with a resultant reduction in vertical dimension, is a common cause of angular cheilosis in the aged.

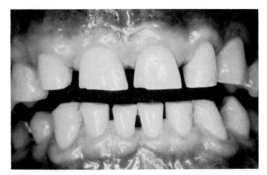

Figure 5–6 Bruxing Habit and Marked Attrition in 43-year-old man.

REFERENCES

1. Andrew, W.: Age Changes in Salivary Glands of Wistar Institute Rats with Particular Reference to the Submandibular Glands. J. Gerontol, 4:95, 1949.
2. Atkinson, P. J., and Woodhead, C.: Changes in Human Mandibular Structure with Age. Arch. Oral Biol., 13:1453, 1968.
3. Baer, P. N., et al.: Alveolar Bone Loss and Occlusal Wear. Periodontics, 1:45, 1963.
4. Baer, P. N., and Bernick, S.: Age Changes in the Periodontium of the Mouse. Oral Surg., Oral Med. & Oral Path., 10:430, 1957.
5. Birren, J. E.: Handbook of Aging and the Individual. Psychological and Biological Aspects. Chicago, University of Chicago Press, 1959.
6. Bourne, S. H.: Structural Aspects of Aging. New York, Hafner Publishing Company, Inc., 1961.
7. Burzynski, N. J.: Relationship Between Age and Palatal Tissue and Gingival Tissue in the Guinea Pig. J. D. Res., 46:539, 1967.
8. Comfort, A.: Aging: The Biology of Senescence. New York, Holt, Rinehart and Winston, Inc., 1964.
9. Coolidge, E.: The Thickness of the Periodontal Membrane. J.A.D.A., 24:1260, 1937.
10. Cowdry, E. V.: Problems of Ageing. 2nd ed. Baltimore, Williams and Wilkins Co., 1942; Chapter 12, T. Wingate Todd, p. 322 (Skeleton and Locomotor System).
11. Figueroa Blamey, J.: Relationship Between Occlusal Disharmonics and Alveolar Atrophy. Clinica de Parodoncia, Facultad de Odontologie Universitad de Chile, 1947.
12. Flieder, D. E.: Cytochemistry of Human Oral Mucosa: Determination of Phospholipids. Protein-Bound Hexoses, Mucoproteins, Collagenous and Non-Collagenous Proteins. J. D. Res., 41:112, 1962.
13. Freeman, J. T.: The Basic Factors of Nutrition in Old Age. Geriatrics, 2:41, 1947.
14. Froehlich, E.: Periodontal Changes in Aging. Deutsche Zahnärtz. Zeitschr., 9:1005, 1965.
15. Gilmore, N., and Glickman, I.: Some Age Changes in the Periodontium of the Albino Mouse, J. D. Res., 38:1195, 1959.
16. Grant, D., and Bernick, S.: Arteriosclerosis in Periodontal Vessels of Aging Humans. J. Periodont., 41:170, 1970.

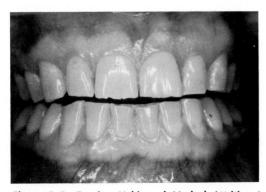

Figure 5–5 Bruxing Habit and Marked Attrition in 25-year-old woman.

17. Greene, A. J.: Study of the Characteristics of Stippling and its Relation to Gingival Health. J. Periodont., *33*:176, 1962.
18. Haim, G., and Baumgartel, R.: Alterations in the Periodontal Ligament Due to Age. Deutsche Zahnärtz. Zeitschr., *23*:340, 1968.
19. Ham, A. W., and Leeson, T. S.: Histology. 4th ed. Philadelphia, J. B. Lippincott Co., 1961, p. 279.
20. Jensen, J. L., and Toto, P. D.: Radioactive Labeling Index of the Periodontal Ligament in Aging Rats. J. D. Res., *47*:149, 1968.
21. Joseph, N. R., Molimard, R., and Bourliere, F.: Aging of Skin I. Titration Curves of Human Epidermis in Relation to Age. Gerontologia, *1*:18, 1957.
22. Kesson, C. M., Morris, N., and McCutcheon, A.: Generalized Osteoporosis in Old Age. Ann. Rheumat. Dis., *6*:146, 1947.
23. Kirk, E., and Kvorning, S. A.: Quantitative Measurements of the Elastic Properties of the Skin and Subcutaneous Tissue in Young and Old Individuals. J. Gerontol., *4*:273, 1949.
24. Klein, A.: Systematic Investigations Concerning the Thickness of the Periodontal Membrane. Zeitschr. f. Stomatol., *26*:417, 1928.
25. Kronfeld, R.: Structure, Function, and Pathology of the Human Periodontal Membrane, New York J. Den., *6*:112, 1936.
26. Kronfeld, R.: Biology of Cementum. J.A.D.A., *25*:1451, 1938.
27. Lansing, A. I.: Calcium Growth in Ageing and Cancer. Science, *106*:187, 1947.
28. Lavelle, C. L. B.: The Effect of Age on the Proliferative Activity of the Periodontal Membrane of the Rat Incisor. J. Periodont. Res., *3*:48, 1968.
29. Manson, J. D., and Lucas, R. B.: A Microradiographic Study of Age Changes in the Human Mandible. Arch. Oral Biol., *7*:761, 1962.
30. Muller, H. S., Little, C. C., and Snyder, L. H.: Genetics, Medicine and Man. Ithaca, N.Y., Cornell Univ. Press, 1947. Chapter IV, Growth and Individuality by C. C. Little, p. 104.
31. Murphy, T. R.: A Biometric Study of the Selicoidal Occlusal Plane of the Worn Australian Dentition. Arch. Oral Biol., *9*:255, 1964.
32. Murphy, T. R.: Reduction of the Dental Arch by Approximal Attrition. Brit. D. J., *116*:483, 1964.
33. Papic, M., and Glickman, I.: Keratinization of the Human Gingiva in the Menstrual Cycle and Menopause. Oral Surg., Oral Med. & Oral Path., *3*:504, 1950.
34. Paunio, K.: The Age Change of Acid Mucopolysaccharides in the Periodontal Membrane of Man. J. Periodont. Res., Suppl. 4, Inter. Conf. Periodont. Res., 32, 1969.
35. Riethe, P.: Surface Changes in the Attached Gingiva in Young and Old People. Deutsche Zahnärzt. Zeitschr., *9*:1028, 1965.
36. Robinson, H. B. G.: Some Clinical Aspects of Intraoral Age Change. Geriatrics, *2*:9, 1947.
37. Robinson, H. B. G., Boling, L. R., and Lischer, B.: Chapter XIII in Cowdry, E. V.: Problems of Ageing. Baltimore, Williams and Wilkins Co., 1942, p. 384.
38. Schei, O., Waerhaug, J., Lovdal, A., and Arno, A.: Alveolar Bone Loss as Related to Oral Hygiene and Age. J. Periodont., *30*:7, 1959.
39. Simms, H. S., and Stolman, A.: Changes in Human Tissue Electrolytes in Senescence. Science, *86*:269, 1937.
40. Skougaard, M. R., Levy, B. M., and Simpson, J.: Collagen Metabolism in Skin and Periodontal Membrane of the Marmoset. J. Periodont. Res., Suppl. 4, Inter. Conf. Periodont. Res., 28, 1969.
41. Soni, N. N.: Quantitative Study of Bone Activity in Alveolar and Femoral Bone of the Guinea Pig. J. D. Res., *47*:584, 1968.
42. Stone, A.: Keratinization of Human Oral Mucosa in the Aged Male. J. D. Med., *8*:69, 1953.
43. Thomas, B. O. A.: Gerondontology. The Study of Changes in Oral Tissue Associated with Ageing. J.A.D.A., *33*:207, 1946.
44. Toto, P. D., and Borg, M.: Effect of Age Changes on the Premitotic Index in the Periodontium of Mice. J. D. Res., *47*:70, 1968.
45. Toto, P. D., Jensen, J., and Sawinski, J.: Sulfate Uptake and Cell Kinetics in Teeth and Bone of Aging Mice. Periodontics, *5*:292, 1967.
46. Volpe, A. R., Manhold, J. H., and Manhold, B. S.: Effect of Age and Other Factors upon Normal Gingival Tissue Respiration. J. D. Res., *41*:1060, 1962.
47. Wentz, F. W., Maier, A. W., and Orban, B.: Age Changes and Sex Differences in the Clinically Normal Gingiva. J. Periodont., *23*:13, 1952.
48. Wood, H. E.: Causal Factors in Shortening Tooth Series with Age. J. D. Res., *17*:1, 1938.

Section Two • Gingival and Periodontal Disease

The term *periodontal disease* is used in a general sense to encompass all diseases of the periodontium, much in the same way as are terms such as "liver disease" or "kidney disease." It is also used in a specific sense to differentiate disease of the supporting periodontal tissues (periodontal ligament, alveolar bone and cementum) from disease confined to the gingiva.

PART I. Gingival disease—disease confined to the gingiva.
General characteristics of gingival disease
Specific gingival diseases

PART II Periodontal disease—disease of the supporting periodontal tissues (periodontal ligament, alveolar bone and cementum).

PART III. The etiology of gingival and periodontal disease.

PART IV. The classification of gingival and periodontal disease.

Part I • Gingival Disease

Chapter 6

GINGIVITIS

THE ROLE OF INFLAMMATION IN GINGIVAL DISEASE

Gingivitis, inflammation of the gingiva, is the most common form of gingival disease. Inflammation is almost always present in all forms of gingival disease, because local irritants which cause inflammation, such as dental plaque, materia alba and calculus, are extremely common, and microorganisms and their injurious products are always present in the gingival environment. The inflammation caused by local irritation gives rise to associated degenerative, necrotic and proliferative changes in the gingival tissues.

There is a tendency to designate all forms of gingival disease as gingivitis, as if inflammation were the only disease process involved. **However, pathologic processes not caused by local irritation, such as atrophy, hyperplasia and neoplasia, also occur in the gingiva.** All cases of gingivitis are not necessarily the same because they present inflammatory changes, and **it is often necessary to differentiate between inflammation and other pathologic processes that may be present in gingival disease.**

The *role of inflammation* in individual cases of gingivitis varies as follows:

1. Inflammation may be the *primary* and *only* pathologic change. This is by far the most prevalent type of gingival disease.

2. Inflammation may be a *secondary* feature, superimposed upon systemically caused gingival disease. For example, inflammation commonly complicates gingival hyperplasia caused by the systemic administration of Dilantin.

3. Inflammation may be the *precipitating factor* responsible for clinical changes in patients with systemic conditions that of themselves do not produce clinically detectable gingival disease. Gingivitis in pregnancy and in leukemia are examples.

COURSE, DURATION AND DISTRIBUTION OF GINGIVITIS

Course and duration

Acute gingivitis: Painful, comes on suddenly and is of short duration.

Subacute gingivitis: A less severe phase of the acute condition.

Recurrent gingivitis: Disease that reappears after having been eliminated by treatment, or that disappears spontaneously and reappears.

Chronic gingivitis: Comes on slowly, is of long duration and is painless unless complicated by acute or subacute exacerbations. Chronic gingivitis is the type most commonly encountered. Patients seldom recollect having had any acute symptoms. **Chronic gingivitis is a fluctuating disease in which inflamed areas persist or become normal and normal areas become inflamed.**[1,2]

Distribution

Localized: Confined to the gingiva in relation to a single tooth or group of teeth.

Generalized: Involving the entire mouth.

Marginal: Involving the gingival margin, but may include a portion of the contiguous attached gingiva.

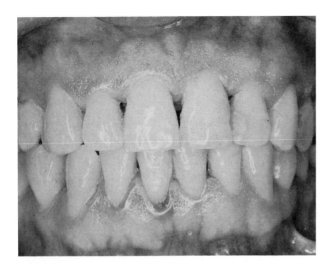

Figure 6–1 Localized Marginal Gingivitis in the mandibular anterior region.

Papillary: Involving the interdental papillae, and often extending into the adjacent portion of the gingival margin. Papillae are more frequently involved than the gingival margin, and the earliest signs of gingivitis most often occur in the papillae.[3]

Diffuse: Involving the gingival margin, attached gingiva and interdental papillae.

The distribution of gingival disease in individual cases is described by combining the above terms as follows:

Localized marginal gingivitis: Confined to one or more areas of the marginal gingiva (Fig. 6–1).

Localized diffuse gingivitis: Extending from the margin to the mucobuccal fold, but limited in area (Fig. 6–2).

Papillary gingivitis: Confined to one or more interdental spaces in a limited area (Fig. 6–3).

Generalized marginal gingivitis: Involvement of the gingival margin in relation to all the teeth. The interdental papillae are usually also involved in generalized marginal gingivitis (Fig. 6–4).

Generalized diffuse gingivitis: Involving the entire gingiva. The alveolar mucosa is usually also affected so that the demarcation between it and the attached gingiva is obliterated (Fig. 6–5). Systemic conditions are involved in the etiology of generalized diffuse gingivitis except in cases caused by acute infection or generalized chemical irritation.

CLINICAL FEATURES OF GINGIVITIS

In evaluating the clinical features of gingivitis it is necessary to be systematic. One must guard against being distracted by the spectacular findings and missing less striking changes which may be of equal, if not greater, diagnostic significance.

A systematic clinical approach requires an orderly examination of the gingiva for the following features: **color, size and shape, consistency, surface texture and position,** and **ease of bleeding and pain.** These clinical characteristics and the microscopic changes responsible for each are discussed in the chapters which follow.

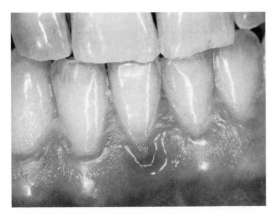

Figure 6–2 Localized Diffuse Gingivitis involving both the marginal and attached gingiva.

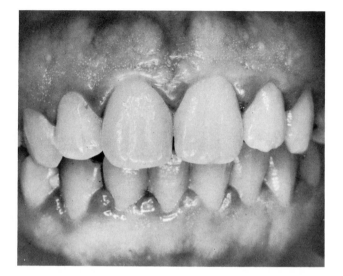

Figure 6–3   Papillary Gingivitis.

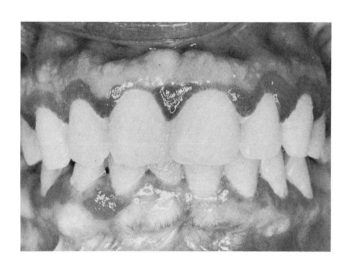

Figure 6–4 Generalized Marginal Gingivitis. The interdental papillae are also involved.

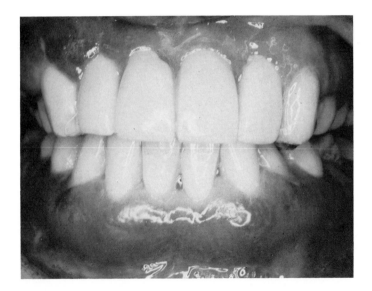

Figure 6–5 Generalized Diffuse Gingivitis. The marginal, interdental and attached gingivae are involved in chronic desquamative gingivitis.

REFERENCES

1. Hoover, D. R., and Lefkowitz, W.: Fluctuation in Marginal Gingivitis. J. Periodont., *36*:310, 1965.
2. Larato, D. C., Stahl, S. S., Brown, R., Jr., and Witkin, G. J.: The Effect of a Prescribed Method of Toothbrushing on the Fluctuation of Marginal Gingivitis. J. Periodont.-Periodontics, *40*:142, 1969.
3. Levin, M. A.: The Interdental Papillae in Gingivitis: A Review Survey. J. Periodont., *37*:230, 1966.

Chapter 7

CHANGES IN THE COLOR OF THE GINGIVA

COLOR CHANGES IN CHRONIC GINGIVITIS

Change in color is a very important clinical sign of gingival disease, and chronic gingivitis is its most common cause. Originating as a slight redness, the color changes through varying shades of red, reddish blue and deep blue with increasing chronicity of the inflammatory process. The changes start in the interdental papillae and gingival margin and spread to the attached gingiva (Fig. 7–1). Proper diagnosis and treatment require an understanding of the tissue changes which alter the color of the gingiva at the clinical level. To attain such understanding it is best to trace the pathology of gingivitis from its inception.

Pathology of chronic gingivitis

Oral microorganisms synthesize potentially harmful products capable of degrading the epithelial intercellular substance and widening intercellular spaces to permit other injurious agents to penetrate into the connective

tissue.[23] The initial response to irritation is erythema; this is marked by dilation of capillaries and increased blood flow, which produce the initial redness. Increased redness results from capillary proliferation, the formation of numerous capillary loops and the development of arterio-venule shunts.[12] As the inflammation becomes chronic, the blood vessels become engorged and congested, venous return is impaired and the blood flow becomes sluggish. The result is tissue anoxemia which superimposes a bluish tinge upon the reddened gingiva. Extravasation of red cells into the connective tissue and breakdown of hemoglobin into its component pigments deepen the color of the gingiva and often cause a blackish hue.

In chronic gingivitis the electron microscope reveals that the intercellular spaces in the crevicular epithelium are enlarged and contain a granular precipitate, cellular fragments, leukocytes, mainly plasma cells and lysosomal granules from disrupted neutrophils (Fig. 7–2). Lysosomes provide acid hydrolases which can destroy collagen and other tissue components. There are bacteria on the surface and under partially desquamated cells but not in the intercellular spaces between the epithelial cells.[9]

With increased widening of the intercellular spaces the intermediate and tight junctions disappear and desmosomes are reduced.[24] In the epithelial cells glycogen granules are increased, mitochondria are swollen and the number of cristae reduced. Disintegration of cytoplasm[6] contents and nucleus precedes cell death.

Neutrophils, lymphocytes, monocytes, mast cells and a predominance of plasma cells, and lysosome granules are present in the connective tissue. Initial disruption of collagen fibers

81

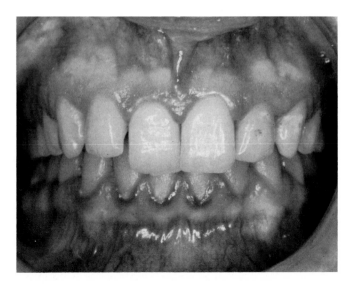

Figure 7–1 Chronic Gingivitis. The marginal and interdental gingivae are smooth, edematous and discolored.

is followed by the formation of focal areas in which collagen is completely destroyed.[13] There is an inverse relationship between the amount of collagen bundles and the number of inflammatory cells.[22] Collagenolytic activity is increased;[1,10] collagenase, normally present in the periodontal tissues, is also produced by bacteria and inflammatory cells.[2]

The basal lamina is at first resistant to erosion; but with more intense inflammation, breaks occur in the continuity through which epithelial cells migrate into the connective tissue. In areas the epithelial connective-tissue interface is obliterated.

Proteolytic activity is increased; the hydrolytic enzymes, alkaline and acid phosphatase,[29] beta-D-glucuronidase, beta-glucosidase, beta-galactosidase total esterase,[14] amino-peptidase[19,21] and cytochrome oxidase[5] are elevated. Lysozyme[4] and sialic acid[25] can be demonstrated, and neutral mucopolysaccharides and RNA are decreased.[27] Plasminogen, the precursor of the fibrinolytic enzyme plasmin, a component of normal gingiva, is found in greatest amounts in mild chronic inflammation and in lesser amounts in moderate to severe inflammation.[11]

Sulfhydryls are increased in proliferating epithelium associated with inflammation and are decreased or absent in degenerated epithelium.[26] Disulfides, absent in proliferating epithelium, are reduced in degenerated epithelium and present in leukocytes. In the connective tissue, sulfhydryls are present in the leukocytes as well as in the normal locations. Glycogen is reduced in inflamed connective tissue[28] and increased in proliferating epithelium. Oxygen consumption is increased when gingivitis is mild and reduced when it is severe.[15]

A shift in the epithelium–connective tissue relationship in chronic inflammation contributes to the color changes seen clinically. The epithelium proliferates and the rete pegs lengthen into the connective tissue. At the same time, the increasing bulk of the inflamed connective tissue presses against the overlying epithelium, causing it to atrophy. The engorged blood vessels of the connective tissue extend to within one or two epithelial cells from the surface.[13] The extensions of inflamed connective tissue close to the surface, separated by deepened epithelial rete pegs, create pinpoint areas of accentuated redness.

Chronic gingivitis is a conflict between destruction and repair. Persistent local irritants injure the gingiva, prolong inflammation and provoke abnormal vascular permeability and exudation.[8] Infiltration by the fluid, cells and enzymes of the inflammatory exudate results in tissue degeneration. At the same time, however, new connective tissue cells and fibers and new blood vessels are formed in a continuous effort to repair the tissue damage. Acid mucopolysaccharides, associated with fibrogenesis, are increased at the periphery of chronically inflamed areas.[18] Ultrastructural regenerative changes in the epithelium include increase in the number and density of cytoplasmic fibers, tonofibrils and ribonu-

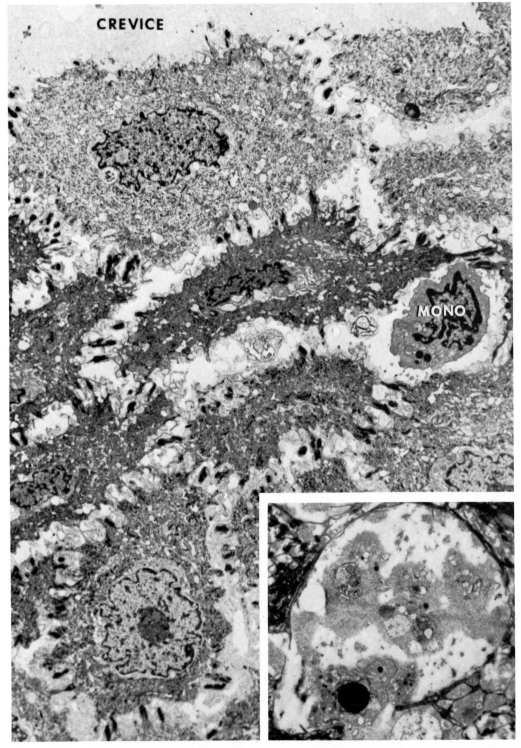

Figure 7–2 Chronic Gingivitis—Crevicular Epithelium. The crevice is at the top. The intercellular spaces are dilated and contain a granular precipitate and cellular fragments. An emigrating monocyte (MONO) is shown between the epithelial cells. × 4400. *Insert,* Cellular fragments and precipitated material in a dilated intercellular space of the crevicular epithelium. Bacteria are not present. × 4036. (From Freedman, H. L., Listgarten, M. A., and Taichman, N. S.[9])

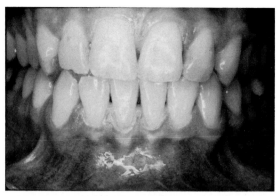

Figure 7–3 "Traumatic Crescents." Crescent-shaped marginal areas of gingival erythema in the mandibular anterior region. Vascular changes produced by trauma from occlusion are the suspected but not proved cause.

cleoprotein particles, reduction in cytoplasmic vacuolization and the return of the intercellular spaces to normal size.[16]

The interaction between the destruction and repair affects the color, size, consistency and surface texture of the gingiva. If increased vascularity, exudation and tissue degeneration predominate, color changes are strikingly apparent; if the dominant features are fibrotic, the color of the gingiva reverts toward normal, despite the existence of prolonged gingivitis.

"TRAUMATIC CRESCENTS." These are small, crescent-shaped, bluish red areas in the marginal gingiva attributed to trauma from occlusion (Fig. 7–3). *They are chronic inflammatory lesions caused by local irritants.* The suspected contributory role of excessive occlusal forces has not been demonstrated.

COLOR CHANGES IN ACUTE GINGIVITIS

Color changes in acute gingival inflammation differ somewhat from those in chronic gingivitis in nature and distribution. The color changes may be marginal, diffuse, or patch-like, depending upon the acute condition. In *acute necrotizing ulcerative gingivitis* the involvement is marginal; in *herpetic gingivostomatitis* it is diffuse, and in *acute reactions to chemical irritation* it is patch-like or diffuse.

Color changes vary with the intensity of the inflammation. In all instances there is an initial bright red erythema. If the condition does not worsen, this represents the only color change until the gingiva reverts to normal. In severe acute inflammation, the red color changes to a shiny slate-gray, which gradually becomes a dull whitish gray. The gray discoloration produced by tissue necrosis is demarcated from the adjacent gingiva by a thin, sharply defined erythematous zone. Detailed descriptions of the clinical features and pathology of the various forms of acute gingivitis are found in Chapter 11.

METALLIC PIGMENTATION

Heavy metals absorbed systemically from therapeutic use or occupational environments may discolor the gingiva and other areas of the oral mucosa.[17] This is different from tattooing produced by the accidental embedding of amalgam or other metal fragments (Fig. 7–4). Bismuth, arsenic and mercury produce a black line in the gingiva

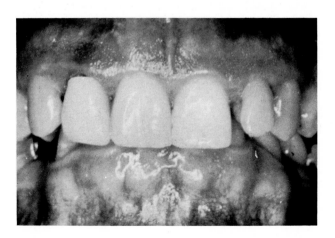

Figure 7–4 Discoloration of Gingiva over lateral incisor caused by embedded metal particles.

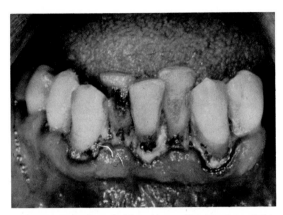

Figure 7–5 Bismuth Line. Linear discoloration of the gingiva in relation to local irritation in a patient receiving bismuth therapy.

which follows the contour of the margin (Fig. 7–5). The pigmentation may also appear as isolated black blotches involving marginal, interdental and attached gingiva. Lead results in a bluish red or deep blue linear pigmentation of the gingival margin (Burtonian line),[7] and silver (argyria) in a violet marginal line, often accompanied by a diffuse bluish gray discoloration throughout the oral mucosa.[20]

Gingival pigmentation from systemically absorbed metals results from **perivascular precipitation of metallic sulfides in the subepithelial connective tissue.** Gingival pigmentation is not an effect of systemic toxicity. It occurs only in areas of inflammation, where the increased permeability of irritated blood vessels permits seepage of the metal into the surrounding tissue. In addition to inflamed gingiva, mucosal areas irritated by biting or abnormal chewing habits such as the inner surface of the lips, the cheek at the level of the occlusal line and the lateral border of the tongue are common pigmentation sites.

Gingival or mucosal pigmentation is eliminated by **removing the local irritating factors and restoring tissue health,** without necessarily discontinuing the metal-containing drugs required for therapeutic purposes. **Temporary correction** is obtained by topical application of concentrated peroxide or by insufflating the gingiva with oxygen to oxidize the dark metallic sulfides. The discoloration reappears unless the procedures are repeated.

CHANGES ASSOCIATED WITH OTHER LOCAL AND SYSTEMIC FACTORS

In Addison's disease the gingiva often presents isolated patches of discoloration, varying from brown to black (Figs. 7–6 and 7–7). Comparable changes are seen in other areas of the oral mucous membrane subject to irritation. The gingiva of patients with blood dyscrasias presents color changes. In *anemia,* the gingiva assumes a diffuse dusky pallor. Diffuse redness of the gingiva is

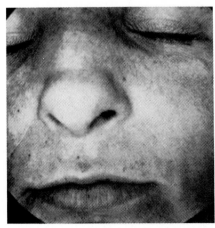

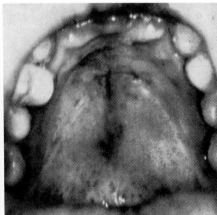

Fig. 7–6   Fig. 7–7

Figure 7–6 Addison's Disease. Diffuse pigmentation of the skin.
Figure 7–7 Addison's Disease. Palate of patient shown in Figure 7–6 with spotty distribution of pigment.

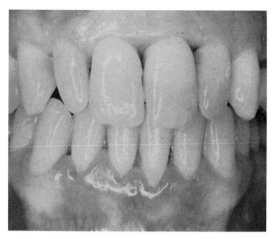

Figure 7–8 Vertical Discoloration of marginal and attached gingiva associated with periodontal pockets.

associated with polycythemia. In leukemia the gingiva is often a deep cyanotic purplish blue. When one realizes that gingival tissues in leukemic individuals are crowded with leukocytes, often with varying degrees of reduction of the red blood cells necessary to supply oxygen to the tissues, the cyanotic appearance of the gingiva is understandable. In hemochromatosis, distinct bronze discoloration of the gingiva is associated with comparable pigmentation of the skin. Yellowish gray discoloration of the gingiva may be a feature of xanthomatous disease. Deficiencies in components of the vitamin B complex may give rise to diffuse bluish red or fiery red discoloration of the gingiva as well as of the remainder of the oral mucosa. Violaceous discoloration of the gingiva has been described in *diabetes*,[30] and raspberry red or diffuse bluish red discoloration is seen in *pregnancy*. Diffuse or spotty red discoloration occurs in desquamative gingivitis, menopausal gingovostomatitis and benign mucous membrane pemphigus (pemphigoid).

Exogenous factors capable of producing color changes in the gingiva include atmospheric irritants, such as coal and metal dust, and coloring agents in food. Green staining of the gingiva and diffuse metallic discoloration are seen in workers dealing with brass and silver respectively. Tobacco causes a gray hyperkeratosis of the gingiva. Isolated zones of discoloration of the gingiva are commonly associated with periodontal pocket formation (Fig. 7–8).

REFERENCES

1. Bennick, A., and Hunt, A. M.: Collagenolytic Activity in Oral Tissues. Arch. Oral Biol., *12*:1, 1967.
2. Beutner, E. H., Triftshauser, C., and Hazen, S. P.: Collagenase Activity of Gingival Tissue from Patients with Periodontal Disease. Proc. Soc. Exp. Biol. & Med., *121*:1082, 1966.
3. Box, H. K.: Signs of Incipient Periodontal Disease. Bulletin Canadian Dental Research Foundation, May, 1925.
4. Burnett, G. M., Gouge, S., and Toye, A. E.: Lysozyme Content of Human Gingiva and Various Rat Tissues. J. Periodont., *30*:148, 1959.
5. Burstone, M. S.: Histochemical Study of Cytochrome Oxidase in Normal and Inflamed Gingiva. Oral Surg., *13*:1501, 1960.
6. Cruz Ortis, F.: Proteolytic Action in Normal and Pathologic Gingival Tissues and in the Granulation Tissue of Periodontal Pockets. Santiago, University of Chile Press, 1946.
7. Dummett, C. O.: Abnormal Color Changes in Gingivae. Oral Surg., Oral Med. & Oral Path., *2*:649, 1949.
8. Egelberg, J.: The Topography and Permeability of Vessels at the Dento-Gingival Junction in Dogs. J. Periodont. Res., Suppl. 1, 1967.
9. Freedman, H. L., Listgarten, M. A., and Taichman, N. S.: Electron Microscopic Features of Chronically Inflamed Human Gingiva. J. Periodont. Res., *3*:313, 1968.
10. Fullmer, H., and Gibson, W.: Collagenolytic Activity in Gingivae of Man. Nature, *209*:728, 1966.
11. Kaslick, R. S., Chasens, A. I., Innerfield, I., and Rowley, G. R.: Tissue Plasminogen in Normal and Inflamed Human Gingiva. J. D. Res., *48*:603, 1969.
12. Kindlova, M.: Changes in the Vascular Bed of the Marginal Periodontium in Periodontitis. J. D. Res., *44*:456, 1965.
13. Levy, B. M., Taylor, A. C., and Bernick, S.: Relationship between Epithelium and Connective Tissue in Gingival Inflammation. J. D. Res., *48*: 625, 1969.
14. Lisanti, V. F.: Hydrolytic Enzymes in Periodontal Tissues. Ann. New York Acad. Sc., 85:461, 1960.
15. Manhold, J. H., and Volpe, A. R.: Effect of Inflammation in the Absence of Proliferation on the Oxygen Consumption of Gingival Tissue. J. D. Res., *42*:103, 1963.
16. Mazzella, W., and Vernick, S.: The Ultrastructure of Normal and Pathologic Human Gingival Epithelium. J. Periodont., *39*:5, 1968.
17. McCarthy, F. P., and Dexter, S. O., Jr.: Oral Manifestations of Bismuth. New England J. Med., *213*:345, 1935.
18. Melcher, A. H.: Some Histological and Histochemical Observations on the Connective Tissue of Chronically Inflamed Human Gingiva. J. Periodont. Res., *2*:127, 1967.
19. Mori, M., and Kishiro, A.: Histochemical Observation of Aminopeptidase Activity in the Normal and Inflamed Oral Epithelium. J. Osaka Univ. D. Sch., *1*:39, 1961.
20. Prinz, H.: Pigmentations of Oral Mucous Membrane. D. Cosmos, *74*:554, 1932.

21. Quintarelli, G.: Histochemistry of the Gingiva. III. The Distribution of Amino-peptidase in Normal and Inflammatory Conditions. Arch. Oral Biol., 2:271, 1960.

22. Schroeder, H. E.: Extraneous Cell Surface Coat in Human Inflamed Crevicular Epithelium. Helv. Odont. Acta, 12:14, 1968.

23. Stallard, R. E., and Awwa, I. A.: The Effect of Alterations in External Environment on the Dento-Gingival Junction. J. D. Res., 48:671, 1969.

24. Thilander, H.: Epithelial Changes in Gingivitis. An Electron Microscopic Study. J. Periodont. Res., 3:303, 1968.

25. Thonard, J. C., and Blustein, R.: Sialic Acid in Human Gingiva. J. D. Res., 44:379, 1965.

26. Turesky, S., Crowley, J., and Glickman, I.: A Histo-chemical Study of Protein-Bound Sulfhydryl and Disulfide Groups in Normal and Inflamed Human Gingiva. J. D. Res., 36:255, 1957.

27. Turesky, S., Glickman, I., and Fisher, B.: The Effect of Physiologic and Pathologic Processes Upon Certain Histochemically Detectable Substances in the Gingiva. J. Periodont., 30:116, 1959.

28. Turesky, S., Glickman, I., and Litwin, T.: A Histo-chemical Evaluation of Normal and Inflamed Human Gingivae. J. D. Res., 30:792, 1951.

29. Winer, R. A., et al.: Enzyme Activity in Periodontal Disease. J. Periodont., 41:449, 1970.

30. Ziskin, D. E., Loughlin, W. C., and Siegel, E. H.: Diabetes in Relation to Certain Oral and Systemic Problems. Part II. Am. J. Ortho. & Oral Surg., 30:758, 1944.

Chapter 8

GINGIVAL ENLARGEMENT

✓*Gingival enlargement,* increase in size, is a common feature of gingival disease. There are many types of gingival enlargement which vary according to the etiologic factors and pathologic processes that produce them.[27]

The term *hypertrophic gingivitis* is not appropriate for pathologic increases in the size of the gingiva. Hypertrophy means "increase in the size of an organ as a result of increase in size of its individual component cells in order to meet increased functional requirements for useful work."[66] Enlargement of the gingiva in gingival disease is not primarily the result of an increase in size of component cells; nor does it generally occur in response to an increased functional requirement for useful work.

CLASSIFICATION OF GINGIVAL ENLARGEMENT

Gingival enlargement is classified according to etiology and pathology as follows:

I. **Inflammatory enlargement**
  A. Chronic
    1. Localized or generalized
    2. Discrete (tumor-like)
  B. Acute
    1. Gingival abscess
    2. Periodontal abscess
II. **Noninflammatory hyperplastic enlargement (gingival hyperplasia)**
  A. Gingival hyperplasia associated with Dilantin therapy
  B. Familial, hereditary or idiopathic hyperplastic gingival enlargement
III. **Combined enlargement**
IV. **Conditioned enlargement**
  A. Hormonal
    1. Enlargement of pregnancy
    2. Enlargement of puberty
  B. Leukemic
  C. Associated with vitamin C deficiency
  D. Nonspecific enlargement
V. **Neoplastic enlargement**
VI. **Developmental enlargement**

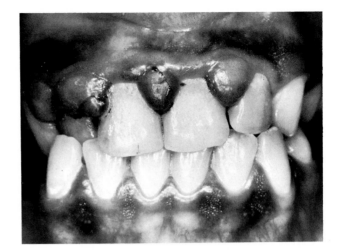

Figure 8-1 Chronic Inflammatory Gingival Enlargement localized to the anterior region, associated with irregularity of teeth.

Location and distribution

Using the criteria of location and distribution, gingival enlargement is designated as follows:

Localized: Limited to the gingiva adjacent to a single tooth or group of teeth.

Generalized: Involving the gingiva throughout the mouth.

Marginal: Confined to the marginal gingiva.

Papillary: Confined to the interdental papilla.

Diffuse: Involving the marginal and attached gingiva and papillae.

Discrete: An isolated sessile or pedunculated "tumor-like" enlargement.

Gingival enlargement is *classified* on the basis of underlying histopathologic changes and etiology as follows:

I. INFLAMMATORY ENLARGEMENT

Gingival enlargement may result from chronic or acute inflammatory changes. The former is by far the more common cause.

Chronic Inflammatory Enlargement

LOCALIZED OR GENERALIZED

Chronic inflammatory gingival enlargement originates as a slight ballooning of the interdental papilla, marginal gingiva, or

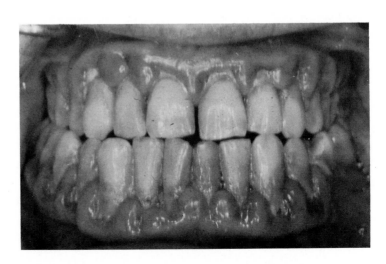

Figure 8-2 Generalized Chronic Inflammatory Gingival Enlargement.

both. In the early stages it produces a life-saver-like bulge around the involved teeth. This bulge increases in size until it covers part of the crowns. The enlargement is generally papillary or marginal, and may be localized (Fig. 8–1) or generalized (Fig. 8–2). It progresses slowly and painlessly unless it is complicated by acute infection or trauma.

DISCRETE (TUMOR-LIKE)

Occasionally, chronic inflammatory gingival enlargement occurs as a discrete sessile or pedunculated mass resembling a tumor. It may be interproximal or on the marginal or attached gingiva (Fig. 8–3). The lesions are slow-growing and usually painless. They may undergo spontaneous reduction in size, followed by reappearance and continued enlargement. Painful ulceration in the fold between the mass and the adjacent gingiva sometimes occurs.

Histopathology

The following features produce chronic inflammatory gingival enlargement (Figs. 8–4 and 8–5): inflammatory fluid and cellular exudate, degeneration of epithelium and con- nective tissue, new capillary formation, vascular engorgement, hemorrhage, proliferation of epithelium and connective tissue, new collagen fibers.

The microscopic components determine the clinical features of the enlargement such as color, consistency and texture. Lesions that consist of a preponderance of inflammatory cells and fluid with associated degenerative changes are deep red or bluish red, soft and friable with a smooth shiny surface; they bleed easily. Lesions predominantly fibrotic with an abundance of fibroblasts and collagen bundles are relatively firm, resilient and pink.

Etiology

Chronic inflammatory gingival enlargement is caused by prolonged local irritation. The following are typical etiologic factors (Hirschfeld[34]): poor oral hygiene (Fig. 8–6), abnormal relationships of adjacent teeth (Fig. 8–7) and opposing teeth, lack of function, cervical cavities (Figs. 8–8 and 8–9), overhanging margins of dental restorations, improperly contoured dental restorations or pontics, food impaction (Fig. 8–10), irritation from clasps or saddle areas of removable prostheses, mouth breathing, nasal obstruction, repositioning of teeth by orthodontic therapy, and habitual pressing of the tongue against the gingiva.[2]

Acute Inflammatory Enlargement

GINGIVAL ABSCESS

A gingival abscess is a localized, painful, rapidly expanding lesion usually of sudden onset. It is generally limited to the marginal gingiva or interdental papilla (Fig. 8–11). In its early stages it appears as a red swelling with a smooth shiny surface. Within 24 to 48 hours, the lesion is usually fluctuant and pointed, with a surface orifice from which a purulent exudate may be expressed. The adjacent teeth are often sensitive to percussion. If permitted to progress, the lesions generally rupture spontaneously.

Histopathology

The gingival abscess consists of a purulent focus in the connective tissue surrounded by

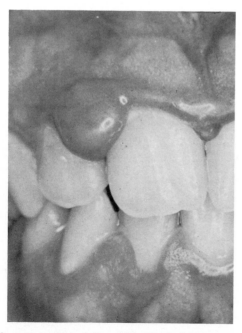

Figure 8–3 Discrete Tumor-like Gingival Enlargement.

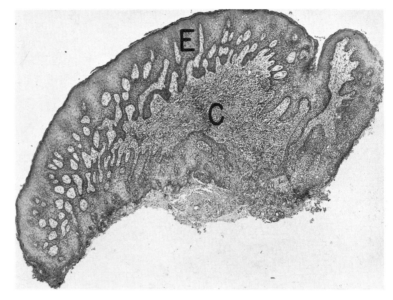

Figure 8–4 Survey Section of Chronic Inflammatory Gingival Enlargement showing the central connective tissue core (C) and thickened epithelium at the periphery (E). Note the ulceration of the epithelial surface at the lower border of the mass that was adjacent to the tooth surface.

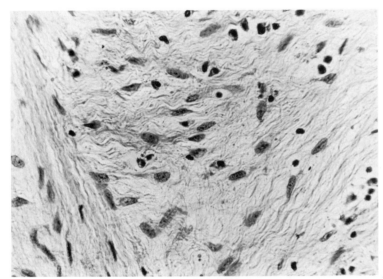

Figure 8–5 High Power Study Showing Young Fibroblasts and collagen fibrils that contribute to the increase in size in chronic inflammatory gingival enlargement.

Figure 8–6 Chronic Inflammatory Gingival Enlargement associated with plaque accumulation around orthodontic appliance.

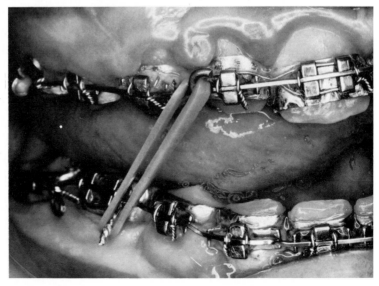

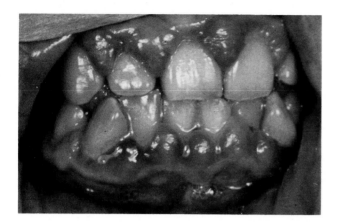

Figure 8-7 Chronic Inflammatory Gingival Enlargement Associated with Irregularity in Tooth Alignment. The difference in the color intensity of the enlarged gingiva and the adjacent comparatively uninvolved attached gingiva is shown in the mandible.

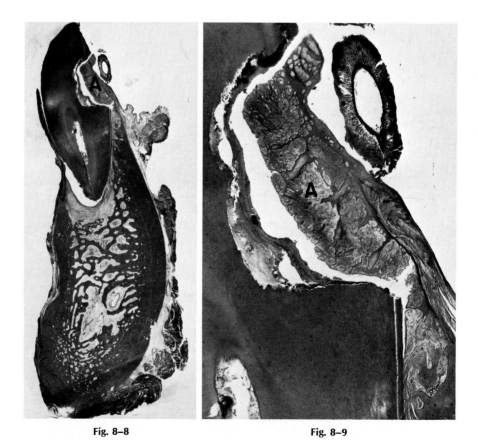

Fig. 8-8   Fig. 8-9

Figure 8-8 Survey section of mandibular canine in situ with cervical carious lesion (A).

Figure 8-9 Detail of Figure 8-8 showing a **Chronic Inflammatory Enlargement** of the gingiva (A) in the carious lesion. Note the continuity between the enlarged mass and the facial gingiva at the lower right.

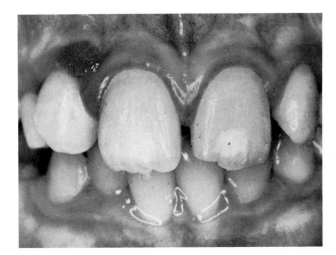

Figure 8–10 Chronic Inflammatory Enlargement Associated With Impaction and Retention of Food in Relation to Malposed Lateral Incisor. Note the extreme vascularity of the lesion.

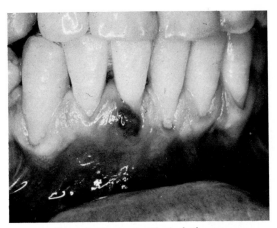

Figure 8–11 Acute Gingival Abscess.

diffuse infiltration of polymorphonuclear leukocytes, edematous tissue and vascular engorgement. The surface epithelium presents varying degrees of intra- and extracellular edema, invasion by leukocytes, and ulceration.

Etiology

Acute inflammatory gingival enlargement is a response to irritation from foreign substances such as a toothbrush bristle, apple core, or lobster shell forcefully embedded into the gingiva. This lesion is confined to the gingiva, and should not be confused with periodontal or lateral abscesses.

PERIODONTAL (LATERAL) ABSCESS

Periodontal abscesses generally produce enlargement of the gingiva but also involve the supporting periodontal tissues. For a detailed description of periodontal abscesses, see Chapter 18.

II. NONINFLAMMATORY HYPERPLASTIC ENLARGEMENT (GINGIVAL HYPERPLASIA)

The term *hyperplasia refers to an increase in the size of tissue or an organ produced by an increase in the number of its component cells. Noninflammatory gingival hyperplasia is produced by factors others than local irritation. It is not common, and occurs most often associated with Dilantin therapy.*

Gingival Hyperplasia Associated with Dilantin Therapy

Enlargement of the gingiva caused by Dilantin sodium* (sodium diphenyl hydantoinate), an anticonvulsant used in the treatment of epilepsy, occurs in some of the patients receiving the drug. Its reported incidence varies from 3 to 62 per cent,[28, 52] with the greater frequencies in younger patients.[3] Its occurrence and severity are not necessarily related to the dosage or duration of drug therapy.

Clinical features

The primary or basic lesion starts as a painless, bead-like enlargement of the facial and lingual gingival margin and interdental papillae (Figs. 8–12 to 8–14). As the condi-

---

*Epanutin in some countries.

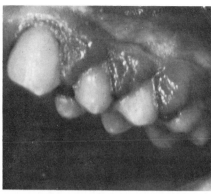

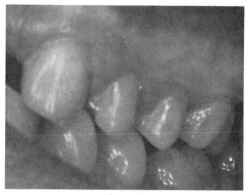

Fig. 8–12   **Fig. 8–13**

Figure 8–12   Gingival Enlargement Associated With Dilantin Therapy. Note the minutely lobulated surface of the enlarged gingiva.

Figure 8–13   Same patient as in Figure 8–12 showing disappearance of the gingival enlargement one month after the cessation of the Dilantin therapy.

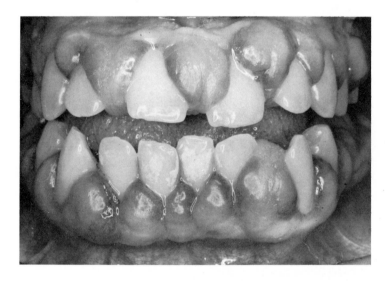

Figure 8–14   Gingival Enlargement Associated With Dilantin Therapy. Note the prominent papillary lesions. The gingiva is firm and nodular. There is marginal inflammation along the crevices deepened by the gingival overgrowth.

Figure 8–15   Massive Hyperplasia Associated With Dilantin Therapy. The teeth are completely covered. The gingiva is firm and dense with a nodular surface.

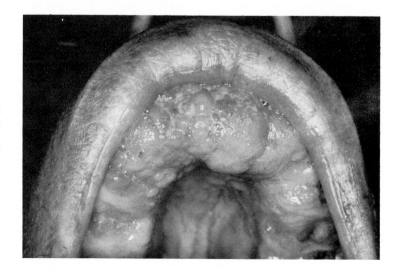

tion progresses, the marginal and papillary enlargements unite, and they may develop into a massive tissue fold covering a considerable portion of the crowns and may interfere with occlusion (Fig. 8–15). When uncomplicated by inflammation, the lesion is mulberry-shaped, firm, pale pink and resilient, with a minutely lobulated surface and no tendency to bleed. The enlargement characteristically appears to project from beneath the gingival margin from which it is separated by a linear groove.

Dilantin-induced hyperplasia may occur in mouths devoid of local irritants, but may be absent in mouths in which local irritants are profuse.

The hyperplasia is usually generalized throughout the mouth, but is more severe in the maxillary and mandibular anterior regions. It occurs in areas in which teeth are present—not in edentulous spaces—and the enlargement disappears in areas from which teeth are extracted. Hyperplasia of the mucosa in edentulous mouths has been reported, but it is rare.[20]

The enlargement is chronic, and slowly increases in size until it interferes with occlusion or becomes unsightly. When surgically removed, it recurs. Spontaneous disappearance occurs within a month after the drug is discontinued.

Local irritants such as plaque, materia alba, calculus, overhanging margins of restorations and food impaction cause inflammation which often complicates gingival hyperplasia caused by the drug. *It is important to distinguish between the increase in size caused by the Dilantin-induced hyperplasia and the complicating inflammation caused by local irritation.* Secondary inflammatory changes add to the size of the lesion caused by Dilantin, produce red or bluish red discoloration, obliterate the lobulated surface demarcations, and create an increased tendency toward bleeding.

Histopathology

The enlargement presents pronounced hyperplasia of connective tissue and epithelium (Fig. 8–16). There is acanthosis of the epithelium, and elongated rete pegs extend deep into the connective tissue which presents densely arranged collagen bundles with an increase in fibroblasts and new blood vessels. Oxytalan fibers are numerous beneath the epithelium and in areas of inflammation.[6] Inflammation is common along the sulcal surfaces of the gingiva. Ultrastructural changes in the epithelium include widening of the intercellular spaces in the basal layer, cytoplasmic edema and rarefaction of desmosomes.[73] The mitotic index is reduced.

Recurrent enlargements appear as granulation tissue composed of numerous young capillaries and fibroblasts and irregularly arranged collagen fibrils with occasional lymphocytes (Figs. 8–17 and 8–18).

Nature of the lesion

The enlargement is basically a hyperplastic reaction initiated by the drug, with inflammation a secondary complicating factor. Some feel that inflammation is a prerequisite for development of the hyperplasia and that it can be prevented by removal of local irritants and fastidious oral hygiene.[31] Others find that toothbrushing reduces the inflammation but does not lessen the hyperplasia or prevent it.[21]

Except in one study,[36] tissue culture experiments indicate that Dilantin stimulates proliferation of fibroblast-like cells[60] and epithelium.[50] Two analogues of Dilantin (1-allyl,5-phenylhydantoinate and 5-methyl,5-phenylhydantoinate) have a similar effect on fibroblast-like cells.[59] Stimulation by Dilantin is inhibited in irradiated cells.[61]

In experimental animals Dilantin causes gingival enlargement independent of local inflammation. It starts as hyperplasia of the connective tissue core of the marginal gingiva, which is followed by proliferation of the epithelium.[39] The enlargement increases by proliferation and expansion of the central core beyond the crest of the gingival margin.

Dilantin occurs in the saliva in amounts correlated with the severity of gingival hyperplasia and the patient's age.[4] But in animals extirpation of the parotid glands does not affect the occurrence of hyperplasia.[7]

Systemic administration of Dilantin accelerates the healing of gingival wounds in nonepileptic humans[63] and increases the tensile strength of healing abdominal wounds in rats.[62]

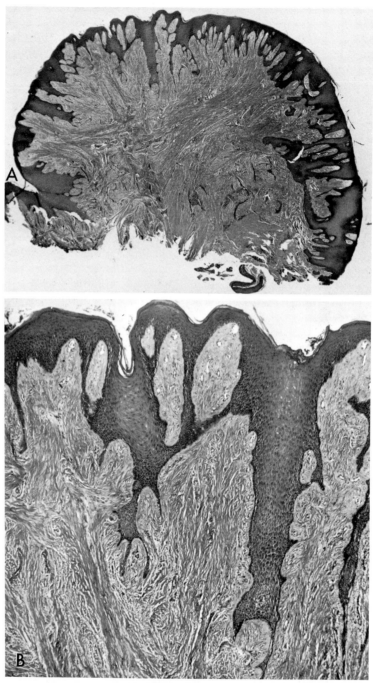

Figure 8–16 Gingival Enlargement Associated With Dilantin Therapy. *A,* Survey section, showing bulbous gingival enlargement. *B,* Detailed view, showing hyperplasia and acanthosis of the epithelium with extension of deep rete pegs into the connective tissue. The connective tissue is densely collagenous. There is little evidence of inflammation.

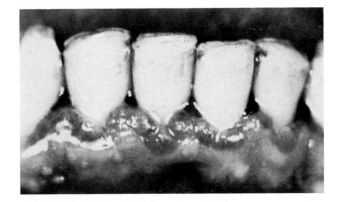

Figure 8–17 Early Recurrence following surgical removal of enlarged gingiva in patient receiving Dilantin therapy.

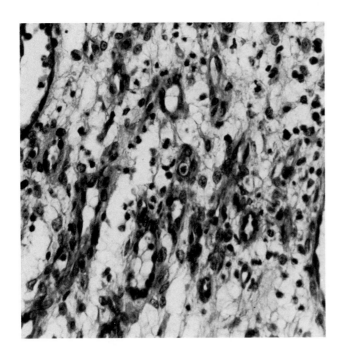

Figure 8–18 Biopsy of Recurrent Gingival Enlargement shown in Figure 8–17. Note the abundance of new blood vessels.

Familial, Hereditary or Idiopathic Hyperplastic Enlargement

✓This is a rare condition of undetermined etiology which has been designated by such terms as gingivomatosis elephantiasis,[5, 41] diffuse fibroma,[16] familial elephantiasis, idiopathic fibromatosis,[79] hereditary or idiopathic hyperplasia,[58] hereditary gingival fibromatosis[77] and congenital familial fibromatosis.

Clinical features

✓The enlargement affects the attached gingiva as well as the gingival margin and interdental papillae, in contrast with Dilantin-induced hyperplasia, which is often limited to the gingival margin and interdental papillae. The facial and lingual surfaces of the mandible and maxilla are generally affected, but the involvement may be limited to either jaw. The enlarged gingiva is pink, firm, almost leathery in consistency, and presents a characteristic minutely "pebbled" surface (Fig. 8–19). In severe cases the teeth are almost completely covered, and the enlargement projects into the oral vestibule. The jaws appear distorted because of the bulbous enlargement of the gingiva. Secondary inflammatory changes are common at the gingival margin.

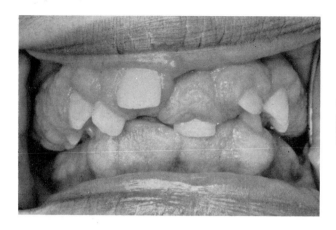

Figure 8–19 Idiopathic Hyperplastic Gingival Enlargement. The gingiva is firm with a nodular pebbled surface. The hyperplastic gingiva deflects the erupting teeth from proper alignment. (From Ball, E. I.[5])

Histopathology

There is a bulbous increase in the amount of connective tissue (Fig. 8–20) that is relatively avascular and consists of densely arranged collagen bundles and numerous fibroblasts. The surface epithelium is thickened and acanthotic with elongated rete pegs.

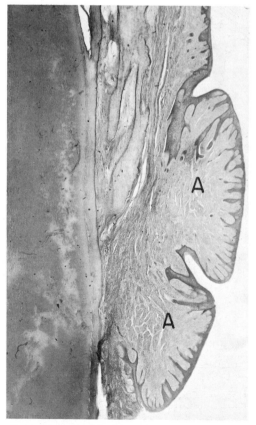

Figure 8–20 Nodular Noninflammatory Hyperplastic Gingival Enlargement (A) involving the attached gingiva.

Etiology

Some cases have been explained on a hereditary basis,[22, 77, 79] but the etiology is unknown, and the hyperplasia is appropriately designated as *idiopathic*. The enlargement usually begins with the eruption of the primary or secondary dentition and may regress after extraction, suggesting the possibility that the teeth may be initiating factors. Nutritional and hormonal etiologies have been explored but have not been substantiated.[51] Local irritation is a complicating factor.

Diffuse gingival hyperplasia should be differentiated from the bulbous distortion in the contour of the jaws associated with marked malocclusion. In the latter condition, the gingiva may be essentially unaltered or may present chronic inflammation of the gingival margin in relation to the malposed teeth (Figs. 8–21 and 8–22). The combination of inflamed marginal gingiva and unaltered attached gingiva on the deformed bone creates the erroneous impression of diffuse gingival enlargement. The dense fibrous consistency and accentuated stippling seen in diffuse hyperplastic enlargement are absent.

III. COMBINED ENLARGEMENT

This condition results when gingival hyperplasia is complicated by secondary inflammatory changes. The development of the combined type of gingival enlargement is depicted in Figure 8–23. Gingival hyperplasia creates conditions favorable for the accumulation of plaque and materia alba by accentuating the depth of the gingival

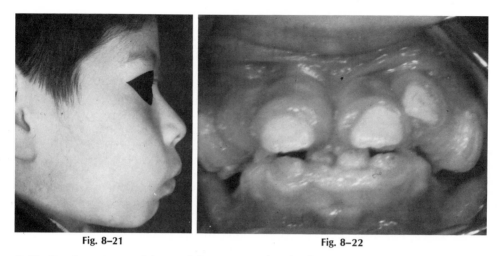

Fig. 8–21   Fig. 8–22

Figure 8–21   Prominent contour of the mouth in a patient with malocclusion.
Figure 8–22   Bulbous distortion of the maxilla and mandible in patient shown in Figure 8–21, aggravated by chronic inflammatory gingival enlargement.

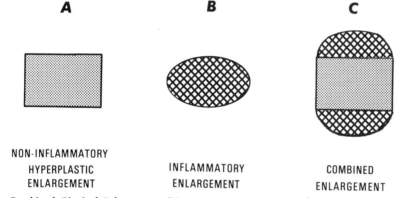

A   **B**   **C**

NON-INFLAMMATORY
HYPERPLASTIC   INFLAMMATORY   COMBINED
ENLARGEMENT   ENLARGEMENT   ENLARGEMENT

Figure 8–23   Combined Gingival Enlargement. Diagrammatic representation showing non-inflammatory hyperplastic enlargement (*A*) complicated by inflammatory enlargement (*B*) to produce combined gingival enlargement (*C*).

sulcus, by interfering with effective hygienic measures, and by deflecting the normal excursive pathways of food. The secondary inflammatory changes (Fig. 8–23, *B*) accentuate the size of the pre-existing gingival hyperplasia (Fig. 8–23, *A*) and produce the combined gingival enlargement (Fig. 8–23, *C*). *In many instances, secondary inflammation obscures the features of the pre-existent noninflammatory hyperplasia to the extent that the entire lesion appears to be inflammatory* (Fig. 8–24).

It is essential that the nature of combined gingival enlargement be understood. It consists of two components: **a primary or basic hyperplasia of connective tissue and epithelium**—the origin of which is unrelated to inflammation—and **a secondary complicating inflammatory component.** The

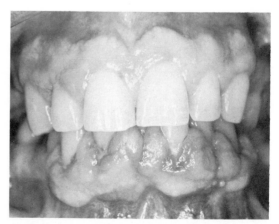

Figure 8–24   Combined Gingival Enlargement in a patient receiving Dilantin therapy. The basic hyperplasia is complicated by secondary inflammatory involvement. Note the edema and discoloration produced by the inflammation.

removal of local irritation eliminates the secondary inflammatory component and the size of the lesion proportionately, but the noninflammatory hyperplasia remains (Fig. 8–23, A). Elimination of the noninflammatory hyperplasia requires correction of the causative factors when possible.

IV. CONDITIONED ENLARGEMENT

This type of enlargement occurs when the systemic condition of the patient is such as to exaggerate or distort the usual gingival response to local irritation, and produces a corresponding modification of the usual clinical features of chronic gingivitis. The specific manner in which the clinical picture of conditioned gingival enlargement differs from chronic gingivitis depends upon the nature of the modifying systemic influence. *Local irritation is necessary for the initiation of this type of enlargement.* The irritation does not, however, solely determine the nature of its clinical features.

There are three types of conditioned gingival enlargement: hormonal, leukemic, and that associated with vitamin C deficiency.

Hormonal Enlargement

ENLARGEMENT IN PREGNANCY

In pregnancy, gingival enlargement may be marginal and generalized or occur as single or multiple tumor-like masses.

Marginal enlargement

The prevalence of marginal gingival enlargement in pregnancy has been reported as 10 per cent[17] and 70 per cent.[78] It results from the aggravation of previously inflamed areas. However, the gingival enlargement does not occur without clinical evidence of local irritation. **Pregnancy does not cause the condition**; the altered tissue metabolism in pregnancy accentuates the response to local irritants.[37]

CLINICAL FEATURES. The clinical picture varies considerably. The enlargement is usually generalized, and tends to be more prominent interproximally than on the facial and lingual surfaces. The enlarged gingiva is bright red or magenta, soft and friable, and has a smooth shiny surface. Bleeding occurs spontaneously or upon slight provocation.

Tumor-like gingival enlargement

The so-called pregnancy tumor is not a neoplasm; it is an inflammatory response to local irritation, and is modified by the patient's condition. It usually appears after the third month of pregnancy, but may occur earlier,[44] and has a reported incidence of 1.8 to 5 per cent.[46]

CLINICAL FEATURES. It appears as a discrete mushroom-like, flattened spherical mass protruding from the gingival margin, or more frequently, from the interproximal space, attached by a sessile or pedunculated

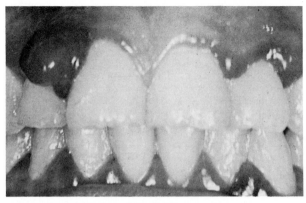

Fig. 8–25

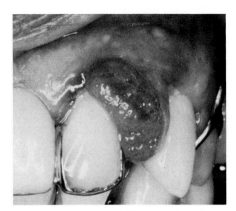

Fig. 8–26

Figure 8–25 **Conditioned Gingival Enlargement** in pregnancy.
Figure 8–26 **Conditioned Gingival Enlargement** in pregnancy associated with local irritation and food impaction.

base (Figs. 8–25 and 8–26). It tends to expand laterally, and pressure from the tongue and cheek perpetuate its flattened appearance. Generally dusky red or magenta, it has a smooth glistening surface that frequently presents numerous deep red pinpoint markings. It is a superficial lesion and ordinarily does not invade the underlying bone. The consistency varies, is usually semifirm, but may present varying degrees of softness and friability. It is usually painless unless its size and shape are such as to foster accumulation of debris under its margin or interfere with the occlusion, in which case painful ulceration may occur.

Histopathology

Both the marginal and tumor-like enlargements consist of a central mass of connective tissue, the periphery of which is outlined by stratified squamous epithelium. The connective tissue consists of numerous diffusely arranged, newly formed and engorged capillaries lined by cuboidal endothelial cells (Fig. 8–27). Between the capillaries there is a moderately fibrous stroma that presents varying degrees of edema and leukocytic infiltration. The stratified squamous epithelium is thickened with prominent rete pegs. The basal epithelium presents some degree of intra- and extracellular edema; there are prominent intercellular bridges and leukocytic infiltration. The surface of the epithelium is generally keratinized. There is generalized chronic inflammatory involvement, usually with a surface zone of acute inflammation.

Gingival enlargement in pregnancy is termed angiogranuloma, which avoids the implication of neoplasm implicit in such terms as fibrohemangioma or pregnancy tumor. Prominent endothelial proliferation with capillary formation and associated inflammation are its characteristic features. The capillary formation exceeds the usual gingival response to chronic irritation and accounts for the enlargement. Although the microscopic findings are characteristic of gingival enlargement in pregnancy, they are not pathognomonic in the sense that they can be used to differentiate between pregnant and nonpregnant patients.[46]

Most gingival disease during pregnancy can be prevented by removal of local irritants and institution of fastidious oral hygiene at the outset. In pregnancy treatment of the gingiva that is limited to the removal of tissue without complete elimination of local irritants is followed by recurrence. Although spontaneous reduction in the size of gingival enlargement commonly follows the termination of pregnancy, the complete elimination of the residual inflammatory lesion requires the removal of all forms of local irritation.

ENLARGEMENT IN PUBERTY

Enlargement of the gingiva is frequently seen during puberty. It occurs in both males

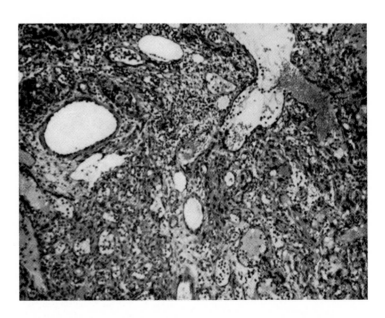

Figure 8–27 Conditioned Gingival Enlargement in pregnancy showing abundance of blood vessels and interspersed inflammatory cells.

and females, and appears in areas of local irritation.

Clinical features

The size of the gingival enlargement is far in excess of that usually seen associated with comparable local factors. It is marginal and interdental, and characterized by prominent bulbous interproximal papillae (Fig. 8–28). Frequently, only the facial gingivae are enlarged; the lingual surfaces are relatively unaltered. This occurs when the mechanical action of the tongue and the excursion of food prevent a heavy accumulation of local irritants on the lingual surface.

In addition to an increase in size, gingival enlargement during puberty presents all of the clinical features generally associated with chronic inflammatory gingival disease. *It is the degree of enlargement and tendency toward massive recurrence in the presence of relatively little local irritation that distinguishes the gingival enlargement of puberty from uncomplicated chronic inflammatory gingival enlargement.* After puberty, the enlargement undergoes spontaneous reduction, but does not disappear until local irritants are removed.

Histopathology

Because the condition is predominantly inflammatory in nature, it is difficult to discern the conditioning systemic influence in terms of specific histologic changes. The microscopic picture is that of chronic inflammation with prominent edema and associated degenerative changes.

Leukemic Enlargement

Clinical features

Leukemic gingival enlargement represents an exaggerated response to local irritation manifested by a dense infiltration of immature and proliferating leukocytes. The clinical picture is more severe than that of simple chronic inflammation. In some leukemic patients gingival enlargement results from chronic inflammation without involvement of leukemic cells and presents the same clinical and microscopic features as in non-leukemic patients.

True leukemic enlargement occurs in acute or subacute leukemia in the presence of local irritation—seldom in chronic leukemia. Clinically, true leukemic enlargement may be diffuse or marginal, localized or generalized. It may appear as a diffuse enlargement of the gingival mucosa (Fig. 8–29), an oversized extension of the marginal gingiva, or a discrete tumor-like interproximal mass. In true leukemic enlargement the gingiva is generally bluish red and has a shiny surface. The consistency is moderately firm, but there is a tendency toward friability and hemorrhage either spontaneously or upon slight irrita-

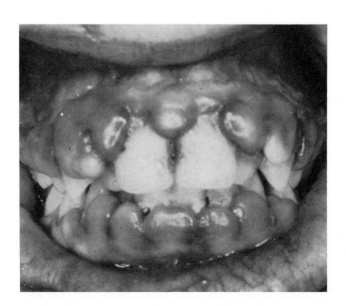

Figure 8–28 Conditioned Gingival Enlargement in puberty in a 13-year-old male.

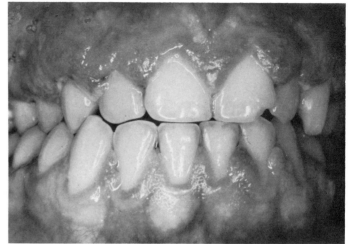

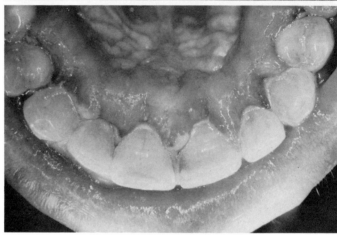

Figure 8–29 Leukemic Gingival Enlargement. *Top,* Leukemic gingival enlargement in a patient with acute myelocytic leukemia. Note that the enlargement is more prominent in the maxilla associated with greater local irritation. *Bottom,* Lingual view of gingival enlargement in a patient with subacute monocytic leukemia, showing bulbous increase in size with discoloration and smooth shiny surface. Note the difference between the enlarged gingiva and the adjacent palatal mucosa.

tion. Acute painful necrotizing ulcerative inflammatory involvement frequently occurs in the crevice formed at the junction of the enlarged gingiva and the contiguous tooth surfaces.

Histopathology

The connective tissue is infiltrated with a dense mass of immature and proliferating leukocytes, the specific nature of which varies with the type of leukemia. Mature leukocytes associated with chronic inflammation are also seen. The capillaries are engorged; the connective tissue is for the most part edematous and degenerated. The epithelium presents varying degrees of leukocytic infiltration with edema. Isolated surface areas of acute necrotizing inflammation with a pseudomembranous meshwork of fibrin, necrotic epithelial cells, polymorphonuclear leukocytes and bacteria are frequently seen.

Enlargement Associated with Vitamin C Deficiency

√Enlargement of the gingiva is generally included in classic descriptions of scurvy. It is important to recognize that such enlargement is essentially a conditioned response to local irritation. Acute vitamin C deficiency does not of itself cause gingival inflammation,[25] but it does cause hemorrhage, collagen degeneration and edema of the gingival connective tissue. These changes modify the response of the gingiva to local irritation to the extent that the normal defensive delimiting reaction is inhibited and the extension of the inflammation exaggerated.[26] The combined effect of acute

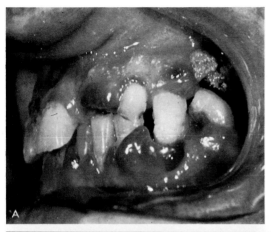

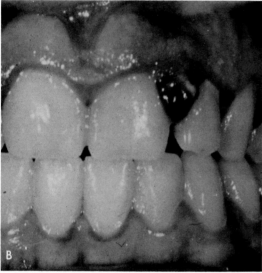

Figure 8–30 A, **Conditioned Gingival Enlargement** in vitamin C deficiency. Note the prominent hemorrhagic areas. B, **Pyogenic granuloma** in a young adult female.

vitamin C deficiency and inflammation produces the massive gingival enlargement in scurvy (Fig. 8–30, A).

Clinical features

Gingival enlargement in vitamin C deficiency is marginal; the gingiva is bluish red, soft and friable, and has a smooth shiny surface. Hemorrhage, either spontaneous or upon slight provocation, and surface necrosis with pseudomembrane formation are common features.

Histopathology

The gingiva presents a chronic inflammatory cellular infiltration with a superficial acute response. There are scattered areas of hemorrhage with engorged capillaries. Marked diffuse edema, collagen degeneration and scarcity of collagen fibrils or fibroblasts are striking findings.

Nonspecific Conditioned Enlargement (Granuloma Pyogenicum)

Granuloma pyogenicum is a tumor-like gingival enlargement considered to be an exaggerated conditioned response to minor trauma (Fig. 8–30, B). The exact nature of the systemic conditioning factor has not been identified.[43]

Clinical features

The lesion varies from that of a discrete spherical tumor-like mass with a pedunculated attachment to a flattened keloid-like enlargement with a broad base. It is bright red or purple, and either friable or firm, depending upon its duration; in the majority of cases it presents surface ulceration and purulent exudation. The lesion tends to involute spontaneously to become a fibroepithelial papilloma, or persists relatively unchanged for years. Treatment consists of removal of the lesions plus the elimination of irritating local factors. The recurrence rate is about 15 per cent.[13] Granuloma pyogenicum is similar in clinical and microscopic appearance to the conditioned gingival enlargement seen in pregnancy.[44] Differential diagnosis depends upon the patient's histoy.

Histopathology

Granuloma pyogenicum appears as a mass of granulation tissue with chronic inflammatory cellular infiltration. Endothelial proliferation and the formation of numerous vascular spaces are the prominent features. The surface epithelium is atrophic in some areas and hyperplastic in others. Surface ulceration and exudation are common features.

V. NEOPLASTIC ENLARGEMENT (GINGIVAL TUMORS)

Benign Tumors of the Gingiva

Epulis is a generic term used clinically to designate all tumors of the gingiva. It serves to locate the tumor, but not to describe it. (Most lesions referred to as epulis are inflammatory rather than neoplastic.) Neoplasms account for a comparatively small proportion of the gingival enlargements, and comprise a small percentage of the total number of oral neoplasms. In a survey of 257 oral tumors,[48] approximately 8 per cent occurred on the gingiva. In another study of 868 growths of the gingiva[9] and palate of which 57 per cent were neoplastic and the remainder inflammatory, the following incidence of tumors was noted: carcinoma, 11.0 per cent; fibroma, 9.3 per cent; giant cell tumor, 8.4 per cent; papilloma, 7.3 per cent; leukoplakia, 4.9 per cent; mixed tumor (salivary gland type), 2.5 per cent; angioma, 1.5 per cent; osteofibroma, 1.3 per cent; sarcoma, 0.5 per cent; melanoma, 0.5 per cent; myxoma, 0.45 per cent; lipoma, 0.3 per cent; fibropapilloma, 0.4 per cent; and adenoma, 0.4 per cent.

FIBROMA

Fibromas of the gingiva arise from the gingival connective tissue or from the periodontal ligament. They are slowly growing, spherical tumors that tend to be firm and nodular but may be soft and vascular. Fibromas are usually pedunculated.

Histopathology

The hard fibroma is composed of densely arranged bundles of well-formed collagen fibers with a scattering of flattened elliptical fibrocytes. It is a relatively avascular tumor. In the soft fibroma, fibroblasts are comparatively more numerous and stellate in shape. Collagen is present but is less densely arranged. Varying degrees of vascularity are also seen. Bone formation within the fibromas is a frequent finding. The bone appears as irregularly arranged trabeculae with osteoblasts and osteoid along the margins. Lipofibroma[47] and myxofibroma[10] of the gingiva and alveolar mucosa have also been described.

NEVUS

The nevus may be pigmented or nonpigmented. It occurs commonly on the skin, but a few cases of gingival nevus have been reported. The lesion is benign and slow growing, varying in color from pale gray to dark brown. It may be flat or raised slightly above the gingival surface, sessile or nodular.[11]

Histopathology

The tumor presents discrete clumps of nevus cells in the submucosa directly beneath the basal cell layer of epithelium and separated from it by connective tissue. The cells may contain melanin or may be pigment-free. In either instance, the nevus cells are demonstrable when stained with dihydroxyphenylalanine (DOPA).

MYOBLASTOMA

Myoblastoma is a benign lesion that is nodular and slightly raised beyond the gingival surface.[30, 42]

Histopathology

It appears as a mass of polyhedral or spindle-shaped cells with prominent acidophilic granular cytoplasm. There is a marked pseudo-epitheliomatous hyperplasia of the covering epithelium. Congenital myoblastoma is sometimes referred to as congenital epulis.

HEMANGIOMA

These are benign blood vessel tumors occasionally seen on the gingiva. They occur as a *capillary* or *cavernous* type, more commonly the former. These tumors are soft, sessile or pedunculated, and painless. They may be smooth or irregularly bulbous in outline. The color varies from deep red to purple, and blanches on the application of pressure. These lesions often appear to arise from the interdental gingival papilla and spread laterally to involve the adjacent teeth.[8] A flat, irregularly outlined, diffuse *congenital form of hemangioma* is also seen, either with or without comparable involvement of the face. Hematomas sometimes occur on the gingiva as the result of trauma (Fig. 8–31).

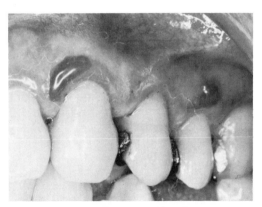

Figure 8–31 **Hematomas** produced by trauma.

PAPILLOMA

Papilloma of the gingiva appears as a hard, wart-like protuberance from the gingival surface (Fig. 8–32). The lesion may be small and discrete, or may appear as broad, hard elevations of the gingiva with minutely irregular surfaces.

Histopathology

The lesion presents a central core of connective tissue with a marked proliferation and hyperkeratosis of the epithelium.

PERIPHERAL GIANT CELL REPARATIVE GRANULOMA

Giant cell lesions of the gingiva arise interdentally or from the gingival margin, occur more frequently on the labial surface, and may be sessile or pedunculated. They vary in appearance from a smooth, regularly outlined mass to an irregularly shaped, multilobulated protuberance with surface indentations (Fig. 8–33). Ulceration of the margin is occasionally seen. The lesions are painless, vary in size, and may cover several teeth. They may be firm or spongy, and the color varies from pink to deep red or purplish blue. There are no pathognomonic clinical features whereby these lesions can be differentiated from other forms of gingival enlargement. Microscopic examination is required for definitive diagnosis (Figs. 8–34 to 8–37).

In the past, giant cell lesions of the gingiva have been referred to as *giant cell epulis* or *peripheral giant cell tumor*. Most often, however, these gingival lesions are essentially responses to local injury and not neoplasms. When they occur on the gingiva they should be referred to as *peripheral giant cell reparative granulomas*[55, 58] to differentiate them from comparable lesions that originate within the jaw bone (central reparative giant cell granuloma).[40]

In some instances, the giant cell reparative granuloma of the gingiva is locally invasive and causes destruction of the underlying bone (Fig. 8–38). Complete removal leads to uneventful recovery.

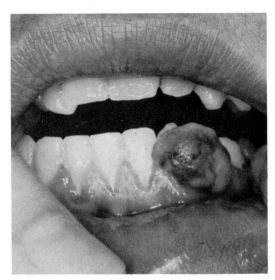

Figure 8–33 **Peripheral Giant Cell Reparative Granuloma.** Comparison of this lesion with the one shown in Figure 8–36 indicates the importance of biopsy for definitive diagnosis.

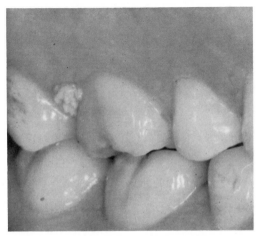

Figure 8–32 **Papilloma** of the gingiva appears as a hard wart-like mass. (Courtesy of Dr. Neal Chilton.)

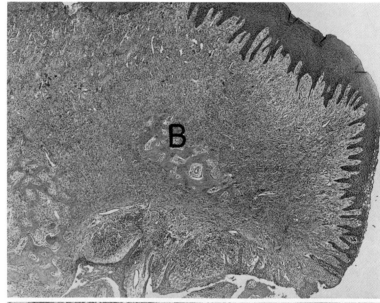

Figure 8–34 Microscopic survey of lesion shown in Figure 8–33. Trabeculae of newly formed bone (B) are contained within the mass.

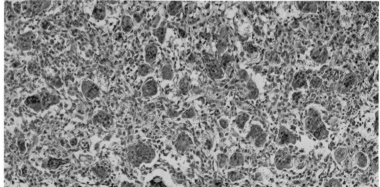

Figure 8–35 High power study of the above lesion demonstrating the giant cells and intervening stroma which comprise the major portion of the mass.

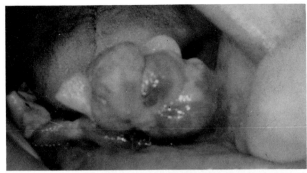

Figure 8–36 Localized gingival enlargement. Microscopic examination reveals it to be a chronic inflammatory lesion. (Compare with Figure 8–33.)

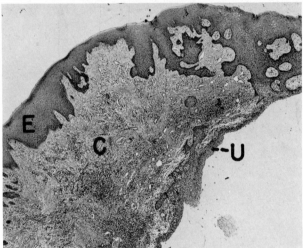

Figure 8–37 Survey section of lesion shown in Figure 8–36. The lesion consists of connective tissue (C) surrounded by stratified squamous epithelium (E). The connective tissue presented marked chronic inflammatory involvement. The surface of the lesion that was in apposition with the teeth is ulcerated (U).

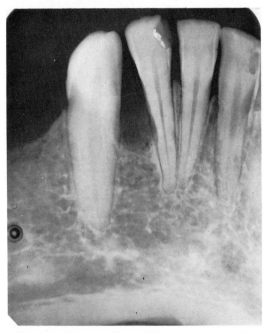

Figure 8–38 Bone Destruction in the interproximal space between the canine and lateral caused by the extension of a peripheral giant cell reparative granuloma of the gingiva. (Courtesy of Dr. Sam Toll.)

Histopathology

The giant cell reparative granuloma presents numerous foci of multinuclear giant cells and hemosiderin particles in a connective tissue stroma. Areas of chronic inflammation are scattered throughout the lesion with acute involvement at the surface. The overlying epithelium is usually hyperplastic with ulceration at the base. Bone formation occasionally occurs within the lesion.

CENTRAL GIANT CELL REPARATIVE GRANULOMA

These lesions arise within the jaws and produce central cavitation. They occasionally create deformity of the jaw such that the gingiva appears enlarged (Fig. 8–39).

Mixed tumors, salivary gland type tumors, eosinophilic granulomas[70] and *plasmacytomas* of the gingiva have also been described but are not often seen.

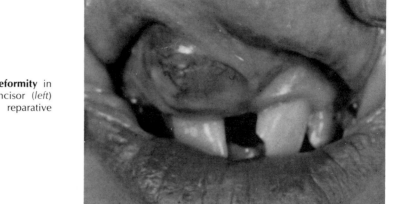

Figure 8–39 Localized Bone Deformity in relation to the maxillary central incisor (*left*) produced by a central giant cell reparative granuloma.

PLASMA CELL GRANULOMA

This is a benign lesion of the marginal interdental or attached gingiva;[14] it usually occurs as a localized mass but may be generalized. It is red, friable, sometimes granular, bleeds easily and is accompanied by focal distribution of adjacent bone. **Microscopically it appears as a dense almost exclusively plasma cell accumulation in solid sheets or a lobular pattern.** Elimination of local irritants by scaling usually suffices as treatment, but surgical removal may be necessary.

LEUKOPLAKIA

Leukoplakia of the gingiva varies in appearance from that of a grayish white flattened scaly lesion to a thick, irregularly shaped, keratinous plaque (Fig. 8–40).

Histopathology

It presents thickening of the epithelium with hyperkeratosis, acanthosis and some degree of dyskeratosis. Inflammatory involvement of the underlying connective tissue is a commonly associated finding. Leukoplakia is caused by chronic irritation. Its capacity for malignant transformation must be borne in mind.

GINGIVAL CYST

Gingival cysts of microscopic proportions are common in the gingiva but they seldom reach a clinically significant size.[49]

When they do, they appear as localized enlargements that may involve the marginal and attached gingiva.[56] They occur in the mandibular canine and premolar areas, most often on the lingual surface. They are painless but with expansion may cause erosion of the surface of the alveolar bone. The cysts develop from odontogenic epithelium or from surface or sulcal epithelium traumatically implanted in the area. Removal is followed by uneventful recovery.

Microscopically they present a cyst cavity lined by stratified squamous epithelium. Small daughter cysts lined with columnar or squamous epithelium may be located in the cyst wall.

Mucus-secreting cysts (mucocele)[35] and *mucous cell metaplasia*[74] have been described as rare findings in the gingiva.

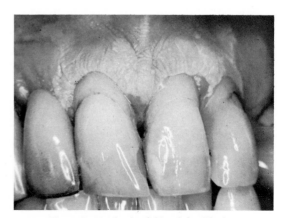

Figure 8–40 Leukoplakia of the Gingiva.

Malignant Tumors of the Gingiva

CARCINOMA

The gingiva is not a common site of oral malignancy. *Squamous cell carcinoma is the most common malignant tumor of the gingiva.* Only 1.9[24] to 5.4 per cent[1] of oral carcinomas occur on the gingiva, with the mandible, usually the molar area, being the most common site. There is often an associated leukoplakia. In patients with multiple primary oral carcinomas, 25 per cent of the tumors were present on the gingiva.[64]

Carcinomas may be *exophytic* or *verrucous*, both of which are outgrowths from the gingival surface, or *ulcerative*, which appear as flat erosive lesions. They are locally invasive, involving the underlying bone and adjacent mucosa. Often symptom-free, they are frequently unnoticed until complicated by painful inflammation. The inflammatory changes may mask the neoplasm. Metastasis is usually confined to the region above the clavicle; however, more extensive involvement may include the lung, liver or bone. A five-year survival rate of 24 per cent has been reported for gingival carcinomas.[65]

MALIGNANT MELANOMA

Malignant melanoma is a rare oral tumor that tends to occur in the gingiva of the anterior maxilla.[7] The malignant melanoma is usually darkly pigmented and is often preceded by the occurrence of localized pigmentation.[18] It may be flat or nodular and is characerized by rapid growth and early metastasis. It arises from melanoblasts in the gingiva, cheek or palate. An unpigmented malignant melanoma of the gingiva has been reported.[45] Infiltration into the underlying bone and metastasis to cervical and axillary lymph nodes are common.

Histopathology

The maglignant melanoma shows some resemblance to the benign nevus; however, the malignant cells vary in morphology. The distribution is irregular and invasive, lacking the clear-cut grouping of benign lesions, and in some areas they are continuous with the surface epithelium. The connective tissue stroma is more often delicate and relatively scarce.

SARCOMA

Fibrosarcoma, lymphosarcoma and *reticulum cell sarcoma* of the gingiva are rare; only isolated cases have been described in the literature.[19, 29, 53] Thoma et al.[71] have described a case of *malignant lymphoma* of the gingiva in a 19 year old female. The lesion was first noticed in an alveolar socket that failed to heal after extraction. The lesion appeared as a persistent raspberry-like protuberance from the surface of the socket associated with suppuration, superficial ulceration and progressive necrosis of the gingiva and underlying bone. Subsequent lesions occurred in other areas of the gingiva followed by denudation of the root surfaces and tooth loss (Figs. 8–41 and 8–42).

METASTASIS

Tumor metastasis to the gingiva is not common. Hardman[32] describes two gingival tumors that metastasized from a *primary chondrosarcoma in the femur.* The gingival tumors resembled fibromas in appearance, and presented secondary inflammatory involvement associated with local irritation. Microscopically, the tumors of the gingiva consisted of a vascular loose network of spindle cells consistent with a diagnosis of *spindle cell sarcoma.* Among other reported cases of metastasis to the gingiva are *adenocarcinoma from the colon,*[38] *carcinoma from the lung,*[76] *chondromyxosarcoma from the axilla,*[57] and *hypernephroma.*[54, 68]

One must not be misled by the low incidence of malignancy of the gingiva. Ulcerations that do not respond to therapy in the usual manner and all gingival tumors and tumor-like lesions must be biopsied (Chap. 33) and submitted for microscopic diagnosis.

VI. DEVELOPMENTAL GINGIVAL ENLARGEMENT

Clinical features

This type of enlargement appears as a bulbous distortion of the labial and marginal contours of the gingiva of teeth in various stages of eruption. It is caused by

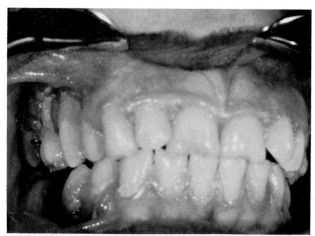

Figure 8–41 Malignant Lymphoma of the Gingiva in a Young Female. The tumor appears as bead-like masses of granulation tissue in the maxillary molar area (*left*).

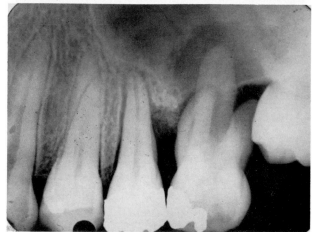

Figure 8–42 Radiograph of patient with malignant lymphoma shown in Figure 8–41. There is extensive loss of bone in relation to the molar and premolar as a result of progressive invasion of the tumor. Note the thickening of the periodontal space around the premolar.

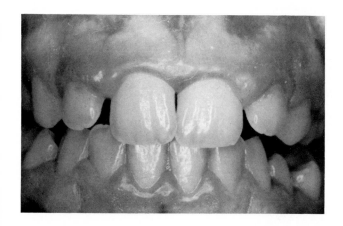

Figure 8–43 Developmental Gingival Enlargement. The normal bulbous contour of the gingiva around the incompletely erupted anterior teeth is accentuated by chronic inflammation.

superimposition of the bulk of the gingiva upon the normal prominence of the enamel in the gingival half of the crown. The enlargement often persists until the epithelial attachment has migrated from the enamel to the cemento-enamel junction.

In a strict sense, developmental gingival enlargement is physiologic and ordinarily presents no problem. However, when it is complicated by marginal inflammation, the composite picture gives the impression of extensive gingival enlargement (Fig. 8–43). Treatment to alleviate the marginal inflammation rather than resection of the "enlargement" is sufficient in these cases.

Histopathology

When uncomplicated by inflammation, developmental enlargement presents no notable pathologic changes. A zone of chronic inflammation at the gingival margin is, however, a common finding.

CHANGES IN GINGIVAL CONTOUR

Changes in gingival contour are for the most part associated with gingival enlargement, but changes in gingival contour may occur in other conditions.

Stillman's clefts

Stillman's clefts are apostrophe-shaped indentations extending from and into the gingival margin for varying distances. The clefts generally occur on the facial surface (Fig. 8–44). One or two may be present in relation to a single tooth. The margins of the clefts are rolled underneath the linear gap in the gingiva and the remainder of the gingival margin is blunt instead of knife-edge. Originally described by Stillman[69] and considered to be the result of occlusal trauma, these clefts were subsequently described by Box[15] as pathologic pockets in which the ulcerative process had extended through to the facial surface of the gingiva. The clefts may repair spontaneously or persist as surface lesions of deep periodontal pockets that penetrate into the supporting tissues. Their association with trauma from occlusion has not been substantiated.

The clefts are divided into: *simple;* cleavage in a single direction (most common), and *compound;* cleavage in more than one direction (Tishler[72]). The length of

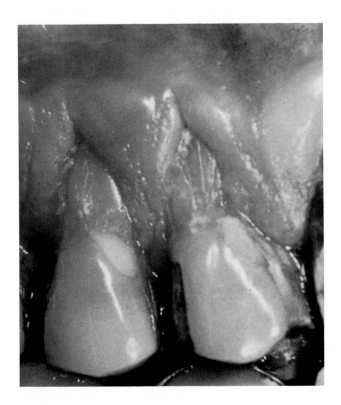

Figure 8–44 "Stillman's Clefts" in the gingiva.

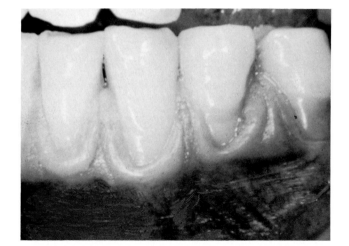

Figure 8–45 "McCall's Festoons" showing characteristic rim-like enlargement of the gingival margin.

the clefts varies from a slight break in the gingival margin to a depth of 5 to 6 mm. or more.

McCall's festoons

McCall's festoons are lifesaver-shaped enlargements of the marginal gingiva that occur most frequently in the canine and premolar areas on the facial surface. In the early stages, the color and consistency of the gingiva are normal. Accumulation of food debris leads to secondary inflammatory changes (Fig. 8–45). Trauma from occlusion and mechanical stimulation are suggested etiologic factors.[23] However, festoons occur on teeth without occlusal antagonists.

REFERENCES

1. Ackerman, L. V., and del Regato, J. A.: Cancer: Diagnosis, Treatment, and Prognosis. St. Louis, C. V. Mosby Co., 1947.
2. Aiguer, J.: Localized Hypertrophic Gingivitis Due To Tongue Habit. J. Periodont., 9:59, 1938.
3. Babcock, J. R.: Incidence of Gingival Hyperplasia Associated with Dilantin Therapy in a Hospital Population. J.A.D.A., 71:1447, 1965.
4. Babcock, J. R., and Nelson, G. H.: Gingival Hyperplasia and Dilantin Content of Saliva. J.A.D.A., 68:195, 1964.
5. Ball, E. I.: Case of Gingivomatosis or Elephantiasis of the Gingiva. J. Periodont., 12:96, 1941.
6. Baratieri, A.: The Oxytalan Connective Tissue Fibers in Gingival Hyperplasia in Patients Treated with Sodium Diphenylhydantoin. J. Periodont. Res., 2:106, 1967.
7. Baxter, H. A., Brown, J. B., and Byars, L. T.: Malignant Melanomas. Am. J. Orth. & Oral Surg., 27:90, 1941.
8. Bellinger, D. H.: Blood and Lymph Vessel Tumors Involving the Mouth. J. Oral Surg., 2:141, 1944.
9. Bernick, S.: Growth of the Gingiva and Palate. II. Connective Tissue Tumors. Oral Surg., Oral Path. & Oral Med., 1:1098, 1948.
10. Bernier, J. L., and Ash, J. E.: Atlas of Dental and Oral Pathology. Washington, D. C., Registry Press, 1948.
11. Bernier, J. L., and Tiecke, R. W.: Nevus of the Gingiva. J. Oral Surg., 8:165, 1950.
12. Bhaskar, S. N., Bernier, J. L., and Godby, F.: Aneurysmal Bone Cyst and Other Giant Cell Lesions of the Jaws. Report of 104 Cases. J. Oral Surg., 17:30, 1959.
13. Bhaskar, S. N., and Jacoway, J. R.: Pyogenic Granuloma—Clinical Features, Incidence, Histology and Result of Treatment. J. Oral Surg., 24:391, 1966.
14. Bhaskar, S. N., Levin, M. P., and Frisch, J.: Plasma Cell Granuloma of Periodontal Tissues. Report of 45 Cases. Periodontics, 6:272, 1968.
15. Box, H. K.: Gingival Clefts and Associated Tracts. New York State D. J., 16:3, 1950.
16. Buckner, H. J.: Diffuse Fibroma of the Gums. J.A.D.A., 24:2003, 1937.
17. Burket, L. W.: Oral Medicine. Philadelphia, J. B. Lippincott Co., 1946, p. 295.
18. Chaudry, A. P., Hampel, A., and Gorlin, R. J.: Primary Malignant Melanoma of the Oral Cavity: A Review of 105 Cases. Cancer, 11:923, 1958.
19. Cook, H. P.: Oral Lymphomas. Oral Surg., Oral Med. & Oral Path., 14:690, 1961.
20. Dallas, B. M.: Hyperplasia of the Oral Mucosa in an Edentulous Epileptic. New Zealand D. J., 59:54, 1963.
21. Elzay, R. P., and Swenson, H. M.: Effect of an Electric Toothbrush on Dilantin Sodium Induced Gingival Hyperplasia. New York J. Den., 34:13, 1964.
22. Emerson, T. G.: Hereditary Gingival Hyperplasia. A Family Pedigree of Four Generations. Oral Surg., Oral Med. & Oral Path., 19:1, 1965.
23. Fuchs, M., and Kurnatowski, A.: Klinische und mikroskopische Untersuchungen der McCall-Girlander. Deutsche Zahnärtz., 17:1125, 1962.
24. Gardner, A. F., Schwartz, F. L., and Pallen, H. S.: Carcinoma of the Oral Regions. Ann. Den., 21:80, 1962.
25. Glickman, I.: The Periodontal Tissues of the

Guinea Pig in Vitamin C Deficiency. J. D. Res., 27:9, 1948.

26. Glickman, I.: The Effect of Acute Vitamin C Deficiency upon the Response of the Periodontal Tissues of the Guinea Pig to Artificially Induced Inflammation. J. D. Res., 27:201, 1948.

27. Glickman, I.: A Basic Classification of Gingival Enlargement. J. Periodont., 21:131, 1950.

28. Glickman, I., and Lewitus, M.: Hyperplasia of the Gingiva Associated with Dilantin (Sodium Diphenyl Hydantoinate) Therapy. J.A.D.A., 28:199, 1941.

29. Goldman, H. M.: Sarcoma. Am. J. Orth. & Oral Surg., 30:311, 1944.

30. Hagen, J. D., Soule, E. H., and Gores, R. J.: Granular-Cell Myoblastoma of the Oral Cavity. Oral Surg., Oral Med. & Oral Path., 14:454, 1961.

31. Hall, W. B.: Dilantin Hyperplasia: A Preventable Lesion. J. Periodont. Res., 4, Suppl. 4:36, 1969.

32. Hardman, F. G.: Secondary Sarcoma Presenting Clinical Appearance of Fibrous Epulis. Brit. D. J., 86:109, 1949.

33. Henefer, E. P., and Kay, L. A.: Congenital Idiopathic Gingival Fibromatosis in the Deciduous Dentition. Oral Surg., 24:65, 1967.

34. Hirschfeld, I.: Hypertrophic Gingivitis — Its Clinical Aspects, J.A.D.A., 19:799, 1932.

35. Hodson, J. J.: Mucous Cell Metaplasia in Human Gingival Epithelium and Its Relation to Certain Mucous Secreting Tumors. Arch. Oral Biol., 5:174, 1961.

36. Hoess, T.: The Effect of 5,5-Diphenylhydantoin (Dilantin) on Fibroblast-like Cells in Culture. J. Periodont. Res., 4:163, 1969.

37. Hugoson, A.: Gingival Inflammation and Female Sex Hormones. J. Periodont. Res., Suppl. 5, 1970.

38. Humphrey, A. A., and Amos, N. H.: Metastatic Gingival Adenocarcinoma from Primary Lesion of Colon. Am. J. Cancer, 28:128, 1936.

39. Ishikawa, J., and Glickman, I.: Gingival Response to the Systemic Administration of Sodium Diphenyl Hydantoinate (Dilantin) in Cats. J. Periodont., 32:149, 1961.

40. Jaffe, H. L.: Giant Cell Reparative Granuloma, Traumatic Bone Cyst, and Fibrous (Fibro-osseous) Dysplasia of the Jaw Bones. Oral Surg., Oral Med. & Oral Path., 6:159, 1953.

41. Kerageorgis, B. P.: Elephantiasis of the Gingivae (Elephantiasis des Gengives). Rev. Chir., Par, 68:308, 1949. Abst. Surg. Gynec. & Obst., 90:461, 1950 (abs).

42. Kerr, D. A.: Myoblastic Myoma. Oral Med., Oral Surg. & Oral Path., 2:41, 1949.

43. Kerr, D. A.: Granuloma Pyogenicum. Oral Surg., Oral Med. & Oral Path., 4:158, 1951.

44. Lee, K. W.: The Fibrous Epulis and Related Lesions. Granuloma Pyogenicum, "Pregnancy Tumor;" Fibro-epithelial Polyp and Calcifying Fibroblastic Granuloma. A Clinico-pathological Study. Periodontics, 6:277, 1968.

45. Loscalzo, L. J.: Unpigmented Melanocarcinoma of the Gingivae. Report of a Case. Oral Surg., Oral Med. & Oral Path., 11:646, 1958.

46. Maier, A. W., and Orban, B.: Gingivitis in Pregnancy. Oral Surg., Oral Med. & Oral Path., 2:334, 1949.

47. Marfino, N. R.: Developing Fibrolipoma of the Free Gingiva. Oral Surg., Oral Med. & Oral Path., 12:489, 1959.

48. McCarthy, F. P.: A Clinical & Pathological Study of Oral Disease. J.A.M.A., 116:16, 1941.

49. Moskow, B. S.: The Pathogenesis of the Gingival Cyst. Periodontics, 4:23, 1966.

50. Nease, W. J.: Effect of Sodium Diphenylhydantoinate on Tissue Cultures of Human Gingiva. J. Periodont., 36:22, 1965.

51. Newby, C. D.: A Report on a Case of Hypertrophied Gum Tissue, J. Canad. D. Assn., 6:183, 1940.

52. Panuska, H. J., Gorlin, R. J., Bearman, J. E., and Mitchell, D. F.: The Effect of Anticonvulsant Drugs Upon the Gingiva. A Series of 1048 Patients. II. J. Periodont., 32:15, 1961.

53. Partsch, C.: Atlas der Zahnheilkunde in Stenokopischen Bilde. Berlin, Julius Springer, 1912.

54. Persson, P. A., and Wallenino, K.: Metastatic Renal Carcinoma (Hypernephroma) in the Gingiva of the Lower Jaw. Acta Odont. Scandinav., 19:289, 1961.

55. Phillips, R. L., and Shafer, W. G.: An Evaluation of the Peripheral Giant Cell Tumor. J. Periodont., 26:216, 1955.

56. Rickles, N. H., and Everett, F. G.: Gingival and Lateral Periodontal Cysts. Parodontol., 14:41, 1960.

57. Robinson, H. B. G.: A Clinic on the Differential Diagnosis of Oral Lesions. Am. J. Orthodont. & Oral Surg., 32:720, 1946.

58. Rushton, M. A.: Hereditary or Idiopathic Hyperplasia of the Gums. D. Practit., 7:136, 1957.

59. Shafer, W. G.: Effect of Dilantin Sodium Analogues on Cell Proliferation in Tissue Culture. Proc. Soc. Exp. Biol. & Med., 106:205, 1960.

60. Shafer, W. G.: Effect of Dilantin Sodium on Various Cell Lines in Tissue Culture. Proc. Soc. Exp. Biol. & Med., 108:694, 1961.

61. Shafer, W. G.: Response of Radiated Human Gingival Fibroblast-like Cells to Dilantin Sodium in Tissue Culture. J. D. Res., 44:671, 1965.

62. Shafer, W. G., Beatty, R. E., and Davis, W. B.: Effect of Dilantin Sodium on Tensile Strength of Healing Wounds. Proc. Soc. Exp. Biol. & Med., 98:348, 1958.

63. Shapiro, M.: Acceleration of Gingival Wound Healing in Non-Epileptic Patients Receiving Diphenylhydantoin Sodium. Exp. Med. & Surg., 16:41, 1958.

64. Sharp, G. S., Bullock, W. K., and Helsper, J. T.: Multiple Oral Carcinomas. Cancer, 14:512, 1961.

65. Sharp, G. S.: Carcinoma of the Gingivae. J. Tenn. S. D. Assn., 29:236, 1959.

66. Smith, L. W., and Gault, E. S.: Essentials of Pathology. 3rd ed. New York, Appleton Century Co., 1948, p. 1925.

67. Soni, N. N., et al.: Mitotic Activity in Human Gingival Epithelium Associated with Dilantin Sodium Therapy. Periodontics, 5:70, 1967.

68. Stein, G.: Hypernephrommetastase als Epulis. Deutsche Ztschr. f. Chir., 219:318, 1929.

69. Stillman, P. R.: Early Clinical Evidences of Disease in the Gingiva and Pericementum. J. D. Res., 3:XXV, 1921.

70. Taddei, G.: Gingival Eosinophilic Granuloma. Arch. Ital. Mal. App. Diger., 19:280, 1953.

71. Thoma, K. H., Holland, D. J., Woodbury, H. W.,

Burrow, J. G., and Sleeper, E. I.: Malignant Lymphoma of the Gingiva. Oral Surg., Oral Med. & Oral Path., *1*:57, 1948.

72. Tishler, B.: Gingival Clefts and Their Significance. D. Cosmos, *49*:1003, 1927.

73. Tollaro, I.: Clinical Statistical Contribution on Gingival Hyperplasia Caused by Anticonvulsants. Riv. Ital. Stomat., *23*:1519, 1968.

74. Traeger, K. A.: Cyst of the Gingiva (Mucocele). Report of a Case. Oral Surg., Oral Med. & Oral Path., *14*:243, 1961.

75. Westphal, P.: Salivary Secretion and Gingival Hyperplasia in Diphenylhydantoin-Treated Guinea Pigs. Svensk. Tandläkane-Tidsskrift, *62*:505, 1969.

76. Willis, R. A.: Pathology of Tumors. St. Louis, C. V. Mosby Co., 1948, p. 376.

77. Zackin, S. J., and Weisberger, D.: Hereditary Gingival Fibromatosis. Oral Surg., Oral Med. & Oral Path., *14*:828, 1961.

78. Ziskin, D. E., Blackberg, S. M., and Stout, A. P.: The Gingivae During Pregnancy. Surg., Gynecol. & Obst., *57*:719, 1933.

79. Ziskin, D. E., and Zegarelli, E.: Idiopathic Fibromatosis of the Gingivae. Ann. Dent., *2*:50, 1943.

Chapter 9

CHANGES IN THE CONSISTENCY, SURFACE TEXTURE AND POSITION OF THE GINGIVA (RECESSION OR GINGIVAL ATROPHY)

CHANGES IN CONSISTENCY

✓Both chronic and acute inflammation produce changes in the normal firm resilient consistency of the gingiva. As noted earlier (page 82), chronic gingivitis is a conflict between destructive and reparative changes, with the consistency of the gingiva determined by the relative balance between the two (Figs. 9–1 and 9–2). Of the

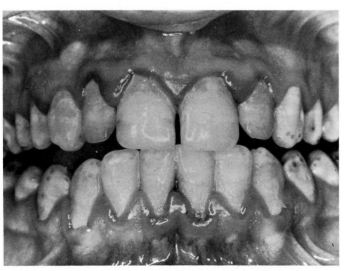

Figure 9–1 Chronic Gingivitis, showing swelling and discoloration produced when inflammatory exudate and tissue degeneration are the predominant microscopic changes. The gingiva is soft, friable and bleeds easily. Note the mottled teeth.

116

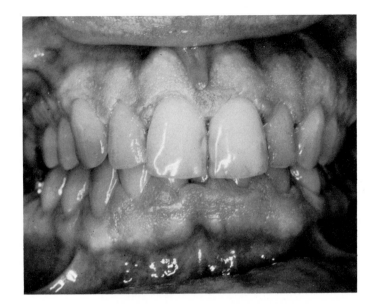

Figure 9–2 Chronic Gingivitis, showing firm gingiva with minutely nodular surface produced when fibrosis predominates in the inflammatory process.

most common types of acute inflammation, acute necrotizing ulcerative gingivitis is primarily a destructive process and acute herpetic gingivostomatis is characterized by vesicle formation. *The clinical alterations in consistency of the gingiva and the microscopic changes which produce them are summarized in Table 9–1.*

CALCIFIED MASSES IN THE GINGIVA

Calcified microscopic masses are frequently seen in the gingiva.[1] They occur singly or in groups, and vary in size, location, shape and structure. Such masses may be calcified material removed from the tooth and traumatically displaced into the gingiva

TABLE 9–1 CLINICAL AND HISTOPATHOLOGIC CHANGES IN GINGIVAL CONSISTENCY

Chronic Gingivitis

Clinical Changes	Underlying Microscopic Features
1. Soggy puffiness that pits on pressure	1. Infiltration by fluid and cells of the inflammatory exudate
2. Marked softness and friability, with ready fragmentation upon exploration with a probe and pinpoint surface areas of redness and desquamation	2. Degeneration of connective tissue and epithelium associated with injurious substances which provoke the inflammation and the inflammatory exudate. Change in the connective tissue–epithelium relationship, with the inflamed, engorged connective tissue expanding to within a few epithelial cells of the surface. Thinning of the epithelium and degeneration associated with edema and leukocytic invasion, separated by areas in which the rete pegs are elongated into the connective tissue
3. Firm, leathery consistency	3. Fibrosis and epithelial proliferation associated with long-standing chronic inflammation

Acute Gingivitis

Clinical Changes	Underlying Microscopic Features
1. Diffuse puffiness and softening	1. Diffuse edema of acute inflammatory origin; fatty infiltration in xanthomatosis
2. Sloughing with grayish flake-like particles of debris adhering to the eroded surface	2. Necrosis with the formation of a pseudomembrane composed of bacteria, polymorphonuclear leukocytes and degenerated epithelial cells in a fibrinous meshwork
3. Vesicle formation	3. Inter- and intracellular edema with degeneration of the nucleus and cytoplasm and rupture of the cell wall

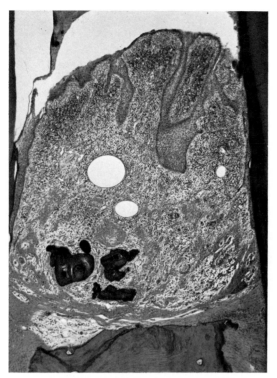

Figure 9–3 **Cementicles** in the gingiva.

during scaling,[6] root remnants, cementum fragments or cementicles (Fig. 9–3). Chronic inflammation and fibrosis and occasionally foreign body giant cell activity occur in relation to these masses. They are sometimes enclosed in an osteoid-like matrix. Crystalline foreign bodies have also been described in the gingiva, but their origin has not been determined.[9]

CHANGES IN SURFACE TEXTURE

Loss of surface stippling is an early sign of gingivitis. In chronic inflammation the surface is either smooth and shiny, or firm and nodular, **depending upon whether the dominant changes are exudative or fibrotic.** Smooth surface texture is also produced by epithelial atrophy in *senile atrophic gingivitis,* and peeling of the surface occurs in *chronic desquamative gingivitis. Hyperkeratosis* results in a leathery texture, and noninflammatory gingival hyperplasia produces a minutely nodular surface.

CHANGE IN POSITION (RECESSION, GINGIVAL ATROPHY)

The "Actual" and "Apparent" Positions of the Gingiva

Recession is *progressive exposure of the root surface by an apical shift in the position of the gingiva.* To understand what is meant by recession one must distinguish between the "actual" and "apparent" positions of the gingiva. The *actual position* is the level of the epithelial attachment on the tooth (Fig. 9–4); whereas the *apparent position* is the level of the crest of the gingival margin. **It is the actual position of the gingiva not the apparent position, which determines the severity of recession. There are two types of recession: visible, which is clinically observable; and hidden, which is covered by gingiva and can only be measured by inserting a probe to the level of epithelial attachment** (Fig. 9–4). For example, in periodontal disease part of the denuded root is covered by the inflamed pocket wall; some of the recession is hidden, and some is visible (Fig. 9–4). The total amount of recession is the sum of the two.

Recession refers to the location of the gingiva, not its condition. Receded gingiva is often inflamed (Figs. 9–5 and 9–6) but

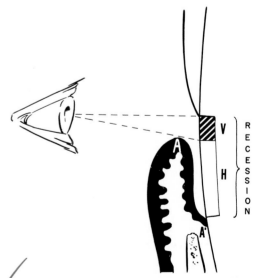

Figure 9–4 Diagram illustrating **Apparent Position of the Gingiva (A), Actual position of the Gingiva (A′), Visible Recession (V), and Hidden Recession (H).**

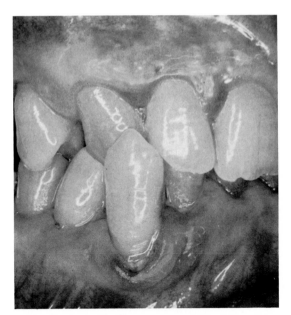

Figure 9–5   Recession on Prominent Canine. Note the severe inflammatory reaction to local irritation.

may be normal except for its position (Fig. 9–7). Recession may be localized to a tooth (Fig. 9–8) or group of teeth, or generalized throughout the mouth (Fig. 9–9).

Etiology

Recession may occur physiologically with age (*physiologic recession*) or under abnormal conditions (*pathologic recession*). The difference is one of degree. Gingival recession increases with age; the incidence varies from 8 per cent in children to 100 per cent after the age of 50.[11]

The causes of gingival recession are faulty toothbrushing (gingival abrasion), tooth malposition, gingivitis and periodontal pocket formation. High frenum attachment may be an aggravating factor. It is suspected, but not proved, that trauma from occlusion aggravates recession by accelerating epithelial proliferation initiated by local irritation.

While toothbrushing is important for gingival health, **faulty toothbrushing causes gingival recession.** Recession tends to be more frequent and severe in patients with comparatively healthy gingiva little dental plaque and good oral hygiene.[2, 7, 8]

Susceptibility to recession is influenced by the position of teeth in the arch,[10] the angle of the root in the bone and the mesiodistal curvature of the tooth surfaces.[5] On rotated, tilted or facially displaced teeth, the bony plate is thinned or reduced in height. Pressure from chewing hard foods or moderate toothbrushing wears away the unsupported gingiva and produces recession.

The effect of the angle of the roots in the bone upon recession is often observed in the maxillary molar area (Fig. 9–10). If the lingual inclination of the palatal root is prominent or the buccal roots flare outward, the bone in the cervical area is thinned or shortened and recession results from wear of the unsupported marginal gingiva (Fig. 9–11). On maxillary molars with flared roots recession is aggravated by occlusal wear. Occlusal wear is accompanied by

Figure 9–6   Recession around malposed anterior teeth. The gingiva is markedly inflamed.

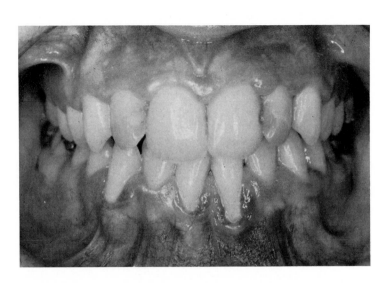

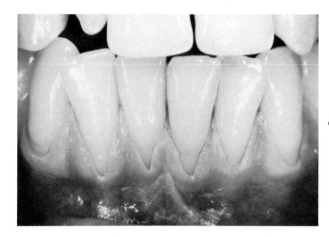

Figure 9-7 Recession on malposed teeth. Note excellent condition of the gingiva.

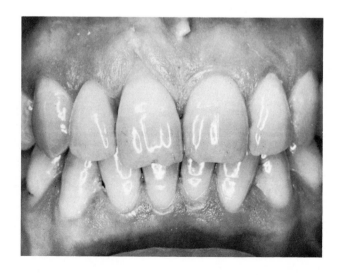

Figure 9-8 Localized Recession on maxillary central incisor associated with aggressive tooth-brushing.

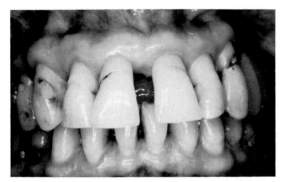

Figure 9–9 Generalized Recession resulting from chronic periodontal disease.

eruption of the tooth and accentuation of its normal buccal inclination. This increases the angulation of the lingual root in the palate, reduces the bone level and furthers recession by lessening the gingival support (Fig. 9–11).

Clinical significance

Several aspects of gingival recession make it clinically significant. Exposed root surfaces are susceptible to caries. Wearing

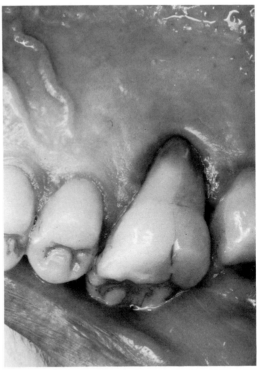

Figure 9–10 Accentuated Recession on a maxillary first molar aggravated by the angulation of the prominent palatal root in the bone.

Figure 9–11 Prominent Palatal Root and Occlusal Wear Aggravating Gingival Recession. *A,* Maxillary first molar with gingiva close to the cervical line. *B,* Maxillary molar with prominent palatal root. The altered root-bone angle results in shortened bone support and gingival recession (R). *C,* Occlusal wear is accompanied by tooth eruption with increase in the normal occlusofacial inclination of the tooth (arrow) and worsening of the palatal root-bone angle (arrow). *D,* Altered palatal root-bone angle following occlusal wear lessens bone support and aggravates gingival recession (R).

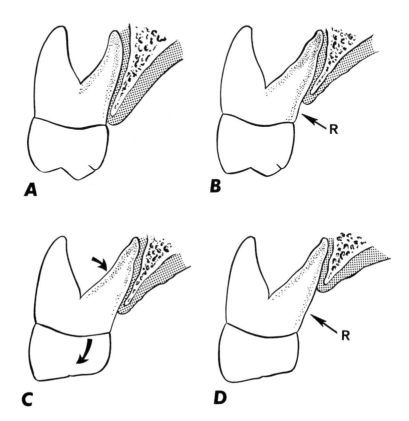

away of the cementum exposed by recession leaves an underlying dentinal surface that is extremely sensitive, particularly to touch. Hyperemia of the pulp and associated symptoms may also result from exposure of the root surface.[4] Interproximal recession creates spaces in which plaque, food and bacteria accumulate.

REFERENCES

1. Barnfield, W. F.: Pathological Calcification in the Gingivae. Am. J. Path., 22:1307, 1946.
2. Gorman, N. J.: Prevalence and Etiology of Gingival Recession. J. Periodont., 38:316, 1967.
3. Hirschfeld, I.: A Study of Skulls in the American Museum of Natural History in Relation to Periodontal Disease. J. D. Res., 5:241, 1923.
4. Merritt, A. A.: Hyperemia of the Dental Pulp Caused by Gingival Recession. J. Periodont., 4:30, 1933.
5. Morris, M. L.: The Position of the Margin of the Gingiva. Oral Surg., Oral Med. & Oral Path., 11:969, 1958.
6. Moskow, B. S.: Calcified Material in Human Gingival Tissues. J. D. Res., 40:644, 1961.
7. O'Leary, T. J., et al.: The Incidence of Recession in Young Males: Relationship to Gingival and Plaque Scores. U.S.A.F. School Aerosp. Med., SAM-TR-67-97:1, November, 1967.
8. O'Leary, T. J., et al.: The Incidence of Recession in Young Males—A Further Study. I.A.D.R. Abstr., 48th General Meeting, 1970, p. 65.
9. Orban, B.: Gingival Inclusions. J. Periodont., 16:16, 1945.
10. Trott, J. R., et al.: An Analysis of Localized Gingival Recession in 766 Winnipeg High School Students. D. Practit., 16:209, 1966.
11. Woofter, C.: The Prevalence and Etiology of Gingival Recession. Periodont. Abstr., 17:45, 1969.

Chapter 10

GINGIVAL BLEEDING

ABNORMAL GINGIVAL BLEEDING CAUSED BY LOCAL FACTORS

Abnormal gingival bleeding is a common sign of gingival disease. It varies in severity, duration, and the ease with which it is provoked.

Chronic and Recurrent Bleeding

The most common cause of abnormal gingival bleeding is chronic inflammation.[2] The bleeding is chronic or recurrent and is provoked by mechanical trauma such as that from toothbrushing, toothpicks or food impaction, or by biting into solid foods such as apples, or by grinding the teeth (bruxism).

Histopathology

The blood vessels of the gingiva are contained in the papillary connective tissue. On the outer surface they are protected from injury by a considerable thickness of keratinized or parakeratinized stratified squamous epithelium. Adjacent to the tooth a plexus of capillaries lies close to the sulcus space, separated from it by a thin layer of semipermeable epithelium.

In gingival inflammation the following alterations result in abnormal gingival bleeding:

Dilation and engorgement of the capillaries increase the susceptibility to injury and bleeding. Injurious agents which initiate the inflammation increase the permeability of the sulcus epithelium by degrading intercellular cement substance and widening the intercellular spaces. As the inflammation becomes chronic, the sulcal epithelium undergoes ulceration. The cellular and fluid exudate and the proliferation of new blood vessels and connective tissue cells create pressure upon the epithelium on the crest and external surface of the marginal and interdental gingiva. The epithelium is thinned and presents varying degrees of degeneration (Figs. 10–1 and 10–2). Because the capillaries are engorged and closer to the surface and the thinned, degenerated epithelium is less protective, stimuli that are ordinarily innocuous cause rupture of the capillaries and gingival bleeding.

The severity of the bleeding and the ease with which it is provoked depend upon the intensity of the inflammation. After the vessels rupture a complex of mechanisms induces hemostasis.[5] The vessel walls contract and blood flow is diminished; blood platelets adhere to the edges of the tissue; a fibrous clot is formed, which contracts and results in approximation of the edges of the injured area. Bleeding recurs, however, when the area is irritated.

Acute Bleeding

Acute episodes of gingival bleeding are caused by injury or occur spontaneously in acute gingival disease. Laceration of the gingiva by aggressive toothbrushing or sharp pieces of hard food causes gingival

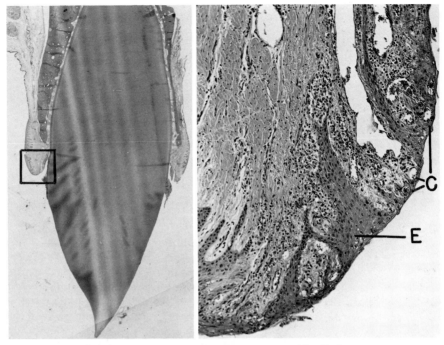

Fig. 10–1   Fig. 10–2

Figure 10–1   Survey section of maxillary canine in situ.

Figure 10–2   High power study from area marked in Figure 10–1 showing the **Inflamed Marginal Gingiva** in relation to the tooth surface. Note the proximity of the capillaries (C) to the surface. There is some thickening of the epithelium (E) but for the most part it is thinned.

bleeding even in the absence of gingival disease. Gingival burns from hot foods or chemicals increase the ease of gingival bleeding.

Spontaneous bleeding or bleeding upon slight provocation occurs in *acute necrotizing ulcerative gingivitis.* **In this condition, engorged blood vessels in the inflamed connective tissue are exposed by desquamation of necrotic surface epithelium.**

ABNORMAL GINGIVAL BLEEDING ASSOCIATED WITH SYSTEMIC DISTURBANCES

There are systemic disorders in which gingival hemorrhage, unprovoked by mechanical irritation, occurs spontaneously, or in which gingival bleeding following irritation is excessive and difficult to control. These are called *hemorrhagic diseases,* and represent a wide variety of conditions that vary in etiology and clinical manifestations.[7] Such conditions have one feature in common; namely, abnormal bleeding in the skin, internal organs and other tissues as well as the oral mucous membrane.

In individual patients the hemorrhagic tendency may be due to failure of one or more of the hemostatic mechanisms.[6] **Hemorrhagic disorders in which abnormal gingival bleeding is encountered include the following:** vascular abnormalities (vitamin C deficiency or allergy such as Henoch-Schönlein's purpura), platelet disorders (idiopathic thrombocytopenic purpura or thrombocytopenic purpura secondary to diffuse injury to the bone marrow), hypoprothrombinemia (vitamin K deficiency resulting from liver disease or sprue), other coagulation defects (hemophilia, leukemia, Christmas disease), deficient platelet thromboplastic factor (PF_3) secondary to uremia[3] and post-rubella purpura.[1] Bleeding may follow the administration of excessive amounts of drugs such as salicylates and the administration of anticoagulants such as Dicumarol and heparin. (Periodontal involvement in hematologic disorders is considered in Chapter 28.)

Cyclical episodes of abnormal gingival bleeding occasionally occur associated with the menstrual period (Chap. 12), and comparatively poor general health and nutritional status have been associated with gingival bleeding following toothbrushing.[4]

REFERENCES

1. Haub, H. P.: Post-rubella Thrombocytogenic Purpura. A Report of Cases with Discussion of Hemorrhagic Manifestations of Rubella. Clin. Pediatr., 7:350, 1968.
2. Milne, A. M.: Gingival Bleeding in 848 Army Recruits. An Assessment. Brit. D. J., 122:111, 1967.
3. Merril, A., et al.: Gingival Hemorrhage Secondary to Uremia. Review and Report of A Case. Oral Surg., 29:530, 1970.
4. Ringsdorf, W., Cheraskin, E., and Clark, J.: Gingival Bleeding and General Health. D. Survey, 44:49, 1968.
5. Sodeman, W. A.: Pathologic Physiology. Mechanisms of Disease. Philadelphia, W. B. Saunders Co., 1950.
6. Stefanini, M., and Dameshek, W.: The Hemorrhagic Disorders. 2nd ed. New York, Grune and Stratton, 1962, p. 78.
7. Wintrobe, M. M.: Clinical Hematology. 5th ed. Philadelphia, Lea & Febiger, 1961, p. 816.

Chapter 11

ACUTE GINGIVAL INFECTIONS

ACUTE NECROTIZING ULCERATIVE GINGIVITIS (ANUG)

The term *acute necrotizing ulcerative gingivitis* (ANUG) connotes an inflammatory destructive disease of the gingiva which presents characteristic signs and symptoms. Other terms by which this condition is known are Vincent's infection, acute ulceromembranous gingivitis, trench mouth, trench gums, phagedenic gingivitis, acute ulcerous gingivitis, acute ulcerative gingivitis, ulcerative gingivitis, ulcerative stomatitis, Vincent's stomatitis, Plaut-Vincent's stomatitis, stomatitis ulcerosa, stomatitis ulcero-membranacea, fusospirillary gingivitis, fusospirillary marginal gingivitis, fusospirillary periodontal gin-

givitis, fusospirillary peridental gingivitis, fusospirillary periodontitis, fetid stomatitis, putrid stomatitis, putrid sore mouth, stomatocace, stomacace, acute septic gingivitis, pseudomembranous angina, and spirochetal stomatitis.

The disease was recognized as far back as the fourth century B.C. by Xenophon, who mentioned that Greek soldiers were affected with "sore mouth" and foul-smelling breath. John Hunter in 1778 described the clinical findings and differentiated it from scurvy and chronic destructive periodontal disease. It occurred in epidemic form in the French army in the nineteenth century, and in 1886 Hersch discussed some of the features associated with the disease, such as enlarged lymph nodes, fever, malaise and increased salivation. In the 1890's Plaut[31] and Vincent[51] described the disease and attributed its origin to fusiform and spirochete bacteria. It was commonly known as *Vincent's infection* during the first half of the twentieth century, but the current designation is acute necrotizing ulcerative gingivitis.

Clinical features

CLASSIFICATION. Necrotizing ulcerative gingivitis most often occurs as an *acute* disease. Its relatively mild and more persistent form is referred to as *subacute*. *Recurrent* disease is marked by periods of remission and exacerbation. Reference is sometimes made to *chronic* necrotizing ulcerative gingivitis. However, it is difficult to justify this designation as a separate entity because most periodontal pockets with ulceration and destruction of gingival

126

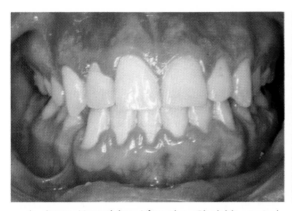

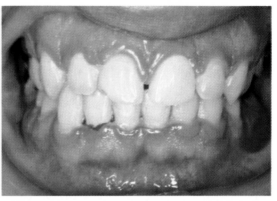

A, **Acute Necrotizing Ulcerative Gingivitis:** typical punched-out interdental papillae.

B, **Acute Necrotizing Ulcerative Gingivitis:** typical lesions with progressive tissue destruction.

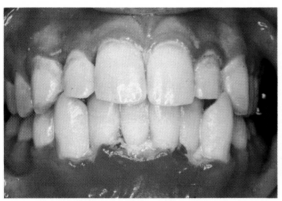

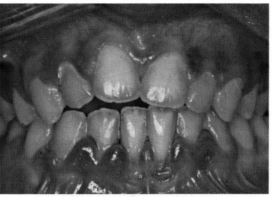

C, **Acute Necrotizing Ulcerative Gingivitis:** typical lesions with spontaneous hemorrhage.

D, **Acute Necrotizing Ulcerative Gingivitis:** superimposed upon underlying chronic periodontal disease.

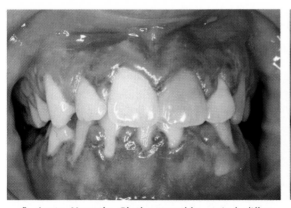

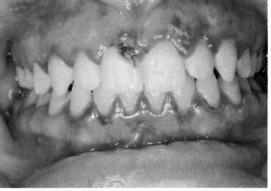

E, **Acute Herpetic Gingivostomatitis:** typical diffuse erythema.

F, **Acute Herpetic Gingivostomatitis:** vesicles on the gingiva.

Figure 11–1

tissue present comparable microscopic and clinical features.

HISTORY. Acute necrotizing ulcerative gingivitis is characterized by *sudden onset*, frequently following an episode of debilitating disease or acute respiratory infection. Occasionally, patients report that it appeared shortly after they had their teeth cleaned. Change in living habits, protracted work without adequate rest, and psychological stress are frequent features of the patient's history.

ORAL SIGNS. *Characteristic lesions are punched-out, crater-like depressions at the crest of the gingiva that involve the interdental papillae, the marginal gingiva or both.* The surface of the gingival craters is covered by a gray, pseudomembranous slough demarcated from the remainder of the gingival mucosa by a pronounced linear erythema (Fig. 11–1, A). In some instances, the lesions are denuded of the surface pseudomembrane, exposing the gingival margin, which is red, shiny and hemorrhagic. The characteristic lesions progressively destroy the gingiva and underlying periodontal tissues (Fig. 11–1, B).

A fetid odor, increased salivation and spontaneous gingival hemorrhage or pronounced bleeding upon the slightest stimulation are additional characteristic clinical signs (Fig. 11–1, C).

Acute necrotizing ulcerative gingivitis occurs in otherwise disease-free mouths or superimposed upon chronic gingivitis (Fig. 11–1, D) or periodontal pockets. Involvement may be limited to a single tooth or group of teeth (Fig. 11–2), or be widespread throughout the mouth. It is rare in edentulous mouths, but isolated spherical lesions occasionally occur on the soft palate.

ORAL SYMPTOMS. The lesions are extremely sensitive to touch, and the patient complains of a constant radiating, gnawing pain that is intensified by spicy or hot foods and mastication. There is a metallic foul taste and the patient is conscious of an excessive amount of "pasty" saliva. **The teeth are characteristically described as feeling like "wooden pegs."**

EXTRA-ORAL AND SYSTEMIC SIGNS AND SYMPTOMS. Patients are usually ambulatory, with a minimum of systemic complications. **Local lymphadenopathy and slight elevation in temperature** are common fea-

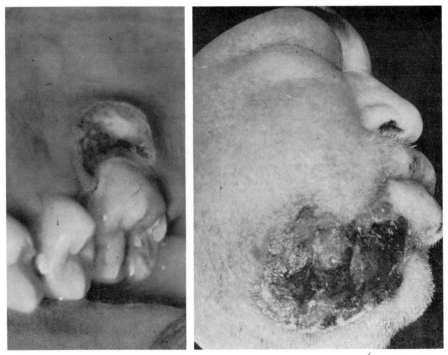

Fig. 11–2   Fig. 11–3

Figure 11–2   Localized Zone of Acute Necrotizing Ulcerative Gingivitis.
Figure 11–3   Noma Following Acute Necrotizing Ulcerative Gingivitis in a 50-year-old male with severe anemia.

tures of the mild and moderate stages of the disease. In severe cases there are marked systemic complications such as high fever, increased pulse rate, leukocytosis, loss of appetite, and general lassitude. Systemic reactions are more severe in children. Insomnia, constipation, gastrointestinal disorders, headache, and mental depression frequently accompany the condition.

Although uncommon, severe sequelae such as the following may occur: noma or gangrenous stomatitis[4] (Fig. 11–3), fusospirochetal meningitis and peritonitis, pulmonary infections,[28] toxemia and fatal brain abscess.[46]

CLINICAL COURSE. The clinical course is indefinite. If untreated, it may result in progressive destruction of the periodontium and denudation of the roots, accompanied by an increase in the severity of toxic systemic complications. It often undergoes a diminution in severity leading to a subacute stage with varying degrees of clinical symptomatology. *The disease may subside spontaneously without treatment.* Such patients generally present a history of repeated remissions and exacerbations. Recurrence of the condition in previously treated patients is also frequent.

Acute necrotizing ulcerative gingivitis and chronic destructive periodontal disease

It is important to understand the relationship between acute necrotizing ulcerative gingivitis and chronic destructive periodontal disease. As pointed out earlier, acute necrotizing ulcerative gingivitis may occur in a mouth devoid of pre-existing gingival disease, or it may be superimposed upon underlying chronic gingivitis and periodontal pockets. **However, it does not usually lead to periodontal pocket formation.** It causes rapid destruction of tissue, in contrast with the chronic inflammatory and proliferative changes which give rise to pocket formation.

Histopathology of the characteristic lesion

Microscopically, the lesion appears as a nonspecific acute, necrotizing inflammation at the gingival margin involving both the stratified squamous epithelium and the underlying connective tissue. The surface epithelium is destroyed and replaced by a pseudomembranous meshwork of fibrin, necrotic epithelial cells, polymorphonuclear leukocytes and various types of microorganisms (Fig. 11–4). This is the zone that appears clinically as the surface pseudomembrane. The underlying connective tissue is markedly hyperemic with numerous engorged capillaries and a dense infiltration of polymorphonuclear leukocytes. This acutely inflamed hyperemic zone appears clinically as the linear erythema beneath the surface pseudomembrane.

The epithelium and connective tissue present alterations in appearance as the distance from the necrotic gingival margin increases. There is a gradual blending of the epithelium from the uninvolved gingiva to the necrotic lesion. At the immediate border of the necrotic pseudomembrane the epithelium is edematous and the individual cells present varying degrees of hydropic degeneration. In addition, there is an infiltration of polymorphonuclear leukocytes in the intercellular spaces. The inflammatory involvement in the connective tissue diminishes as the distance from the necrotic lesion increases until it blends in appearance with the uninvolved connective tissue stroma of the normal gingival mucosa.

It is noteworthy that the microscopic appearance of acute necrotizing ulcerative gingivitis is nonspecific. Comparable changes result from trauma, chemical irritation or the application of escharotic drugs.

The relation of bacteria to the characteristic lesion has been studied with the light microscope and electron microscope. With the former it appears that the exudate on the surface of the necrotic lesion contains cocci, fusiform bacilli and spirochetes.[48] The layer between necrotic and living tissue contains enormous numbers of fusiform bacilli and spirochetes in addition to leukocytes and fibrin. Spirochetes invade the underlying living tissue;[5, 10, 48] other organisms seen on the surface are not found there. Some investigators feel the spirochetes are pushed into the tissue when gingival specimens are removed for microscopic study.[12]

Electron microscopic examination reveals that in acute necrotizing ulcerative gingivitis, the gingiva is divisible into the following four zones, which blend with each other and may not all be present in every case:[25]

Zone 1: *Bacterial zone,* most superficial, consists of varied bacteria, including a few spirochetes of small, medium and large types.

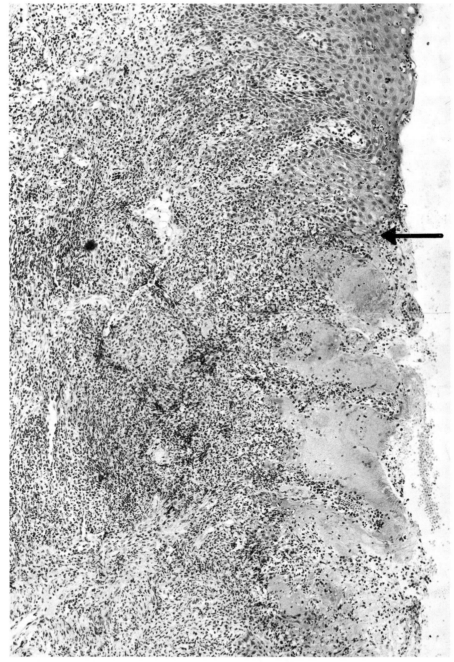

Figure 11–4   Survey Section of the Gingiva in Acute Necrotizing Ulcerative Gingivitis. The portion of the section below the arrow is the accumulation of leukocytes, fibrin and necrotic tissue which form the gray marginal pseudomembrane.

Zone 2: *Neutrophil-rich zone*, contains numerous leukocytes, predominantly neutrophils, with bacteria, including many spirochetes of various types between the leukocytes.

Zone 3: *Necrotic zone*, consists of disintegrated tissue cells, fibrillar material, remnants of collagen fibers, numerous spirochetes of the intermediate and large type, with few other organisms.

Zone 4: *Zone of spirochetal infiltration*, consists of well preserved tissue infiltrated with intermediate and large spirochetes, without other organisms.

In no instance are spirochetes deeper than 300 microns from the surface. The majority of spirochetes in the deeper zones are morphologically different from cultivated strains of *Borrelia vincentii*. They occur in non-necrotic tissue ahead of other types of bacteria and may be present in high concentrations intercellularly in the epithelium adjacent to the ulcerated lesion and in the connective tissue.

The bacterial flora

Smears taken of the lesions (Fig. 11–5) present scattered bacteria, predominantly spirochetes and fusiform bacilli, desquamated epithelial cells and occasional polymorphonuclear leukocytes. A smear consisting of only spirochetes and fusiform bacilli is rarely seen. Usually these two organisms are seen together with other oral spirochetes, vibrios, streptococci and filamentous organisms. The Borrelia and other spirochetal organisms form a light-staining, conspicuous, interlacing network throughout the microscopic field. The fusiform bacilli stain darkly with gentian violet and present a granular appearance.

For a long time it was felt that *Borrelia vincentii* was the predominant spirochete in acute necrotizing ulcerative gingivitis. Recent electron microscopic studies indicate that **the spirochetes may be classified into three morphologic groups: "small,"** 7 to 39 per cent of the total spirochetes

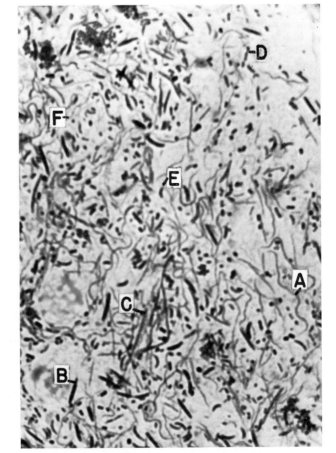

Figure 11–5 Bacterial Smear from Lesion in Acute Necrotizing Ulcerative Gingivitis. *A,* Spirochete. *B,* Bacillus fusiformis. *C,* Filamentous organism (Actinomycetes or Leptotrichia). *D,* Streptococcus. *E,* Vibrio. *F,* Treponema microdentium.

present; "**intermediate,**" 43.9 to 90 per cent and "**large,**" 0 to 20 per cent.[26] It was also suggested that "intermediate" spirochetes other than *Borrelia vincentii* (also in the "intermediate" group) are present in greater numbers in pooled scrapings from acute necrotizing ulcerative gingivitis, and are found in greater percentages in the deeper portion of the lesions.

The mean fusiform count in the saliva of patients with acute necrotizing ulcerative gingivitis is higher than in "normal" patients.[19] *Fusobacterium nucleatum* accounts for 75 per cent of the total fusiforms in both groups.

SMEAR PREPARATION. The following is a simple procedure for preparation of a stained bacterial smear:

1. A sample of exudate is obtained with a platinum wire loop, which is previously flamed to red heat and permitted to cool.
2. The involved area is first cleared of obvious superficial debris by gently wiping with cotton pellet soaked in sterile water or saline. This will facilitate obtaining a sample close to the surface of living cells. The loop is gently scraped along the involved surface and, where possible, into the periodontal pockets.
3. The material is spread thinly on a clear glass slide. A thick smear is often impossible to read properly. The smear is allowed to dry in air. This requires approximately one minute.
4. The smear is fixed by passing the slide, filmside upwards, over a flame several times until the slide is warm. Overheating is undesirable.
5. After cooling, the slide is stained. The smear is covered with a half saturated aqueous solution of gentian (crystal) violet and allowed to remain for one minute. The slide is then washed with tap water.
6. After drying in air, a drop of immersion oil is placed on the stained film and the slide examined with the oil immersion lens of the microscope. The smear may be kept for a considerable time without alteration. For greater permanence, however, the smear should be covered with a glass cover slip mounted in Canadian balsam.

Diagnosis

Diagnosis is based upon clinical findings. A bacterial smear may be used to corroborate the clinical diagnosis, but it is not necessary or definitive because the bacterial picture is not appreciably different from that in marginal gingivitis, periodontal pockets, pericoronitis or herpetic gingivostomatitis.[36]

Bacterial studies are useful, however, in the differential diagnosis between acute necrotizing ulcerative gingivitis and specific infections of the oral cavity such as diphtheria, thrush, actinomycosis and streptococcal stomatitis.

Microscopic examination of the biopsied tissue is not sufficiently specific to be diagnostic. It can be used to differentiate acute necrotizing ulcerative gingivitis from specific infections such as tuberculosis or from neoplastic disease, but it does not differentiate between acute necrotizing ulcerative gingivitis and other acute necrotizing conditions of nonspecific origin such as those produced by trauma or escharotic drugs.

Differential diagnosis

Necrotizing ulcerative gingivitis should be differentiated from other conditions that resemble it in some respects, such as acute herpetic gingivostomatitis (Table 11–1), chronic periodontal pockets, desquamative gingivitis (Table 11–2), streptococcal gingivostomatitis, aphthous stomatitis, gonococcal gingivostomatitis, diphtheritic and syphilitic lesions (Table 11–3), tuberculous gingival lesions, moniliasis, agranulocytosis, dermatoses (pemphigus, erythema multiforme, lichen planus) and stomatitis venenata.

STREPTOCOCCAL GINGIVOSTOMATITIS, GONOCOCCAL STOMATITIS, AGRANULOCYTOSIS, VINCENT'S ANGINA. *Steptococcal gingivostomatitis* is a rare condition characterized by a diffuse erythema of the gingiva and other areas of the oral mucosa. In some instances it is confined as a marginal erythema with marginal hemorrhage. Necrosis of the gingival margin is not a feature of this disease, nor is there a notably fetid odor. Bacterial smears show a predominance of streptococcal forms, which upon culture appear as *Streptococcus viridans*.

Gonococcal stomatitis is rare and is caused by *Neisseria gonorrheae*. The oral mucosa is covered with a grayish membrane that sloughs off in areas exposing an underlying raw bleeding surface.[14] It is most common in the newborn, caused by infection from the maternal passages; but cases in adults caused by direct contact have been described.

Agranulocytosis is characterized by ul-

TABLE 11-1 DIFFERENTIATION BETWEEN ACUTE NECROTIZING ULCERATIVE GINGIVITIS AND ACUTE HERPETIC GINGIVOSTOMATITIS

Acute Necrotizing Ulcerative Gingivitis	Acute Herpetic Gingivostomatitis
Etiology not established (possibly fusospirochetal)	Specific viral etiology
Necrotizing condition	Diffuse erythema and vesicular eruption
Punched-out gingival margin. Pseudomembrane that peels off leaving raw areas. Marginal gingiva affected, other oral tissues rarely	Vesicles rupture and leave slightly depressed oval or spherical ulcer
	Diffuse involvement of gingiva, may include buccal mucosa and lips
Relatively uncommon in children	Occurs more frequently in children
No definite duration	Duration of 7 to 10 days
No demonstrated immunity	An acute episode results in some degree of immunity
Contagion not demonstrated	Contagious

ceration and necrosis of the gingiva, which resemble that of acute necrotizing ulcerative gingivitis. The oral condition in agranulocytosis is primarily necrotizing. Because of the diminished defense mechanism in agranulocytosis, the clinical picture is not marked by the severe inflammatory reaction seen in acute necrotizing ulcerative gingivitis. Blood studies serve to differentiate between necrotizing ulcerative gingivitis and the gingival necrosis in agranulocytosis.

Vincent's angina is a fusospirochetal infection of the oropharynx and throat, as distinguished from acute necrotizing ulcerative gingivitis, which affects the marginal gingiva. In Vincent's angina there is a painful membranous ulceration of the throat with edema and hyperemic patches breaking down to form ulcers covered with pseudomembranous material. The process may extend to the larynx and middle ear.

ACUTE NECROTIZING ULCERATIVE GINGIVITIS IN LEUKEMIA. Leukemia, per se, does not produce acute necrotizing ulcerative gingival inflammation. However, acute necrotizing ulcerative gingivitis commonly occurs superimposed upon gingival tissues altered by leukemia.

The differential diagnosis consists not in distinguishing between acute necrotizing ulcerative gingivitis and leukemic gingival changes, but rather in determining whether leukemia is a *predisposing factor* in a

TABLE 11-2 DIFFERENTIATION BETWEEN ACUTE NECROTIZING ULCERATIVE GINGIVITIS, CHRONIC DESQUAMATIVE GINGIVITIS AND CHRONIC PERIODONTAL DISEASE

Acute Necrotizing Ulcerative Gingivitis	Desquamative Gingivitis	Chronic Destructive Periodontal Disease
Bacterial smears show fusospirochetal complex	Bacterial smears reveal numerous epithelial cells, few bacterial forms	Bacterial smears show fusospirochetal complex
Marginal gingiva affected	Diffuse involvement of the marginal and attached gingiva and other areas of the oral mucosa	Marginal gingiva affected
Acute history	Chronic history	Chronic history
Painful	May or may not be painful	Painless if uncomplicated
Pseudomembrane	Patchy desquamation of the gingival epithelium	No desquamation generally but purulent material may appear from pockets
Papillary and marginal necrotic lesions	Papillae do not undergo necrosis	Papillae do not undergo notable necrosis
Affects adults of both sexes, occasionally children	Affects adults, most often females	Generally in adults, occasionally in children
Characteristic fetid odor	None	Some odor present but not strikingly fetid

TABLE 11-3 DIFFERENTIATION BETWEEN ACUTE NECROTIZING ULCERATIVE GINGIVITIS, DIPHTHERIA AND SECONDARY STAGE OF SYPHILIS

Acute Necrotizing Ulcerative Gingivitis	Diphtheria	Secondary Stage of Syphilis (Mucous Patch)
Etiology not established (possibly fusospirochetal)	Specific bacterial etiology: *Corynebacterium diphtheriae*	Specific bacterial etiology: *Treponema pallidum*
Affects marginal gingiva	Very rarely affects marginal gingiva	Rarely affects marginal gingiva
Membrane removal very easy	Membrane removal difficult	Membrane not detachable
Painful condition	Less painful	Not very painful
Marginal gingiva affected	Throat, fauces, tonsils affected	Any part of mouth affected
Serology negative	Serology negative	Serology positive (Wassermann, Kahn tests)
Immunity not conferred	Immunity conferred by an attack	Immunity not conferred
Doubtful contagiousness	Very contagious	Only direct contact will communicate the disease
Antibiotic therapy relieves symptoms	Antibiotic treatment has little effect	Antibiotic therapy has excellent results

mouth in which acute necrotizing ulcerative gingivitis is present. For example, if a patient with acute necrotizing involvement of the gingival margin also presents generalized diffuse discoloration and edema of the attached gingiva, the possibility of an *underlying, systemically induced gingival change* should be considered. Leukemia is one of the conditions which would have to be ruled out.

ERYTHEMA MULTIFORME, EROSIVE LICHEN PLANUS, LUPUS ERYTHEMATOSUS, PEMPHIGUS, TUBERCULOUS ULCER, MONILIASIS, STOMATITIS VENENATA AND CHEMICAL BURNS. For descriptions of the above conditions that may be useful in differentiating between them and acute necrotizing ulcerative gingivitis, see Chapter 13.

Etiology

THE ROLE OF BACTERIA. Plaut[31] and Vincent,[51] in 1894 and 1896 respectively, introduced the concept that acute necrotizing ulcerative gingivitis was caused by specific bacteria, namely, the fusiform bacillus and a spirochetal organism.

Opinions still differ regarding whether bacteria are the primary causative factors in acute necrotizing ulcerative gingivitis. Several observations encourage the concept of primary etiology: **Spirochetal organisms and Bacillus fusiforms are always found in the disease;** other organisms are also involved. Rosebury, MacDonald and Clark[36] describe a fusospirochetal complex consisting of *Treponema microdentium,* inter-mediate spirochetes, *Borrelia buccalis,* vibrios, fusiform bacilli and filamentous organisms in addition to the fusiform bacillus and *Borrelia vincentii.* The fact that necrotizing ulcerative gingivitis occurs in groups, suggesting contagion, encourages the concept of bacterial origin. Immunity tests on patients with necrotizing ulcerative gingivitis show definite reactions to cultures of fusiform bacilli, suggesting pathogenicity of the organisms.[48]

Bacteria and their products do participate in the tissue destruction in acute necrotizing ulcerative gingivitis. However, the concept that these organisms are the primary etiologic factors meets with considerable resistance, predicated upon the following facts: (1) Fusospirochetal organisms in essentially the same proportions[2] are found in many common oral conditions such as chronic destructive periodontal disease, marginal gingivitis and pericoronitis. Additional factors may be required to produce the rapid destruction in acute necrotizing ulcerative gingivitis. There are quantitative differences between the bacterial flora in these conditions and acute necrotizing ulcerative gingivitis, but their significance has not been established. The organisms, in small numbers, are found in normal sulci. (2) Acute necrotizing ulcerative gingivitis has not been produced experimentally in humans or animals by inoculation of bacterial exudates from the lesions. Exudates from acute necrotizing ulcerative gingivitis produce fusospirochetal abscesses when inoculated subcutaneously in experimental animals, and the infection is freely transmissible in series.[35] Local intracutaneous injection of a hyaluronidase and chondroitinase-containing cell-free filtrate of an oral microaerophilic diphtheroid bacillus aggravated spirochetal lesions produced by oral treponemes.[20] Only in one animal experiment has the transmission of lesions comparable to those seen in man been reported.[1]

The specific etiology of acute necrotizing ulcerative gingivitis has not been established. The prevalent opinion is that it is one of a group of *fusospirochetal* diseases, caused by a complex of bacterial organisms, but requiring underlying tissue changes to facilitate the pathogenic activity of the bacteria. In addition to the fusiform bacillus and *Borrelia vincentii*, other types of spirochetes, vibrios and streptococci are invariably included in the complex of bacteria isolated from the lesions in this group of diseases. The other diseases in the group are Vincent's angina, cancrum oris, genital fusospirochetosis, pulmonary fusospirochetosis and tropical ulcer.

LOCAL PREDISPOSING FACTORS. **Pre-existing gingivitis, injury to the gingiva and smoking are important predisposing factors.** Although necrotizing ulcerative gingivitis may appear in an otherwise disease-free mouth, it most often occurs *superimposed upon pre-existing chronic gingival disease and periodontal pockets.* Chronic inflammation entails circulatory and degenerative alterations that increase the susceptibility to infection. Any local factors capable of inducing chronic gingival inflammation may predispose to acute necrotizing ulcerative gingivitis. Deep periodontal pockets and pericoronal flaps are particularly vulnerable areas for the occurrence of the disease because they offer a favorable environment for the proliferation of the fusospirochetal complex. Box[3] refers to such locations as *"incubation zones."*

Areas of the gingiva traumatized by opposing teeth in malocclusion, such as the palatal surface behind maxillary incisors and the labial gingival surface of mandibular incisors, are frequent sites of acute necrotizing ulcerative gingivitis.

SYSTEMIC PREDISPOSING FACTORS. Acute necrotizing ulcerative gingivitis is often superimposed upon gingiva altered by severe systemic disease.

Nutritional Deficiency. Necrotizing gingivitis has been produced by placing animals on nutritionally deficient diets. Goldberger and Wheeler[17] described a deficiency state in dogs simulating human pellagra with oral symptoms consisting of erythema progressing to superficial necrosis of the mucosa of cheeks, tongue, soft palate and gingiva. Underhill and Mendel[50] produced a similar ulcerative condition in dogs on diets deficient in vitamin A and carotene. The fusospirochetal bacterial complex was found in the oral lesions induced by nutritional deficiency by Smith,[42] Miller and Rhoads,[28] and others.[22] The theory offered to explain their finding was invasion by oral fusospirochetal organisms secondary to lowered tissue resistance caused by deficiency of niacin or vitamin A.

Topping and Fraser[47] found that necrotizing gingivitis occurred in monkeys deficient in vitamin C or B complex with or without nicotinic acid and riboflavin supplements. However, only the animals in the B complex deficient group developed ulceration at the gingival margin. Fusospirochetal organisms were found in all the experimental animals, but no correlation was made between the bacteria and the clinical lesions. Chapman and Harris[6] confirmed the findings of Topping and Fraser that monkeys maintained on vitamin deficient diets develop a tendency to oral lesions including necrotizing gingivitis. Animals on diets deficient in vitamin B complex in particular developed severe oral ulcerating lesions. They also found an accompanying increase in the fusospirochetal flora in the mouths of the experimental animals, but the bacteria were regarded as opportunists, proliferating only when the tissues were altered by the vitamin deficiency. Clinical observations have been presented that suggest that low vitamin intake[24] or vitamin C deficiency[33] predisposes to acute necrotizing ulcerative gingivitis.

The Conditioning Effect of Nutritional Deficiency Upon Bacterial Pathogenicity. Nutritional deficiencies (vitamin C) accentuate the severity of the pathologic changes induced when the fusospirochetal bacterial complex is injected into animals.[42] Necrotizing lesions have been produced by injecting fusospirochetal organisms into vitamin B_2-deficient rats.[23] A correlation between vitamin C deficiency and intestinal fusospirochetosis has been reported in humans and animals.[54] Fusospirochetes may gain a foothold in the intestines in small breaks in the mucosa caused by vitamin C-deficiency-induced mucosal hemorrhages.

Debilitating Disease. Debilitating systemic disease may predispose the gingiva to acute necrotizing ulcerative gingivitis. Included among such systemic disturbances are metallic intoxication, cachexia caused by such chronic diseases as syphilis or cancer, severe gastrointestinal disorders such as ulcerative colitis, blood dyscrasias such as the leukemias and anemia, influenza and the common cold.[7] Nutritional deficiency secondary to debilitating disease may be an additional predisposing factor. Fusospirochetal abscesses and gingival bleeding[52] have been produced in experimental animals by injecting scillaren B, a mixture of glucosides derived from squill which lowers tissue resistance by reducing the leukocytes.[45, 49] An ulcerative gangrenous stomatitis occurred in animals with experimentally induced leukopenia.[28, 44] Necrotizing gingivitis and stomatitis occurred in 74 per cent of animals with experimentally produced renal insufficiency.[21]

PSYCHOSOMATIC FACTORS. Psychological factors appear to be important in the etiology of acute necrotizing ulcerative gingivitis. The disease often occurs under stress situations such as induction into the army and school examinations.[11, 16] Psychological disturbances are common in patients with the disease,[18] along with increased adrenocortical secretion.[39] Significant correlation between two personality traits, dominance and abasement, suggest the presence of an acute necrotizing ulcerative gingivitis–prone personality.[13] The mechanisms whereby psychologic factors create or predispose to gingival damage have not been established, but alterations in digital and gingival capillary responses suggestive of increased autonomic nervous activity have been demonstrated in patients with acute necrotizing ulcerative gingivitis.[15]

Epidemiology and prevalence

Acute necrotizing ulcerative gingivitis often occurs in groups in an epidemic pattern. At one time it was considered contagious, but this has not been substantiated.[37]

The prevalence of acute necrotizing ulcerative gingivitis appears to have been rather low in the United States and Europe prior to 1914. In World Wars I and II there were numerous "epidemics" among the Allied troops, but Germans did not seem to be similarly affected. There have also been epidemic-like outbreaks among civilian populations.

Acute necrotizing ulcerative gingivitis occurs at all ages,[8] with the highest prevalence reported as between ages 20 and 30[9, 43] and between ages 15 and 20.[23] It is not common in children in the United States, Canada and Europe, but in India 54[27] and 58 per cent[30] of the patients in two studies were under 10 years old. In a random school population in Nigeria it occurred in 11.3 per cent of children between the ages of 2 and 6,[40] and in a Nigerian hospital population it was present in 23 per cent of children under 10 years old.[11] In low socio-economic groups it has been reported in several members of the same family. Opinions differ as to whether it is more common during the winter,[29, 32] summer or fall,[23, 41] or whether there are no peak seasons.[9, 53]

COMMUNICABILITY. Distinction must be made between communicability and transmissibility when referring to the characteristics of disease. The term *transmissible* denotes a capacity for the maintenance of an infectious agent in successive passage through a susceptible animal host.[34] The term *communicable* signifies a capacity for the maintenance of infection by natural modes of spread such as direct contact through drinking water, food and eating utensils, via the airborne route or by means of arthropod vectors. A disease that is communicable is described as contagious. It has been demonstrated that disease associated with the fusospirochetal bacterial complex is transmissible; *however, it has not been shown to be communicable or contagious.*

Attempts have been made to spread acute necrotizing ulcerative gingivitis from human to human without success.[38] King[22] traumatized an area in his gingiva and introduced debris from a severe case of acute necrotizing ulcerative gingivitis. There was no response until he happened to fall ill shortly thereafter, and subsequent to his illness observed the characteristic lesion in the experimental area. It may be inferred with reservation from this experiment that systemic debility is a prerequisite for the contagion of acute necrotizing ulcerative gingivitis.

It is a common impression that, because acute necrotizing ulcerative gingivitis often occurs in groups using the same kitchen facilities, the disease is spread by bacteria on eating utensils. There is no evidence to substantiate this assumption. Growth of fusospirochetal organisms requires extremely carefully controlled conditions and an anaerobic environment; they do not ordinarily survive on eating utensils.[20] Even if organisms commonly persist on eating utensils, it is necessary to demonstrate that organisms cause the disease before its spread by eating utensils can be presumed.

The occurrence of the disease in epidemic-like outbreaks does not necessarily mean that it is contagious. The affected groups may be afflicted by the disease because of common predisposing factors rather than because of its spread from person to person.

REFERENCES TO ACUTE NECROTIZING ULCERATIVE GINGIVITIS

1. Berke, J. D.: Experimental Study of Acute Ulcerative Stomatitis. J.A.D.A., 63:86, 1961.
2. Berman, K. S., and Gibbons, R. J.: Bacteriologic Census of Debris Obtained from Vincent's Infection. I.A.D.R. Abstract 267, Forty-Third General Meeting, 1965.
3. Box, H. K.: Necrotic Gingivitis. Toronto, University of Toronto Press, 1930.
4. Cadham, F. T.: Vincent's Disease; Infection due to Fuso-spirillary Invasion. J. Canad. M. A., 17:556, 1927.
5. Cahn, L. R.: The Penetration of the Tissue by Vincent's Organisms. A Report of a Case. J. D. Res., 9:695, 1929.
6. Chapman, O. D., and Harris, A. E.: Oral Lesions Associated with Dietary Deficiencies in Monkeys. J. Infect. Dis., 69:7, 1941.
7. Coutley, R. L.: Vincent's Infection. Brit. D. J., 74:34, 1943.
8. Daley, F. H.: Studies of Vincent's Infection at the Clinic of Tufts College Dental School from October, 1926 to February, 1928. J. D. Res., 8:408, 1928.
9. Dean, H. T., and Singleton, J. E., Jr.: Vincent's Infection—A Wartime Disease. Am. J. Pub. Health, 35:433, 1945.
10. Ellerman: Vincent's Organisms in Tissue. Z. Hyg. Infekt. Pr., 56:453, 1907.
11. Emslie, R. D.: Cancrum Oris. D. Practit., 13:481, 1963.
12. Fish, E. W.: Parodontal Disease. London, Eyre and Spottiswoode, Ltd., 1946.
13. Formicola, A. J., Witte, E. T., and Curran, P. M.: A Study of Personality Traits and Acute Necrotizing Ulcerative Gingivitis. J. Periodont., 41:36, 1970.
14. Frazer, A. D., and Menton, J.: Gonococcal Stomatitis. Brit. Med. J., 1:1020, 1931.
15. Giddon, D. B.: Psychophysiology of the Oral Cavity. J. D. Res. (suppl. to #6), 45:1627, 1966.
16. Giddon, D. B., Zackin, S. J., and Goldhaber, P.: Acute Necrotizing Gingivitis in College Students. J.A.D.A., 68:381, 1964.
17. Goldberger, J., and Wheeler, G. A.: Experimental Blacktongue of Dogs and Its Relation to Pellagra. U.S. Public Health Report, 43:172, 1928.
18. Goldhaber, P., and Giddon, D. B.: Present Concepts Concerning the Etiology and Treatment of Acute Necrotizing Ulcerative Gingivitis. Internat. D. J., 14:468, 1964.
19. Hadi, A. W., and Russell, C.: Quantitative Estimations of Fusiforms in Saliva from Normal Individuals and Cases of Acute Ulcerative Gingivitis. Arch. Oral Biol., 13:1371, 1968.
20. Hampp, E. G., and Mergenhagen, S. E.: Experimental Infection with Oral Spirochetes. J. Infect. Dis., 109:43, 1961.
21. Holman, R. L.: Necrotizing Arteritis in Dogs Related to Diet and Renal Insufficiency. Am. J. Path., 19:993, 1943.
22. King, J. D.: Nutritional and Other Factors in Trench Mouth with Special Reference to the Nicotinic Acid Component of Vitamin B Complex. Brit. D. J., 74:113, 1943.
23. Kirkpatrick, R. M., and Clements, F. W.: Diet in Relation to Vincent's Infection. D. J. Australia, 6:371, 1934.
24. Lapira, E.: Ulcerative Stomatitis Associated with Avitaminosis in Malta. Brit. D. J., 74:257, 1943.
25. Listgarten, M. A.: Electron Microscopic Observations on the Bacterial Flora of Acute Necrotizing Ulcerative Gingivitis. J. Periodont., 36:328, 1965.
26. Listgarten, M. A., and Lewis, D. W.: The Distribution of Spirochetes in the Lesion of Acute Necrotizing Ulcerative Gingivitis: An Electron Microscopic and Statistical Survey. J. Periodont., 38:379, 1967.
27. Miglani, D. C., and Sharma, O. P.: Incidence of Acute Necrotizing Gingivitis and Periodontosis Among Cases Seen at the Government Hospital, Madras. J. All Ind. D. Assn., 37:183, 1965.
28. Miller, D. K., and Rhoads, C. P.: The Experimental Production in Dogs of Acute Stomatitis Associated with Leukopenia and a Maturation Defect of the Myeloid Elements of the Bone Marrow. J. Exp. Med., 61:173, 1935.
29. Pedler, J. A., and Radden, B. G.: Seasonal Influence of Acute Ulcerative Gingivitis. D. Pract. & D. Rec., 8:23, 1957.
30. Pindborg, J. J., et al.: Occurrence of Acute Necrotizing Gingivitis in South Indian Children. J. Periodont., 37:14, 1966.
31. Plaut, H. C.: Studien zur bakteriellen Diagnostik der Diphtherie und der Anginen. Deutsch. Med. Wchnschr., 20:920, 1894.
32. Proske, H. O., and Sayers, R. R.: Pulmonary Fusospirochetal Infection. U.S. Public Health Reports, 49:839, 1934.
33. Radusch, D. F.: Nutrition and Dental Health. J. Periodont., 17:27, 1946.
34. Rosebury, T.: Is Vincent's Infection a Communicable Disease? J.A.D.A., 29:823, 1942.

35. Rosebury, T., and Foley, G.: Experimental Vincent's Infection. J.A.D.A., 26:1798, 1939.
36. Rosebury, T., MacDonald, J. B., and Clark, A.: A Bacteriologic Survey of Gingival Scrapings from Periodontal Infections by Direct Examination, Guinea Pig Inoculation and Anaerobic Cultivation. J. D. Res., 29:718, 1950.
37. Schluger, S.: Necrotizing Ulcerative Gingivitis in the Army. Incidence, Communicability, and Treatment. J.A.D.A., 38:174, 1949.
38. Schwartzman, J., and Grossman, L.: Vincent's Ulceromembranous Gingivostomatitis. Arch. Pediat., 58:515, 1941.
39. Shannon, I. L., Kilgore, W. G., and Leary, T. J.: Stress as a Predisposing Factor in Necrotizing Ulcerative Gingivitis. J. Periodont.-Periodontics, 40:240, 1969.
40. Sheiham, A.: An Epidemiological Study of Oral Disease in Nigerians. J. D. Res., 44:1184, 1965.
41. Skach, M., Zabrodsky, S., and Mrklas, L.: A Study of the Effect of Age and Season on the Incidence of Ulcerative Gingivitis. J. Periodont. Res., 5:187, 1970.
42. Smith, D. T.: Spirochetes and Related Organisms in Fusospirochetal Disease. Baltimore, Williams & Wilkins, 1932.
43. Stammers, A. F.: Vincent's Infection. Brit. D. J., 76:171, 1944.
44. Swenson, H. M.: Induced Vincent's Infection in Dogs. J. D. Res., 23:190, 1944.
45. Swenson, H. M., and Muhler, J. C.: Induced Fusospirochetal Infection in Dogs. J. D. Res., 26:161, 1947.
46. Thompson, L. E.: A Fatal Case of Brain Abscess from Vincent's Angina. D. Digest, 35:821, 1929.
47. Topping, N. H., and Fraser, H. F.: Mouth Lesions Associated with Dietary Deficiencies in Monkeys. U.S. Pub. Health Reports, 54:431, 1939.
48. Tunnicliff, R., Fink, E. B., and Hammond, C.: Significance of Fusiform Bacilli and Spirilla in Gingival Tissue. J.A.D.A., 23:1959, 1936.
49. Tunnicliff, R., and Hammond, C.: Abscess Production by Fusiform Bacilli in Rabbits and Mice by the Use of Scillaren-B or Mucin. J. D. Res., 16:479, 1937.
50. Underhill, F. P., and Mendel, L. B.: Further Experiments on the Pellagra-like Syndrome in Dogs. Am. J. Physiol., 83:589, 1928.
51. Vincent, H.: Sur l'étiologie et sur les lésions anatomopathologiques de la pourriture d'hôpital. Ann. de l'Inst. Pasteur, 10:448, 1896.
52. Wallace, H., Wallace, E. W., and Robertson, O. H.: The Production of Experimental Plaut-Vincent's Angina in the Dog. J. Clin. Invest., 12:909, 1933.
53. Wilkie, R.: An Etiology of Vincent's Gingivitis. Brit. D. J., 78:65, 1945.
54. Woolsey, F. M., and Black, S. R.: Vitamin C Deficiency and Intestinal Fusospirochetoses. Arch. Pathol., 28:503, 1939.

ACUTE HERPETIC GINGIVOSTOMATITIS

Etiology

Acute herpetic gingivostomatitis is an infection of the oral cavity caused by the herpes simplex virus.[6, 10, 13] Secondary bacterial infection frequently complicates the clinical picture. Acute herpetic gingivostomatitis occurs most frequently in infants and children below the age of 6,[13] but it is also seen in adolescents and adults. It occurs with equal frequency in males and females.

Clinical features

ORAL SIGNS. The condition appears as a diffuse, erythematous, shiny involvement of the gingiva and the adjacent oral mucosa with varying degrees of edema and gingival bleeding (Fig. 11–1, *E*). In its initial stage, it is characterized by the presence of discrete spherical gray vesicles (Fig. 11–1, *F*), which may occur on the gingiva, the labial and buccal mucosa, the soft palate, the

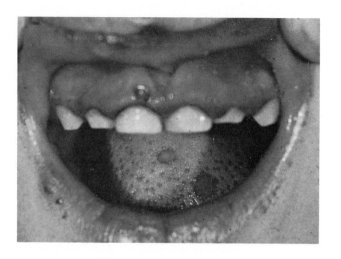

Figure 11–6 Vesicles on Tongue in Acute Herpetic Gingivostomatitis.

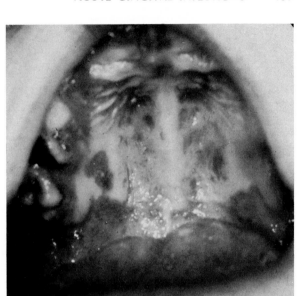

Figure 11-7 Involvement of the Palate in Acute Herpetic Gingivostomatitis.

pharynx, the sublingual mucosa and the tongue (Fig. 11-6). After approximately 24 hours the vesicles rupture and form painful small ulcers with a red, elevated halo-like margin and a depressed yellowish or grayish white central portion. These occur either in widely separated areas or in clusters where confluence occurs (Fig. 11-7).

Occasionally, acute herpetic gingivitis may occur without overt vesiculation. Diffuse erythematous shiny discoloration and edematous enlargement of the gingivae with a tendency toward bleeding comprise the clinical picture.

The course of the disease is limited to 7 to 10 days. The diffuse gingival erythema and edema that appear early in the disease persist for several days after the ulcerative lesions have healed. Scarring does not occur in the areas of healed ulcerations.

Acute herpetic gingivostomatitis may appear in a *localized* form following operative procedures in the oral cavity. Surfaces of the oral mucosa traumatized by cotton rolls or vigorous application of digital pressure in the course of operative procedures are the sites of predilection. The condition appears one or two days after the trauma, and the in-

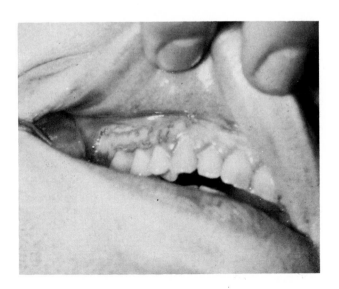

Figure 11-8 Acute Herpetic Involvement Following Surface Trauma With a Cotton Roll.

volvement presents a diffuse shiny erythema with numerous pinpoint vesicles confined to an area that can be clearly demarcated from adjacent uninvolved mucosa (Fig. 11–8). The vesicles rupture and form painful ulcerations. The duration of the involvement is 7 to 10 days, followed by uneventful healing.

ORAL SYMPTOMS. The disease is accompanied by generalized "soreness" of the oral cavity, which interferes with eating or drinking. The ruptured vesicles are the focal sites of pain, and are particularly sensitive to touch, thermal changes and condiments, fruit juices and the excursive action of coarse foods. In infants the disease is marked by irritability and refusal to take food.

EXTRA-ORAL AND SYSTEMIC SIGNS AND SYMPTOMS. Herpetic involvement of the lips or face (herpes labialis, "cold sore") with vesicles and surface scab formation may accompany the intraoral disease (Fig. 11–9). Cervical adenitis, fever as high as 101 to 105° F. and generalized malaise are common.

HISTORY. Recent acute infection is a common feature of the history of patients with acute herpetic gingivostomatitis.[7] The condition frequently occurs during and immediately after an episode of such febrile disease as pneumonia, meningitis, influenza and typhoid. It also tends to occur in periods of anxiety, strain or exhaustion and during menstruation. A history of exposure to patients with herpetic infection of the oral cavity of lips may also be elicited.

Acute herpetic gingivostomatitis often occurs in the early stage of infectious mononucleosis.[11]

Histopathology

The discrete ulcerations of herpetic gingivostomatitis that result from rupture of the vesicles present a central portion of acute inflammation with ulceration and varying degrees of purulent exudate surrounded by a zone rich in engorged blood vessels. The microscopic picture of the vesicles is characterized by extra- and intracellular edema and degeneration of the epithelial cells. The cell cytoplasm appears liquefied and clear; the cell membrane and nucleus stand out in relief. The nucleus later degenerates, loses its affinity for stain and finally disintegrates. The vesicle formation results from fragmentation of the degenerated epithelial cells.

The fully developed vesicle is a cavity in the epithelial cells with occasional polymorphonuclear leukocytes. The base of the vesicle is formed by edematous epithelial cells of the basal and prickle cell layers. The superficial surface of the vesicle is formed by compressed upper layers of prickle cells of the stratum granulosum and the stratum corneum. Occasionally, rounded eosinophilic inclusion bodies[12] are found in the nuclei of epithelial cells bordering vesicles. According to present theories, inclusion bodies may be either a colony of virus particles, degenerated protoplasm remnants of the affected cell, or a combination of both.[12]

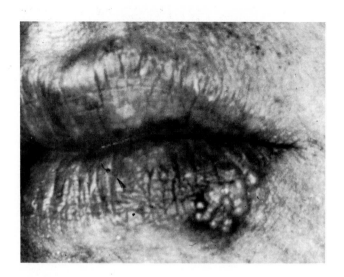

Figure 11–9 Cluster of Herpetic Vesicles ("Cold Sore").

Diagnosis

The diagnosis is usually established from the patient's history and the clinical findings. Material may be obtained from the lesions and submitted to the laboratory for confirmatory tests.

TISSUE CULTURE. Material is obtained from the lesion on a sterile cotton-tipped applicator and sent to the laboratory in skimmed milk. This is then inoculated into cultures of susceptible cells and incubated for 24 hours. Degenerative cellular changes preventable by antibody to herpes simplex virus constitute a positive finding.

DETERMINATION OF ANTIBODY TITER OF PATIENT'S SERUM DURING CONVALESCENCE. If a specimen of blood is collected when the patient is first seen and examined for neutralizing antibodies, none will be found. Successive specimens taken during the convalescent period, however, will show a rising titer of neutralizing antibodies that will remain high permanently.

CULTURE ON CHORIO-ALLANTOIC MEMBRANE OF THE CHICK EMBRYO. Material is removed from the suspected lesion with a cotton swab and placed in salivary solution or thioglycollate media for submission to the laboratory. Small amounts of the material are injected into ten-day-old embryonated eggs; after 48 hours the egg is opened and the chorio-allantoic membrane is inspected for pocks or viral colonies.

TZANC TEST. If the vesicle is intact, the top is removed and the fluid is allowed to escape. The base of the lesion is scraped with a sharp instrument such as the end of a scalpel blade or the sharp edge of a broken throat stick. The tissue obtained is smeared out on a glass slide, allowed to dry, and then stained with a polychrome stain such as Wright's or Giemsa's. A characteristic multinucleated giant cell is observed that is seen in no other disease. If the vesicle has already ruptured, the base is scraped in the manner described above.

PAUL TEST. Material obtained by gently wiping a sterile cotton-tipped applicator over the vesicle is applied to a freshly scarified rabbit cornea. Herpes simplex virus produces an encephalitis in 48 to 72 hours. In 24 hours small blisters appear along the lines and points of scarification. Inclusion bodies first described by Lipschutz may be seen microscopically in the cells of the cornea. These small rod-shaped inclusion bodies, 0.1 to 0.2 or 0.5 micron, were also described by Nicolau and Kopciowska.[12] This test is not commonly employed because of its doubtful reliability.

BIOPSY. Stained sections of the vesicles of acute herpetic gingivostomatitis, herpes

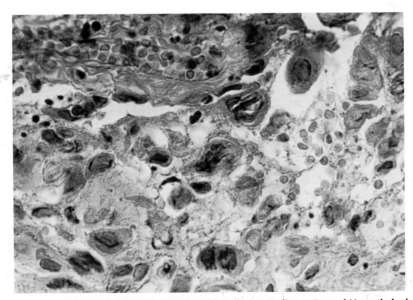

Figure 11–10   Biopsy Showing Giant Cells With Inclusion Bodies at Base of Herpetic Lesion.

zoster, and varicella (chicken pox) reveal eosinophilic intranuclear inclusion bodies in the peripheral cells (Fig. 11–10).

HEMATOLOGIC STUDIES. It has not been possible to demonstrate alterations in the hematologic picture of patients with acute herpetic gingivostomatitis.

Differential diagnosis

Acute herpetic gingivostomatitis should be differentiated from the following conditions:

1. ACUTE NECROTIZING ULCERATIVE GINGIVITIS. (See page 133.)

2. ERYTHEMA MULTIFORME. The vesicles in erythema multiforme are generally more extensive than those in acute herpetic gingivostomatitis and upon rupture present a tendency toward pseudomembrane formation. In addition, the tongue in the former condition usually is markedly involved, with infection of the ruptured vesicles resulting in varying degrees of ulceration. Oral involvement in erythema multiforme may be accompanied by skin lesions. The duration of erythema multiforme may be comparable to that of acute herpetic gingivostomatitis, but prolonged involvement for a period of weeks is not uncommon.

The Stevens-Johnson Syndrome. This is a comparatively rare form of erythema multiforme, characterized by vesicular hemorrhagic lesions in the oral cavity, hemorrhagic ocular lesions and bullous skin lesions.

3. BULLOUS LICHEN PLANUS. This painful condition, characterized by large blisters on the tongue and cheek that rupture and undergo ulceration, runs a prolonged, indefinite course. Patches of linear gray lace-like lesions of lichen planus are often interspersed among the bullous eruptions. Coexistent involvement of the skin affords a basis of differentiation between bullous lichen planus and acute herpetic gingivostomatitis.

4. DESQUAMATIVE GINGIVITIS. This condition is characterized by diffuse involvement of the gingiva with varying degrees of "peeling" of the epithelial surface and exposure of the underlying tissue. It is a chronic condition.

5. APHTHOUS STOMATITIS (CANKER SORE). This is a condition characterized by the appearance of discrete spherical vesicles that rupture after 1 or 2 days and form depressed spherical ulcers. The ulcers consist of a saucer-like red or grayish red central portion and an elevated rim-like periphery (Fig. 11–11). The lesions may occur anywhere in the oral cavity, the mucobuccal fold and the floor of the mouth being common sites. Aphthous stomatitis is painful. It may occur as single lesions or scattered throughout the mouth. The duration of each lesion is 7 to 10 days. As a rule, the lesions are larger than those seen in acute herpetic gingivostomatitis.

Aphthous stomatitis occurs in the following forms:

Occasional Aphthae. In this condition a single lesion occurs occasionally, at intervals that vary from months to years. Healing of the lesion is followed by uneventful recovery.

Acute Aphthae. This condition is characterized by an acute episode of aphthae, which may persist for weeks. During this period, lesions appear in different areas of the mouth, replacing others that are healing or healed. Such acute episodes are often seen in children with acute gastrointestinal disorders and may also occur in adults under comparable conditions. Remission of the gastrointestinal disturbance is generally accompanied by cessation of the acute episode of aphthae.

Chronic Recurrent Aphthae. This is a perplexing condition in which one or more oral lesions are always present. The involvement may extend over a period of years. In rare instances, lesions on the

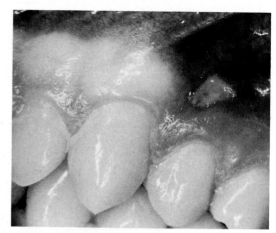

Figure 11–11 Aphthous Lesion in the Mucobuccal Fold. The depressed gray center is surrounded by an elevated red border.

genital, anal and conjunctival mucosa accompany the oral aphthae. One or more oral lesions are always present. The duration of involvement with chronic aphthae may be a period of years.

The etiology of aphthous stomatitis is unknown. Herpes simplex virus was suspected to be the cause, but antibody[16] and tissue culture[14] studies discourage this opinion. Other factors suggested as causing or predisposing to aphthous stomatitis include hormonal disturbances, allergic phenomena,[2] gastrointestinal disorders and psychosomatic factors.[1]

Aphthous stomatitis is a different clinical entity from acute herpetic gingivostomatitis.[5,17] The ulcerations may appear the same in both conditions, but diffuse erythematous involvement of the gingiva and acute toxic systemic symptoms do not occur in aphthous stomatitis.

Communicability

Acute herpetic gingivostomatitis is contagious.[4,9] Most adults have developed immunity to herpes simplex virus as the result of infection during childhood,[3] which in most instances is subclinical. For this reason acute herpetic gingivostomatitis occurs most often in infants and children. Although recurrent herpetic gingivostomatitis has been reported,[8] it does not ordinarily recur unless immunity is destroyed by debilitating systemic disease. Herpetic infection of the skin such as herpes labialis does recur.[15]

REFERENCES TO ACUTE HERPETIC GINGIVOSTOMATITIS

1. Alexander, F., and French, W.: Studies in Psychosomatic Medicine. Chicago. University of Chicago Press, 1948.
2. Brink, O.: Clinical Observations on the Etiology of Stomatitis Aphthosa. Paradentium, 11:192, 1939.
3. Burnet, F. M., and Williams, S. W.: Herpes Simplex: New Point of View. M. J. Australia, 1:637, 1939.
4. Chilton, N. W.: Herpetic Stomatitis. Am. J. Orth. & Oral Surg., 30:335, 1944.
5. Dodd, R., and Ruchman, J.: Herpes Simplex Virus not the Etiologic Agent of Recurrent Stomatitis. Pediatrics, 5:833, 1950.
6. Dodd, K., Johnston, L. M., and Buddingh, G. J.: Herpetic Stomatitis. J. Pediat., 12:95, 1938.
7. Greenberg, M. S., Brightman, V. J., and Ship, I. I.: Clinical and Laboratory Differentiation of Recurrent Intraoral Herpes Simplex Virus Infections Following Fever. J. D. Res., 48:385, 1969.
8. Griffin, J. W.: Recurrent Intraoral Herpes Simplex Virus Infection. Oral Surg., 19:209, 1965.
9. Levine, H. D., et al.: Vesicular Pharyngitis and Stomatitis. J.A.M.A., 112:2020, 1939.
10. McNair, S. T.: Herpetic Stomatitis. J. D. Res., 29:647, 1950.
11. Nathanson, I., and Morin, G. E.: Herpetic Stomatitis. An Aid in the Early Diagnosis of Infectious Mononucleosis. Oral Surg., Oral Med. & Oral Path., 6:1284, 1953.
12. Nicolau, S., and Kopciowska, L.: Inclusion Bodies in Experimental Herpes. Ann. Inst. Pasteur, 60:401, 1938.
13. Scott, T. F. M., Steigman, A. S., and Convey, J. H.: Acute Infectious Gingivostomatitis: Etiology, Epidemiology, and Clinical Picture of Common Disorders Caused by Virus of Herpes Simplex. J.A.M.A., 117:999, 1941.
14. Ship, I. I., Ashe, W. K., and Scherp, H. W.: Recurrent "Fever Blister" and "Canker Sore": Test for Herpes Simplex and Other Viruses with Mammalian Cell Cultures. Arch. Oral. Biol., 3:117, 1961.
15. Ship, I. I., Brightman, V. J., and Laster, L. L.: The Patient with Recurrent Aphthous Ulcers and the Patient with Recurrent Herpes Labialis: A Study of Two Population Samples. J.A.D.A., 75:645, 1967.
16. Stark, M. M., Kibbrick, S., and Weisberger, D.: Studies on Recurrent Aphthae. Evidence that Herpes Simplex is not the Etiologic Agent with Further Observations on the Immune Responses in Herpetic Infection. J. Lab. & Clin. Med., 44:261, 1954.
17. Weathers, D. R., and Griffin, J. W.: Intraoral Ulcerations of Recurrent Herpes Simplex and Recurrent Aphthae: Two Distinct Clinical Entities. J.A.D.A., 81:81, 1970.

PERICORONITIS

The term *pericoronitis* refers to inflammation of the gingiva in relation to the crown of an incompletely erupted tooth (Fig. 11–12). It occurs most frequently in the mandibular third molar area.[1,4,5] Pericoronitis may be acute, subacute or chronic.

Clinical features

The partially erupted or impacted mandibular third molar is the most common site of pericoronitis. The space between the crown of the tooth and the overlying gingival flap is an ideal area for the accumulation of food debris and bacterial growth (Fig. 11–13). Even in patients with no clinical signs or symptoms, the gingival flap is often chronically inflamed and infected

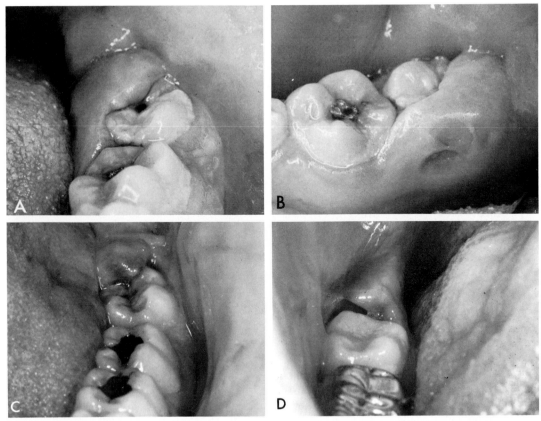

Figure 11–12 **Pericoronitis.** *A,* Third molar partially covered by infected flap. *B,* Lingual view showing sinus draining from infected flap. *C,* Swollen flap with suppuration at the tip. *D,* Opening into pericoronal abscess.

and presents varying degrees of ulceration along its inner surface. Acute inflammatory involvement is a constantly imminent possibility.

Acute pericoronitis is identified by varying degrees of involvement of the pericoronal flap and adjacent structures as well as systemic complications. Influx of inflammatory fluid and cellular exudate results in an increase in the bulk of the flap, which interferes with complete closure of the jaws. The flap is traumatized by contact with the opposing jaw and the inflammatory involvement is aggravated. **The resultant clinical picture is that of a markedly red, swollen, suppurating lesion that is exquisitely tender, with radiating pains to the ear, throat, and floor of the mouth.** In addition to the pain, the patient is extremely uncomfortable because of a foul taste and an inability to close the jaws. Swelling of

the cheek in the region of the angle of the jaw and lymphadenitis are common findings. The patient may also present toxic systemic complications such as fever, leukocytosis and malaise.

Complications

The involvement may become localized in the form of a pericoronal abscess. It may spread posteriorly into the oropharyngeal area and medially to the base of the tongue, making it difficult for the patient to swallow. Depending upon the severity and extent of the infection, there is lymph node involvement of the submaxillary, posterior cervical, deep cervical and retropharyngeal lymph nodes.[2,3] Peritonsillar abscess formation, cellulitis and Ludwig's angina are infrequent but nevertheless potential sequelae of acute pericoronitis.

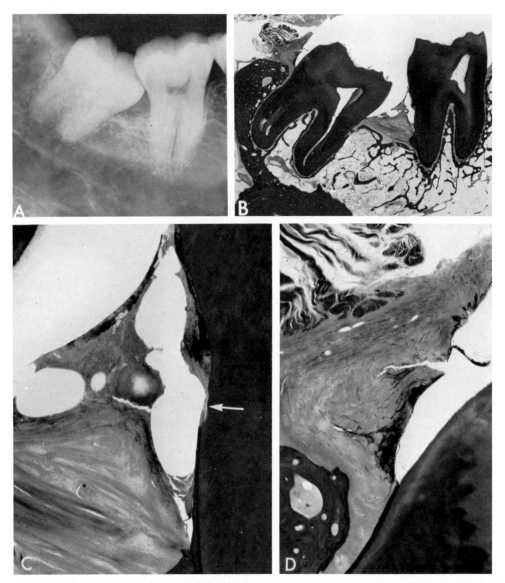

Figure 11–13 Pericoronitis Around Impacted Third Molar. *A,* Radiograph of impacted *mandibular* third molar. *B,* Survey section of molar area. *C,* Plaque, bacteria and calculus between the second and third molars. Note the resorption of cementum and dentin on the distal surface of the second molar *(arrow). D,* Inflamed gingiva on the distal surface of the third molar.

REFERENCES TO PERICORONITIS

1. Blair, V. P.: The Gingival Operculum and the Erupting Lower Third Molar. Arch. Clin. Oral Path., *4*:283, 1940.
2. Jacobs, M. H.: Pericoronal and Vincent's Infections: Bacteriology and Treatment. J.A.D.A., *30*:392, 1943.
3. Perkins, A. E.: Acute Infections Around Erupting Mandibular Third Molar. Brit. D. J., *76*:199, 1944.
4. Robinson, R. A.: Clinical Aspects of Diseases Associated with Impacted Mandibular Third Molars. Arch. Clin. Oral Path., *4*:348, 1940.
5. Salman, I.: Pericoronal Infection. D. Outlook, *26*: 460, 1939.

Chapter 12

GINGIVAL CHANGES IN PUBERTY, MENSTRUATION AND PREGNANCY: CHRONIC DESQUAMATIVE GINGIVITIS AND MENOPAUSAL GINGIVOSTOMATITIS

There are several types of gingival disease in which modification of the sex hormones is considered to be either the initiating or complicating factor.

THE GINGIVA IN PUBERTY

Puberty is frequently accompanied by an exaggerated response of the gingiva to local irritation.[22, 23] Pronounced inflamma-
tion, bluish red discoloration, edema and enlargement result from local irritants that would ordinarily elicit a comparatively mild gingival response (Fig. 12–1). Excessive anterior overbite aggravates these cases because of the complicating effects of food impaction and injury to the gingiva on the labial aspect of the mandibular teeth and palatal aspect in the maxilla.[7]

As adulthood is approached, the severity of the gingival reaction diminishes even when local irritants are still present. Complete return to normal requires their removal. Although the prevalence and severity of gingival disease are increased in puberty, it should be understood that *gingivitis is not a universal occurrence during this period; with proper care of the mouth it can be prevented.*

GINGIVAL CHANGES ASSOCIATED WITH THE MENSTRUAL CYCLE

As a general rule, the menstrual cycle is not accompanied by notable gingival changes, but occasional problems do occur. During the menstrual period the preva-

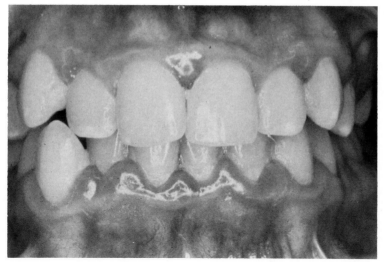

Figure 12–1 **Puberty,** showing gingivitis with edema, discoloration and enlargement.

lence of gingivitis increases[24] and patients may complain of bleeding gums or a bloated-tense feeling in the gums in the days preceding menstrual flow. Horizontal tooth mobility is increased between the third and fourth weeks of the menstrual cycle.[4] The salivary bacterial count is increased during menstruation and at ovulation 11 to 14 days earlier.[38] The exudate from inflamed gingiva is increased during menstruation, suggesting that existent gingivitis is aggravated by menstruation, but crevicular fluid of normal gingiva is unaffected.[18]

A variety of oral changes have been reported associated with the menstrual cycle, which usually appear several days before the menstrual period. These include ulcerations of the oral mucosa that seem to have a familial trend,[10, 36] aphthae and vesicular lesions and *vicarious bleeding* in the oral cavity,[44] "menstruation gingivitis" characterized by periodic recurrent hemorrhage with bright red and rose-colored proliferations of the interdental papillae, and persistent ulceration of the tongue and buccal mucosa that worsens just before the menstrual period. **Microscopic examination of the gingiva in a patient with a cyclical recurrent gingivitis revealed desquamation of epithelial cells from the stratum granulosum and the surface.**[34]

Periodically recurring ulcers of the mouth and occasionally of the vulva may accompany or precede the menstrual period. The oral lesions heal in 3 to 4 days and the vaginal tenderness disappears after menstruation and for the remainder of the cycle. The lesions do not appear if the patient becomes pregnant, but recur post partum. Improvement has been reported with systemic estrogen[21] or anterior pituitary hormone.[50]

An oral syndrome, termed *periodic transitory menogingivitis*,[46] has been described, consisting of discomfort, sensitiveness, redness and congestion of the gingiva with bleeding under the normal stress of mastication. The condition was observed just prior to menstruation, in amenorrheas of different types, post-hysterectomy, prior to and after ruptured ectopic pregnancy, and during and after menopause. Soreness of the mouth and tongue that appeared a few days prior to menstruation and increased in severity for several days was reported as relieved by systemic estrogen and recurred when the drug was withdrawn.[17] *Periodic agranulocytic leukopenia, which may be a factor in the production of oral changes, has also been associated with the menstrual cycle.*[20]

Cyclical gingival changes associated with menstruation have been attributed to hormonal imbalances and in some instances are accompanied by a history of ovarian dysfunction.[6] Rhythmic changes in capillary fragility associated with the menstrual cycle and increased tendency to capillary hemorrhage immediately before and during menstruation[2] may affect bleeding of the gingiva.

GINGIVAL DISEASE IN PREGNANCY

Pregnancy itself does not cause gingivitis. Gingivitis in pregnancy is caused by local irritants, just as it is in nonpregnant individuals. Pregnancy accentuates the gingival response to local irritants and produces a clinical picture different from that which occurs in nonpregnant individuals (Figs. 12–2 to 12–4). No notable changes occur in the gingiva in pregnancy in the absence of local irritants. Local irritants cause the gingivitis; pregnancy is a secondary modifying factor.

The severity of gingivitis is increased during pregnancy beginning from the second to third month. Patients with slight chronic gingivitis which attracted no particular attention before pregnancy become aware of the gingiva because previously inflamed areas become excessively enlarged and edematous and more noticeably discolored. Patients with a slight amount of gingival bleeding before pregnancy become concerned about an increased tendency to bleed.

Gingivitis becomes most severe by the eighth month and decreases during the ninth, and plaque accumulation follows a similar pattern.[28] Some report the greatest severity between the second and third trimesters.[8] The correlation between gingivitis and the quantity of plaque is closer after parturition than during pregnancy. This suggests that pregnancy introduces other factors which aggravate the gingival response to local irritants.

The prevalence of gingivitis in pregnancy (38 per cent,[1] 45.4 per cent,[30] 52 per cent,[29] 53.8 per cent,[14] 85.9 per cent,[17] 100 per cent[28]) varies according to the group studied. The prevalence appears to be increased in pregnancy,[42] but this is a difficult determination to make. Pregnancy affects the severity of previously inflamed areas; it does not alter healthy gingiva. Impressions of increased prevalence may be created by aggravation of previously inflamed but unnoticed areas.[41, 44] Also increased in pregnancy are tooth mobility,[39] pocket depth and gingival fluid.[19, 25]

Clinical features

Pronounced vascularity is the most striking clinical feature. The gingiva is inflamed and varies in color from a bright red to a bluish red sometimes described as "old rose."[33, 51, 52] The marginal and interdental gingiva is edematous, pits on pressure, appears smooth and shiny, is soft and friable, and sometimes presents a raspberry-like appearance. The extreme redness results from marked vascularity, and there is an increased tendency to bleed. The gingival changes are usually painless unless complicated by acute infection, marginal ulceration and pseudomembrane formation. In some cases the inflamed gingiva forms discrete "tumor-like" masses, referred to as "pregnancy tumors" (described in Chapter 8).

There is partial reduction in the severity

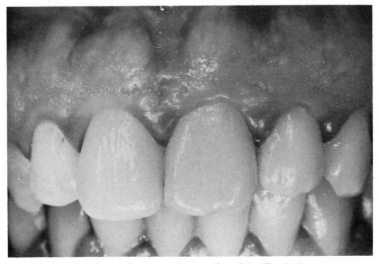

Figure 12–2   Early Changes in the Interdental Papillae in Pregnancy.

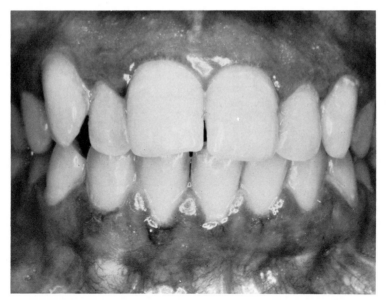

Figure 12–3 **Pregnancy,** showing edema, discoloration and bleeding.

of gingivitis by two months post partum, and after one year the condition of the gingiva is comparable to that in patients who have not been pregnant.[9] However, the gingiva does not return to normal so long as local irritants are present. Also reduced following pregnancy are horizontal tooth mobility, gingival fluid and pocket depth. Some report a loss of periodontal attachment during pregnancy which is not completely restored post partum.[8]

Histopathology

The microscopic picture[30, 52] of gingival disease in pregnancy is one of nonspecific vascularizing proliferative inflammation. There is marked inflammatory cellular infiltration with edema and degeneration of the gingival epithelium and connective tissue. The epithelium is hyperplastic, with accentuated rete pegs and varying degrees of intracellular and extracellular edema and infiltration by leukocytes.

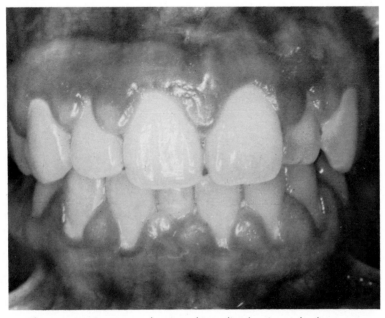

Figure 12–4 **Pregnancy,** showing edema, discoloration and enlargement.

Newly formed, engorged capillaries are present in abundance. Surface ulcerations or pseudomembrane formation is an occasional finding.

Histochemical studies reveal abnormal amounts of water- and alcohol-insoluble glycoprotein residues in the inflamed gingiva.[12] Comparable findings are observed in gingivitis in puberty, in menstruation, and in severe desquamative gingivitis. In an effort to differentiate changes caused by the pregnancy from those caused by local irritation, Turesky et al.[48] studied the attached gingiva that was uninvolved by inflammation, as distinguished from inflamed marginal and interdental areas. They reported that in pregnancy there is diminished surface keratinization, increase in rete peg length, and increase in glycogen in the epithelium. In the connective tissue, the basement layer is thinned and the carbohydrate-protein complexes and glycogen in the ground substance are reduced in density. Electrometric studies indicate a *decrease in the density of glycoprotein* in the gingiva in the early months of pregnancy, which *returns to normal several months after parturition.*[15]

The effect of pregnancy upon the gingival response to local irritants is explained on a hormonal basis. There is a marked increase in estrogen and progesterone during pregnancy and a reduction after parturition. The severity of gingivitis varies with the hormonal levels in pregnancy.[19] The aggravation of gingivitis has been attributed principally to the increased progesterone which produces dilatation and tortuosity of the gingival microvasculature, circulatory stasis and increased susceptibility to mechanical irritation—all of which favor leakage of fluid into perivascular tissues.

It has also been suggested that the accentuation of gingivitis in pregnancy occurs in two peaks: (1) during the first trimester, when there is overproduction of gonadotropins and (2) during the third trimester, when estrogen and progesterone levels are highest.[28] Destruction of gingival mast cells by the increased sex hormones and the resultant release of histamine and proteolytic enzymes may also contribute to the exaggerated inflammatory response to local irritants.[27]

Hormonal contraceptives and the gingiva

Hormonal contraceptives aggravate the gingival response to local irritants in a manner similar to pregnancy,[11, 26] and in an extremely small number of patients produce gingival changes comparable to those observed in pregnancy.

CHRONIC DESQUAMATIVE GINGIVITIS (GINGIVOSIS)

Chronic desquamative gingivitis is a term used to describe a *relatively uncommon gingival disturbance*, which in its severe form presents rather striking clinical features.[32] Reference to chronic desquamative gingivitis appeared as far back as 1897, when it was described by Tomes.[47] Under the term "chronic diffuse desquamative gingivitis," Prinz[37] described a condition he felt was similar to that referred to by Magitot in 1868 as "gingivite funguose."

Chronic desquamative gingivitis occurs most often in females, usually after age 30, but it may occur any time after puberty, and also in males. It is seen in edentulous mouths as well as in those with natural dentitions.[35, 43]

Chronic desquamative gingivitis occurs in varying degrees, which may be grouped as follows:

MILD FORM. In its mildest form there is diffuse erythema of the marginal, interdental and attached gingiva; the condition is usually painless and comes to the attention of the patient or dentist because of the over-all discoloration. The mild form occurs most frequently in young females between 17 and 23 years of age, usually without systemic indication of a hormonal disturbance.

MODERATE FORM. This is a more advanced form. It presents a patchy distribution of bright red and gray areas involving the marginal and attached gingiva (Fig. 12–5, A). The surface is smooth and shiny, and the normally resilient gingiva becomes *soft*. There is slight pitting upon pressure, and the epithelium is not firmly adherent to the underlying tissues. Massaging of the gingiva with the finger results in *peeling of the epithelium* and exposure of the underlying bleeding connective tissue surface.

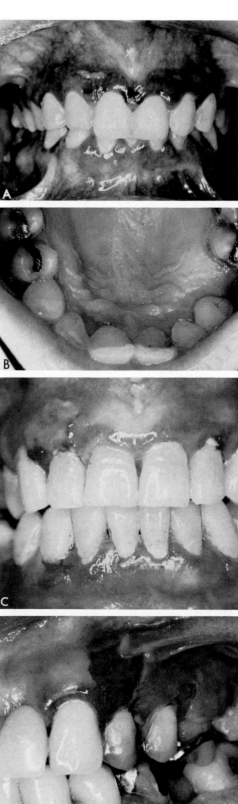

Figure 12–5 Chronic Desquamative Gingivitis of Varied Severity. *A,* Moderate. Generalized edema and erythema associated with inflammation and exposure of underlying connective tissue. *B,* Lingual view of patient shown in *A.* Aside from slight marginal erythema, there is little evidence of change in the gingiva and adjacent mucosa. *C,* Severe. Scattered, irregularly shaped denuded areas produce a mosaic appearance. Note the ulceration between the right maxillary lateral and canine. *D,* Severe. Complete denudation of the epithelium with exposure of underlying erythematous inflamed connective tissue.

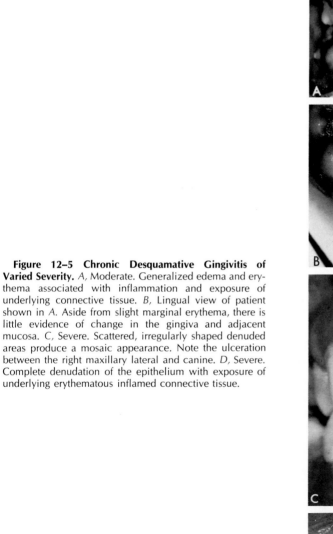

The oral mucosa in the remainder of the mouth is extremely smooth and shiny. This condition is seen most frequently in persons between 30 and 40 years of age. Patients complain of a burning sensation and sensitivity to thermal changes. *Inhalation of air is painful.* The patient cannot tolerate condiments, and toothbrushing causes painful denudation of the gingival surface.

SEVERE FORM. In this and other forms of desquamative gingivitis the lingual surface is usually less severely involved than the labial (Fig. 12–5, *B*) because the tongue and friction from food excursion reduce the accumulation of local irritants and limit the inflammation. This form is characterized by scattered, irregularly shaped areas in which the gingiva is denuded and strikingly red in appearance (Fig. 12–5, *C*). Since the gingiva separating these areas is grayish blue, in over-all appearance the gingiva seems *speckled.* The surface epithelium is shredded and friable and can be peeled off in *small patches* (Fig. 12–5, *D*).

There are occasionally surface vessels which rupture, releasing a thin, aqueous fluid and exposing an *underlying surface* that is red and raw. A *blast of air* directed at the gingiva *causes elevation of the epithelium* and the consequent formation of a bubble. The areas of involvement seem to shift to different locations on the gingiva. The mucous membrane other than the gingiva is smooth and shiny and may present a fissuring in the cheek adjacent to the line of occlusion.

The condition is *extremely painful.* The patient cannot tolerate coarse foods, condiments or temperature changes. There is a constant, *dry* burning sensation throughout the oral cavity which is accentuated in the denuded gingival zones.

Histopathology

The pathologic changes vary among different individuals, and can be grouped into two principal types:[16]

(1) *Bullous* type of chronic desquamative gingivitis, characterized by massive replacement of the papillary and reticular connective tissue with an inflammatory exudate of edema,

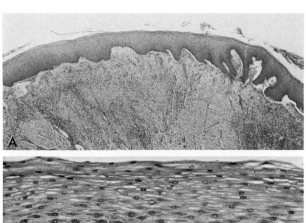
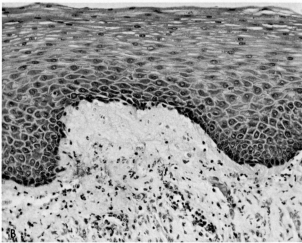

Figure 12–6 Chronic Desquamative Gingivitis—Bullous Type. *A,* There is massive replacement of the papillary and reticular connective tissue by inflammatory exudate, disruption of the epithelial-connective tissue junction and the formation of large subepithelial bullae. *B,* Detailed view showing blunting of epithelial rete pegs and inflammatory exudate of edema, fibrin and leukocytes which have replaced the connective tissue.

fibrin and leukocytes (Fig. 12–6). Large sub-epithelial bullae form at the epithelium–connective tissue junction, elevating the epithelium from the connective tissue. In the areas of the bullae, the basement membrane is destroyed, the epithelial rete pegs are blunted, there is intercellular edema in the basal epithelial layer and the remainder of the epithelium appears unchanged.

(2) *Lichenoid type* of desquamative gingivitis. This type is characterized by a dense subepithelial band of chronic inflammatory exudate in which lymphocytes predominate. The epithelium is either (a) atrophic without a well-formed sinous layer or rete pegs or (2) atrophic with isolated spike-like rete pegs (Fig. 12–7). Infiltration of leukocytes and edema into the epithelium results in separation and vacuolization in the cells in the basal layer and one or two layers above it. There is a junctional vesicle formation with thinning and disintegration of the basement membrane and separation of the epithelium from the connective tissue. Where the basement membrane

persists, it adheres to the connective tissue side of the vesicle.

Electron microscopy reveals that the most striking alterations occur at the epithelial–connective tissue interface.[3] There are intercellular edema and intracellular degeneration of the basal epithelial layer associated with inflammation and formation of subepithelial vesicles or bullae. The basal lamina exhibits irregularities in density and width, disruption from degenerated basal epithelial cells and a tendency to adhere to the connective tissue which forms the floor of the bullae. In some bullae the basal lamina is absent.

The bullae contain granular material, cytoplasmic debris, red blood cells and free nuclei presumably derived from lipid cells.[45] Fine fibrillar material and granular material contained in vesicle-like areas are found in the connective tissue.

The surface epithelial cells are parakeratinized but the progression of condensation is disturbed.[45]

The ultrastructural changes are comparable to other bullous conditions,[49] and it is difficult to determine whether the initial changes take place in the basal epithelial layer or the basal lamina.

Histochemical studies reveal fragmentation or clumping of PAS-positive material, increased staining intensity and thinning or absence of the basement membrane.[13] Glycogen is present and disulfides are decreased in the epithelium in areas of inflammation and overlying bullae and vesicles. With toluidine blue, the inflamed connective tissue stains metachromatic, granular and fibrillar; in uninflamed areas the papillary layer is orthochromatic, with slight metachromasia in the reticular layer.

Etiology

The most severe changes in chronic desquamative gingivitis are inflammatory and occur on the facial surface associated with local irritants. However, there is a continuing suspicion, as yet unsubstantiated, that it is primarily a systemically caused degenerative condition, and the inflammatory changes are secondary. This is the reason it is sometimes referred to as *gingivosis*. Hormonal imbalance,[13] deficiency of estrogen in the female or testosterone in the male[53] and nutritional deficiency[5] are suggested etiologic factors.

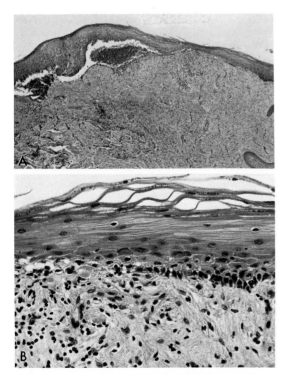

Figure 12–7 Chronic Desquamative Gingivitis—Lichenoid Type. *A,* The epithelium is atrophic, the connective tissue is inflamed and the epithelium is separated from the connective tissue by a subepithelial vesicle. *B,* Detailed view, showing atrophic parakeratotic epithelium with vacuolization of the basal cells and microvesicle formation at the epithelium–connective tissue junction.

There is some question as to whether chronic desquamative gingivitis is (1) a single disease entity; (2) a variant of bullous and vesicular dermatologic disorders such as lichen planus, erythema multiforme or benign mucous membrane pemphigoid; or (3) a nonspecific gingival response to a variety of causes. Its origin may be systemic, but local irritants and the inflammation they produce account for many of its clinical and microscopic features.

MENOPAUSAL GINGIVOSTOMATITIS (SENILE ATROPHIC GINGIVITIS)

This condition occurs during the menopause or in the postmenopausal period. Mild signs and symptoms sometimes appear associated with the earliest menopausal changes. Menopausal gingivostomatitis is not a common condition. Its designation has led to the erroneous impression that it invariably occurs associated with the menopause, whereas the opposite is true. Oral disturbances are not a common feature of the menopause.

Clinical features

The gingiva and remaining oral mucosa are *dry and shiny*, vary in color from abnormal paleness to redness, and bleed easily. There is fissuring in the mucobuccal fold in some cases,[40] and comparable changes may occur in the vaginal mucosa. The patient complains of a dry, burning sensation throughout the oral cavity, associated with *extreme sensitivity* to thermal changes, abnormal taste sensations described as "salty," "peppery" or "sour,"[31] and difficulty with removable partial prostheses.

Histopathology

Microscopically, the gingiva presents atrophy of the germinal and prickle cell layers of the epithelium and, in some instances, areas of ulceration.

When menopausal gingivostomatitis occurs in *edentulous patients*, they cannot tolerate dentures very well. Normally, when full dentures are inserted there is an initial period of adaptation of the oral mucosa.

Thickening of the epithelium is part of the physiologic adaptation that makes toleration of the denture possible. In patients with menopausal gingivostomatitis, the thin, atrophic epithelium offers very little protection. Consequently the oral mucosa bruises easily in the presence of even slight surface abrasion. Thickening of the epithelium to accommodate the denture does not develop because of the atrophic tendency governing the epithelium. As a result, the patient is continually uncomfortable, even with well-fitting dentures in proper functional relation. The outline of the denture is clearly demarcated by the fiery red and shiny appearance of the underlying sore mucosa.

The signs and symptoms of menopausal gingivostomatitis are in some degree comparable to those of chronic desquamative gingivitis. The prevailing opinion is that both these conditions arise from an atrophy and diminished keratinization of the oral epithelium associated with a diminution in estrogen or a disturbance in its utilization. Signs and symptoms similar to those of menopausal gingivostomatitis occasionally occur following ovariectomy or sterilization by radiation in the treatment of malignant neoplasms.

REFERENCES

1. Biro, S.: Studies Regarding the Influence of Pregnancy Upon Caries. Vierteljahr. f. Zahnheilk., *14*: 371, 1898.
2. Brewer, J. L.: Rhythmic Changes in the Skin Capillaries and their Relations to Menstruation. Am. J. Obst. & Gynec., *36*:597, 1938.
3. Brusati, R., and Bracchetti, A.: Electron Microscopic Study of Chronic Desquamative Gingivitis. J. Periodont.-Periodontics, *40*:388, 1969.
4. Burdine, J. T., and Friedman, L. A.: Horizontal Tooth Mobility and the Menstrual Cycle. I.A.D.R. Abstracts, 48th Annual Meeting, 1970, p. 64, #62.
5. Calman, L. R.: Pathology of the Oral Cavity. Baltimore, The Williams & Wilkins Co., 1941, p. 154.
6. Calman, A. S.: Oral Complications of Pregnancy. D. Outlook, *17*:2, 1930.
7. Cohen, M.: The Gingiva at Puberty. J. D. Res., *34*:679, 1955.
8. Cohen, D. W., Friedman, L., Shapiro, J., and Kyle, G. C.: A Longitudinal Investigation of the Periodontal Changes During Pregnancy. J. Periodont.-Periodontics, *40*:563, 1969.
9. Cohen, D. W., Shapiro, J., Friedman, L., and Kyle, G. C.: Periodontal Observations During Pregnancy and One Year Post Partum—II. I.A.D.R. Abstracts, 48th Annual Meeting, 1970, p. 63, #60.
10. Dayton, A. C.: Case of Metastasis of Menstrual

Secretion from the Uterus to Mouth. Am. J. D. Sc., 10:42, 1949.

11. El-Ashiry, G. M., et al.: Comparative Study of the Influence of Pregnancy and Oral Contraceptives on the Gingivae. Oral Surg., Oral Med. & Oral Path., 30:472, 475.

12. Engel, M. B.: Hormonal Gingivitis. J.A.D.A., 44:691, 1952.

13. Engel, M., Ray, H. G., and Orban, B.: The Pathogenesis of Desquamative Gingivitis. J. D. Res., 29:410, 1950.

14. Fraser, G. A.: Pregnancy Gingivitis. S. African D. J., 10:138, 1944.

15. Gans, B. J., Engel, M. B., and Joseph, N. R.: Electrometric Studies of Human Gingiva in Pregnancy. J. D. Res., 35:566, 1956.

16. Glickman, I., and Smulow, J. B.: Histopathology and Histochemistry of Chronic Desquamative Gingivitis. Oral Surg., Oral Med. & Oral Path., 21:325, 1966.

17. Heinemann, M., and Anderson, B. G.: Oral Manifestations of Certain Systemic Disorders. Yale J. Biol. & Med., 17:583, 1945.

18. Holm-Pedersen, P., and Löe, H.: Flow of Gingival Exudate as Related to Menstruation and Pregnancy. J. Periodont. Res., 2:13, 1967.

19. Hugoson, A.: Gingival Inflammation and Female Sex Hormones. J. Periodont. Res., Suppl. 5, 1970.

20. Jackson, H., Jr., and Merril, D.: Agranulocytic Angina Associated with the Menstrual Cycle. New England J. Med., 210:175, 1934.

21. Jones, O. V.: Cyclical Ulcerative Vulvitis and Stomatitis. J. Obst. & Gynæc. Brit. Emp., 47:557, 1940.

22. Knapp, E.: An Unusual Case of Periodontitis Marginalis Progressiva Chronica in a Thirteen Year Old Girl. Deutsch. Zahnärtz. Wochenschr., 38:1080, 1935.

23. Kutzleb, H. J.: Changes in the Oral Mucosa in Ovarian Disturbances. Deutsch. Zahnärtz. Wochenschr., 42:906, 1939.

24. Larato, D., Stahl, S., Brown, R., Jr., and Witkin, G.: The Effect of a Prescribed Method of Toothbrushing on the Fluctuation of Marginal Gingivitis. J. Periodont.-Periodontics, 40:142, 1969.

25. Lindhe, J., and Attström, R.: Gingival Exudation During the Menstrual Cycle. J. Periodont. Res., 2:194, 1967.

26. Lindhe, J., and Björn, A. L.: Influence of Hormonal Contraceptives on the Gingiva of Women. J. Periodont. Res., 2:1, 1967.

27. Lindhe, J., and Brånemark, P. I.: Changes in Microcirculation after Local Application of Sex Hormones. J. Periodont. Res., 2:185, 1967.

28. Löe, H.: Periodontal Changes in Pregnancy. J. Periodont., 36:209, 1965.

29. Looby, J. P.: cited by Burket, L. W.: Oral Medicine. Philadelphia, J. B. Lippincott Co., 1946, p. 294.

30. Maier, A. W., and Orban, B.: Gingivitis in Pregnancy. Oral Surg., Oral Med. & Oral Path., 2:234, 1949.

31. Massler, M., and Henry, J.: Oral Manifestations

During the Female Climacteric. The Alpha Omegan, p. 105, Sept. 1950.

32. McCarthy, F. P., McCarthy, P. L., and Shklar, G.: Chronic Desquamative Gingivitis: A Reconsideration. Oral Surg., Oral Med. & Oral Path., 13:1300, 1960.

33. Monash, S.: Proliferative Gingivitis of Pregnancy. Surg., Gynec. & Oral Obst., 42:794, 1926.

34. Muhlemann, H. R.: Gingivitis Intermenstrualis. Schweiz. Monatschr. f. Zahnh., 58:865, 1948.

35. Oles, R.: Chronic Desquamative Gingivitis. J. Periodont., 38:485, 1967.

36. Pappworth, M. H.: Cyclical Mucosal Ulceration. Brit. M. J., 1:271, 1941.

37. Prinz, H.: Chronic Diffuse Desquamative Gingivitis. D. Cosmos, 74:331, 1932.

38. Prout, R. E. S., and Hopps, R. M.: A Relationship Between Human Oral Bacteria and the Menstrual Cycle. J. Periodont., 41:98, 1970.

39. Rateitschak, K. H.: Tooth Mobility Changes in Pregnancy. J. Periodont. Res., 2:199, 1967.

40. Richman, M. J., and Abarbanel, A. R.: Effects of Estradiol, Testosterone, Diethylstilbestrol and Several of their Derivatives Upon the Human Mucous Membrane. J.A.D.A., 30:913, 1943.

41. Ringsdorf, W. M., Powell, B. J., Knight, L. A., and Cheraskin, E.: Periodontal Status and Pregnancy. Am. J. Obst. & Gynec., 83:258, 1962.

42. Schour, I.: Endocrines and Teeth. J.A.D.A., 21:322, 1934.

43. Scopp, I. W.: Desquamative Gingivitis. J. Periodont., 35:149, 1964.

44. Shelmire, B.: Certain Diseases of Oral Mucous Membrane and Vermilion Border of Lips. Internat. J. Orthodont., 14:817, 1928.

45. Stern, I. B.: Electron Microscopic Observations of Desquamative Gingivitis. I.A.D.R. Abstracts, 48th Annual Meeting, 1970, p. 199, #602.

46. Stoloff, C. I.: Periodic Transitory Meno-gingivitis Incidental in Women: A New Non-Pathological Classification of Gingival Disturbance. J. D. Res., 13:190, 1933.

47. Tomes, J.: A System of Dental Surgery. Revised by Tomes, C. S. L., 4th edition. P. Blackiston's Son and Company, 1897, p. 638.

48. Turesky, S., Fisher, B., and Glickman, I.: A Histochemical Study of the Attached Gingiva in Pregnancy. J. D. Res., 37:1115, 1958.

49. Whitten, J., Jr.: The Fine Structure of Desquamative Stomatitis. J. Periodont., 39:75, 1968.

50. Ziserman, A. J.: Ulcerative Vulvitis and Stomatitis of Endocrine Origin. J.A.M.A., 104:826, 1935.

51. Ziskin, D. E., and Blackberg, S. N.: A Study of the Gingivae During Pregnancy. J. D. Res., 13:253, 1933.

52. Ziskin, D. E., Blackberg, S. N., and Stout, A.: The Gingivae During Pregnancy; An Experimental Study and a Histopathological Interpretation. Surg., Gynec. & Obst., 57:719, 1933.

53. Ziskin, D. E., and Nesse, G. J.: Pregnancy Gingivitis, History, Classification, Etiology. Am. J. Orth. & Oral Surg., 32:390, 1946.

Chapter 13

THE ORAL MUCOSA IN DERMATOLOGIC DISEASE[*]

---

[*]Original draft by Francis P. McCarthy, M.D., and Philip L. McCarthy, M.D.

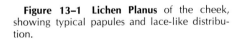

Oral and skin lesions often occur together in dermatologic disease.[34] Furthermore, changes in the oral cavity may mark the onset of the disease and precede the skin lesions by months or years. In many conditions such as lichen planus, erythema multiforme and pyostomatitis vegetans, oral lesions may constitute the only manifestation. Oral manifestations in the absence of skin involvement often result from drugs capable of causing dermatoses. Gingival involvement in dermatologic disorders presents a challenging diagnostic and therapeutic problem.

LICHEN PLANUS (LICHEN RUBER PLANUS)

Lichen planus is an inflammatory disease of the skin characterized by glistening violaceous angulated papules. When the disease is confined to the skin it may be acute, subacute or chronic; oral involvement is usually chronic. The etiology is not known, but psychosomatic factors seem to be involved in a large percentage of cases.

Oral lesions

Lichen planus may occur only in the oral cavity or on the skin, but in most cases lesions eventually develop in both locations.[49] Frictional factors play a role in determining the location of these lesions. The most common locations are the buccal mucosa in relation to the occlusal plane of the teeth, the tongue, the facial surface of the gingiva, hard palate and lower lip.[1] **The lesions are usually symmetrical and tend to be dendritic and papular. The dendritic lesions consist of grayish white, linear, lacelike elevations composed of individual papules (Figs. 13–1 to 13–3).**

The papules are usually the size of a pinhead. The lesions frequently present erosion at the sites of frictional trauma. These

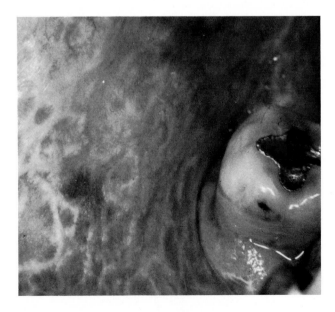

Figure 13–1 Lichen Planus of the cheek, showing typical papules and lace-like distribution.

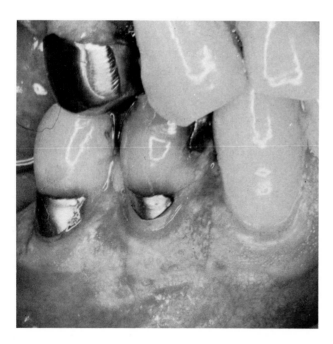

Figure 13–2 Lichen Planus of the gingiva with prominent papules.

areas are bright red, and apt to cause symptoms such as dryness and pain.

Bullous or vesicular lichen planus is a less common form of the disease. Although often confined to the skin or oval cavity, it may involve both. The initial oral involvement may be papular and dendritic, or occur as *vesicular* or *bullous* lesions that are soon followed by the characteristic minute papules with linear markings. **The bullae rupture, with the formation of bright red,**

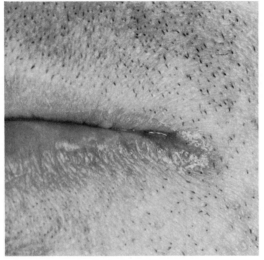

Figure 13–3 Lichen Planus at the labial commissure showing typical papules.

eroded lesions that are extremely painful and easily irritated by hot or spicy foods. The disease tends to run a chronic or subacute course, with eroded lesions involving the buccal mucosa, tongue, lips and gingiva. The duration varies from several months to many years.

Histopathology

Microscopically, lichen planus is characterized by thickening of the epithelium, leukocytic infiltration in the immediately subjacent connective tissue and associated degenerative changes in the basal portion of the epithelium. The thickened epithelium presents hyperkeratosis and acanthosis (Fig. 13–4). There is hydropic degeneration with intra- and intercellular edema and leukocytic infiltration in the basal portion of the epithelium and destruction of the basement membrane. In the underlying connective tissue there is a dense lymphocytic infiltration, characteristically confined to a broad zone immediately beneath the epithelium. Involvement of the epithelium by inflammatory cells and fluid results in epithelial degeneration and a partial obliteration of the clear-cut demarcation between the epithelium and connective tissue (Fig. 13–5). In cases of pronounced edema, liquefaction of the ruptured epithelial cells results in vesicle formation.

Fig. 13–4

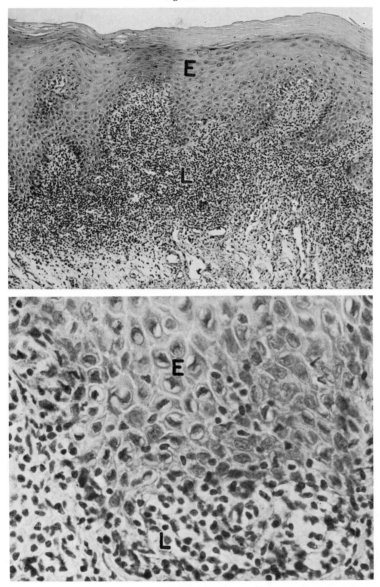

Fig. 13–5

Figure 13–4   Microscopic Appearance of Lichen Planus. Biopsy from lesion on the gingiva showing hyperkeratosis and acanthosis of the epithelium (E). There is dense lymphocytic infiltration of the lamina propria (L) confined to a broad zone immediately beneath the epithelium.

Figure 13–5   High power view of Fig. 13–4 showing edema and degeneration in the basal portion of the epithelium (E) with leukocytic infiltration in the lamina propria (L).

Electron microscopic studies indicate that lichen planus can be divided into three stages. The earliest stage is degeneration of the cytoplasm of the epithelial cells with aggregation of particulate material. The intercellular spaces are enlarged, accompanied by lymphocytic infiltration. In the second stage there is loss of collagen fibers in the superficial lamina propria. The final stage shows degeneration and necrosis of the basal and lower spinous layers of the epithelium with the exception of the desmosomes, which are for the most part structurally unaltered. The superficial lamina propria is also degenerated and necrotic and the basement lamina is no longer visible. Secondary bacterial involvement of the necrotic tissue is often observed.[55]

Differential diagnosis

Among the conditions to be considered in the differential diagnosis of lichen planus are linear leukoplakia, lupus erythematosus, pemphigus vulgaris and benign mucous membrane pemphigus.

LINEAR LEUKOPLAKIA. Leukoplakia occurs in patches (Fig. 13–6) of varied size or in linear form. The linear lesions are usually asymmetrical and may show erythematous margins, but they require microscopic study to differentiate them from lichen planus. A local cause can usually be demonstrated, such as friction from faulty occlusion or irritation from tobacco or a dental appliance.

WHITE SPONGE NEVUS (WHITE FOLDED GINGIVOSTOMATITIS). This is a benign, painless familial condition which may be present at birth or appear during childhood. It occurs in the oral cavity in both males and females, with rectal and/or vaginal involvement. The surface of the oral mucosa is white, thickened and in minute folds with papillary projections (Fig. 13–7). Involvement may be patchy or generalized.

Microscopically, the epithelium is thickened and parakeratotic with vacuolization of cells and pyknotic nuclei. There is moderate plasma cell and lymphocytic infiltration of the underlying connective tissue.

LUPUS ERYTHEMATOSUS. Since skin lesions are present in practically all of these cases, the differential diagnosis should be made readily, but in the rare instance of a purely oral case of lupus erythematosus, biopsy is necessary for accurate diagnosis.

PEMPHIGUS VULGARIS. Pemphigus vulgaris may simulate chronic oral bullous lichen planus. In *pemphigus* the lesions tend to *heal* and *recur* while in *lichen planus* they tend to *remain fixed*. Diagnosis is confirmed by biopsy.

BENIGN MUCOUS MEMBRANE PEMPHIGUS (PEMPHIGOID). See page 165.

Treatment

Lichen planus tends to resist treatment, and oral lesions may persist for years. The

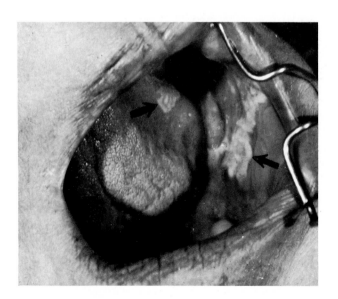

Figure 13–6 Leukoplakia of the buccal mucosa and lateral aspect of tongue. Note raised white lesions.

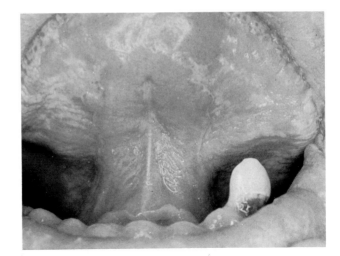

Figure 13–7 White Sponge Nevus (white folded gingivostomatitis), showing thickened epithelium with minute surface folds on the tongue and lips.

possibility of psychogenic etiology should be explored. Bismuth (sodium bismuth triglycollamate), two tablets three times daily, is a popular form of treatment, but a toxic reaction with gastrointestinal upset and headache occurs in some cases. Tranquilizing drugs, vitamins and antibiotics have also been used with some success. Corticosteroids, systemically and topically applied, afford symptomatic relief of bullous lesions.

PEMPHIGUS

Pemphigus is an acute or chronic skin disease that usually presents oral lesions. Of the several types of the condition, pemphigus vulgaris is the most common.

Pemphigus Vulgaris[13]

The duration of the disease varies and is apt to be more chronic in older persons. A typical case of pemphigus runs a course of several years with periods of spontaneous remission, and is characterized by successive crops of bullae, which tend to heal in the early stages of the disease and leave pigmented macular areas.

The etiology is unknown, but it has been suggested that autoimmunity may be a factor. The intercellular antibodies in pemphigus are autoantibodies, which have also been demonstrated before the appearance of the characteristic lesion, and the severity of the lesions is proportional to the autoantibody titer.[7]

Oral lesions

The oral lesions of pemphigus vulgaris may precede the skin lesions by as much as two years or longer,[14] or may occur later in the disease. **The characteristic picture is that of *primary bullous lesions* in the mucous membrane. The thin-walled lesions rupture promptly, leaving a raw area that is subsequently covered with a *membranous exudate* (Fig. 13–8).**

The initial bullae are usually as large as the thumb nail. In the early stages of the disease, they tend to be discrete and few; individual lesions usually heal within ten days to two weeks. As the disease progresses, the oral lesions coalesce with deeper ulcerations, so that relatively little

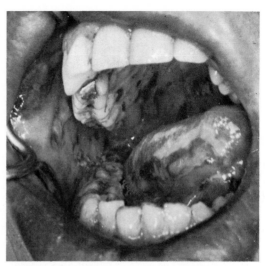

Figure 13–8 Pemphigus of the oral cavity. (Courtesy of Dr. Kurt H. Thoma.)

normal mucosa remains. Involvement of the pharynx, larynx and trachea may ensue. Pain is severe; chewing and swallowing are extremely difficult.

Histopathology

The microscopic picture in pemphigus vulgaris is diagnostic. *Acantholysis and intraepithelial vesicles are the pathognomonic changes (Fig. 13-9).* **Suprabasal clefts are created in the epithelium. The basal layer remains attached to the connective tissue, which is inflamed.**

Electron microscopic studies indicate breakdown of the epithelial intercellular cement substance as the first stage in the development of acantholysis (Figs. 13-9 and 13-10);[23] **others feel that the destruction starts in the tonofilaments**[56] **or the desmosomes.**[9]

Differential diagnosis

The oral lesions of erythema multiforme are frequently similar to those seen in pemphigus. In the former condition, however, there are recurrent active episodes of comparatively short duration followed by long intervals without skin or oral lesions.

Bullous lichen planus must also be considered in the differential diagnosis. The primary lesion of pemphigus may be of a bullous character, followed by erosion with associated pain and discomfort. In lichen planus, however, the *characteristic dendritic lesions are always found associated with the bullae.* Biopsy studies are usually sufficient to differentiate this condition from pemphigus.

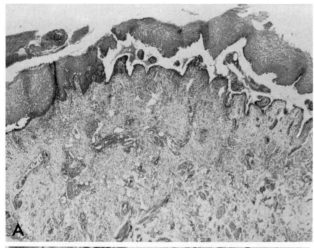

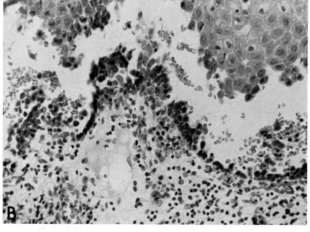

Figure 13-9 Pemphigus Vulgaris. *A,* Oral mucosa showing acantholysis and intra-epithelial vesicle. *B,* Detailed view of intra-epithelial vesicle in pemphigus.

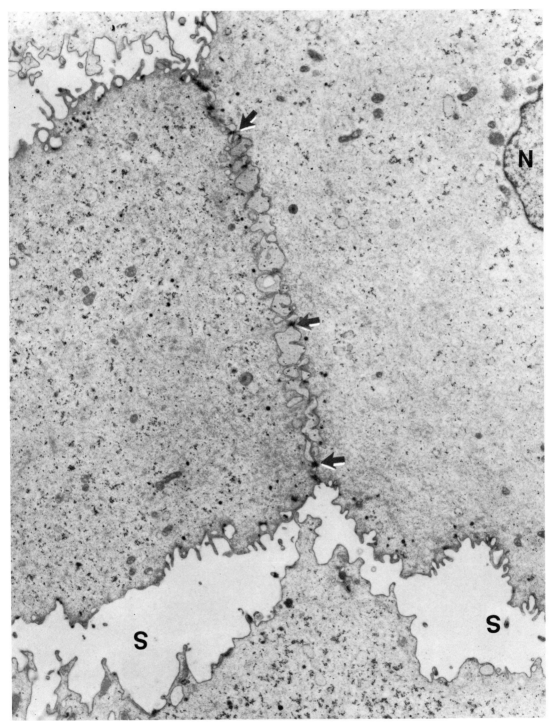

Figure 13–10   Oral Pemphigus Vulgaris. Cellular junctions are disrupted and adjoining cells are detached except for one junction which is still connected through remaining desmosomes (arrows). S = Spaces between disrupted cells; N = nucleus. ×8500. (Courtesy of Dr. K. Hashimoto.)

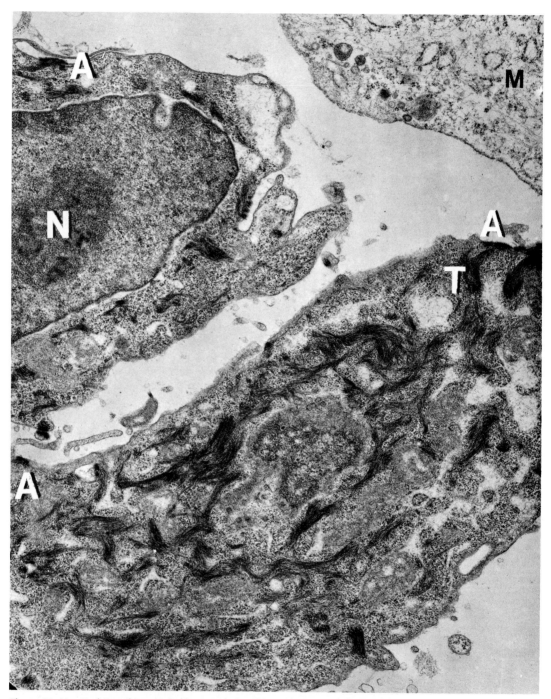

Figure 13–11 Oral Pemphigus Vulgaris. Acantholysed keratinocytes. In spite of disruption of cell to cell junction and detachment of desmosomes, cell membranes are intact and tonofibrils (T) are still attached to the attachment plaques (A) of acantholyzed desmosomes. M = Migrating macrophage; N = nucleus. ×20,000. (Courtesy of Dr. K. Hashimoto.)

Prognosis and treatment

Patients can be maintained and the lesion controlled with systemic corticosteroids, but the drug side effects may be severe.

Pemphigus Vegetans

Pemphigus vegetans may be considered a subacute form of pemphigus vulgaris with comparable but somewhat less severe clinical features. This form of the disease may be confined to the oral cavity for several weeks or months before the skin is involved. In the vegetative type of pemphigus, oral lesions dominate the picture, with crusted lesions of the skin being seen in intertriginous areas.

BENIGN MUCOUS MEMBRANE PEMPHIGUS (PEMPHIGOID)

This rare condition resembles pemphigus vulgaris clinically, but its microscopic appearance differentiates it from the true pemphigus group. For this reason the term *pemphigoid* has been suggested.[30] It is characterized by *bullous lesions* confined to the oral mucous membrane. Ocular and vaginal lesions sometimes accompany the oral changes. Skin lesions are not common.[48] The disease begins as *flaccid bullae that rupture* and leave slowly healing erosions.

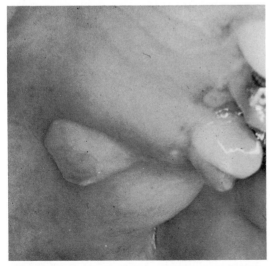

Figure 13–12 Benign Mucous Membrane Pemphigus (Pemphigoid) showing bulla on the palate.

It differs from pemphigus vulgaris in that the oral lesions are milder but may be intermittent and of many years duration.

There is usually widespread involvement of the marginal and attached gingiva, and in some instances other areas of the oral mucosa (Figs. 13–12 and 13–13). The gingiva presents a diffuse redness, may or may not be painful, and bleeds readily. The epithelium can be separated from the underlying inflamed connective tissue by a blast of warm air or with an instrument. The symptoms and the severity of oral involvement undergo unexplained remissions and exacerbations. Oral hygiene is impaired, and chronic gingivitis complicates the clinical picture.

Histopathology

The microscopic appearance is nonspecific but differs from the true pemphigus group. It is characterized by dense leukocytic infiltration of the connective tissue. There is subepithelial vesicle formation and separation of the epithelium from the inflamed connective tissue. The epithelium is degenerated, but acantholysis and intraepithelial vesicles observed in pemphigus vulgaris are not present. In areas without bullae the epithelium is thinned and presents varying degrees of degeneration.

Treatment

The etiology is unknown. Systemic corticosteroid therapy may be effective, but sometimes only partially so, and the drug side effects may be more troublesome than the oral lesions. Oral lesions tend to be more resistant to therapy than those on the skin.[47]

Topical corticosteroid ointments (Kenalog), reduce the symptomatology, partly by their protective action, but the effects cannot be predicted. Temporary relief from pain, particularly to enable the patient to eat, can be obtained from the use of 0.5 per cent Dyclone (dyclonin hydrochloride), diluted one half with water, as a mouth wash. The anesthetic effect usually lasts 40 minutes or longer.[54]

The condition is considerably improved by eliminating the complicating effects of marginal gingival inflammation caused by local irritation. Local periodontal therapy is indicated for this purpose. Attention

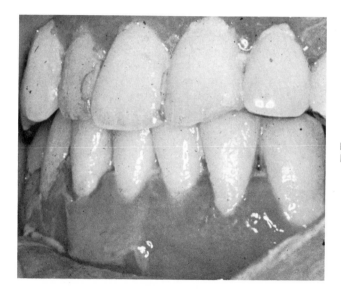

Figure 13–13 Benign Mucous Membrane Pemphigus. Note remnant of ruptured bullous lesion in lower left area.

should be given to the fit and design of removable prostheses. Slight irritation from such appliances results in exaggerated ulcerations.

ERYTHEMA MULTIFORME

Erythema multiforme is an acute inflammatory eruptive disease involving the skin and oral cavity. More than 80 per cent of the patients with skin involvement present oral lesions,[8] and in rare instances it may be confined to the mouth.[32] **The pathognomonic skin lesions are of a target or iris variety with a *central vesicle* or *bulla* surrounded by an *urticarial zone*.**

Erythema multiforme is usually a *recurrent disease*. It may be ushered in with fever preceded by a chill, and the duration of the average episode is from ten days to several weeks. The frequency of involvement varies from three or more attacks per year to a single attack every few years.

Oral lesions

The oral lesions consist of *purplish red macules* or *papules* with interspersed *bullous lesions*. The *tongue* usually presents *severe involvement*, with erosion of the bullae followed by ulceration. The lesions are painful so that chewing and swallowing are impaired.

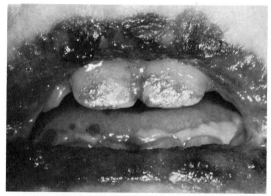

Fig. 13–14

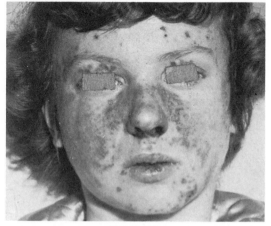

Fig. 13–15

Figure 13–14 Stevens-Johnson Syndrome. Note the crusting of the lips and vesicular eruption on the tongue.

Figure 13–15 Lupus Erythematosus showing butterfly distribution of lesions on the face and crusting of the lips.

Microscopically, there is liquefaction degeneration of the upper epithelium with the development of intra-epithelial vesicles, without acantholysis which occurs in pemphigus. Degenerative changes also occur in the basement membrane.[46]

Treatment

There is no specific treatment. Steroid therapy suppresses the symptoms while the disease runs its course.

The Stevens-Johnson Syndrome

The Stevens-Johnson syndrome is a rare form of erythema multiforme, characterized by *erythematous, hemorrhagic*, and *bullous lesions*. The oral cavity, conjunctivae and genitals are involved as well as other areas of the skin (Fig. 13–14). This hemorrhagic type of erythema multiforme is associated with high fever and prostration, and may be fatal in a small percentage of cases. The oral lesions appear as purpuric vesicles or bullae. Suppurating superficial and deep erosions of the gingiva are also seen.

Treatment

Steroid therapy is the treatment of choice.

LUPUS ERYTHEMATOSUS

Lupus erythematosus, one of the so-called collagen diseases,[25] may be divided into a *chronic discoid type* and an *acute disseminated type*. The incidence of oral involvement in lupus erythematosus varies, depending upon the acuteness of the disease. Although not more than 10 per cent of the chronic discoid type present oral lesions, as many as 75 per cent of the acute disseminated type have some oral manifestation before death. The *characteristic "butterfly" distribution* of the lesions *on the face* is a diagnostic aid in this disease (Fig. 13–15). Lupus erythematosus may occur on the oral mucous membrane without skin lesions in extremely rare instances.

Chronic discoid type[19, 39]

In the oral cavity the disease appears as *well-defined, slightly elevated* and *in-filtrated lesions* with a *bluish or dark red areola*.[42] The lesions are usually localized and are seen more often on the buccal mucosa. At the border of the lesion there may be numerous dilated blood vessels having a radial arrangement extending into the surrounding tissue, coupled with whitish pin-head papules. In the early stages, the center of the lesion is slightly depressed and eroded, and covered with a bluish red epithelial surface showing scarring. In older lesions, the erythematous border becomes less elevated and is transformed into a whitish or bluish white peripheral zone of thickened epithelium. The dilated vessels are replaced by white lines having the same diverging radial arrangement. On the tongue the disease occurs as circumscribed, smooth, reddened areas in which the papillae are lost, or as patches with whitish sheen resembling leukoplakia.

On the lip, the lesions are somewhat similar to those in the mouth and, in most cases, the lip is involved by direct extension from perioral skin lesions. Localized patches may be present or the entire lip may be involved. Early in the disease, the lip is swollen, bluish red, and often everted. The lip lesions may be covered with adherent scales and crusts remaining localized and rarely diffuse (Fig. 13–15). At the margins of the patches, dilated capillaries or fine branching radial lines may be seen. The lip is tender and sensitive and on removal of the adherent scales, bleeding from the raw surface is noted. Depressed scars may follow the healed deeper lesions.

Microscopically, the epithelial changes in the chronic discoid type consists of keratinization, keratotic plugging, acanthosis, atrophy, pseudocarcinomatous hyperplasia and liquefaction degeneration of the basal cell layer.[2]

Periods of activity and quiescence occur. The lesions enlarge by peripheral extension, accompanied by the occurrence of fresh erosions and superficial ulcerations, followed by atrophic changes. Some burning sensation occurs in the erosions and deeper ulcerations.

Acute disseminated type

In the disseminated variety, the oral lesions are more *acute*, and *greater destruction* occurs. The lesions are characterized by soft, irregular, superficial or moderately deep erosions, usually covered with a necrotic, grayish pseudomembrane.

Differential diagnosis

Diagnosis usually depends upon the identification of the accompanying skin lesions. The diagnosis of discoid lupus erythematosus confined to the oral cavity is very difficult to make, even by microscopic examination. The acute disseminated variety may present a variety of oral lesions that are essentially nonspecific and erosive in nature. *Erythema multiforme* and *pemphigus* may sometimes appear quite similar. Biopsy, although not definitive, will aid in differentiating between *lupus erythematosus* and *erosive leukoplakia* or *lichen planus.*

Treatment

The treatment of lupus erythematosus is nonspecific. Systemic bismuth and gold have been used in the past. Corticotropin (ACTH) and corticosteroids are used currently for the systemic varieties of the disease, and the antimalarial drugs are very

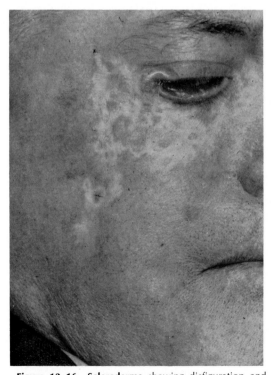

Figure 13–16 Scleroderma showing disfiguration and induration of the skin.

successful in controlling the chronic discoid variety, but in disseminated lupus erythematosus these drugs have no effect.

SCLERODERMA

Scleroderma[41, 53] is characterized by a primary induration and edema of the skin in localized patches or diffuse areas, and later with atrophy and pigmentation (Fig. 13–16). There are three distinct forms: diffuse scleroderma, acrosclerosis and circumscribed scleroderma (morphea). The etiology is obscure, although it is considered by many investigators to be of neurotrophic origin. In all types of the disease the first sign is usually a moderate induration of the skin gradually followed by the atrophic stage, which results in permanent disfiguration. Ulceration can occur, but it is rare and is seen only in advanced cases. Hemiatrophy is fairly common in cases of facial involvement, sometimes being accompanied by false ankylosis of the temporomandibular joint.

Oral lesions[4, 10, 33]

The diffuse and acrosclerotic types frequently involve the oral cavity. Although the entire mucous membrane may be involved, it is the tongue that is most commonly observed to show pathologic changes, followed in frequency by the buccal mucosa and gingiva. There may be painful induration of the tongue and gingiva.[45] The usual symptom is a minor speech defect due to impaired mobility of the tongue. The progress of scleroderma of the mucous membranes is chronic, but reportedly more rapid than that of the skin lesions.

In the acrosclerotic variety, the lips become thin and rigid, and their movements are greatly restricted. The opening of the oral cavity is usually materially reduced. Difficulty in eating and talking may follow. Obliterative endarteritis may result in avascularity with increased susceptibility to infection.[17]

In acrosclerosis and diffuse scleroderma, Stafne and Austin[50] have described a characteristic roentgenographic picture consisting of an increase in the width of the periodontal space. This widening was found in 8 of 127 cases of acrosclerosis and in one case of diffuse scleroderma, with the findings much less marked in the latter condition. In acrosclerosis the authors noted that the amount of widening varies. All of the teeth may not be affected, and the posterior teeth are involved more often than the anterior teeth. Radiographically the periodontal space in relation to the entire root is widened to an almost uniform thickness.[38] The increase in width of the periodontal spaces occurs at the expense of the alveolar bone. The lamina dura is obliterated. Clinically the teeth are firm. **Microscopically, the continuity of the periodontal fibers from the cementum to the alveolar bone is broken near the cementum.**

Treatment

There is no effective treatment; however, use of an immunosuppressive agent (Azathioprine) has been described.[24]

PYOSTOMATITIS VEGETANS

This rare disease may be confined to the oral cavity or associated with skin lesions.

Oral lesions

In the oral cavity the primary lesions appear as *multiple small pustules* with a *yellowish tip* and a *reddened base*[35] (Fig. 13–17). The process spreads within a very few weeks to involve the entire oral cavity and creates a diffuse granular surface. As the oral lesions become chronic, the buccal mucosa proliferates to form folds, and the miliary abscesses are found on the summits of the rugae and in the deep invaginations. Oral involvement is accompanied by a mild degree of pain.

Histopathology

Microscopically, there is pronounced hyperkeratosis and acanthosis with broadening and elongation of the rete pegs (Fig. 13–18). The connective tissue presents a granulomatous inflammatory process with unruptured miliary abscesses. Degeneration of the epithelium and focal areas of surface necrosis are also seen.

Treatment

The disease tends to be chronic and resistant to therapy. Because it is frequently associated with an ulcerative colitis, both of these conditions must be treated simultaneously. Iron, liver and vitamin therapy are of value, but no specific therapy has been discovered to date.

EPIDERMOLYSIS BULLOSA DYSTROPHICA

This is a rare hereditary disease characterized by generalized bullous eruption involving the skin and oral mucosa. Dys-

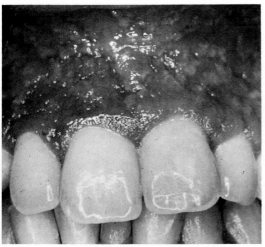

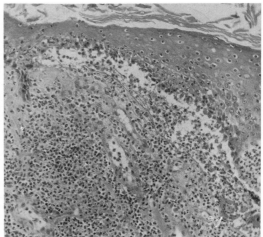

Fig. 13–17   Fig. 13–18

Figure 13–17   Pyostomatitis Vegetans. Multiple small abscesses create granular appearance of the gingiva and adjacent mucosa.

Figure 13–18   Pyostomatitis Vegetans, section showing hyperkeratosis of the epithelium and granulomatous inflammation in the connective tissue.

trophic changes occur in the nails, and enamel formation is defective.

The slightest friction or trauma is followed by the development of large bullae, which rupture, ulcerate and form a scar. The oral lesions are apt to be constant, serious and complicated by inflammatory periodontal changes. Toothbrushing, hard foods and dental care precipitate the eruption of bullae. Mobility of the tongue may be impaired by scar tissue, and cicatricial bands in the oropharynx may interfere with deglutition. Several variants of the disease have been described.[31]

Microscopically, bullae occur deep in the epidermis or at the junction with the underlying connective tissue. Elastic tissue is reduced or absent, and the connective tissue is moderately inflamed. Leukoplakia and carcinoma are described as possible sequelae of mucous membrane bullae.[40]

Treatment

There is no specific treatment.

DERMATOMYOSITIS

Dermatomyositis is a rare acute, subacute or chronic disease of unknown etiology characterized by muscle pains and weakness, edema, dermatitis and inflammation and degeneration of muscles. Any skeletal muscle may become involved, including the tongue, and extreme tenderness, pain and weakness may be noted. Edema may be a prominent feature during the early stages of the disease; atrophy is a late manifestation. **Various forms of stomatitis have been described, ranging from diffuse erosive processes to lesions indistinguishable from lupus erythematosus.** The course of the disease is extremely variable, ranging from a rapidly fatal variety to chronic forms that may undergo spontaneous remission.

Treatment

Corticosteroid therapy is used for the disease.

SYPHILIS

Syphilis is a chronic, specific infection of the body by the spirochete, *Treponema*

pallidum, which results in many cutaneous and mucous membrane manifestations. The disease is divided into the following stages.

Primary Stage

This stage is marked by the appearance of the chancre and ends with its disappearance. The chancre or primary lesion of syphilis develops at the point of inoculation, usually in a period of two to six weeks after entrance of the spirochete.

From 5 to 10 per cent of chancres are found in places other than on the genitalia, and about 70 per cent of these extragenital lesions are found on the lips or within the oral cavity. The lips are more frequently involved and multiple primary lesions may occur.

Oral lesions

Lip and intra-oral chancres *vary from small, slightly indurated lesions to deep indolent ulcerations.* Chancres of the oral cavity may be divided into two general types: erosive and ulcerative. Lymph node enlargement is noted in the cervical region, and if the lesion is in or near the median line, the cervical adenopathy may be bilateral. The ulcerative type of mucous membrane chancre may vary from a relatively small ulcer the size of a fingernail, to a large ulcerating nodule. The base and border of the lesion are markedly indurated, and there may be evidence of secondary pyogenic infection.

These lesions tend to have an adherent crust when present on the lip, but within the oral cavity they show a broad, ulcerating, granulating surface. **As a rule, the primary lesion is relatively painless, but those with associated secondary infection may be very tender and painful.**

On the *tongue* the chancre is more often located near the tip and is usually markedly indurated and shows early ulceration. Chancre of the gingiva is comparatively rare. It appears as an indurated ulcer, which may be covered with a pseudomembrane (Fig. 13–19). Recession of the gingival tissue exposing the tooth root occurs if the lesions begin at the gingival margin. Chancres of the gingiva may also be of the nodular type, with superficial erosion varying in size from that of a split pea to larger

Fig. 13–19

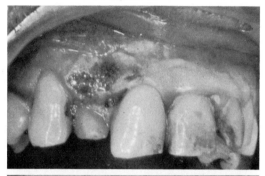

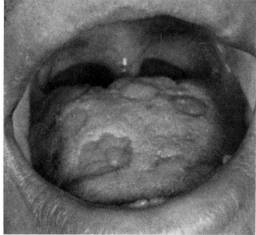

Fig. 13–20

Figure 13–19   Primary Stage of Syphilis. Chancre of the gingiva.

Figure 13–20   Secondary Stage of Syphilis. Patchy denudation of the tongue.

lesions, involving the gingiva in relation to several teeth.

Differential diagnosis

In *differential diagnosis* one should consider the possibility of an *aphthous lesion* that has been secondarily infected or aggravated by overtreatment with chemical irritants. *Epidermoid carcinoma* also may resemble a chancre, but these lesions do not show cervical lymph node enlargement in the early stage.

Darkfield examination of the deep serum from the chancre reveals *Treponema pallidum* if no specific medication has previously been given. One should not rely on darkfield examination of intraoral lesions, as normally occurring spirochetes may be very difficult to differentiate from *T. pallidum.*

Chancre of the gingiva tends to grow rapidly and is apt to be more painful than the slower growing tubercular lesions.

Secondary Stage

The secondary stage is characterized by *cutaneous eruption* and *mucous patches* in the *oral cavity.* The mucous patch is the most *contagious lesion of syphilis,* as its surface is covered with an abundance of spirochetes. *Accidental infection* of the *dentist's fingers* may occur in untreated cases of syphilis with active mucous patches. Mucous patches are slightly elevated, well demarcated, gray-white lesions with a smooth glistening surface surrounded by an erythematous margin.

There is a *macular type of syphilid* involving the oral cavity early in the secondary stage, which represents a manifestation of the generalized skin eruption. The tongue and palate are most commonly involved, but the *tongue shows the more classic picture of this type of lesion* (Fig. 13–20). These lesions are seen on the tongue as *reddish, round, multiple, symmetrical nonindurated plaques.* Slow denudation of the normal coating of the tongue occurs with shedding of the filiform papillae. The lesions are usually smooth and nonerosive early in their development, and may assume a grayish color and either disappear or develop into a true mucous patch.

A papular type of syphilid is a rare form seen on the dorsum of the tongue or the external commissures of the labial orifice. These lesions are about the size of a split pea, and at the angles of the mouth show a split arrangement with one half of the papule on the upper lip and the other half on the lower lip. Such lesions must be differentiated from the common intertrigo labialis or maceration due to other causes.

Differential diagnosis

Among the lesions to be considered in the differential diagnosis of mucous patches are the denuded areas found on the tongue in *glossitis areata migrans (geographical tongue).* In this condition, the individual lesions are characterized by a slight, yellowish, peripheral margin, and tend to clear and reappear at new areas from day to day.

Acute necrotizing ulcerative inflammation produces localized necrotic and gangrenous lesions. In rare cases, acute necrotizing ulcerative inflammation may be superimposed upon a secondary syphilitic mucous patch and confuse the diagnosis. Severe *aphthous stomatitis* with deep lesions is found in the *periadenitis necrotica* type, which may simulate erosive secondary syphilis.

Tertiary Stage

The tertiary stage of syphilis includes visceral, cutaneous and oral lesions. The two types of tertiary luetic infection in the oral cavity are gummatous and interstitial. Both conditions tend to leave secondary changes, namely, perforations of the hard and soft palate and atrophic interstitial glossitis respectively.

THE GUMMATOUS REACTION. The *tongue* is a common site of a single or multiple gummatous process (Fig. 13–21). **The gumma is characterized by a growth of epithelioid tissue in which the spirochete is absent. It usually develops slowly as a relatively painless nodule that may grow to a rather large mass.** It tends to ulcerate, with the production of a thick sanguineous secretion. Healing of the gumma results in the formation of cicatricial tissue, producing a lobulated appearance of the tongue, known as *lingua lobulata.* Other locations of gummata are the *hard and soft palate.*

THE INTERSTITIAL REACTION. More commonly, the tongue is involved in a *sclerosing process*, with the development of the atrophic glossitis of tertiary syphilis referred to as "bald tongue." **The tongue is smooth, red and glistening in its entirety or may present isolated patches of normal papillae.** The tongue may be shriveled, owing to replacement of the musculature by connective tissue.

The production of this lesion may be explained by a sequence of related pathologic changes. The tongue, a mobile organ subject to mild trauma, receives a large dose of spirochetes in the secondary stage, and if the disease is untreated or inadequately treated, **endarteritis of the smaller vessels results. Later, owing to the interstitial sclerosing process, together with the resulting decrease in the blood supply, the papillae undergo atrophy with the production of patchy smooth bald areas on the surface.** *Leukoplakia* is a common secondary feature, usually as the result of irritation from the products of combustion and heat from smoking. Because the leukoplakic lesions may undergo malignant change, the incidence of carcinoma of the tongue in patients with syphilitic glossitis is high (Fig. 13–22).

Histopathology

The gumma appears microscopically as a granulomatous process with epithelioid tissue and giant cells and areas of coagulation necrosis. The *T. pallidum* is not demonstrable in the lesion. The diagnosis is confirmed by serologic tests.

Biopsy of syphilitic interstitial glossitis reveals a wide subepithelial zone in which there is disorganization of the musculature caused by an interstitial proliferation of connective tissue. Marked narrowing of the lumina of the efferent arteries is also noted. Atrophy of the epithelial surface and filiform papillae is pronounced in the smooth areas noted clinically on the surface of the tongue.

Congenital Syphilis

In congenital syphilis, acute moist papules with fissuring may occur at the ex-

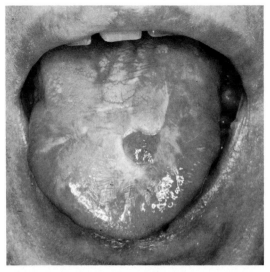

Figure 13–21   Gumma and Leukoplakia of the Tongue.

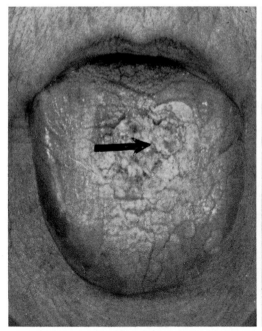

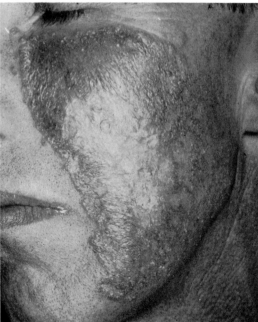

Fig. 13–22   Fig. 13–23

Figure 13–22   Tertiary Stage of Syphilis. Interstitial glossitis with verrucous epidermoid carcinoma (*arrow*).
Figure 13–23   Lupus Vulgaris.

ternal labial commissures with subsequent healing and scarring and the formation of *radiating "ragades."* The Hutchinson incisor with the characteristic notching is another oral feature of congenital syphilis. The *deformed central incisor, interstitial keratitis* and *deafness* comprise *Hutchinson's triad of congenital syphilis.* These do not always occur together but one or more features are usually demonstrable with other manifestations of congenital syphilis such as "saddle nose" or "saber shins."

TUBERCULOSIS

Tuberculous involvement of the oral cavity is relatively rare and seen more often in males. Although the lesions may involve any area of the oral mucous membrane, the site of involvement is usually the tongue.

Tuberculous lesions of the oral cavity include (1) lupus vulgaris, (2) tuberculous ulcer, (3) disseminated miliary tuberculosis, and (4) tuberculosis cutis orificialis.

Lupus Vulgaris

Lupus vulgaris begins usually before adolescence and tends to be chronic. The face is the most common site of involvement. The small, soft, yellowish or brownish nodules coalesce to form a single lesion. On pressure with the diascope, a characteristic "apple jelly" color is seen which is pathognomonic of the disease. There is a tendency for the lesion to ulcerate, forming an indolent granulomatous ulcer with cicatrizing areas and crusting (Fig. 13–23).

Oral lesions

The oral cavity is rarely involved and, if so, usually by *continuity from the lips.* When the upper lip is involved, it first becomes swollen, fissured, and crusted, with the formation of granulation tissue extending into the cavity. After healing, marked deformity from the resulting scars may occur. In the oral cavity, lupus vulgaris begins as a *soft nodule with subsequent ulceration.* The nodules are soft, slightly

elevated, red or yellowish white. The con-
fluent nodules tend to form livid plaques,
which are apt to bleed readily.

Histopathology

**Microscopically, lupus vulgaris presents
typical tubercle formation consisting of nests
of epithelioid cells in the upper and middle
zones of the corium, showing the central giant
cell of the Langhans type and a peripheral
zone of lymphocytes.**

Differential diagnosis

As primary involvement of the oral cavity
with lupus vulgaris is extremely rare, the
diagnosis is usually made by the characteristic lesions on the skin or lip which, by
continuity, involve the oral mucosa. Definitive diagnosis is made by biopsy.

Treatment

Treatment with calciferol (vitamin D),
and more recently with streptomycin,
isonicotinic acid hydrazide (isoniazid) and
para-aminosalicylic acid, has revolutionized
the treatment of all tuberculous skin, mucous membrane, and lymph node lesions.
The use of these preparations, either singly
or combined, has been particularly effective
in lupus vulgaris.

Tuberculous Ulcer

Two types of tuberculous ulcers are seen
in the oral cavity, primary and secondary.
The primary type of lesion occurs in non-
tuberculous individuals, principally children, and involves the lip or tongue. The
lesion resembles the primary lesion of
syphilis, beginning as an *indurated, sharply
defined lesion*, followed by ulceration with
lymph node involvement. The diagnosis is
made by a biopsy showing typical granula-
tomatous process, with the demonstration
of tubercle bacilli in the tissues.

The secondary type of tuberculous ulcer
is seen more frequently. It occurs in individuals with tuberculosis and may be subdivided into *nodular, ulcerative and
verrucous types* (Fig. 13-24). The nodular
type is more often found at the tip of the
tongue, although it may occur elsewhere in

Fig. 13-24

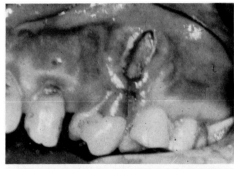

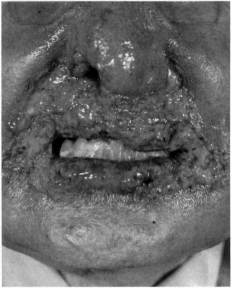

Fig. 13-25

**Figure 13-24   Ulcerative Tuberculous Lesion on the
Gingiva.** (Courtesy Dr. Irving Meyer.)
Figure 13-25   Tuberculosis Cutis Orificialis.

the oral cavity. It is characterized by a
slowly developing, relatively painless
nodule, which may enlarge to a considerable size without showing any appreciable
evidence of ulceration. This lesion resembles a syphilitic gumma, especially if
located on the tongue. Considering the
number of cases of pulmonary tuberculosis,
this type of lesion is rare.

The verrucous type of tuberculous lesion
in the oral cavity is the rarest of this group.
Its usual location is on the dorsum of the
tongue in the region of the circumvallate
papillae, or on the lips. The lesion may
simulate the verrucous type of epidermoid
carcinoma.

Disseminated Miliary Tuberculosis

Oral involvement in disseminated miliary tuberculosis occurs in the terminal stage of the disease. The oral lesions tend to break down and produce multiple painful shallow ulcerations, which occur anywhere in the oral cavity. Systemic streptomycin has been particularly effective in the relief of this type of involvement.

Tuberculosis Cutis Orificialis

This type of tubercular process is usually secondary to pulmonary tuberculosis of many years standing. It tends to involve the nasal, oral and genital regions, beginning as a *localized granulation tissue with ulceration*. It is generally complicated by secondary infection with pyogenic organisms. The process is slow but progressive and involves the lips, tongue, gingiva and buccal mucosa (Fig. 13–25). The involvement may be superficial or deep. It is generally painful and appears as an irregularly outlined mass of granulation tissue bathed in a mucopurulent exudate.

Histopathology

Microscopically, tuberculosis cutis orificialis presents numerous miliary tubercles deep in the cutis. Necrosis and ulceration occur early, and numerous tubercle bacilli are present in the lesions.

Treatment

The chemotherapeutic agents referred to under lupus vulgaris are also used in the treatment of this condition.

ORAL MANIFESTATIONS OF VIRUS DISEASES

Recurrent Herpes Labialis

This is a recurrent herpetic infection that takes the form of the so-called "cold-sore" or "fever blister." The lips are the most common site but any part of the integument may be involved. The individual lesions last from 7 to 10 days. The over-all duration of the disease varies from a few months to

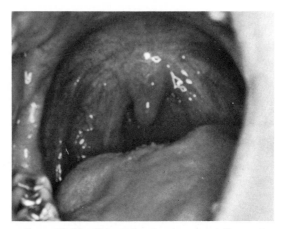

Figure 13–26 Herpangina showing acute inflammation of the oropharynx with vesicle formation.

two years or more. Diagnosis is established by isolation of the virus.

Acute Herpetic Gingivostomatitis

This is an acute infection of the oral cavity produced by the herpes simplex virus. (This disease is described in Chapter 11.)

Herpes Zoster

Herpes zoster is an *inflammation of the posterior root ganglion of the spinal nerves* or an *extramedullary ganglion of a cranial nerve*. It is characterized by pain and burning and vesicle formation along the distribution of the involved nerve.

The etiologic agent is a filtrable virus closely related in morphology and physiology to the virus of herpes simplex and varicella. In some cases, trauma and leukemic infiltration may be predisposing factors. It occurs most frequently in the fifth and seventh decades, although occasionally the disease is found in children. As a general rule, the disease is more severe in older patients.

The herpetic eruption is usually preceded by pain or burning along the distribution of the involved nerve, which may last for 24 to 48 hours before the *typical vesicular eruption* appears. The vesicles, which are surrounded by a distinct *erythematous base*, appear in groups. They rupture and heal gradually in 5 to 10 days. The lesions are characteristically *unilateral*, although *bilateral* involvement has been reported.

Oral lesions

The *fifth cranial nerve* is involved in about 15 per cent of the cases. When the maxillary and mandibular divisions of the fifth cranial nerve are involved, lesions occur on the skin, oral mucosa or both. The anterior portion of the tongue, soft palate, and cheek are the most frequent intra-oral sites. Burket[10] states that the oral lesions are of shorter duration than the dermal involvement.

Treatment

Besides palliative local treatment, the many different types of parenteral therapy include the use of posterior pituitary extract, dihydroergotamine, protamide and convalescent serum. The large number of such agents and their wide differences of action are indications of their ineffectiveness. Antibiotics are used but their value is limited to controlling secondary infection.

Molluscum Contagiosum

Molluscum contagiosum is a virus disease of the epithelium that very rarely involves mucous membranes and is characterized by *small, nodular lesions*, which usually have *minute, rounded surface orifices.*

Oral lesions

The lesions may range from pin-head to pea size and develop slowly. At first they are *globular* in shape with broad bases, but as they enlarge they become *flattened* and *umbilicated.* They may be discrete or grouped. Their most common location in the oral cavity is on the dorsal surface of the *tongue*, although they have been reported on other areas, especially the lips,

Histopathology

Microscopically, molluscum contagiosum is characterized by the presence of "molluscum bodies," which are degenerating epithelial cells. The prickle cells increase in size as the surface of the lesion is approached, and inclusion bodies develop adjacent to the nuclei. Nearer the surface, the cells lose their nuclei but retain the inclusion bodies. At the surface, the inclusion bodies are no longer present and the cells appear as a homogeneous mass.

Treatment

The lesions are very amenable to local therapy. Piercing them with a sharp instrument usually stops their growth, and in a few days they deteriorate and drop off the surface. Electrodesiccation, cauterization or "shelling out" with a blunt instrument may be employed in resistant cases.

Verruca Vulgaris

Oral lesions

Verruca vulgaris is a small lesion 2 to 6 mm. in size, commonly located on the *tongue, vestibule* or *buccal mucosa.* It is usually grayish white in color and may bleed profusely if traumatized.

Histopathology

Microscopically, verruca vulgaris presents marked acanthosis and some hyperkeratosis of the epithelium. The lesion is confined to the epithelium without extending into the underlying tunica propria.

Treatment

Treatment consists of elimination by electrodesiccation or electrocautery. In addition, podophyllin in alcohol when applied topically to mucous membrane warts is an effective medication.

Lymphopathia Venereum (Lymphogranuloma Venereum)

This is the only venereal disease caused by a virus. The initial lesion is a *small papule* or *vesicle*, which soon disappears and is usually insignificant. It is soon followed, however, by painful regional adenopathy. The nodes may suppurate and chronic scarring results.

Oral lesions

Oral lesions of lymphopathia venereum are very rare. Coutts and Banderas[15] described a triad consisting of *iritis, aphthous lesions of the mouth and genitals, and a positive Frei test,*[*18] which they attributed to the virus of lymphogranuloma venereum.

The oral lesion consists of a small, slightly painful, *superficial ulceration* with *nonindurated* borders. A softened red palate with small erythematous granulomatous lesions and regional lymphadenopathy and dysphagia are associated findings. The diagnosis of the oral lesions can be made on the basis of the history and findings of anogenital lesions and a positive Frei test.

Treatment

Systemic Aureomycin, 250 mg. four times a day, or sulfonamides, 2.0 gm. a day for 10 to 14 days.

Foot and Mouth Disease

Epizootic stomatitis is an acute contagious disease characterized by fever, chills, malaise, and the formation of *vesicles* on the fingers, toes, oral mucosa and the lips. The disease is rare in the United States. Dairymen, farmers and butchers are most commonly affected. Direct contamination from infected animal secretions, such as raw milk, is the common method of transmission.

Oral lesions

The primary vesicles appear at the point of entry of the virus, most often on the lips, oral mucosa or fingers. The vesicles, which vary in size, develop rapidly, rupture and heal—usually without leaving a trace of their existence. There is an initial dryness of the mouth followed by a marked increase in salivation, generalized pruritus[44] and adenopathy. The disease usually starts to clear in 7 to 10 days, but 3 to 4 weeks will elapse before all lesions have disappeared. There is no specific treatment.

Frei test: 0.1 cc. of vaccine prepared from the purulent material of a lesion is injected intradermally. In a positive reaction, an erythematous infiltrated papule surrounded by a zone of erythema appears in 48 hours.

Herpangina

In 1920, Zaharsky[57] first described this disease, which is marked by an uncomplicated brief course and a *sore throat* characterized by *vesicular* and *aphthous lesions in the faucial areas.* It occurs in epidemics and involves children in most cases, although adults are occasionally affected.

The disease is characterized by an initial high fever and moderately severe constitutional symptoms, such as headache, nausea, and vomiting, and occasionally in young children by convulsions.

Group A, type 2 Coxsackie virus has been isolated as the etiologic agent.

Oral lesions

The throat and the posterior part of the oral cavity show minute *vesicles* or, if these have ruptured, *small punched-out ulcers.* They occur on the anterior pillar of the fauces, the tonsils, the pharynx, and the edge of the soft palate. The number of the lesions varies from 2 to 20. Dysphagia is often marked. The general and local symptoms disappear in a few days.

Diagnosis

The disease appears to be quite similar to herpetic stomatitis except that only the posterior aspect of the oral cavity is involved; the constitutional symptoms are not as severe, and the course of the disease is shorter.

Treatment

There is no specific treatment.

DRUG ERUPTIONS

An increase in the incidence of skin and oral manifestations of hypersensitivity to drugs has been noted since the advent of the sulfonamides, barbiturates and the various antibiotics. The eruptive skin and oral lesions are attributed to the fact that the drug acts as an *allergen,* either alone or in combination, *sensitizing* the tissues and then causing the allergic reaction.

Eruptions in the oral cavity resulting

from sensitivity to drugs that have been taken by mouth or parenterally are termed stomatitis medicamentosa. The local reaction from the use of a medicament in the oral cavity, such as a so-called "aspirin burn" and the stomatitis resulting from topical penicillin, is referred to as stomatitis venenata or contact stomatitis. Such changes may result from either the irritating local action of the drug or from drug sensitivity. In many cases skin eruptions may accompany the oral lesions.

In general, drug eruptions in the oral cavity are *multiform. Vesicular* and *bullous lesions* occur commonly, but *pigmented or nonpigmented macular lesions* are frequently observed. Erosions, often followed by deep ulceration with purpuric lesions, may also occur. The lesions are seen in different areas of the oral cavity, with the gingiva frequently being affected.

There are hundreds of drugs capable of producing skin eruptions with or without mouth lesions. Constitutional symptoms may be severe or entirely absent. Only a few of the important and most commonly used drugs that may be associated with skin and oral eruptions will be considered here.

Agranulocytosis characterized by *necrotic oral lesions, sore throat* and *leukopenia* may follow the use of gold salts, arsphenamine, aminopyrine, phenacetin, sulfonamides and antibiotics. The barbiturates[28] and salicylates[11] (Fig. 13–27) occasionally produce vesicular or bullous lesions followed by erosions in the oral cavity. Phenolphthalein, found in many proprietary laxatives, may produce bullous lesions followed by erosions (usually confined to a single lesion) on the skin and in the oral cavity (Fig. 13–28).

Iodides and bromides may give rise to bullous and hemorrhagic eruptions in the oral cavity and, on the skin, acne, urticaria, or suppurating and vegetating lesions. The sulfonamides are responsible for a variety of skin and oral lesions, including vesicles, bullae and ulceration. Sulfonamide ointment has been a factor in producing sensitization in a large percentage of cases.[52] A so-called "fixed eruption" of mucous membrane and skin caused by sulfadiazine[12] has been reported. Atabrine (quinacrine hydrochloride), used in the prevention and treatment of malaria in World War II, produced a skin eruption called atypical lichenoid dermatitis characterized by lesions resembling lichen planus on the skin and oral mucosa (Fig. 13–29).

Skin and oral eruptions and acute monilial infection have been associated with the widespread use of antibiotics (Figs. 13–30 and 13–31).

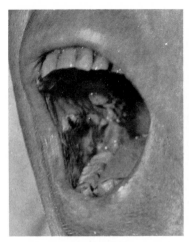

Fig. 13–27

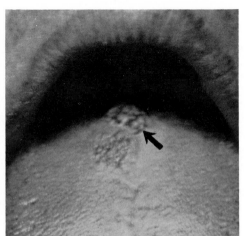

Fig. 13–28

Figure 13–27 **Stomatitis Medicamentosa** resulting from bismuth salicylate showing necrosis of the buccal mucosa with pigmentation.

Figure 13–28 **Fixed Eruption Due to Phenolphthalein.** Note the bullous lesion on dorsum of tongue.

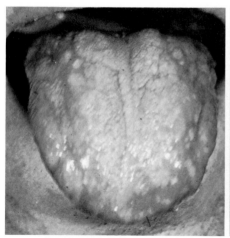 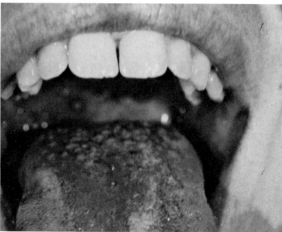

Fig. 13–29   Fig. 13–30

Figure 13–29 **Stomatitis Medicamentosa.** Atrophic tongue due to Atabrine.
Figure 13–30 **Stomatitis Medicamentosa Due to Penicillin.** Note irregularly outlined denudation on the surface of the tongue.

FUNGUS DISEASES OF THE ORAL CAVITY

Although fungus disease of the oral cavity is relatively uncommon, the following conditions are occasionally seen.

Acute Moniliasis (Candidiasis, Thrush)[29, 37]

Acute infection with *Candida albicans* is the most common of the fungus diseases involving the oral cavity. Moniliasis is essentially a disease of infancy, although adults, particularly those who are debilitated or diabetic, may be affected. Moniliasis of the oral cavity is seen in some patients under systemic antibiotic therapy. In infants, epidemics may occur in nurseries from contaminated nipples, articles of clothing and bedding. There is also a significantly higher incidence in children born of mothers with monilial vaginitis.

Oral lesions

The oral lesions may appear anywhere on the mucosal surface as a simple patch, but usually the lesions are multiple. The *characteristic lesions are creamy-white, simulating coagulated milk, adherent and, when forcibly removed, give rise to bleeding points* (Figs. 13–32 and 13–33). Intertriginous maceration at the labial commissures both in children and adults may reveal *C. albicans.*

Diagnosis

The diagnosis is based upon the history, clinical appearance of the lesions and microscopic study of smears of scrapings from them. The spores of *C. albicans* are round to oval, 2 to 4 mμ in size (Fig. 13–34), smaller than red blood corpuscles, and readily stained with dyes such as methylene blue and gentian violet. The smear on the slide is flooded with 10 per cent potassium hydroxide solution and heated gently before the stain is applied.

Swabs from the exudate on Sabouraud's culture medium at room temperature give rise to characteristic colonies of the fungus. The colonies grow in 3 to 5 days as creamy-white, medium-sized moist colonies with a definite odor of yeast. Thick suspensions in salt solution injected into the ear vein of the rabbit cause death in 4 to 5 days. Multiple abscesses of the kidneys reveal the characteristic spores of *C. albicans.*

Clinically, thrush may simulate *diphtheria, macerated epithelium* of the buccal mucosa from chronic irritation (biting habit), *leukoplakia* and possibly *lichen planus.* These conditions are readily ruled out by any of the above laboratory procedures.

Fig. 13–31

Fig. 13–32

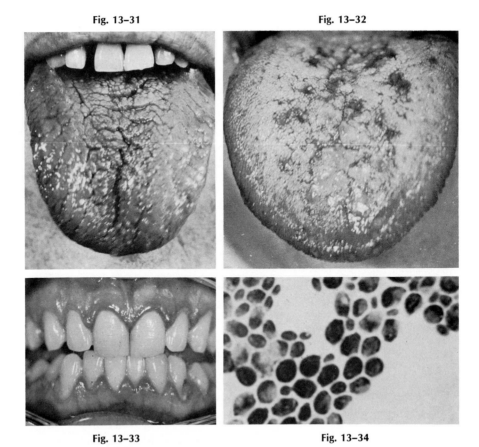

Fig. 13–33

Fig. 13–34

Figure 13–31   Prominent Papillae and Discoloration of the Tongue Associated With the Local Use of Penicillin.
Figure 13–32   Acute Moniliasis of the Tongue.
Figure 13–33   The Gingiva in Acute Moniliasis.
Figure 13–34   Smear from Lesion of Acute Moniliasis Showing Spores of Candida Albicans.

Chronic Moniliasis

This is a rare type of *C. albicans* infection resulting in a *granulomatous lesion* that begins in infancy or early childhood and may persist for several years.[29] The oral lesions are often accompanied by involvement of the nails and skin (Figs. 13–35 to 13–37). In contrast to the mild, superficial acute forms of monilial infection, monilial granuloma[20] manifests itself by a deep inflammatory reaction with the production of granulation tissue. Ultimate involvement of the lungs with multiple abscesses, often associated with kidney lesions, results in death in a high percentage of cases.

Diagnosis

The diagnosis is confirmed by laboratory studies as for acute moniliasis.

Treatment

Nystatin and amphotericin B used topically or systemically are effective in the treatment of moniliasis. Older nonspecific remedies such as the use of gentian violet and Lugol's solution are still popular.

Actinomycosis

Actinomycosis, caused by Actinomyces, (*A. bovis* and *A. israelii*), is a disease that involves many parts of the body and is most frequently seen about the oral cavity. The Actinomyces are classified as an intermediate group between the fungi and bacteria, and may be considered as bacteria-like fungi. Actinomyces are common normal habitants of the oral cavity.

Approximately 90 per cent of the cases of actinomycosis are of the cervicofacial type,[43] and a large percentage of these follow extraction of teeth. One of the characteristics of actinomycosis is the lack of immediate tissue reaction following invasion of the Actinomyces. Clinically, as described by Lamb et al.,[27] the cervicofacial type of actinomycosis presents the following features: **dark-red discoloration of the skin, slate-blue elevated lesions, multiple nodules with formation of ridges and furrows in the creases of the skin and neck, distinct board-like induration and multiple sinuses with both macroscopic and microscopic granules in the purulent discharge. Pain is usually mild and sometimes absent.**

The *tongue* is occasionally the primary site of the disease. It starts as a deep-seated *painless nodule* that grows slowly and eventually breaks through the mucosa, discharging a *yellowish purulent material.* On the *gingiva,* the picture is somewhat similar. It takes about 4 to 6 weeks for an actinomycotic nodule to soften and discharge its contents.

Differential diagnosis

A large group of conditions may simulate actinomycosis. Among them are *tuberculosis, syphilitic gummas, blastomycosis,*

Fig. 13–35   **Fig. 13–36**

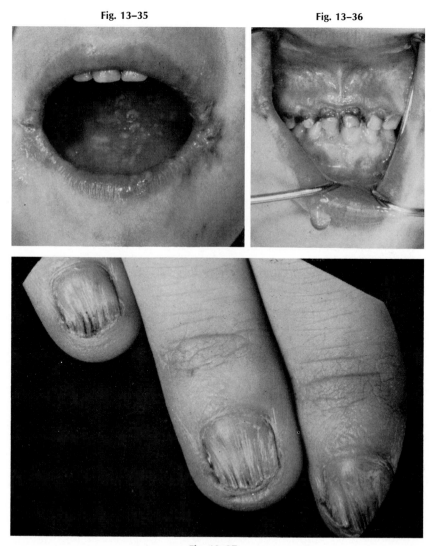

Fig. 13–37

Figure 13–35   Chronic Moniliasis Showing Involvement of the Tongue and Lips. (Courtesy of Dr. David Weisberger.)
Figure 13–36   Chronic Moniliasis Showing Involvement of the Marginal Gingiva in the Maxilla. (Courtesy of Dr. David Weisberger.)
Figure 13–37   Chronic Moniliasis Showing Involvement of the Nails. (Courtesy of Dr. David Weisberger.)

lymphogranuloma venereum or *malignancy,* usually of the *lymphomatous type,* and *lupus vulgaris.*

Diagnosis

The purulent exudate from the lesions is collected from the draining sinuses and examined grossly for the yellow sulfur granules. **Microscopically, the granules appear as lobulated bodies composed of delicate branching, intertwined filaments. The organism can be grown anaerobically in thioglycollate medium.**

Treatment

Surgical drainage of the lesion is effective; filtered x-ray irradiation, systemic penicillin, amphotericin B, and other antibiotics and sulfa drugs are also used.

Histoplasmosis

Histoplasmosis,[42] one of the rare fungus diseases of man, shows cutaneous or mucomembranous lesions in one half of the cases reported to date. Darling[16] first reported cases in Panama and originally named the causative agent *Histoplasma capsulatum.* The method of transmission of this fungus to man is not definitely known; the dog may be the intermediate host, as *H. capsulatum* has been isolated from that animal.

Oral lesions occurred in 28 of 88 cases compiled by Miller.[36] The lesions may occur anywhere in the oral cavity, but the *tongue* is the most common site. The most common form is a *very indurated ulcer,* although *nodular lesions* are almost as common as ulcers. The lesion also presents as verrucous or granular masses.[6] Purpuric, macular areas may accompany the ulcerations.

The skin lesions may be multiform in character and include papules, ulcerations, purpuric lesions, impetiginous eruptions and generalized scaling dermatosis. The disease presents systemic manifestations as well as cutaneous and oral lesions. The symptoms include elevated temperature, anemia and leukopenia. Lymph node and pulmonary involvement resembling both lymphoblastoma and pulmonary tuberculosis occur in many cases.

Histopathology

Microscopically, histoplasmosis is classified among the chronic infectious granulomas and cannot be definitely differentiated on the basis of cellular changes from other members of the group. Multinucleated macrophages containing the yeast-like fungi are diagnostic. The fungi are seen in large mononuclear cells and appear as small oval bodies 1 to 4 microns in diameter surrounded by a nonstaining capsule. The organism has to be differentiated from the Leishmania protozoan parasites. Lymphocytic and plasma cell infiltration may be associated with focal areas of necrosis. Epithelial hyperplasia and fibrosis occur around the necrotic areas, and typical Langhans' giant cells are often present.

REFERENCES

1. Andreasen, J. O.: Oral Lichen Planus. I. A Clinical Evaluation of 115 Cases. Oral Sur., 25:31, 1968.
2. Andreasen, J. O., and Poulsen, H. E.: Oral Manifestations in Discoid and Systemic Lupus Erythematosus. 2. Histologic Investigation. Acta Odont. Scandinav., 22:389, 1964.
3. Baldridge, G. D., and Blank, H.: Effect of Aureomycin on the Herpes Simplex Virus in Embryonated Eggs. Proc. Soc. Exp. Med. & Biol., 72:506, 1949.
4. Barber, H. W.: Circumscribed Scleroderma of the Buccal Mucosa. Proc. Roy. Soc. Med., 37:73, 1944.
5. Barcaglia, A.: Hemilateral Scleroderma with Hemiatrophy and Vitiligo in a Boy Four Years of Age. Pediatria, 45:533, 1937.
6. Bennett, D. E.: Histoplasmosis of the Oral Cavity and Larynx. Arch. Int. Med. (Chicago), 120:417, 1967.
7. Beutner, E. H., et al.: The Immunopathology of Pemphigus and Bullous Pemphigoid. J. Invest. Derm., 51:63, 1968.
8. Brantzaeg, P.: Erytheme Multiforme Exudatium. Odont. T., 72:363, 1964.
9. Braun-Falco, O., and Vogell, W.: Elektronen-Mikroskopische Untersuchungen zur Dynamik der Akantholyse bei Pemphigus Vulgaris. II Mitteilung. Die Akantholytische Blase. Arch. Klin. Exp. Derm., 223:533, 1965.
10. Burket, L. W.: Oral Medicine. Philadelphia, J. B. Lippincott Co., 1946, p. 151.
11. Claman, H. N.: Mouth Ulcers Associated with Prolonged Chewing of Gum Containing Aspirin. J.A.M.A., 202:651, 1967.
12. Cole, L. W.: Fixed Eruption of Mucous Membrane and Skin Caused by Sulfadiazine. Arch. Derm. & Syph., 54:675, 1946.
13. Combes, F. L., and Canizares, O.: Pemphigus Vulgaris, a Clinicopathological Study of One Hundred Cases. Arch. Derm. & Syph., 62:786, 1950.
14. Cooke, B. E. D.: Diagnosing Features of Pemphigus Affecting the Oral Mucosa, J. D. Res., 40: 1281, 1961.

15. Coutts, W. E., and Banderas, B. T.: Lymphogranulomatosis Venerea and Its Clinical Syndromes. Urol. & Cutan. Rev., 38:263, 1934.
16. Darling, S. T.: The Morphology of the Parasite (Histoplasma Capsulatum) and Lesions of Histoplasmosis, a Fatal Disease of Tropical America. J. Exp. Med., 11:515, 1909.
17. Foster, T. D., et al.: Dental Involvement in Scleroderma. Brit. D. J., 124:353, 1968.
18. Frei, W.: On the Skin Test in Lymphogranuloma Inguinale. J. Invest. Derm., 1:367, 1938.
19. Gahan, E.: Lupus Erythematosus. Clinical Observations in 443 Cases. Arch. Derm. & Syph., 45:685, 1942.
20. Hanser, P. V., and Rothman, S.: Monilial Granuloma, Report of Case. Arch. Derm. & Syph., 61:297, 1950.
21. Haselden, F. G.: Bullous Lichen Planus. Oral Surg., 24:472, 1967.
22. Hashimoto, K.: Lichen Ruber Planus of the Mouth Mucosa. J. Jap. Stomat. Soc., 36:48, 1969.
23. Hashimoto, K., and Lever, W.: An Electronmicroscopic Study of Pemphigus Vulgaris of the Mouth and Skin with Special Reference to the Intercellular Cement. J. Invest. Derm., 48:540, 1967.
24. Jansen, G. T., et al.: Generalized Scleroderma. Treatment with Immunosuppressive Agents. Arch. Derm., 97:690, 1968.
25. Klemperer, P.: The Concept of Collagen Diseases. Am. J. Path., 26:505, 1950.
26. Komori, A., Welton, N. A., and Kelln, E. E.: The Behavior of the Basement Membrane of Skin and Oral Lesions in Patients with Lichen Planus, Erythema Multiforme, Lupus Erythematosus, Pemphigus Vulgaris, Pemphigoid, and Epidermolysis Bullosa. Oral Surg., 22:752, 1966.
27. Lamb, J. H., Lain, E., and Jones, P.: Actinomycosis of Face and Neck. J.A.M.A., 134:351, 1947.
28. Lawson, B. F.: Severe Stomatitis Associated with Barbiturate Ingestion. J. Oral Med., 24:13, 1969.
29. Lehner, T.: Chronic Candidiasis. Brit. D. J., 116:539, 1964.
30. Lever, W. F.: Pemphigus. Medicine, 32:1, 1953.
31. Levy, B. P., Reeve, C. M., and Kierland, R. R.: The Oral Aspects of Epidermolysis Bullosa Dystrophica: A Case Report. J. Periodont. 40:431, 1970.
32. Lighterman, I.: Erythema Multiforme Limited to the Oral Cavity—Report of a Case. Oral Surg., Oral Med. & Oral Path., 11:1237, 1958.
33. Looby, J. P., and Burket, L. W.: Scleroderma of the Face with Involvement of the Alveolar Process. Am. J. Orthodont. & Oral Surg., 28:493, 1942.
34. McCarthy, F. P.: A Clinical and Pathologic Study of Oral Disease Based on 2300 Consecutive Cases. J.A.M.A., 116:16, 1941.
35. McCarthy, F. P.: Pyostomatitis Vegetans. Arch. Derm. & Syph., 60:750, 1949.
36. Miller, H. E., et al.: Histoplasmosis, Cutaneous and Mucomembranous Lesions. Arch. Derm. & Syph., 56:715, 1947.
37. Miller, J. L.: Moniliasis. Arch. Derm. & Syph., 54:484, 1946.
38. Mitchell, D. F., and Chaudhry, A. P.: Roentgenographic Manifestations of Scleroderma. Oral Surg., Oral Med. & Oral Path., 10:307, 1957.
39. Monash, S.: Oral Lesions of Lupus Erythematosus. D. Cosmos, 73:511, 1931.
40. Montgomery, H.: Dermatopathology. New York, Harper and Row, 1967, p. 84.
41. O'Leary, P. A., and Nomland, R.: A Clinical Study of One Hundred and Three Cases of Scleroderma. Am. J. M. Sc., 180:95, 1930.
42. Parsons, R. G., and Zarofonetis, C. J. D.: Histoplasmosis in Man. Arch. Int. Med., 75:1, 1945.
43. Rud, J.: Cervicofacial Actinomycosis. J. Oral Surg., 25:229, 1967.
44. Schlosser, S.: Foot and Mouth Disease: Oral Manifestations in Man. D. Abstracts, 6:693, 1961.
45. Scópp, I. W., and Schlagel, E.: Scleroderma: Its Orofacial Manifestations. Oral Surg., Oral Med. & Oral Path., 15:1510, 1962.
46. Shklar, G.: Oral Lesions of Erythema Multiforme, Histologic and Histochemical Observations. Arch. Derm. (Chicago), 92:495, 1965.
47. Shklar, G., et al.: Oral Lesions in Bullous Pemphigoid. Arch. Derm. (Chicago), 99:663, 1970.
48. Shklar, G., and McCarthy, P. L.: Oral Manifestations of Benign Mucous Membrane Pemphigus (Mucous Membrane Pemphigoid). Oral Surg., Oral Med. & Oral Path., 12:950, 1959.
49. Shklar, G., and McCarthy, P. L.: The Oral Lesions of Lichen Planus. Oral Surg., Oral Med. & Oral Path., 14:164, 1961.
50. Stafne, E. C., and Austin, L. T.: A Characteristic Dental Finding in Acrosclerosis and Diffuse Scleroderma. Am. J. Orthodont. & Oral Surg., 30:25, 1944.
51. Sugarman, M. M.: Lupus Erythematosus. Oral Surg., Oral. Med. & Oral Path., 6:836, 1953.
52. Sulzberger, M. B., Kanof, A., Baer, R. L., and Lowenberg, C.: Sensitization by Topical Application of Sulfonamides. J. Allergy, 18:92, 1947.
53. Templeton, H. J.: Localized Scleroderma with Bullae. Arch. Derm. & Syph., 43:360, 1941.
54. Weisberger, D.: Treatment of Some Diseases of the Soft Tissues of the Mouth. D. Clin. North America, March 1960, p. 215.
55. Whitten, J. B., Jr.: Intra-oral Lichen Planus Simplex: An Ultrastructure Study. J. Periodont., 41:261, 1970.
56. Wilgram, G. F., Caulfield, J. B., and Lever, W. F.: An Electron Microscopic Study of Acantholysis in Pemphigus Vulgaris. J. Invest. Derm., 36:373, 1961.
57. Zaharsky, J.: Herpetic Sore Throat. Southern M. J., 13:871, 1920.

Part II • Periodontal Disease

THE PERIODONTAL POCKET

A periodontal pocket is a pathologically deepened gingival sulcus; it is one of the important clinical features of periodontal disease. Progressive pocket formation leads to destruction of the supporting periodontal tissues, and loosening and exfoliation of the teeth.

SIGNS AND SYMPTOMS

The only reliable method of locating periodontal pockets and determining their extent is careful probing of the gingival margin along each tooth surface.

The following clinical signs indicate the presence of periodontal pockets:

1. Enlarged, bluish red marginal gingiva with a "rolled" edge separated from the tooth surface (Fig. 14–1).

2. A reddish blue vertical zone from the gingival margin to the attached gingiva, and sometimes into the alveolar mucosa (Fig. 14–2).

3. A break in the faciolingual continuity of the interdental gingiva.

4. Shiny, discolored and puffy gingiva associated with exposed root surfaces (Fig. 14–3).

5. Gingival bleeding.

6. Purulent exudate at the gingival margin (Fig. 14–4), or its appearance in response to digital pressure on the lateral aspect of the gingival margin (Fig. 14–5).

7. Looseness, extrusion and migration of teeth.

8. The development of diastemata where none had existed (Fig. 14–6).

Periodontal pockets are generally painless but may give rise to the following symptoms:

Localized pain or a sensation of pressure after eating, which gradually diminishes; a foul taste in localized areas; a tendency to suck material from the interproximal spaces; radiating pain "deep in the bone," which is worse on rainy days; a "gnawing" feeling or feeling of itchiness in the gums, sometimes described as feeling like "worms"; the urge to dig a pointed instrument into the gums with relief from the resultant bleeding; complaints that food "sticks between the teeth," the teeth "feel loose," or prefer-

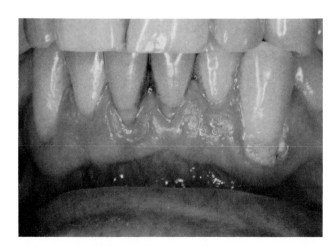

Figure 14–1 Periodontal Pockets around the central incisors and left canine, showing rolled margins and separation from the tooth surfaces. Note the materia alba on the canine.

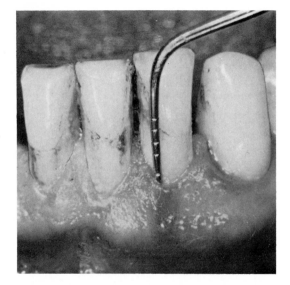

Figure 14–2 Periodontal Pocket with vertical discolored zone extending to the alveolar mucosa.

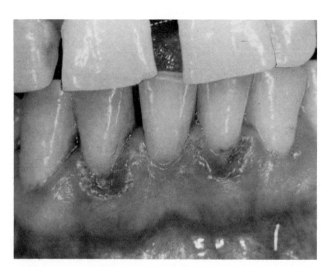

Figure 14–3 Periodontal Pockets with puffy discolored gingiva and exposed root surfaces.

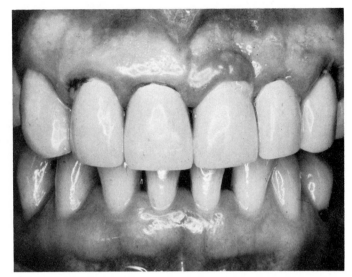

Figure 14–4 Purulent Exudate from periodontal pocket on the maxillary left central incisor.

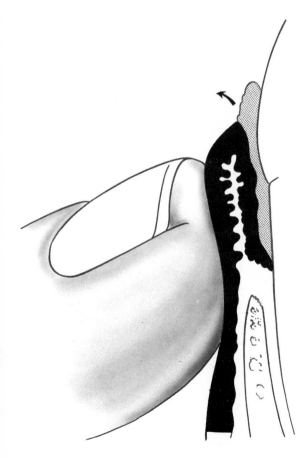

Figure 14–5 Purulent Exudate Expressed from Periodontal Pocket by Digital Pressure.

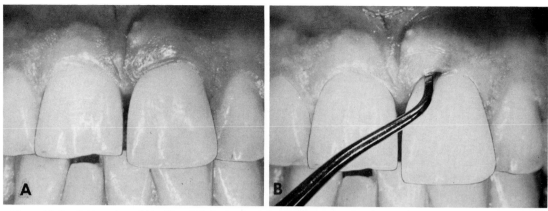

Figure 14–6 *A,* **Extrusion of Maxillary Left Incisor** and diastema associated with periodontal pocket. *B,* Entire length of periodontal probe inserted to the base of periodontal pocket on central incisor.

ence to "eat on the other side"; sensitivity to heat and cold; toothache in the absence of caries.

CLASSIFICATION

Periodontal pockets are classified according to morphology and their relationship to adjacent structures as follows:

Gingival pocket (relative)

A gingival pocket is formed by gingival enlargement without destruction of the underlying periodontal tissues. The sulcus is deepened because of the increased bulk of the gingiva (Fig. 14–7).

Periodontal pocket (absolute)

This is the type of pocket that occurs in periodontal disease. The gingiva is diseased and the sulcus is deepened; there is destruction of the supporting periodontal tissues (Fig. 14–7). Absolute pockets are of two types: (1) suprabony (supracrestal), in which the bottom of the pocket is coronal to the underlying alveolar bone, and (2) infrabony (intrabony, subcrestal or intraalveolar), in which the bottom of the pocket is apical to the level of the adjacent alveolar bone. In this type the lateral pocket wall

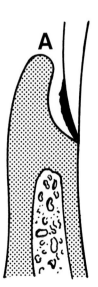
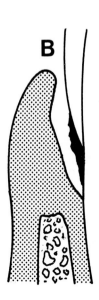
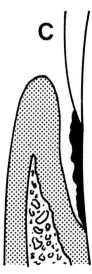

Figure 14–7 Different Types of Periodontal Pockets. *A,* Gingival pocket. There is no destruction of the supporting periodontal tissues. *B,* Suprabony pocket. The base of the pocket is coronal to the level of the underlying bone. *C,* Infrabony pocket. The base of the pocket is apical to the level of the adjacent bone.

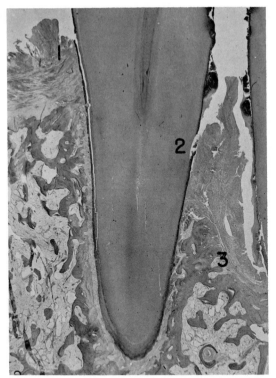

Figure 14–8 Suprabony Pockets of different depths on the distal (1) and mesial (2) surfaces of second premolar. Interdental space with suprabony pocket (2) and **Infrabony Pocket** (3) on the approximating tooth surfaces.

lies between the tooth surface and the alveolar bone (Fig. 14–7).

Pockets of different depths and types may occur on different surfaces of the same tooth and on approximating surfaces of the same interdental space (Fig. 14–8).

Classification by number of surfaces involved

Classification according to the number of surfaces involved is as follows:

SIMPLE. One tooth surface (Fig. 14–9).

COMPOUND. Two or more tooth surfaces. The base of the pockets is in direct communication with the gingival margin along each of the involved surfaces (Fig. 14–9).

COMPLEX. This is a spiral-type pocket that originates on one tooth surface and twists around the tooth to involve one or more additional surfaces (Figs. 14–9 and 14–10). The only communication with the gingival margin is at the surface where the pocket originates. To avoid missing the compound or complex types, all pockets should be probed laterally as well as vertically.

PATHOGENESIS

Periodontal pockets are caused by local irritants (microorganisms and their products, food remnants which furnish nutrients to the microorganisms and food impaction) which produce pathologic tissue changes and deepening of the gingival sulcus. **There are no systemic conditions which initiate periodontal pockets.** On the basis of depth alone, it is sometimes difficult to differentiate between a deep normal sulcus and a shallow periodontal pocket. In such borderline cases pathologic changes in the gingiva differentiate the two conditions.

Figure 14–9 Classification of Pockets According to Involved Tooth Surfaces. A, Simple pocket. B, Compound pocket. C, Complex pocket.

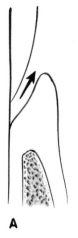

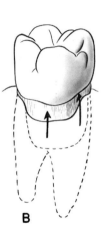

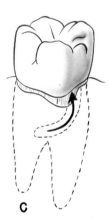

A   B   C

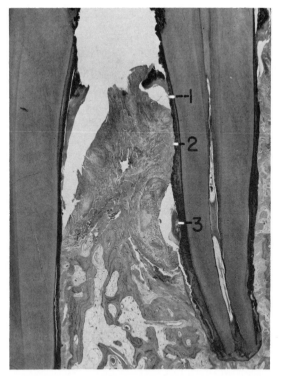

Figure 14–10 Complex Pocket. The base of pocket is shown at 3. The pocket then spirals around onto another surface of the tooth and communicates with the oral cavity at 1. In the area marked 2, the periodontal ligament is attached to the tooth.

Deepening of the gingival sulcus may occur by (1) movement of the gingival margin in the direction of the crown (this produces a "gingival" rather than a periodontal pocket; sulcus depth is increased by enlargement of the gingiva without destruction of supporting tissues); (2) migration of the epithelial attachment apically and its separation from the tooth surface; or (3) what is usually the case, a combination of both processes. In a sense, pocket formation may be likened to the stretching of an accordion in that distance is increased by movement in opposite directions (Fig. 14–11).

The sequence of changes involved in transition from the normal gingival sulcus to the pathologic periodontal pocket is as follows:

Pocket formation starts as an inflammatory change in the connective tissue wall of the gingival sulcus caused by local irritation. The cellular and fluid inflammatory exudate causes degeneration of the surrounding connective tissue, including the gingival fibers. In association with the inflammation, the epithelial attachment proliferates along the root in the form of finger-like projections two or three cells in thickness. The coronal portion of the

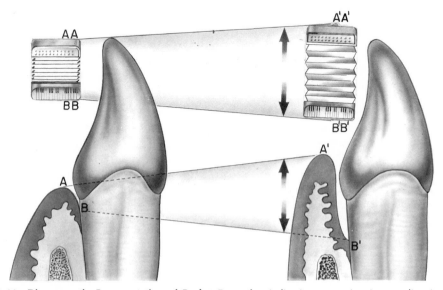

Figure 14–11 Diagrammatic Representation of Pocket Formation indicating expansion in two directions from the normal gingival sulcus *AB* to the periodontal pocket *A'B'*. Note comparison with expanding accordion *AA, BB* to *A'A', B'B'*.

epithelial attachment detaches from the root as the apical portion migrates.

With continued inflammation the gingiva increases in bulk and the crest of the gingival margin extends toward the crown. The epithelial attachment continues to migrate along the root and separate from it. The epithelium of the lateral wall of the pocket proliferates to form bulbous and cord-like extensions into the inflamed connective tissue. Leukocytes and edema from the inflamed connective tissue infiltrate the epithelium lining the pocket, resulting in varying degrees of degeneration and necrosis.

HISTOPATHOLOGY

The Suprabony Pocket

Once formed, the periodontal pocket is a chronic inflammatory lesion complicated by proliferative and degenerative changes. It presents the following microscopic features:

The soft tissue wall

The connective tissue is edematous and densely infiltrated with plasma cells (approximately 80 per cent)[42] and lymphocytes and a scattering of polymorphonuclear leukocytes. The blood vessels are increased in number, dilated and engorged. The connective tissue presents varying degrees of degeneration. Single or multiple necrotic foci are occasionally present.[27] In addition to exudative and degenerative changes, the connective tissue presents proliferation of the endothelial cells with newly formed capillaries, fibroblasts and collagen fibers (Fig. 14–12).

The epithelial attachment at the base of the pocket varies in the length, width and in the condition of the epithelial cells. The variations range from the extremes of a long narrow band to a comparatively short wide clump of cells (Fig. 14–13). The cells may be well formed and in good condition, or present slight to marked degeneration (Fig. 14–14).

Special note should be made of the fact that extension of the epithelial attachment along the root requires the presence of healthy epithelial cells. Degeneration of the epithelial attachment would retard rather than accelerate pocket formation. Degenerative changes are seen in the epithelial attachment at the base of periodontal pock-

ets, but they are usually less severe than those in the epithelium of the lateral pocket wall. Since migration of the epithelial attachment requires healthy viable cells, it is reasonable to assume that the degenerative changes seen in this area occur after the epithelial attachment reached its position on the cementum.

The severest degenerative changes in the periodontal pocket occur along the lateral wall. The epithelium of the lateral wall of the pocket presents striking proliferative and degenerative changes.[5] Epithelial buds or interlacing cords of epithelial cells project from the lateral wall into the adjacent inflamed connective tissue and frequently extend farther apically than the epithelial attachment. These epithelial projections, as well as the remainder of the lateral epithelium, are densely infiltrated by leukocytes and edema from the inflamed connective tissue. The cells undergo vacuolar degeneration and rupture to form vesicles. Progressive degeneration and necrosis of the epithelium leads to ulceration of the lateral wall, exposure of the underlying markedly inflamed connective tissue, and suppuration. In some cases acute inflammation is superimposed upon the underlying chronic changes.

The severity of the degenerative changes is not necessarily related to pocket depth. Ulceration of the lateral wall may occur in shallow pockets. Deep pockets are occasionally observed in which the lateral epithelium is intact and presents only slight degeneration (Fig. 14–15).

The epithelium at the crest of the periodontal pocket is generally intact and thickened, with prominent rete pegs. When acute inflammation occurs on the surface of the periodontal pocket, however, the crest of the gingiva undergoes degeneration and necrosis.

Periodontal pockets are healing lesions

Periodontal pockets are chronic inflammatory lesions, and as such are constantly undergoing repair.

The condition of the soft tissue wall of the periodontal pocket results from a balance between destructive and constructive tissue changes. The destructive changes consist of the fluid and cellular inflammatory exudate and the associated degenerative changes stimu-

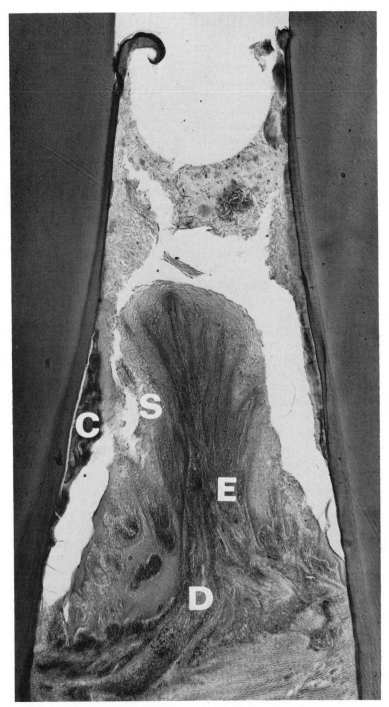

Figure 14–12 Interdental Papilla with Suprabony Pockets on Proximal Tooth Surfaces. D, Densely inflamed connective tissue; E, proliferating pocket epithelium; S, ulceration of lateral wall with pus exuding adjacent to calculus (C).

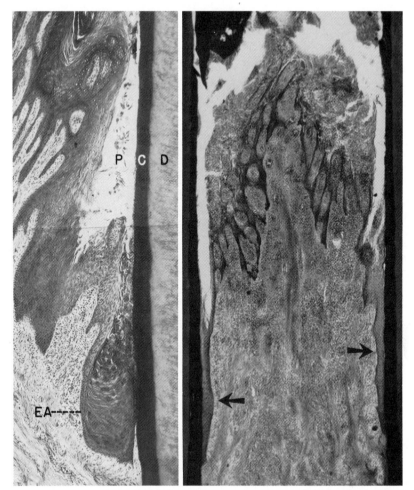

Figure 14–13 Varied Conformations of Epithelial Attachment. *Left,* Hyperkeratotic nodular epithelial attachment (EA) at the base of pocket (P), cementum (C), dentin (D). *Right,* Interdental papilla showing lengthy epithelial attachment (arrows) in two proximal pockets.

lated by the local irritation. The constructive changes consist of the formation of connective tissue cells, collagen fibers and blood vessels in an effort to repair the tissue damage caused by inflammation.

Healing does not go to completion because of the persistence of local irritants. These irritants continue to stimulate fluid and cellular exudate, which in turn causes degeneration of the new tissue elements formed in the continuous effort at repair.

The balance between exudative and constructive changes determines the color, consistency, and surface texture of the pocket wall. If the inflammatory fluid and cellular exudate predominate, the pocket wall is bluish red, soft, spongy and friable, with a smooth shiny surface. If there is a relative predominance of newly formed connective tissue cells and fibers, the pocket wall is firm and pink. At the clinical level the former is generally referred to as an edematous pocket, the latter as fibrotic.

Edematous and fibrotic pockets represent opposite extremes of the same pathologic process rather than different disease entities. They are subject to constant modification, depending upon the relative predominance of exudative and constructive changes.

The outer appearance of a periodontal pocket may be misleading because it is not necessarily a true indication of what is taking place throughout the pocket wall. The severest degenerative changes in periodontal pockets occur along the inner

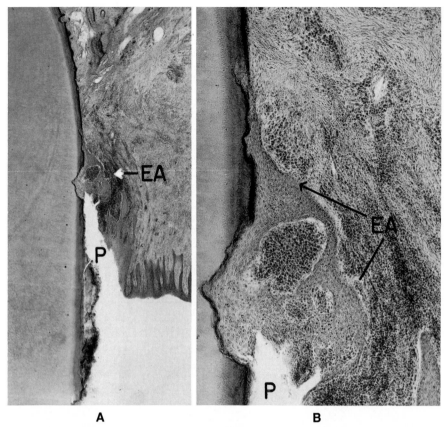

A   **B**

Figure 14–14 *A,* **Low-Power Section of Periodontal Pocket** (*P*). The location of the epithelial attachment is indicated by the arrow (*EA*). The lateral epithelial wall is ulcerated. *B,* **Detailed Study of Epithelial Attachment** (*EA*) at the base of the pocket (*P*). Note extension of well-formed epithelial cells (arrow) along the resorbed root surface. There is a dense accumulation of leukocytes enclosed within the epithelium.

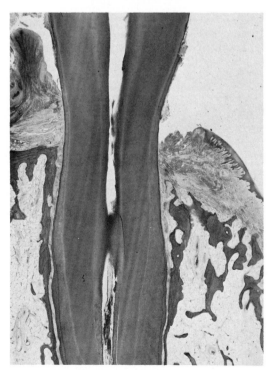

Figure 14–15 **Shallow Ulcerated Pocket in Relation to One Surface of a Tooth** (*right*) in contrast with intact deeper pocket in relation to other tooth surface (*left*).

aspect. In some cases inflammation and ulceration on the inside of the pocket are walled off by fibrous tissue on the outer aspect (Fig. 14–16). Outwardly the pocket appears pink and fibrotic despite the degeneration taking place within.

The contents

Periodontal pockets contain debris which is principally microorganisms and their products (enzymes, endotoxins and other metabolic products),* dental plaque, gingival fluid, food remnants, salivary mucin, desquamated epithelial cells and leukocytes. Plaque-covered calculus usually projects from the tooth surface (Fig. 14–17). If a purulent exudate is present, it consists of living, degenerated and necrotic leukocytes (predominantly polymorphonuclear), living and dead bacteria, serum and a scant

---

*Micoorganisms and their products, and their significance in periodontal disease, are discussed in detail in Chapter 23.

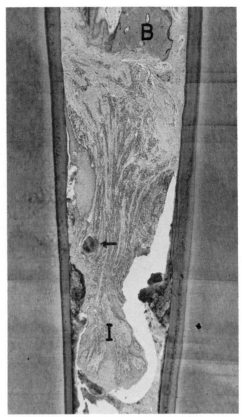

Figure 14–17 Interdental Papilla (I) with ulcerated suprabony periodontal pockets on its mesial and distal aspects. Calculus is present on the approximal tooth surfaces and within the gingiva (*arrow*). The bone is shown at B.

amount of fibrin[25] (Fig. 14–18). The contents of periodontal pockets filtered free from organisms and debris have been demonstrated to be toxic when injected subcutaneously into experimental animals.[20]

The significance of pus formation

There is a tendency to overemphasize the importance of the purulent exudate and equate it with the severity of periodontal disease. Because it is a dramatic clinical finding, early observers assumed it was responsible for the loosening and exfoliation of the teeth. *Pus is a common feature of periodontal disease, but it is only a secondary sign.* The presence of pus or the ease with which it can be expressed from the pocket merely reflects the nature of the inflammatory changes in the pocket wall. It

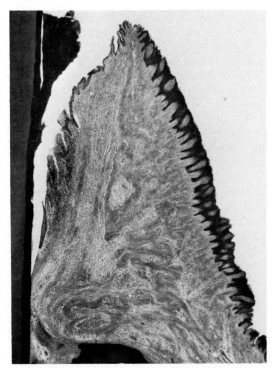

Figure 14–16 Periodontal Pocket Wall. The inner half is inflamed and ulcerated, the outer half is densely collagenous.

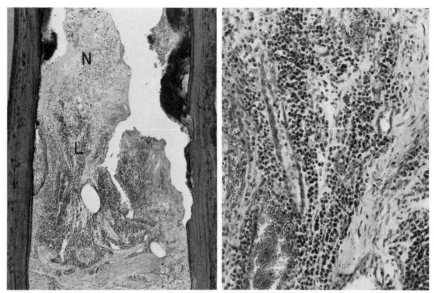

Figure 14–18 *Left,* **Pus Formation** (*N*) at the crest of a necrotic interdental papilla. There is a dense underlying leukocytic infiltration. *Right,* Detailed study of dense leukocytic infiltration and distended engorged capillaries.

is no indication of the depth of the pocket or the severity of destruction of the supporting tissues. Extensive pus formation may occur in shallow pockets, while deep pockets may present little or no pus.

The root surface wall

The root surface wall of periodontal pockets often undergoes changes that are significant because they may *cause pain* and *complicate periodontal treatment.* The following types of changes may occur in the root surface:

DECALCIFICATION AND REMINERALIZATION OF CEMENTUM. As the pocket deepens, the cementum undergoes decalcification plus, in some instances, the removal of matrix collagen and loss of cementum.[34] These changes accompany the degradation of periodontal ligament fibers which occur in the path of the advancing pocket. Upon exposure to the oral cavity an exchange of minerals and organic components may occur at the cementum-saliva interface, producing a hypermineralized surface zone of cementum.[33]

The hypermineralized zone is detectable by electron microscope, but microhardness tests indicate that the hardness of cementum is unaltered as compared with normal.[31, 40] It may even be softened,[23] along with the dentin.[10]

Cementum hardness varies in different areas on the same tooth almost as much as it does from tooth to tooth. The microhardness of calculus also varies but it is generally greater than that of cementum.

The permeability of the cemental pocket wall is altered, the calcium and magnesium content is increased, and phosphorus may be increased or diminished.[35, 36] Pathologic granules occur in the cementum and dentin,[4] and there may be disintegration of the cementum at the cementodentinal junction.[39]

ROOT CARIES. Exposure to oral fluids and bacterial plaque result in proteolysis of the embedded remnants of Sharpey's fibers; the cementum may be softened and undergo fragmentation and cavitation.[21] **Involvement of the cementum is followed by bacterial penetration of the dentinal tubules, resulting in destruction of the dentin (Fig. 14–19). In severe cases, large sections of necrotic cementum become detached from the tooth and separated from it by masses of bacteria (Fig. 14–20).**

The tooth may not be painful, but exploration of the root surface reveals the presence of a defect; penetration of the involved area with a probe elicits pain.

Caries of the root may lead to *pulpitis,* sensitivity to sweets and thermal changes, or severe pain. Pathologic exposure of the pulp occurs in severe cases. **It is well to bear in mind that root caries may be the**

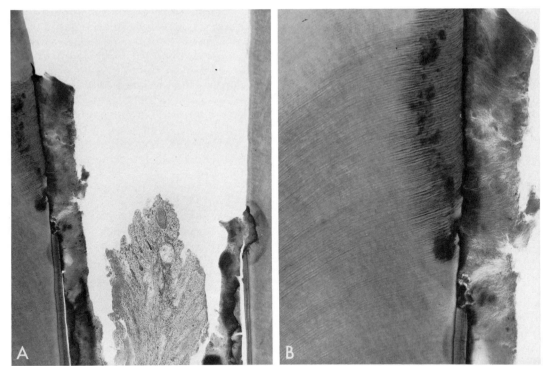

Figure 14–19   Caries on Root Surfaces Exposed by Periodontal Disease. *A,* Interdental space, showing inflamed gingiva and caries on proximal tooth surfaces. *B,* Caries of cementum and dentin, showing bacterial invasion of dentinal tubules. Note the filamentous structure of the dental plaque and darker staining of calculus adherent to the root.

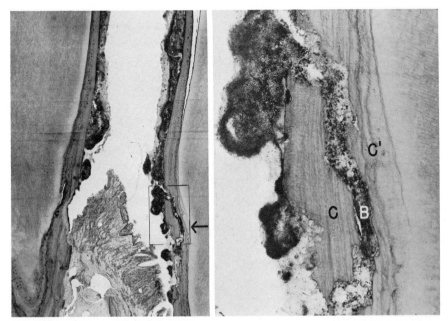

Figure 14–20   *Left,* Mesiodistal section through an interdental space in a patient with extensive periodontal destruction. An area of **Cementum Necrosis** is enclosed within the rectangle designated by the arrow.

Right, Detailed section of area enclosed in the rectangle showing **Necrotic Fragment of Cementum** (*C*) separated from lamellated cementum (*C'*) by clumps of bacteria (*B*).

cause of toothache in patients with periodontal disease without evidence of coronal decay.

Caries of the cementum requires special attention when the pocket is treated. The necrotic cementum must be removed by scaling and root planing until firm tooth surface is reached, even if this entails extension into the dentin.

CELLULAR RESORPTION. Areas of cellular resorption of cementum and dentin are common in roots uninvolved with periodontal disease. These are of no particular significance because they are symptom-free, and so long as the root is covered by the periodontal ligament, they are apt to undergo repair. However, if the root is exposed by progressive pocket formation before repair of such areas occurs, they appear as isolated cavitations that penetrate into the dentin. These areas can be differentiated from caries of the cementum by their clear-cut outline and hard surface. Once exposed to the oral cavity, they may be sources of considerable pain and require restoration.

Pulp changes associated with periodontal pockets

Spread of infection from periodontal pockets may cause pathologic changes in the pulp.[7] *Such changes may give rise to painful symptoms or adversely affect the response of the pulp to restorative procedures.* **Involvement of the pulp in periodontal disease occurs either through the apical foramen or lateral canals in the root after spreading from the pocket through the periodontal ligament. Atrophy or hypertrophy of the odontoblastic layer, hyperemia, leukocytic infiltration, interstitial calcification and fibrosis are the types of pulp changes that occur in such cases.**

The pulpal changes are correlated with the severity of periodontal involvement,[43] but not in all cases.[24] In experimental animals artificially induced pulp inflammation spread to the furcation area (10 to 15 per cent), probably through lateral canals;[32] and injury to the gingiva led to formation of secondary dentin.[38]

Gingival recession and pocket depth

Pocket formation causes recession of the gingiva and denudation of the root surface.

The severity of recession is generally, but not always, correlated with the depth of the pocket. This is because *the degree of recession depends upon the location of the base of the pocket on the root surface, whereas the depth is the distance between the base of the pocket and the crest of the gingiva.* Pockets of the same depth may be associated with different degrees of recession (Fig. 14-21), and pockets of different depths may be associated with the same amount of recession (Fig. 14-22).

Exposure of the roots after pockets are eliminated depends upon the amount of recession before treatment is instituted. A realistic appraisal of recession associated with periodontal pockets will prevent the erroneous impression that it is caused by the treatment.

Relation of pocket depth to alveolar bone destruction

Severity of bone loss may generally be correlated with pocket depth—but not always. Extensive bone loss may be associated with shallow pockets, and slight loss with deep pockets. Destruction of alveolar bone may occur in the absence of periodontal pockets associated with trauma from occlusion and in periodontosis.

The area between the base of the pocket and the alveolar bone

Normally, the distance between the epithelial attachment and the alveolar bone is relatively constant. In periodontal disease, however, this distance varies considerably. **In some instances, the base of the pocket is close to the bone and separated from it by only a band of collagen fibers. In others, the base of the pocket is separated from the bone by a broad zone of granulation tissue.**

The Infrabony Pocket

In infrabony pockets the base is apical to the level of the alveolar bone, and the pocket wall lies between the tooth and bone. Infrabony pockets most often occur interproximally, but may be located on the facial and lingual tooth surfaces. Most often the pocket spreads from the surface on which it originates to one or more contiguous surfaces. Statistical information regarding the

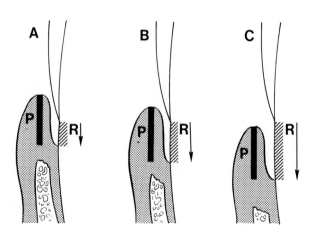

Figure 14–21 Same Pocket Depth—Different Amounts of Recession. *A,* Pocket depth (P), recession (R). *B,* Pocket depth (P) same as in *A,* more recession (R). *C,* Pocket depth (P) same as in *A,* still more recession (R).

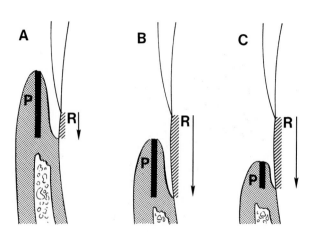

Figure 14–22 Difference Between Pocket Depth and Amount of Recession. *A,* Deep pocket (P), slight recession (R). *B,* Deep pocket (P), marked recession (R). *C,* Shallow pocket (P), marked recession (R).

TABLE 14–1 CORRELATION OF CLINICAL AND HISTOPATHOLOGIC FEATURES OF THE PERIODONTAL POCKET

Clinical Features	Histopathologic Features
1. The gingival wall of the periodontal pocket presents varying degrees of bluish red discoloration, flaccidity, a smooth shiny surface, and pitting on pressure.	1. The discoloration is caused by circulatory stagnation; the flaccidity, by destruction of the gingival fibers and surrounding tissues; the smooth, shiny surface, by the atrophy of the epithelium and edema; the pitting on pressure, by edema and degeneration.
2. Less frequently the gingival wall may be pink and firm.	2. In such cases fibrotic changes predominate over exudation and degeneration, particularly in relation to the outer surface of the pocket wall. However, despite the external appearance of health, the inner wall of the pocket invariably presents some degeneration, and is often ulcerated (Fig. 14–16).
3. Bleeding is elicited by gently probing the soft tissue wall of the pocket.	3. Ease of bleeding results from increased vascularity, thinning and degeneration of the epithelium, and the proximity of the engorged vessels to the inner surface.
4. When explored with a probe the inner aspect of the periodontal pocket is generally painful.	4. Pain upon tactile stimulation is due to ulceration of the inner aspect of the pocket wall.
5. In many cases pus may be expressed by applying digital pressure.	5. This occurs in pockets with suppurative inflammation of the inner wall.

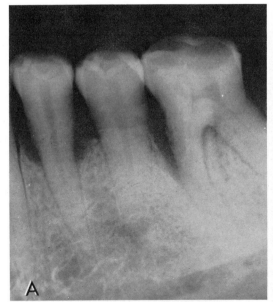

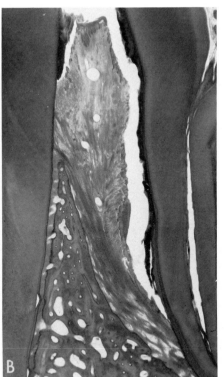

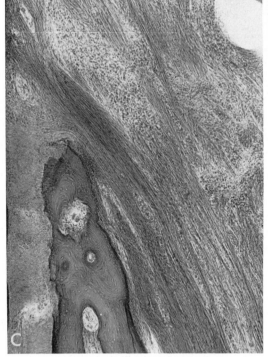

Figure 14–23 Infrabony Pocket on Mesial Surface of Molar. *A,* Radiograph showing deep angular defect on the mesial surface of the first molar. The bifurcation is also involved. There are shallower, broader defects on the first premolar. Note the calculus on the mesial surface of the molar. *B,* Interdental space between the second premolar with a suprabony pocket (*left*) and the first molar with an infrabony pocket. Note the following: the transseptal fibers which extend from the base of the infrabony pocket along the bone to the root of the premolar; the relationship of the epithelial lining of the pocket to the transseptal fibers; the calculus on the root. *C,* Transseptal fibers extending from the distal surface of the premolar over the crest of the bone into the infrabony pocket. Note the leukocytic infiltration of the transseptal fibers.

prevalence of infrabony pockets is not available. It has been suggested that 25 per cent of periodontal pockets are of the infrabony type,[8] and that the pockets are deeper on the pressure side of the teeth (the side toward which the teeth are tilted). *The inflammatory, proliferative and degenerative changes in infrabony and suprabony pockets are the same, and both lead to destruction of the supporting periodontal tissues.*

Differences between infrabony and suprabony pockets

The principal differences between infrabony and suprabony pockets are the relationship of the soft tissue wall of the pocket to the alveolar bone, the pattern of bone destruction, and the direction of the transseptal fibers of the periodontal ligament (Fig. 14–23).

The distinguishing features of suprabony

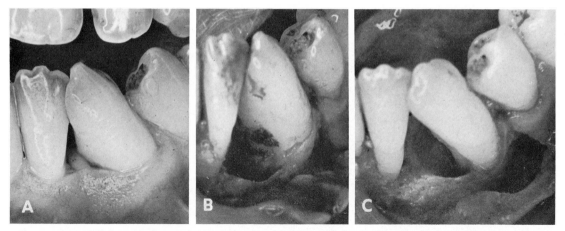

Figure 14–24 Infrabony Pocket on the Mesial Surface of the Mandibular Canine. *A,* Rolled gingival margin and space between gingiva and canine suggest presence of periodontal pocket. *B,* Flap reflected to show calculus on root and three wall bone defect. *C,* Bone defect, calculus removed.

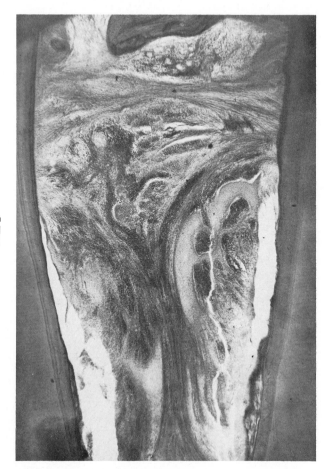

Figure 14–25 Two Suprabony Pockets in an Interdental Space between the maxillary cuspid and lateral incisor. Note the normal horizontal arrangement of the transseptal fibers.

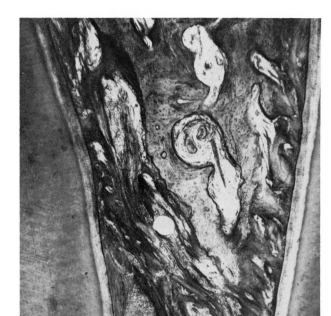

Figure 14–26 Early Infrabony Pocket on Maxillary Incisor (*left*). Note the oblique arrangement of the transseptal fibers.

TABLE 14–2 DISTINGUISHING FEATURES OF SUPRABONY AND INFRABONY POCKETS

Suprabony Pocket	Infrabony Pocket
1. The base of the pocket is coronal to the level of the alveolar bone.	1. The base of the pocket is apical to the crest of the alveolar bone, so that the bone is adjacent to part or all of the soft tissue wall (Fig. 14–7).
2. The pattern of destruction of the underlying bone is horizontal.	2. The bone destructive pattern is vertically angular or crater-like, creating an inverted deformity in the bone (Fig. 14–24).
3. Interproximally, the transseptal fibers that are restored during progressive periodontal disease are arranged horizontally in the space between the base of the pocket and the alveolar bone (Fig. 14–25).	3. Interproximally, the transseptal fibers are oblique rather than horizontal.[9] They extend from the cementum beneath the base of the pocket along the bone, and over the crest to the cementum of the adjacent tooth (Fig. 14–26).
4. On the facial and lingual surfaces, the periodontal ligament fibers beneath the pocket follow their normal horizontal-oblique course between the tooth and the bone.	4. On the facial and lingual surfaces, the periodontal ligament fibers follow the angular pattern of the adjacent bone. They extend from the cementum beneath the base of the pocket along the bone and over the crest to join with the outer periosteum.

and infrabony pockets are summarized in Table 14–2. The morphologic features of the infrabony pocket are important because they reflect a difference in etiology and necessitate modification in treatment techniques (see Chap. 44).

Classification of infrabony pockets

Infrabony pockets are classified in different ways; often used features are the *number of walls*[29] in the osseous defect (Fig. 14–27) and its *depth and width*, because they are important factors which influence the outcome of treatment. Infrabony defects may have one wall (Fig. 14–28), two walls, or three or four walls (Fig. 14–29). They are sometimes referred to as "**intrabony pockets**" when the osseous defect has three walls. When the number of walls in the apical portion of the defect is different from the number in the occlusal portion, the term *combined osseous defect* is used (Fig. 14–30).

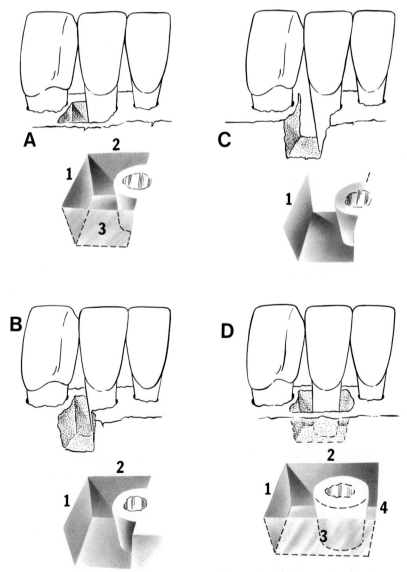

Figure 14–27   One-, Two-, Three- and Four-Walled Infrabony Defects on right lateral incisor. *A,* Three bony walls: (1) distal, (2) lingual and (3) facial wall. *B,* Two-wall defect: (1) distal and (2) lingual walls. *C,* One-wall defect: (1) distal wall only. *D,* Four-wall defect completely surrounds the root: (1) distal, (2) lingual, (3) facial and (4) mesial walls.

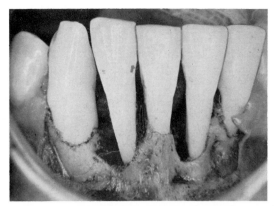

Figure 14–28 One-Wall Infrabony Defect on the mesial surface of the left lateral incisor and 1½-wall defect (distal wall and one half of the labial wall) on the distal surface of the right lateral.

Infrabony pockets are classified according to depth and width as follows:

Type 1. Shallow narrow

Type 2. Shallow wide (Fig. 14–31)

Type 3. Deep narrow (Fig. 14–32)

Type 4. Deep wide (Fig. 14–32)

Infrabony pockets generally occur in forms which represent gradients of the aforementioned types.

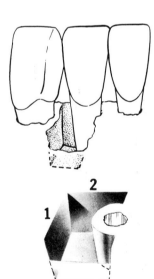

Figure 14–30 Combined Type of Osseous Defect. Because the facial wall is one half the height of the distal (1) and lingual (2) walls, this is an osseous defect with three walls in its apical half and two walls in the occlusal half.

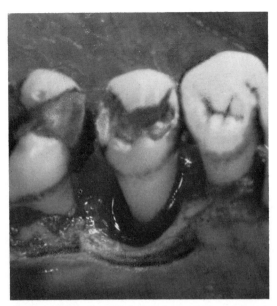

Figure 14–29 Four-Wall Infrabony Defect Viewed From the Lingual Surface, consisting of facial, lingual, mesial and distal walls in relation to the second premolar. The facial bony wall is obscured by the tooth.

The etiology of infrabony pockets

Infrabony pockets are caused by the same local irritants as suprabony pockets, plus trauma from occlusion.[8] The trauma adds to the effect of the inflammation in the following ways:[12, 13, 30] (1) By altering the alignment of the transseptal periodontal fibers, it diverts the inflammation directly into the periodontal ligament space rather than into the interdental septum. (2) By injuring the periodontal ligament fibers, it aggravates the destruction produced by inflammation. This further reduces the obstruction to the proliferating pocket epithelium. Instead of remaining coronal to the bone, the epithelium extends between the root and the bone (Fig. 14–33), creating an infrabony pocket. (3) By causing bone resorption lateral to the periodontal ligament, it worsens the bone loss caused by inflammation alone and leads to the creation of the osseous defect associated with infrabony pockets.

There are still differing opinions regarding the etiology of infrabony pockets.[30] The causative role of inflammation combined with trauma from occlusion has been studied extensively* but this does not rule out

---

*This subject is discussed in detail in Chapter 24.

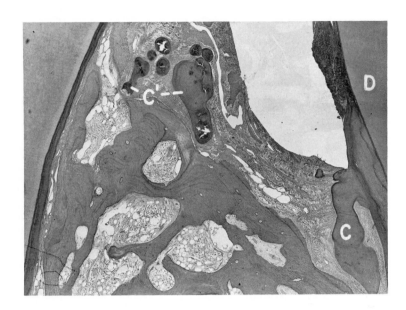

Figure 14–31 Shallow, Broad Infrabony Pocket. Cementicles in the pocket wall (C') represent an infrequent complication which may occur in any type of periodontal pocket. The epithelium at the base of the pocket is attached to a cementicle (C) which is adherent to the tooth (D).

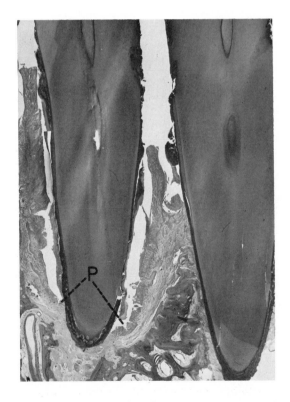

Figure 14–32 Deep Narrow Infrabony Pocket (P) on the mesial surface of the mandibular lateral incisor (*left*). Deep wide infrabony pocket (P) on the distal surface (*right*).

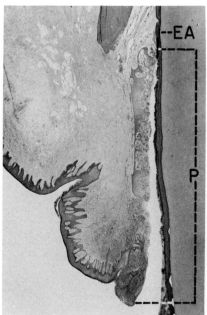
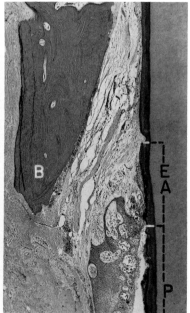

Figure 14–33 Transition from Suprabony Pocket to Infrabony Pocket. *Left,* Deep pocket (P) on the facial surface of a maxillary tooth. The epithelial attachment is shown at EA. *Right,* Base of the pocket. The epithelial attachment (EA) has migrated beyond the crest of the bone (B) and started to change the suprabony pocket to an infrabony pocket. At this early stage, the base of the pocket (P) is still coronal to the bone.

other etiologic factors that have not as yet been researched. Food impaction and infrabony pockets often occur together,[28] but it has not been established whether the food impaction produces the pockets or aggravates infrabony pockets caused by other factors.

THEORIES ON THE PATHOGENESIS OF PERIODONTAL POCKETS

The histopathology of the periodontal pocket is well documented; however, it has been subjected to varied interpretations. The following theories regarding how periodontal pockets develop are presented as useful background information for the interpretation of current and future concepts.

I. Destruction of the gingival fibers is a prerequisite for the initiation of pocket formation.

This concept focuses attention upon the migration of gingival fibers. The contention is that proliferation of the epithelial attachment along the root can take place only if the underlying gingival fibers are destroyed.[11] These fibers are considered a barrier to the normal migratory tendency of the epithelium at the base of the

sulcus,[14] and it is believed that their degeneration and necrosis occur secondary to gingival inflammation or the action of bacterial enzymes such as hyaluronidase.[2] As soon as the topmost fiber is digested and absorbed, the epithelium proliferates along the root until a healthy fiber is reached.

Gottlieb and Orban[19] have questioned this concept. They point to areas of repaired idiopathic tooth resorption immediately beneath the epithelial attachment, and note that since the resorption of the tooth entailed detachment of the gingival fibers, repair would not have been possible had the epithelium proliferated simply because the fibers had been destroyed. They also point out that when the epithelial attachment is attached to the enamel, and is separated from the cementum by unattached connective tissue rather than fibers embedded in the tooth, pathologic migration of the epithelial attachment does not occur.

II. The initial change in pocket formation occurs in the cementum.

In seeking an explanation for pocket formation, Gottlieb stresses the changes in tooth surface rather than the gingiva. He envisions downgrowth of the epithelial attachment as a physiologic phenomenon that is part of the process of continuous eruption of teeth throughout life.[17, 18] Under physiologic conditions, the continuous deposition of new cementum acts as a barrier that prevents accelerated migration of the epithelial attachment. So long as continuous cementum deposition is not disturbed, migration of the epithelial attachment at a pathologic rate cannot occur.[15,16] However, if the tooth surface is of low resistance, or if the normal deposition of cementum is impaired, inflammation or trauma can do additional harm by destroying either the cementum or the gingiva, or both. This dissolves the organic connection between the two, and the epithelium proliferates along the root until it meets undisturbed connective tissue fibers and cementum. Death of the cementum does not necessary occur under such circumstances, as evidenced by the fact that epithelium attaches itself to cementum after its organic connection with the periodontal ligament fibers is destroyed.

III. Stimulation of the epithelial attachment by inflammation rather than destruction of gingival fibers is the prerequisite for the initiation of the periodontal pocket.

Destruction of the underlying gingival fibers is not a prerequisite for epithelial migration.[1] Stimulated by inflammation, the epithelium migrates along the root without preceding destruction of the gingival fibers. In such instances the epithelial cells burrow between the intact gingival fibers and attach themselves farther apically on the cementum in bundle-free areas. The epithelial attachment may move between healthy connective tissue fibers, enmesh them in an epithelial network, and produce secondary fiber degeneration.

IV. Pathologic destruction of the epithelial attachment due to infection or trauma is the initial histologic change in pocket formation.

According to Skillen,[37] the epithelial attachment has few protective qualities for safeguarding the underlying connective tissue against spread of infection. It is the normal downgrowth of the oral epithelium behind the epithelial attachment that protects the underlying connective tissue. The epithelial attachment is an area of low resistance subject to infection. In experimental animals, pocket formation occurs because of pathologic dissolution of the epithelial attachment due to infection or trauma, or both. Accumulation of debris in the pocket may be secondary—after the pocket is formed by dissolution of the epithelial attachment.

V. The periodontal pocket is initiated by invasion of bacteria at the base of the sulcus or the absorption of bacterial toxins through the epithelial lining of the sulcus.

According to Box,[6] either because of imperfect junction of the epithelial cells and the cementum or extreme thinness of the epithelium, the base of the sulcus offers a poor defense against bacteria. In the evolution of a pocket, initial invasion of bacteria at the base of the sulcus leads to the following changes: inflammation in the underlying connective tissue, ulceration at the base of the crevice, sloughing of the epithelium and loss of attachment to the cementum, progressive loss of connective tissue, and penetration of the pocket into the deeper tissues. Specific infective agents possibly related to *Leptothrix falciformis* are capable of deepening the periodontal pocket. Also Arnim and Holt[3] consider the epithelial lining of the sulcus a poor barrier against bacterial toxins, which initiate inflammatory changes leading to pocket formation.

VI. Pocket formation is initiated in a defect in the sulcus wall.

According to Becks,[5] the formation and maintenance of the normal 1 mm.-deep sulcus results from the coordination of degeneration of the enamel epithelium, proliferation of the oral epithelium, and atrophy of the gingival papilla. Disturbance of this correlation, whether by inflammation or injury, leads to pathologic pocket formation.

Pocket formation occurs between the oral epithelium and the enamel epithelium, rather than by separation of enamel epithelium from the cuticle. If degeneration of the enamel epithelium takes place rapidly without being covered by the oral epithelium, a defect occurs in the lateral sulcus wall. This defect constitutes a "locus minoris resistentiae" which is a portal of entry for bacteria with resultant inflammation. This induces proliferation of the basal cells of the enamel epithelium and the oral epithelium, a protective mechanism for the connective tissue. Inflammation is a stimulant to oral epithelium proliferation, which shuts off nutrition from enamel epithelium, hastens its degeneration, and increases the pocket depth.

In some cases, pathologic pocket formation may be initiated without inflammation appearing to play a role. In such instances there is an accelerated degeneration of the enamel epithelium, possibly of systemic origin. This is followed by proliferation of the oral epithelium to cover the defect.

VII. Proliferation of the epithelium of the lateral wall, rather than the epithelium at the base of the sulcus, is the initial change in the formation of the periodontal pocket.

Wilkinson[41] regards epithelial proliferation as the primary change in pocket formation. He describes the following sequence of changes: Proliferation and downgrowth of the oral epithelium or proliferation of the epithelial attachment result in a thickening of the epithelial lining of the sulcus. The cause of this proliferation is not known. Because of the increased thickness, the cells along the inner aspect of the sulcus, are deprived of nutrition and undergo degeneration and necrosis. The degenerated and necrotic epithelial cells become calcified (serumal calculus). Separation of the calcified masses from the adjacent normal epithelium produces a pocket or trough. These changes are followed by proliferation of the epithelium along the cementum, and detachment of its coronal portion from the root surface. The epithelial changes that initiate pocket formation are not caused by infection. Inflammatory changes in pocket formation are secondary to the epithelial changes. Wilkinson suggests that vitamin A deficiency may be an important factor in initiating pocket formation.

VIII. Two-stage pocket formation.

James and Counsell[22] disagree with the concept that proliferation of epithelial attachment followed by separation from cementum forms a pocket. Instead, they feel pocket formation occurs in two stages:

The first stage is proliferation of the subgingival epithelium (epithelial attachment). The second stage is loss of the superficial layers of the proliferated epithelium, which produces a space or pocket. The rate of proliferation of the epithelium at the base is such that it precedes the destruction of the superficial epithelium, and the pocket is therefore always lined with epithelium.

IX. Inflammation is the initial change in the formation of the periodontal pocket.

According to this concept periodontal pockets start as inflammatory lesions.[26] The first reaction is a vascular change in the underlying connective tissue.

Inflammation in the connective tissue stimulates the following changes in the epithelial lining of the sulcus and in the epithelial attachment: increased mitotic activity in the basal epithelial layer, and sometimes in the prickle cell layer; increased production of keratin with desquamation. The cellular desquamation adjacent to the tooth surface tends to deepen the pocket.

The epithelial cells of the basal layer at the bottom of the sulcus and in the area of attach-

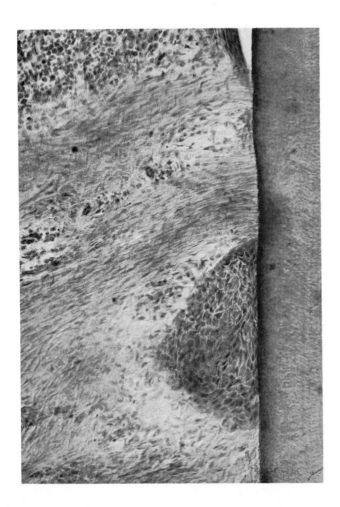

Figure 14–34 Section Showing Finger-Like Projection of Epithelium which has proliferated along the root surface into space created by destruction of gingival fibers. Some fibers still remain between the proliferated epithelium and the base of the pocket (*top*). Note inflammatory cells among the gingival fibers.

ment proliferate into the underlying connective tissue and break up the gingival fibers. The dissolution of connective tissue results in the formation of what is described as an *open lesion*. It is the repair of the lesion in the absence of treatment that establishes the periodontal pocket. Granulation tissue fills in the defect created by the open lesion, and the epithelium proliferates inward. This forms a lining of the repaired open lesion to a point where the connective tissue is attached to the root. In pocket formation, the epithelium does not proliferate along the root; instead it proliferates from the gingival surface to cover the connective tissue lesion created by inflammation, and thereby forms the lining of the pocket.

X. Pathologic epithelial proliferation occurs secondary to noninflammatory degenerative changes in the periodontal membrane.

Under the term "periodontosis" a condition has been described which is characterized by generalized noninflammatory degeneration of the collagen fibers embedded in the cementum. Under such conditions, the normal barrier afforded by the gingival fibers is diminished. This facilitates the migration of the epithelial attachment along the root and pocket formation, in the presence of local irritation.

Comment regarding pocket formation

The following salient facts regarding pocket formation are worthy of special note:

Local irritation is required for the initiation and progress of pocket formation.

Proliferation of the epithelial attachment along the root and degeneration of the underlying gingival fibers are primary changes in pocket formation.

Proliferation of the epithelial attachment is stimulated by local irritation. Inflammation caused by local irritation produces degeneration of the gingival fibers, making it easier for the epithelium to move along the root (Fig. 14–34).

Systemic disorders do not initiate pocket formation, but they may affect pocket depth by causing degeneration of gingival and periodontal fibers.

REFERENCES

1. Aisenberg, M. S., and Aisenberg, A. D.: A New Concept of Pocket Formation. Oral Surg., Oral Med. & Oral Path., *1*:1047, 1948.
2. Aisenberg, M. S., and Aisenberg, A. D.: Hyaluroni- dase in Periodontal Disease. Oral Surg., Oral Med. & Oral Path., *4*:317, 1951.
3. Arnim, S. S., and Holt, R. T.: The Defense Mechanism of the Gingiva. J. Periodont., *26*:79, 1955.
4. Bass, C. C.: A Previously Undescribed Demonstrable Pathologic Condition in Exposed Cementum and the Underlying Dentine. Oral Surg., Oral Med. & Oral Path., *4*:641, 1951.
5. Becks, H.: Normal and Pathologic Pocket Formation, J.A.D.A., *16*:2167, 1929.
6. Box, H. K.: New Aspects of Periodontal Research. J. Canad. D. Assn., *13*:3, 1941.
7. Seltzer, S., Bender, I. B., and Ziontz, M.: The Interrelationship of Pulp and Periodontal Disease. Oral Sur., Oral Med. & Oral Path., *16*:1474, 1963.
8. Carranza, F. A., and Erausquin, R.: Our First Periodontal Findings. Revista Odontologica. Buenos Aires, *27*:485, 1939.
9. Carranza, F. A., Jr., and Glickman, I.: Some Observations on the Microscopic Features of the Infrabony Pockets. J. Periodont., *28*:33, 1957.
10. Emslie, R. D., and Stack, M. V.: The Micro Hardness of Roots of Teeth with Periodontal Disease. D. Practit., *9*:101, 1958.
11. Fish, E. W.: Surgical Pathology of the Mouth. London, Isaac Pitman & Sons, 1948, p. 316.
12. Glickman, I., and Smulow, J. B.: Alterations in the Pathway of Gingival Inflammation into the Underlying Tissues Induced by Excessive Occlusal Forces. J. Periodont., *33*:7, 1962.
13. Glickman, I., and Smulow, J. B.: The Combined Effects of Inflammation and Trauma from Occlusion in Periodontitis. Internat. D. J., *19*:393, 1969.
14. Goldman, H. M.: The Relationship of the Epithelial Attachment to the Adjacent Fibers of the Periodontal Membrane. J. D. Res., *23*:177, 1944.
15. Gottlieb, B.: The Formation of the Pocket; Diffuse Alveolar Atrophy. Proc. 7th Int. D. Cong., *2*:1631, 1926.
16. Gottlieb, B.: Tissue Changes in Pyorrhea. J.A.D.A., *14*:2178, 1927.
17. Gottlieb, B.: Continuous Deposition of Cementum. J.A.D.A., *30*:842, 1943.
18. Gottlieb, B.: The New Concept of Periodontoclasia. J. Periodont., *17*:7, 1946.
19. Gottlieb, B., and Orban, B.: Biology and Pathology of the Tooth (Translated by M. Diamond). New York, The Macmillan Co., 1938, p. 64.
20. Graham, J. W.: Toxicity of Sterile Filtrate from Parodontal Pockets. Proc. Roy. Soc. Med., *30*:1165, 1937.
21. Herting, H. C.: Electron Microscope Studies of the Cementum Surface Structures of Periodontally Healthy and Diseased Teeth. J. D. Res., *46*: Supplement, 1247, 1967.
22. James, W., and Counsell, A.: A Histological Investigation into "So-Called Pyorrhea Alveolaris." Brit. D. J., *48*:1237, 1927.
23. Masi, P. L., and Benini, A.: Richerche su la Microdurezza del Dente Umano Parodontosico. Riv. Ital. Stomatol., *18*:293, 1963.
24. Mazur, B., and Massler, M.: Influences of Periodontal Disease on the Dental Pulp. Oral Surg., Oral Med. & Oral Path., *17*:592, 1964.
25. McMillan, L., Burrill, D. Y., and Fosdick, L. S.: An Electron Microscope Study of Particulates in Periodontal Exudate. J. D. Res., *37*:51, 1958. (Abst.)

26. Nuckolls, J., and Dienstein, B., in collab. with Bell, D. G., and Rule, R. W., Jr.: The Periodontal Lesions — The Development of the Lesion and the Establishment and Treatment of the Periodontal Pocket. J. Periodont., *21*:7, 44, 1950.
27. Orban, B., and Ray, A. G.: Deep Necrotic Foci in the Gingiva. J. Periodont., *19*:91, 1948.
28. Prichard, J.: A Technique for Treating Infrabony Pockets Based on Aveolar Process Morphology. D. Clin. North America, March, 1960, p. 85.
29. Prichard, J.: The Infrabony Technique as a Predictable Procedure. J. Periodont., *28*:202, 1957.
30. Proceedings, World Workshop in Periodontics. The University of Michigan, 1966, p. 272.
31. Rautiola, C. A., and Craig, R. G.: The Micro Hardness of Cementum and Underlying Dentin of Normal Teeth and Teeth Exposed to Periodontal Disease. J. Periodont., *32*:113, 1961.
32. Seltzer, S., Bender, I., Nazimov, H., and Sinai, I.: Pulpitis-Induced Interradicular Periodontal Changes in Experimental Animals. J. Periodont., *38*:124, 1967.
33. Selvig, K. A.: Biological Changes at the Tooth-Saliva Interface in Periodontal Disease. J. D. Res., *48*:Supplement, Part 1, 846, 1969.
34. Selvig, K. A.: Ultrastructural Changes in Cementum and Adjacent Connective Tissue in Periodontal Disease. Acta Odont. Scandinav., *24*:459, 1966.
35. Selvig, K. A., and Zander, H. A.: Chemical Analysis and Microradiography of Cementum and Dentin from Periodontally Diseased Human Teeth. J. Periodont., *33*:303, 1962.
36. Simpson, Zuniga, Jorge: Spectrographic Analysis of Normal and Pathologic Teeth. Santiago, Chile, University of Chile Press, 1946.
37. Skillen, W. G.: Normal Characteristics of the Gingiva and Their Relation to Pathology. J.A.D.A., *17*:1088, 1930.
38. Stahl, S. S.: Pulpal Response to Gingival Injury in Adult Rats. Oral Surg., Oral Med. & Oral Path., *16*:1116, 1963.
39. Thilander, H.: Some Structural Changes in Periodontal Disease. D. Practit., *11*:191, 1961.
40. Warren, E. B., Hansen, N. M., Swartz, M. L., and Phillips, R. W.: Effects of Periodontal Disease and of Calculus Solvents on Microhardness of Cementum. J. Periodont., *35*:505, 1964.
41. Wilkinson, F. C.: A Patho-Histological Study of the Tissue Tooth Attachment. D. Record, *55*:105, 1935.
42. Wittwer, J. W., Dickler, E. H., and Toto, P. D.: Comparative Frequencies of Plasma Cells and Lymphocytes in Gingivitis. J. Periodont., *40*:274, 1969.
43. Zilkens, K.: Some Observations Regarding the Pulp in Periodontal Disease. Fortschritte der Zahnheilk., *3*:289, 1927.

Chapter 15

EXTENSION OF INFLAMMATION FROM THE GINGIVA TO THE SUPPORTING PERIODONTAL TISSUES

The extension of inflammation from the marginal gingiva into the supporting periodontal tissues marks the transition from *gingivitis* to *periodontitis*. The term *marginal periodontitis* is also used to connote the destruction of periodontal tissues produced by the extension of inflammation from the gingiva.

For many years opinion differed regarding the pathway of gingival inflammation into the supporting tissues. Some considered it to be by way of the lymphatics of the periodontal ligament (Talbot,[11] Fish,[5] Black[2]); some felt that the inflammation extended along the fibers of the periodontal ligament or the outer periosteum of the alveolar bone (Noyes[10] and Coolidge[4]); while others maintained that the inflammation spread from the gingiva into the alveo-

lar bone and that it rarely, if ever, extended directly into the periodontal ligament (Box,[3] Kronfeld,[8] and Thoma and Goldman[14]). The findings of Weinmann[13] led to a general acceptance of the latter concept; namely, that gingival inflammation follows the course of the blood vessels through the loosely arranged tissues around them into the alveolar bone. **The pathway of the spread of inflammation is critical, because it affects the pattern of the bone destruction in periodontal disease.**

THE PATHWAYS OF GINGIVAL INFLAMMATION

Local irritation causes inflammation in the marginal gingiva and interdental papillae. The inflammation penetrates and destroys the gingival fibers, usually at a short distance from their attachment into the cementum (Fig. 15–1). It then spreads into the supporting tissues along the following pathways (Fig. 15–2):

Interproximal pathways

Interproximally, inflammation spreads in the loose connective tissue around the blood vessels through the transseptal fibers and then into the bone through vessel channels which perforate the crest of the

211

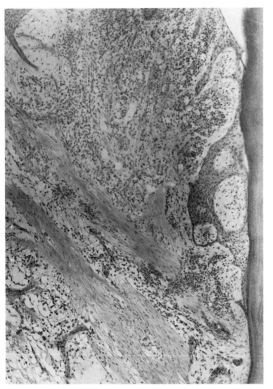

Figure 15–1 Destruction of Gingival Fibers associated with the extension of inflammation from the gingiva into the supporting periodontal tissues.

interdental septum. **The location at which the inflammation enters the bone depends upon the location of the vessel channels.** It may enter the interdental septum at the center of the crest (Fig. 15–3), toward the side (Fig. 15–4) of the crest or at the angle of the septum (Fig. 15–5), and it may enter the bone through more than one channel (Fig. 15–5). After reaching the marrow spaces, the inflammation may return from the bone into the periodontal ligament (Fig. 15–2). Less frequently, the inflammation spreads from the gingiva directly into the periodontal ligament and from there into the interdental septum (Fig. 15–2).[1]

Facial and lingual pathways

Facially and lingually, inflammation from the gingiva spreads **along the outer periosteal surface of the bone** (Fig. 15–2) and penetrates into the **marrow spaces through vessel channels in the outer cortex.**

Reestablishment of transseptal fibers

In its course from the gingiva to the bone, the inflammation destroys the transseptal

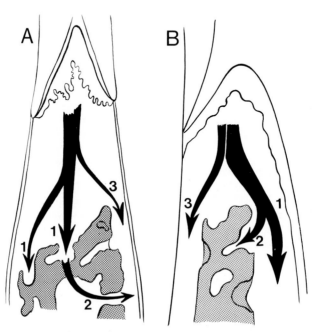

Figure 15–2 Pathways of Inflammation From the Gingiva into the Supporting Periodontal Tissues in Periodontitis. *A,* **Interproximally.** (1) From the gingiva into the bone, (2) from the bone into the periodontal ligament, (3) from the gingiva into the periodontal ligament. *B,* **Facially and Lingually.** (1) From the gingiva along the outer periosteum, (2) from the periosteum into the bone, (3) from the gingiva into the periodontal ligament.

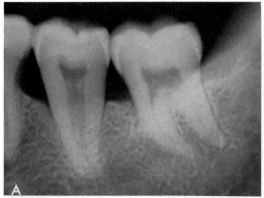

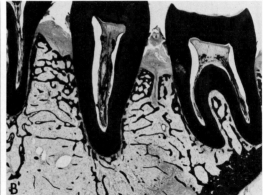

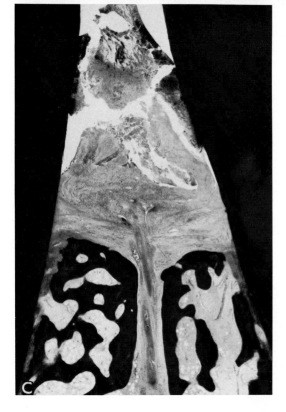

Figure 15–3 Extension of Inflammation into the Center of the Interdental Septum.
A, Molar region showing periodontal bone loss. B, Survey section of the second and third molars. C, Inflammation from the gingiva penetrates the transseptal fibers and enters the bone around blood vessel in the center of the septum.

fibers and reduces them to disorganized granular fragments interspersed among the inflammatory cells and edema (Figs. 15–6 and 15–4 B). However, there is a continuous tendency to recreate transseptal fibers across the crest of the interdental septum further along the root as the bone destruction progresses. As a result, transseptal fibers are present even in cases of extreme periodontal bone loss (Fig. 15–7).[6]

The dense transseptal fibers are of clinical significance when surgical procedures are employed for the eradication of perio-

dontal pockets. They form a firm covering over the bone, which is encountered after the superficial granulation tissue is removed.

ALTERATIONS IN THE PATHWAY OF INFLAMMATION CAUSED BY EXCESSIVE OCCLUSAL FORCES

The usual pathways of inflammation from the gingiva into the supporting periodontal tissues have been described above. **Just as**

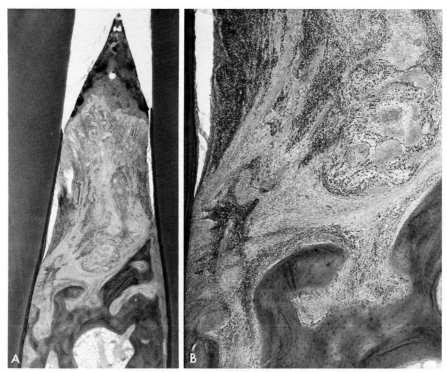

Figure 15–4 Inflammation Enters the Interdental Septum at the Center of the Crest and Near the Crestal Angle. *A,* Interdental periodontal pockets with inflammation extending into the bone. *B,* Inflammation enters the crest of the interdental bone at two areas. Note the granular necrosis of the collagen fibers in the inflamed area above the bone.

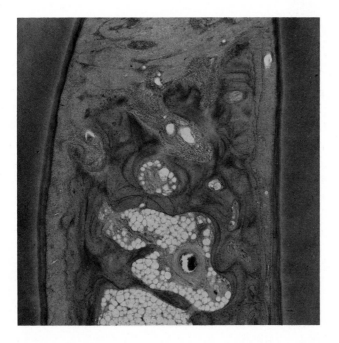

Figure 15–5 Inflammation Enters the Interdental Bone at the Angle of the Crest and in two other areas.

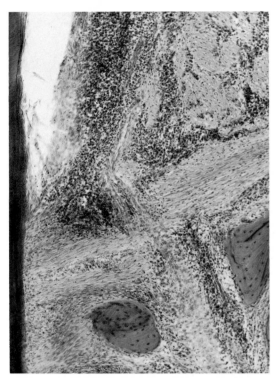

Figure 15–6 Penetration and Destruction of Transseptal Fibers as Inflammation Extends into the Bone.

the pathway of inflammation is affected by anatomical factors, it is also influenced by occlusal forces. Excessive occlusal forces may alter the supporting tissues in such a way as to divert the inflammation from its usual course.[7] In so doing it alters the pattern of bone destruction produced by the inflammation so that instead of horizontal destruction, angular bony defects and craters with infrabony pockets may result.

Excessive pressure affects the alignment of the transseptal fibers so that they become angular instead of horizontal. It also causes compression, degeneration and realignment of the periodontal ligament fibers so that they are more parallel than perpendicular to the tooth and bone. Instead of following its usual interdental course into the interdental bone, the inflammatory exudate is channeled between the transseptal fibers directly into the periodontal ligament (Fig. 15–8).

Inflammation occasionally enters directly into the periodontal ligament when the occlusal forces are normal. But when excessive forces are the responsible factor, the effects are more pronounced. There is a funnel-shaped widening of the periodontal ligament space, aggravated by the increased bone resorption caused by the excessive occlusal pressure (Fig. 15–8). Excessive occlusal forces also alter the pathway of inflammation on the facial and lingual surfaces, but infrabony defects occur there less frequently.

Excessive tension also affects the pathway of inflammation. It causes stretching and unraveling of the principal fiber bundles of the periodontal ligament, reducing the barrier provided by the intact bundles and permitting the inflammation direct access to the periodontal ligament.[9]

CLINICAL ASPECTS OF INFLAMMATION IN THE PERIODONTAL LIGAMENT

Regardless of whether it extends directly from the gingiva or indirectly through the alveolar bone, inflammation is often present in the periodontal ligament in periodontal disease, contributing to tooth mobility and pain.

Tooth mobility

Inflammation in the periodontal ligament is one of the factors responsible for pathologic tooth mobility, along with loss of alveolar bone and trauma from occlusion. The inflammatory exudate reduces tooth support by causing degeneration and destruction of the principal fibers and a break in the continuity between the root and the bone. The extent to which inflammation in the periodontal ligament contributes to tooth mobility is dramatically demonstrated when the inflammation is eliminated by treatment and the tooth becomes firm.

Pain

Inflammation in the periodontal ligament is usually chronic and asymptomatic. However, superimposed acute inflammation is frequently the cause of considerable pain. With the influx of the acute exudate, the tooth becomes elevated in its socket and there is a desire on the part of the patient to "grind" on it. Repeated contact with the opposing teeth causes the tooth to become sensitive to percussion. The condition may develop into an acute periodontal abscess unless the irritating agents are removed.

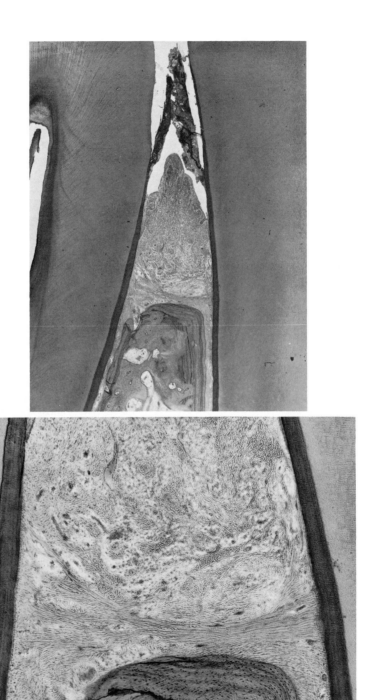

Figure 15–7 Reformation of the Transseptal Fibers in Periodontal Disease. *Top,* Mesiodistal section through the interdental septum showing gingival inflammation with pocket formation and bone loss. *Bottom,* Bone margin showing recreated transseptal fibers of the periodontal ligament just above the bone. Note pronounced degeneration of the connective tissue above the transseptal fibers.

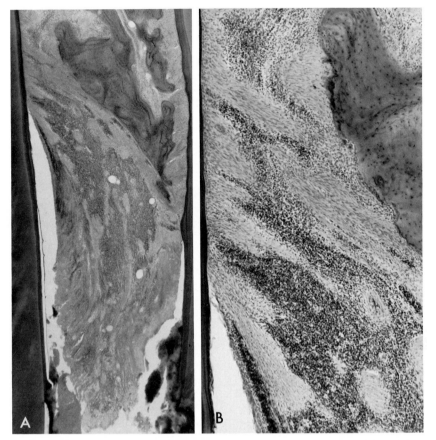

Figure 15–8   Inflammation Extends Directly into the Periodontal Ligament. *A,* Infrabony pocket on the mesial surface of maxillary premolar (*left*). *B,* Inflammation at the base of infrabony pocket extends directly into the periodontal ligament. Note the funnel-shaped widening of the periodontal ligament space and the osteoclastic resorption along the bone surface.

REFERENCES

1. Akiyoshi, M., and Mori, K.: Marginal Periodontitis: A Histological Study of the Incipient Stage. J. Periodont., *38*:45, 1967.
2. Black, G. V.: Operative Dentistry. Chicago, Medical-Dental Publishing Co., 1936, p. 165.
3. Box, H. K.: Twelve Periodontal Studies. Toronto, University of Toronto Press, 1940.
4. Coolidge, E. D.: Inflammatory Changes in the Gingival Tissue Due to Local Irritation. J.A.D.A., *18*:2255, 1931.
5. Fish, E. W.: Bone Infection. J.A.D.A., *26*:691, 1939.
6. Fullmer, H. M.: A Histochemical Study of Periodontal Disease in the Maxillary Alveolar Process of 135 Autopsies. J. Periodont., *32*:206, 1961.
7. Glickman, I., and Smulow, J. B.: Alterations in the Pathway of Gingival Inflammation into the Underlying Tissues Induced by Excessive Occlusal Forces. J. Periodont., *33*:7, 1962.
8. Kronfeld, R.: Histopathology of the Teeth and Their Surrounding Structures. Philadelphia, Lea & Febiger, 1939, p. 315.
9. Macapanpan, L. C., and Weinmann, J. P.: The Influence of Injury to the Periodontal Membrane on the Spread of Gingival Inflammation. J. D. Res., *33*:263, 1954.
10. Noyes, F. B.: A Review of the Work on the Lymphatics of Dental Origin. J.A.D.A., *14*:714, 1927.
11. Talbot, E. S.: Interstitial Gingivitis. Philadelphia, S. S. White Manufacturing Co., 1899.
12. Thoma, K. H., and Goldman, H. M.: The Classification & Histopathology of Parodontal Disease. J.A.D.A., *24*:1915, 1937.
13. Weinmann, J. P.: Progress of Gingival Inflammation into the Supporting Structures of the Teeth. J. Periodont, *12*:71, 1941.

Chapter 16

BONE LOSS AND PATTERNS OF BONE DESTRUCTION IN PERIODONTAL DISEASE

The crux of the problem of chronic destructive periodontal disease lies in the changes that occur in the bone. Changes in the other tissues of the periodontium are important, but in the final analysis it is the destruction of bone that is responsible for loss of the teeth.

PHYSIOLOGIC ALVEOLAR BONE EQUILIBRIUM

The height of the alveolar bone is normally maintained by a constant equilibrium between bone formation and bone resorption,[3] which is regulated by local and systemic influences (Fig. 16–1). When resorption exceeds formation, bone height is reduced. Reduction in the height of the alveolar bone occurs physiologically with age and is termed *physiologic* or *senile atrophy*.

Bone destruction in periodontal disease exceeds the physiologic reduction in bone height. The bone equilibrium is altered so that resorption exceeds formation, with normal bone formation remaining unaltered. Any factor or combination of factors that changes the physiologic bone equilibrium so that resorption exceeds formation results in loss of alveolar bone.

Bone loss in periodontal disease may re-

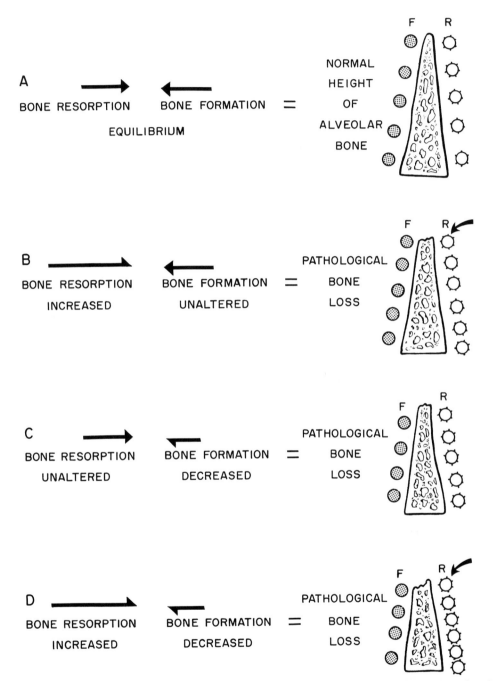

Figure 16–1 Diagrammatic Representation of Bone Formative–Bone Resorptive Relationships in Periodontal Health and Disease. *A,* Physiologic equilibrium between bone resorption (R) and bone formation (F) responsible for the maintenance of normal alveolar bone height. *B,* Pathological bone loss produced when bone resorption is increased (arrow). *C,* Pathological bone loss produced when bone formation is decreased. *D,* Pathological bone loss produced when bone resorption is increased (arrow) and bone formation decreased.

sult from any of the following changes (Fig. 16–1):

1. Increased resorption in the presence of normal or increased formation.
2. Decreased formation in the presence of normal resorption.
3. Increased resorption combined with decreased formation.

MECHANISMS OF BONE RESORPTION

The biological systems responsible for bone resorption have been studied extensively,[20] but their precise nature has not been established. The following types of bone resorption have been described:

Lacunar resorption (osteoclasis)

The destruction of bone results from the action of osteoclasts, which are usually multinuclear but may be mononuclear. The following explanations of the manner in which osteoclasts resorb bone have been offered:

1. Initial decalcification of the mineral salts of the bone caused by a local drop in the pH.
2. Proteolytic action upon the organic matrix, resulting in liberation of calcium salts.
3. Simultaneous destruction of the inorganic and organic components.[16]
4. Phagocytosis of the organic matrix after the inorganic salts are removed as the result of alterations in the local physico-chemical equilibrium.[1,11]

Halisteresis (osteolysis)

In this process the bone disintegrates into its separate components without the action of osteoclasts. Theories offered in explanation of noncellular destruction of bone include: softening and liquefaction of the organic matrix followed by a leaching out of the inorganic components;[23] loss of the inorganic components caused by disturbances in the normal physicochemical equilibrium,[15] followed by the reversion of the organic component to connective tissue. Opinions differ as to whether bone resorption can occur without the action of osteoclasts.[22]

Increased vascularity

Increased osteoclastic resorption of bone has been attributed to pressure from hyperemia. According to Leriche and Policard,[15] increased circulation within bone favors resorption, whereas blood or lymphatic stasis favors bone formation. Jaffe[11] describes a "vascular resorption" in which dilatation and an increase in the number of blood vessels are basic factors underlying the bone destruction. The vascular changes are made possible by decalcification of the contiguous bone matrix caused by alterations in the electrolyte balance by local and systemic factors.

BONE DESTRUCTION IN PERIODONTAL DISEASE

Bone destruction in periodontal disease is caused principally by local factors. It may also be caused by systemic factors, but their role has not been defined. If all the local factors responsible for bone destruction in periodontal disease were to be classified, it would be found that they fall into two groups: those that cause *gingival inflammation*, and those that cause *trauma from occlusion*. Acting singly or together, inflammation and trauma from occlusion are responsible for the locally caused bone destruction in periodontal disease and determine its destruction, severity and pattern (Fig. 16–2).

Bone Destruction Caused by Chronic Inflammation

Chronic inflammation is the most common cause of bone destruction in periodontal disease.

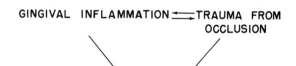

Figure 16–2 Local Factors responsible for bone destruction in periodontal disease.

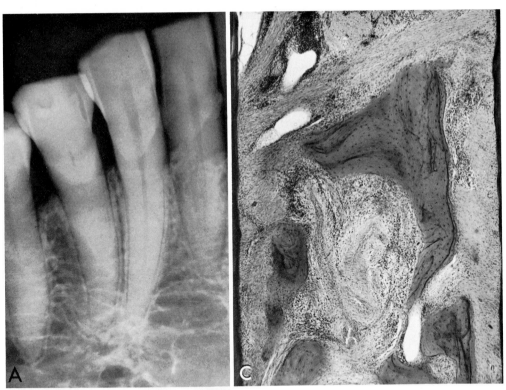

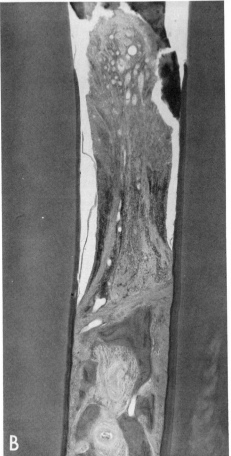

Figure 16–3 Early Periodontal Bone Destruction. *A,* Early periodontal bone loss in the canine and premolar areas. *B,* Interdental space between the canine and first premolar, showing calculus and periodontal pockets. *C,* Interdental septum beneath the periodontal pockets. The inflammation has invaded the marrow space, and there is lacunar resorption of the surrounding bone surface. Note the inflammation in the periodontal ligament on the right side.

Histopathology

Inflammation reaches the bone by extension from the gingiva (Chap. 15). It spreads into the marrow spaces and replaces the marrow with a leukocytic and fluid exudate, new blood vessels and proliferating fibroblasts (Fig. 16–3). Multinuclear osteoclasts and mononuclear phagocytes are increased in number[6] and the bone surfaces are lined with cove-like resorption lacunae (Fig. 16–4). In the marrow spaces resorption proceeds from within, causing first a thinning of the surrounding bone trabeculae and enlargement of the marrow spaces, followed by destruction of the bone and reduction in bone height.

The inflammation also stimulates bone formation immediately adjacent to active bone resorption (Fig. 16–5) and along trabecular surfaces removed from the inflammation in an apparent effort to reinforce the resorbing bone (buttressing bone formation) (Fig. 16–6).

Mechanisms Whereby Inflammation Destroys Bone in Periodontal Disease

The process of bone resorption has been studied extensively.[17, 20] "Resorption stimulating factors" (parathyroid extract, crystalline vitamins A and D), described by Goldhaber,[7, 8] lead to bone resorption in tissue culture. Their activity is dependent upon and regulated by oxygen tension.

Other substances, one of which is heparin, enhance the activity of resorption stimulating factors and are termed "bone resorption stimulating co-factors." Bone resorption is increased by the addition of human gingival fragments to tissue culture.[7] Many explanations have been considered, but the mechanisms of bone destruction in inflammatory periodontal disease have not as yet been determined.

Inflammation in periodontal disease is accompanied by an increase in osteoclasts and mononuclear phagocytes, both of which resorb bone by removing the mineral crystals and digesting the exposed collagen. The increased vascularity associated with inflammation may also cause bone resorption by stimulating an increase in osteoclasts[11, 15] and by elevating the local oxygen tension. The lowered pH of the inflammatory process may also affect bone resorption.[21]

Proteolytic enzymes in the periodontal tissues or produced by gingival bacteria may also participate in bone resorption.[9] Collagenase is present in the normal periodontium and increased in inflamed gingiva; it is also produced by oral bacteria. Collagenolytic activity is produced in resorbing bone *in vitro*, but the collagen content is not correlated with the severity of bone loss.[4] By breaking down the bone matrix ground substance, hyaluronidase produced by oral bacteria may influence the resorp-

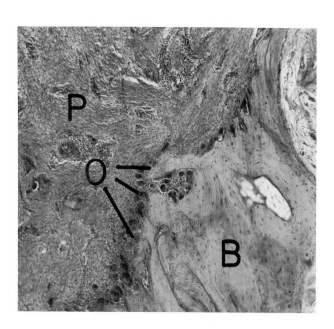

Figure 16–4 Pronounced Osteoclastic Activity. Osteoclasts (O) along the bone (B) surface adjacent to inflammation in a periodontal pocket (P).

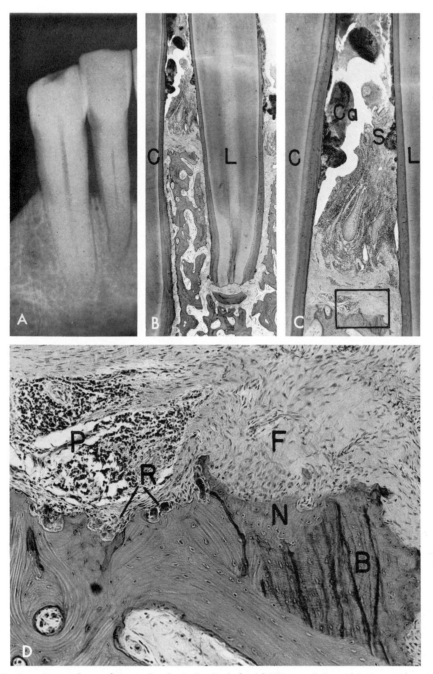

Figure 16-5   Bone Resorption and Formation in Active Periodontal Disease. *A,* Lateral incisor and canine with bone loss. *B,* Survey section of lateral (L) and canine (C). *C,* Interdental space between lateral (L) and canine (C), showing calculus (Ca) and periodontal pockets with suppuration (S). A detailed view of the bone margin within the rectangle is shown in C.

D, Bone margin beneath the periodontal pockets. Note the following: osteoclastic resorption (R) beneath the inflammation (P), and newly formed bone (N) with a thin surface layer of osteoid and osteoblasts adjacent to the resorption. The new bone is separated from the lamellated bone (B) by an irregular resorption line. An area of fibrosis is shown at F.

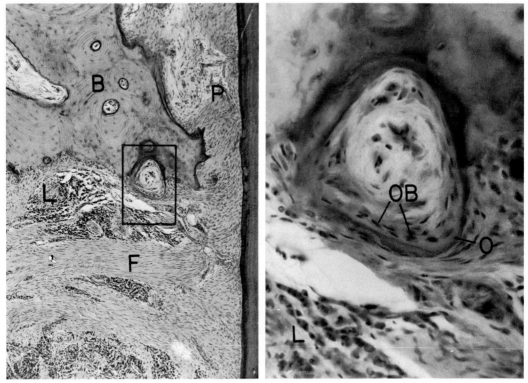

Figure 16–6   Central Buttressing Bone Formation in Chronic Periodontal Disease. *Left,* Survey section of crest of interdental bone (B) beneath inflamed connective tissue (L). The periodontal ligament is shown at P, the transseptal fibers at F. *Right,* High-power study of area in rectangle showing osteoblasts (OB) and layer of osteoid buttressing thinned remnant of resorbed bone (O). Leukocytic infiltration is shown at L.

tive process. The possibility that bacterial endotoxins stimulate resorption by attracting osteoclasts has also been suggested.[19]

The bone destruction caused by inflammation in periodontal disease is not a process of bone necrosis.[6,12] It entails the activity of *living cells* along *viable bone.* When tissue necrosis and pus are present in periodontal disease, they occur in the soft tissue walls of periodontal pockets, not along the resorbing margin of the underlying bone. The severity of bone loss is not necessarily correlated with the depth of periodontal pockets, the severity of ulceration of the pocket wall, or the presence or absence of pus.

Bone Formation in Periodontal Disease

It is significant that the response of alveolar bone to inflammation includes bone formation as well as resorption. It means that **bone loss in periodontal disease** is not simply a destructive process but results from the predominance of resorption over formation. New bone formation retards the rate of bone loss, compensating in some degree for the bone destroyed by inflammation. Newly formed osteoid is more resistant to resorption than mature bone.[10] Because of the interaction between bone resorption and bone formation, **bone loss in periodontal disease is not necessarily continuous. It is a progressive process, but its rate cannot be predicted.**

Occasionally in autopsy specimens of untreated disease, there are areas where bone resorption has ceased and new bone is being formed on the previously eroded bone margin. **This indicates that bone resorption in periodontal disease *may occur as an intermittent process* with periods of remission and exacerbation.** This is consistent with the varied rates of progress observed clinically in untreated periodontal disease.

The microscopic bone formation in response to inflammation varies in amount and distribution. It is governed by the severity and distribution of the inflammation and by systemic influences. In this way systemic factors which affect the metabolic processes involved in bone formation influence the bone loss in periodontal disease.

The presence of bone formation in response to inflammation in active periodontal disease has a bearing on the outcome of treatment. Elimination of inflammation to remove the stimulus to bone resorption and the establishment of conditions conducive to healing are basic aims in periodontal treatment. Healing of the periodontium following treatment depends upon the body's reparative processes, one of which is the formation of new bone. An active tendency toward bone formation in untreated disease could benefit healing if carried over into the post-treatment period.

The radiograph is extremely useful in diagnosis, but it does not detect microscopic resorptive and formative activities. Sometimes, endosteal bone formation in periodontal disease produces increased radiodensity (condensing osteitis) adjacent to eroded bone margins. However, there may be bone formation in periodontal disease without any radiographic suggestion of its presence (Fig. 16–7).

Bone Destruction Caused by Trauma from Occlusion

Inflammation is the more common cause of periodontal destruction, the other being trauma from occlusion.* Trauma from occlusion can produce bone destruction in the absence of inflammation or combined with it.

Trauma in the absence of inflammation

In the absence of inflammation, the changes in trauma from occlusion vary from increased compression and tension of the periodontal ligament and increased osteoclasis of alveolar bone, to necrosis of the periodontal ligament and bone and resorption of bone and tooth structure. These

---

*For a detailed discussion of trauma from occlusion see Chapter 24.

changes are reversible in that they are repaired if the offending forces are removed. However, persistent trauma from occlusion causes funnel-shaped widening of the crestal portion of the periodontal ligament with resorption of the adjacent bone. These changes represent adaptation of the periodontal tissues to "cushion" increased occlusal force, but they produce defects in the bone which weaken tooth support and cause tooth mobility.

Trauma combined with inflammation

When combined with inflammation, trauma from occlusion acts as a co-destructive factor in periodontal disease. It aggravates the bone destruction caused by the inflammation, and causes bizarre bone patterns and infrabony pockets.

Bone Destruction Caused by Systemic Disorders

Alveolar bone loss has been produced in experimental animals by various types of systemic disturbances (see Chaps. 26, 27 and 28) without other features of periodontal disease, such as inflammation and pocket formation. It is also possible to aggravate the bone destruction caused by local factors by systemic means. However, in humans the situation is not quite as clear.

Theoretically any systemic disturbance which adversely affects one or more of the supporting periodontal tissues could, if it were severe enough, cause loss of alveolar bone. Such cases have been described and referred to by the term *periodontosis* (Chap. 30) or *diffuse atrophy of alveolar bone* or *negative bone factor*. When systemic disorders are suspected as the cause of bone loss, it is usually difficult to identify them.

Bone-destructive processes in systemically caused periodontal disease are described as degenerative (hence the term periodontosis) rather than inflammatory. It has also been suggested[6] that systemically caused bone loss may result from a process called *halisterisis* or *osteolysis*,[2] in which the minerals are withdrawn and the bone reverts to connective tissue.[2] However, opinions differ regarding whether bone resorption can occur without osteoclasts.[22]

Periodontal bone resorption may occur in

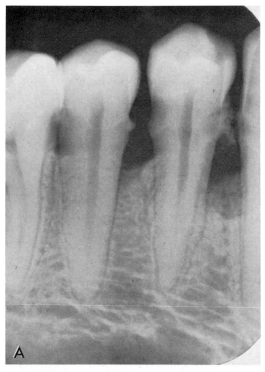

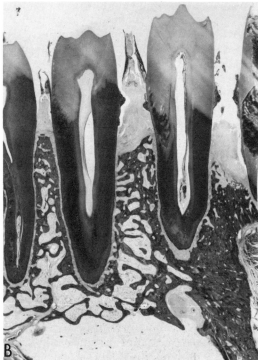

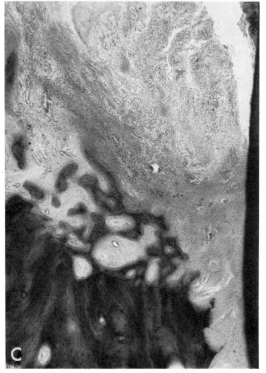

Figure 16–7 Bone Formation in Untreated Periodontal Disease. *A,* Radiograph showing bone destruction in the mandibular premolar areas. Note the heavy calculus deposits. *B,* Survey section of the distal surface of the canine (*right*), the first and second premolars and the mesial surface of the first molar, showing periodontal disease with bone loss. *C,* Interdental space between the canine and first premolar, showing inflammation and newly formed bone trabeculae on the previously resorbed bone margin.

generalized skeletal disturbances such as hyperparathyroidism or Hand-Schüller-Christian disease (see Chap. 33). In such patients the locally caused inflammatory bone destruction is superimposed upon the resorptive changes caused by the systemic disorder.

Comment

Bone loss in periodontal disease has been described above as being caused by three separate conditions—inflammation, trauma from occlusion and systemic disorders. This separation is an artificial one made to facilitate analysis of the problem. In reality, their effects upon the periodontal tissues are interrelated.

BONE LOSS AND TOOTH MOBILITY

Loss of alveolar bone in periodontal disease is an important cause of tooth mobility, but other factors are involved. As a result the degree of tooth mobility in periodontal disease is not necessarily correlated with the amount of bone loss. (For a discussion of tooth mobility and the factors which cause it, see Chapter 19.)

FACTORS DETERMINING BONE MORPHOLOGY IN PERIODONTAL DISEASE

Normal variation in the morphology of alveolar bone

There is considerable normal variation in the morphology of alveolar bone (Chap. 4), and it affects the osseous contours produced by periodontal disease. The bone features that significantly affect the bone destructive pattern in periodontal disease are the *thickness, width,* and *crestal angulation of the interdental septa, the thickness of the facial and lingual alveolar plates, the presence of fenestrations* and *dehiscences on the root surfaces, thickening of the alveolar bone margins to accommodate functional demands* and the *alignment of the teeth.*

For example, angular osseous defects cannot form in thin facial or lingual alveolar plates, which have little or no cancellous bone between the outer and inner cortical layers. In such instances, the entire crest of the plate is destroyed and the height of the bone is reduced.

Exostoses

Exostoses are outgrowths of bone of varied size and shape. They occur more often on the facial surface than on the lingual, and apparently serve no useful purpose. The cervical margin of the alveolar bone is often thickened in response to increased functional demands so that it is sometimes difficult to differentiate between linear exostoses and functional adaptation.

The pathway of inflammation

Because chronic inflammation is an important cause of bone destruction, its pathway in the supporting tissues is a significant determinant of the bone morphology produced by periodontal disease.

Trauma from occlusion

Trauma from occlusion is a critical factor in determining the dimension and shape of bone deformities. Together with inflammation, it is a co-destructive factor that changes the bone destructive pattern by altering the pathway of inflammation. In the absence of inflammation it produces angular defects at the bony crest by injuring the periodontal ligament and causing resorption of the adjacent bone.

Food impaction

Interdental bone defects often occur where the proximal contact is abnormal or absent. Pressure and irritation from food impaction contribute to the inverted bone architecture. In some instances the poor proximal relationship may be the result of a shift in tooth position because of extensive bone destruction that preceded food impaction. In such cases food impaction is a complicating factor, rather than the initial cause of the bone defect.

Buttressing bone formation (lipping)

Bone formation sometimes occurs in an attempt to buttress bone trabeculae weakened by resorption. When it occurs within the jaw it is termed *central buttressing bone formation;*[5] when it occurs on the external surface it is referred to as *peripheral buttressing bone.* The latter may cause bulging of the bone contour, termed *lipping,* which sometimes accompanies the formation of osseous craters and infrabony defects (Fig. 16–8).

Systemic type of periodontal disease (periodontosis)

Vertical or angular destruction of alveolar bone is considered typical of systemically caused periodontal disease (periodontosis). The bone destructive pattern is attributed to degenerative changes in the periodontal tissues caused by systemic disturbances.

BONE DESTRUCTIVE PATTERNS IN PERIODONTAL DISEASE

In addition to reducing bone height, periodontal disease alters the morphology of the bone. An understanding of the nature and pathogenesis of these alterations is essential for effective diagnosis and treatment.

Horizontal bone loss

This is the most common pattern of bone loss in periodontal disease. The bone is reduced in height and the bone margin is horizontal or slightly angulated. Interdental septa and the facial and lingual plates are affected, but not necessary to an equal degree around the same tooth (Fig. 16–9).

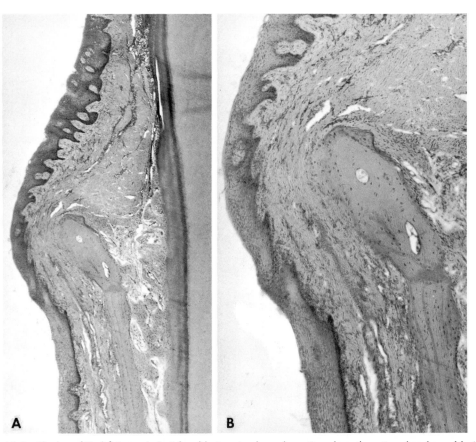

Figure 16–8 Lipping of Facial Bone. *A,* Peripheral buttressing bone formation along the external surface of facial bony plate and at the crest. Note the deformity in the bone produced by the buttressing bone formation and the bulging of the mucosa. *B,* Detailed view showing "lipping" and deformity produced by buttressing bone formation.

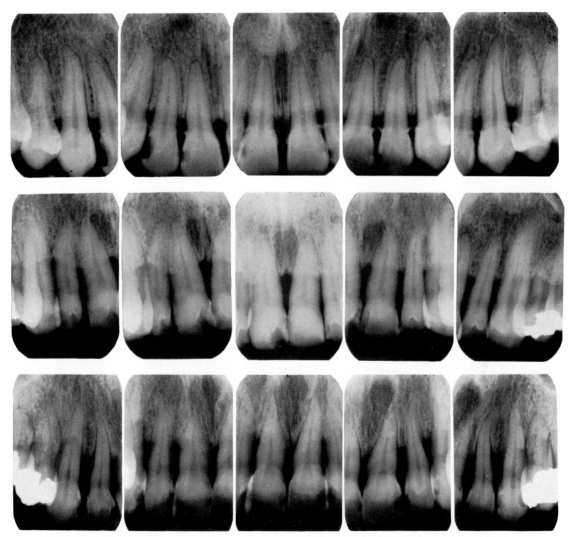

Figure 16–9 **Horizontal Bone Loss.** Three patients with different degrees of destruction in the anterior maxilla.

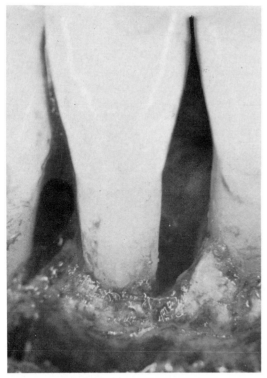

Figure 16–10 **Interdental Crater** between the facial and lingual alveolar plates.

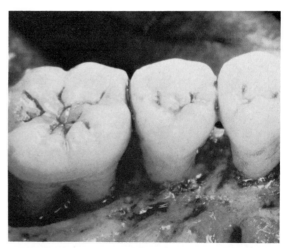

Figure 16–11 **Osseous Crater** around mandibular first molar.

Bone deformities (osseous defects)

The following are types of bone deformities produced by periodontal disease.[18] They usually occur in adults but have been reported in human skulls with deciduous dentitions.[14] Their presence may be suggested by the radiograph, but **careful probing and surgical exposure of the area are required to determine their conformation and dimensions.**

OSSEOUS CRATERS. These are concavities in the crest of the interdental bone confined within facial and lingual walls (Fig. 16–10), and less frequently between the tooth surface and facial or lingual bony plate (Fig. 16–11).

INFRABONY DEFECTS. Such defects are hollowed-out troughs in the bone alongside one or more denuded root surfaces enclosed within one, two, three or four bony walls (Fig. 16–12). The base of the defect is

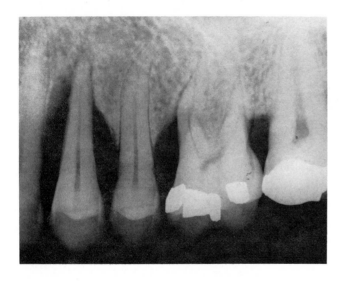

Figure 16–12 **Angular Defects** of different depths.

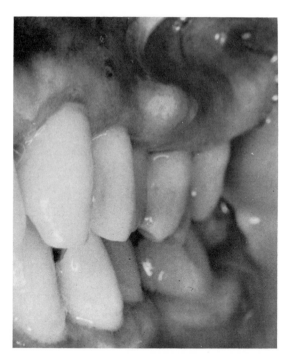

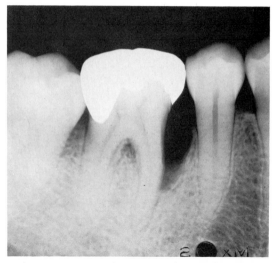

Figure 16–14 Hemiseptum on the Distal Surface of the Second Premolar. Note the furcation involvement of the molar.

Figure 16–13 Exostoses.

located apical to the surrounding bone (Chap. 14).

In human skulls it was observed that intrabony defects (a term reserved by some for three-walled infrabony defects) are most common on the mesial surface of the maxillary and mandibular second and third molars; that they are present in an increasing percentage of individuals from age two to 44 when the maximum is reached; and that the number of defects per individual is greatest after age 60.[13]

BULBOUS BONE CONTOURS. These are bony enlargements caused by exostoses, adaptation to function or buttressing bone formation (Fig. 16–13).

HEMISEPTA. The remaining portion of an interdental septum after the mesial or

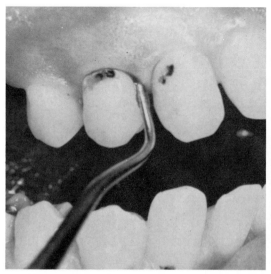

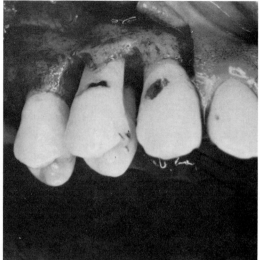

Figure 16–15 Irregular Bone Margin. *Left,* Probe in deep infrabony pocket on the mesial surface of maxillary premolar. *Right,* Elevated flap shows irregular bone margin with notching of interdental bone.

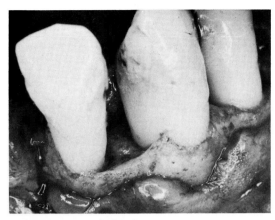

Figure 16–16 **Labial Ledge** produced by interproximal resorption.

distal portion has been destroyed by disease is termed a hemiseptum (Fig. 16–14).

INCONSISTENT MARGINS. These are angular or U-shaped defects produced by resorption of the facial or lingual alveolar plate, or abrupt differences between the height of the facial or lingual margins and the height of the interdental septa (Fig. 16–15).

LEDGES. Ledges are plateau-like bone margins caused by resorption of thickened bony plates (Fig. 16–16).

REFERENCES

1. Albright, F., and Reifenstein, E. C.: The Parathyroid Glands and Metabolic Bone Disease. Baltimore, Williams & Wilkins Co., 1948, p. 5.
2. Belanger, L. F.: *In* The Parathyroid Glands (P. J. Gaillard, R. V. Talmage, and A. M. Budy, Eds.). Chicago, University of Chicago Press, 1965, pp. 137–143.
3. Carranza, F. A., Jr., and Cabrini, R. L.: Histormetric Studies of Periodontal Tissues. Periodontics, 5:308, 1967.
4. Fullmer, H. M., et al.: Collagenase and Gingival Disease. *Proceedings, First Pan-Pacific Congress of Dental Research*, 1970, pp. 167–171.
5. Glickman, I., and Smulow, J. B.: Buttressing Bone Formation in the Periodontium. J. Periodont., 36:365, 1965.
6. Glickman, I., and Wood, H.: Bone Histology in Periodontal Disease. J. D. Res., 21:35, 1942.
7. Goldhaber, P.: Enhancement of Bone Resorption in Tissue Culture by Human Gingival Fragments. Inter. Assn. for Dent. Res. Program, No. 45 1967, p. 178.
8. Goldhaber, P.: Some Chemical Factors Influencing Bone Resorption. *In* Tissue Culture in Mechanisms of Hard Tissue Destruction (R. F. Sognnaes, Ed.) Washington, D.C., American Academy for the Advancement of Science, 1963, pp. 609–636.
9. Irving, J. T.: Factors Concerning Bone Loss Associated with Periodontal Disease. J. D. Res., 49:262, 1970.
10. Irving, J. T., and Heeley, J. D.: Tissue Reaction to the Implantation of Labeled Isogenous Bone. Abstract. I.A.D.R. Program and Abstracts of Papers, 1969, 224.
11. Jaffe, H. L.: The Resorption of Bone. Arch. Surg., 20:355, 1930.
12. Kronfeld, R.: Condition of Alveolar Bone Underlying Periodontal Pockets. J. Periodont., 6:22, 1935.
13. Larato, D. C.: Intrabony Defects in the Dry Human Skull. J. Periodont., 41:496, 1970.
14. Larato, D. C.: Periodontal Bone Defects in the Juvenile Skull. J. Periodont., 41:473, 1970.
15. Leriche, R., and Policard, A.: The Normal and Pathological Physiology of Bone. Chap. IV. St. Louis, C. V. Mosby Co., 1928.
16. McLean, F. C., and Urist, M. R.: Bone. An Introduction to the Physiology of the Skeletal System. 2nd ed. Chicago, University of Chicago Press, 1961, p. 97.
17. Melcher, A. H., and Eastoe, J. E.: Biology of the Periodontium. New York, Academic Press, 1969, pp. 315–319.
18. Prichard, J. F.: Periodontal Surgery. Practical Dental Monographs. Chicago, Year Book Publishers, Inc., Nov., 1961, pp. 16–19.
19. Rizzo, A. A., and Mergenhagen, S. E.: Histopathologic Effects of Endotoxin Injected into Rabbit Oral Mucosa. Arch. Oral Biol., 9:659, 1964.
20. Sognnaes, R. F., Editor: Mechanisms of Hard Tissue Destruction. American Association for the Advancement of Science. Washington, D.C., 1963, pp. 371–662.
21. Swenson, O., and Claff, L. C.: Changes in the Hydrogen Ion Concentration of Healing Fractures. Proc. Soc. Exper. Biol. & Med., 61:151, 1946.
22. Urist, M. R.: The Problem of Osteoporosis. Clin. Res., 6:377, 1958.
23. Von Recklinghausen, F.: Untersuchungen über Rachitis und Osteomalacie. Gustav Fischer: Jena, 1910.

Chapter 17

FURCATION INVOLVEMENT

The term *furcation involvement* refers to commonly occurring conditions in which the bifurcation and trifurcation of multi-rooted teeth are denuded by periodontal disease.[1,2] The mandibular first molars are the most common sites, and the maxillary premolars the least common; the number of furcation involvements increases with age.[3]

CLINICAL FEATURES

The denuded bifurcation or trifurcation may be visible or obscured by the inflamed wall of a periodontal pocket. The extent of involvement is determined by exploration with a blunt probe, with a simultaneous blast of warm air to facilitate visualization. The tooth may or may not be mobile and is usually symptom-free, but there may be painful complications. These include **sensitivity to thermal changes** caused by caries or lacunar resorption of the root in the furcation area, **recurrent or constant throbbing pain** caused by pulp changes, and **sensitivity to percussion** from acute inflammatory involvement of the periodontal ligament. Furcation involvement may result in acute periodontal or periapical abscess formation, with all the symptoms that accompany such lesions (Figs. 17–1 and 17–2).

MICROSCOPIC FEATURES

Microscopically, furcation involvement presents no unique pathologic features. It is simply a phase in the rootward extension of the periodontal pocket. In its early stages, it presents widening of the periodontal space with cellular and fluid inflammatory exudation (Fig. 17–3), followed by epithelial proliferation into the bifurcation area from an adjoining periodontal pocket (Fig. 17–4). Extension of the inflammation into the bone leads to resorption and reduction in bone height (Fig. 17–5). Bone formation is often present adjacent to areas of resorption and along adjoining medullary

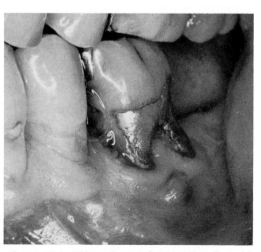

Figure 17–1 Bifurcation Involvement Complicated by Periodontal Abscess.

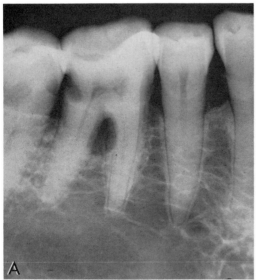

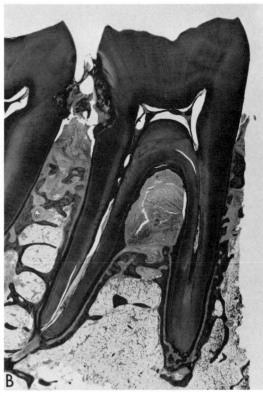

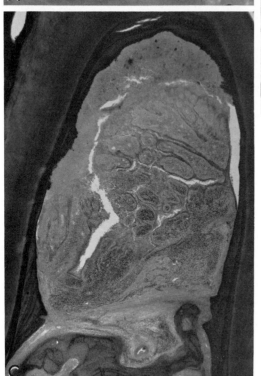

Figure 17–2 Furcation Involvement Complicated by Abscess Formation. *A,* Bifurcation involvement of mandibular first molar. Also note caries. *B,* Section through mandibular first molar showing periodontal disease with bifurcation involvement. Note the caries. *C,* Abscess in the bifurcation. Note extension of the inflammation into the bone and thickened blood vessel.

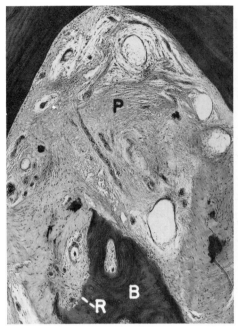

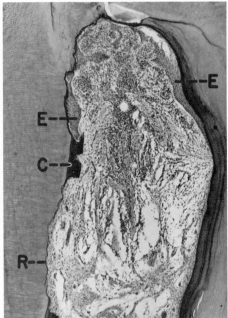

Fig. 17-3   Fig. 17-4

Figure 17-3   **Bifurcation Area in a Mandibular Molar.** The periodontal space is widened. There is edema, degeneration and slight leukocytic infiltration of the periodontal ligament, and an area of resorption (R) at the margin of the bone (B).

Figure 17-4   **Bifurcation Area** showing proliferation of epithelium (E), edema and degeneration of connective tissue, bone loss and destruction of cementum (C) and dentin with irregularly hollowed-out lacunae along the dentinal surface (R).

spaces (Fig. 17-6). **The bone destructive pattern may be horizontal or may produce angular osseous defects associated with infrabony pockets (Fig. 17-7).** Plaque, calculus and bacterial debris occupy the denuded furcation space. Findings that complicate furcation involvement and account for painful symptoms include caries of cementum and dentin with involvement of the dentinal tubules (Fig. 17-8); idiopathic tooth resorption in which cementum is absent and the dentin presents a clear-cut, irregular margin with hollowed-out lacunae (Fig. 17-4); and abscess formation in the furcation area.

ETIOLOGY

Bifurcation and trifurcation involvement are stages of progressive periodontal disease and have the same etiology. **However, of all areas of the periodontium, the bifurcation and trifurcation are the most sensitive to injury from excessive occlusal forces.**[3] Trauma from occlusion should be particularly suspect as a contributing etiologic factor in cases of furcation involvement

with crater-like or angular deformities in the bone, especially when bone destruction is localized to one of the roots.

RADIOGRAPHIC FEATURES

Definitive diagnosis of furcation involvement is made by **clinical examination which includes careful probing.** Radiographs are helpful but present artefacts which make it possible for furcation involvement to be present without detectable radiographic changes.

For example, in Figure 17-9, the trifurcation of the maxillary first molar appears involved, whereas that of the second molar does not. Microscopic sections of the autopsied jaw indicate that both the first (Fig. 17-10) and second (Fig. 17-11) molars are involved. The opaque palatal root of the second molar hides the bone loss in the trifurcation.

Variations in radiographic technique may obscure the presence and extent of furcation involvement. A tooth may present marked bifurcation involvement in one film

(Text continued on page 242.)

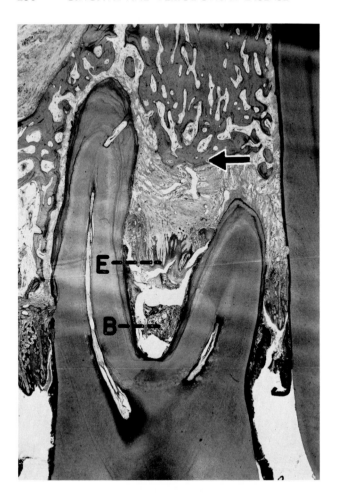

Figure 17–5 Trifurcation Involvement.
Maxillary first molar showing pronounced bone loss, inflammation and epithelial proliferation (E). Bacterial debris is shown at B. The area indicated by the arrow is shown in Figure 17–6.

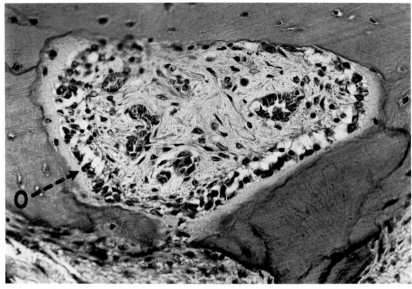

Figure 17–6 Detail of Figure 17–5 (*arrow*) showing osteoblasts (O) and pale staining osteoid lining medullary space adjoining bone margin undergoing resorption.

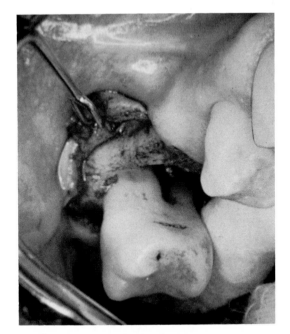

Figure 17–7 Crater-like Osseous Defect in Trifurcation of Molar.

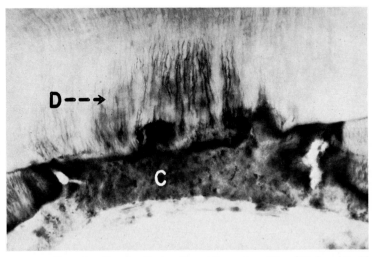

Figure 17–8 Trifurcation Showing Destruction of Cementum (C) and Caries of Dentin (D).

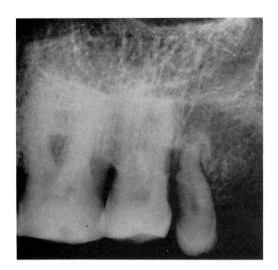

Figure 17–9 Radiograph Showing Trifurcation Involvement of the Maxillary First Molar. The second molar does not appear to be involved. Compare with Figures 17–10 and 17–11.

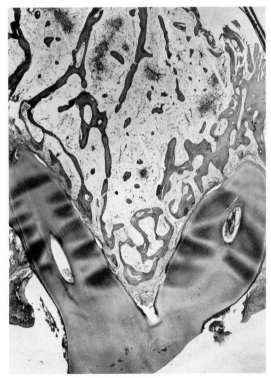

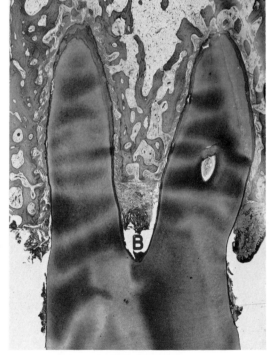

Fig. 17–10

Fig. 17–11

Figure 17–10 Buccopalatal section through the **Maxillary First Molar** shown in Figure 17–9. The trifurcation is involved and there are periodontal pockets on the buccal (*left*) and palatal roots (*right*).

Figure 17–11 Buccopalatal section through the **Maxillary Second Molar** shown in Figure 17–9. There is involvement of the trifurcation at B, which is not visible radiographically.

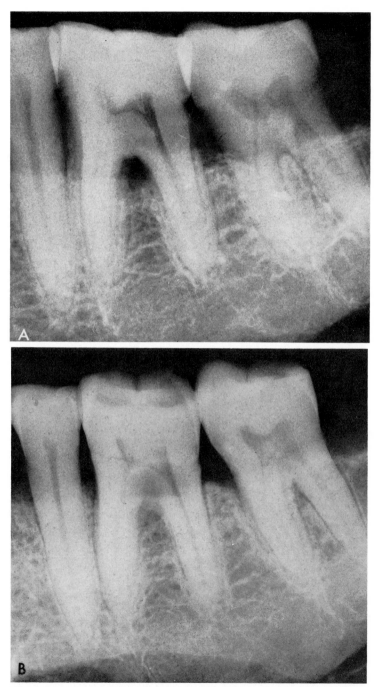

Figure 17–12 *A,* **Bifurcation Involvement** indicated by triangular radiolucence in bifurcation area of mandibular first molar. The second molar presents only a slight thickening of the periodontal space in the bifurcation area. *B,* Same area, different angulation. The triangular radiolucence in the bifurcation of the first molar is obliterated and involvement of the second molar bifurcation is apparent.

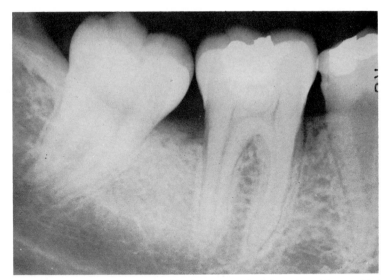

Figure 17–13 Early Furcation Involvement suggested by fuzziness in the bifurcation of the mandibular first molar, particularly when associated with bone loss on the roots.

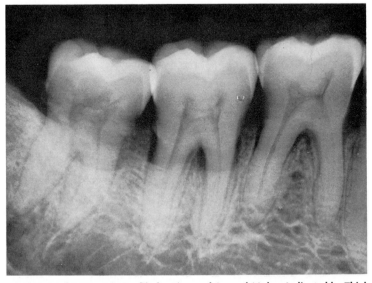

Figure 17–14 Bifurcation Involvement of Mandibular First and Second Molars Indicated by Thickening of Periodontal Space in Bifurcation Area. The bifurcation of the third molar is also involved but the thickening of the periodontal space is partially obscured by the external oblique line.

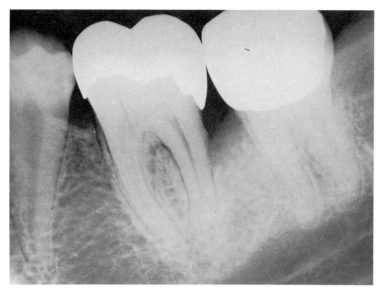

Figure 17–15 **Bifurcation Involvement** of first molar, associated with bone loss on the distal root.

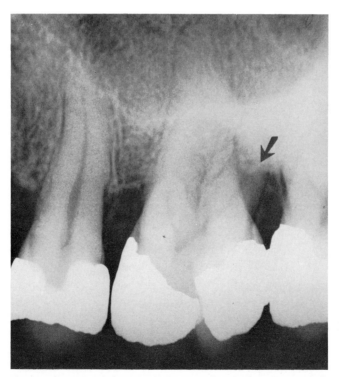

Figure 17–16 **Trifurcation Involvement of the First Molar Partially Obscured by the Radiopaque Lingual Root.** The horizontal line across the distobuccal root demarcates the apical portion, which is covered by bone, from the remainder of the root where the bone has been destroyed.

(Fig. 17–12, A), but appear uninvolved in another (Fig. 17–12, B). Films should be taken at different angles to reduce the risk of missing furcation involvement.

Aids in radiographic interpretation

The recognition of large, clearly defined radiolucency in the furcation area presents no problem (Fig. 17–12, A), but less clearly defined radiographic changes produced by furcation involvement are often overlooked. To assist in the radiographic detection of furcation involvement the following criteria are suggested:

1. The slightest radiographic change in the furcation area should be investigated clinically, especially if there is bone loss on adjacent roots (Fig. 17–13).

2. Diminished radiodensity in the furcation area in which outlines of bone trabeculae are visible (Fig. 17–14).

3. Whenever there is marked bone loss in relation to a single molar root, it may be assumed that the furcation is also involved (Figs. 17–15 and 17–16). This is an extremely important rule. Treatment limited to the root with extensive bone loss may seal the infected bifurcation or trifurcation, prevent drainage, and lead to formation of a periodontal abscess.

REFERENCES

1. Easley, J. R., and Drennan, G. A.: Morphological Classification of the Furca. J. Canad. D. Assn., 35: 104, 1969.
2. Glickman, I.: Bifurcation Involvement in Periodontal Disease. J.A.D.A., 40:528, 1950.
3. Glickman, I., Stein, R. S., and Smulow, J. B.: The Effects of Increased Functional Forces Upon the Periodontium of Splinted and Non-Splinted Teeth. J. Periodont., 32:290, 1961.
4. Larato, D. C.: Furcation Involvements: Incidence and Distribution. J. Periodont., 41:499, 1970.

Chapter 18

THE PERIODONTAL ABSCESS

A periodontal abscess is a localized purulent inflammation in the periodontal tissues. It is also known as a *lateral* or *parietal abscess.* Periodontal abscess formation may occur as follows:

1. Deep extension of infection from a periodontal pocket into the supporting periodontal tissues, and localization of the suppurative inflammatory process along the lateral aspect of the root.

2. Lateral extension of inflammation from the inner surface of a periodontal pocket into the connective tissue of the pocket wall. Localization of the abscess results when drainage into the pocket space is impaired (Fig. 18–1).

3. In a pocket that describes a tortuous course around the root (complex pocket), a periodontal abscess may form in the cul-de-sac, the deep end of which is shut off from the surface.

4. Incomplete removal of calculus during treatment of a periodontal pocket. In this instance, the gingival wall shrinks, occluding the pocket orifice, and a periodontal abscess occurs in the sealed-off portion of the pocket.

5. A periodontal abscess may occur in the absence of periodontal disease, following

trauma to the tooth or perforation of the lateral wall of the root in endodontic therapy.

Classification

Periodontal abscesses are classified according to location as follows:

1. *Abscess in the supporting periodontal tissues* along the lateral aspect of the root. In this condition, there is generally a sinus in the bone, which extends laterally from the abscess to the external surface (Fig. 18–2).

2. *Abscess in the soft tissue wall of a deep periodontal pocket* (Figs. 18–3 and 18–4).

Clinical features

Periodontal abscesses may be *acute* or *chronic.* Acute lesions often subside but persist in the chronic state, whereas chronic lesions may exist without their having been acute. Chronic lesions frequently undergo acute exacerbations.

ACUTE ABSCESS. The acute periodontal abscess is accompanied by symptoms such as **throbbing radiating pain, exquisite tenderness of the gingiva to palpation, sensitivity of the tooth to percussion, tooth mobility, lymphadenitis and systemic effects such as fever, leukocytosis and malaise.**

The acute periodontal abscess appears as an ovoid elevation of the gingiva along the lateral aspect of the root (Figs. 18–5 and 18–6). The gingiva is edematous and red, with a smooth, shiny surface. The shape and consistency of the elevated area vary. It

243

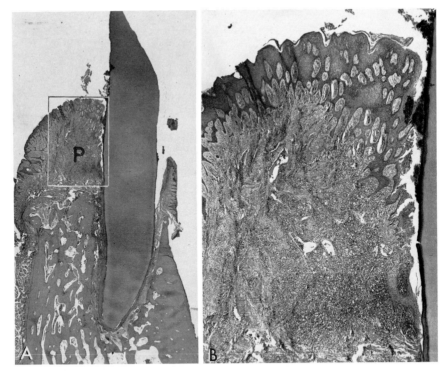

Figure 18–1 *A,* **Periodontal Abscess (P) on the Lingual Surface of Mandibular Incisor** (abscess enclosed in rectangle). *B,* Detailed view of periodontal abscess showing dense leukocytic infiltration and suppuration.

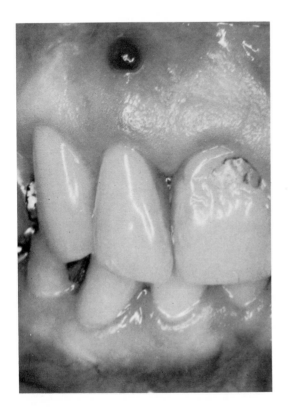

Figure 18–2 Periodontal Abscess deep in the periodontium showing hemorrhagic tissue at the sinus orifice.

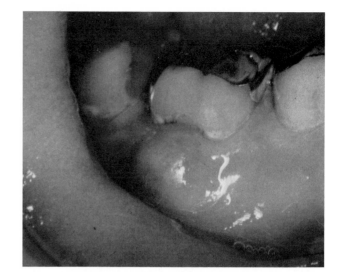

Figure 18–3 Chronic Periodontal Abscess in the Wall of a Deep Pocket.

may be dome-like and relatively firm, or pointed and soft. In most instances, pus may be expressed from the gingival margin by gentle digital pressure. Occasionally, the patient may present symptoms of an acute periodontal abscess *without any notable clinical lesion or radiographic changes.*

CHRONIC ABSCESS. The chronic periodontal abscess usually presents a sinus that opens onto the gingival mucosa somewhere along the length of the root. There may be a history of intermittent exudation (Fig. 18–7). The orifice of the sinus may appear as a difficult to detect pinpoint opening, which when probed reveals a sinus tract deep in the periodontium (Fig. 18–8). The sinus may be covered by a small, pink, bead-like mass of granulation tissue (Fig. 18–9).

The chronic periodontal abscess is usually asymptomatic. The patient may report episodes characterized by **dull gnawing**

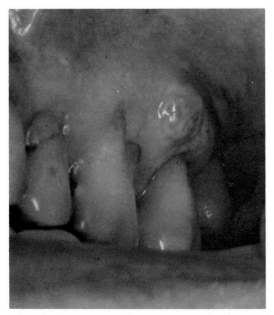

Figure 18–4 Periodontal Abscess on Maxillary Second Molar.

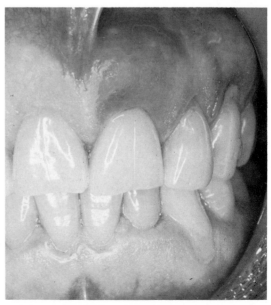

Figure 18–5 Acute Periodontal Abscess on Maxillary Left Central Incisor.

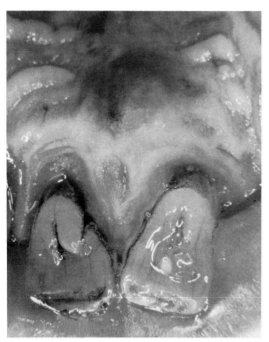

Figure 18–6 Acute Periodontal Abscess on the Lingual Surface.

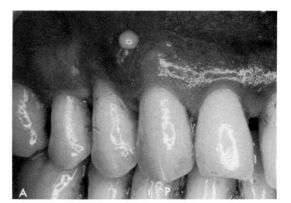

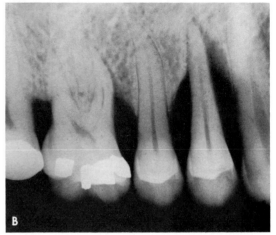

Figure 18–7 Suppuration from a Chronic Periodontal Abscess. *A,* Suppurative draining sinus between the canine and first premolar. *B,* Radiograph showing extensive bone destruction in the area of the draining sinus.

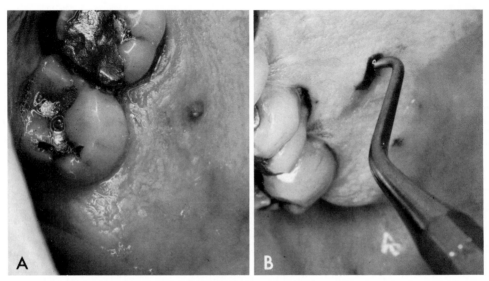

Figure 18–8 Pinpoint Orifice of Sinus from Palatal Periodontal Abscess. *A,* Pinpoint orifice on the palate indicative of sinus from periodontal abscess. *B,* Probe extends into abscess deep in the periodontium.

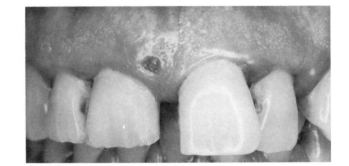

Figure 18–9 Granulation Tissue at the orifice of sinus from periodontal abscess.

pain, slight elevation of the tooth, and a desire to bite down and grind the tooth. The chronic periodontal abscess often undergoes acute exacerbations with all the associated symptoms.

Radiographic appearance

The typical radiographic appearance of the periodontal abscess is that of a discrete area of radiolucence along the lateral aspect of the root (Figs. 18–10 and 18–11). However, the radiographic picture is not always typical (Fig. 18–12) because of many variables such as:

1. The stage of the lesion. In the early stages the acute periodontal abscess is extremely painful but presents no radiographic changes.

2. The extent of bone destruction and the morphology of the bone.

3. The location of the abscess.

Lesions in the soft tissue wall of a periodontal pocket are less likely to produce radiographic changes than those deep in the supporting tissues.

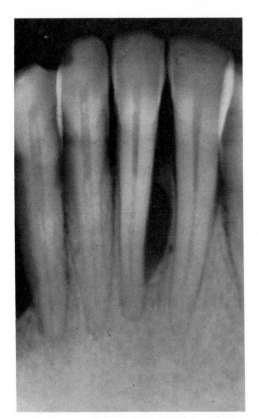

Figure 18–10 Radiolucent Area on the lateral aspect of root with chronic periodontal abscess.

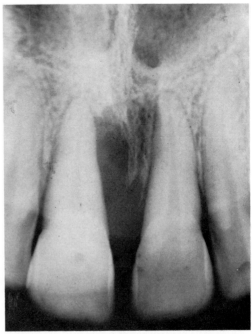

Figure 18–11 Typical Radiographic Appearance of Periodontal Abscess on Right Central Incisor.

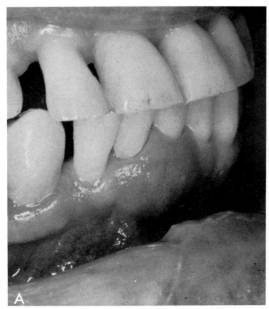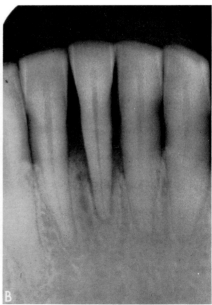

Figure 18–12 Chronic Periodontal Abscess. *A,* Periodontal abscess in the right central and lateral incisor area. *B,* Extensive bone destruction and thickening of the periodontal ligament space around the right central incisor.

Abscesses on the facial or lingual surface are obscured by the radiopacity of the root; interproximal lesions are more likely to be visualized radiographically.

The radiograph alone cannot be relied upon for the diagnosis of a periodontal abscess.

Diagnosis

Diagnosis of the periodontal abscess requires correlation of the history and clinical and radiographic findings. **Continuity of the lesion with the gingival margin is clinical evidence of the presence of a periodontal abscess.** The suspected area should be probed carefully along the gingival margin in relation to each tooth surface for the presence of a channel from the marginal area to the deeper periodontal tissues. **The abscess is not necessarily located on the same surface of the root as the pocket from which it is formed.** A pocket on the facial or lingual surface may give rise to a periodontal abscess interproximally. It is common for a periodontal abscess to be localized on a root surface other than that along which the pocket originated because impairment of drainage is more likely to occur when a pocket follows a tortuous course.

Differential diagnosis between a periodontal and periapical abscess

The following are useful guides in the differential diagnosis between a *periodontal* and *periapical* abscess:

If the tooth is nonvital, the lesion is most likely periapical. In severe cases a periodontal abscess may extend to the apex and cause pulp involvement and necrosis. Except in such cases, however, periodontal abscesses do not cause devitalization of teeth.

An apical abscess may spread along the lateral aspect of the root to the gingival margin, but when the apex and lateral surface of a root are involved by a single lesion that can be probed directly from the gingival margin, it is more likely to have originated as a periodontal abscess.

Radiographic findings are helpful in differentiating between a periodontal and periapical lesion, but their usefulness is limited. Early acute periodontal and periapical abscesses present no radiographic changes. Ordinarily an area of radiolucence along the lateral surface of the root suggests the presence of a periodontal abscess, whereas apical rarefaction suggests a periapical abscess. **However, acute periodontal** abscesses that show no radiographic changes frequently cause symptoms in teeth with long-standing radiographically detectable periapical lesions that are not contributing to the patient's complaint. Clinical findings such as the presence of extensive caries, pocket formation, tooth vitality, and the existence of a continuity between the gingival margin and the abscess area, often prove to be of greater diagnostic value than radiographs.

A draining sinus on the lateral aspect of the root suggests periodontal rather than apical involvement, whereas a sinus from a periapical lesion is more likely to be located further apically. However, sinus location is not conclusive. In many instances, particularly in children, the sinus from a periapical lesion drains on the side of the root rather than at the apex.

The periodontal abscess and the gingival abscess

The principal differences between the periodontal abscess and the gingival abscess are location and history. (Described under Acute Inflammatory Gingival Enlargement, Chapter 8.) The gingival abscess is confined to the marginal gingiva, and it often occurs in previously disease-free areas. It is usually an acute inflammatory response to foreign material forced into the gingiva. In rare instances it results from infection of an epithelial-lined gingival cyst.[2] The periodontal abscess involves the supporting periodontal tissues and generally occurs in the course of chronic destructive periodontal disease.

The periodontal cyst

This is an uncommon lesion which produces localized destruction of the periodontal tissues along a lateral root surface, most often in the mandibular canine–premolar area.[3] It is believed to be an odontogenic cyst caused by proliferation of the epithelial rests of Malassez, but the stimulus initiating the cellular activity is not understood. Other theories regarding its origin suggest that (a) it may be a lateral dentigerous cyst retained in the jaw after the tooth erupted, that (b) it may be caused by traumatic implantation of oral epithelium, or that (c) it may result from stimulation of the epithelial rests of the periodontal ligament by infection from a periodontal abscess or from the pulp through an accessory root canal. A periodontal cyst is usually asymptomatic and without grossly detectable changes, or it may present a localized tender swelling. Radiographically, when located interproximally it appears on the side of the root as a radiolucent area bordered by a radiopaque line, which cannot be differentiated from the radiographic appearance of a periodontal abscess.

REFERENCES

1. Cross, W. G.: Lateral Periodontal Cyst: Report of a Case. J. Periodont., 25:287, 1954.
2. Ritchey, B., and Orban, B.: Cysts of the Gingiva. Oral Surg., Oral Med. & Oral Path., 6:765, 1952.
3. Standish, S. N., and Shafer, W. G.: The Lateral Periodontal Cyst. J. Periodont., 29:27, 1958.

Chapter 19

PATHOLOGIC MIGRATION (WANDERING); TOOTH MOBILITY

PATHOLOGIC MIGRATION

Pathologic migration refers to tooth movement that results when the balance among the factors which maintain physiologic tooth position are disturbed by periodontal disease. Pathologic migration is common and may be the earliest sign of disease, or it may occur associated with gingival inflammation and pocket formation as the disease progresses.

Pathologic migration occurs most frequently in the anterior region, but posterior teeth may also be affected. The teeth move in any direction, usually accompanied by mobility and rotation. Pathologic migration in the occlusal or incisal direction is termed extrusion or elongation, the former term being preferred. All degrees of pathologic migration are encountered, and one or more teeth may be affected (Fig. 19–1). It is important to detect it in its early stages (Fig. 19–2) and to prevent more serious involvement by eliminating the causative factors. Even in the early stage, some degree of bone loss has occurred.

Pathogenesis

Pathologic migration represents the cumulative effect of a combination of factors. The normal position of the teeth in the arch is maintained by an equilibrium between many factors, such as the health of the periodontal tissues, the forces of occlusion, presence of a full complement of teeth, tooth morphology and cuspal inclination, pressure from the lips, cheeks and tongue, the physiologic tendency toward mesial migration, the nature and location of contact point relationships, approximal, incisal and occlusal attrition and the axial inclination of the teeth. Alterations in any of these factors start an interrelated sequence of changes in the environment of a single tooth or group of teeth that results in pathologic migration.

Pathologic migration occurs under the following conditions:

Inflammatory periodontal disease (periodontitis)

Pathologic migration consists of two components: (1) *destruction of tooth-supporting*

250

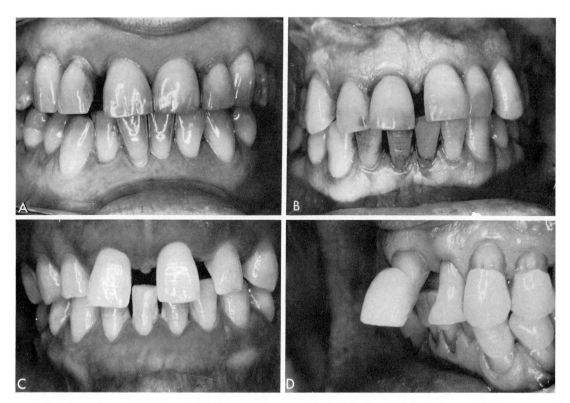

Figure 19–1 Stages in Pathologic Migration. *A,* Migration of right maxillary lateral incisor. *B,* Labial migration of maxillary central incisors and left canine, and mesial migration of right lateral. *C,* Migration and extrusion of maxillary and mandibular incisors. *D,* Severe migration of maxillary central incisor.

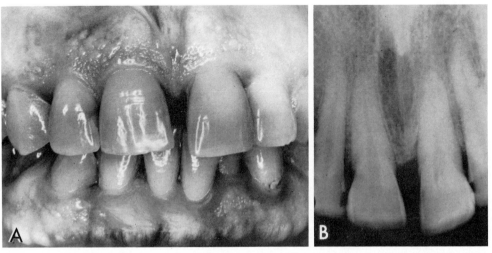

Figure 19–2 *A,* **Pathologic Migration and Early Extrusion** of maxillary central incisor. *B,* Radiograph showing bone loss on extruded central incisor.

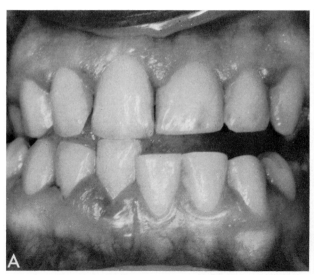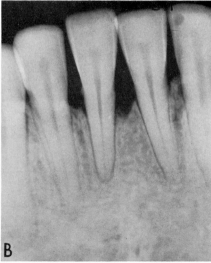

Figure 19–3 Pathologic Migration Aggravated by Excessive Occlusal Force. A, Mandibular central incisor extruded beyond the line of occlusion. Note that the maxillary central incisor is also extruded. B, Thickening of the periodontal ligament space around the central incisor, and angular bone destruction pattern typical of injury produced by excessive occlusal forces.

tissues by periodontal disease and (2) a force to move the weakened tooth. Destruction of the periodontal tissues creates an imbalance between the tooth and the occlusal and muscular forces it is ordinarily called upon to bear. The weakened tooth is unable to maintain its normal position in the arch and moves away from the force, unless it is restrained by proximal contact. The force that moves the weakened tooth may be created by a variety of factors such as occlusal contacts, the tongue or the food bolus.

It is important to understand that **the abnormality in pathologic migration rests with** **the weakened periodontium.** The force itself need not be abnormal. Forces that are acceptable to the intact periodontium become injurious when periodontal support is reduced. An example of this is the tooth with abnormal proximal contacts. Abnormally located proximal contacts convert the normal anterior component of force to a wedging force, which forces the tooth occlusally or incisally. The wedging force, withstood by the intact periodontium, causes the tooth to extrude when the periodontal support is weakened by disease. **As its position changes, the tooth is subjected to abnormal occlusal forces which aggravate**

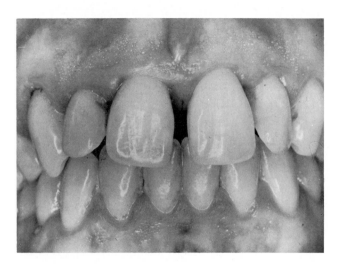

Figure 19–4 Pathologic migration continues despite absence of contact between mandibular and maxillary incisors.

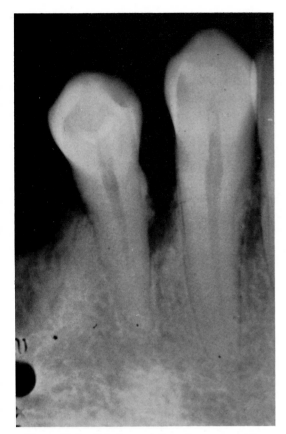

Figure 19–5 Calculus and Bone Loss on mesial surface of canine that has drifted distally.

the destruction and the migration (Fig. 19–3).

Pathologic migration may continue after a tooth no longer contacts its antagonist (Fig. 19–4). Pressure from the tongue, from the food bolus in mastication and from proliferating granulation tissue provide the force.

Drifting following failure to replace missing teeth

Drifting of teeth often occurs into the spaces created by unreplaced missing teeth. **Drifting differs from pathologic migration in that it does not result from destruction of the periodontal tissues.** However, drifting usually creates conditions that lead to periodontal disease, so that the initial tooth movement becomes aggravated by loss of periodontal support (Fig. 19–5).

Drifting generally occurs in a mesial direction, combined with tilting or extrusion beyond the occlusal plane. The premolars frequently drift distally (Figs. 19–6 and 19–7). Although drifting is a common sequel of unreplaced missing teeth, it does not always occur (Fig. 19–8).

FAILURE TO REPLACE FIRST MOLARS. *The pattern of changes that may follow failure to replace missing first molars is characteristic.* In extreme cases it consists of the following:

1. Tilting of the second and third molars, resulting in a decrease in vertical dimension (Fig. 19–9).

2. The premolars move distally and the mandibular incisors tilt or drift lingually. The mandibular premolars, while drifting distally, lose their intercuspating relationship with the maxillary teeth and may tilt distally.

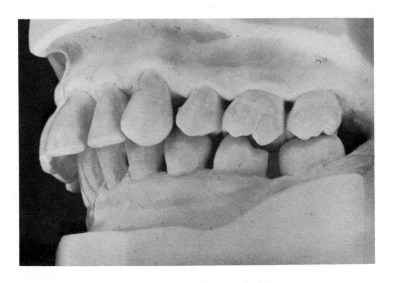

Figure 19–6 Maxillary First Molar Tilted and Extruded into space created by missing mandibular tooth.

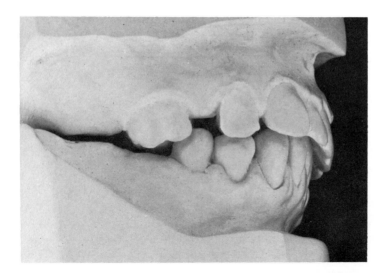

Figure 19–7 Distal Drifting of Maxillary and Mandibular Premolars. The maxillary molar is extruded and tilted.

3. Anterior overbite is increased. The mandibular incisors strike the maxillary incisors near the gingiva or traumatize the gingiva.

4. The maxillary incisors are pushed labially and laterally (Fig. 19–10).

5. The anterior teeth extrude because the incisal apposition has largely disappeared.

6. Diastemata are created by the separation of the anterior teeth (Fig. 19–9).

The disturbed proximal contact relationships lead to food impaction, gingival inflammation and pocket formation, followed by bone loss and tooth mobility. Occlusal disharmonies created by the altered tooth positions traumatize the supporting tissues of the periodontium and aggravate the destruction caused by the inflammation. Reduction in periodontal support leads to further migration of the teeth and mutilation of the occlusion.

Periodontosis (diffuse atrophy of alveolar bone)

Pathologic migration is an early sign of periodontosis (diffuse atrophy of the alveolar bone). The teeth are weakened by

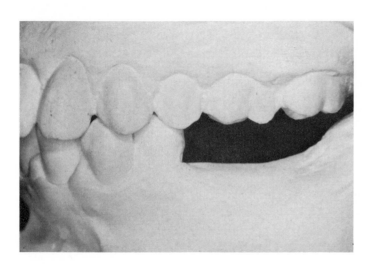

Figure 19–8 No Drifting or Extrusion despite four year's absence of mandibular teeth.

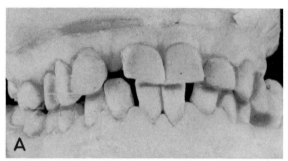

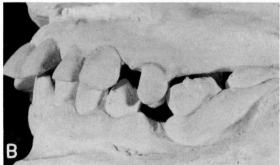
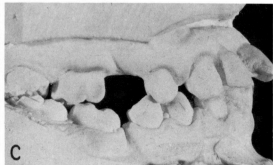

Figure 19-9 Mutilation of Occlusion Associated with Unreplaced Missing Teeth. Note pronounced pathologic migration, disturbed proximal contacts and functional relationships with "closing of the bite."

loss of periodontal support. The maxillary and mandibular anterior incisors drift labially, rotate and extrude, and create diastemata between the teeth (Fig. 19–11).

Trauma from occlusion

Trauma from occlusion may cause a shift in tooth position either by itself, or combined with inflammatory or degenerative periodontal disease. The direction of movement depends upon the occlusal force.

Tongue pressure

Pressure from the tongue may cause drifting of the teeth in the absence of periodontal disease or contribute to pathologic

Figure 19-10 Maxillary Incisors Pushed Labially in Patient with bilateral unreplaced mandibular molars. Note extrusion of the maxillary molars.

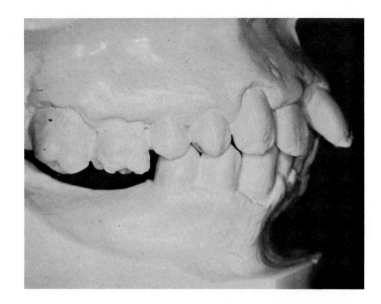

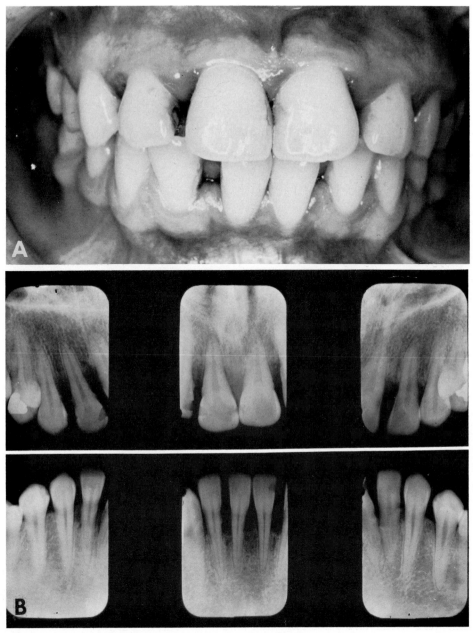

Figure 19–11 *A,* **Pathologic Migration** of maxillary and mandibular teeth in patient with **Periodontosis.** *B,* Radiographs showing bone loss around the anterior teeth.

migration of teeth with reduced periodontal support (Fig. 19–12).

Pressure from chronic inflammatory granulation tissue[2]

In teeth weakened by periodontal destruction, pressure from the granulation tissue of periodontal pockets may contribute to pathologic migration. The teeth may return to their original positions after the pockets are eliminated, but, if there has been more destruction on one side of a tooth than the other, the healing tissues tend to pull in the direction of the lesser destruction.

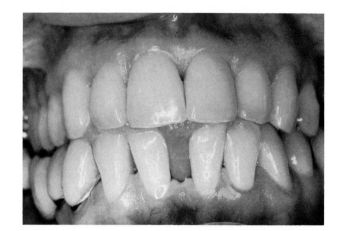

Figure 19–12 Pathologic Migration associated with tongue pressure.

Disturbance in the synchronism between active and passive eruption

Gottlieb[1] considered pathologic migration to be caused by a disturbance in the balance between active and passive eruption. It is produced when the teeth do not erupt at an even rate and some are worn down more by attrition than others. Teeth with least attrition must bear the entire biting force and are most susceptible to pathologic migration.

TOOTH MOBILITY

Normal Mobility

Teeth normally have a certain range of mobility, single rooted teeth more than multirooted, and the incisors have the most.* The mobility is principally in a horizontal direction; it also occurs axially but to a much lesser degree.[7] The range of physiologic tooth mobility varies among individuals and from hour to hour in individual teeth in the same person. It is highest upon arising, possibly because of slight extrusion in the absence of function during the night, and diminishes during the day, possibly from intrusion by pressure from chewing and swallowing. The 24-hour variations in tooth mobility are less in patients

*For a comprehensive review of the subject of mobility, including an excellent bibliography, the reader is referred to the article by H. R. Mühlemann.[4]

with a healthy periodontium and greater in patients with periodontal disease or occlusal habits such as bruxing and clenching.[6]

Tooth mobility occurs in two stages: (1) **The initial or intrasocket stage,** in which the tooth moves within the confines of the periodontal ligament. This is associated with viscoelastic distortion of the ligament and redistribution of periodontal fluids, interbundle content and fibers.[3] (2) **The secondary stage,** which occurs gradually and entails elastic deformation of the alveolar bone in response to increased horizontal forces.[5] The tooth itself is also deformed by the impact of a force applied to the crown, but not to a clinically significant degree.

Elastic recoil, slow recovery and periodontal pulse[4]

When a force such as that normally applied to teeth in occlusion is discontinued, the teeth return to their original position in two stages; the first is an *immediate spring-like elastic recoil;* the second is a slow *asymptomatic recovery movement.* The recovery movement is pulsating and apparently associated with the normal pulsation of the periodontal vessels which occurs in synchrony with the cardiac cycle.

Abnormal (Pathologic) Mobility

Mobility beyond the physiologic range is termed abnormal or pathologic. It is pathologic in the sense that it exceeds the limits of normal mobility values, rather than that the periodontium is necessarily diseased at the time of examination. Pathologic mobility is caused by one or more of the following factors:

1. **Loss of alveolar bone and periodontal ligament and support.** The amount of mobility depends upon the severity and distribution of the tissue loss on individual root surfaces, the length and shape of the roots and the root size compared to the crown. A tooth with short tapered roots is more likely to loosen than one with normal-sized or bulbous roots with the same amount of bone loss. Because bone loss is not the sole cause of tooth mobility and tooth mobility usually results from a combination of factors, the severity of tooth mobility does not necessarily correspond with the amount of bone loss.

2. **Trauma from occlusion.** Injury produced by excessive occlusal forces and incurred during abnormal occlusal habits such as bruxing and clenching which are aggravated by emotional stress is a common cause of tooth mobility. Mobility is also increased by hypofunction.[5]

3. **The extension of inflammation from the gingiva into the periodontal ligament results in degenerative changes which increase mobility.** The changes usually occur in periodontal disease which has advanced beyond the early stages, but tooth mobility is sometimes observed in severe gingivitis. The spread of inflammation from an acute periapical abscess produces a temporary increase in tooth mobility in the absence of periodontal disease.

Tooth mobility is increased in pregnancy, and sometimes associated with the menstrual cycle or the use of hormonal contraceptives. It occurs in patients with or without periodontal disease, presumably because of physicochemical changes in the periodontal tissues.

Mobility is also temporarily increased for a short period after periodontal surgery.

REFERENCES

1. Gottlieb, B.: Formation of the Pocket; Diffuse Atrophy of Alveolar Bone. J.A.D.A., *15*:462, 1928.
2. Hirschfeld, I.: The Dynamic Relationship between Pathologically Migrating Teeth and Inflammatory Tissue in Periodontal Pockets: a Clinical Study. J. Periodont., *4*:35, 1933.
3. Kurashima, K.: Viscoelastic Properties of Periodontal Tissue. Bull. Tokyo Med. D. Univ., *12*:240, 1965.
4. Mühlemann, H. R.: Tooth Mobility: A Review of Clinical Aspects and Research Findings. J. Periodont., *38*:686, 1967.
5. Mühlemann, H. R., Savdir, S., and Rateitschak, K. H.: Tooth Mobility—Its Causes and Significance. J. Periodont., *36*:148, 1965.
6. O'Leary, T. J.: Tooth Mobility. Dent. Clin. North America, *13*:567, 1969.
7. Parfitt, G. J.: Measurement of the Physiologic Mobility of Individual Teeth in an Axial Direction. J. D. Res., *39*:608, 1960.

Chapter 20

GINGIVAL AND PERIODONTAL DISEASE IN CHILDHOOD

The terminal effects of periodontal disease observed in adults have their inception earlier in life. Gingival disease in childhood may progress to jeopardize the periodontium of the adult. The increasing awareness of the prevalence of gingival and periodontal disease in children,[29] coupled with the need for more information regarding the early stages of periodontal disease, have focused attention upon the periodontium in childhood.[5, 10, 24, 27, 44]

The developing dentition and certain systemic metabolic patterns are peculiar to childhood. There are also gingival and periodontal disturbances that occur more frequently in childhood and are, therefore, identified with this period. Consequently, some degree of coherence is provided by grouping the facts regarding gingival and periodontal problems in childhood in a separate chapter.

THE PERIODONTIUM OF THE DECIDUOUS DENTITION

The *gingiva* in the deciduous dentition is pale-pink, firm and either smooth or stippled (in 35 per cent of children in the 5 to 13 age group[39]) (Fig. 20–1). The interdental gingiva is broad faciolingually and tends to be relatively narrow mesiodistally in conformity with the contour of the approximal tooth surfaces. It is comparable to

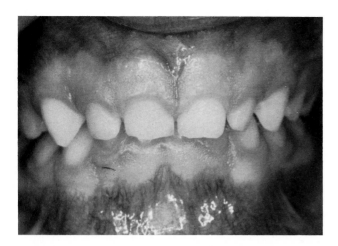

Figure 20–1 Deciduous Dentition with Stippled Gingiva.

that of the adult in that it consists of a facial and lingual papilla with an intervening depression or *col*. The mean gingival sulcus depth for the primary dentition is 2.1 mm. ± 0.2.[36]

Microscopically, the stratified squamous epithelium of the gingiva presents well-differentiated rete pegs with a parakeratinized (Fig. 20–2) or keratinized surface, the latter correlated with stippling. The connective tissue is predominantly fibrillar and is differentiated into papillary and reticular layers. The well-differentiated collagen bundles seen in the adult are not present in childhood. The epithelium initially covering the col is odontogenic, rather than oral, in origin. It is a few cells thick and nonkeratinized. The *periodontal ligament* of the deciduous teeth is wider than that of the permanent dentition. During eruption the principal fibers are parallel to the long axis of the teeth; the bundle arrangement seen in the adult dentition occurs when the teeth encounter their functional antagonists.

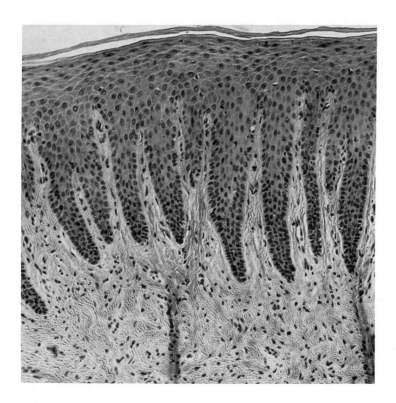

Figure 20–2 Normal Gingiva in a Four-Year-Old Patient Showing Stratified Squamous Epithelium with Rete Pegs and Surface Keratinization. The papillary arrangement of the underlying connective tissue can also be seen.

The *alveolar bone* in relation to the deciduous dentition shows a prominent lamina dura radiographically, in the crypt stage and during eruption. The trabeculae of the alveolar bone are fewer but thicker, and the marrow spaces tend to be larger than in the adult. The crests of the interdental septa are flat.[7]

PHYSIOLOGIC GINGIVAL CHANGES ASSOCIATED WITH TOOTH ERUPTION

During the transitional period in the development of the dentition, changes occur in the gingiva associated with eruption of the permanent teeth. It is important to recognize these physiologic changes and differentiate them from gingival disease that often accompanies tooth eruption. The following are physiologic changes in the gingiva associated with tooth eruption:

PRE-ERUPTION BULGE. Before the crown appears in the oral cavity, the gingiva presents a bulge which is firm, may be slightly blanched, and conforms to the contour of the underlying crown.

FORMATION OF THE GINGIVAL MARGIN. The marginal gingiva and sulcus develop as the crown penetrates the oral mucosa. In the course of eruption the gingival margin is usually edematous, rounded and slightly reddened (Fig. 20–3).

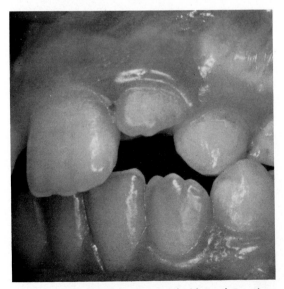

Figure 20–3   Gingivitis Associated with Tooth Eruption. Prominent rolled gingival margin which is slightly inflamed and edematous around erupting maxillary lateral incisor.

NORMAL PROMINENCE OF THE GINGIVAL MARGIN. During the period of the mixed dentition it is normal for the marginal gingiva around the permanent teeth to be quite prominent, particularly in the maxillary anterior region. At this stage in tooth eruption the gingiva is still attached to the crown, and it appears prominent when superimposed upon the bulk of the underlying enamel (Fig. 20–4).

GINGIVAL DISEASE

Chronic marginal gingivitis

This is the most prevalent type of gingival change in childhood. The gingiva presents all the changes in color, size, consistency and surface texture characteristic of chronic inflammation. Fiery red surface discoloration is often superimposed upon underlying chronic changes.

ETIOLOGY. In children, as in adults, the most common cause of gingivitis is local irritation, as well as local conditions which lead to the accumulation of local irritants.

Most gingivitis in children is caused by *poor oral hygiene, dental plaque** and *materia alba*[28] (Fig. 20–5). Dental plaque appears to form more rapidly in children (aged 8 to 12) than in adults.

Calculus, another source of gingival irritation, is uncommon in infants,[6] occurs in approximately 9 per cent of children between the ages of 4 and 6, 18 per cent at ages 7 to 9, and 33 to 43 per cent at ages 10 to 15.[15] In children with *cystic fibrosis,* calculus formation is more common (77 per cent at ages 7 to 9, 90 per cent at ages 10 to 15), and more severe, probably related to increased concentrations of phosphate, calcium and protein in the saliva.[31]

Gingivitis Associated with Tooth Eruption. The frequency with which gingivitis occurs around erupting teeth has given rise to the term *eruption gingivitis.* However, tooth eruption per se does not cause gingivitis. The inflammation results from local irritants that accumulate around erupting teeth. The inflammatory changes accentuate the normal prominence of the gingival mar-

*For detailed discussions of dental plaque, materia alba and calculus, see Chapter 22.

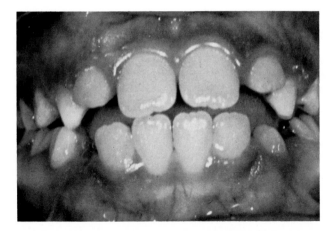

Figure 20–4 Prominent Marginal Gingiva on the cervical third of partially erupted maxillary anterior teeth.

Figure 20–5 Chronic Marginal Gingivitis associated with materia alba.

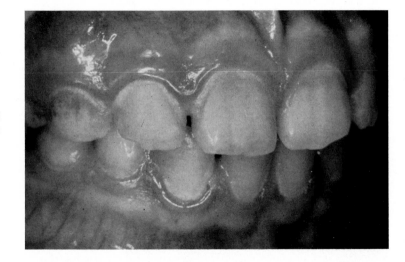

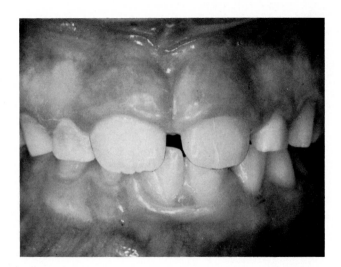

Figure 20–6 Developmental Gingival Enlargement caused by inflammation superimposed upon the normal prominence of the gingiva at this stage of tooth eruption.

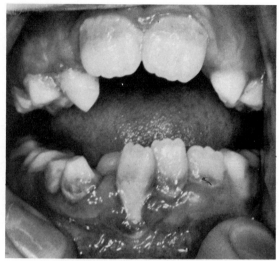

Figure 20–7 Severe Gingivitis associated with accumulation of irritants and food impaction around malposed teeth.

gin and create the impression of a marked gingival enlargement (Fig. 20–6).

Loose and Carious Teeth. Partially exfoliated loose deciduous teeth frequently cause gingivitis. Irritation by the eroded margin of partially resorbed teeth causes gingival changes varying from slight discoloration and edema to abscess formation with suppuration. Other sources of gingival irritation are food impaction and plaque and materia alba accumulation around teeth partially destroyed by caries. Children frequently develop *unilateral chewing habits* to avoid loose or carious teeth, aggravating the accumulation of irritants on the non-chewing side.

Malposed Teeth and Malocclusion. Gingivitis occurs more frequently and with greater severity around malposed teeth because of the increased tendency toward accumulation of plaque and materia alba. Severe changes include gingival enlargement, bluish red discoloration, ulceration (Fig. 20–7) and the formation of deep pockets from which pus can be expressed. Gingival health and contour are restored by correction of the malposition (Figs. 20–8 and 20–9), elimination of local irritants and, when necessary, surgical removal of the enlarged gingiva.

Gingivitis is increased in children with *excessive overbite* and *overjet,* in *nasal obstruction* and in *mouth breathing.*[38] *Pyogenic granulomas* and *peripheral giant-cell reparative granulomas* occasionally occur in the gingiva.[3] (For a description of these lesions, see Chapter 8.)

Localized gingival recession

Gingival recession around individual teeth or groups of teeth is a common source of concern. The gingiva may be inflamed or free of disease, depending upon the presence or absence of local irritants. There are many causes of gingival recession (see Chapter 9), but in children the *position of the tooth in the arch is the most important.*[35] Gingival recession occurs on teeth in labial version (Fig. 20–10) or on those which are tilted or rotated so that the roots project labially. The recession may be a transitional phase in tooth eruption and may correct itself when the teeth attain proper alignment, or it may be necessary to realign the teeth orthodontically.

Acute gingival infections

ACUTE HERPETIC GINGIVOSTOMATITIS. This is the most common type of acute gingival infection in childhood. It often occurs as a sequel of upper respiratory tract infection. (It is described in Chapter 11.)

MONILIASIS (THRUSH). This is a mycotic infection of the oral cavity caused by the fungus *Candida albicans,* and is most often *acute* (Fig. 20–11) but may be *chronic.* (It is described in Chapter 13.)

ACUTE NECROTIZING ULCERATIVE GINGIVITIS. The incidence of acute necrotizing ulcerative gingivitis in childhood is low. (It is described in Chapter 11.) Acute herpetic gingivostomatitis, which is more common in childhood, is occasionally

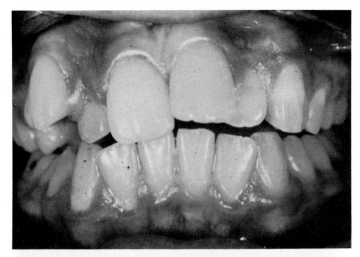

Figure 20–8 Gingival Enlargement in relation to malposed maxillary lateral and canine (*left*). (Courtesy of Dr. Coenraad F. Moorrees, Forsyth Dental Center, Boston.)

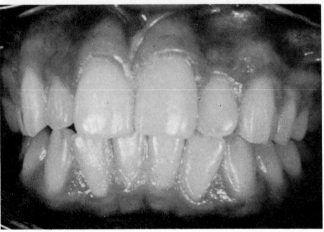

Figure 20–9 Disappearance of gingival enlargement shown in Figure 20–8 following orthodontic correction of the malposed teeth. (Courtesy of Dr. Coenraad F. Moorrees.)

Figure 20–10 Gingival Recession on labially positioned mandibular central incisors.

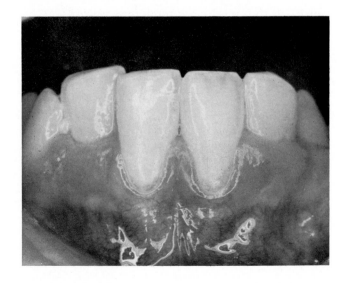

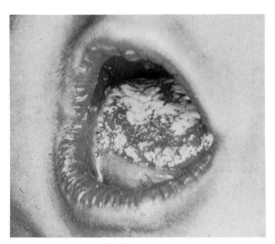

Figure 20–11   Acute Moniliasis (Thrush).

erroneously diagnosed as acute necrotizing ulcerative gingivitis.

PERIODONTAL DISEASE

Periodontitis occurs occasionally in the deciduous dentition,[20] and in 5 per cent of teenagers. There are also situations of severe rapid periodontal destruction and premature tooth loss in children and teenagers which are considered to be primarily degenerative diseases of the periodontium, with inflammation a secondary destructive factor.[2] These are infrequent; they are usually referred to as periodontosis* and appear to be divisible into the following groups:

I. Periodontosis (Advanced Alveolar Bone Loss in Adolescence)

In these patients periodontal destruction occurs around more than a single tooth, but the entire dentition is not necessarily involved. The first permanent molars and anterior teeth are usually affected first, the bone destruction is vertical (angular) rather than horizontal and there is pathologic migration of the anterior teeth (Fig. 20–12). Bone loss is severe, but teeth can often be retained by comprehensive periodontal treatment.

In a study of 2050 adolescents 14 cases were reported, in an approximate ratio of three females to one male. Some cases appear to be hereditary and follow a familial pattern with siblings often affected.[2,8] A systemic etiology has been suspected, but none has been identified.

II. Palmoplantar Hyperkeratosis with Premature Periodontal Destruction (Periodontosis) (Papillon-Lefèvre Syndrome)

This is a syndrome* characterized by **hyperkeratosis of the palms and soles, premature severe destruction of the periodontium (periodontosis) and in some cases calcification of the dura.** The skin and periodontal changes usually appear together before the age of four with the deciduous dentition lost by five years of age. The permanent dentition erupts normally, but because of the active periodontal destruction the teeth are exfoliated within two to three years after they erupt. Patients are edentulous by 12 to 15 years of age.[9] The third molars are also lost a few years after eruption.

The microscopic changes include chronic inflammation of the gingiva and supporting periodontal tissues, with destruction of the epithelial attachment, and degeneration of periodontal ligament fibers with resorption of bone, cementum and dentin.

The syndrome is inherited and appears to follow an **autosomal recessive pattern.**[3] Parents are not affected and both must carry the autosomal genes for the syndrome to appear in the offspring. It may occur in siblings; males and females are equally affected. The estimated frequency is one to four per million; a total of approximately 53 cases have been reported.

III. Severe Idiopathic Periodontal Destruction in Children

This is an extremely rare condition of unknown etiology unrelated to any syndrome.[26] Periodontal destruction is severe and generalized, with some teeth com-

---

*For a detailed discussion of Periodontosis, see Chapter 30.

*For literature, reviews and case reports, see Gorlin, R. J., et al.,[18] and Galanter, D. R., and Bradford, S.[17]

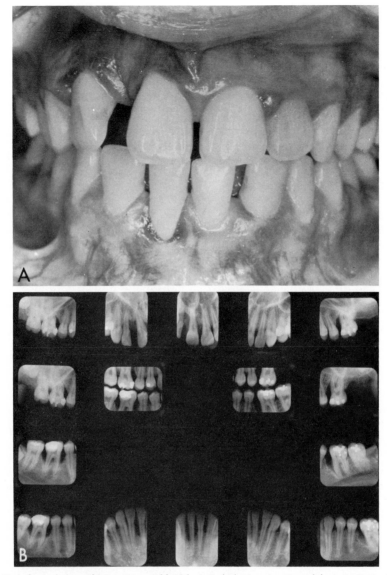

Figure 20–12   Periodontosis in a Thirteen-Year-Old Girl. *A,* Pathologic migration of the anterior teeth considered to be characteristic of periodontosis. *B,* "Typical" distribution of bone destruction in the first molar and anterior regions. Note the angular pattern of the bone loss.

pletely denuded of bone (Figs. 20–13 and 20–14), accompanied by tooth mobility and pathologic migration. There is also generalized severe gingival inflammation, with gingival enlargement and purulent periodontal pockets. Medical history, examination and laboratory tests are essentially negative, with no notable changes in other bones.

IV. Precocious Advanced Alveolar Atrophy

Miller, Wolf and Siedler[30] described periodontal bone loss in young patients and designated it *precocious advanced alveolar atrophy.* It is usually associated with elevated serum cholesterol and calcium levels and a flattened sugar tolerance curve. The patients favor a high carbohydrate diet.

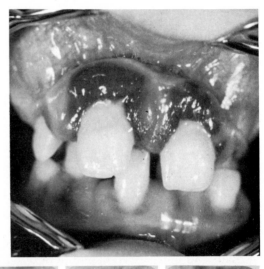

Figure 20–13 Pronounced Gingival Inflammation and pathologic migration in an eight-year-old patient. (Courtesy of Drs. P. Losch and C. Boyes, Children's Hospital, Boston.)

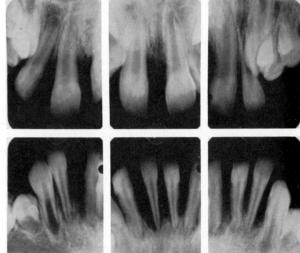

Figure 20–14 Radiographs of patient shown in Figure 20–13 showing pronounced generalized bone loss.

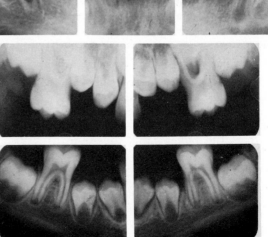

Severest changes occur around the first permanent molars and incisors. It is suspected that unidentified systemic factors weaken the periodontium around these teeth when they erupt, so that the tissues are destroyed by normal occlusal forces. Teeth which erupt later may be well supported by bone. Treatment entails extraction of extensively involved first molars to prevent jeopardizing the second molars and premolars.

TRAUMATIC CHANGES IN THE PERIODONTIUM

Traumatic changes may occur in the periodontal tissues of deciduous teeth under the following conditions:

In shedding deciduous teeth, resorption of teeth and bone weakens the periodontal support so that the existing functional forces are injurious to the remaining supporting tissues.[3]

Excessive occlusal forces may be produced by malalignment, mutilation, loss or extractions of teeth or dental restorations.

In the mixed dentition, the periodontium of the permanent teeth may be traumatized because they bear an increased occlusal load when the adjacent deciduous teeth are shed. The periodontal ligament of an erupting permanent tooth may be injured by occlusal forces transmitted through the deciduous tooth it is replacing.[19]

Microscopically,[1, 25, 32, 33] the least severe traumatic changes consist of compression, ischemia and hyalinization of the periodontal ligament. With severe injury there is crushing and necrosis of the periodontal ligament with the formation of hemorrhagic cysts.

In most instances the injuries are repaired and tooth loss does not result. However, such traumatized teeth may be sore or loose. Repair may result in *ankylosis* of the tooth to the bone, fixing the tooth in situ. When the permanent dentition erupts, ankylosed deciduous teeth appear to be *submerged.*

ORAL MANIFESTATIONS OF SYSTEMIC DISEASE

Certain childhood diseases present specific alterations in the oral cavity.[4, 21, 43]

Among these are the communicable diseases.

CHICKENPOX (VARICELLA). Successive papillary eruptions and vesicles appear on the buccal mucosa as well as on the face and remainder of the cutaneous body surface (Fig. 20–15). On the buccal mucosa the vesicles break down to become small ulcerated craters with surrounding erythema resembling the lesions of acute herpetic stomatitis. Comparable but more extensive oral lesions are seen in *smallpox (variola).*

MEASLES (RUBEOLA). Koplik spots are pathognomonic of measles and are found in 97 per cent of patients. They are seen two to three days before the rash appears (Fig. 20–16). They occur most often on the buccal mucosa opposite the first molars or on the inner aspect of the lower lip, and appear as bluish white specks—pin-point in size—surrounded by a bright red areola. They are best seen in daylight. At first only a few are present, but later they become numerous and coalesce. In addition to these specific lesions, measles may also be accompanied by erythema and edema of the gingiva and remainder of the oral mucosa, and discrete bluish red discolored areas on the soft palate.

SCARLET FEVER (SCARLATINA). Diffuse fiery-red discoloration of the oral mucosa occurs in scarlet fever. Characteristic tongue changes include (1) "raspberry tongue," a bright red, shiny discoloration with prominent papillae (Fig. 20–17), and (2) "strawberry tongue," a coated surface covering an underlying bright red discoloration with prominent papillae (Fig. 20–18).

DIPHTHERIA. Diphtheria is characterized by pseudomembrane formation in the oropharynx that appears as a gray, friable, curtain-like extension in the area of the anterior faucal pillars. Diffuse erythema of the oral mucous membrane with vesicle formation is also commonly seen in this condition (Fig. 20–19).

CONGENITAL HEART DISEASE. Gingival disease and other oral symptoms may occur in children with congenital heart disease.[23] In cases of *tetralogy of Fallot* which is characterized by pulmonary stenosis, right side ventricular enlargement, a defect in the interventricular septum, or malposition of the aorta to the right, the oral changes include purplish red discoloration of the lips and severe marginal gin-

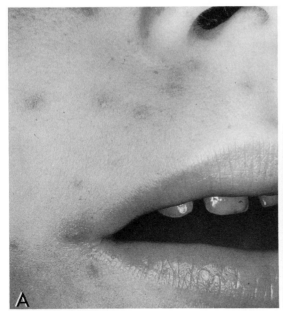

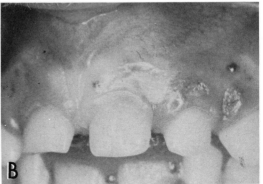

Figure 20–15 Chickenpox (Varicella). *A,* Skin lesions. *B,* Vesicles on gingiva.

Fig. 20–16   Fig. 20–17

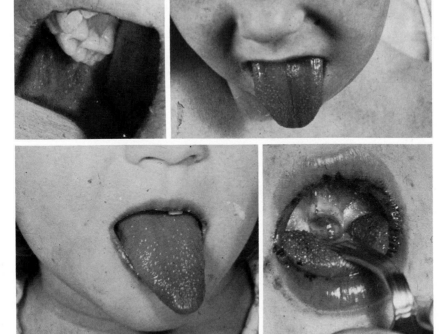

Fig. 20–18   Fig. 20–19

Figure 20–16 Koplik spots on the buccal mucosa in measles. (Courtesy Dr. Louis Weinstein, Tufts University Medical School.)

Figure 20–17 "Raspberry tongue" in scarlet fever showing smooth shiny discoloration with prominent papillae. (Courtesy Dr. Louis Weinstein, Tufts University Medical School.)

Figure 20–18 "Strawberry tongue" of scarlet fever with moderately coated tongue and prominent papillae. (Courtesy Dr. Louis Weinstein, Tufts University Medical School.)

Figure 20–19 Diphtheritic membrane, forming curtain-like projection in the oropharynx. (Courtesy Dr. Louis Weinstein, Tufts University Medical School.)

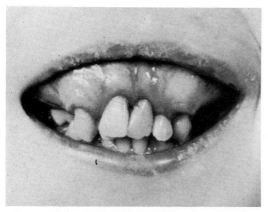

Figure 20–20   Erythroblastic Anemia. Note the prominence of the maxilla and pallor of the gingival mucosa. (Courtesy of Dr. M. M. Cohen and Dr. J. M. Baty, Floating Hospital, Boston.)

givitis. The tongue is coated, fissured and edematous, and there is extreme reddening of the fungiform and filiform papillae. There is an increased number of subepithelial capillaries, which approaches the normal value following cardiac surgery.[16]

In cases of *tetralogy of Eisenmenger* there is pulmonary insufficiency and a diastolic murmur; the lips, cheeks and buccal mucous membranes are cyanotic but less markedly so than in the tetralogy of Fallot. Severe generalized marginal gingivitis is a common finding. In cases where there is *transposition of the aorta and superior vena cava vessels,* cyanotic discoloration and marginal gingivitis of a lesser degree are noted. In *coarctation of the aorta* there is a narrowing of the vessel in the

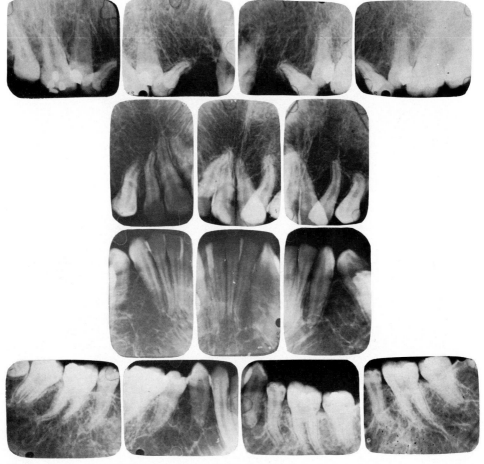

Figure 20–21   Radiographs of Patient with Erythroblastic Anemia. There is generalized rarefaction of the bone and enlarged irregularly arranged medullary spaces. (Courtesy Dr. M. M. Cohen and Dr. J. M. Baty.)

region where it is joined by the ductus arteriosus. These cases show marked inflammation of the gingiva in the anterior part of the mouth.

ERYTHROBLASTIC ANEMIA (COOLEY'S ANEMIA). This is an inherited disorder characterized by a hemolytic anemia, splenomegaly, nucleated red blood cells in the peripheral blood and generalized skeletal lesions.[13] Skeletal changes are absent or minimal during the first year of life. The osteoporosis characteristic of the disease occurs during early childhood and is followed by sclerosis. The most characteristic bony changes are noted in the metacarpals and femurs. Pneumatization of the paranasal sinuses is retarded.

Oral changes[11] include pallor and cyanosis of the mucous membrane and marked malocclusion owing to overgrowth of the alveolar ridge of the maxilla (Fig. 20–20). There is an associated spreading of the teeth with creation of large interproximal spaces.

Radiographic examination reveals generalized rarefaction of the jaws with an alteration in trabecular pattern characterized by an irregularly arranged heterogenous lattice, with obliteration of the lamina dura in some areas (Fig. 20–21).

ACUTE AND SUBACUTE LEUKEMIA. These diseases in children are accompanied by gingival changes (Fig. 20–22). (See Chap. 28.)

LIPID DISTURBANCES. Gingival manifestations of diseases such as *Hand-Schüller-Christian, Gaucher, Niemann-Pick* and *disseminated xanthomatosis* include enlargement with yellow discoloration and fatty nodules (Fig. 20–23).

NUTRITIONAL DEFICIENCIES. Oral changes associated with deficiencies in components of the vitamin B complex and vitamin C (Fig. 20–24) sometimes occur secondary to gastrointestinal disorders. (Oral changes in vitamin deficiencies are described in Chapter 26.)

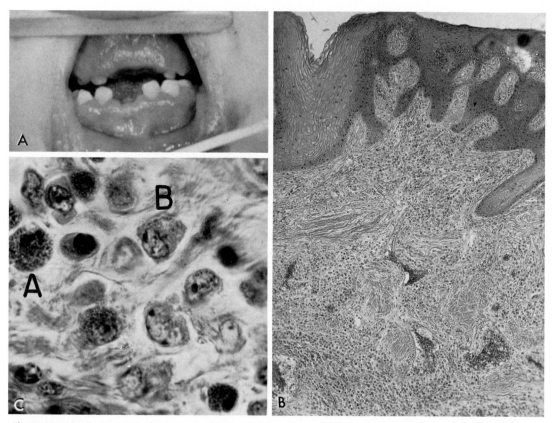

Figure 20–22 *A,* **Acute Myelogenous Leukemia,** showing diffuse gingival enlargement. *B,* Section of gingival biopsy, showing dense leukocytic infiltration. *C,* Detailed study of myeloid cells in gingival biopsy. Myelocytes are shown at A and B.

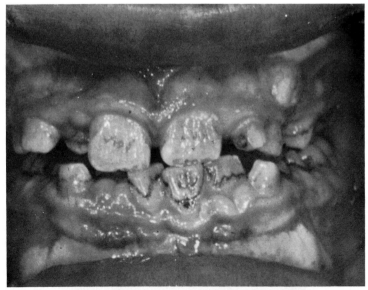

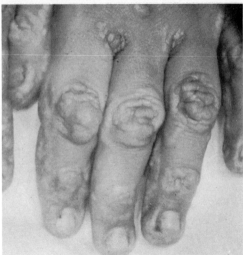

Figure 20–23 *Top,* **Fatty Infiltration of the Gingiva** in disseminated xanthomatosis. *Bottom,* Same patient showing fatty nodules on the hand. (Courtesy of Dr. M. M. Cohen.)

DIABETES. In childhood, uncontrolled diabetes may be accompanied by marked destruction of alveolar bone.[37] Although gingival inflammation is a frequent finding in such cases, the extent of alveolar bone loss is in excess of that generally seen in children with comparable gingival involvement.

MONGOLISM (DOWN'S SYNDROME). Mongolism is a congenital disease caused by a chromosomal abnormality (trisomy 21) and characterized by mental deficiency and retardation of growth. The prevalence of periodontal disease is high and, although plaque, calculus and periodontal pockets are present, the severity of periodontal destruction exceeds that explainable by local factors alone (Fig. 20–25).[12, 22, 42]

CEREBRAL PALSY. Hypoplasia, attrition, malocclusion and temporomandibular dys-

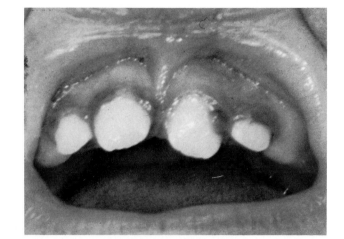

Figure 20–24 Scorbutic Child with discoloration and enlargement of the gingiva.

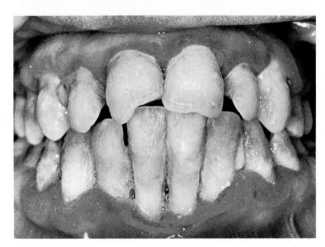

Figure 20–25 Mongoloid Child with severe periodontal destruction. (Courtesy of Dr. Stanley Schwartz.)

function are increased in cerebral palsy.[41] Because oral hygiene is a problem, the prevalence of periodontal disorders and caries may be high.

REFERENCES

1. Bauer, W.: Ueber traumatische Schädigungen des Zementmantels der Zahne mit einem Beitrag zur Biologie des Zementes. Deutsch. Monatsch. f. Zahnhk., 45:769, 1927.
2. Benjamin, S. D., and Baer, P. N.: Familial Patterns of Advanced Aveolar Bone Loss in Adolescence (Periodontosis). Periodontics, 5:82, 1967.
3. Bernick, S., and Freedman, N.: Microscopic Studies of the Periodontium of the Primary Dentitions of Monkeys. II. Posterior Teeth During the Mixed Dentitional Period. Oral Surg., Oral Med. & Oral Path., 7:322, 1954.
4. Blackstone, C. H.: A Clinical and Roentgenographic Study of Periodontic Problems in Children with Systemic Disease. J.A.D.A., 29:1664, 1942.
5. Bradley, R. E.: Periodontal Lesions of Children— Their Recognition and Treatment. D. Clin. North America, Nov., 1961, p. 671.
6. Brauer, J. C.: Periodontal Problems in the Child Patient. J. Periodont., 11:7, 1940.
7. Brauer, J. C., Higley, L. B., Massler, M., and Schour, I.: Dentistry for Children. Chap. 7. 2nd ed. Philadelphia, The Blakiston Company, 1947.
8. Butler, J.: A Familial Pattern of Juvenile Periodontitis (Periodontosis). J. Periodont.-Periodontics, 40:115, 1969.
9. Carvel, R. I.: Palmar-Plantar Hyperkeratosis and Premature Periodontal Destruction. J. Oral Med., 24:73, 1969.
10. Cohen, D. W., and Goldman, H. M.: Periodontal Disease in Children, P.D.M., July, 1962, p. 3.
11. Cohen, M. M., and Baty, J. M.: Oral Manifestations of Erythroblastic Anemia. J.A.D.A., 32:1396, 1945.
12. Cohen, M. M., Winer, R. A., Schwartz, S., and Shklar, G.: Oral Aspects of Mongolism. Part I. Periodontal Disease in Mongolism. Oral Surg. Oral Med. & Oral Path., 14:92, 1961.
13. Cooley, T. B., Witwer, E. R., and Lee, P.: Anemia in Children with Splenomegaly and Peculiar Changes in Bones. Am. J. Dis. Child., 34:347, 1927.
14. Eichel, R. A.: A Clinical Television Evaluation of Plaque Formation in Children. Internat. Assn. for Dent. Res. Program and Abstracts, 48th General Meeting, 1970, p. 171.

15. Everett, F. G., Tuchler, H., and Lu, K. H.: Occurrence of Calculus in Grade School Children in Portland, Oregon. J. Periodont., *34*:54, 1963.

16. Forsslund, G.: Occurrence of Subepithelial Gingival Blood Vessels in Patients with Morbus Caeruleus (Tetralogy of Fallot). Acta Odont. Scandinav., *20*:301, 1962.

17. Galanter, D. R., and Bradford, S.: Hyperkeratosis Palmoplantaris and Periodontosis: The Papillon-Lefèvre Syndrome. J. Periodont.-Periodontics, *40*:40, 1969.

18. Gorlin, R. J., Sedano, H., and Anderson, V. E.: The Syndrome of Palmar-Plantar Hyperkeratosis and Premature Periodontal Destruction of the Teeth. J. Pediat., *65*:895, 1964.

19. Grimmer, E. A.: Trauma in an Erupting Premolar. J. D. Res., *18*:267, 1939.

20. Harndt, E.: Marginal Periodontal Disease in the Deciduous Dentition. A.R.P.A. Internat., *13*:1, 1955.

21. Jacobs, M. H.: Oral Lesions in Childhood. Oral. Surg., Oral Med. & Oral Path., *9*:871, 1956.

22. Johnson, N. P., and Young, M. A.: Periodontal Disease in Mongols. J. Periodont., *34*:41, 1963.

23. Kaner, A., Losch, P., and Green, H.: Oral Manifestations of Congenital Heart Disease. J. Pediat., *29*:269, 1946.

24. Kerr, D. A.: Stomatitis and Gingivitis in the Adolescent and Preadolescent. J.A.D.A., *44*:27, 1952.

25. Kronfeld, R., and Weinmann, J.: Traumatic Changes in the Periodontal Tissues of Deciduous Teeth. J. D. Res., *19*:441, 1940.

26. Losch, P., and Boyers, C.: Personal communication.

27. McCall, J. D.: Gingival and Periodontal Disease in Children. J. Periodont., *9*:7, 1938.

28. McCombie, F., and Stothard, D.: Relationships Between Gingivitis and Other Dental Conditions. J. Canad. D. Assn., *30*:506, 1964.

29. McIntosh, W. G.: Gingival and Periodontal Disease in Children. J. Canad. D. Assn., *20*:12, 1954.

30. Miller, S. C., Wolf, A., and Seidler, B. B.: Generalized Rapid Alveolar Atrophy. J. D. Res., *19*:306, 1940.

31. Notman, S., Mandel, I. D., and Mercadante, J.: Calculus in Normal Children and Children with Cystic Fibrosis. Internat. Assn. for Dent. Res. Program and Abstracts, 48th General Meeting, 1970, p. 64.

32. Oppenheim, A.: Histologische Befunde beim Zahnwechsel. Ztschr. f. Stomat., *20*:543, 1922.

33. Orban, B., and Weinmann, J.: Signs of Traumatic Occlusion in Average Human Jaws. J. D. Res., *13*:216, 1933.

34. Papillon, M. M., and Lefevre, P.: Deux Cas de Kératodermie Palmaire et Plantaire Symetrique Familiale (Maladie de Meleda) chez le Frère et la Soeur. Coexistance dans les Deux Cas d'Alterations Dentaires Graves. Soc. Franç. Derm. et Syph., *31*:82, 1924.

35. Parfitt, G. J., and Mjor, I. A.: A Clinical Evaluation of Local Gingival Recession in Children. J. D. Child., *31*:257, 1964.

36. Rosenblum, F. N.: Clinical Study of the Depth of the Gingival Sulcus in the Primary Dentition. J. D. Child., *5*:289, 1966.

37. Rutledge, C. E.: Oral and Roentgenographic Aspects of the Teeth and Jaws of Juvenile Diabetics. J.A.D.A., *27*:1740, 1940.

38. Somjen, I.: Seltene Fälle von Gingivitis. Korrespond. f. Zahnärtzte., *57*:122, 1933.

39. Soni, N. N., Silberkweit, M., and Hayes, R. L.: Histological Characteristics of Stippling in Children. J. Periodont., *34*:31, 1963.

40. Standish, S. M., and Shafer, W. G.: Gingival Reparative Granulomas in Children. J. Oral Surg., Anes. & Hosp. D. Serv., *19*:367, 1961.

41. Sznajder, N.: Oral Diseases in Cerebral Palsy Children. Rev. Assoc. Odont. Argentina, *52*:96, 1964.

42. Sznajder, N., Carraro, J. J., Otero, E., and Carranza, F. A., Jr.: Clinical Periodontal Findings in Trisomy 21 (Mongolism). J. Periodont. Res., *3*:1, 1968.

43. Teuscher, G. W.: Systemic Disease in Children of Interest to the Dentist. D. Clin. North America, July, 1958, p. 481.

44. Thomas, B. O. A.: The Child Patient as a Future Periodontal Problem. J.A.D.A., *35*:763, 1947.

CHAPTER 21

THE EPIDEMIOLOGY OF GINGIVAL AND PERIODONTAL DISEASE

Periodontal disease is one of the most widespread diseases of mankind. No nation and no area of the world is free from it and in most it has a high prevalence, affecting in some degree approximately half the child population and almost the entire adult population....

World Health Organization[110]

Periodontal Disease—A Public Health Problem

Indices for the Epidemiologic Study of Gingival and Periodontal Disease
 P.M.A. Index (Schour and Massler)
 Gingival Recession Index (Stahl and Morris)
 Periodontal Index (Russell)
 Gingival-Bone Count (Dunning and Leach)
 Periodontal Disease Index (Ramjford)
 Periodontal Disease Rate
 Gingival Periodontal Index (O'Leary, Gibson, Shannon, Scheussler and Nabers)
  Gingival Status
  Periodontal Status
  Irritation Index
 Simplified Oral Hygiene Index (Greene and Vermillion)
  Debris Index
  Calculus Index
 Plaque Index (Quigley and Hein)
 Gingival Index (Löe and Silness)
 Plaque Index (Silness and Löe)
 Retention Index (Bjorby and Löe)
 Calculus Surface Index (Ennever, Sturzenberger and Radike)
 Calculus Index (Volpe, Mandel and Hogan)

Prevalence of Gingivitis

Prevalence of Periodontal Disease

Factors Affecting the Prevalence and Severity of Gingivitis and Periodontal Disease
 Age
 Oral Hygiene

 Sex
 Race
 Occupation
 Education
 Professional Dental Care
 Geographic Location
 Social Customs and Nutrition
 Fluoride

Distribution of Gingivitis and Periodontal Disease in Different Areas of the Oral Cavity

The Relationship Between Periodontal Disease and Caries

Epidemiologic surveys conducted throughout the world point to the universal distribution of gingival and periodontal disease.[23, 83, 87] From the earliest times, disease of the supporting structures of the teeth has been recognized in almost every culture. Paleontologic studies indicate that periodontal disease existed in early man.[80, 109]

PERIODONTAL DISEASE—A PUBLIC HEALTH PROBLEM[3, 30, 79]

Statistics vary in different populations, but it is the consensus that periodontal dis-

275

ease is the major cause of tooth loss in the adult population.[2, 75, 91] Caries is responsible for most tooth extractions up to the age of approximately 35, after which periodontal disease becomes the major factor (Fig. 21–1). Approximately 60 to 70 per cent of the tooth loss in the United States after age 40 is caused by periodontal disease,[40] whereas in India periodontal disease is responsible for about 80 per cent of teeth extracted after age 30.[66] Some figures indicate that caries and periodontal disease equally share the responsibility for tooth loss between the ages of 40 to 50, after which periodontal disease becomes the principal cause.[105] It has been shown that periodontal disease is responsible for approximately 50 per cent of the total tooth loss after age 15, and caries for approximately 37 per cent, with the remainder of teeth lost by other cause such as accidents, impactions and prosthetic or orthodontic reasons (Fig. 21–2).

Reports from varied sources agree on the widespread prevalence and seriousness of periodontal disease. For example, it has been estimated that in a target population of 111 million adults in the United States 20 million would have lost all their natural teeth, and gingivitis or periodontal disease would be present in 75 per cent of the remainder;[95] that two thirds of the young adults, 80 per cent of the middle age population and 90 per cent of the people over 65 suffer from periodontal disorders;[38] and that of the 90 million men and women in the United States with at least one permanent tooth, three out of four individuals have had some form of periodontal disease.[50]

Periodontal disease becomes the major cause of tooth loss after age 35, but **periodontal disease is not primarily a disease of adults.** It starts a long time before it necessitates tooth extraction. By 15 years of age four out of five people have gingivitis, and in 4 per cent (higher in some populations) periodontitis is already present. **All the gingivitis of early life does not necessarily develop into periodontal disease, but with infrequent exceptions periodontal disease which destroys adult dentitions starts as gingivitis.**

INDICES FOR THE EPIDEMIOLOGIC STUDY OF GINGIVAL AND PERIODONTAL DISEASE

Study of the epidemiology of periodontal disease requires uniform and precise criteria for assessing and recording the periodontal status of individuals and populations. Methods which express clinical observations in numerical values are known as *indices*. There are many indices for recording and quantitating periodontal disorders which can be used with reproducible accuracy.[94] Although subject to some limitations, they provide valuable data regarding many epidemiologic aspects of gingival and periodontal disease.

P.M.A. index (Schour and Massler[93])

This index is used to record the prevalence and severity of gingivitis. The gingiva mesial to each tooth on the facial surface is divided into three units: the interdental papilla (P), the gingival margin (M) and the attached gingiva (A). Each unit is scored as to the presence (1) or absence (0) of inflammation. P, M and A values are totaled

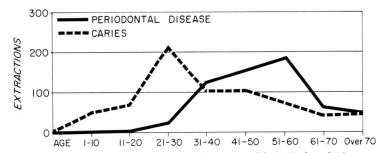

Figure 21–1 Age Factor in the Number of Dental Extractions Caused by Periodontal Disease and Caries. (Modified from Allen, E. F.[2])

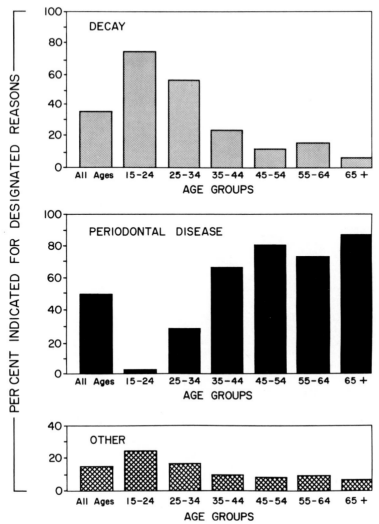

Figure 21-2 Tooth Loss Caused by Decay, Periodontal Disease and Other Causes from Ages 15 to 65. The first bar in each graph is the average for the total period. (Pelton, J. J., Pennell, E. H., and Druzina, A.[75])

separately, added together, and expressed in one figure (the P.M.A. index). The index is computed from findings in the maxillary and mandibular incisors, canines and premolars, which have been found to represent 82 to 85 per cent of the gingival inflammation in the entire mouth.[59, 62]

Gingival recession index (Stahl and Morris[101])

This index is a modification of the P.M.A. (above) in that it assesses gingival recession rather than the condition of the attached gingiva. Abnormalities of the gingival papilla (P) and gingival margin (M) in relation to each tooth are recorded, plus gingival recession (R) if the root is exposed.

The recession index expressed in percentage is obtained by dividing the number of affected teeth by the total number of teeth present and multiplying by 100. Similar determination can be made for papillary and marginal gingival disease.

Periodontal index, P.I. (Russell[82])

This method for scoring gingival and periodontal disease uses the criteria shown in Table 21-1. Since it uses the more obvious signs of disease as criteria, the prevalence and severity as expressed by the periodontal index tend to be understated in comparison with some other scoring methods.

TABLE 21–1   THE PERIODONTAL INDEX (RUSSELL)

Score	Criteria and Scoring for Field Studies	Additional X-ray Criteria Followed in the Clinical Test
0	NEGATIVE. There is neither overt inflammation in the investing tissues nor loss of function due to destruction of supporting tissues.	Radiographic appearance is essentially normal.
1	MILD GINGIVITIS. There is an overt area of inflammation in the free gingivae, but this area does not circumscribe the tooth.	
2	GINGIVITIS. Inflammation completely circumscribes the tooth, but there is no apparent break in the epithelial attachment.	
4	(Used when radiographs are available.)	There is early, notchlike resorption of the alveolar crest.
6	GINGIVITIS WITH POCKET FORMATION. The epithelial attachment has been broken and there is a pocket (not merely a deepened gingival crevice due to swelling in free gingivae). There is no interference with normal masticatory function, the tooth is firm and has not drifted.	There is horizontal bone loss involving the entire alveolar crest, up to half of the length of the tooth root.
8	ADVANCED DESTRUCTION WITH LOSS of MASTICATORY FUNCTION. The tooth may be loose; may have drifted; may sound dull on percussion with a metallic instrument; may be depressible in its socket.	There is advanced bone loss, involving more than one-half of the length of the tooth root, or a definite infrabony pocket with widening of the periodontal ligament. There may be root resorption, or rarefaction at the apex.

RULE: When in doubt, assign the lesser scores.

$$\text{Periodontal Index}° = \frac{\text{Sum of individual scores}}{\text{Number of teeth present}}$$

°The index for individuals with clinically normal gingiva is from 0 to 0.1 or 0.2; for those with a clinical diagnosis of gingivitis, from 0.1 to 1.0; for those with severe gingivitis with incipient destructive disease, from 0.5 to 1.9; for those with established destructive disease, from 1.5 to 5.0; and for those with severe terminal destructive disease, from about 4.0 to 8.0.

Gingival-bone count (Dunning and Leach[31])

This index records the gingival condition and the level of condition of the crest of the alveolar bone. The bone level is assessed by clinical examination, but radiographs are recommended for greater accuracy. The gingival-bone count is scored as shown in Table 21–2.

Periodontal disease index (Ramfjord[77])

This index is based upon examination of six teeth: the maxillary left central incisor, left first bicuspid, and right first molar; and the mandibular right central incisor, right first bicuspid and left first molar.

When no sulci extend beyond the cemento-enamel junction, the gingivitis on each tooth is graded as 0 (absent), 1, 2 or 3 (most severe). When a sulcus or pocket is present and extends up to 3 mm. apical to the cemento-enamel junction, the gingival score is disregarded and a score of 4 assigned to that particular tooth. When the pockets are 3 to 6 mm. and over 6 mm. apical to the cemento-enamel junction, the assigned scores are 5 and 6 respectively. Totaling the scores and dividing by the number of teeth examined (a maximum of 6) gives the periodontal disease index for the individual.

Periodontal disease rate

This index records the number of periodontally diseased teeth in one mouth and computes the disease rate as follows:

$$\text{Periodontal Disease Rate} = \frac{\text{Number of teeth affected by periodontal disease}}{\text{Total number of teeth}} (\times 100 \text{ for percentage})$$

TABLE 21–2 THE GINGIVAL-BONE COUNT (DUNNING AND LEACH)

Gingival score (One score is assigned to each tooth studied. A mean is then computed for the whole mouth.)
Negative... 0
Mild gingivitis involving the free gingiva (margin, papilla or both)... 1
Moderate gingivitis involving both free and attached gingivia 2
Severe gingivitis with enlargement and easy hemorrhage... 3

Bone score (One score is assigned to each tooth studied. A mean is then computed for the whole mouth.)
No bone loss 0
Incipient bone loss or notching of the alveolar crest.. 1
Bone loss approximating one fourth of root length or pocket formation one side not over one half root
   length.. 2
Bone loss approximating one half of root length or pocket formation one side not over three fourths root
   length; mobility slight° 3
Bone loss approximating three fourths of root length or pocket formation one side to apex; mobility
   moderate° 4
Bone loss complete; mobility marked° 5
Maximum possible GB count per person 8

°If mobility or impairment of masticatory function varies considerably from that to be expected with bone loss seen, the score may be altered up or down one point.

Gingival periodontal index, G.P.I. (O'Leary, Gibson, Shannon, Scheussler and Nabers[72])

The mandible and maxilla are each divided into one anterior and two posterior segments. The gingival status and periodontal status for each segment are evaluated and scored as follows:

GINGIVAL STATUS

0 = Tissue tightly adapted to the teeth, firm consistency with physiologic architecture.

1 = Slight to moderate inflammation as indicated by changes in color and consistency, involving one or more teeth in the same segment but not completely surrounding any one tooth.

2 = If the above changes singly or combined completely encircle one or more teeth in a segment.

3 = Marked inflammation as indicated by loss of surface continuity (ulceration), spontaneous hemorrhage, loss of faciolingual continuity of any interdental papilla, marked deviation from normal contour, such as gross thickening or enlargement covering more than one third of the anatomic crown, recession, and clefts.

The area with the highest score is the gingival score for the entire segment, and the *gingival status* for the mouth is obtained by dividing the total score by the number of segments.

PERIODONTAL STATUS. The periodontal status of each segment is assessed with a periodontal probe, using the cemento-enamel junction as a fixed reference. Only on teeth which have erupted to the occlusal plane, the probe is inserted at the mesial and distal line angles of proximal surfaces and in the center of facial and lingual surfaces. Periodontal status is scored as follows:

0 = If the probe does not extend apical to the cemento-enamel junction (the gingival score is used for such areas).

4 = Up to 3 mm. apical to the cemento-enamel junction.

5 = Three to 6 mm. apical to the cemento-enamel junction.

6 = Six mm. or more apical to the cemento-enamel junction.

The area with the highest score is the periodontal score for the entire segment, and the *periodontal status* for the mouth is obtained by dividing the total score by the number of segments.

IRRITATION INDEX. The teeth in each segment are dried; the facial and lingual surfaces are checked with a sickle-shaped explorer for materia alba, supra- and subgingival calculus and overhanging margins of restorations. The irritation index is scored as follows:

0 = No detectable materia alba or calculus.

1 = Slight amount of materia alba or calculus, extending not more than 2 mm. from the gingival margin.

2 = Materia alba covering up to one half of the clinical crown or gross supragingival calculus.

3 = Materia alba or supragingival calculus covering more than one half of the clinical crown, or subgingival calculus or overhanging restorations detectable by probing.

The area with the highest score is the score for the entire segment, and the *irritation index* for the mouth is obtained by dividing the total score by the number of segments.

Simplified oral hygiene index, OHI-S (Greene and Vermillion[43])

The simplified oral hygiene index is a combination of the debris index and the calculus index.

DEBRIS INDEX (DI-S). The following six teeth are scored: the facial surface of the first fully erupted molar in the right and left maxilla; the facial surface of the maxillary right central incisor and the mandibular left central incisor; and the lingual surface of the first fully erupted molar on the right and left sides of the mandible. Debris is scored from 0 to 3, using the criteria shown in Figure 21–3. The amount of debris is determined by scraping a No. 23 explorer across the tooth surface. The *debris index* is

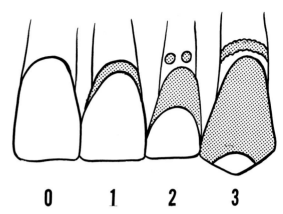

Figure 21–4 Criteria for Scoring Calculus.
0 – No calculus present.
1 – Supragingival calculus covering not more than one-third of the exposed tooth surface.
2 – Supragingival calculus covering more than one-third but not more than two-thirds of the exposed tooth surface or the presence of individual flecks of subgingival calculus around the cervical portion of the tooth or both.
3 – Supragingival calculus covering more than two-thirds of the exposed tooth surface or a continuous heavy band of subgingival calculus around the cervical portion of tooth or both.

obtained by totaling the scores and dividing by six.

CALCULUS INDEX (CI-S). Calculus is scored on the same six tooth surfaces, using the criteria indicated in Figure 21–4. The extent of calculus is determined visually and by probing with an explorer. The scores are totaled and divided by six to obtain the *calculus index.*

Plaque index, P.I. (Quigley and Hein[76])

This is a method for assessing disclosed plaque (by using a dye-containing rinse or wafer). A score of 0 to 5 is assigned to each facial and lingual nonrestored surface of all teeth except third molars, as follows:

0 = No plaque.

1 = Separate flecks of plaque at the cervical margin of the tooth.

2 = A thin continuous band of plaque (up to 1 mm.) at the cervical margin of the tooth.

3 = A band of plaque wider than 1 mm. but covering less than one third of the crown of the tooth.

4 = Plaque covering at least one third but

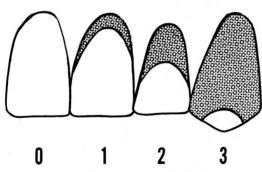

Figure 21–3 Criteria for Scoring Oral Debris.
0 – No debris or stain present.
1 – Soft debris covering not more than one-third of the tooth surface, or the presence of extrinsic stains without other debris regardless of surface area covered.
2 – Soft debris covering more than one-third but not more than two-thirds, of the exposed tooth surface.
3 – Soft debris covering more than two-thirds of the exposed tooth surface.

less than two thirds of the crown of the tooth.

5 = Plaque covering two thirds or more of the crown of the tooth.

The *plaque index* for the entire mouth is determined by dividing the total score by the number of examined surfaces.

Gingival index, G.I.
(Löe and Silness[57])

This is a system for assessing the quality, severity and location (quantity) of gingival disease. The circumference of the gingival margin is divided into four areas (buccal, lingual, mesial and distal). Each of the four areas is scored from 0 to 3, according to the following criteria:

0 = Normal gingiva.

1 = Mild inflammation, slight change in color, slight edema; no bleeding on probing.

2 = Moderate inflammation; redness edema and glazing; bleeding on probing.

3 = Severe inflammation; marked redness and edema; ulceration; tendency to spontaneous bleeding.

The scores around each tooth are totaled and divided by four to determine the gingival index for the tooth. Totaling all the indices and dividing by the number of teeth in the mouth provides the gingival index for the individual. The gingival index may be obtained for a segment of the mouth or group of teeth in the same way.

Plaque index, P.I.
(Silness and Löe[57])

This index is obtained in the same way as the gingival index above, except that it records plaque instead of the condition of the gingiva, using the following criteria:

0 = No plaque in the gingival area.

1 = A film adhering to the free gingival margin and adjacent area of the tooth. The plaque may only be recognized by running a probe across the tooth surface.

2 = Moderate accumulation of soft deposits within the gingival pocket on the gingival margin and/or adjacent tooth surface which can be seen by the naked eye.

3 = Abundance of soft matter within the gingival pocket and/or on the gingival margin and adjacent tooth surface.

Retention index
(Bjorby and Löe[57])

This index was created for the assessment of retentive factors on the tooth surface adjacent to the gingival margin. It follows the same principles as the gingival index and the plaque index above, except that it uses the following criteria:

0 = No caries, no calculus, no imperfect margin of dental restoration in a gingival location.

1 = Supragingival cavity, calculus or imperfect margin of dental restoration.

2 = Subgingival cavity, calculus or imperfect margin of dental restoration.

3 = Large cavity, abundance of calculus or grossly insufficient marginal fit of dental restoration in a supra- and/or subgingival location.

Calculus surface index
(Ennever, Sturzenberger
and Radike[36])

This index is used for short-term studies of calculus accumulation. The four mandibular incisors are graded for presence (1) or absence (0) of calculus on each of four surfaces (lingual, facial, mesial, and distal). The total number of surfaces with calculus is the index. (The maximum possible score is 16.)

Calculus index (Volpe,
Manhold and Hazen[106])

The height of calculus on the lingual surface of the six mandibular anteriors is measured with a probe. Three measurements in millimeters are made on each tooth surface (two diagonal and one perpendicular); each measurement is scored from 0 to 3, making 9 the maximum possible for each tooth. The calculus index is the total score for the six teeth.

PREVALENCE OF GINGIVITIS

Most surveys of gingivitis have been conducted in children, adolescents and young adults because in older persons gingival inflammation has usually advanced to periodontitis and is not recorded separately as gingivitis. Surveys of the prevalence and severity of gingivitis vary with the populations studied and are summarized in Table 21–3.

TABLE 21–3 PREVALENCE OF GINGIVITIS IN CHILDREN AND YOUNG ADULTS

Investigators	Year	Group Studied	No. Children in Group	Age Group	Percentage of Persons Affected with Gingivitis
Ainsworth and Young	1925	School children in England and Wales	4063	2–14 yrs.	40
McCall	1933	New York	4600	1–14 yrs.	98
Messner et al.	1938	Children in twenty-six states of U.S.	1,438,318	6–14 yrs.	3.5–8.6
Marshall-Day and Tandan	1940	Middle class children in Lahore, India	756	approx. 13 yrs.	68
Marshall-Day	1940	Fluoride endemic area in Northern India	203	5–18 yrs.	59.6
King	1940	Isle of Lewis	2280	6–15 yrs.	90
Campbell and Cook	1942	Dundee Hospital in Scotland	1924		2.2
Marshall-Day	1944	Boys in Kangra district of India (poor nutrition)	200	approx. 13 yrs.	81
Marshall-Day and Shourie	1944	Low-middle class school children	613	5–15 yrs.	80
King, Franklyn and Allen	1944	English boys	403	11–14 yrs. Group A Group B	77.4 87.6
	1944	Gibraltar evacuees in England	135	10–14 yrs.	85.2
King	1945	Primary school children in Dundee, Scotland	103	12–14 yrs.	90
	1945	Harpenden Institution, England	170	11–14 yrs.	Groups vary 56.4–97.5
Marshall-Day and Shourie	1947	Low to middle class male school children in Lahore, India	1054	9–17 yrs.	99.4
Marshall-Day and Shourie	1947	Girls of high socio-economic level at Lahore, India	179	9–17 yrs.	73.7
Schour and Massler	1947	Four communities in Italy suffering from malnutrition	682 721	6–10 yrs. 11–20 yrs.	40.3 55.3
Marshall-Day et al.	1948	Puerto Rico	1648	6–18 yrs.	60–79
Massler, Schour, and Chopra	1950	Suburban Chicago school children	804	5–14 yrs.	64.3
Marshall-Day and Shourie	1950	Virgin Island (91% Negro population)	823 860	6–18 yrs. 5–13 yrs.	57.0 26.9
Stahl and Goldman	1953	School children in Massachusetts	1300	13–17 yrs.	29.0
Russell	1957	Urban United States	White 6682 15,922 4031	5–9 yrs. 10–14 yrs. 15–19 yrs.	10.8 25.5 37.3
			Negro 37 494	5–9 yrs. 10–19 yrs.	8.1 28.7
Greene	1960	School boys in low socio-economic area of India	1613	11–17 yrs.	96.9
		School boys in low socio-economic area of Atlanta, Georgia	577	11–17 yrs.	92.0
Zimmerman and Baker	1960	White children from Maryland	529	6–12 yrs.	35
		Negro children from Texas	442	6–12 yrs.	67
		White children from Texas	435	6–12 yrs.	79
Jamison	1963	Tecumseh, Michigan (deciduous teeth only)	159	5–14 yrs.	99.4
McHugh et al.	1964	Dundee, Scotland, boys and girls	2905	13 yrs.	99.4
Dutta	1965	Calcutta, India, boys and girls	1424	6–12 yrs.	89.8
Wade	1966	Iraq	200	13–15 yrs.	97.0
		London	222	13–15 yrs.	
Sheiham	1968	Nigeria	1620	10 yrs. and older	99+
Sheiham	1969	Surrey	756	11–17 yrs.	99.7
Murray	1969	West Hartlepool, 1.5–2.0 ppm. fluoride			
		Boys	211	15 yrs.	94.8
		Girls	175	15 yrs.	86.3
		York, 0.2 ppm. fluoride			
		Boys	202	15 yrs.	95.5
		Girls	179	15 yrs.	85.5

The prevalence and severity of gingivitis in children and young adults appear to follow a pattern. Gingivitis does not ordinarily occur until the age of four or five (McCall[63]). By the age of 14 nearly all children show some involvement.

Both the prevalence and severity increase with age (Ainsworth and Young[1]), with a sharp rise at seven to eight years associated with the eruption of permanent teeth (Fig. 21–5) (Massler, Schour and Chopra[62]). This rise is continued until the maximum is reached at puberty, which occurs earlier in girls. Following puberty there is a slight decline in the prevalence of gingivitis, and a sharp decline in the severity (Parfitt[74]). The prevalence begins to rise again in young adults and continues until, by age 26, 80 to 90 per cent of persons are affected.[28, 58] A prevalence of 100 per cent has been reported in male groups aged 17 to 22.[8, 56]

The reported prevalence of gingivitis in children ranges from highs of 98 (McCall[63]) and 92 per cent in the United States, 97 (Greene[42]), and 99.4 per cent (Marshall-Day[25]) in India, and 99+ per cent (Sheiham[97]) in Nigeria, to lows of 3.5 to 8.6 per cent in the United States (Messner et al.[67]) and 2.2 per cent in Scotland (Campbell and Cook[16]).

PREVALENCE OF PERIODONTAL DISEASE

Periodontal disease is generally considered a disease of adults;[73] however, it has been reported at earlier ages, as follows: 9 per cent of children in the 11 to 15 age group;[69] and 4 per cent between the ages of 13 and 15.[28]

The prevalence and severity of periodontal disease increase with age.[33, 44] The periodontal index (Russell) rises from a mean of 0.02 at ages five to nine, to 2.35 at ages over 60, with periodontal pockets present in 0.09 per cent in the former age group and 53.2 per cent in the latter.[86] The incidence in the 19 to 25 year age group is from 10 to 29 per cent.[28, 39, 90] *By age 45, 97 to 100 per cent have periodontal disease.*[11, 28, 69] Lesser figures set the prevalence of periodontal disease at 75 per cent in white persons and 90 per cent in Negroes at age 60.[86] The increasing severity of periodontal disease with age is reflected by the observations from metropolitan areas in the United States that one fourth of alveolar bone support was lost by ages 46 to 48 years and one third by age 60[20] (Fig. 21–6). Clinically demonstrable suppuration occurred in 40 per cent of individuals at age

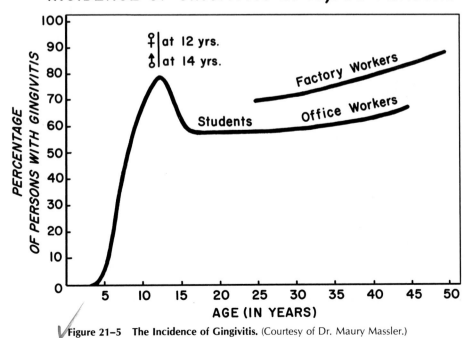

Figure 21–5 The Incidence of Gingivitis. (Courtesy of Dr. Maury Massler.)

AVERAGE ALVEOLAR BONE RESORPTION

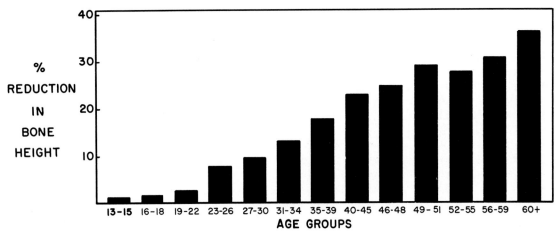

Figure 21–6   Increase in Alveolar Bone Resorption with Age. (Marshall-Day, C. D.[23])

40, and in approximately 50 per cent in older persons; abnormal tooth mobility increased from 25 per cent between the ages of 35 and 39, to 79 per cent at age 60.[28]

FACTORS AFFECTING THE PREVALENCE AND SEVERITY OF GINGIVITIS AND PERIODONTAL DISEASE

AGE. The prevalence and severity of gingival and periodontal disease increase with age and also appear to be related to other factors, as follows:

ORAL HYGIENE. **Poor oral hygiene, because it leads to the accumulation of** *plaque, materia alba* **and** *calculus,* **is the most important factor which affects the prevalence and severity of gingival and periodontal disease.**[83, 90] Other etiologic factors may be significant, but so far as can be determined by existing epidemiologic methods, their influence is obscured by an overwhelming effect of poor oral hygiene.

SEX. The sex difference in the incidence of gingivitis and periodontal disease is not striking. Up to the age of 14, girls seem to be affected more than boys[62, 74] (approximately 90 per cent in girls and 88.4 per cent in boys in primary school, and 97.5 per cent in girls and 92.5 per cent in boys in the 12 to 14 year group[53]). Beyond the age of 14, the incidence is slightly greater in males.[59]

The prevalence and severity of periodontal disease and the prevalence of periodontal pockets tend to be greater in males than females at almost all ages[49] (Table 21–4). Yet to be determined is whether the difference is sex-linked or the result of difference in oral hygiene habits or other factors.

RACE. Comparisons of the prevalence and severity of gingivitis in Negro and Caucasian children give varied results from which firm conclusions cannot be drawn.[14, 61, 86, 102, 111]

Periodontal disease tends to be more prevalent and more severe in Negroes than in Caucasians at all age levels.[86] At the ages of 20 to 29, the periodontal index (Russell) in Negroes is 0.48 and periodontal pockets are present in 13.6 per cent. In Caucasians at the same age the index is 0.44, with pockets in 8.1 per cent. Beyond the age of 60 years the periodontal index for Negroes is 3.67, with pockets present in 77.7 per cent; the findings in Caucasians are 2.34 and 53.2 per cent.

OCCUPATION. Gingival inflammation appears to be less frequent and less severe in occupations which require greater skills and more educational background.[89] The incidence of gingivitis is lower in office personnel than in factory workers.[5, 60]

EDUCATION. In children with superior intelligence quotients,[111] and adults with a higher educational background the prevalence and severity of gingival and periodontal disease are less and the oral hygiene better regardless of race.[46, 81, 89]

PROFESSIONAL DENTAL CARE. The incidence and severity of periodontal disorders are lower in individuals under regular dental care.[89, 108] The prevalence and severity of disease increase with neglect.

GEOGRAPHIC LOCATION. In the United States, there are regional differences in the incidence and severity of gingival and periodontal disease. Factors other than oral hygiene that may account for such differences have not been investigated. Gingivitis is more prevalent in rural areas than in urban areas.[12] It is higher in Texas[111] and Chicago[61] than in Maryland and Philadelphia, respectively.

The prevalence of periodontal disease is similar in cities such as New York, Chicago and Baltimore, but higher in Birmingham. Below the age of 35 the incidence of periodontal disease is higher in Canada than in Boston.[87]

Gingival disease and periodontal disease are global problems, and their prevalence and severity in most parts of the world thus far surveyed are greater than in the United States (Table 21–5).[9, 83, 88] Comparisons made between similar oral hygiene groups indicated that boys (11 to 17 years of age) in India had significantly higher periodontal scores than those in the state of Georgia.[42] In India[45, 78] and Singapore[64] periodontal disease with bone loss occurs in children[27] and is almost universal after the age of 16.

In Norway periodontal bone loss appears to be of the same order as in Boston, Massachusetts.[87]

SOCIAL CUSTOMS AND NUTRITION. Social customs and group habits such as food selection and methods of preparation, use of tobacco,[4, 5, 103] and betel nut chewing[7] influence the prevalence and severity of periodontal disease.[18] Surveys in various parts of the world demonstrate no relationship between population nutritional status and periodontal disease except for a tendency toward increased prevalence and severity in areas of vitamin A deficiency and protein malnutrition.[85]

FLUORIDE. Some investigators claim that the concentration of fluoride in drinking water does not affect the prevalence and severity of gingivitis in children,[35, 47, 70, 71] whereas others report that periodontal disease is less severe in fluoride areas,[34] and that the prevalence of gingival disorders in children using 1.0 to 1.2 ppm. fluoride in the water is less than in those using 0.1 ppm.[6, 84]

DISTRIBUTION OF GINGIVITIS AND PERIODONTAL DISEASE IN DIFFERENT AREAS OF THE ORAL CAVITY

The oral regions most commonly affected with gingival disease are, in descending

TABLE 21–4 PERIODONTAL STATUS OF ADULTS, BY AGE AND SEX, UNITED STATES, 1960–62*

Age in Years	Average PI†	Per Cent With Periodontal Pockets	Average OHI-S‡
Men			
18–24	0.62	10	1.5
25–34	0.92	22	1.6
35–44	1.27	30	1.7
45–54	1.62	37	1.9
55–64	2.15	46	2.1
65–74	2.50	58	2.5
75–79	2.91	60	2.2
Women			
18–24	0.48	10	1.2
25–34	0.60	12	1.2
35–44	0.82	21	1.2
45–54	1.23	30	1.5
55–64	1.56	36	1.6
65–74	1.62	33	1.6
75–79	2.94	54	1.9

*From Johnson, E. S., Kelly, J. E., and Van Kirk, L. E.[49]
†Periodontal index (Russell[82]).
‡Simplified oral hygiene index (Greene and Vermillion[43]).

TABLE 21–5 AVERAGE PERIODONTAL INDEX IN CIVILIANS (BOTH SEXES), AGED 40–49 YEARS, SURVEYED BY EXAMINERS OF THE NATIONAL INSTITUTE OF DENTAL RESEARCH, UNITED STATES*

Population Group	Average Periodontal Index
Baltimore, Maryland (white)	1.03
Colorado Springs, Colorado	1.04†
Alaska; primitive Eskimos	1.17‡
Ecuador	1.85
Ethiopia	1.86
Baltimore, Maryland (Negro)	1.99
Uganda[99]	2.50§
Vietnam; Vietnamese	2.18
Colombia	2.21
Alaska; urban Eskimos	2.31‡
Chile	2.74
Lebanon; Lebanese	2.98
Thailand	3.30
Lebanon; Palestinian refugees	3.52
Burma	3.58
Jordan; Jordanian civilians	3.96
Vietnam; Hill Tribesmen	3.97
Trinidad	4.21
Jordan; Palestinian refugees	4.41

*Modified from Russell, A. L.[83]
†Ages 40–44 only.
‡Males only.
§Age over 40.

order of frequency, the facial surfaces of the maxillary anterior, mandibular anterior, maxillary molar and premolar and mandibular molar and premolar areas; and the lingual surfaces of the maxilla and the mandible. In older persons the lingual surface in the mandible is involved more frequently than that in the maxilla.[20]

The severity of bone loss is greater interproximally than facially and lingually. The incisor and molar areas are more severely involved than the canine and premolar areas,[27, 37, 69, 90, 104] with least bone loss in the mandibular canine and premolar region. Bone loss in the maxilla is generally more severe than in the mandible,[10] except for the anterior region, in which the situation is reversed.[27, 108] The sequence of tooth eruption, the position of teeth in the arch, growth changes, the age at which periodontal disease begins, the distribution of local irritants, occlusal factors, as well as factors not yet completely understood, all influence the location and severity of bone loss in periodontal disease.

THE RELATIONSHIP BETWEEN PERIODONTAL DISEASE AND CARIES

Numerous investigations have attempted to determine a relationship between the occurrence of periodontal disease and caries.[17, 41, 51, 55] Some consider them antagonistic processes with the presence of one precluding the occurrence of the other.[15, 41, 51] Statistical studies suggest a positive correlation between caries and gingival disease,[13, 96] but this has not been substantiated.[21, 53, 108]

A clear-cut positive or negative relationship between the occurrence of periodontal disease and caries has not been established; they should be considered as independent processes.[68] However, it should be noted that there are individuals who are relatively caries-free and predisposed to periodontal disease and others who are comparatively immune to periodontal destruction and susceptible to caries. The mandibular anterior region, which is least susceptible to caries, is an area most severely affected by periodontal disease. On the other hand, carious areas predispose to the accumulation of local irritants and food impaction, which in turn lead to gingivitis.

REFERENCES

1. Ainsworth, N. J., and Young, M.: The Incidence of Dental Disease in Children. Med. Res. Council, Special Report Series No. 97. London, His Majesty's Stationery Office, 1925.
2. Allen, E. F.: Statistical Study of the Primary Causes of Extraction. J. D. Res., 23:453, 1944.
3. Andrews, G., and Krogh, H. W.: Permanent Tooth Mortality. D. Progress, 1:130, 1961.
4. Arno, A., Schei, O., Lovdal, A., and Waerhaug, J.: Alveolar Bone Loss as a Function of Tobacco Consumption. Acta Odont. Scandinav., 17:3, 1959.
5. Arno, A., Waerhaug, J., Lovdal, A., and Schei, O.: Incidence of Gingivitis as Related to Sex, Occupation, Tobacco Consumption, Toothbrushing and Age. Oral Surg., Oral Med. & Oral Path., 11:587, 1958.
6. Ast, D. B., and Schlesinger, E. R.: The Conclusion of a Ten-Year Study of Fluoridation. Am. J. Pub. Health, 46:265, 1956.
7. Balendra, W.: The Effect of Betel Chewing on the Dental and Oral Tissues and Its Possible Relationship to Buccal Carcinoma. Brit. D. J., 87:83, 1949.
8. Barnard, P. D., and Bradley, D. I.: Dental Conditions of Senior Dental Students. Australian D. J., 11:338, 1966.

9. Barros, L., and Witkop, C. S. J.: Oral and Genetic Study of Chileans—1960—III. Periodontal Disease and Nutritional Factors. Arch. Oral Biol., 8:195, 1963.

10. Beagrie, G. S., and James, G. A.: The Association of Posterior Tooth Irregularity and Periodontal Disease. Brit. D. J., 113:239, 1962.

11. Belting, C. M., Massler, M., and Schour, I.: Prevalence and Incidence of Alveolar Bone Disease in Men. J.A.D.A., 47:190, 1953.

12. Benjamin, E. M., Russell, A. L., and Smiley, R. D.: Periodontal Disease in Rural Children of 25 Indian Countries. J. Periodont., 28:294, 1957.

13. Black, G. V.: Something of the Etiology and Early Pathology of the Diseases of the Periodontal Membrane with Suggestions as to Treatment. D. Cosmos, 55:1219, 1913.

14. Bolden, T. E.: Gingivitis in Negro School Children. Quarterly Nat. D. A., 21:129, 1963.

15. Broderick, F. W.: Antagonism Between Dental Caries and Pyorrhea. Am. D. Surg., 49:103, 1929.

16. Campbell, H. G., and Cook, R. P.: Incidence of Gingivitis at Dundee Dental Hospital. Year Book of Dentistry. Chicago, Year Book Publishers, 1942.

17. Citron, J.: About the Question of the Internal Etiology of Paradentosis. Zahnärztl. Rdsch., 37:1319, 1928.

18. Davies, G. N.: Social Customs and Habits and Their Effect on Oral Disease, J. D. Res., 42:209, 1963.

19. Day, C. D. Marshall-: Chronic Endemic Fluorosis in Northern India. Brit. D. J., 68:409, 1940.

20. Day, C. D. Marshall-: The Epidemiology of Periodontal Disease. J. Periodont., 22:13, 1951.

21. Day, C. D. Marshall-: Nutritional Deficiencies and Dental Caries in Northern India. Brit. D. J., 76:115, 143, 1944.

22. Day, C. D. Marshall-: Oral Conditions in the Famine District of Hissar. J.A.D.A., 31:52, 1944.

23. Day, C. D. Marshall-: Periodontal Disease: Present Status and Interpretation of Epidemiological Research. In Muhler, J. C., and Hine, M. K.: A Symposium on Preventive Dentistry. St. Louis, C. V. Mosby Co., 1956, p. 174.

24. Day, C. D. Marshall-, and Shourie, K. L.: Gingival Disease in the Virgin Islands. J.A.D.A., 40:175, 1950.

25. Day, C. D. Marshall-, and Shourie, K. L.: Hypertrophic Gingivitis in Indian Children and Adolescents. Ind. J. Med. Res., 35(4):261, 1947.

26. Day, C. D. Marshall-, and Shourie, K. L.: The Incidence of Periodontal Disease in the Punjab. Ind. J. Med. Res., 32:47, 1944.

27. Day, C. D. Marshall-, and Shourie, K. L.: A Roentgenographic Study of Periodontal Disease in India. J.A.D.A., 39:572, 1949.

28. Day, C. D. Marshall-, Stephens, R. G., and Quigley, L. F.: Periodontal Disease: Prevalence and Incidence. J. Periodont, 26:185, 1955.

29. Day, C. D. Marshall-, and Tandan, G. C.: The Incidence of Dental Caries in the Punjab. Brit. D. J., 69:389, 1940.

30. Dummett, C. O.: The Relation of Periodontal Disease to Public Health. J.A.D.A., 54:49, 1957.

31. Dunning, J. M., and Leach, L. B.: Gingival-Bone Count: A Method for Epidemiological Study of Periodontal Disease. J. D. Res., 39:506, 1960.

32. Dutta, A.: A Study on Prevalence of Periodontal Disease and Dental Caries Amongst the School-going Children in Calcutta. J. All Ind. D. Assn., 37:367, 1965.

33. Emslie, R. D.: A Dental Health Survey in the Republic of the Sudan. Brit. D. J., 120:167, 1966.

34. Englander, H. R., Kesel, R. G., and Gupta, O. P.: Comparison of Periodontal Health of Adult Lifetime Residents of Fluoride and Fluoride Deficient Cities (Abst). I.A.D.R., 40:33, 1962.

35. Englander, H. R., and White, C. L.: Periodontal and Oral Hygiene Status of Teenagers in Optimum and Fluoride-Deficient Cities. J.A.D.A., 68:173, 1964.

36. Ennever, J., Sturzenberger, C. P., and Radike, A. W.: Calculus Surface Index for Scoring Clinical Calculus Studies. J. Periodont., 32:54, 1961.

37. Fleming, W. C.: Localization of Pyorrhea Involvement. D. Cosmos, 54:538, 1926.

38. Galagan, D. J.: Dental Health and the Need for Prevention. Proceedings, Symposium—Applied Preventive Dentistry, Washington, D.C. Columbia, Mo., the Curators, University of Missouri, 1965, p. 1.

39. Goldhush, A.: Oral Aspects of Aviation Medicine. In Burket, L.: Oral Medicine. Philadelphia, J. B. Lippincott Co., 1946.

40. Goldman, H. M.: Prevalence of Parodontal (Periodontal) Disease. 4. In the United States. Internat. D. J., 5:458, 1955.

41. Gottlieb, B.: Zur Atiologie und Therapie der Alveolarpyorrhoe. Zeitschr. f. Stomatol., 18:59, 1920.

42. Greene, J. C.: Periodontal Disease in India: Report of an Epidemiological Study. J. D. Res., 39:302, 1960.

43. Greene, J. C., and Vermillion, J. R.: Oral Hygiene Index: A Method for Classifying Oral Hygiene Status, J.A.D.A., 61:172, 1960.

44. Grewe, J. M., Gorlin, R. J., and Meskin, L. H.: Human Tooth Mortality: A Clinical-Statistical Study. J.A.D.A., 72:106, 1966.

45. Gupta, O. P.: Epidemiological Studies of Dental Diseases in the State of Kerala. I. Prevalence and Severity of Periodontal Disease. J. All Ind. D. Assn., 35:45, 1962.

46. Horton, J. E., and Sumnicht, R. W.: Relationships of Educational Levels to Periodontal Disease and Oral Hygiene with Variables of Age and Geographic Regions. J. Periodont., 38:335, 1967.

47. James, P. M. C., et al.: Gingival Health and Dental Cleanliness in English School Children. Arch. Oral Biol., 3:57, 1960.

48. Jamison, H. C.: Prevalence of Periodontal Disease of the Deciduous Teeth. J.A.D.A., 66:207, 1963.

49. Johnson, E. S., Kelly, J. E., and VanKirk, L. E.: Selected Dental Findings in Adults by Age, Race and Sex, United States 1960–1962. Washington, D.C., U.S. Department of Health, Education and Welfare, National Center for Health Statistics, Series 11, No. 7, 1965.

50. Kelly, J. E., and VanKirk, L. E.: U.S. Department of Health, Education and Welfare: Periodontal Disease in Adults. Publication No. 1000, Series 11, No. 12, 1966.

51. Kesel, R. G.: Are Dental Caries and Periodontal Disease Incompatible? J. Periodont., 21:30, 1950.

52. King, J. D.: Dental Disease in the Isle of Lewis. Medical Research Council, Special Report Series, No. 241. London, His Majesty's Stationery Office, 1940.

53. King, J. D.: Gingival Disease in Dundee. D. Record, 65:9, 32, 55, 1945.

54. King, J. D., Franklyn, A. B., and Allen, I.: Gingival Disease in Gibraltar Evacuee Children. Lancet, 1:495, 1944.

55. Landgraph, E., Banhigyi, S.: Untersuchungen über den Cholesterin-, Bilirubin- und Reservealkaligehalte des Blutes bei Paradentosekranken. Zeitschr. f. Stomatol., 29:11, 1931.

56. Lightner, L. M., et al.: The Periodontal Status of Incoming Air Force Academy Cadets. J.A.D.A., 75:111, 1967.

57. Löe, H.: The Gingival Index, the Plaque Index and the Retention Index Systems. J. Periodont., 38:610, 1967.

58. Lovdal, A., Arno, A., and Waerhaug, J.: Incidence of Clinical Manifestations of Periodontal Disease in Light of Oral Hygiene and Calculus Formation. J.A.D.A., 56:21, 1958.

59. Massler, M., and Savara, B. S.: Relation of Gingivitis to Dental Caries and Malocclusion in Children 14 to 17 Years of Age. J. Periodont., 22:87, 1951.

60. Massler, M., and Schour, I.: The P-M-A Index of Gingivitis. J. D. Res., 28:634, 1949 (Abstract).

61. Massler, M., Cohen, A., and Schour, I.: Epidemiology of Gingivitis in Children. J.A.D.A., 45:319, 1952.

62. Massler, M., Schour, I., and Chopra, B.: Occurrence of Gingivitis in Suburban Chicago School Children. J. Periodont., 21:146, 1950.

63. McCall, J. O.: The Periodontist Looks at Children's Dentistry. J.A.D.A., 20:1518, 1933.

64. McCombie, F., and Chua, S. C.: Dental Epidemiology in Malaya. Part II, A Survey of Chinese, Malay and Indian Young Adult Males in Singapore. J. Canad. D. Assn., 23:687, 1957.

65. McHugh, W. D., McEven, J. D., and Hitchin, A. D.: Dental Disease and Related Factors in 13-Year Old Children in Dundee. Brit. D. J., 117: 246, 1964.

66. Mehta, F. S., Sanjana, M. K., Shroff, B. C., and Doctor, R. H.: Relative Importance of the Various Causes of Tooth Loss. J. All Ind. D. Assn., 30: 211, 1958.

67. Messner, C. T., Gafaver, W. M., Cady, F. C., and Dean, H. T.: Dental Survey of School Children Ages 6 to 14 Years Made in 1933–1934 in 26 States. Public Health Bulletin 226. Washington, D.C., U.S. Printing Office, 1938.

68. Miller, S. C., and Seidler, B. B.: A Correlation between Periodontal Disease and Caries. J. D. Res., 19:549, 1940.

69. Miller, S. C., and Seidler, B. B.: Relative Alveoloclastic Experience of the Various Teeth. J. D. Res., 21:365, 1942.

70. Moore, R. M., Muhler, J. C., and McDonald, R. E.: A Study of the Effect of Water Fluoride Content and Socio-Economic Status on the Occurrence of Gingivitis in School Children. J. D. Res., 43:782, 1964.

71. Murray, J. J.: Gingivitis in 15-Year Old Children from High Fluoride and Low Fluoride Areas. Arch. Oral Biol., 14:951, 1969.

72. O'Leary, T., Gibson, W. A., Shannon, I. L., Schuessler, C. F., and Nabers, C. L.: A Screening Examination for Detection of Gingival and Periodontal Breakdown and Local Irritants. Periodontics, 1:167, 1963.

73. O'Rourke, J. T.: An Analysis of the Personnel Resources of the Dental Profession. J.A.D.A., 30:997, 1943.

74. Parfitt, G. J.: A Five Year Longitudinal Study of the Gingival Condition of a Group of Children in England. J. Periodont., 28:26, 1957.

75. Pelton, W. J., Pennell, E. H., and Druzina, A.: Tooth Morbidity Experience of Adults. J.A.D.A., 49:439, 1954.

76. Quigley, G. A., and Hein, J. W.: Comparative Cleansing Efficiency of Manual and Power Brushing. J.A.D.A., 65:26, 1962.

77. Ramfjord, S. P.: Indices for Prevalence and Incidence of Periodontal Disease. J. Periodont., 30:51, 1959.

78. Ramfjord, S. P.: The Periodontal Status of Boys 11 to 17 Years Old in Bombay, India. J. Periodont., 32:237, 1961.

79. Resolution of the American Public Health Association. J.A.D.A., 50:232, 1955.

80. Ruffer, M. A.: Studies in the Palaeopathology of Ancient Egypt. Chicago, University of Chicago Press, 1921.

81. Russell, A. L.: A Social Factor Associated with the Severity of Periodontal Disease. J. D. Res., 36: 922, 1957.

82. Russell, A. L.: A System of Classification and Scoring for Prevalence Surveys of Periodontal Disease. J. D. Res., 35:350, 1956.

83. Russell, A. L.: Epidemiology of Periodontal Disease. Internat. D. J., 17:282, 1967.

84. Russell, A. L.: Fluoride, Domestic Water and Periodontal Disease. Am. J. Pub. Health, 47:688, 1957.

85. Russell, A. L.: International Nutrition Surveys: A Summary of Preliminary Dental Findings. J. D. Res., 42:233, 1963.

86. Russell, A. L.: Some Epidemiological Characteristics of Periodontal Disease in a Series of Urban Populations. J. Periodont., 28:286, 1957.

87. Russell, A. L.: The Geographical Distribution and Epidemiology of Periodontal Disease. World Health Organization Expert Committee on Dental Health (Periodontal Disease). WHO/DH/ 34. Geneva, 1960.

88. Russell, A. L.: World Epidemiology and Oral Health. In Kreshover, S. J., and McClure, F. J. (eds.): Environmental Variables in Oral Disease. Washington, D.C., American Association for the Advancement of Science, 1966, pp. 21–39.

89. Russell, A. L., and Ayers, P.: Periodontal Disease and Socio-Economic Status in Birmingham, Ala. Am. J. Pub. Health, 50:206, 1960.

90. Schei, O., Waerhaug, J., Lovdal, A., and Arno, A.: Alveolar Bone Loss as Related to Oral Hygiene and Age. J. Periodont., 30:7, 1959.

91. Scherp, H. W.: Current Concepts in Periodontal Disease Research: Epidemiological Contributions. J.A.D.A., 68:667, 1964.

92. Schour, I., and Massler, M.: Gingival Disease in Postwar Italy (1945). I. Prevalence of Gingivitis in Various Age Groups. J.A.D.A., 35:475, 1947.

93. Schour, I., and Massler, M.: Survey of Gingival Disease Using the PMA Index. J. D. Res., 27: 733, 1948.

94. Schroeder, Von, H. E., and Muhlemann, J. R.: Indexmethode und Epidemiologie der Parodontalen Erkrankungen. Schweiz. Mschr. Zahnheilk., 74:7, 1964.

95. Selected Dental Findings in Adults by Age, Race and Sex, United States, 1962, by National Center for Health Statistics, U.S.P.H.S., U.S. Department of Health, Education and Welfare. Washington, D.C., U.S. Government Printing Office, 1965, Series 11, No. 7.

96. Shay, H., and Smart, G. A.: The Association of Local Factors with Gingivitis. Brit. D. J., 78:135, 1945.

97. Sheiham, A.: The Epidemiology of Chronic Periodontal Disease in Western Nigerian Children. J. Periodont. Res., 3:257, 1968.

98. Sheiham, A.: The Prevalence and Severity of Periodontal Disease in Surrey School Children. D. Practit., 19:232, 1969.

99. Skougard, M. R., Pindborg, J. J., and Roed-Petersen, B.: Periodontal Conditions in 1934 Ugandans. Arch. Oral Biol., 14:707, 1969.

100. Stahl, D. G., and Goldman, H. M.: Incidence of Gingivitis Among a Sample of Massachusetts School Children. Oral Surg., Oral Med. & Oral Path., 6:707, 1953.

101. Stahl, S. S., and Morris, A. L.: Oral Health Conditions Among Army Personnel at the Army Engineering Center. J. Periodont., 26:180, 1955.

102. Sterling, E. B.: Health Studies of Negro Children. U. S. Pub. Health Rep., 43:2713, 1928.

103. Summers, C., and Oberman, A.: Association of Oral Disease with Twelve Selected Variables: I. Periodontal Disease. J. D. Res., 47:457, 1968.

104. Tenenbaum, B., Karshan, M., Ziskin, D., and Nahoun, K. I.: Clinical and Microscopic Study of the Gingivae in Periodontosis. J.A.D.A., 40: 302, 1950.

105. Trott, J. R., and Cross, H. G.: An Analysis of the Principal Reasons for Tooth Extractions in 1813 Patients in Manitoba. D. Practit., 17:20, 1966.

106. Volpe, A. R., Manhold, J. H., and Hazen, S. P.: In Vivo Calculus Assessment: A Method and Its Reproducibility. J. Periodont., 36:292, 1965.

107. Wade, A. B.: Validity of Anterior Segment Gingival Scores in Epidemiologic Studies. J. Periodont., 37:55, 1966.

108. White, C. L., and Russell, A. L.: Some Relations Between Dental Caries Experience and Active Periodontal Disease in Two Thousand Adults. New York J. Den., 32:211, 1962.

109. Wilkinson, F. C., Adamson, K. T., and Knight, F.: A Study of the Incidence of Dental Disease in the Aborigines, From the Examination of 65 in the Collection Found in the Melbourne University. Australian J. Den., 33:109, 1929.

110. World Health Organization: Technical Report Series, No. 207, 1961, p. 3.

111. Zimmerman, E. R., and Baker, W. A.: Effect of Geographic Location and Race on Gingival Disease in Children. J.A.D.A., 61:542, 1960.

Part III • The Etiology of Gingival and Periodontal Disease

The etiology of gingival and periodontal disease is customarily classified into local and systemic factors, but their effects are interrelated. *Local factors* are those in the immediate environment of the periodontium, and *systemic factors* result from the general condition of the patient. **Most gingival and periodontal disease is caused by local factors, usually more than one.**

Local factors cause inflammation, which is the principal pathologic process in gingival and periodontal disease. Systemic factors monitor the periodontal response to local factors, so that the effect of local irritants is often dramatically aggravated by the systemic condition of the patient. Conversely, local factors intensify periodontal tissue changes produced by systemic conditions.

The causes for gingival and periodontal disease are the same, with one exception. Injury produced by excessive occlusal forces (trauma from occlusion) does not cause gingivitis, but it often contributes to destruction of the supporting tissues in periodontal disease.

Chapter 22

DENTAL PLAQUE, ACQUIRED PELLICLE, MATERIA ALBA, FOOD DEBRIS, DENTAL CALCULUS AND DENTAL STAINS

Many types of deposits accumulate on the tooth surface. They are classified as soft and hard; tenacious, adherent or loosely adherent; colored or colorless; transparent or opaque. In the past they were designated by a variety of terms, often with the same term applied to different deposits (Table 22–1). More recently there has been increasing interest in identifying distinguishing features of the deposits and their disease-producing potential.

DENTAL PLAQUE

Dental plaque* **is a soft amorphous granular deposit which accumulates on the surfaces of teeth, dental restorations and dental calculus.** It adheres firmly to the underlying surface, from which it can only be detached by mechanical cleansing. Rinsing and air or water sprays will not entirely remove it. In small amounts plaque

---

*The terms dental plaque and plaque are used interchangeably.

TABLE 22–1 HISTORICAL REVIEW OF TERMINOLOGY USED FOR SOFT ORAL DEPOSITS[*]

1897	J. C. Williams	A thick felt-like mass of acid-forming microorganism
1897	G. V. Black	Gelatinous layers of micro-organisms
1898	G. V. Black	Gelatinous microbial plaque
1898	J. C. Williams	Microbic plaques
1899	G. V. Black	Gelatinous microbic plaque—transparent gelatin layers produced by microbes
1902	W. D. Miller	Bacterial plaque
1941	W. Wild	Plaque—adheres to the surface in the habitually unclean spaces of the dentition, and is composed of finely distributed food debris (carbohydrate, protein, fat) saliva (mucin, desquamated epithelial cells) and various bacteria
1953	R. M. Stephan	Plaque—the sum total of all soft, exogenous material which adheres to dental surfaces
1961	World Health Organization	Plaque—primarily microorganisms; materia alba—oral debris, microorganisms, epithelial and blood cells and little food debris
1963	C. Dawes, G. N. Jenkins, C. H. Tongue	Dental plaque—all soft deposits, exclusive of food debris
1969	R. S. Schwartz, M. Massler[155]	Classified soft deposits as follows: 1. Acquired pellicle—a noncellular thin film 2. Dental plaque—an organized transparent deposit which is primarily composed of bacteria and their products 3. Material alba—soft, whitish deposit, with no specific architecture, which can be removed with water spray 4. Food debris—retained food, which is usually removed by saliva and oral muscular action

[*]Abstracted from Schroeder, H. E.[151] with additions.

is not visible unless it is discolored by pigments from within the oral cavity or is stained by disclosing solutions or wafers (Figs. 22–1, A and B).[*] As it accumulates it becomes a visible globular mass with a pin-

---

[*]The use of disclosing solutions and wafers is described in Chapter 32.

point nodular surface which varies from gray to yellowish-gray to yellow in color.

Plaque occurs supragingivally, mostly on the gingival third of the teeth,[174] and subgingivally,[49] with a predilection for surface cracks, defects and roughness,[18, 117] and overhanging margins of dental restorations. It forms to an equal degree on the mandible and maxilla, more on posterior teeth than anterior, more on proximal surfaces,[158] in lesser amounts facially, and least on the lingual surface.[86, 96, 173]

Dental Plaque and the Acquired Pellicle (Acquired Cuticle)[35]

Dental plaque is usually deposited on a previously formed acellular film called the acquired pellicle (Fig. 22–2),[90, 118] but it may form directly on the tooth surface (Fig. 22–3).[47] Both situations may occur in adjacent areas on the same tooth. As the plaque matures, the underlying pellicle may persist, undergo bacterial degradation or become calcified.[90] **The acquired pellicle is a thin, smooth, colorless, translucent film diffusely distributed on the crown with slightly greater amounts near the gingiva.** On the crown it is continuous with subsurface enamel components. When stained with disclosing agents, pellicle appears as a thin, pale, staining surface sheen in contrast with the deeper staining granular plaque (Fig. 22–1, C).

Pellicle forms on a cleaned tooth surface within minutes,[91] is from 0.05 to 0.8 micron thick,[108, 167] is firmly adherent to the tooth surface and continuous with enamel rods beneath it.[121] The acquired pellicle is a product of the saliva. It is bacteria-free,[113] periodic acid–Schiff (PAS) positive, and contains glycoproteins,[142] derivatives of glycoproteins,[88] polypeptides and lipids.

Plaque Formation

Plaque formation begins by the apposition of a monolayer of bacteria[47] on the acquired pellicle or tooth surface. The organisms are "attached" to the tooth (1) by an adhesive interbacterial matrix,[156] or (2) by an affinity of the hydroxyapatite of the enamel for glycoproteins, which adsorbs acquired pellicle and bacteria to the tooth. Plaque grows by (1) the addition of new bacteria, (2) the multiplication of bacteria and (3) the

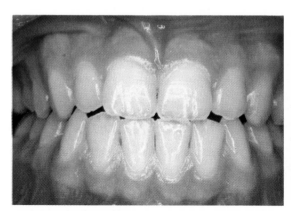

A, **Unstained Dentition.**

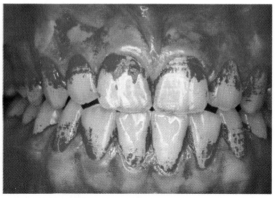

B, **Teeth Stained** with basic fuchsin disclosing solution, showing dental plaque on gingival third of tooth surface.

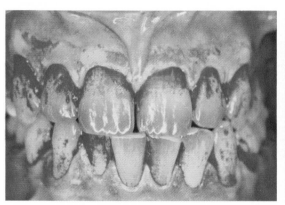

C, **Teeth Stained** with disclosing solution, showing diffuse pale staining pellicle contrasted with darker staining plaque.

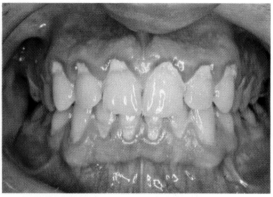

D, **Materia Alba** generalized throughout the mouth with heaviest accumulation near the gingiva. Note the associated gingivitis.

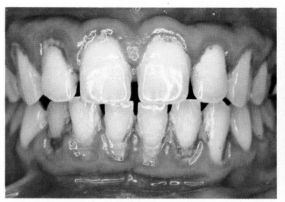

E, **Supragingival Calculus** in a patient with gingival inflammation.

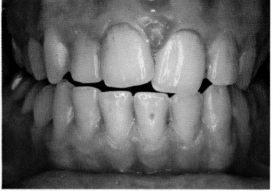

F, **Green Stain** on anterior teeth. Note inflamed, enlarged interdental papilla between overlapped maxillary incisors.

Figure 22–1 Deposits on Tooth Surfaces.

accumulation of bacterial products. The bacteria are held together in the plaque by an adhesive interbacterial matrix and by an adhesive surface coating which they produce.[50]

Measurable amounts of plaque may occur within six hours after teeth are thoroughly cleaned,[40] with maximum accumulation reached in approximately 30 days. The rate of formation and the location vary between individuals, on different teeth in the same mouth, and on different areas of individual teeth.[72]

Composition of Dental Plaque

Dental plaque consists principally of proliferating microorganisms and a scattering of epithelial cells, leukocytes, and macrophages in an adherent intercellular matrix. Organic and inorganic solids form about 20 per cent of the plaque; the remainder is water.[34] Bacteria constitute approximately 70 per cent of the solid material and the rest is intercellular matrix.[45, 54] Plaque stains periodic acid–Schiff (PAS) positive and orthochromatic with toluidine blue.[174]

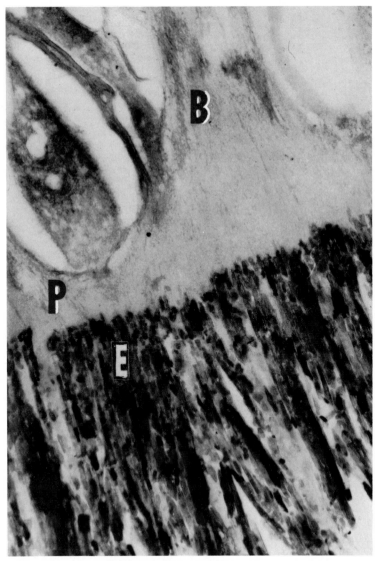

Figure 22–2 Dental Plaque Forming on Pellicle. Electromicrograph of undecalcified incisor, showing bacterial plaque (B) and acquired pellicle (P) on enamel surface (E). × 36,000. (Courtesy of Leach, S. A., and Saxton, C. A.[90])

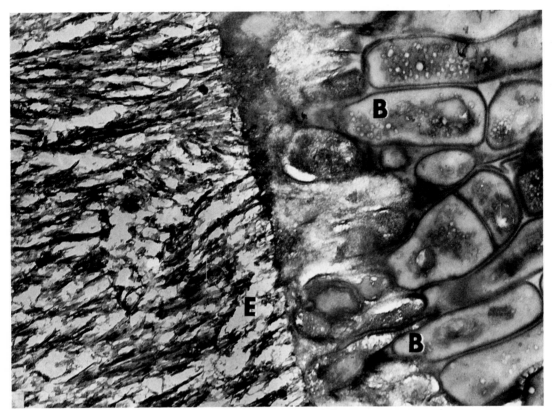

Figure 22–3 Plaque Formed Directly on Enamel Surface. Electromicrograph of decalcified noncarious enamel surface, showing remnants of enamel matrix (E) and bacteria in plaque (B), without intervening pellicle. (Courtesy of Frank, R. M., and Brendel, A.[47])

Plaque matrix

ORGANIC CONTENT. The organic matrix consists of a polysaccharide-protein complex of which the principal components are carbohydrates and proteins, approximately 30 per cent each, and lipids, approximately 15 per cent, with the nature of the remainder unclear.[110] They represent extracellular products of plaque bacteria, their cytoplasmic and cell membrane remnants, ingested foodstuff and derivatives of salivary glycoproteins. The carbohydrate present in greatest amount in the matrix is dextran, a bacteria-produced polysaccharide which forms approximately 9.5 per cent of the total plaque solid (Table 22–2). Other matrix carbohydrates are levan, another polysaccharide bacterial product (approximately 4 per cent), galactose (approximately 2.6 per cent), and methylpentose in the form of rhamnose. Bacterial remnants provide muramic acid, lipids and some matrix protein, for which salivary glycoproteins are the principal source.[110, 160]

INORGANIC CONTENT. The principal inorganic components of plaque matrix are calcium and phosphorus, with small amounts of magnesium, potassium and sodium.[61, 106] They are bound to the organic components of the matrix.[52, 159] The inorganic content is higher on the mandibular anterior teeth than in the remainder of the mouth and is also generally higher on lingual surfaces.[152] The total inorganic content

TABLE 22–2 CARBOHYDRATE CONTENT OF PLAQUE MATRIX*

	Percentage of Lyophilized Matrix Weight	
	Mean	Range
Dextran (polymer of glucose)	9.5%	8–10%
Hexosamine	4%	3–6%
Methylpentose	3.1%	2–4%
Galactose	2.6%	1.7–4.4%
Levan (polymer of fructose)	0.4%	0.1–0.7%

*Modified from Mandel, I. D.[110]

of early plaque is small, with the greatest increase occurring in plaque which is transformed to calculus (see page 305). Fluoride topically applied to the teeth[61] and in drinking water[33] becomes incorporated in the plaque.

Plaque bacteria

✓Dental plaque is a living and productive substance with many microcolonies of organisms in various stages of growth. As plaque develops, the bacterial population changes from an initial predominance of cocci (principally gram-positive) to a more complex one that contains many filamentous and nonfilamentous rods, as follows (Table 22–3):

At the outset: The bacteria consist almost entirely of facultative cocci and rods (Neisseria, Nocardia and Streptococcus).[139] Streptococci form approximately 50 per cent of the bacterial population, with *Streptococcus sanguis* the predominant organism.[23] As the plaque increases in thickness, anaer-

TABLE 22–3 PLAQUE BACTERIA—RELATIVE PERCENTAGES AS PLAQUE MATURES*

Organisms	Day 1	2	3	4	5	7	9	14	21	28	Over 28 days
Gram-positive facultative cocci											28
Streptococci	46	50	69	39	53	51	36	43	39	50	17–27
S. mutans											
S. sanguis											
Others				1		3		4		1	
Staphylococci											few
Gram-positive facultative rods											24
Corynebacterium (diphtheroidal filamentous)	3		1		6	8	9				
Nocardia (aerobic diphtheroidal)	6		0.5		1	0.2	0.1				23
Odontomyces viscosus											
Gram-negative facultative cocci											3.5
Neisseria	9	12	8	17	6	10	2	5	11	4	2–3
Gram-negative facultative rods											0
None											
Gram-positive, anaerobic cocci											13
Peptostreptococci											
Gram-positive anaerobic rods											18–
Leptotrichia buccalis (filamentous)		3		1.5		1.5		2	4	4	6
Actinomyces (filamentous diphtheroid)	0		1		6	18	23				
A. naeslundi		1		1			0	1	14	11.5	
A. israeli		0		0			0	1	0	2	2
Corynebacterium (diphtheroid filamentous)											
Propionibacterium (diphtheroidal)											
Gram-negative anaerobic cocci											6
Veillonella	1.4		3.7		15.5	14	12.5				6
Gram-negative anaerobic rods		15		13		2		17	4	7	10
Spirillum											
Vibrio											
Fusobacterium (filamentous)	0	1.4	0.1	1	0.3	1.2	0.8	3	2	2	2–4
Bacteroides (filamentous)											4
Spirochetes—gram-negative anaerobic											<0.1

*Compiled from References 54, 70, 76, 103, 139 and 166.

obic conditions are created within it and the flora changes accordingly. The surface organisms probably derive their nourishment from the oral environment, whereas the deeper organisms utilize in addition the metabolic products of other plaque bacteria and plaque matrix components.

Second to third day: Gram-negative cocci and rods increase in numbers and percentage (from approximately 7 to 30 per cent),[103, 166] of which approximately 15 per cent are anaerobic rods.

Fourth to fifth day: Fusobacterium, Actinomyces, and Veillonella, all strict anaerobes, increase in number with Veillonella comprising approximately 16 per cent of the flora.[139]

As the plaque matures: After seven days spirella and spirochetes appear in small numbers, especially in the gingival crevice area. Filamentous organisms continue to increase in percentage and number, with the greatest increase in *Actinomyces naeslundi*, from 1 to 14 per cent from the fourteenth to the twenty-first day.[70]

Twenty-eighth to ninetieth day: Streptococci diminish from approximately 50 per cent to 30 to 40 per cent. Rods, particularly the filamentous forms, increase to approximately 40 per cent.

Mature plaque contains approximately 2.5×10^{11} bacteria per gram (by total microscopic count). Cultivable anaerobes comprise 4.6×10^{10} per gm. of organisms and 2.5×10^{10} per gm. of plaque. The facultative and anaerobic bacteria consist of approximately 40 per cent gram-positive cocci, 10 per cent gram-negative cocci, 40 per cent gram-positive rods and 10 per cent gram-negative rods.[54] *Bacteroides melaninogenicus* and spirochetes which are normally found in the gingival sulcus are present in only small numbers.[53] The bacterial populations of subgingival and supragingival plaque are quite similar, except that there is a greater proportion of vibrios and fusobacteria subgingivally.[133] Plaque in most individuals contains the same principal groups of bacteria. However, the proportion and even the species of organisms within each group vary, as well as the proportion of the groups themselves. The variation occurs from individual to individual, tooth to tooth, and even on different areas of the same tooth.

Plaque Architecture

In the first few days plaque appears as a dense meshwork of cocci with occasional rod forms almost to the exclusion of other organisms.[118, 174] As the plaque matures, filaments and threads gradually increase while coccal forms decrease. On the inner surface, they are aligned in a perpendicular palisade arrangement in tuft-like groups separated by cocci (Fig. 22–4). As the surface is approached, the filaments and threads appear singly and less regularly arranged,[112, 117] and colonies of cocci accumulate on the surface.

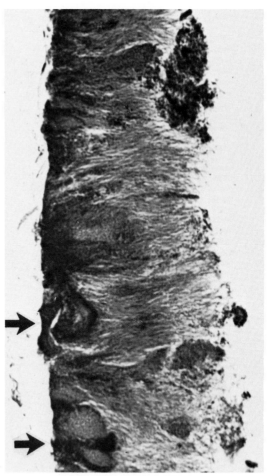

Figure 22–4   Five-Day Plaque, showing spherical calcification foci (*arrows*), and perpendicular alignment of filamentous organisms along the inner surface and colonies of cocci on the outer surface. (From Turesky, S., Renstrup, G., and Glickman, I.[174])

The Role of Saliva in Plaque Formation

Saliva contains a mixture of glycoproteins collectively called mucin.[88] All salivary glycoproteins have not been identified, but they consist of proteins combined with various carbohydrates (oligosaccharides) such as sialic acid, fucose, galactose, glucose, mannose, and two hexosamines: N-acetylgalactosamine and N-acetylglucosamine. Enzymes (glycosidases) produced by oral bacteria split off carbohydrates which they utilize as nutrients. Plaque contains some of the protein but very little of the carbohydrate from the salivary glycoproteins (Fig. 22–5).[89]

One of the glycosidases is the enzyme neuraminidase[136] which separates sialic acid from salivary glycoprotein. Sialic acid and fucose, carbohydrates always present in salivary glycoprotein, are absent in plaque. Loss of sialic acid results in reduced salivary viscosity and the formation of a precipitate considered to be a factor in the formation of plaque.[88]

The Role of Ingested Nutrients in Plaque Formation

Plaque is not a food residue, but plaque bacteria utilize ingested nutrients to form components of the matrix. The most readily utilized nutrients are those which diffuse easily into the plaque, such as the soluble sugars: sucrose, glucose, fructose, maltose, and lesser amounts of lactose. Starches, which are larger, less diffusible molecules, also commonly serve as bacterial substrates.[27]

Several types of plaque bacteria have the capacity to produce extracellular products from ingested nutrients (Fig. 22–5). The principal extracellular products are the polysaccharides, dextran and levan. Of these dextran is the more important because

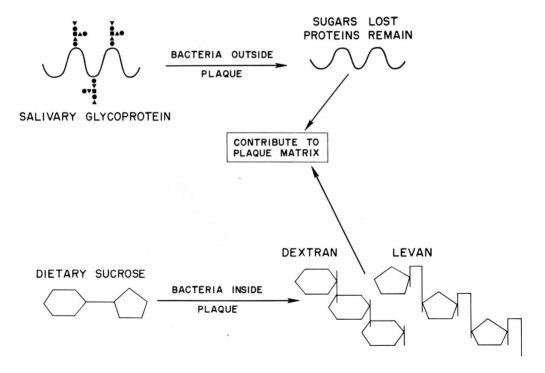

FORMATION OF THE PRINCIPAL PROTEIN
AND CARBOHYDRATE COMPONENTS OF
THE DENTAL PLAQUE

Figure 22–5   Formation of the Principal Protein and Carbohydrate Components of Dental Plaque from salivary glycoproteins and dietary sucrose. (From Leach, S. A.[88])

of its greater quantity, its adhesive properties which may attach the plaque to the tooth, and its relative insolubility and resistance to destruction by bacteria.[32, 45] Dextran is produced from sucrose by streptococci, principally *S. mutans* and *S. sanguis*.[23, 85, 187] Dextran is also formed from other sugars and starches but in much smaller quantities.

Levan, a much smaller component of the plaque matrix, is formed by *Odontomyces viscosus*, a gram-positive aerobic filament,[76] and by certain streptococci.[51] Itself a bacterial product, levan is used as a carbohydrate nutrient by plaque bacteria in the absence of exogenous sources.[32]

Diet and Plaque Formation

Dental plaque is not a food residue, and the rate of plaque formation is not related to the amount of food consumption. Some investigators feel that neither the presence or absence of food in the oral cavity nor the frequency of meals affects the development of plaque.[39] Others report that plaque formation is diminished in patients nourished by stomach tube.[102] Dental plaque forms more rapidly during sleep, when no food is ingested, than following meals.[88] This may be because the mechanical action of food and the increased salivary flow during mastication may deter plaque formation. The consistency of the diet affects the rate of plaque formation. Plaque forms rapidly on soft diets, whereas hard chewy foods retard it.[38] (For additional discussion of food consistency and plaque formation, see Chapter 32.)

In man and in some laboratory animals, dietary supplements of sucrose increase plaque formation[24, 39] and affect its bacterial composition.[19] This is attributed to extracellular polysaccharides produced by bacteria. Glucose supplements do not have a similar effect; and plaque formation occurs on high protein fat diets and carbohydrate-free diets, but in small amounts.

Significance of Dental Plaque

Plaque is the principal etiologic factor in caries, gingivitis and periodontal disease, and it forms the initial stage of dental calculus (see page 305).

Plaque in the etiology of gingival and periodontal disease

There are many local causes for gingival and periodontal disease, but poor oral hygiene overshadows all others.[22, 58, 145] **There is a high correlation between poor oral hygiene,[67, 71, 148] the presence of plaque[2, 26, 131] and the prevalence and severity of gingival and periodontal disease.[97, 101, 104, 116, 120, 146, 161]** In human experiments when oral hygiene procedures are discontinued, plaque accumulates and gingivitis results within 10 to 21 days; the severity of gingival inflammation is correlated with the rate of plaque formation. When oral hygiene procedures are reinstated, plaque is removed from most tooth surfaces within 48 hours and gingivitis disappears one to eight days later (Fig. 22–6).[103, 166]

The principal significance of dental plaque in the etiology of gingival and periodontal disease lies in its concentration of bacteria and their products.[37] Bacteria con-

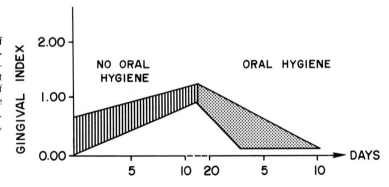

Figure 22–6 Accumulation of Plaque and Development of Gingivitis within 10 to 21 days after cessation of oral hygiene procedures (left side), followed by disappearance of plaque and gingivitis after oral hygiene procedures are reinstated (right side). (Löe, H., Theilade, E., and Jensen, S. B.[103])

tained in the plaque and in the region of the gingival sulcus are capable of causing tissue damage and disease, but the mechanisms whereby they produce gingival and periodontal disease in humans have not been established. The role of microorganisms in the etiology of gingival and periodontal disease is discussed in detail in Chapter 23.

The multipotential of dental plaque

The morphology, metabolic activity and pH levels of dental plaque vary on different teeth and in different areas on the same tooth surface.[44] There is considerable interest in identifying the factors in dental plaque which determine its cariogenic, calculogenic, and gingival disease-producing activity. "Acid" plaques and "basic" plaques have been linked to caries and periodontal disease respectively.[83, 105] Plaque which occurs on the crowns of rodent teeth in which *dextran-forming streptococci* predominate[36, 85, 187] causes dental caries, in contrast with subgingival plaque containing *levan-forming Odontomyces viscosus* and *streptococci* which produce root caries and periodontal disease.[51, 76] Dissolution of inorganic crystals within the plaque[47] and reduced levels of calcification[147] have been suggested as distinguishing features of cariogenic plaque.

MATERIA ALBA

Materia alba* is a local irritant which is a common cause of gingivitis. It is a yellow or gray-white soft and sticky deposit somewhat less adherent then dental plaque (Fig. 22–1, *D*).[151, 155] Materia alba is clearly visible without using disclosing solutions and it is deposited on tooth surfaces, restorations, calculus and on the gingiva.[108, 124] It tends to accumulate on the gingival third of the teeth and on malposed teeth (Fig. 22–1, *D*). It can form on previously cleaned teeth within a few hours, and during periods when no food is ingested.[135] Materia alba can be flushed away with a water spray, but

mechanical cleansing is required to assure complete removal.

Long considered to consist of stagnant food debris, materia alba is now recognized to be a concentration of microorganisms, desquamated epithelial cells, leukocytes, and a mixture of salivary proteins and lipids,[108, 151, 188] with few or no food particles.[135] It lacks a regular internal pattern such as is observed in plaque.[155] The irritating effect of materia alba upon the gingiva is most likely caused by bacteria and their products. Materia alba has also been demonstrated to be toxic when injected into experimental animals after the bacterial component was destroyed by heat.[15]

FOOD DEBRIS

Most food debris is rapidly liquefied by bacterial enzymes and cleared from the oral cavity within five minutes after eating, but some remains on the teeth and mucous membrane.[17, 135] Salivary flow, mechanical action of the tongue, cheek and lips, and form and alignment of the teeth and jaws affect the rate of food clearance, which is accelerated by increased chewing and low viscosity of saliva.[28, 87] Although it contains bacteria, food debris is different from plaque and materia alba and is easier to remove. Dental plaque is not a derivative of food debris, nor is food debris an important cause of gingivitis.[39] Food debris should be differentiated from fibrous strands trapped interproximally in areas of food impaction.*

The rate of clearance from the oral cavity varies with the type of food and the individual. Liquids are cleared more readily than solids. For example, traces of sugar ingested in aqueous solution remain in the saliva for approximately 15 minutes, whereas sugar consumed in solid form is present as long as 30 minutes after ingestion.[176] Sticky foods, such as figs, bread, toffee, and caramel, may adhere to tooth surfaces for over an hour, whereas coarse foods and raw carrots and apples are quickly cleared. Plain bread is cleared faster than bread with butter,[17] brown rye bread faster than white[87] and cold foods slightly faster than hot.

---

*Materia alba is a traditional clinical term for a material which is essentially a heavy accumulation of plaque.

---

*Food impaction is discussed in Chapter 25.

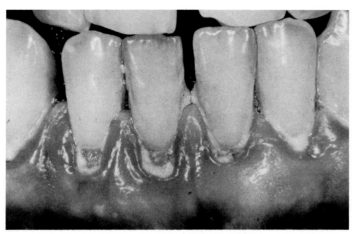

Figure 22–7   Supragingival Calculus.

CALCULUS

Calculus was recognized as a clinical entity in some way related to periodontal disease as far back as the tenth century. Albucasis of Cordova,[185] an Arabian physician, designed a set of scaling instruments for removing calculus in patients afflicted with periodontal disease. Fauchard,[43] in 1728, termed it tartar or slime, and referred to it as "a substance which accumulates on the surface of the teeth and which becomes, when left there, a stony crust of more or less considerable volume. The most common cause of the loss of teeth is the negligence of these people who do not clean their teeth when they might, and that they perceive the lodgment of this foreign substance which produces diseases of the gums."

Supragingival and Subgingival Calculus

Calculus is an adherent, calcified or calcifying mass that forms on the surface of natural teeth and dental prostheses (Fig. 22–1, E). It is classified according to its relation to the gingival margin as follows:

Supragingival calculus (visible calculus) refers to calculus coronal to the crest of the gingival margin and visible in the oral cavity (Fig. 22–7). Supragingival calculus is usually white or white-yellow, of hard, clay-like consistency, and easily detached from the tooth surface with a scaler. The color is affected by such factors as tobacco or food pigment. It may occur on a single tooth or a group of teeth, or be generalized throughout the mouth. Supragingival calculus occurs most frequently and in greatest quantity on the buccal surfaces of the maxillary molars opposite Stensen's duct (Fig. 22–8), the lingual surfaces of the mandibular anterior teeth opposite Wharton's duct, and more on the central incisors than on the laterals (Fig. 22–9).[172] In extreme cases calculus may form a bridge-like

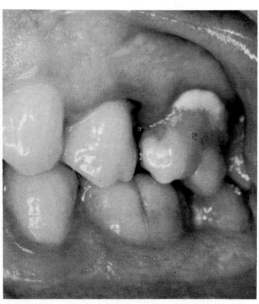

Figure 22–8   Calculus on Molar Opposite Stensen's Duct.

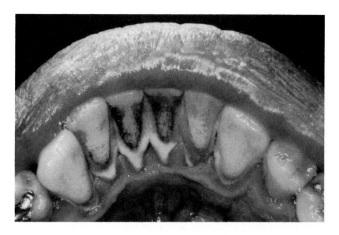

Figure 22–9 Calculus and Stain on lingual surface in relation to orifice of submaxillary and sublingual glands.

structure along adjacent teeth (Fig. 22–10) or cover the occlusal surface of teeth without functional antagonists (Fig. 22–11).

Subgingival calculus refers to calculus below the crest of the marginal gingiva, usually in periodontal pockets, not visible upon oral examination. Determination of the location and extent of subgingival calculus requires careful probing with an explorer (Fig. 22–12). It is usually dense and hard, dark brown or green-black, flint-like in consistency, and firmly attached to the tooth surface. Supragingival and subgingival calculus generally occur together, but one may be present without the other.

Supragingival calculus is also referred to as *salivary,* and subgingival calculus as *serumal*—predicated on the assumption that the former is derived from the saliva and the latter from the blood serum. This concept, overshadowed for a long time by the feeling that saliva was the sole source of all calculus, has been revised. It is the current consensus that the minerals for the formation of supragingival calculus come from the saliva, whereas the gingival fluid which resembles serum is the mineral source for subgingival calculus.[73, 164]

Supra- and subgingival calculus usually appear in the early teens and increase with age.[59, 97, 138] The supragingival type is more common; subgingival calculus is rare in children, and supragingival calculus is uncommon up to the age of 9. The reported prevalence of both types of calculus at different ages varies considerably, according to the examination criteria of different investigators and in different population groups. Between the ages of 9 and 15, supragingival calculus has been reported in from 37[42] to 70 per cent[92] of the individuals studied; in the 16 to 21 age group it ranges from 44[154] to 88 per cent,[96] and in 86[10] to 100 per cent after age 40.[101] The prevalence

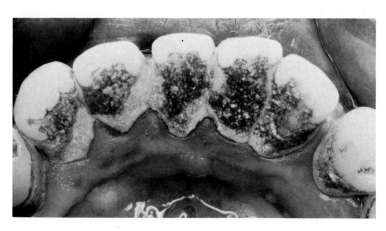

Figure 22–10 Calculus forming a bridge-like structure on the lingual surface of the mandibular anterior teeth.

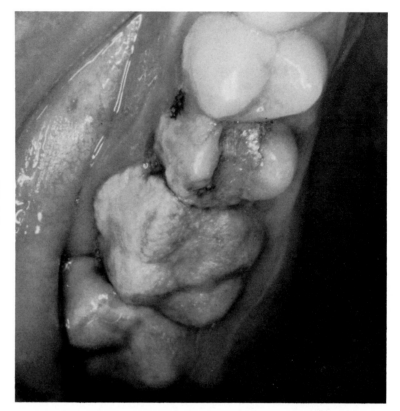

Figure 22–11 Calculus covering nonfunctioning maxillary molars and part of the second premolar. Compare with the first premolar which has functional antagonists.

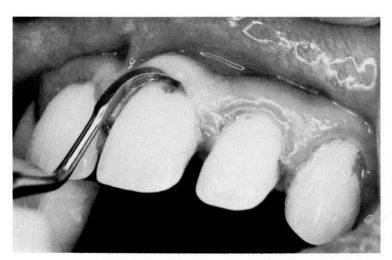

Figure 22–12 Subgingival Calculus revealed by deflecting the pocket wall. Note the inflammation on adjacent lateral incisor and canine associated with supra- and subgingival calculus.

of subgingival calculus is generally slightly lower than the supragingival type, but it approaches a range of from 47 to 100 per cent of individuals after the age of 40.

Composition of Calculus

Inorganic content

Supragingival calculus consists of inorganic (70 to 90 per cent)[56] and organic components. The inorganic portion consists of calcium phosphate, $Ca_3(PO_4)_2$, 75.9 per cent; calcium carbonate, $CaCO_3$, 3.1 per cent; and magnesium phosphate, $Mg_3(PO_4)_2$, with trace amounts of other metals. The principal inorganic components are calcium, 39 per cent; and phosphorus, 19 per cent, with 0.8 per cent magnesium and 1.9 per cent carbon dioxide and trace amounts of Na, Zn, Sr, Br, Cu, Mn, W, Au, Al, Si, Fe, and F.[127] At least two thirds of the inorganic component is crystalline in structure.[95] The four main crystal forms and their

percentages are hydroxyapatite, $Ca_{10}(OH)_2(PO_4)_6$, approximately 58 per cent; brushite, $CaHPO_4 \cdot 2H_2O$, approximately 9 per cent; and magnesium whitlockite, $Ca_9(PO_4)_6 \times PO_4 \cdot (X = Mg^{11} \cdot F^{11})$, and octacalcium-phosphate $Ca_4H(PO_4)_3 \cdot 2H_2O$, approximately 21 per cent each.[144] Generally two or more crystal forms occur in a calculus sample, with hydroxyapatite and octacalcium phosphate being the most common (in 97 to 100 per cent of all supragingival calculus) and in the greatest amounts. Brushite is more common in the mandibular anterior region and whitlockite in the posterior areas. The incidence of the four crystal forms varies with the age of the deposit.[153]

Organic content

The organic component of calculus consists of a mixture of protein-polysaccharide complexes, desquamated epithelial cells, leukocytes and various types of microorganisms (Fig. 22–13);[65, 109] 1.9 to 9.1 per cent of the organic component is carbohydrate,

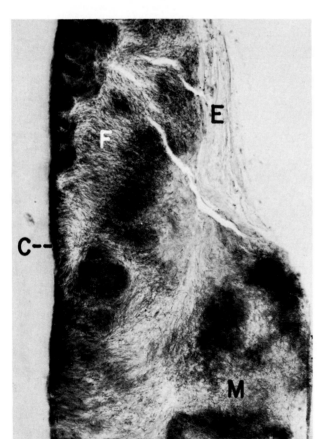

Figure 22–13 Detailed Study of Calculus showing an inner cuticle-like structure (C), filamentous organisms (F), cocci (M) and desquamated epithelial cells (E).

which consists of galactose, glucose, rhamnose, mannose, glucuronic acid, galactosamine, and sometimes arabinase, galacturonic acid, and glucosamine, all of which are present in salivary glycoprotein, except arabinase and rhamnose.[80, 98, 162] Protein derived from the saliva accounts for 5.9 to 8.2 per cent, and includes most of the amino acids.[98, 109, 162] Lipids account for 0.2 per cent of the organic content in the forms of neutral fats, free fatty acids, cholesterol, cholesterol esters, and phospholipids.[99]

SUBGINGIVAL CALCULUS. The composition of subgingival calculus is similar to supragingival, with some differences. It has the same hydroxyapatite content,[169] more magnesium whitlockite, and less brushite and octacalcium phosphate.[144] The ratio of calcium to phosphate is higher subgingivally, and the sodium content increases with the depth of periodontal pockets.[100] Salivary proteins present in supragingival calculus are not found subgingivally.[12] Dental calculus, salivary duct calculus and calcified dental tissues are similar in inorganic composition.

Bacterial content

The percentage of gram-positive and gram-negative filamentous organisms is greater within calculus than in the remainder of the oral cavity. The microorganisms at the periphery are predominantly gram-negative rods and cocci. Most of the organisms within calculus are nonviable. Bibby[16] and Yardeni[189] presented the following regarding the bacterial composition of calculus:

BIBBY
Calculus divided into external, middle and internal portions.
Supragingival Calculus.
1. Predominance of gram-positive filaments.
2. Next in frequency; gram-negative filaments and cocci.
3. Gram-positive cocci seen in calculus about which suppuration had taken place.
Subgingival Calculus.
1. Superficial layers: gram-negative filaments most numerous.
2. Deep and middle zones: gram-positive filaments predominant.
YARDENI
Calculus divided into three zones: calculus itself, the zone peripheral to the calculus, and the inner calculus surface.

1. Calculus itself. A great number of gram-positive filaments of the actinomyces type. Some gram-positive threads, which could be identified as leptotrichia. Numerous borrelia in individual cases. Gram-negative cocci were scarce.
2. The internal surface of the calculus was almost sterile.
3. A zone encircling or adjacent to the calculus with predominantly gram-negative cocci and rods.

Attachment of Calculus to the Tooth Surface

Differences in the manner in which calculus is attached to the root affect the relative ease or difficulty encountered in its removal. The intercellular substance[156] and/or bacteria[84] attach calculus to the tooth surface in one or more of the following ways:

1. By means of the acquired pellicle.[167, 180, 190]

2. By penetration into the cementum and dentin (Figs. 22–14 and 22–15).

3. In areas of unrepaired cemental and dentinal resorption that become exposed by gingival recession.

4. By interlocking of inorganic crystals of calculus with those of the tooth structure.

5. In spaces created by cemental separation.

How Calculus Is Formed

Calculus is dental plaque which has undergone mineralization, so that the formation of calculus begins with the dental plaque. The soft plaque is hardened by precipitation of mineral salts which usually starts any time from the second to the fourteenth day of plaque formation, but calcification has been reported as early as four to eight hours.[170] Calcifying plaques become 50 per cent mineralized in two days and 60 to 90 per cent in 12 days.[124, 152, 157]

All plaque does not necessarily undergo calcification. Early plaque contains a small amount of inorganic material which increases as plaque develops into calculus. Plaque which does not develop into calculus reaches a plateau of maximum mineral content by two days.[124, 152, 157]

Saliva is the mineral source for supragingival calculus, and the gingival fluid most likely furnishes the minerals for subgingival calculus. Plaque has the ability to concentrate calcium two to 20 times its level in saliva.[34] Early plaque of heavy calculus formers contains more calcium and three times more phosphorus and less potassium than that of nonformers, suggesting that phosphorus may be more critical than calcium in plaque mineralization.[106]

Calcification entails binding of calcium ions to the carbohydrate-protein complexes of the organic matrix,[107] and the precipitation of crystalline calcium phosphate salts. Crystals initially form in the intercellular matrix and on the bacterial surfaces, and finally within the bacteria.[57, 191]

Calcification begins along the inner surface of the plaque adjacent to the tooth in separate foci of cocci which increase in size and coalesce to form solid masses of calculus (Fig. 22–4). It is accompanied by alterations in the bacterial content and staining qualities of the plaque. With the occurrence of calcification, filaments and threads increase in number beyond that of the other organisms. In the calcification foci there is a change from basophilia to eosinophilia; the staining intensity of periodic acid-Schiff positive groups and sulfhydryl and amino groups is reduced; and staining with toluidine blue, initially orthochromatic, becomes metachromatic and disappears.[174] Calculus is formed in layers often separated by a thin cuticle which becomes embedded in it as calcification progresses.[112]

Rate of formation and accumulation

The starting time and rate of calcification and accumulation of calculus vary from person to person and in different teeth and at different times in the same person.[126, 171] Based on these differences, individuals may be classified as heavy, moderate or slight calculus formers or as nonformers. The

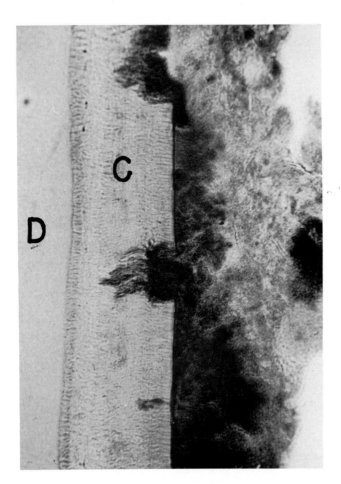

Figure 22–14 Calculus on Tooth Surface Embedded within the Cementum (C). Note the early stage of penetration shown in the lower portion of the illustration. The dentin is at D.

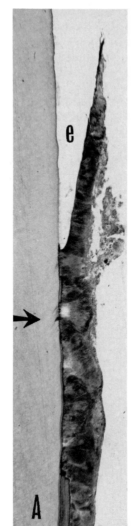

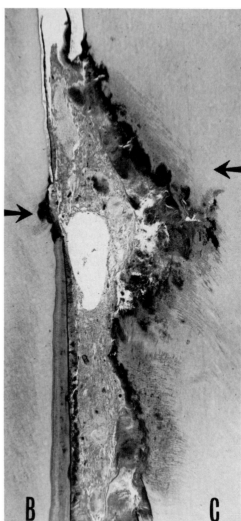

Figure 22–15 Calculus. *A,* Calculus attached to pellicle on enamel surface (e). The enamel was removed in preparation of the specimen. Also note calculus attached to dentin and associated penetration of dental tubules (*arrow*). *B* and *C,* Proximal surfaces with early and advanced root caries and with calculus attached to carious surfaces (*arrows*).

average daily increment in calculus formers is from 0.10 to 0.15 mg. of dry weight.[157, 172] The calculus on the lingual surface of the mandibular anterior teeth is a reliable indication of the amount in the entire dentition.[177] **Ninety per cent of all the calculus occurs on the mandibular anterior teeth.**[111]

Calculus formation continues until it reaches a maximum from which it may be reduced in amount. The time required to reach the maximum level has been reported as ten weeks,[30] 18 weeks[115] and six months.[178] The decline from maximum accumulation (reversal phenomenon)[125, 178] may be explained by the vulnerability of bulky calculus to mechanical wear from food and the cheeks, lips and tongue.

Theories regarding the mineralization of calculus

Theories regarding the mechanisms whereby plaque is mineralized to form calculus fit into two principal concepts:[127]

"BOOSTER CONCEPT." According to this concept *mineral precipitation results from a local rise in the degree of saturation of calcium and phosphate ions* which may be brought about in several ways: (1) A rise in pH of the saliva causes precipitation of calcium phosphate salts by lowering the precipitation constant. The pH may be elevated by the loss of carbon dioxide, by the formation of ammonia by dental plaque and bacteria, or by protein degradation during stagnation.[16, 68, 128] (2) Colloidal proteins in saliva bind calcium and phosphate ions and maintain a supersaturated solution with respect to calcium phosphate salts. With stagnation of saliva colloids settle out; the supersaturated state is no longer maintained, leading to precipitation of calcium phosphate salts.[66, 137] (3) Phosphatase liberated from dental plaque, desquamated epithelial cells or bacteria is believed to play a role in the precipitation of calcium phosphate by hydrolyzing organic phosphates in saliva and thus increasing the concentration of free phosphate ions.[29, 186] Another enzyme, esterase, present in the cocci, filamentous organisms, leukocytes, macrophages and desquamated epithelial cells of dental plaque, may initiate calcification by hydrolyzing fatty esters into free fatty acids.[6] The fatty acids form soaps with calcium and magnesium that are converted later into the less soluble calcium phosphate salts.

"EPITACTIC CONCEPT." According to this concept, seeding agents induce small foci of calcification, which enlarge and coalesce to form a calcified mass.[129] The seeding agents in calculus formation are not known, but it is suspected that the intercellular matrix of plaque plays an active role.[112, 123, 184] The carbohydrate-protein complexes may initiate calcification by removing calcium from the saliva (chelation) and binding with it to form nuclei that induce subsequent deposition of minerals.[107, 179] Plaque bacteria have also been implicated as possible seeding agents (discussed in the following section).

Role of microorganisms in the mineralization of calculus

Mineralization of plaque starts extracellularly around both gram-positive and gram-negative organisms, but may start intracellularly in some gram-positive bacteria.[156] It spreads until the matrix and bacteria are calcified.[57, 141, 191] Some feel that plaque bacteria actively participate in the mineralization of calculus, by forming phosphatases, changing the plaque pH or inducing mineralization,[41, 107] but the prevalent opinion is that they are only passively involved[57, 140, 184] and are simply calcified along with other plaque components. The occurrence of calculus-like deposits in germ-free animals

encourages this opinion.[55, 63] However, other experiments suggest that transmissible factors are involved in calculus formation, and that penicillin in the diet reduces calculus formation.[7] Nonviable bacteria calcify more readily than viable organisms, and it has been suggested that nonviable organisms are essential to the mineralization process, but bacterial metabolic activity is not.[141]

SYSTEMIC FACTORS — DIET AND NUTRITION. The significance of diet in calculus formation depends more upon its consistency than upon its content. Calculus deposition is retarded by coarse detergent foods[78, 132, 183] and hastened by soft[64, 165] and finely ground diets.[168] Calculus forms in the absence of food intake in tube-fed animals.[77]

In experimental animals increased calculus formation has been associated with deficiencies of vitamin A,[79] niacin or pyridoxine,[14] and with increases in dietary calcium, phosphorus, bicarbonate, protein[9, 165] and carbohydrates.[8] Opinions differ regarding the effect of high-fat diets on calculus formation. Sucrose-enriched diets which result in increased plaque do not appear to affect the formation of calculus.[8, 82] The mean nutrient intake and the dietary content of vitamin A and calcium are higher in calculus formers than in nonformers, but the dietary ascorbic acid is lower.[163]

Increased calculus formation has been associated with disturbed emotional states.[5]

CALCULUS INHIBITION BY SALIVA. It has been suggested that an inhibitory mechanism in saliva controls the rate of calculus formation. An inverse relationship has been reported between the amount of calculus and the pyrophosphate content of parotid saliva.[46] Some question the presence of pyrophosphate in saliva[74] and its ability to inhibit calculus formation.[81]

The Relative Etiologic Significance of Plaque and Calculus

Plaque is more important than calculus in the etiology of gingival and periodontal disease.[69, 138] Gingivitis occurs in the absence of calculus,[114] and the formation of plaque leads to gingivitis which disappears when the plaque is removed.[149, 166] It is difficult to separate the effects of calculus and plaque upon the gingiva, because calculus is always covered with a nonmineralized layer of plaque.[150] There is a positive correlation between calculus and the prevalence of gingivitis,[138] but it is not as high as between plaque and gingivitis.[158] The development of calculus leads to only a slight increase in gingivitis over that associated with soft plaque alone.[134] In young individuals the periodontal condition is more closely related to plaque accumulation than to calculus, but the situation is reversed with age.[58, 97]

Calculus, gingivitis and periodontal disease increase with age. It is extremely rare to find a periodontal pocket without subgingival calculus, although in some cases it may be of microscopic proportions; and the severest inflammation in the pocket wall is adjacent to the calculus (Fig. 22–16). The

nonmineralized plaque on the calculus surface is the principal irritant,[1] but the underlying calcified portion is a significant contributing factor. It does not irritate the gingiva directly, but it provides a fixed nidus for the continued accumulation of irritating surface plaque and holds the plaque against the gingiva.

Subgingival calculus may be the product rather than the cause of periodontal pockets. Plaque initiates the gingival inflammation which starts pocket formation, and the pocket provides a sheltered area for plaque and bacterial accumulation. Increased flow of gingival fluid associated with gingival inflammation provides the minerals which convert the continually accumulating plaque into subgingival calculus.

Regardless of its primary or secondary relationship in pocket formation and although the principal irritating feature of calculus is surface plaque, rather than its calcified interior, calculus is a significant pathogenic factor in periodontal disease. It perpetuates inflammation, which is responsible for deepening of periodontal pockets and destruction of supporting periodontal tissues.

DENTAL STAINS

Pigmented deposits on the tooth surface are called *stains*. They are esthetic problems but may also cause gingival irritation. Stains result from the pigmentation of ordinarily colorless developmental and acquired dental cuticles (see Chap. 1) by chromogenic bacteria, food and chemicals. They vary in color and composition, and in the firmness with which they adhere to the tooth surface.

BROWN STAIN. This is a thin translucent acquired, usually bacteria-free, pigmented pellicle.[113, 175] It occurs in individuals who do not brush sufficiently or use a dentifrice with inadequate cleansing action. It is found most commonly on the buccal surface of the maxillary molars and on the lingual surface of the mandibular incisors.

TOBACCO STAINS. Tobacco produces dark brown or black tenacious surface deposits and brown discoloration of tooth substance. Staining results from coal tar combustion products and penetration of pits and fissures, enamel, and dentin by tobacco

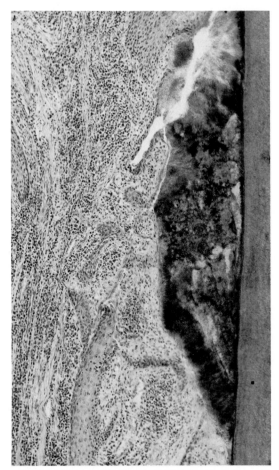

Figure 22–16 Suppurative Inflammation in periodontal pocket wall adjacent to uncalcified plaque on calculus surface.

juices. Staining is not necessarily proportional to the tobacco consumed, but depends to a considerable degree upon preexistent dental cuticles which attach the tobacco products to the tooth surface.

BLACK STAIN. This usually occurs as a thin black line on the teeth facially and lingually near the gingival margin, and as a diffuse patch on the proximal surfaces. It is firmly attached, tends to recur after removal, is more common in women and may occur in mouths with excellent hygiene. Chromogenic bacteria are the probable cause.

GREEN STAIN. This is a green or green-yellow stain, sometimes of considerable thickness, which is common in children (Fig. 22–1, F). It is considered to be the stained remnants of the enamel cuticle, but this has not been substantiated.[3] The discoloration has been attributed to fluorescent bacteria, and fungi such as Penicillium and Aspergillus.[4] Green stain usually occurs on the facial surface of the maxillary anterior teeth, in the gingival half, more often in boys (65 per cent) than in girls (43 per cent).[93] A high incidence has been reported in children with tuberculosis of cervical lymph nodes and other tuberculous lesions.

ORANGE STAIN. Orange stain is less common than green or brown stains. It may occur on both the facial and lingual surfaces of anterior teeth. Serratia marcescens and Flavobacterium lutescens[11] have been suggested as the responsible chromogenic organisms.

METALLIC STAINS. Metals and metallic salts may be introduced into the oral cavity in metal-containing dust inhaled by industrial workers, or through orally administered drugs. The metals combine with dental cuticle, producing a surface stain, or penetrate the tooth substance and cause permanent discoloration. Copper dust produces a green stain, and iron dust a brown stain. Iron-containing medicines cause a black iron sulfite deposit. Other occasionally seen metallic stains are manganese (black), mercury (green-black), nickel (green), and silver (black).

REFERENCES

1. Allen, D., and Kerr, D.: Tissue Response in the Guinea Pig to Sterile and Non-Sterile Calculus. J. Periodont., 36:121, 1965.

2. Ash, M. M., Gitlin, B. N., and Smith, W. A.: Correlation Between Plaque and Gingivitis. J. Periodont., 35:424, 1964.
3. Ayers, P.: Green Stains. J.A.D.A., 26:3, 1939.
4. Badanes, B. B.: The Role of Fungi in Deposits Upon the Teeth. D. Cosmos, 75:1154, 1933.
5. Badanes, B. B., and Parodneck, C. B.: The Influence of Emotional States Upon Tartar Formation. J.A.D.A., 24:1421, 1937.
6. Baer, P. N., and Burstone, M. S.: Esterase Activity Associated with Formation of Deposits on Teeth. Oral Surg., Oral Med. & Oral Path., 12: 1147, 1959.
7. Baer, P. N., Keyes, P. H., and White, C. L.: Studies on Experimental Calculus Formation in the Rat. XII. On the Transmissibility of Factors Affecting Dental Calculus. J. Periodont., 39:86, 1968.
8. Baer, P. N., Stephan, R. M., and White, C. L.: Studies on Experimental Calculus Formation in the Rat. I. Effect of Age, Sex, Strain, High Carbohydrate, High Protein Diets. J. Periodont., 32: 190, 1961.
9. Baer, P. N., and White, C. L.: Studies on Experimental Calculus Formation in the Rat. IX. The Effect of Varying the Protein and Fat Content of the Diet on Calculus Deposition and Alveolar Bone Loss. J. Periodont., 37:113, 1966.
10. Barros, L., and Witkop, C. P.: Oral and Genetic Study of Chileans, 1960. III. Periodontal Disease and Nutritional Factors. Arch. Oral Biol., 8:195, 1963.
11. Bartels, H. A.: A Note on Chromogenic Micro-Organisms from an Organic Colored Deposit of the Teeth. Int. J. Orthodont., 25:795, 1939.
12. Baumhammers, A., and Stallard, R. E.: A Method for the Labeling of Certain Constituents in the Organic Matrix of Dental Calculus. J. D. Res., 45:1568, 1966.
13. Beck, D. J., et al.: A Simple Method for Public Health Dental Survey in Developing Countries. New Zealand D. J., 60:274, 1964.
14. Becks, H., Wainwright, W. W., and Morgan, A. F.: Comparative Study of Oral Changes in Dogs Due to Deficiencies of Pantothenic Acid, Nicotinic Acid and Vitamin B Complex. Am. J. Orthodont. & Oral Surg., 29:183, 1943.
15. Beckwith, T. D., and Williams, A.: Materia Alba as Toxic Material. Am. D. Surg., 49:73, 1929.
16. Bibby, B. G.: The Formation of Salivary Calculus. D. Cosmos, 77:668, 1935.
17. Bibby, B. G., Goldberg, H. J. V., and Chen, E.: Evaluation of Caries-Producing Potentialities of Various Foodstuffs. J.A.D.A., 42:491, 1951.
18. Björn, H., and Carlsson, J.: Observations on a Dental Plaque Morphogenesis. Odont. Rev., 15:23, 1964.
19. Bowen, W. H., and Cornick, D.: Effects of Carbohydrate Restriction in Monkeys (M. irus) with Active Caries. Helv. Odont. Acta, 11:27, 1967.
20. Bowen, W. H., and Gilmour, M. N.: Actinomyces and Calculus Formation (Abst.). J. D. Res., 38: 709, 1959.
21. Boyle, P. E.: Kronfeld's Histopathology of the Teeth and Their Surrounding Structures. 2nd ed. Philadelphia, Lea & Febiger, 1950, p. 470.
22. Brandtzaeg, P., and Jamison, H.: A Study of

Periodontal Health and Oral Hygiene in Norwegian Army Recruits. J. Periodont., 35:302, 1964.

23. Carlsson, J.: Presence of Various Types of Non-Hemolytic Streptococci in Dental Plaque and in Other Sites of the Oral Cavity of Man. Odont. Revy, 18:55, 1967.

24. Carlsson, J., and Egelberg, J.: Effect of Diet on Early Plaque Formation in Man. Odont. Revy, 16:112, 1965.

25. Carlsson, J., and Egelberg, J.: Local Effect of Diet on Plaque Formation and Development of Gingivitis in Dogs. II. Effect of High Carbohydrate Versus High Protein-Fat Diets. Odont. Revy, 16:42, 1965.

26. Chawla, T. N., Nanda, R. S., and Mathur, M. N.: Bacterial Plaque and Its Relation to Periodontal Disease. All-India D. Assn. J., 31:121, 1959.

27. Ciba Foundation Symposium: Caries Resistant Teeth. Boston, Little, Brown and Company, 1965, p. 292.

28. Ciba Foundation Symposium: Caries Resistant Teeth. Boston, Little, Brown and Company, 1965, p. 296.

29. Citron, S.: The Role of Actinomyces Israeli in Salivary Calculus Formation. J. D. Res., 24:87, 1945.

30. Conroy, C., and Sturzenberger, O.: The Rate of Calculus Formation in Adults. J. Periodont., 39:142, 1968.

31. Critchley, P., Wood, J. M., Saxton, C. A., and Leach, S. A.: The Polymerisation of Dietary Sugars by Dental Plaque. Caries Res., 1:112, 1967.

32. da Costa, T., and Gibbons, R. J.: Hydrolysis of Levan by Human Plaque Streptococci. Arch. Oral Biol., 13:609, 1968.

33. Dawes, C., et al.: The Relation Between the Fluoride Concentrations in the Dental Plaque and in Drinking Water. Brit. D. J., 119:164, 1965.

34. Dawes, C., and Jenkins, G. N.: Some Inorganic Constituents of Dental Plaque and Their Relationship to Early Calculus Formation and Caries. Arch. Oral Biol., 7:161, 1962.

35. Dawes, C., Jenkins, G. N., and Tonge, C. H.: The Nomenclature of the Integuments of the Enamel Surface of Teeth. Brit. D. J., 115:65, 1963.

36. De Stopelaar, J. D., Van Houte, J., and De Moor, C. E.: The Presence of Dextran-Forming Bacteria Identified as Streptococcus bovis and Streptococcus sanguis in Human Dental Plaque. Arch. Oral Biol., 12:1199, 1967.

37. Dornan, D. C.: Dental Plaque: Its Inflammatory Potential. Periodont. Abstr., 16:138, 1968.

38. Egelberg, J.: Local Effect of Diet on Plaque Formation and Development of Gingivitis in Dogs. Part I. Effect of Hard and Soft Diets. Odont. Revy, 16:31, 1965.

39. Egelberg, J.: Local Effect of Diet on Plaque Formation and Development of Gingivitis in Dogs. III. Effect of Frequency of Meals and Tube Feeding. Odont. Revy, 16:50, 1965.

40. Eichel, R. A.: A Clinical Television Evaluation of Plaque Formation in Children. I.A.D.R. Abstracts, 1970, No. 491, p. 171.

41. Ennever, J.: Microbiologic Mineralization: A Calcifiable Cell-free Extract from a Calcifiable Microorganism. J. D. Res., 41:1383, 1962.

42. Everett, F. G., Tuchler, H., and Lu, K. H.: Occurrence of Calculus in Grade School Children in Portland, Oregon, J. Periodont., 34:54, 1963.

43. Fauchard, P.: The Surgeon Dentist—Translated by Lilian Lindsay from the 1746 Edition. London, Butterworth & Co., 1946, p. 66.

44. Fitzgerald, R. J.: Plaque Microbiology and Caries. Ala. J. Med. Sc., 5:239, 1968.

45. Fitzgerald, R. J., and Jordan, H. V.: Polysaccharide Producing Bacteria and Dental Caries. In Harris, R. S. (Ed.): The Art and Science of Dental Caries Research. New York, Academic Press, 1968.

46. Vogel, J. J., and Amdur, B. H.: Inorganic Pyrophosphate in Parotid Saliva and Its Relation to Calculus Formation. Arch. Oral Biol., 12:159, 1967.

47. Frank, R. M., and Brendel, A.: Ultrastructure of the Approximal Dental Plaque and the Underlying Normal and Carious Enamel. Arch. Oral Biol., 11:883, 1966.

48. Freeman, I. A.: Removal of Deposits upon Teeth. Den. Rev., 11:379, 1897.

49. Fundak, C. P., and Ash, M.: Correlation Between Supragingival Plaque, Subgingival Plaque and Gingival Crevice Depth. I.A.D.R. Abstracts, 1969, No. 349, p. 128.

50. Gibbons, R. J.: Dental Plaque. Edited by W. D. McHugh. London, E. & S. Livingstone Co., 1970, p. 207.

51. Gibbons, R. J., and Banghart, S. B.: Induction of Dental Caries in Gnotobiotic Rats with a Levan Forming Streptococcus and a Streptococcus Isolated From Subacute Bacterial Endocarditis. Arch. Oral Biol., 13:297, 1968.

52. Gibbons, R. J., and Banghart, S. B.: Synthesis of Extracellular Dextran by Cariogenic Bacteria and Its Presence in Human Dental Plaque. Arch. Oral Biol., 12:11, 1967.

53. Gibbons, R. J., Kapsimalis, B., and Socransky, S. S.: The Source of Salivary Bacteria. Arch. Oral Biol., 9:101, 1964.

54. Gibbons, R. J., Socransky, S. S., De Araujo, W. C., et al.: Studies of the Predominant Cultivable Microbiota of Dental Plaque. Arch. Oral Biol., 9:365, 1964.

55. Glas, J. E., and Krasse, B.: Biophysical Studies on Dental Calculus from Germ Free and Conventional Rats. Acta. Odont. Scandinav., 20:127, 1962.

56. Glock, G. E., and Murray, M. M.: Chemical Investigation of Salivary Calculus. J. D. Res., 17:257, 1938.

57. Gonzales, F., and Sognnaes, R. F.: Electromicroscopy of Dental Calculus. Science, 131:156, 1960.

58. Greene, J. C.: Oral Hygiene and Periodontal Disease. Am. J. Pub. Health, 53:913, 1963.

59. Greene, J. C., and Vermillion, J. R.: The Oral Hygiene Index. J.A.D.A., 68:7, 1964.

60. Gressly, F.: Experimental Calculus Formation. Periodontics, 1:53, 1963.

61. Grøn, P., Yao, K., and Spinelli, M.: A Study of Inorganic Constituents in Dental Plaque. J. D. Res., 48:799, 1969.

62. Grossman, L. I.: Effect of Chemical Agents on a Calculus Substitute. Oral Surg., Oral Med. & Oral Path., 7:484, 1954.

63. Gustafsson, B. E., and Krasse, B.: Dental Calculus in Germ Free Rats. Acta Odont. Scandinav., 20: 135, 1962.

64. Haber, G. G.: The Effect of the Differences in the

Quality of Bread upon Nutrition and the Development of Dental Caries and Tartar in Germany and Switzerland, 1932–1937. Brit. D. J., 68:142, 1940.

65. Hampar, B., Mandel, I. D., and Ellison, S. A.: The Carbohydrate Components of Supragingival Calculus. (Absts.) J. D. Res., 40:752, 1961.

66. Herrenknecht, W., and Becks, H.: Oral Hygiene. Fortschr. Zahnhk., 4:736, 1928.

67. Heylings, R. T.: Study of the Prevalence and Severity of Gingivitis in Undergraduates at Leeds University (1960). D. Practit., 12:129, 1961.

68. Hodge, H. C., and Leung, S. W.: Calculus Formation. J. Periodont., 21:211, 1950.

69. Hoover, D. R., and Robinson, H. B. G.: Effect of Automatic and Hand Toothbrushing on Gingivitis. J.A.D.A., 65:361, 1962.

70. Howell, A., Rizzo, A., and Paul, F.: Cultivable Bacteria in Developing and Mature Human Dental Calculus. Arch. Oral Biol., 10:307, 1965.

71. James, P. M. C., et al.: Gingival Health and Dental Cleanliness in English Schoolchildren. Arch. Oral Biol., 3:57, 1960.

72. Jenkins, G. N.: The Chemistry of Plaque. Ann. New York Acad. Sci., 131:786, 1965.

73. Jenkins, G. N.: The Physiology of the Mouth. Oxford, Blackwell Scientific Publications, 1966, p. 495.

74. Jenkins, G. N., Ferguson, D. B., and Edgar, W. M.: Fluoride and the Metabolism of Salivary Bacteria. Helv. Odont. Acta, 11:2, 1967.

75. Jensen, A. T., and Danø, M.: Crystallography of Dental Calculus and Precipitation of Certain Calcium Phosphates. J. D. Res., 33:741, 1954.

76. Jordan, H. V., Keyes, P. H., and Lim, S.: Plaque Formation and Implantation of Odontomyces viscosus in Hamsters Fed Different Carbohydrates. J. D. Res., 48:(Suppl.)824, 1969.

77. Kakehashi, S., Baer, P. N., White, C., and Gluck, G.: Studies on Experimental Calculus Formation in the Rat. VI. Effect of Diet Intubation, Meal Feeding and Nibbling. J. Periodont., 34:513, 1963.

78. King, J. D.: Experimental Investigation of Periodontal Disease in the Ferret and in Man, with Special Reference to Calculus Formation. D. Practit., 4:157, 1954.

79. King, J. D., and Gimson, A. P.: Experimental Investigations of Parodental Disease in the Ferret and Related Lesions in Man. Brit. D. J., 83:126, 1947.

80. King, J. D., and Glover, R. E.: The Relative Effects of Dietary Constituents and Other Factors Upon Calculus Formation and Gingival Disease in the Ferret. J. Path. & Bact., 57:353, 1945.

81. Kinoshita, S., and Mühlemann, H. R.: Effect of Sodium Ortho- and Pyrophosphate on Supragingival Calculus. Helv. Odont. Acta, 10:46, 1966.

82. Kinoshita, S., Schait, A., Brebou, M., and Mühlemann, H. R.: Effect of Sucrose on Early Dental Calculus and Plaque. Helv. Odont. Acta, 10:134, 1966.

83. Kleinberg, I., and Jenkins, G. N.: The pH of Dental Plaques in Different Areas of the Mouth Before and After Meals and Their Relationship to the pH and Rate of Flow of Resting Saliva. Arch. Oral Biol., 9:493, 1964.

84. Kopczyk, R., and Conroy, C.: The Attachment of Calculus to Root Planed Surfaces. Periodontics, 6:78, 1968.

85. Krasse, B.: Human Streptococci and Experimental Caries in Hamsters. Arch. Oral Biol., 11:429, 1966.

86. Kupczak, L. J., Volpe, A. R., and King, W. J.: Dental Plaque: Relationship Between Accumulation Patterns in Human Adult Dentition and Clinical Investigations. I.A.D.R. Abstracts, 1969, No. 642, p. 201.

87. Lanke, L. S.: Influence on Salivary Sugar of Certain Properties of Foodstuffs and Individual Oral Conditions. Acta Odont. Scandinav., 15:3, Suppl. 23, 1957.

88. Leach, S. A.: Plaque Chemistry and Caries. Ala. J. Med. Sc., 5:247, 1968.

89. Leach, S. A., Critchley, P., Kolendo, A. B., and Saxton, C. A.: Salivary Glycoproteins as Components of the Enamel Integuments. Caries Res., 1:104, 1967.

90. Leach, S. A., and Saxton, C. A.: An Electron Microscopic Study of the Acquired Pellicle and Plaque Formed on the Enamel of Human Incisors. Arch. Oral Biol., 11:1081, 1966.

91. Lenz, H., and Mühlemann, H. R.: Repair of Etched Enamel Exposed to the Oral Environment. Helv. Odont. Acta, 7:47, 1963.

92. Leung, S. W.: Role of Calculus Deposits in Periodontal Disease. In A Symposium on Preventive Dentistry. St. Louis, C. V. Mosby Company, 1956, p. 206.

93. Leung, S. W.: Naturally Occurring Stains on the Teeth of Children. J.A.D.A., 41:191, 1950.

94. Leung, S. W.: The Uneven Distribution of Calculus in the Mouth. J. Periodont., 22:7, 1951.

95. Leung, S. W., and Jensen, A. T.: Factors Controlling the Deposition of Calculus. Internat. D. J., 8:613, 1958.

96. Lightner, L. M., et al.: The Periodontal Status of Incoming Air Force Academy Cadets. U.S.A.F. School of Aerospace Medicine, SAM-TR-66-66, August, 1966, p. 1.

97. Lilienthal, B., Amerena, V., and Gregory, G.: An Epidemiological Study of Chronic Periodontal Disease. Arch. Oral Biol., 10:553, 1965.

98. Little, M. F., Bowman, L., Casciani, C. A., and Rowley, J.: The Composition of Dental Calculus. III. Supragingival Calculus—the Amino Acid and Saccharide Component. Arch. Oral Biol., 11:385, 1966.

99. Little, M. F., Bowman, L. M., and Dirksen, T. R.: The Lipids of Supragingival Calculus. J. D. Res., 43:836, 1964.

100. Little, M. F., and Hazen, S. P.: Dental Calculus Composition. 2. Subgingival Calculus: Ash, Calcium, Phosphorus and Sodium. J. D. Res., 43:645, 1964.

101. Littleton, N. W.: Dental Caries and Periodontal Disease Among Ethiopian Civilians. Pub. Health Rep., 78:631, 1963.

102. Littleton, N. W., Carter, C. H., and Kelly, R. T.: Studies of Oral Health in Persons Nourished by Stomach Tube. J.A.D.A., 74:119, 1967.

103. Löe, H., Theilade, E., and Jensen, S. B.: Experimental Gingivitis in Man. J. Periodont., 36:177, 1965.

104. Lovdal, A., Arno, A., Schei, O., and Waerhaug, J.: Combined Effect of Subgingival Scaling and Controlled Oral Hygiene on the Incidence of Gingivitis. Acta Odont. Scandinav., 19:537, 1961.

105. Lovdal, A., Arno, A., and Waerhaug, J.: Incidence of Clinical Manifestations of Periodontal Disease

in Light of Oral Hygiene and Calculus Formation. J.A.D.A., 56:21, 1958.

106. Mandel, I. D.: Biochemical Aspects of Calculus Formation. J. Periodont. Res., 4:(Suppl. 4)7, 1969.

107. Mandel, I. D.: Calculus Formation. The Role of Bacteria and Mucoprotein. Dental Clinics of North America, 1960, p. 731.

108. Mandel, I. D.: Dental Plaque: Nature, Formation, and Effects. J. Periodont., 37:357, 1966.

109. Mandel, I. D.: Histochemical and Biochemical Aspects of Calculus Formation. Periodontics, 1:43, 1963.

110. Mandel, I. D.: Plaque and Calculus. Ala. J. Med. Sc., 5:313, 1968.

111. Mandel, I. D.: Plaque and Calculus Measurements—Rate of Formation and Pathologic Potential. J. Periodont., 38:721, 1967.

112. Mandel, I. D., Levy, B. M., and Wasserman, B. H.: Histochemistry of Calculus Formation. J. Periodont., 28:132, 1957.

113. Manly, R. S.: A Structureless Recurrent Deposit on Teeth. J. D. Res., 22:479, 1943.

114. Marshall-Day, C. D., and Shourie, K. L.: Gingival Disease in the Virgin Islands. J.A.D.A., 40:175, 1950.

115. Matt, M. M., Stout, F. W., and Swancar, J. R.: Deposition Curves of In Vivo Calculus Formation. I.A.D.R. Abstracts, 1970, No. 705, p. 225.

116. McCombie, F., and Stothard, D.: Relationship Between Gingivitis and Other Dental Conditions. J. Canad. D. Assn., 30:506, 1964.

117. McDougall, W. A.: Studies on the Dental Plaque. I. The Histology of the Dental Plaque and Its Attachment. Australian D. J., 8:261, 1963.

118. McDougall, W. A.: Studies on the Dental Plaque. II. The Histology of the Developing Interproximal Plaque. Australian D. J., 8:398, 1963.

119. McDougall, W. A.: Studies on the Dental Plaque. IV. Levans and the Dental Plaque. Australian D. J., 9:1, 1964.

120. McHugh, W. D., McEwen, J. D., and Hitchin, A. D.: Dental Disease and Related Factors in 13-year-old Children in Dundee. Brit. D. J., 117:246, 1964.

121. Meckel, A. H.: The Formation and Properties of Organic Films on Teeth. Arch. Oral Biol., 10:585, 1965.

122. Moskow, B. S.: Calculus Attachment in Cemental Separations. J. Periodont., 40:125, 1969.

123. Mühlemann, H. R., and Schneider, U. K.: Early Calculus Formation. Helv. Odont. Acta, 3:22, 1959.

124. Mühlemann, H. R., and Schroeder, H.: Dynamics of Supragingival Calculus Formation. Adv. Oral Biol., 1:175, 1964.

125. Mühlemann, H. R., and Villa, P. R.: The Marginal Line Calculus Index. Helv. Odont. Acta, 11:175, 1967.

126. Muhler, J. C., and Ennever, J.: Occurrence of Calculus Through Several Successive Periods in a Selected Group of Subjects. J. Periodont., 33:22, 1962.

127. Mukherjee, S.: Formation and Prevention of Supragingival Calculus. J. Periodont. Res., Suppl. 2, 1968.

128. Naeslund, C.: A Comparative Study of the Formation of Concretions in the Oral Cavity and in the Salivary Glands and Ducts. D. Cosmos, 68:1137, 1926.

129. Neuman, W. F., and Neuman, M. W.: The Chemical Dynamics of Bone Mineral. Chicago, University of Chicago Press, 1958, p. 209.

130. Niles, E. S.: Odontolithus Influenced by Calcic and Phosphatic Diathesis (Salivary Calculus). D. Cosmos, 23:203, 242, 502, 1881.

131. O'Leary, T. J., Shannon, I. L., and Prigmore, J. R.: Clinical Correlation and Systemic Status in Periodontal Disease. J. Periodont., 33:243, 1962.

132. O'Rourke, J. T.: The Relation of the Physical Character of the Diet to the Health of the Periodontal Tissues. Am. J. Orthodont. & Oral Surg., 33:687, 1947.

133. Oshrain, H. I., Salkind, A., and Mandel, I. D.: Studies of the Histology and Bacteriology of Subgingival Plaque and Calculus. J. Periodont. Res., Suppl. 4, 1969, p. 9.

134. Parfitt, G. J.: A Survey of the Oral Health of Navajo Indian Children. Arch. Oral Biol., 1:193, 1959.

135. Parfitt, G. J.: Summary of the Problem of the Prevention of Periodontal Disease. Ala. J. Med. Sc., 5:395, 1968.

136. Perlitsh, M. J., and Glickman, I.: Salivary Neuraminidase. III. Its Relation to Oral Disease. J. Periodont., 38:189, 1967.

137. Prinz, H.: The Origin of Salivary Calculus. D. Cosmos, 63:231, 369, 503, 619, 1921.

138. Ramfjord, S. P.: The Periodontal Status of Boys 11 to 17 Years Old in Bombay, India. J. Periodont., 32:237, 1961.

139. Ritz, H. L.: Microbial Population Shifts in Developing Human Dental Plaque. Arch. Oral Biol., 12:1561, 1967.

140. Rizzo, A. A., Martin, G. R., Scott, D. B., and Mergenhagen, E. E.: Mineralization of Bacteria. Science, 135:439, 1962.

141. Rizzo, A. A., Scott, D. B., and Bladen, H. A.: Calcification of Oral Bacteria. Ann. New York Acad. Sci., 109:14, 1963.

142. Rolla, G., Kornstad, L., Mathiesen, P., and Povatong, L.: Selective Adsorption of an Acidic Glycoprotein from Human Saliva to Tooth Surfaces. J. Periodont. Res., Suppl. 4, Inter. Conf. Periodont. Res., 8, 1969.

143. Rosebury, T., and Karshan, M.: Salivary Calculus. Dental Science and Dental Art. Philadelphia, Lea & Febiger, 1938.

144. Rowles, S. L.: The Inorganic Composition of Dental Calculus. In Blackwood, H. J. J. (ed.): Bone and Tooth. Oxford, Pergamon Press, 1964, pp. 175–183.

145. Russell, A. L.: International Nutrition Surveys: A Summary of Preliminary Dental Findings. J. D. Res., 42:233, 1963.

146. Russell, A. L., Leatherwood, E. C., Consolazio, C. F., and Van Reen, R.: Periodontal Disease and Nutrition in South Vietnam. J. D. Res., 44:775, 1965.

147. Sandham, H. J., Lopez, H., Zuniga, M. A., and Koulourides, T.: Relation Between Location, Composition and Demineralizing Potential of Dental Plaque. I.A.D.R. Abstracts, 1970, No. 614, p. 202.

148 and 149. Schei, O., Waerhaug, J., Lovdal, A., and Arno, A.: Alveolar Bone Loss as Related to Oral Hygiene and Age. J. Periodont., 30:7, 1959.

150. Schroeder, H. E.: Crystal Morphology and Gross Structures of Mineralizing Plaque and of Calculus. Helv. Odont. Acta, 9:73, 1965.

151. Schroeder, H. E.: Formation and Inhibition of Dental Calculus. Berne, Stuttgart and Vienna, Hans Huber Publ., 1969, pp. 12–15.

152. Schroeder, H. E.: Inorganic Content and Histology of Early Dental Calculus in Man. Helv. Odont. Acta, 7:17, 1963.

153. Schroeder, H. E., and Bambauer, H. U.: Stages of Calcium Phosphate Crystallization During Calculus Formation. Arch. Oral Biol., *11*:1, 1966.

154. Schroeder, H. E., and Marthaler, T.: In Schroeder, H. E.: Formation and Inhibition of Dental Calculus. Berne, Stuttgart, and Vienna, Hans Huber Publ., 1969, p. 22.

155. Schwartz, R. S., and Massler, M.: Tooth Accumulated Materials: A Review and Classification. J. Periodont.-Periodontics, *40*:407, 1969.

156. Selvig, K. A.: The Formation of Plaque and Calculus on Recently Exposed Tooth Surfaces. J. Periodont. Res., Suppl. 4, *4*:10, 1969.

157. Sharawy, A., Sabharwal, K., Socransky, S., and Lobene, R.: A Quantitative Study of Plaque and Calculus Formation in Normal and Periodontally Involved Mouths. J. Periodont., *37*:495, 1966.

158. Silness, J., and Löe, H.: Periodontal Disease in Pregnancy. Acta Odont. Scandinav., *22*:121, 1964.

159. Silverman, G., Kay, M., and Kleinberg, I.: Chemical Binding Between the Macromolecular Constituents of Dental Plaque. I.A.D.R. Abstracts 1965, p. 136.

160. Silverman, G., and Kleinberg, I.: Fractionation of Human Dental Plaque and the Characterization of Its Cellular and Acellular Components. Arch. Oral Biol., *12*:1387, 1967.

161. Simaan, C., and Skach, M.: Clinical and Histological Evaluation of Gingival Massage in the Treatment of Chronic Gingivitis. J. Periodont., *37*:383, 1966.

162. Standford, J. W.: Analysis of the Organic Portion of Dental Calculus. J. D. Res., *45*:128, 1966.

163. Stanton, G.: The Relation of Diet to Salivary Calculus Formation. J. Periodont., *40*:167, 1969.

164. Stewart, R. T., and Ratcliff, P. A.: The Source of Components of Subgingival Plaque and Calculus. Periodont. Abstr., *14*:102, 1966.

165. Stewart, W. H., and Burnett, G. W.: The Relationship of Certain Dietary Factors to Calculus-Like Formation in Albino Rats. J. Periodont., *31*:7, 1960.

166. Theilade, E., Wright, W. H., Jensen, S. B. and Löe, H.: Experimental Gingivitis in Man. II. A Longitudinal Clinical and Bacteriological Investigation. J. Periodont. Res., *1*:1, 1966.

167. Theilade, J.: Electron Microscopic Study of Calculus Attachment to Smooth Surfaces. Acta Odont. Scandinav., *22*:379, 1964.

168. Theilade, J., and Fitzgerald, R. J.: Dental Calculus in the Rat: Effect of Diet and Erythromycin. Acta Odont. Scandinav., *21*:571, 1963.

169. Theilade, J., and Schroeder, H. E.: Recent Results in Dental Calculus Research. Internat. D. J., *16*:205, 1966.

170. Tibbetts, L. S., and Kashiwa, H. K.: A Histochemical Study of Early Plaque Mineralization. I.A.D.R. Abst. 1970, No. 616, p. 202.

171. Turesky, S., et al.: Effects of Changing the Salivary Environment on Progress of Calculus Formation. J. Periodont., *33*:45, 1962.

172. Turesky, S., Gilmore, N. D., and Glickman, I.: Calculus Inhibition by Topical Application of the Chloromethyl Analogue of Victamine C. J. Periodont., *38*:142, 1967.

173. Turesky, S., Gilmore, N. D., and Glickman, I.: Reduced Plaque Formation by the Chloromethyl Analogue of Victamine C. J. Periodont., *41*:41, 1970.

174. Turesky, S., Renstrup, G., and Glickman, I.: Histologic and Histochemical Observations Regarding Early Calculus Formation in Children and Adults. J. Periodont., *32*:7, 1961.

175. Vallotton, C. F.: An Acquired Pigmented Pellicle of the Enamel Surface. J. D. Res., *24*:161, 171, 183, 1945.

176. Volker, J. F., and Pinkerton, D. M.: Acid Production in Saliva-Carbohydrates. J. D. Res., *26*:229, 1947.

177. Volpe, A. R., Kupczak, L. J., and King, W. J.: In Vivo Calculus Assessment: Part III. Scoring Techniques, Rate of Calculus Formation, Partial Mouth Exams. vs. Full Mouth Exams and Intraexaminer Reproducibility. Periodontics, 5:184, 1967.

178. Volpe, A. R., Kupczak, L. J., King, W. J., Goldman, H., and Schulmann, S. M.: In Vivo Calculus Assessment. Part IV. Parameters of Human Clinical Studies. J. Periodont., *40*:76, 1969.

179. Von der Fehr, F., and Brudevold, F.: In Vitro Calculus Formation. J. D. Res., *39*:1041, 1960.

180. Voreadis, E. G., and Zander, H. A.: Cuticular Calculus Attachment. Oral Surg., Oral Med. & Oral Path., *11*:1120, 1958.

181. Waerhaug, J.: Effect of Rough Surfaces Upon Gingival Tissue. J. D. Res., *35*:323, 1956.

182. Waerhaug, J.: The Source of Mineral Salts in Subgingival Calculus. J. D. Res., *34*:563, 1955.

183. Wallace, J. S.: The Newer Knowledge of Hygiene in Diet. J.A.D.A., *18*:1322, 1931.

184. Wasserman, B. H., Mandel, J. D., and Levy, B. M.: In Vitro Calcification of Calculus. J. Periodont., *29*:145, 1958.

185. Weinberger, B. W.: An Introduction to the History of Dentistry. St. Louis, C. V. Mosby Co., 1948, p. 203.

186. Wilkinson, F. C.: A Patho-Histological Study of the Tissue of Tooth Attachment. D. Record, *55*:105, 1935.

187. Wood, J. M., and Critchley, P.: The Extracellular Polysaccharide Produced from Sucrose by a Cariogenic Streptococcus. Arch. Oral Biol., 11: 1039, 1966.

188. World Health Organization: Periodontal Disease: Report of an Expert Committee on Dental Health. Internat. D. J., *11*:544, 1961.

189. Yardeni, J.: Dental Calculus. J. D. Res., *27*:532, 1948.

190. Zander, H. A.: The Attachment of Calculus to Root Surfaces. J. Periodont., *24*:16, 1953.

191. Zander, H. A., Hazen, S. P., and Scott, D. B.: Mineralization of Dental Calculus. Proc. Soc. Exper. Biol. & Med., *103*:257, 1960.

Chapter 23

THE ROLE OF MICROORGANISMS IN THE ETIOLOGY OF GINGIVAL AND PERIODONTAL DISEASE

Microorganisms are important in the etiology of periodontal disease, as initiating, perpetuating or complicating factors. The exact manner in which they participate in the disease process and their relationship to other etiologic factors are under intensive study.*

NORMAL ORAL FLORA

The oral cavity is sterile at birth, but a simple, primarily aerobic flora becomes established within six to ten hours.[12] Anaerobes appear in some mouths within the first ten days, and are present in nearly all by five months of age, before the teeth erupt, and in 100 per cent of mouths when the incisors appear.[58] The anaerobes increase with age but the facultative types remain numerically predominant. Microscopic counts in saliva range from 43 million to 5.5 billion organisms per milliliter, with an average of 750 million.[16] A representative census of the salivary bacterial population is shown in Table 23–1. Also present in healthy mouths are fungi, including Can-

---

*For an analysis of research developments, the reader is referred to the report of the Conference on Specific Questions Related to Periodontal Disease, in the Journal of Dental Research, 49:191, 1970.

TABLE 23-1 INDIGENOUS FLORA OF HUMAN SALIVA*

Bacterial Group	Predominant Isolates of the Group	Percentage
Gram-positive facultative cocci	Streptococci represent 41 per cent of all isolates and are composed of S. salivarius, S. mitis, and small numbers of enterococci; the remainder are staphylococci	46.2
Gram-negative anaerobic cocci	Veillonella	15.9
Gram-positive anaerobic cocci	Peptostreptococcus or Peptococcus	13.0
Gram-positive facultative rods	Diphtheroids	11.8
Gram-negative anaerobic rods	*Vibrio sputorum*, Bacteroides, Fusobacterium	4.8
Gram-positive anaerobic rods	Corynebacterium or propionibacteria, Actinomyces	4.8
Gram-negative facultative rods	Unidentified	2.3
Gram-negative facultative cocci	Unidentified	1.2

*Modified from Gordon, D. F., Jr., and Jong, B. B.: Appl. Microbiol., *16*:428, 1968.

dida, Cryptococcus and Saccharomyces;[8] protozoa such as *Entamoeba gingivalis* and *Trichomonas tenax*;[127] and in some instances viruses.

Most of the salivary bacteria are derived from the dorsum of the tongue, from which they are detached by mechanical action; lesser amounts come from the remainder of the oral mucous membrane. The oral microbial population is relatively constant but varies from patient to patient and at different times in the same area.[57] The number of microorganisms increases temporarily during sleep, and decreases after eating or toothbrushing. The oral flora is also affected by age, diet, composition and rate of flow of saliva, and systemic factors.[69]

THE SALIVA

Because saliva* serves as the culture medium and constant environment of oral microorganisms it affects their metabolic activity and the condition of the oral tissues.

Contents of the saliva

The saliva (pH 6.2 to 7.4) is 99.5 per cent water and 0.5 per cent organic and inorganic solids. Its composition is described in detail by Jenkins.[59] In addition to ingested foods, the principal organic components are proteins in the form of glycoproteins (see Chap. 22). Serum albumin, gamma globulins, and carbohydrates derived principally from the glycoproteins are also present. The principal inorganic components are calcium, phosphorus, sodium, potassium and magnesium, plus traces of numerous other elements. Saliva also contains the gases carbon dioxide, oxygen and nitrogen in solution and a bicarbonate buffering system.

SALIVARY ENZYMES. The enzymes normally found in the saliva[19] (Table 23–2) are derived from the salivary glands, bacteria, leukocytes, oral tissues and ingested substances. Certain salivary enzymes are increased in periodontal disease; they are hyaluronidase and lipase,[76] β-glucuronidase and chondroitin sulfatase,[108] amino acid decarboxylases,[47] catalase and peroxidase[72] and collagenase.[26, 103]

ANTIBACTERIAL FACTORS. Saliva contains antibacterial factors such as lysozyme[62] which exerts a lytic effect on micrococci and sarcinae, enzymes effective against lysozyme-resistant organisms[64] and against most transient organisms,[11] and an enzyme[86] that hydrolyzes mucopolysaccharides and may affect organisms such as Pneumococcus. Factors which inhibit growth of diphtheria bacilli ("inhibin")[29] and *Lactobacillus casei*[27] and *mutines*, which render some pathogenic organisms nonpathogenic,

---

*A comprehensive review of the literature dealing with saliva has been prepared by Afonsky.[1]

have also been described. Systemically administered antibiotics may also be secreted into the saliva.[128] Parotid secretion contains antibodies against indigenous oral bacteria,[71] and saliva also contains *gamma globulins* capable of antibody activity.[70]

COAGULATION FACTORS. Several factors (VIII, IX, X, PTA and the Hageman factor) that hasten blood coagulation and protect wounds from bacterial invasion have been identified[28] in saliva, and the presence of an active fibrinolytic enzyme has been suggested.[123]

VITAMINS. Thiamine, riboflavin, niacin, pyridoxine, pantothenic acid, biotin, folic acid, and vitamin B_{12}[30] are the principal vitamins found in saliva; vitamin C and vitamin K[67] have also been reported. Suggested sources of the vitamins are microbial synthesis and secretion by salivary glands, food

debris, degenerating leukocytes and exfoliated epithelial cells.

LEUKOCYTES. In addition to desquamated epithelial cells, the saliva contains all forms of leukocytes, of which the principal cells are the polymorphonuclear granulocytes. The number of leukocytes varies from person to person and at different times of the day, and is increased in gingivitis. They reach the oral cavity by migrating through the lining of the gingival sulcus. Living polymorphonuclear granulocytes in saliva are sometimes referred to as *orogranulocytes (OGC's)*, and their rate of migration into the oral cavity as the *orogranulocytic migratory rate (OMR)*. Some feel that the rate of migration is correlated with the severity of gingival inflammation and is therefore a reliable index for assessing gingivitis;[114] others disagree.[104]

TABLE 23–2 SALIVARY ENZYMES AND THEIR SOURCES*

| Enzyme | Source Indicated by X | | |
	Glands	Microorganisms	Leukocytes
Carbohydrases			
Amylase	X	—	—
Maltase	—	X	X
Invertase	—	X	—
Beta-glucuronidase	X	X	X
Beta-D-galactosidase	—	X	X
Beta-D-glucosidase	—	X	—
Lysozyme	X	—	X
Hyaluronidase	—	X	—
Mucinase	—	X	—
Esterases			
Acid phosphatase	X	X	X
Alkaline phosphatase	X	X	X
Hexosediphosphatase	—	X	—
Aliesterase	X	X	X
Lipase	X	X	X
Acetylcholinesterase	X	—	X
Pseudo-cholinesterase	X	X	X
Chondrosulfatase	—	X	—
Arylsulfatase	—	X	—
Transferring enzymes			
Catalase	—	X	—
Peroxidase	X	—	X
Phenyloxidase	—	X	—
Succinic dehydrogenase	X	X	X
Hexokinase	—	X	X
Proteolytic enzymes			
Proteinase	—	X	X
Peptidase	—	X	X
Urease	—	X	—
Other enzymes			
Carbonic anhydrase	X	—	—
Pyrophosphatase	—	X	—
Aldolase	X	X	X

*From Chauncey, H. H.: J.A.D.A., 63:360, 1961.

MICROORGANISMS IN GINGIVAL AND PERIODONTAL DISEASE

Periodontal health is maintained by a symbiotic balance among the oral microorganisms and between the organisms and the host. The organisms live in a state of parasitism with the human host and ordinarily produce no pathologic changes, but they have the potential to cause disease.

Disease results from a disturbance of the balance (1) among the bacteria or (2) between the bacteria and the host, or from both conditions. Disturbance of the symbiotic balance among the microorganisms leads to mucosal disease if it produces an overwhelming overgrowth of a single pathogenic organism. For example, in patients under prolonged antibiotic therapy the growth of many bacteria is depressed, but the nonsensitive fungus *Candida albicans* proliferates and produces oral moniliasis.

The balance between micoorganisms and the host is disturbed by an increase in the number and virulence of bacteria or a decrease in host resistance or both. *Dental plaque concentrates bacteria and their products in the gingival area and shifts the balance in favor of the organisms.* Irritants other than bacteria, such as food impaction and mechanical, chemical and thermal extremes, injure the gingiva and lower the resistance to infection. They also cause gingival inflammation, which deepens the gingival sulcus and provides a protected environment for the concentration of bacteria and their products.

Resistance factors in the gingival area

The resistance of the gingiva to microbial infection is affected by local and systemic factors. Brandtzaeg[13] divides the local factors into two groups, as follows:*

GROUP 1. PHYSICAL AND BIOCHEMICAL GINGIVAL RESISTANCE FACTORS

1. *The crestal and outer epithelium of the marginal gingiva is thick and keratinized or parakeratinized* and is a barrier against bacteria and their products.

2. *Renewal of the sulcal epithelium acts as a self-cleansing mechanism.*[115] Continuous outward migration and desquamation of

the sulcal epithelium at the orifice removes bacteria which are attached to the surface epithelial cells.

3. *Sulcal epithelium produces plasma proteins which help maintain adhesion to the tooth.* The epithelium of the gingival sulcus is thin and acts as a semipermeable membrane of little protective value. Its vulnerability to bacteria is reduced by adhesion to the tooth, which is aided by plasma proteins produced by the sulcal epithelium,[120] and by pressure from gingival fibers and pressure in the blood vessels. Proteolytic enzymes, particularly proteases,[111] produced by bacteria or by disintegrating leukocytes, destroy plasma proteins and reduce adhesion and cause detachment of the epithelium. Plasma proteins produced by the sulcal epithelium and also contained in the gingival fluid renew the epithelial adhesion.

4. *Flow of gingival fluid washes particulate matter from the sulcus and dilutes injurious substances.* It contains the enzyme lysozyme which has a lytic effect on bacterial cell walls. Disintegration of leukocytes may be the source of lysozyme in the gingival fluid and in the gingival tissue. Gingival fluid also contains a fibrinolytic enzyme system[49] which may be protective. As the gingival fluid is increased in inflammation,[15, 54] its contribution to local resistance increases.

5. *Saliva exerts a protective effect by cleansing bacteria from the gingival surface and by the antibacterial factors it contains (see page 316).*

6. *The indigenous oral flora may protect the gingiva against infection by specific antagonisms against exogenous bacteria which make it difficult for them to survive.*[99]

GROUP II. IMMUNOLOGIC AND PHAGOCYTIC GINGIVAL RESISTANCE FACTORS

A local immune reaction protects the periodontium against bacteria and their products. Antibodies are resistance factors formed by the host in response to specific foreign substances called antigens, several of which are contained in oral bacteria and their products. The three main groups of serum proteins which may act as antibodies and are called immunoglobulins are γG-, γA- and γM-globulins.*

Antibodies against antigens of plaque and

---

*For an extensive discussion of this subject the reader is referred to Brandtzaeg's presentation.[13]

*Also designated as IgG, IgA and IgM.

sulcal bacteria are released in the gingiva by plasma cells,[14, 25] which are the predominant cells in chronic inflammation, and by lymphocytes. Immunoglobulins are also present in the serum and gingival fluid in approximate ratios of 12:4:1, and in lower concentrations and different proportions in the saliva.[12]

The local gingival immune response activates inflammation, which is also important to resistance against bacteria. It attracts polymorphonuclear leukocytes which phagocytize antigenic material, immunologically competent cells (lymphocytes which initiate a specific immune response), and macrophages which digest disintegrated polymorphonuclear leukocytes and antigenic material; increases capillary permeability and the exudation of plasma and gingival fluid; concentrates serum immune factors and antibodies; and forms a fibrin meshwork[14] which limits bacterial invasion, provides pathways for migration of polymorphonuclear leukocytes and facilitates the entrapment and the phagocytosis of bacteria.

SYSTEMIC CONDITIONS WHICH AFFECT HOST RESISTANCE. Systemic conditions, such as starvation, malnutrition, severe vitamin deficiency, and debilitating disease, impair local tissue metabolism and reduce gingival resistance to infection. Leukopenia reduces the availability of antibody formation and phagocytic cells which combat bacteria; and oral fusopirochetal organisms are increased in vitamin C and vitamin B deficiencies.[18] Agammaglobulinemia prevents the host from protecting itself against invading antigens.[98]

Bacteria in the normal gingival sulcus

The composition of the normal sulcus flora is presented in Table 23–3.[118] The concentration of bacteria in the gingival sulcus and dental plaque is much greater than in saliva, but these areas contribute only a minute portion of the total salivary count.[48] The percentage distribution of bacteria in the sulcus and plaque differs from that in the saliva.[41] *Bacteroides melaninogenicus* constitute 4.5 per cent of the cultivable bacteria in the sulcus, 0.42 per cent in the saliva and 0.32 per cent in plaque. *Streptococcus salivarius*, the predominant organism on the tongue, repre-

sents only 0.47 per cent of the cultivable bacteria in the sulcus, and 0.67 per cent in the plaque.[41]

The debris found in the area of the normal gingival sulcus consists almost entirely of bacteria, with a total microscopic count of approximately 1.7×10^{11} organisms per wet weight gram of sulcus contents. The majority of organisms are anaerobes, with an average total viable count of 4×10^{10}, as compared with 1.6×10^{10} of aerobic organisms.[*43, 119]

Bacteria in diseased periodontal pockets

The total number of organisms in diseased periodontal pockets is greater than in normal gingival sulci. However, the types of bacteria and their relative percentages are not significantly altered, except for a slight relative increase in spirochetes,[24, 39, 43, 66, 119] and possibly gram-negative cocci.[109] Despite the differences in the clinical features of chronic gingivitis and acute necrotizing ulcerative gingivitis (see Chap. 11), their bacterial flora is the same.[101, 102]

EVIDENCE IN SUPPORT OF THE ROLE OF BACTERIA IN THE ETIOLOGY OF PERIODONTAL DISEASE

Socransky[118] has documented the following facts which strongly support a significant bacterial role in the etiology of gingival and periodontal disease:

1. Topical or systemic antibiotics alleviate the severity of acute necrotizing ulcerative gingivitis and reduce gingival exudation in humans.

2. Dietary antibiotics reduce periodontal inflammation and bone destruction in animals. The severity of gingivitis is correlated with the amount of gingival debris which consists almost entirely of bacteria.

3. Cessation of toothbrushing and the resultant accumulation of bacterial plaque leads to gingivitis, which disappears when the plaque is removed.

4. Mechanical irritants such as overhanging fillings and rough surfaces in contact

---

*Using a technique which limited the cultivable organisms to 25 per cent of the total number observed microscopically.[118]

TABLE 23–3 ORGANISMS OF THE HUMAN GINGIVAL CREVICE REGION[*]

Group	Approximate Percentage of Cultivable Microbiota	Genera and/or Species Commonly Found in this Site
Gram-positive facultative cocci	28.8	Staphylococci Enterococci S. mutans S. sanguis "S. mitis"
Gram-positive anaerobic cocci	7.4	Peptostreptococcus
Gram-positive facultative rods	15.3	Corynebacterium Lactobacillus Nocardia O. viscosus B. matruchotii
Gram-positive anaerobic rods	20.2	A. bifidus A. israeli A. naeslundi A. odontolyticus P. acnes L. buccalis Corynebacterium
Gram-negative facultative cocci	0.4	Neisseria
Gram-negative anaerobic cocci	10.7	V. alcalescens V. parvula
Gram-negative facultative rods	1.2	
Gram-negative anaerobic rods	16.1	B. melaninogenicus B. oralis V. sputorum F. nucleatum S. sputigenum
Spiral organisms	1 to 3	T. denticola T. oralis T. macrodentium B. vincentii

[*]From Socransky, S. S.: J. D. Res., 49:203, 1970.

with the gingiva produce little or no inflammation until bacterial plaque accumulates around them.

5. Calculus which forms in germ-free animals generally does not create gingival inflammation, pockets or bone loss, which are produced by introducing bacteria in the absence of calculus. Silk sutures inserted interdentally in germ-free animals produces little change, but inflammatory periodontal disease results when bacteria are added.

Periodontal bone loss occurs in germ-free animals,[6] but its rate is accelerated by the introduction of a mixture of gingival bacteria.[42]

Pure cultures of certain human oral streptococci[40] and gram-positive rods (*Odontomyces viscosus*) initiate a periodontal syndrome in germ-free animals, and periodontal disease is transmissible by bacterial transfer in experimental animals.[65]

Pathogenicity of oral microorganisms

Bacteria indigenous to the gingival sulcus and their products are potentially pathogenic in that they result in infection when introduced in experimental animals, and human bites cause infection in man. Exudates[56, 80, 102] or gingival scrapings from the lesions of periodontal disease, inoculated subcutaneously into rabbits or guinea pigs, induce necrotic lesions which are serially transmissible in animals. A mixture of fusiform and spirochetal organisms of the original flora persists through the repeated transfers. The fusospirochetal complex has also been identified in human bite wounds,[81] lung abscesses[92] and tropical ulcer.[2,117]

A group of four oral organisms has been isolated that can produce transmissible subcutaneous abscesses in animals.[78] This group consists of two *Bacteroides* species, one of which is *B. melaninogenicus* and the other unidentified, a motile gram-negative anaerobic bacillus, and a facultative diphtheroid. Together they produce collagenase, fibrinolysin, deoxyribonuclease and ribonuclease.[79]

MECHANISMS WHEREBY MICROORGANISMS MAY CAUSE GINGIVAL AND PERIODONTAL DISEASE

The disease-producing potential of oral bacteria and their products has been demonstrated, but the manner in which they cause gingival and periodontal disease is still hypothetical. Among the many possible mechanisms are the following:

Bacterial invasion

Bacteria are present in the gingiva in acute necrotizing ulcerative gingivitis,[77] but though opinions differ, it is the consensus that they do not penetrate the tissues in chronic gingivitis.[36,50,106,121,129] Bacterial products appear to be more important than the bacteria themselves in causing inflammation.[79]

Enzymes

Bacteria in plaque and in the area of the gingival sulcus produce many enzymes—some of them listed in Table 23–4—which are potentially destructive or can act as spreading factors for infection and injurious agents.[107] Many of the components of the gingiva (see Chap. 1) are substrates for these enzymes, but the initiation of periodontal disease by the interaction of bacterial enzymes with gingival substrate has not been demonstrated.[124]

Hyaluronidase introduced experimentally into the gingiva causes disruption and edema of the connective tissue and proliferation of epithelium,[1a,87,110] but does not produce inflammation.[23] There appears to

TABLE 23–4*

Bacteria	Enzyme(s) Produced	Substrate
Staphylococci	Hyaluronidase	Hyaluronic acid
	Coagulase	Clotting of plasma
	Gelatinase	Gelatine
	Hemolysins	Erythrocytes
Streptococci	Hyaluronidase	Hyaluronic acid
	Streptokinase	Fibrin, fibrinogen
	Hemolysins	Erythrocytes
	B-glucuronidase	Glucuronidic linkages
	Proteases	Various proteins
Diphtheroids	Hyaluronidase	Hyaluronic acid
	Chondroitinase	Chondroitin sulfate
Fusobacteria	Protease(s)	Various proteins
	Sulfatase	Aryl sulfates
B. melaninogenicus	Collagenase	Reconstituted collagen
Spirochetes	Protease(s)	Various proteins
Gram-negative cocci	Protease(s)	Various proteins

*From Schultz-Haudt, S. D.: Internatl. D. J., *14*:398, 1964.

be no difference in the hyaluronidase content of gingival debris from "normal" and "periodontally diseased" subjects.[22]

Collagenase, produced by *Bacteroides melaninogenicus*, is also formed by and present in normal gingiva (in slight amounts) and chronically and acutely inflamed gingiva (in greater amounts).[38] By enzymatic digestion of collagen, collagenase causes hemorrhage of gingival vessels, particularly small arterioles.[35]

Plasma cells which are abundant in inflamed gingiva and provide antibodies also produce large quantities of acid hydrolases, specifically acid phosphatase, esterase, aminopeptidase, aryl sulfatase and beta glucuronidase, which could be significant in the breakdown of gingival tissues.[23]

Lysosomes contained within bacteria and leukocytes[122] are liberated upon their destruction and are potentially injurious to the periodontal tissues.[51]

Endotoxins

Endotoxins are lipopolysaccharide-protein complexes in the cell walls of numerous strains of gram-negative oral bacteria which are released upon their destruction. Endotoxins are injurious to periodontal tissues and cause inflammation, possibly by activating a local immune reaction. In experimental animals, endotoxins cause necrosis of oral mucosa and bone in previously sensitized areas (Shwartzman phenomenon),[60, 83, 96] and they depress bone growth in tissue culture.[90]

Endotoxins are present in saliva[131] and in bacteria in the gingival sulcus and plaque.[43, 82, 84] The endotoxin activity of saliva and gingival debris[131] and the level of antibodies to oral endotoxin are higher in periodontal disease than in periodontal health.[31] The endotoxin content of the gingival sulcus is correlated with the severity of gingival inflammation.[113] Endotoxins from oral bacteria appear to penetrate damaged or ulcerated gingival epithelium rather than intact surfaces, suggesting a secondary rather than initiating role in gingival disease.[94]

Toxins

It has been suggested that gingivitis is caused by toxins formed by bacteria[33] and by degeneration of surface epithelial cells.[93] However, no *exotoxins* have been demonstrated in the oral cavity except in association with specific infectious diseases such as diphtheria.

Spirochetes, vibrios, fusiforms, Veillonella and some bacteroides (not *B. melaninogenicus*),[95] anaerobic bacteria commonly found in periodontal pockets, are capable of producing hydrogen sulfide, which is caustic and can cause tissue necrosis. It is absent in normal sulci but is common in the apical areas of deep pockets associated with increased inflammation. Oral bacteria also produce ammonia, a potential irritant which has been associated with periodontal disease.[37]

Local immune reaction*

Components of oral bacteria and their products may act as antigens which elicit a

---

*For additional information on this subject the reader is referred to the Proceedings of the Conference on the Implications of Immune Reactions in the Pathogenesis of Periodontal Disease, published in J. Periodont., *41*:195, 1970.

local immune reaction in the gingiva. The purpose of the immune reaction is primarily protective, but because it can also trigger a local inflammatory response, it may be a factor in the development of gingivitis.[10, 85] Inflammation adds to local resistance (see page 319), but it also causes periodontal damage. Vascular stasis in gingival inflammation impairs the tissue nutrition and increases susceptibility to infection. The inflammatory fluid and cellular exudate cause degeneration of gingival epithelium and connective tissue, and prolongation of the inflammation leads to periodontitis with pocket formation and bone resorption.

It has not been established that bacterial antigens cause periodontal disease, but there is considerable evidence of immunologic responses in diseased periodontal tissues. Immunoglobulins and specific antibodies to oral bacterial antigens are present in inflammatory cells and tissues in gingivitis.[105, 125] Plasma cells and to a lesser extent lymphocytes, which are the predominant types in chronic gingivitis,[25] are antibody-producing cells. Antigens produced by *Streptococcus mitis* are present in gingivitis, but not in healthy gingiva.[130] The serum antibody level to Fusobacterium is elevated in patients with periodontal disease[32] (not correlated with disease severity),[73] and circulating antibodies are produced in response to endotoxin extracts from *Bacteroides melaninogenicus*.[21]

Bacterial allergy

Allergy (hypersensitivity) is a "specific acquired, usually deleterious reactivity of an individual to a substance which in similar amounts does not provoke a similar reaction in the majority of the previously unexposed members of the same species."[17] The possibility that an immediate or delayed allergic response is a factor in gingival inflammation is suggested by the following findings: the presence of localized eosinophilia in some cases of gingivitis[55, 91] (not confirmed by other investigators),[75] the demonstration in humans of hypersensitivity to antigens of plaque bacteria,[88] and the production of chronic allergic inflammation by sensitizing the gingiva of experimental animals with ovalbumin.[97]

The possibility that autoimmunity, sensitization to components of the host's own tissues, might be a complicating etiologic factor in periodontal disease has been explored, without positive results.[14]

Viruses in the etiology of gingival and periodontal disease

Viruses cause acute herpetic gingivostomatitis (page 138) and other oral infections (page 175), but they have not been associated with chronic gingival and periodontal disease in humans. The following periodontal changes have been described in experimental animals inoculated with viruses: developmental abnormalities;[3] intranuclear inclusion bodies in fibroblasts of the periodontal ligament; nuclear fragmentation, and fragmentation and complete absence of principal fibers; absence of supporting bone; round cell infiltration in periodontal space; root resorption; ankylosis (rat virus);[4] alveolar bone loss and apical migration of the epithelial attachment (rat virus);[5] noninflammatory degeneration of the periodontium, resembling periodontosis (polyoma virus);[34] severe periodontal disease with suppurating periodontal pockets; and extensive resorption of alveolar bone (polyoma virus).[112]

HISTORICAL BACKGROUND REGARDING THE ETIOLOGIC ROLE OF ORAL MICROORGANISMS

Early observations regarding the bacteriology of periodontal disease are presented here as background information for the interpretation of recent developments.

One of the earliest complete studies of the bacterial flora associated with periodontal disease was performed by Goadby.[46] He found various streptococci, *Bacillus fusiformis* and spirochetes, and a great number of other organisms. His conclusion was that lowered resistance resulting from insufficient production of substances immune to the oral flora was the primary factor in the etiology of the disease. He was interested in autogenous vaccines made from the organisms of the periodontal lesions to assist in curing the disease. Glynn[45] considered the nonhemolytic streptococci to be the chief pathogenic aerobic organisms in periodontal infections. According to Hart-

zell,[53] the leading role in the etiology of periodontal disease was played by the streptococci, which, being the first to penetrate the tissues and create the initial lesion, prepared the way for other organisms.

Another early investigator of the bacteria in pathologic pockets was Noguchi.[89] He isolated in pure culture the particular spirochete, which he called *Treponema mucosum*, from the exudate in periodontal pockets. The organisms apparently thrived on injured or impaired tissue but did not grow on healthy or intact tissue. He also recognized the presence in chronic periodontal disease of streptococci, staphylococci, and pneumococci, but believed that specific oral spirochetes were directly responsible for the disease. He also noted the presence of other spiral forms, as well as the fusiform bacillus. Since Noguchi was one of the first bacteriologists to perfect techniques for the cultivation of spirochetes, he tended to place much emphasis upon their presence. Actually, Leeuwenhoek, in the late seventeenth century, was the first to record the existence of oral spirochetes. The discovery of the oral spirochetes was the initial step in the development of the field of general bacteriology.

Kritchevsky and Séguin[74] recovered spirochetal forms of bacteria from every case of chronic destructive periodontal disease that they studied. Considering the bacteria a possible cause, they treated their cases with intravenous salvarsan, but obtained only temporary results unless careful scaling of the teeth was included in the treatment. They assumed that the spirochetes were secondary invaders because they flourished in the debris and microaerophilic environment of the periodontal pocket. Hemmens and Harrison[56] found little difference between the bacterial flora of normal gingiva and of suppurative lesions. They believed bacteria in periodontal disease to be secondary invaders, possibly responsible for the suppurative phase. Smith,[116] however, concluded that *Treponema microdentium* and the fusiform bacillus, as well as anaerobic streptococcus and the vibrio, could together cause suppurative periodontal disease in the absence of any other factors. Tunnicliff et al.[126] found that a combination of fusiform bacilli and spirilla became pathogenic when the vitality of the tissue was impaired. Gins[44] believed that all gingival disease was caused by spirilla and should therefore be designated "spirillosis."

At one time there was considerable interest in the amebae as causative factors in periodontal disease. Barrett[7] and Bass and Johns[9] considered *Entamoeba gingivalis* and *E. buccalis* of such etiologic significance that they recommended the amebicide emetine for the treatment of periodontal disease. Glynn[45] found the ameba *E. buccalis* abundant in mouths with poor oral hygiene. It was present in periodontal pockets, but not consistently so. It was not found in healthy periodontal tissues, and emetine had no effect upon it. Hartzell[52] also studied the use of emetine in the treatment of periodontal disease and became convinced of its uselessness. Keilty[63] found *E. gingivalis* present in direct smears in 95.5 per cent of 201 cases of destructive periodontal disease, and absent in control cases. He concluded that it is a harmless parasite. Jirovec[61] demonstrated amebae and trichomonads in periodontal disease but considered them of no pathogenic significance.

Conant and Rosebury[20] discussed the presence of actinomycetes in the oral cavity and Rosebury[100] reviewed the subject in considerable detail. These are a varied group of filamentous microorganisms with characteristics between bacteria and molds. They are found in the normal gingival sulcus and in calculus. *Actinomyces bovis* is a true parasite of mucous membrane and occurs in the presence of low-grade, nonspecific, inflammatory processes in the gingiva. The accepted concept is that it may produce disease as an endogenous infection, comparable with *S. viridans* in endocarditis or *E. coli* in cystitis. The disease, however, is not periodontal disease but actinomycosis.

REFERENCES

1. Afonsky, D.: Saliva and Its Relation to Oral Health. Univ. of Alabama Press, 1961.
1a. Aisenberg, M. S., and Aisenberg, A. D.: Hyaluronidase in Periodontal Disease. Oral Surg., Oral Med. & Oral Path., 4:317, 1951.
2. Apostoleides, A. G.: Note on the Recent Epidemic of Tropical Septic Ulcer in Palestine (Tropical Sloughing Phagedena). J. Trop. Med. & Hyg., 25:81, 1922.
3. Baer, P. N., and Kilham, L.: A Comparison of the Effects of Four Viruses on the Periodontium of the Syrian Hamster. J. Periodont., 36:127, 1965.
4. Baer, P. N., and Kilham, L.: Rat Virus and Periodontal Disease. III. The Histopathology of the Early Lesion in the First Molar. Oral Surg., Oral Med. & Oral Path., 17:116, 1964.
5. Baer, P. N., and Kilham, L.: Rat Virus and Periodontal Disease. IV. The Aged Hamster. Oral Surg., Oral Med. & Oral Path., 18:803, 1964.
6. Baer, P. N., and Newton, W. L.: Studies on Periodontal Disease in the Mouse: III. The Germfree Mouse and Its Conventional Control. Oral Surg., Oral Med. & Oral Path., 13:1134, 1960.
7. Barrett, M. T.: Clinical Report upon Amoebic Pyorrhea. D. Cosmos, 56:1345, 1914.
8. Bartels, H. A., and Blechman, H.: Survey of the Yeast Population in Saliva and an Evaluation of Some Procedures for Identification of Candida Albicans, J. D. Res., 41:1386, 1962.
9. Bass, C. C., and Johns, M.: Pyorrhea Dentalis and Alveolaris—Specific Cause and Treatment. J.A.M.A., 64:553, 1915.
10. Berglund, S. E.: Introduction to Conference on the Implications of Immune Reactions in the Pathogenesis of Periodontal Disease. J. Periodont., 41:195, 1970.
11. Bibby, B. G., Van Kesteren, M., and Berry, G. P.: Antibacterial Factors in Saliva. J. Bact., 43:573, 1942.
12. Brandtzaeg, P.: Immunochemical Comparison of Proteins in Human Gingival Pocket Fluid, Serum and Saliva. Arch. Oral Biol., 10:795, 1965.
13. Brandtzaeg, P.: Local Factors of Resistance in the Gingival Area. J. Periodont. Res., 1:19, 1966.
14. Brandtzaeg, P., and Kraus, F. W.: Autoimmunity and Periodontal Disease. Odont. T., 73:285, 1965.
15. Brill, N.: The Gingival Pocket Fluid. Studies of its Occurrence, Composition, and Effect. Acta Odont. Scandinav., 20: Suppl. 32, 1962.
16. Burnett, G. W., and Scherp, H. W.: Oral Microbiology and Infectious Disease. 3rd ed. Baltimore, Williams and Wilkins Co., 1968, Chapter 20.
17. Burnett, G. W., and Scherp, H. W.: Oral Microbiology and Infectious Disease. 3rd ed. Baltimore, Williams and Wilkins Co., 1968, p. 255.
18. Chapman, O. D., and Harris, A. E.: Oral Lesions and Dietary Deficiencies in Monkeys. J. Inf. Dis., 69:7, 1941.
19. Chauncey, H. H.: Salivary Enzymes. J.A.D.A., 63:360, 1961.
20. Conant, N. F., and Rosebury, T.: The Actinomycetes. In Dubois, R.: Bacterial and Mycotic Infections of Man. Philadelphia, J. B. Lippincott Co., 1948.
21. Courant, P. R., and Gibbons, R. J.: Studies on the Immunology of *Bacteroides melaninogenicus*. I.A.D.R. Abstr., No. 153, 1966.
22. Courant, P. R., Paunio, I., and Gibbons, R. J.: Infectivity and Hyaluronidase Activity of Debris from Healthy and Diseased Gingiva. Arch. Oral Biol., 10:119, 1965.
23. Cowley, G. C.: The Initiation of Gingival Inflammation. J. Periodont. Res., 4:21, Suppl. No. 4, 1969.
24. Crawley, M. C., Beppler, W. A., and Ramfjord, S. P.: The Bacterial Flora of the Normal Gingival Sulcus. J. Periodont., 35:502, 1964.
25. Dalbow, M. H., Thonard, J. C., Crosby, R. C., and Beutner, H. E.: Immune Response to Intragingival Antigenic Stimulation Detected by Im-

munofluorescence. I.A.D.R. Abstr., No. 270, Gen. Meeting, 1965, p. 104.

26. Dewar, M. R.: Bacterial Enzymes and Periodontal Disease. J. D. Res., 37:100, 1958.

27. Dogon, I. L., Kerr, A. C., and Amdur, B. H.: Characterization of an Antibacterial Factor in Human Parotid Secretions, Active Against Lactobacillus Casei. Arch. Oral Biol., 7:81, 1962.

28. Doku, H. C., and Taylor, R. G.: Thromboplastin Generation by Saliva. Oral Surg., Oral Med. & Oral Path., 15:1295, 1962.

29. Dold, H., and Weigmann, F.: Ueber die Wirkung des Menschlichen Speichels auf Diphtheriebacillen. Ztschr. f. Hyg. Infektionskr., 116:158, 1934.

30. Dreizen, S., and Hampton, J. K., Jr.: Radioisotopic Studies of the Glandular Contribution of Selected B Vitamins in Saliva. J. D. Res., 48:579, 1969.

31. Evans, R. T., and Mergenhagen, S. W.: Occurrence of Natural Antibacterial Antibody in Human Parotid Fluid. Proc. Soc. Exper. Biol., 119:815, 1965.

32. Evans, R. T., Spaeth, S., and Mergenhagen, S. E.: Bacterial Antibody in Mammalian Serum to Obligatorily Anaerobic Gram-Negative Bacteria. J. Immunology, 97:112, 1966.

33. Fish, E. W.: Surgical Pathology of the Mouth. London, Sir Isaac Pitman & Sons, 1948, p. 306.

34. Fleming, H. S., and Soni, N. N.: S.E. Polyoma Virus and the Periodontium. Periodontics, 2:115, 1964.

35. Folke, L. E. A.: Microvascular Effects of Collagenase. J. Periodont. Res., 4:29, Suppl. 4, 1969.

36. Freedman, H. L., Listgarten, M. A., and Taichman, N. S.: Electron Microscopic Features of Chronically Inflamed Human Gingiva. J. Periodont. Res., 3:313, 1968.

37. Frostell, G.: Studies in Oral Biochemical Bacteriology. Acta Odont. Scandinav., 18(Suppl. 29): 7, 1960.

38. Fullmer, H. M., Baer, P., and Driscoll, E.: Correlation of Collagenase Production to Periodontal Disease. J. Periodont. Res., 4:30, Suppl. 4, 1969.

39. Gibbons, R. J.: Some Aspects of the Bacteriology of Periodontal Disease. Internat. D. J., 14: 407, 1964.

40. Gibbons, R. J., Berman, K. S., Knoettner, P., and Kapsimalis, B.: Dental Caries and Alveolar Bone Loss in Gnotobiotic Rats Infected with Capsule Forming Streptococci of Human Origin. Arch. Oral Biol., 11:549, 1966.

41. Gibbons, R. J., Kapsimalis, B., and Socransky, S. S.: The Source of Salivary Bacteria. Arch. Oral Biol., 9:101, 1964.

42. Gibbons, R. J., and Socransky, S. S.: Enhancement of Alveolar Bone Loss in Gnotobiotic Mice Harbouring Human Gingival Bacteria. Arch. Oral Biol., 11:847, 1966.

43. Gibbons, R. J., Socransky, S. S., Sawyer, S., Kapsimalis, B., and Macdonald, J. B.: The Microbiota of the Gingival Crevice Areas of Man. II. The Predominant Cultivable Organisms. Arch. Oral Biol., 8:281, 1963.

44. Gins, H. A.: The Significance of Spirillosis for the Pathogenesis of the Periodontal Disturbances. Deutsche Zahnärzt. Ztschr., 2:282, 1947.

45. Glynn, E. E.: The Organisms Found in Periodontal Infections and Their Relations to the Toxemia. Brit. D. J., 44:601, 1923.

46. Goadby, K.: Diseases of the Gums and Oral Mucous Membrane. New York, Oxford University Press, 1928.

47. Gochman, N., Meyer, R. K., Blackwell, R. Q., and Fosdick, L. S.: The Amino Acid Decarboxylase of Salivary Sediment. J. D. Res., 38:998, 1959.

48. Gordon, D. F., Jr., and Jong, B. B.: Indigenous Flora from Human Saliva. Appl. Microbiol., 16:428, 1968.

49. Gustafsson, G. T., and Nilsson, I. M.: Fibronolytic Activity in Fluid from Gingival Crevice. Proc. Soc. Exp. Biol., 106:277, 1961.

50. Haberman, S.: Inflammatory and Non-Inflammatory Responses to Gingival Invasions by Microorganisms. J. Periodont., 30:190, 1959.

51. Hampp, S., and Folke, L.: The Lysosomes and Their Possible Role in Periodontal Disease. Odont. T., 76:353, 1968.

52. Hartzell, T. B.: The Use of Emetine in the Treatment of Periodontal Disease. J. Allied D. Soc., 2:143, 1915.

53. Hartzell, T. B.: Etiology of Pyorrhea Alveolaris with Simplified Treatment. J.A.D.A., 12:1452, 1925.

54. Harvey, P. M.: Elimination of Extraneous Material from the Gingival Crevice. J. Periodont., 33:231, 1962.

55. Healy, J. C., Daley, F. H., and Sweet, M. H.: Medical Aspects of Periodontoclasia and Gingivitis. J. Lab. & Clin. Med., 21:698, 1936.

56. Hemmens, E. S., and Harrison, R. W.: Studies on the Anaerobic Bacterial Flora of Suppurative Periodontitis. J. Infect. Dis., 70:131, 1942.

57. Hine, M. K., and Bibby, B. G.: Variations in the Oral Flora from Time to Time. J. D. Res., 18:61, 1939.

58. Hurst, V.: Fusiforms in the Infant Mouth. J. D. Res., 36:513, 1957.

59. Jenkins, G. N.: The Physiology of the Mouth. 3rd ed. Philadelphia, F. A. Davis Co., 1966, pp. 288–357.

60. Jensen, S. B., Jackson, F. V., and Mergenhagen, S. W.: Alterations in Type and Bactericidal Activity of Mouse Peritoneal Phagocytes After Intraperitoneal Administration of Endotoxin. Acta Odont., 22:71, 1964.

61. Jirovec, O.: Contribution à la microbiologie de la cavité buccale humaine. Paradontologie, 2:117, 1948.

62. Jolles, P., and Petit, J. F.: Purification and Analysis of Human Saliva Lysozyme. Nature, 200:168, 1963.

63. Keilty, R. A.: Focal Infection. A Bacteriological Study of the Gums in 200 Cases. J. Med. Res., 43:377, 1922.

64. Kerr, A. C., and Wedderburn, D. L.: Antibacterial Factors in the Secretions of Human Parotid and Submaxillary Glands. Brit. D. J., 105:321, 1958.

65. Keyes, P. H., and Jordan, H. V.: Periodontal Lesions in the Syrian Hamster: III. Findings Related to an Infectious and Transmissible Component. Arch. Oral Biol., 9:377, 1964.

66. Klein, H. S.: Spirochetes in Normal Mouths, Gingivitis, and Suppurative Periodontitis. Acta Odont. Scandinav., 7:92, 1946.

67. Klinkhamer, J. M.: Saliva. In Lazzari, E.: Dental Biochemistry. Philadelphia, Lea and Febiger, 1968, Chapter 9.

68. Klinkhamer, J. M., and Zimmerman, S.: The Function and Reliability of the Orogranulocytic

Migratory Rate as a Measure of Oral Health. J. D. Res., *48*:709, 1969.

69. Kraus, F. W.: Microbiology of the Oral Cavity and Its Systemic Significance. D. Clin. North America, July 1958, p. 309.

70. Kraus, F. W., and Konno, J.: Antibodies in Saliva. Ann. N.Y. Acad. Sc., *106*:311, 1963.

71. Kraus, F. W., and Konno, J.: The Salivary Secretion of Antibody. Ala. J. Med. Sc., 2:15, 1965.

72. Kraus, F. W., Perry, W. I., and Nickerson, J. F.: Salivary Catalase and Peroxidase Values in Normal Subjects and in Persons with Periodontal Disease. Oral Surg., Oral Med. & Oral Path., *11*:95, 1958.

73. Kristoffersen, T., and Hofstad, T.: Antibodies in Humans to an Isolated Antigen from Oral Fusobacteria, and Their Possible Role in Bacterial Inflammation. J. Periodont. Res., 4:17, Suppl. 4, 1969.

74. Kritchevsky, B., and Séguin, P.: The Unity of Spirochetes of the Mouth. D. Cosmos, *66*:511, 1924.

75. Kutscher, A. H., Chilton, N. W., Bacher, B. J., and Foord, A.: Local Eosinophil Count in Gingival Disease. J. Periodont., 23:102, 1952.

76. Lisanti, V. F.: Hydrolytic Enzymes in Periodontal Tissues. Ann. N.Y. Acad. Sc., 85:461, 1960.

77. Listgarten, M. A.: Electron Microscopic Observations on the Bacterial Flora of Acute Necrotizing Ulcerative Gingivitis. J. Periodont., 36:328, 1965.

78. Macdonald, J. B., and Gibbons, R. J.: The Relationship of Indigenous Bacteria to Peridontal Disease. J. D. Res., 41 (Suppl. to No. 1):320, 1962.

79. Macdonald, J. B., Socransky, S. S., and Gibbons, R. J.: Aspects of the Pathogenesis of Mixed Anaerobic Infections of Mucous Membrane. J. D. Res., *42*:529, 1963.

80. Macdonald, J. B., Sutton, R. M., and Knoll, M. L.: The Production of Fusospirochetal Infections in Guinea Pigs with Recombined Pure Cultures. J. Infect. Dis., *95*:275, 1954.

81. McMaster, P.: Human Bite Infections. Am. J. Surg., *45*:60, 1939.

82. Mergenhagen, S. E., and Varah, E.: Serologically Specific Lipopolysaccharides from Oral Veillonella. Arch. Oral Biol., 8:31, 1963.

83. Mergenhagen, S. E.: Nature and Significance of Somatic Antigens of Oral Bacteria. J. D. Res., *46*:46, 1967.

84. Mergenhagen, S. E., Hampp, E. G., and Scherp, H. W.: Preparation and Biological Activities of Endotoxins from Oral Bacteria. J. Infect. Dis., *108*:304, 1961.

85. Mergenhagen, S. E., Tempel, T. R., and Snyderman, R.: Immunologic Reactions and Periodontal Inflammation. J. D. Res., 49:256, 1970.

86. Meyer, K.: Mucolytic Enzymes. In Green, D. E.: Currents in Biochemical Research. New York, Interscience Publishers, 1946.

87. Murphy, P. J., and Stallard, R. E.: An Altered Gingival Attachment Epithelium; A Result of the Enzyme Hyaluronidase. Periodontics, 6:105, 1968.

88. Nisengard, R., Beutner, E. H., and Hazen, S. P.: Immunologic Studies of Periodontal Disease. IV. Bacterial Hypersensitivity and Periodontal Disease. J. Periodont., 39:329, 1968.

89. Noguchi, H.: Treponema Mucosum (new species)

90. Norton, L. A., Moore, R. R., and Proffit, W. R.: Effects of Whole Oral Flora and *B. melaninogenicus* upon Bone Growth in Organ Culture. I.A.D.R. Abstr., No. 107, 1969, p. 67.

91. Orban, B.: Eosinophile Leukocytes in the Pulp and Gingiva. J. D. Res., *19*:537, 1940.

92. Proske, H. O., and Sayers, R. R.: Pulmonary Fusospirochetal Infection. Pub. Health Rep., *49*:839, 1934.

93. Ray, H. G., and Orban, B.: Deep Necrotic Foci in the Gingiva. J. Periodont., *19*:91, 1948.

94. Rizzo, A.: Absorption of Bacterial Endotoxin into Rabbit Gingival Pocket Tissue. Periodontics, 6:65, 1968.

95. Rizzo, A.: Possible Role of Hydrogen Sulfide in Human Periodontal Disease. Periodontics, 5:233, 1967.

96. Rizzo, A., and Mergenhagen, S.: Histopathologic Effects of Endotoxin Injected into Rabbit Oral Mucosa. Arch. Oral Biol., 9:659, 1964.

97. Rizzo, A. A., and Mitchell, C. T.: Chronic Allergic Inflammation Induced by Repeated Deposition of Antigen in Rabbit Gingival Pockets. Periodontics, 4:5, 1966.

98. Robbins, S. L.: Pathology. 3rd ed. Philadelphia, W. B. Saunders Co., 1967, p. 242.

99. Rosebury, T.: Microorganisms Indigenous to Man. New York, McGraw-Hill Book Co., 1962, p. 371.

100. Rosebury, T.: The Parasitic Actinomycetes and Other Filamentous Microorganisms of the Mouth: A Review. Bact. Rev., 8:189, 1944.

101. Rosebury, T.: The Nature and Significance of Infection in Periodontal Disease. Am. J. Orthodont. & Oral Surg., *33*:658, 1947.

102. Rosebury, T., Macdonald, J. B., and Clark, A.: A Bacteriologic Survey of Gingival Scrapings from Periodontal Infections by Direct Examination, Guinea Pig Inoculation, and Anaerobic Cultivation. J. D. Res., *29*:718, 1950.

103. Roth, G. D., and Meyers, H. I.: Hide Powder and Collagen Lysis by Organisms From the Oral Cavity. Oral Surg., Oral Med. & Oral Path., 9: 1172, 1956.

104. Schiott, C. R., and Loe, H.: The Origin and Variation in the Number of Leukocytes in the Human Saliva. J. Periodont. Res., Suppl. 4:24, 1969.

105. Schneider, T. F., et al.: Specific Bacterial Antibodies in the Inflamed Human Gingiva. Periodontics, 4:53, 1966.

106. Schneider, T. F., Toto, P. D., Gargiulo, A. W., and Pollock, R. J.: Specific Bacterial Antibodies in the Inflamed Human Gingiva. Periodontics, 4:53, 1966.

107. Schultz-Haudt, S. D.: Biochemical Aspects of Periodontal Disease. Internat. D. J., *14*:398, 1964.

108. Schultz-Haudt, S., Bibby, B. G., and Bruce, M. A.: Tissue Destructive Products of Gingival Bacteria from Nonspecific gingivitis. J. D. Res., *33*:624, 1954.

109. Schultz-Haudt, S., Bruce, M. A., and Bibby, B. G.: Bacterial Factors in Nonspecific Gingivitis. J. D. Res., *33*:454, 1954.

110. Schultz-Haudt, S., Dewar, M., and Bibby, B. G.:

a Mucous Producing Spirochete from Pyorrhea Alveolaris, Grown in Pure Culture. J. Exp. Med., *16*:194, 1912.

Effects of Hyaluronidase on Human Gingival Epithelium. Science, 117:653, 1953.

111. Schultz-Haudt, S. D., Waerhaug, J., From, S. H., and Attramadal, A.: On the Nature of Contact Between Gingival Epithelium and the Tooth Enamel Surface. Am. Soc. Perio., 1:103, 1963.

112. Shklar, G., and Cohen, M. M.: The Development of Periodontal Disease in Experimental Animals Infected with Polyoma Virus. Periodontics, 3:281, 1965.

113. Simon, B. I., et al.: The Role of Endotoxin in Periodontal Disease. II. Correlation of the Quantity of Endotoxin in Human Gingival Exudate with the Clinical Degree of Inflammation. J. Periodont., 41:81, 1970.

114. Skougaard, M. R., Bay, I., and Klinkhamer, J. M.: Correlation Between Gingivitis and Orogranulocytic Migratory Rate. J. D. Res., 48:716, 1969.

115. Skougaard, M. R., and Beagrie, G. S.: Renewal of Gingival Epithelium in Marmosets (*Callithrix jacchus*) as Determined Through Autoradiography with Thymidine-H³. Acta Odont. Scandinav., 20:467, 1962.

116. Smith, D. T.: Spirochetes and Related Organisms in Fuso-Spirochetal Disease. Baltimore, Williams & Wilkins Co., 1932.

117. Smith, E. C.: Cultivation of the Spirochetes Associated with Tropical Ulcer. Proc. Roy. Soc. Med. Section of Tropical Diseases and Parasitology, 24:1, 1930–31.

118. Socransky, S. S.: Relationship of Bacteria to the Etiology of Periodontal Disease. J. D. Res., 49:203, 1970.

119. Socransky, S. S., Gibbons, R. J., Dale, A. C., Bortnick, L., Rosenthal, E., and Macdonald, J. B.: The Microbiota of the Gingival Crevice Area of Man—I. Total Microscopic and Viable Counts and Counts of Specific Organisms. Arch. Oral Biol., 8:275, 1963.

120. Stallard, R. E., Diab, M. A., and Zander, H. A.: The Attaching Substance Between Enamel and Epithelium—A Product of the Epithelial Cells. J. Periodont., 36:130, 1965.

121. Sussman, H., Bartels, H. A., and Stahl, S. S.: The Potential of Microorganisms to Invade the Lamina Propria of Human Gingival Tissues. J. Periodont., 40:210, 1969.

122. Taichman, N. S., Freedman, H. L., and Urihara, T.: Inflammation and Tissue Injury. Arch. Oral Biol., 11:1385, 1966.

123. Taylor, R. G., Doku, H. C., and Romero, J.: Direct Determination of Fibrinolytic Activity of Human Saliva. J. D. Res., 43:86, 1964.

124. Thonard, J. C.: The Microbiology of Periodontal Disease. Ala. J. Med. Sc., 5:302, 1968.

125. Thonard, J. C., Crosby, R. C., and Dalbow, M. H.: Detection of IgM and IgA Immunoglobulins in Diseased Human Periodontal Tissue. I.A.D.R. Abstr., No. 328, 1966.

126. Tunnicliff, R., et al.: Fusiform Bacilli and Spirilla in Gingival Tissue. J.A.D.A., 23:1959, 1936.

127. Wantland, W. W., Wantland, E. M., and Winquist, D. L.: Collection, Identification, and Cultivation of Oral Protozoa. J. D. Res., 42:1234, 1963.

128. Watase, R. K., Bahn, A. N., and Haga, C.: Penicillin-Resistant Streptococci from the Saliva. J. D. Res., 45:243, 1966.

129. Winford, T., and Haberman, S.: Isolation of Aerobic Gram Positive Filamentous Rods from Diseased Gingiva. J. D. Res., 45:1159, 1966.

130. Wittwer, J. W., Toto, P. D., and Dickler, E. H.: Streptococcus Mitis Antigens in Inflamed Gingiva. J. Periodont., 40:639, 1969.

131. Zwemer, J. D., and Steinman, R. R.: The Endotoxic Activity of Human Saliva. J. D. Res., 39:1074, 1960.

Chapter 24

TRAUMA FROM OCCLUSION IN THE ETIOLOGY OF PERIODONTAL DISEASE

Occlusal forces affect the condition and structure of the periodontium. Periodontal health is not a static state. It depends upon a balance between an internal systemically controlled milieu that governs periodontal metabolism and the external environment of the tooth, of which occlusion is an important component.

To remain structurally and metabolically sound, the periodontal ligament and alveolar bone require the mechanical stimulation of occlusal forces. An inherent "margin of safety" common to all tissues permits some variation in occlusion without the periodontium being adversely affected. However, when function is insufficient the periodontium atrophies, and when occlusal forces exceed the adaptive capacity of the tissues, they are injured. The injury is called trauma from occlusion.

THE FUNCTIONAL COMPONENT IN PERIODONTAL HEALTH

To understand the role of trauma from occlusion in periodontal disease it is necessary to understand the relationship of occlusion to periodontal health. This starts with the development of the tooth. When the crown of the tooth is completed, it is contained within a bony crypt in the jaw, protected from external environmental factors. As the tooth erupts into the oral cavity, it becomes confronted with an entirely new world. Pressure from the lips and the tongue, the cheeks, the child's fingers, the pacifier, and food are thrust upon it. To enable the crown to withstand such forces the root is built as the tooth erupts and the periodontium develops around the root to hold it in the jaw. **The periodontium is custom built to meet the functional demands of the tooth; support of the tooth is the only reason for its existence.**

OCCLUSION — THE SUSTAINING FORCE

Just as the tooth depends upon the periodontal tissues to keep it in the jaw, so do the periodontal tissues depend upon the functional activity of the tooth to remain healthy. When there is insufficient functional stimulation the periodontal tissues atrophy; when the tooth is extracted the periodontium disappears. **Occlusion is the lifeline of the periodontium.** In periodontal health, it provides the mechanical stimulation which marshals the complex biologic mechanisms responsible for the well-being of the periodontium.

PHYSIOLOGIC ADAPTIVE CAPACITY OF THE PERIODONTIUM TO OCCLUSAL FORCES

When there is an increased functional demand upon it, the periodontium tries to accommodate the demand. The adaptive capacity varies in different persons and in the same person at different times. The effect of occlusal forces upon the periodontium is influenced by their **severity, direction, frequency** and **duration.**

When the *severity of occlusal forces* is increased, the periodontium responds by a thickening and increase in the fibers in the periodontal ligament and increase in the density of alveolar bone. Changing the direction of occlusal forces causes a reorientation of the stresses and strains within the periodontium.[19]

The principal fibers of the periodontal ligament are arranged so that they can best accommodate occlusal forces in the long axis of the tooth. When *axial forces* are increased there is viscoelastic distortion of the periodontal ligament and ultimate compression of the periodontal fibers and resorption of bone in the apical areas. The fibers in relation to the remainder of the root are placed under tension, and new bone is formed.[45] **In designing dental restorations and prostheses every effort is made to direct occlusal forces axially in order to benefit from the greater tolerance of the periodontium to forces in this direction.**

Lateral or horizontal forces are ordinarily accommodated by bone resorption in areas of pressure and bone formation in areas of tension (Fig. 24–1). The most advantageous point of application of a lateral force is near the cervical line. As the point of application is moved coronally, the distance from the center of rotation or lever arm is lengthened

and the force upon the periodontal ligament increases.[56]

Torques or rotational forces cause both tension and pressure which, under physiologic conditions, result in bone formation and bone resorption respectively.[46] Torques are the type of force most likely to injure the periodontium.

Duration and **frequency** affect the response of alveolar bone to occlusal forces.[37] Constant pressure on bone causes resorption, whereas intermittent force favors bone formation. The time lapse between pressure applications apparently influences the bone response. Recurrent forces over short intervals of time have essentially the same resorbing effect as constant pressure.

When the occlusal forces exceed the adaptive capacity of the periodontium, tissue injury results.[1, 13, 27, 29, 31, 33, 40, 42]

TRAUMA FROM OCCLUSION

Periodontal tissue injury caused by occlusal forces is called trauma from occlusion.* **Trauma from occlusion is the tissue injury — not the occlusal force.** An occlusion which produces such injury is called a traumatic occlusion.[4] Excessive occlusal forces may also disrupt the function of the masticatory musculature and *cause painful spasms, injure the temporomandibular joints* or *produce excessive tooth wear*, but the term trauma from occlusion is generally used in connection with injury in the periodontium.

Trauma from occlusion may be *acute* or *chronic. Acute trauma from occlusion* results from an abrupt change in occlusal force such as that produced by a restoration or prosthetic appliances which interfere with the occlusion or alter the direction of occlusal forces on the teeth. The results are pain, sensitivity to percussion and increased tooth mobility. If the force is dissipated by a shift in the position of the tooth or by wearing away or correction of the restoration, the injury heals and the symptoms subside. Otherwise, periodontal injury may

---

*This term is used throughout the text to designate periodontal tissue injury produced by occlusal forces. It is also known as "traumatism"[41] and "occlusal trauma."

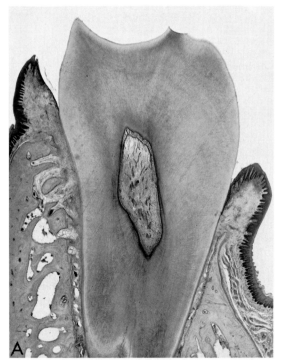

A

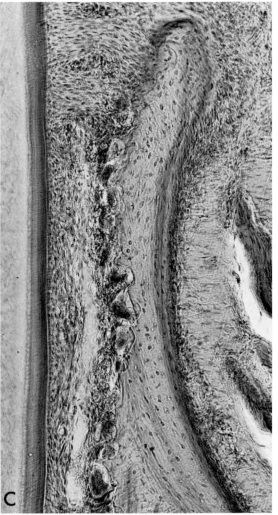

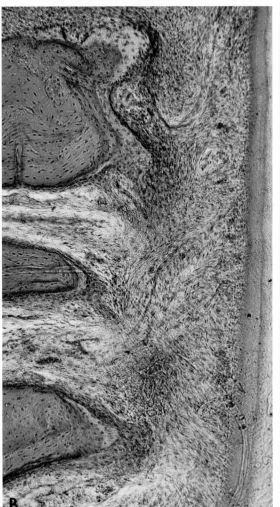

B

C

Figure 24–1   Periodontal Accommodation to Lateral Forces. *A,* Mandibular premolar. *B,* Lingual surface, showing new bone formation in response to tension on the periodontal ligament. Note the pale-staining osteoid bordered by osteoblasts and the incremental lines indicative of previous additions to the bone. *C,* Facial surface shows compression of the periodontal ligament and osteoclastic resorption of the bony plate. Note the new bone formed on the external surface. This is **Peripheral Buttressing Bone,** which reinforces the resorbing facial plate. Note, too, that the buttressing bone has produced a bulge in the bony contour.

worsen and develop into necrosis with periodontal abscess formation, or it may persist as a chronic condition.

Chronic trauma from occlusion is more common than the acute form and is of greater clinical significance. It most often develops from gradual changes in the occlusion produced by tooth wear, drifting and extrusion of teeth, combined with parafunctional habits such as bruxing and clenching, rather than as a sequel to acute periodontal trauma. The features of chronic trauma from occlusion and their significance are discussed below.

Three stages of trauma from occlusion

Trauma from occlusion occurs in three stages. The first is **injury**, the second is **repair**, and the third is a **change in the morphology of the periodontium**. Tissue injury is produced by excessive occlusal forces. Nature attempts to repair the injury and restore the periodontium. This can occur if the force is diminished or the tooth drifts away from it. If, however, the offend-

ing force is chronic, the periodontium is remodeled to cushion its impact. The ligament is widened at the expense of the bone, angular bone defects occur without periodontal pockets and the tooth becomes loose.

Stage I: Injury. The severity, location and pattern of the tissue damage depend upon the severity, frequency and direction of the injurious forces. *Slightly excessive pressure* **stimulates increased osteoclastic resorption of the alveolar bone, with a resultant widening of the periodontal ligament space.** *Slightly excessive tension* **causes elongation of the periodontal ligament fibers and apposition of alveolar bone. In areas of increased pressure the blood vessels are numerous and reduced in size; in areas of increased tension they are enlarged.**[60]

Greater pressure produces **a gradation of changes in the periodontal ligament, starting with compression of the fibers with thrombosis of the blood vessels and hemorrhage, and advancing to hyalinization and necrosis of the ligament. There is also excessive resorption of alveolar bone (Fig. 24–2) and, in some instances, resorption of tooth substance.** *Severe tension* **causes widening of the periodontal**

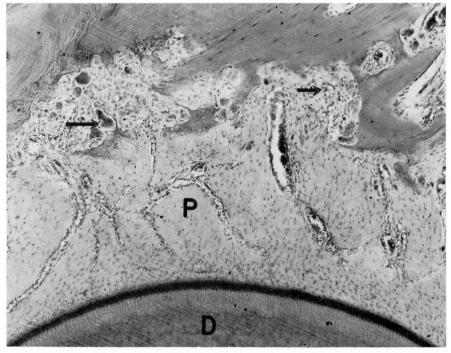

Figure 24–2 Trauma from Occlusion at Root Apex. Note bone resorption with prominent osteoclasts (*arrow*). The periodontal ligament (P) is widened as the result of bone resorption, and the blood vessels are engorged. The root is shown at D.

ligament, thrombosis, hemorrhage, tearing of the periodontal ligament and resorption of alveolar bone.

Pressure severe enough to force the root against bone causes **necrosis of the periodontal ligament and bone. The bone is resorbed by cells from viable periodontal ligament adjacent to the necrotic area and from the marrow spaces, a process called "undermining resorption."**

The bifurcation and trifurcation are the areas of the periodontium most susceptible to injury from excessive occlusal forces.[26]

With injury to the periodontium there is a temporary depression in mitotic activity and in the rate of proliferation and differentiation of fibroblasts,[54] **collagen and bone formation,**[10, 47] **which return to normal following dissipation of the force.**

Stage II: Repair. Repair is constantly going on in the normal periodontium. In trauma from occlusion the injured tissues stimulate increased reparative activity. **The damaged tissues are removed, and new connective tissue cells and fibers, bone and cementum are formed in an attempt to restore the injured periodontium (Fig. 24–3).** A force remains traumatic only so long as the damage it produces exceeds the reparative capacity of the tissues. Cartilage sometimes develops in the periodontal ligament spaces as an aftermath of the trauma.[16]

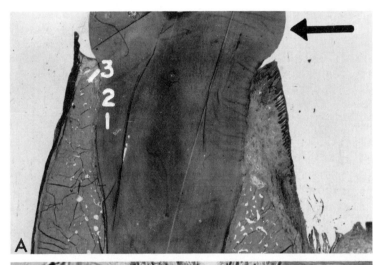

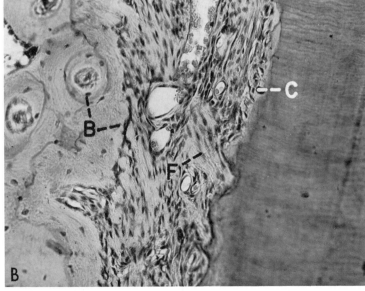

Figure 24–3 *A,* Faciolingual survey section of mandibular tooth of dog, subjected to **Excessive Lateral Force** *(arrow)* that injured periodontium in area marked 1,2,3.

B, **Reversibility of Trauma from Occlusion.** Healing in area marked 1,2,3, one month after cessation of force. There is new bone formation (B) in relation to the periodontal ligament and endosteal bone margins. Cementum (C) is being deposited along the eroded dentinal surface. Note the fibroblasts with collagen fibers (F) being embedded in the cementum and extending into the newly formed bone.

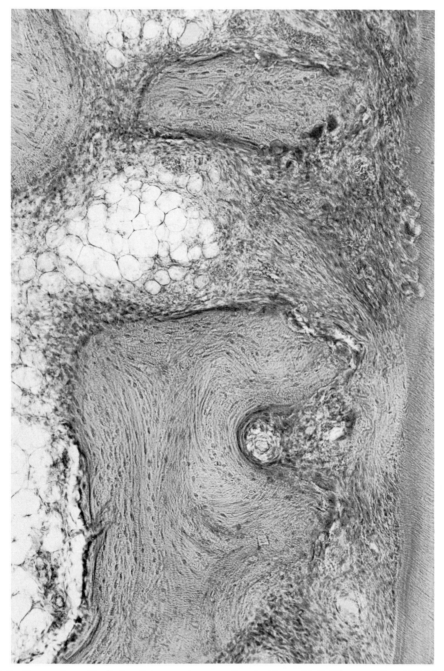

Figure 24–4   Trauma from Occlusion. Injury more severe than in Figure 24–2. The cementum (*right*) is undergoing resorption, the periodontal ligament is compressed and necrotic, and the bone is undergoing resorption. Note the osteoblasts and new bone (central buttressing bone formation) on the trabecular margins adjacent to the marrow.

BUTTRESSING BONE FORMATION. When bone is resorbed by excessive occlusal forces nature attempts to reinforce the thinned bone trabeculae with new bone (Fig. 24–4). This attempt to compensate for lost bone is called buttressing bone formation and is an important feature of the reparative process associated with trauma from occlusion.[22] It also occurs when bone is destroyed by inflammation or osteolytic tumors.

Buttressing bone formation occurs within the jaw (central) and on the bone surface (peripheral). In central buttressing bone formation the endosteal cells deposit new bone which restores the bone trabeculae and reduces the size of the marrow spaces (Fig. 24–5).

Peripheral buttressing bone formation occurs on the facial and lingual surfaces of the alveolar plate. Depending upon its severity, it may produce a shelf-like thickening of the alveolar margin referred to as *lipping* (Fig. 24–1), or a pronounced bulge in the contour of the facial and lingual bone (see Chap. 16).

Stage III: Adaptive Remodeling of the Periodontium. If the repair cannot keep pace with the destruction caused by the occlusion, the periodontium is remodeled in an effort to create a structural relationship in which the forces are no longer injurious to the tissues. To cushion the impact of the offending forces the periodontal ligament is widened and the adjacent bone loss is resorbed.[20] The involved teeth become loose.[59] **The results are a thickened periodontal ligament, funnel-shaped at the crest, and angular defects in the bone.**

Effects of insufficient occlusal force

Insufficient occlusal force may also be injurious to the supporting periodontal tissues.[12] Insufficient stimulation causes **degeneration of the periodontium manifested by thinning of the periodontal ligament, atrophy of the fibers, osteoporosis of the alveolar bone and reduction in bone height.** Hypofunction results from an open bite relationship, absence of functional antagonists, or unilateral chewing habits that neglect one side of the mouth.

Reduced function also deprives the gingiva of surface cleansing from deter-

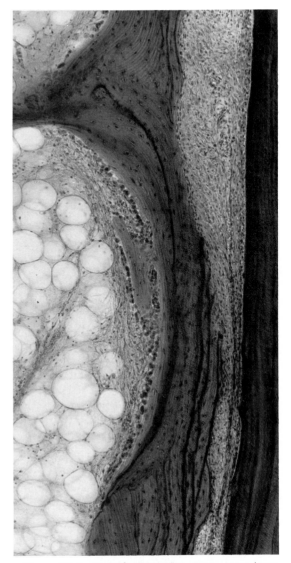

Figure 24–5 Central Buttressing Bone. New bone formation on the marrow side of alveolar bone which is undergoing resorption on the side of the periodontal ligament.

gent foods. This leads to an accumulation of plaque and bacteria which cause gingival inflammation.

Trauma from occlusion is reversible

Trauma from occlusion is reversible. When trauma is artificially induced in experimental animals, the teeth move away or are intruded into the jaw. The impact of the artificially created force is relieved and the tissues undergo repair. The fact that trauma from occlusion is reversible under such conditions does not mean that it always corrects itself and therefore is temporary and of limited clinical significance. **The injurious force must be relieved in order for repair to occur.**[26] If conditions in humans do not permit the teeth to escape from or adapt to excessive occlusal force, periodontal damage persists[13, 33] until the excessive forces are corrected by the clinician.

THE ROLE OF TRAUMA FROM OCCLUSION IN THE ETIOLOGY OF GINGIVITIS AND PERIODONTAL DISEASE

Everything in the life of the periodontium bears the touch of the occlusion. Just as the occlusion is a critical environmental factor in the life of the healthy periodontium, its influence continues in periodontal disease. **Inflammation in the periodontium cannot separate it from the influence of occlusion.** Because occlusion is the constant monitor of the condition of the periodontium, it affects the response of the periodontium to inflammation and becomes a factor in all cases of periodontal disease.

The role of trauma from occlusion in gingivitis and periodontitis is best understood if the periodontium is considered as consisting of two zones (Fig. 24–6): *the zone of irritation* and the *zone of co-destruction.*

The zone of irritation

The zone of irritation consists of the marginal and interdental gingiva with its boundary formed by the gingival fibers (Fig. 24–6). This is where gingivitis and periodontal pockets start. They are caused by local irritation from plaque, bacteria, calculus and food impaction. With few exceptions,[5, 55] researchers agree that trauma from occlusion does not cause gingivitis or periodontal pockets.[4, 26, 27, 32, 43, 57, 59, 61]

The local irritants which start gingivitis and periodontal pockets affect the marginal gingiva, but trauma from occlusion occurs in the supporting tissues and does not affect the gingiva. The marginal gingiva is unaffected by trauma from occlusion because its blood supply is sufficient to maintain it even when the vessels of the periodontal ligament are obliterated by excessive occlusal forces.[28]

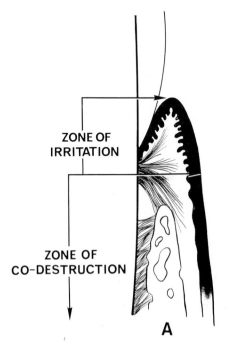

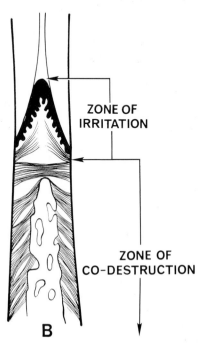

Figure 24–6   Zones of Irritation and Co-destruction in Periodontal Disease. *A,* Facial or lingual surface. *B,* Interproximal area.

So long as inflammation is confined to the gingiva it is not affected by occlusal forces. When it extends from the gingiva into the supporting periodontal tissues (that is, when gingivitis becomes periodontitis), inflammation enters the zone of co-destruction.

The zone of co-destruction

The zone of co-destruction begins with the transseptal fibers interproximally and the alveolar crest fibers facially and lingually (Fig. 24–6). It consists of the supporting periodontal tissues, the periodontal ligament, alveolar bone and cementum. When inflammation reaches the supporting periodontal tissues, **its pathway and the destruction it causes come under the influence of the occlusion.**

This means that occlusion is a factor in all cases of periodontal disease; it may be favorable or unfavorable. If the occlusion is favorable, that is, if it provides the functional stimulation that the periodontal tissues require, inflammation is the sole local destructive factor in periodontitis. If occlusion is unfavorable, that is, if it is excessive or inadequate, it alters the environment and pathway of inflammation, produces periodontal injury and becomes a co-destructive factor which affects the pattern and severity of tissue destruction in periodontal disease.[24]

How Occlusal Forces Affect Inflammation in the Zone of Co-destruction. The pathway of inflammation from the gingiva into the supporting structures in periodontitis is described in Chapter 15. The inflammatory exudate passively follows the path of least resistance, and its direction is affected by the alignment of the transseptal and alveolar crest fibers. Trauma from occlusion changes the tissue environment around the inflammatory exudate in two ways; it does not alter the inflammatory process. (1) Excessive occlusal forces alter the alignment of the transseptal and alveolar crest fibers and change the pathway of the inflammation so that it extends directly into the periodontal ligament.[21] (2) Excessive occlusal forces produce periodontal ligament damage and bone resorption which aggravate the tissue destruction caused by inflammation.[11] Combined with inflammation, trauma from occlusion leads to infrabony pockets, angular and crater-like osseous defects, and excessive tooth mobility.[3, 15, 23, 24, 58]

There is considerable variability in the response of the periodontium to the combination of inflammation and trauma from occlusion. Inflammation from the gingiva may reach the periodontal ligament through vessel channels in the bone in the absence of trauma from occlusion;[2] the combination of tilting or excessive occlusal forces and inflammation does not necessarily lead to infrabony pockets,[14, 17, 49] and angular bone destruction may occur beneath suprabony pockets.[24]

The existence of a co-destructive relationship between inflammation and trauma from occlusion does not rule out the possibility that both may be present without the production of infrabony pockets and angular defects. The inflammation or the trauma may not be severe enough, or the anatomy of the tooth or bone may not be conducive to their formation. For example, if the facial or lingual bone is very thin, it may undergo resorption before an angular defect can develop. For similar reasons the absence of infrabony pockets and osseous defects does not rule out the presence of trauma from occlusion. **Such periodontal lesions may be produced by etiologic factors other than the combination of inflammation and trauma from occlusion, but they have not as yet been demonstrated.**

Changes produced by trauma from occlusion alone

In the absence of local irritants severe enough to produce periodontal pockets, trauma from occlusion may cause excessive loosening of teeth, widening of the periodontal ligament, and angular (vertical) defects in the alveolar bone without pockets.

Radiographic signs of trauma from occlusion

The radiographic signs of trauma from occlusion are shown in Figures 24–7 and 24–8. They include (1) widening of the periodontal space, often with thickening of the lamina dura in the following areas: along the lateral aspect of the root, in the apical region and in bifurcation and trifurcation areas: (2) "vertical" rather than

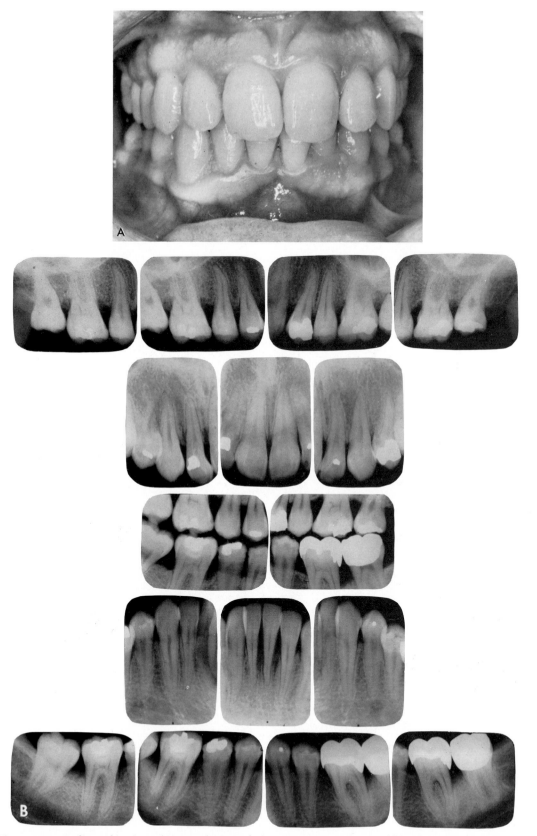

Figure 24–7   Radiographic Signs of Trauma from Occlusion. *A,* Twenty-seven year old female with only slight clinical evidence of periodontal disease. Little suggestion of the bone destruction shown radiographically. *B,* Radiographs show typical signs of trauma from occlusion: widening of the periodontal space in the mandibular anterior region, early angular bone destruction and furcation involvement in the molar areas.

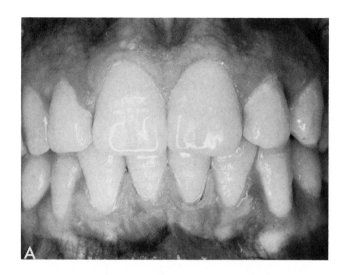

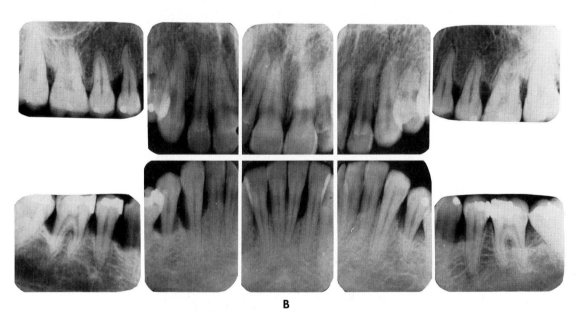

Figure 24–8 Radiographic Signs of Trauma from Occlusion. *A,* Thirty year old female with slight gingival disease. *B,* Radiographs show typical signs of trauma from occlusion: thickening of lamina dura, varied degrees of angular bone destruction and furcation involvement.

"horizontal" destruction of the interdental septum, with the formation of infrabony defects; (3) radiolucence and condensation of the alveolar bone and (4) root resorption.

It should be understood that widening of the periodontal space and thickening of the lamina dura do not necessarily indicate destructive changes. They may result from thickening and strengthening of the periodontal ligament and alveolar bone, which constitute a favorable response to increased occlusal forces (Fig. 24–9).

Other clinical changes attributed to trauma from occlusion

A wide variety of clinical changes has been attributed to trauma from occlusion,[39] *based upon clinical impressions rather than substantiated evidence*. These are summarized below as a matter of interest:

Food impaction
Abnormal habits
Obscure facial pain
Erosion
Recession
Gingival bleeding
Cheek biting
Sensitiveness of the occlusal and incisal surfaces
Chronic necrotizing ulcerative gingivitis
Hyperplasia of the gingiva
Pericementitis
Bruxism
Unilateral mastication
Limited excursion of the mandible (insufficient wear)
Unlimited excursion of the mandible (excessive wear)
Interproximal caries[48]
Formation of subgingival calculus and gingivitis[53]
Tendency toward epulis formation
Blanching of the gingiva upon the application of occlusal force
Pulp: hyperemia resulting in hypersensitivity to cold; pulpitis; pulp necrosis; pulp stones
Box[6] and Stillman[52] considered trauma to be the causative factor for the following incipient signs of periodontal disease:
Traumatic crescent. A crescent-shaped, bluish red zone of gingiva confined to about 1/6 of the circumference of the root.
Congestion, ischemia or *hyperemia* of the marginal gingiva.
Recession of the gingiva, which may be asymmetrical, associated with resorption of the alveolar crest.

Stillman's clefts. Indentations in the gingival margin, generally on one side of the tooth. Two clefts frequently occur on the same tooth. Intermittent compressions of the periodontal ligament followed by abnormal flushing of the gingival capillaries and enlargement and engorgement of the gingival vessels were considered to be the mechanism responsible for the cleft.
McCall's festoons. Discrete semilunar enlargement of the marginal gingiva.
Absence of stippling. This is interpreted as evidence of edema secondary to trauma.
Injection of the blood vessels in the marginal gingiva.
Sharply demarcated linear depressions in the alveolar mucosa, parallel to the long axis of the root and overlying the septal bone.
Distended veins in the oral mucosa.

The effects of excessive occlusal forces on the dental pulp

The effects of excessive occlusal forces upon the dental pulp have not been established. Some clinicians report the disappearance of pulp symptoms following correction of occlusal forces. Pulp reactions have been noted in animals subjected to increased occlusal forces,[14a, 57] but not when the forces were light and over short periods.[35]

The causes of trauma from occlusion

Trauma from occlusion may be caused by (1) alterations in occlusal forces, (2) reduced capacity of the periodontium to withstand occlusal forces, or a combination of both.

The criterion which determines whether an occlusion is traumatic is whether it produces injury, rather than how the teeth occlude. Any occlusion which produces periodontal injury is traumatic. Malocclusion is not necessary to produce trauma; it may occur when the occlusion appears "normal."[38] The dentition may be anatomically and esthetically acceptable, but functionally injurious. Conversely, not all malocclusions are necessarily injurious to the periodontium. Occlusal relationships which are traumatic are referred to by such terms as "occlusal disharmony," "functional imbalance" or occlusal dystrophy. This is because of their effect upon the periodontium, not because of the position

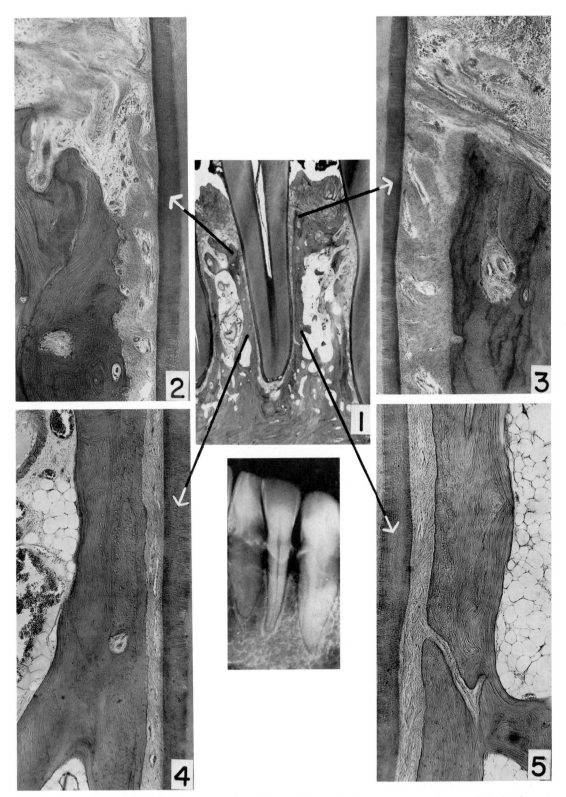

Figure 24–9 Widened Periodontal Space Produced by Two Types of Tissue Response to Increased Occlusal Forces.
Radiograph shows thickening of periodontal space and lamina dura around the lateral incisor. *1,* Survey microscopic section of lateral incisor. *2,* Mesial surface-widening of the periodontal space has resulted from resorption of alveolar bone associated with pressure. *3,* Distal surface-widening of the periodontal space has resulted from thickening of the periodontal ligament which is a favorable response to increased tension. *4 and 5,* Thinned periodontal ligament at axis of rotation, one-third the distance from the apex.

of the teeth. Since trauma from occlusion refers to the tissue injury rather than the occlusion, **an increased occlusal force is not traumatic if the periodontium can accommodate it.**

Trauma from occlusion is sometimes described as being a *primary* or *secondary* (complicating) factor in the etiology of periodontal destruction. Periodontal inflammation and trauma from occlusion so often occur together that it is difficult to determine which came first.

Primary trauma from occlusion

Trauma from occlusion may be considered the primary etiologic factor in periodontal destruction if the only local alteration to which a tooth is subjected is one of occlusion. Examples are periodontal injury produced around teeth *with a previously healthy periodontium* (1) following insertion of a "high filling," (2) following insertion of a prosthetic replacement which creates excessive forces on abutment and antagonistic teeth, (3) following the drifting or extrusion of teeth into spaces created by unreplaced missing teeth and (4) following the orthodontic movement of teeth into functionally unacceptable positions.

Secondary (complicating) trauma from occlusion

Trauma from occlusion is considered a secondary (complicating) cause of periodontal destruction when the adaptive capacity of the periodontium to withstand occlusal forces is impaired. The periodontium becomes vulnerable to injury and **previously physiologic occlusal forces become traumatic.**

Factors which impair the capability of the periodontium to withstand occlusal forces

Inflammation of the periodontal ligament in periodontal disease leads to degeneration of principal fibers, and impairs the capacity of the periodontal ligament to withstand occlusal forces and transmit them to the bone.

When *alveolar bone and periodontal fibers* are destroyed by periodontal disease, the burden upon the remaining tissues is increased, because (1) there is less tissue to withstand the forces and (2) the leverage upon the remaining tissues is increased.

When teeth with inflammatory periodontal disease migrate (pathologic migration) into positions in which they are subjected to excessive occlusal forces, the occlusion injures the periodontium and aggravates the migration of the teeth.

Teeth loosened by periodontal disease move in their sockets so that they are tilted in relation to opposing teeth and encounter injurious lateral occlusal forces. Back and forth movement of loose teeth interferes with the normal "wear and tear" repair so that otherwise acceptable occlusal forces become injurious.

Hypofunction results in atrophy of the periodontal ligament and alveolar bone which impairs the initial responsiveness of the periodontium when occlusion is restored.

Age[30] *and systemic disorders* which inhibit the anabolic activity or induce degenerative changes in the periodontium lessen the capacity to withstand occlusal forces.[25, 39, 44]

SUMMARY

Trauma from occlusion is an important etiologic factor in periodontal disease. Understanding its effect upon the periodontium is useful in the clinical management of periodontal problems.

Trauma from occlusion is an integral part of the destructive process in periodontal disease. It does not start gingivitis or periodontal pockets, but it affects the progress and severity of periodontal pockets started by local irritation.

Trauma from occlusion and inflammation are different pathologic processes which occur in the same disease, periodontitis. They are not different diseases.

Inflammation starts in the gingiva and spreads into the supporting periodontal tissues; trauma from occlusion starts in the supporting periodontal tissues—both cause tissue destruction. They become interrelated co-destructive factors capable of producing the recognizable clinical and radiographic changes in the periodontium described in this chapter.

Because individuals vary in their periodontal response to local oral factors and because inflammation and trauma from occlusion occur in combinations of varied severity, they may not always produce infrabony pockets with angular or crater-like osseous defects. However, when such lesions are present the combination of inflammation and trauma from occlusion is the likely cause. There may be other etiologic factors, but they have not as yet been identified.

REFERENCES

1. Adrion, W.: Structural Changes in the Paradontium in Traumatic Influence. Deutsch. Monat. f. Stomat., 3:97, 1933.
2. Akiyoshi, M., and Mori, K.: Marginal Periodontitis: A Histologic Study of the Incipient Stage. J. Periodont., 38:45, 1967.
3. Balfe, R., Carranza, F. A., and Erausquin, R.: The Periodontal Structures in Case Number 8. Revista Odontológica, Buenos Aires, July, 1938.
4. Bhaskar, S. N., and Orban, B.: Experimental Occlusal Trauma. J. Periodont., 26:270, 1955.
5. Box, H. K.: Experimental Traumatogenic Occlusion in Sheep. Oral Health, 25:9, 1935.
6. Box, H. K.: Signs of Incipient Periodontal Disease. J.A.D.A., 12:1150, 1925.
7. Box, H. K.: Traumatic Occlusion and Traumagenic Occlusion. Oral Health, 20:642, 1930.
8. Box, H. K.: Twelve Periodontal Studies. University of Toronto Press, 1940, p. 55.
9. Breitner, C.: Tissue Changes Caused by So-Called Bite-Raising Plate Acting on the Front Teeth. Ztschr. f. Stomatol., 30:1185, 1932.
10. Carranza, F. A., Jr., and Cabrini, R. L.: Histometric Studies of Periodontal Tissues. Periodontics, 5:308, 1967.
11. Carranza, F. A., Jr., Simes, R. J., and Cabrini, R. L.: Effect of Combined Etiologic Factors in Experimental Periodontal Lesions. J. Periodont. Res., Suppl. 4, Abst. 28, p. 33, 1969.
12. Cohn, S. A.: Disuse Atrophy of the Periodontium in Molar Teeth of Mice. J. D. Res., 40:707, 1961.
13. Coolidge, E. D.: Traumatic and Functional Injuries Occurring in the Supporting Tissues of Human Teeth. J.A.D.A., 25:343, 1938.
14. Comar, M. D., Kollar, J. A., and Gargiulo, A. W.: Local Irritation and Occlusal Trauma as Co-Factors in the Periodontal Disease Process. J. Periodont., 40:193, 1969.
14a. Cooper, M. B., Landay, M. A., and Seltzer, S.: The Effects of Excessive Occlusal Forces on the Pulp. II. Heavier and Longer Term Forces. J. Periodont., 42:353, 1971.
15. Erausquin, R., and Carranza, F. A.: Primeros Hallazgos Paradentosicos. Rev. Odont. (Buenos Aires), 27:486, 1939.
16. Everett, F. G., and Bruckner, R. J.: Cartilage in the Periodontal Ligament Space. J. Periodont., 41:165, 1970.
17. Ewen, S. J., and Stahl, S. S.: The Response of the Periodontium to Chronic Gingival Irritation and Long Term Tilting Forces in Adult Dogs. Oral Surg., Oral Med., & Oral Path., 15:1426, 1962.
18. Glickman, I.: Occlusion and the Periodontium. J. D. Res., 46, Supplement 53, 1967.
19. Glickman, I., Roeber, F., Brion, M., and Pameijer, J.: Photoelastic Analysis of Internal Stresses in the Periodontium Created by Occlusal Forces. J. Periodont., 41:30, 1970.
20. Glickman, I., and Smulow, J. B.: Adaptive Alterations in the Periodontium of the Rhesus Monkey in Chronic Trauma from Occlusion. J. Periodont., 39:101, 1968.
21. Glickman, I., and Smulow, J. B.: Alterations in the Pathway of Gingival Inflammation into the Underlying Tissues Induced by Excessive Occlusal Forces. J. Periodont., 33:7, 1962.
22. Glickman, I., and Smulow, J. B.: Buttressing Bone Formation in the Periodontium. J. Periodont., 36:365, 1965.
23. Glickman, I., and Smulow, J. B.: Effect of Excessive Occlusal Forces upon the Pathway of Gingival Inflammation in Humans. J. Periodont., 36:141, 1965.
24. Glickman, I., and Smulow, J. B.: The Combined Effects of Inflammation and Trauma from Occlusion in Periodontitis. Internat. D. J., 19:393, 1969.
25. Glickman, I., Smulow, J. B., and Moreau, J.: Effect of Alloxan Diabetes upon the Periodontal Response to Excessive Occlusal Forces. J. Periodont., 37:146, 1966.
26. Glickman, I., Stein, R. S., and Smulow, J. B.: The Effects of Increased Functional Forces Upon the Periodontium of Splinted and Non-Splinted Teeth. J. Periodont., 32:290, 1961.
27. Glickman, I., and Weiss, L.: Role of Trauma from Occlusion in Initiation of Periodontal Pocket Formation in Experimental Animals. J. Periodont., 26:14, 1955.
28. Goldman, H.: Gingival Vascular Supply in Induced Occlusal Traumatism. Oral Surg., Oral Med. & Oral Path., 9:939, 1956.
29. Gottlieb, B., and Orban, B.: Changes in the Tissue Due to Excessive Force Upon the Teeth. Leipzig, G. Thieme, 1931.
30. Gottlieb, B., and Orban, B.: Tissue Changes in Experimental Traumatic Occlusion with Special Reference to Age and Constitution. J. D. Res., 11:505, 1931.
31. Grohs, R.: Changes in the Human Periodontal Membrane Due to Overstress. Ztschr. f. Stomatol., 29:386, 1931.
32. Itoiz, M. E., Carranza, F. A., Jr., and Cabrini, R. L.: Histologic and Histometric Study of Experimental Occlusal Trauma in Rats. J. Periodont., 34:305, 1963.
33. Karolyi, M.: Beobachtungen über Pyorrhea Alveolaris. Oest. ung. Viertel jschr. Zahnheilk., 17:279, 1901.
34. Kemper, W. W., Johnson, J. F., and Van Huysen, G.: Periodontal Tissue Changes in Response to High Artificial Crowns. J. Pros. Dent., 20:160, 1968.
35. Landay, M. A., Nazimov, H., and Seltzer, S.: The Effects of Excessive Occlusal Forces on the Pulp. J. Periodont., 41:3, 1970.
36. Macapanpan, L. C., and Weinmann, J. P.: The Influence of Injury to the Periodontal Membrane on the Spread of Gingival Inflammation. J. D. Res., 33:263, 1954.

37. Massoni, J., Gonzales, V., Haskel, E., and Sales, G.: Effect of Traumatic Forces Applied on the Molars of the Rat. Odont. Uruguaya, 20:5, 1964.
38. McCall, J. O.: Traumatic Occlusion. J.A.D.A., 26:519, 1939.
39. Miller, S. C.: Textbook of Periodontia. 3rd ed., Philadelphia, Blakiston Co., 1950, p. 350.
40. Orban, B.: Tissue Changes in Traumatic Occlusion. J.A.D.A., 15:2090, 1928.
41. Orban, B.: Classification of Periodontal Diseases. Paradentologie, 3:159, 1949.
42. Orban, B., and Weinmann, J.: Signs of Traumatic Occlusion in Average Human Jaws. J. D. Res., 13:216, 1933.
43. Ramfjord, S. P., and Kohler, C. A.: Periodontal Reaction to Functional Occlusal Stress. J. Periodont., 30:95, 1959.
44. Rothblatt, J. M., and Waldo, C. M.: Tissue Response to Tooth Movement in Normal and Abnormal Metabolic States. J. D. Res., 32:678, 1953.
45. Schwarz, A. M.: Movement of Teeth Under Traumatic Stress. D. Items Int., 52:96, 1930.
46. Skillen, W. C., and Reitan, K.: Tissue Changes Following Rotation of Teeth in the Dog. Angle Orthodont., 10:140, 1940.
47. Solt, C. W., and Glickman, I.: A Histologic and Radioautographic Study of Healing Following Wedging Interdental Injury in Mice. J. Periodont., 39:249, 1968.
48. Sorrin, S.: Traumatic Occlusion: Its Detection and Correction. D. Digest, 40:170, 1934.
49. Stahl, S. S.: The Responses of the Periodontium to Combined Gingival Inflammation and Occluso-Functional Stresses in Four Human Surgical Specimens. Periodontics, 6:14, 1968.
50. Stahl, S. S., Miller, S. C., and Goldsmith, E. D.: The Effects of Vertical Occlusal Trauma on the Periodontium of Protein Deprived Young Adult Rats. J. Periodont., 28:87, 1957.
51. Stallard, R. E.: The Effect of Occlusal Alterations on Collagen Formation Within the Periodontium. Periodontics, 2:49, 1964.
52. Stillman, P. R.: Differential Diagnosis of Early Periodontal Lesions. Bull. Ont. Dent. Assoc., 1925.
53. Stillman, P. R.: Early Clinical Evidences of Disease in the Gingiva and Pericementum. J. D. Res., 3:xxv, 1921.
54. Stillman, P. R., and McCall, J. O.: Textbook of Clinical Periodontia. New York, The Macmillan Company, 1937, p. 116.
55. Stones, H. H.: An Experimental Investigation Into the Association of Traumatic Occlusion with Paradontal Disease. Proc. Roy. Soc. Med., 31:479, 1938.
56. Thurow, R. C.: The Periodontal Membrane in Function. Angle Orthodont., 15:18, 1945.
57. Waerhaug, J.: Pathogenesis of Pocket Formation in Traumatic Occlusion. J. Periodont., 26:107, 1955.
58. Waerhaug, J., and Hansen, E. R.: Periodontal Changes Incidental to Prolonged Occlusal Overload in Monkeys. Acta Odont. Scandinav., 24:91, 1966.
59. Wentz, F. M., Jarabak, J., and Orban, B.: Experimental Occlusal Trauma Imitating Cuspal Interferences. J. Periodont., 29:117, 1958.
60. Zaki, A. E., and Van Huysen, G.: I.A.D.R. Abstracts of the 40th General Meeting, 1962, p. 4.
61. Zander, H. A., and Mühlemann, H. R.: The Effect of Stresses on the Periodontal Structures. Oral Surg., Oral Med. & Oral Path., 9:380, 1956.

Chapter 25

FOOD IMPACTION, HABIT AND OTHER LOCAL FACTORS IN THE ETIOLOGY OF PERIODONTAL DISEASE

FOOD IMPACTION

Food impaction is the forceful wedging of food into the periodontium by occlusal forces. It may occur interproximally or in relation to the facial or lingual tooth surfaces. Food impaction is a very common cause of gingival and periodontal disease. Far too frequently, failure to recognize and eliminate food impaction is responsible for the unsuccessful outcome of an otherwise thoroughly treated case of periodontal disease.

The Mechanism of Food Impaction

The forceful wedging of food normally is prevented by the integrity and location of the proximal contact, the contour of the marginal ridges and developmental grooves and the contour of the facial and lingual surfaces. An intact, firm proximal contact relationship prevents the forceful wedging of food interproximally. The location of the contact is also important in protecting the tissues against food impaction. The optimal cervico-occlusal location of the contact is at the longest mesiodistal diameter of the tooth, close to the crest of the marginal ridge. The proximity of the contact point to the occlusal plane reduces the tendency toward food impaction in the smaller occlusal embrasure. The absence of contact or the presence of an unsatisfactory proximal relationship is conducive to food impaction (Fig. 25–1).

The contour of the occlusal surface estab-

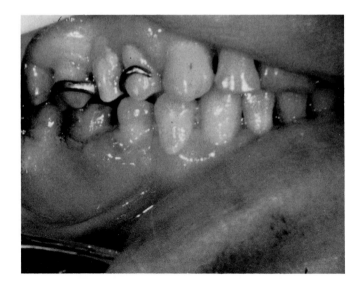

Figure 25–1 Gingival Inflammation and Abscess Formation associated with food impaction between the mandibular second premolar and molar.

lished by the marginal ridges and related developmental grooves normally serves to deflect food away from the interproximal spaces (Fig. 25–2). As the teeth wear down and flattened surfaces replace the normal convexities, the wedging effect of the opposing cusp into the interproximal space is exaggerated (Fig. 25–2), and food impaction results. Cusps that tend to forcibly wedge food interproximally are known as *plunger cusps*. The plunger cusp effect may occur with wear as indicated above, or may be the result of a shift in tooth position following the failure to replace missing teeth.

Excessive anterior overbite is a common cause of food impaction. The forceful wedging of food into the gingiva on the facial surfaces of the mandibular anterior teeth and the lingual surfaces of the maxillary teeth produces varying degrees of periodontal involvement. Gingival changes in the mandibular anterior region, associated with excessive anterior overbite, are easily detectable (Fig. 25–3). Unless they are severe, however, the effects of food impaction on the lingual surface of the maxilla are often overlooked. It should be stressed that inflammation caused by lingual food impaction may spread to the contiguous facial gingival margin. The possibility that lingual food impaction may be a contributory factor should always be explored when the etiology of gingival disease in the anterior maxilla is being considered.

In a classic dissertation on the subject, Hirschfeld[21] **presented the following classification of factors causing food impaction:**

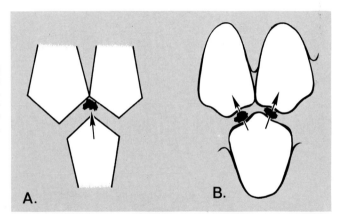

Figure 25–2 Food Impaction. *A,* Wedging effect upon food bolus (*arrow*) which results from wearing away of normal occlusal convexities and protective marginal ridges (after Hirschfeld). *B,* Food impaction corrected by restoring occlusal convex surfaces and marginal ridges and directing food onto the occlusal surface (*arrows*).

A.

B.

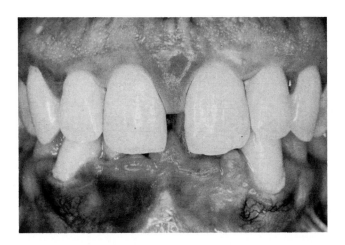

Figure 25–3 Inflammatory Gingival Enlargement in the mandibular anterior region associated with overbite and food impaction.

Class I. Occlusal wear

Type A. Wedging action produced by the transformation of occlusal convexities into oblique facets (Fig. 25–4).

Type B. Remaining obliquely worn cusp of a maxillary tooth overhanging the distal surface of its functional antagonist (Fig. 25–5).

Type C. Obliquely worn mandibular tooth overlapping the distal surface of its functional antagonist (Fig. 25–6).

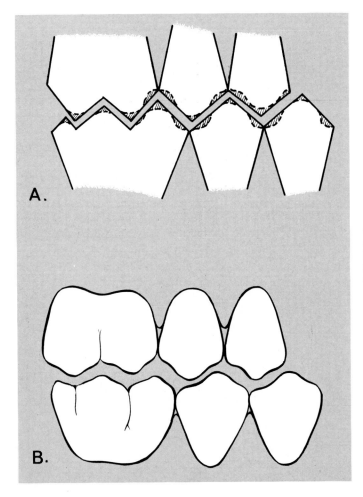

Figure 25–4 Correction of Food Impaction in Worn Dentition. *A*, Flattened occlusal surfaces result in food impaction. Dotted lines show recontouring of occlusal surfaces necessary to correct food impaction. *B*, Recontoured occlusal surfaces.

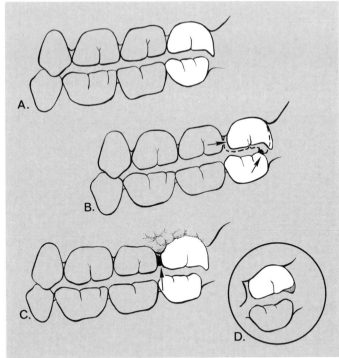

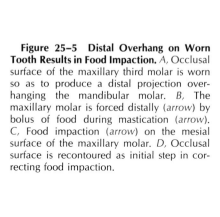

Figure 25-5 **Distal Overhang on Worn Tooth Results in Food Impaction.** *A,* Occlusal surface of the maxillary third molar is worn so as to produce a distal projection overhanging the mandibular molar. *B,* The maxillary molar is forced distally (*arrow*) by bolus of food during mastication (*arrow*). *C,* Food impaction (*arrow*) on the mesial surface of the maxillary molar. *D,* Occlusal surface is recontoured as initial step in correcting food impaction.

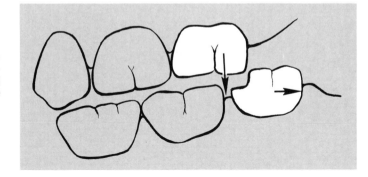

Figure 25-6 **Food Impaction.** Mandibular third molar forced distally (*arrow*) because of notch created by attrition. Food impaction (*arrow*) on the mesial surface is the result.

Class II. Loss of proximal support

Type A. Loss of distal support through the removal of a distally adjacent tooth (Fig. 25-7).

Type B. Loss of mesial support due to extraction.

Type C. Oblique drifting due to non-replacement of a missing tooth.

Type D. Permanent occlusal openings to interdental spaces.

1. Drifting after extraction.
2. Habits forcing teeth out of position.
3. Periodontal disease.
4. Caries (Fig. 25-8).

Class III. Extrusion beyond the occlusal plane

Type A. Extrusion of a tooth retaining contiguity with the adjacent mesial and distal members.

Class IV. Congenital morphologic abnormalities

Type A. Position of a tooth in torsion (Figs. 25-9 and 25-10).

Type B. Emphasized embrasures between thick-necked teeth.

Type C. Buccolingual tilting.

Type D. Lingual or buccal position of a tooth (Fig. 25-11).

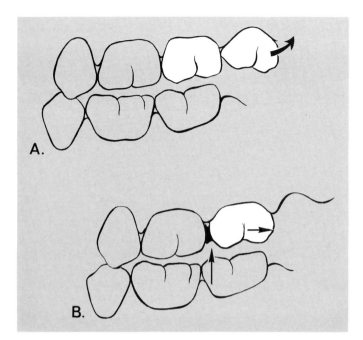

A.

B.

Figure 25–7 Food Impaction. *A,* Removal of maxillary third molar (*arrow*) permits second molar to be forced distally when teeth contact in occlusion. *B,* Bolus of food forced interproximally (*arrow*) as maxillary second molar is wedged distally (*arrow*).

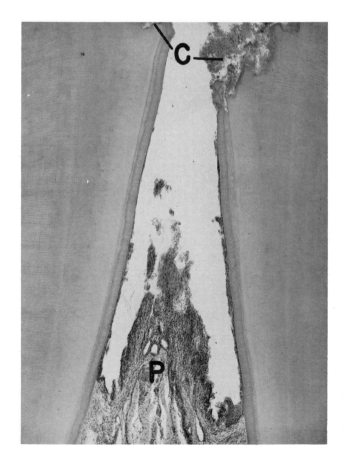

Figure 25–8 Mesiodistal section through mandibular premolars showing loss of proximal contact because of caries (C) which results in food impaction and inflammation of the interdental gingiva (P).

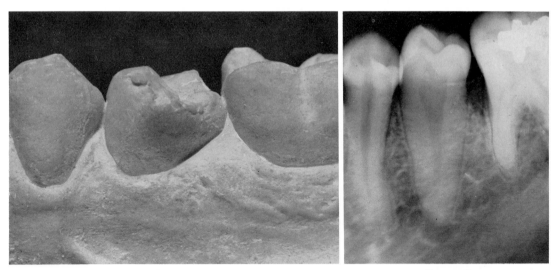

Fig. 25–9   Fig. 25–10

Figure 25–9   Improper Proximal Contact Relationship Associated with Malposed Premolar. Note inclined "plateau" which directs food from occlusal surface of the premolar into the distal interdental space.

Figure 25–10   Bone Loss in area of food impaction associated with improper contact between mandibular second premolar and molar.

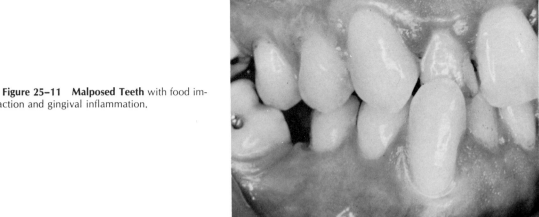

Figure 25–11   Malposed Teeth with food impaction and gingival inflammation.

Class V. Improperly constructed restorations

Type A. Omission of contact points (Fig. 25–12).

Type B. Improper location of contact points.

Type C. Improper occlusal contour.

Type D. Improperly constructed cantilever restorations.

Type E. Scalloped cervical bevels on the tissue-borne areas of prosthetic restorations.

Lateral food impaction

In addition to food impaction by occlusal forces, lateral pressure from the lips, cheeks and tongue may force food interproximally. This is more likely to occur when the gingival embrasure is enlarged by tissue destruction in periodontal disease or by recession. Impaction results when food forced into such an embrasure during mastication is retained instead of passing through.

Sequelae of Food Impaction

Food impaction serves to initiate gingival and periodontal disease and aggravates the severity of pre-existent pathologic changes. The following signs and symptoms occur associated with food impaction:

1. **Feeling of pressure and the urge to dig the material from between the teeth.**

2. **Vague pain, which radiates deep in the jaws.**

3. **Gingival inflammation with bleeding and a foul taste in the involved area.**

4. **Gingival recession.**

5. **Periodontal abscess formation.**

6. **Varying degrees of inflammatory involvement of the periodontal ligament with an associated elevation of the tooth in its socket, prematurity in functional contact and sensitivity to percussion.**

7. **Destruction of alveolar bone.**

8. **Caries of the root.**

UNREPLACED MISSING TEETH

Failure to replace extracted teeth initiates a series of changes producing varying degrees of periodontal disease.[12, 22] In isolated cases, spaces created by tooth extraction may not cause undesirable sequelae. However, the frequency with which periodontal disease results from the failure to replace one or more missing teeth points to the advisability and prophylactic value of early prosthesis.

The ramifications of the failure to replace the first molar are sufficiently consistent to be recognized as a clinical entity. **When the mandibular first molar is missing, the initial change is a mesial drifting and tilting of the mandibular second and third molars and extrusion of the maxillary molar. The distal cusps of the mandibular second molar are elevated and act as plungers impacting food**

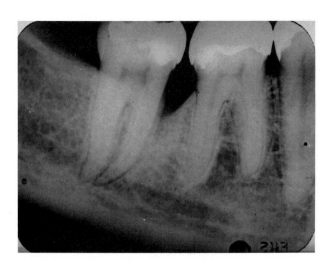

Figure 25–12 **Food Impaction** and bone loss associated with restorations that fail to restore and maintain proximal contact.

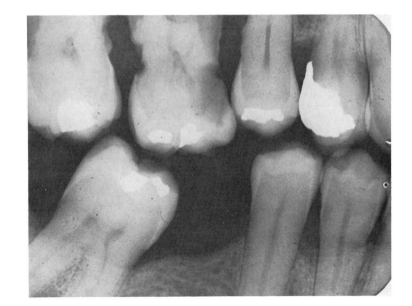

Figure 25–13 Tilted Mandibular Molar and Extruded Maxillary Molar associated with unreplaced tooth. Note caries in maxillary molar.

into the interproximal space between the extruded maxillary first molar and the maxillary second molar (Fig. 25–13). If there is no maxillary third molar, the distal cusps of the mandibular second molar act as a wedge which breaks the contact between the maxillary first and second molars and deflects the maxillary second molar distally. This results in food impaction, gingival inflammation and bone loss in the interproximal area between the maxillary first and second molars. Tilting of the mandibular molars and extrusion of the maxillary molars alter the respective contact relationships of these teeth, thereby favoring food impaction. Bone loss and pocket formation are commonly seen in relation to the extruded and tilted teeth (Figs. 25–14 to 25–16).

Tilting of the posterior teeth also results in reduction in the vertical dimension and accentuation of the anterior overbite. The mandibular anterior teeth slide gingivally along the palatal surfaces of the maxillary anterior teeth, resulting in a distal shift in the position of the mandible. In addition, there is food impaction and pocket formation in relation to the anterior teeth and a tendency toward labial migration and diastema formation in the maxilla. Distal drifting of the second premolar with food impaction and pocket formation in relation to the opened interproximal space between the premolars may be further complica-

tions. The aforementioned changes are accompanied by alterations in the functional relationships of the inclined cusps with resultant occlusal disharmonies injurious to the periodontium.

The combination of changes associated with the unreplaced mandibular first molar does not occur in all cases, nor are all the changes identified with failure to replace other teeth in the arch. In general, however, drifting and tilting of the teeth, with alterations in proximal contact, result from failure to replace teeth that have been extracted. These changes are common factors in the etiology of periodontal disease.

HABIT

Habit is an important factor in the initiation and progress of periodontal disease. Frequently, the presence of an unsuspected habit is revealed in cases that have failed to respond to periodontal therapy. Habits of significance in the etiology of periodontal disease have been classified as follows by Sorrin:[53]

1. *Neuroses*, such as lip biting and cheek biting, which lead to extrafunctional positioning of the mandible; toothpick biting and wedging between the teeth, "tongue-thrusting," fingernail biting, pencil and fountain pen biting and occlusal neuroses.

2. *Occupational habit*, such as the hold-

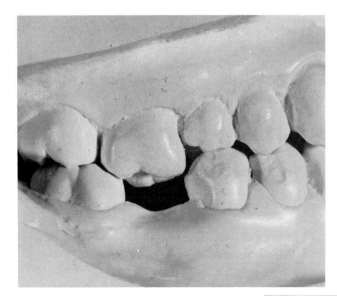

Figure 25–14 Extrusion of Maxillary First Molar into space created by unreplaced mandibular molar.

Figure 25–15 Extruded Maxillary First Molar with Trifurcation Involvement.

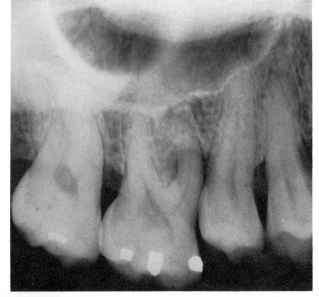

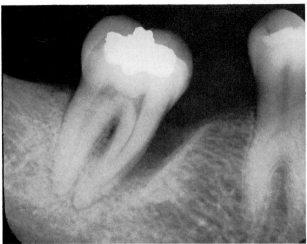

Figure 25–16 Angular Bone Loss on the Mesial Surface of Tilted Molar.

ing of nails in the mouth as practised by cobblers, upholsterers or carpenters, thread biting and pressure of a reed during the playing of certain musical instruments.

3. *Miscellaneous*, such as pipe (Fig. 25–17) or cigarette smoking, tobacco chewing, incorrect methods of toothbrushing, mouth breathing and thumb sucking.

Tongue-Thrusting

Special mention should be made of "tongue-thrusting" because it is so frequently undetected. It entails persistent forceful wedging of the tongue against the teeth, particularly in the anterior region. **Instead of placing the dorsum of the tongue**

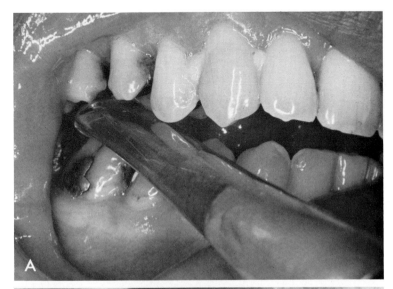

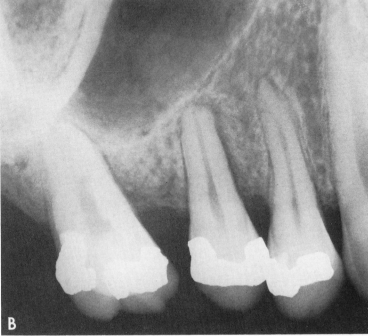

Figure 25–17   Trauma Associated with Holding Pipe in Fixed Position. *A,* Pipe held by maxillary first and second premolars and molar. Note the intruded second premolar and tilted molar. *B,* Radiograph showing intruded second premolar with apical resorption and widened periodontal ligament and angular bone destruction on the mesial surface. Note the widened periodontal ligament on the first premolar and the tilted molar.

against the palate with the tip behind the maxillary teeth during swallowing, the tongue is thrust forward against the mandibular anterior teeth which tilt and also spread laterally (Fig. 25–18).

Ray and Santos[43] divide patients with tongue-thrusting into two groups: (1) those in whom tongue-thrusting is part of a syndrome including a *hyposensitive palate and macroglossia*, and (2) those in whom the tongue-thrusting is a habit acquired in childhood or adult life. Tongue-thrusting is generally associated with abnormal swallowing habits (reverse swallow). These habits usually develop in infancy, and some[1, 55] suspect that they arise from bottle feeding with improperly designed nipples. Nasopharyngeal disease and allergy have also be implicated as possible causes of tongue-thrusting.

Tongue-thrusting causes excessive lateral pressure, which may be traumatic to the periodontium.[11, 13, 50] It also causes spreading and tilting of the anterior teeth,

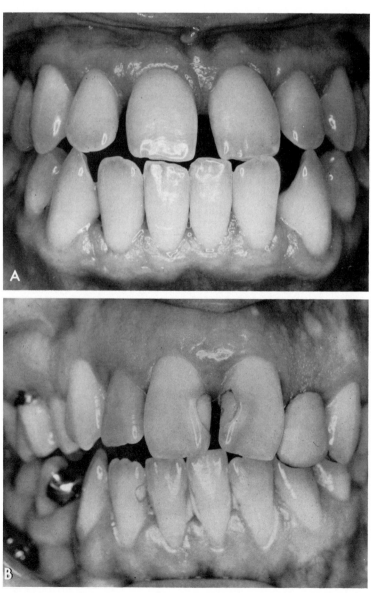

Figure 25–18 Tongue Thrusting. *A,* Tilting and spreading of anterior teeth associated with tongue thrusting. *B,* Hypo-occlusion of lateral incisor, canine and premolar associated with tongue thrusting.

with an open bite, anteriorly, posteriorly or in the premolar area (Fig. 25–18).

Numerous secondary sequelae may develop from tongue-thrusting. The altered inclination of the maxillary anterior teeth results in a change in the direction of the functional forces so that lateral pressure against the crowns is increased. This aggravates the labial drift and undesirable labiolingual rotational forces. The antagonism between forces that direct the tooth labially, and inward pressure from the lip, may lead to tooth mobility. The altered inclination of the teeth also interferes with food excursion and favors the accumulation of food debris at the gingival margin. The loss of proximal contact leads to food impaction. Tongue-thrusting is an important contributing factor responsible for pathologic migration.[9, 12]

Bruxism, Clenching and Tapping

Bruxism consists of aggressive, repetitive or continuous grinding or gritting of the teeth during the day or night[44] or both—most frequently by adults but also by children. *Clenching* is continuous or intermittent closure of the jaws under pressure, and *tapping* is repetitive tooth contacts made on isolated prominent tooth surfaces or dental restorations. Bruxism, clenching and tapping are different occlusal habits which should be considered together because their etiology is the same and they may produce comparable symptoms.

Patients are usually unaware of the habit, but may complain of pain or a tired feeling in the jaws or muscles, particularly upon arising in the morning, which may radiate to the head and neck, a burning sensation in the muscles[46] or headache.[37]

The aforementioned habits represent perversions of occlusion that are potentially injurious to the periodontal tissues, the masticatory muscles and the temporomandibular joint. They are referred to by the term *"parafunction"* which designates tooth contacts in other than chewing and swallowing.[14]

Etiology

The etiology of bruxism and related occlusal habits is not known, but they are usually attributed to occlusal abnormalities and/or emotional tension.[29, 36] It is felt that the habits are triggered by occlusal disharmonies such as occlusal prematurities, and represent struggling movements of the mandible in an attempt to wear away or push aside the offensive tooth surfaces.[16] This opinion is supported by the finding that bruxism is accompanied by abnormal muscle activity, and both disappear when occlusal disharmonies are corrected.[42] There is also evidence that emotional tension, anxiety and deep-seated aggression could cause or aggravate bruxism, clenching and tapping.[57–59]

The relative significance of occlusal disharmonies and emotional factors in the etiology of bruxing, clenching and tapping is not clear. Almost everybody has some form of occlusal disharmony, but there is no indication of how severe it must be to trigger an occlusal habit. People differ in their reaction to occlusal disharmonies. This is where the emotional factors enter the picture. Emotional tension may alter the individual threshold to tolerate the annoyance caused by an occlusal disharmony. A bruxing habit would be the result. Comparable occlusal disharmonies may trigger occlusal habits in some patients and not in others, and the response of a given individual to an occlusal disharmony may vary according to his emotional status.

The effects of bruxism, clenching and tapping habits

Bruxism causes excessive tooth wear characterized by facets on tooth surfaces not ordinarily reached by functional movements, and exaggerated facets in normal functional areas, widening of the occlusal surfaces, and in severe cases reduction in the vertical dimension (Chap. 55). Bruxism does not necessarily cause alveolar destruction.[6] The periodontium often responds favorably to the increased function by thickening of the periodontal ligament and increased density of alveolar bone.

However, the repetitive impact created by bruxism and clenching may injure the periodontium by depriving it of function-free periods necessary for normal repair. By traumatizing the periodontium, occlusal habits aggravate existing periodontal disease and lead to tooth mobility.[8, 24, 28] **Periodontal injury is most severe around teeth** in premature contact. Tapping habits which concentrate on isolated teeth or sections of the arch are more likely to produce injury than are generalized bruxing and clenching.

Occlusal habits may also cause temporomandibular joint disorders secondary to hypertonicity of the masticatory muscles, or reduction in vertical dimension from excessive wear uncompensated for by passive eruption.

Tobacco

Ordinarily, smoking does not lead to striking gingival changes. Heat and accumulated products of combustion are local irritants particularly undesirable in periods of post-treatment healing. The following oral changes may occur in smokers:

1. Brownish, tar-like deposits and discoloration of tooth structure.

2. Diffuse grayish discoloration and leukoplakia of the gingiva.

3. "Smoker's palate," characterized by prominent mucous glands with inflammation of the orifices and a diffuse erythema, or wrinkled "cobblestone" surface.

4. Holding a pipe in a fixed location may cause tooth wear, with the formation of an elliptical space between the teeth, drifting and intrusion of teeth, and traumatic changes in the supporting periodontal tissues.

Increased prevalence of chronic gingivitis and acute necrotizing ulcerative gingivitis,[3] as well as increased prevalence and severity of periodontal disease,[2, 51, 56] has been reported in smokers; in addition, plaque accumulation is increased in smokers,[7] with more calculus in pipe smokers than cigarette smokers.[18, 39, 40] It has been noted that women from the ages of 20 to 39 and men from ages 30 to 59 who smoke cigarettes have about twice the chance of having periodontal disease or becoming edentulous as do nonsmokers.[52]

A specific type of gingivitis termed "gingivitis toxica,"[40] characterized by destruction of the gingiva and underlying bone, has been attributed to the chewing of tobacco.

Keratinized cells in the gingiva are increased in smokers,[10] but no changes other than altered oxygen consumption can be detected in the buccal mucosa. The mucosal response to irritation from tobacco may be modified by experimentally induced systemic disturbance.[27] Daily application of cigarette smoke to the cheek pouch of hamsters for up to 20 months failed to produce any significant change other than occasional slight epithelial hyperplasia.[47]

Betel Chewing

The chewing of betel, common in tropical Asiatic countries, leads to an increased incidence of periodontal disease.[32, 60] The betel fragments lodge interproximally and cause gingivitis and periodontal pockets with bone loss.

MOUTH BREATHING

Gingivitis is often seen associated with mouth breathing.[30] The gingival changes include erythema, edema, enlargement, and a diffuse surface shininess in the exposed areas. The maxillary anterior region is the common site of such involvement. In many cases the altered gingiva is clearly demarcated from the adjacent unexposed normal mucosa (Fig. 25–19). The exact manner in which mouth breathing affects gingival changes has not been demonstrated. Its harmful effect is generally attributed to irritation from surface dehydration. However, comparable changes could not be produced by "air drying" the gingiva of experimental animals.[26]

TOOTHBRUSH TRAUMA

Alterations in the gingiva as well as abrasion of the teeth may result from aggressive brushing in a horizontal or rotary fashion. The deleterious effect of abusive brushing is accentuated when excessively abrasive dentifrices are used.

The gingival changes attributable to toothbrush trauma may be acute or chronic. The acute changes are varied in appearance and duration and include scuffing of the epithelial surface with denudation of the underlying connective tissue to form a painful gingival bruise (Fig. 25–20). Punctate lesions are produced by penetration of

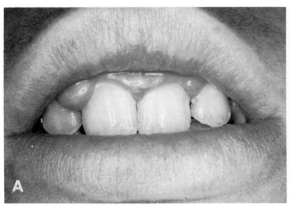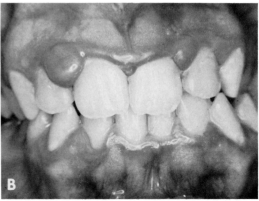

Figure 25–19 Gingivitis in Mouth Breather. *A,* High lip line in mouth breather. *B,* Gingivitis and inflammatory gingival enlargement in exposed area of gingiva.

the gingiva by perpendicularly aligned bristles. Painful vesicle formation in traumatized areas is also seen. Diffuse erythema and denudation of the attached gingiva throughout the mouth may be a striking sequel of overzealous brushing. The acute gingival changes noted above commonly occur when the patient transfers to a new brush. A toothbrush bristle forcibly embedded and retained in the gingiva is a common cause of the acute gingival abscess (Chap. 8).

Chronic toothbrush trauma results in gingival recession with denudation of the root surface. Often the gingival margin is enlarged and appears "piled up" as if it were molded in conformity with the strokes of the toothbrush. Linear grooves may be present that extend from the margin to the attached gingiva. The gingiva in such areas is usually pink and firm.

Improper use of dental floss, toothpicks or wooden interdental stimulators may result in gingival inflammation. The creation of interproximal spaces by destruction of the gingiva from overzealous use of toothpicks leads to the accumulation of debris and inflammatory changes.

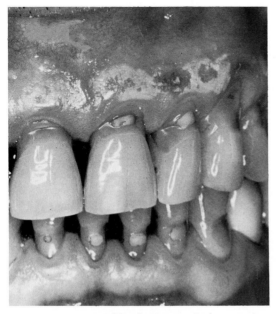

Figure 25–20 Toothbrush Trauma. Surface erosions and hyperkeratosis caused by abusive tooth brushing.

CHEMICAL IRRITATION

Acute gingival inflammation may be caused by chemical irritation, either as the result of sensitivity or nonspecific tissue injury. In allergic inflammatory states, the gingival changes range from simple erythema to painful vesicle formation and ulceration. Severe reactions to ordinarily innocuous mouth washes or dentifrices or denture materials are often explainable on this basis.

Acute inflammation with ulceration may be produced by the nonspecific injurious effect of chemicals upon the gingival tissues (Chap. 51). The indiscriminate use of strong mouth washes (Figs. 25–21 and 25–22), the application of aspirin tablets (Fig. 25–23) to alleviate toothache, injudicious use of escharotic drugs, and accidental contact with drugs such as phenol or silver nitrate are representative of the manner in which

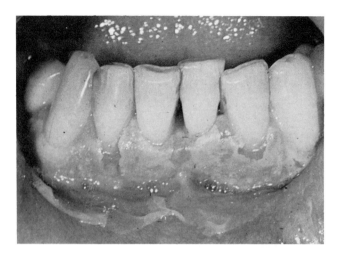

Figure 25–21   Chemical Burn. Necrosis and sloughing produced by undiluted mouth wash.

chemical irritation to the gingiva commonly is produced.

Gingival irritation is also seen in workers in various industries in which chemicals are employed.[48] Gases such as ammonia, chlorine, bromine, acid fumes, and metallic dust are common offenders. The chemical irritation in such occupations is usually of long duration and not necessarily productive of spectacular gingival changes. However, in patients with persistent gingival disease that is refractory to treatment, the occupational background should always be explored.

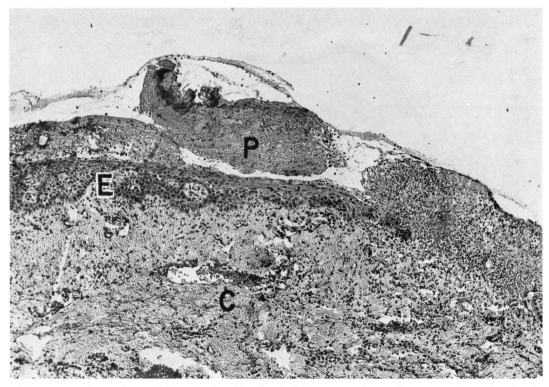

Figure 25–22   Biopsy of Necrotic Area Produced by Chemical Burn. Note inflammed connective tissue (C) and surface pseudomembrane (P). Of particular clinical importance is the newly formed sheet of epithelial cells (E) which undermines the necrotic pseudomembrane and separates it from the underlying connective tissue. This is an important feature of the healing process.

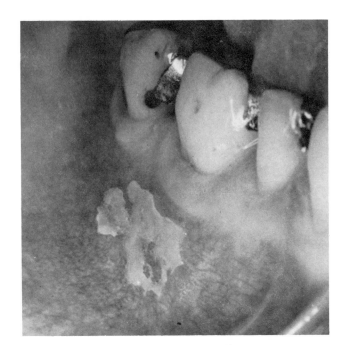

Figure 25–23 Aspirin Burn. Necrosis of mucosa produced by repeated use of aspirin tablets to relieve toothache.

MALOCCLUSION

Depending upon its nature, malocclusion exerts a varied effect in the etiology of gingivitis and periodontal disease.[34, 41, 45] Irregular alignment of teeth results in accumulation of irritating food debris and food impaction. Gingival recession is associated with facially displaced teeth (Fig. 25–24). Occlusal disharmony associated with malocclusion results in injury to the periodontium.[35, 38] The incisal edges of the anterior teeth often cause irritation to the gingiva in the opposing jaw in patients with severe overbite. Open bite relationships lead to unfavorable periodontal changes caused by accumulation of plaque and an absence or diminution in function (Fig. 25–25).[9, 25] The prevalence and severity of periodontal disease are increased in children with bimaxillary protrusions.[23]

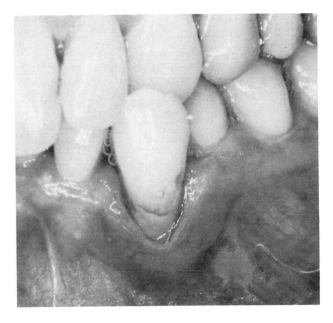

Figure 25–24 Gingival Recession and Inflammation on Malposed Canine.

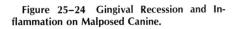

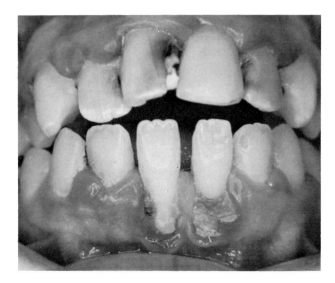

Figure 25–25 Chronic Gingivitis associated with "open bite" and accumulation of plaque and food debris.

FAULTY DENTAL RESTORATIONS

Faulty dental restorations[61] and prostheses are common causes of gingivitis and periodontal disease (Figs. 25–26 to 25–28). Overhanging margins provide ideal locations for the accumulation of plaque and the multiplication of bacteria, which give rise to enzymes and other injurious substances. Accumulation of plaque in partially "washed out" synthetic porcelain restorations close to the gingival margin is a common source of irritation to the gingiva. Restorations that do not reproduce the contour of the buccal surfaces of molars deflect food into the gingival margin with resultant inflammation. Inadequate or improperly located proximal contacts, and failure to reproduce the normal protective anatomy of the occlusal marginal ridges and developmental grooves, lead to food impaction. Failure to re-establish adequate interproximal embrasures fosters the accumulation of irritants. Restorations that do not conform with occlusal wear patterns cause occlusal disharmonies that may be injurious to the supporting periodontal tissues.

Further analysis of the significance of faulty restorative dentistry in the etiology of gingival and periodontal disease is presented in Chapter 54.

Fig. 25–26

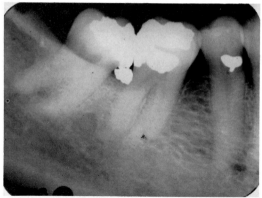

Fig. 25–27

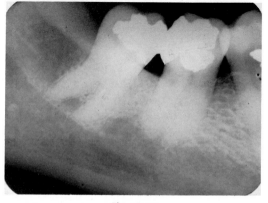

Figure 25–26 Amalgam Excess which is source of irritation to the gingiva.

Figure 25–27 Amalgam Excess Removed.

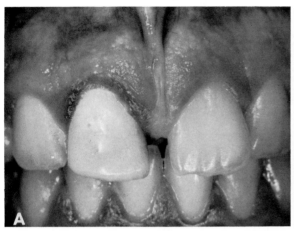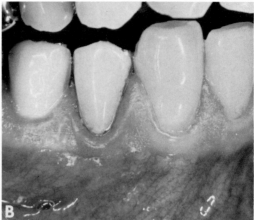

Figure 25–28 *A,* **Gingival Inflammation and Recession** associated with accumulated irritants on rough margin of crown. *B,* **Inadequate Mesioproximal Contour on First Premolar Restoration** leads to accumulation of irritants and gingival inflammation.

DENTAL PROCEDURES

The use of rubber dam clamps, copper bands, matrix bands and disks in such a manner as to lacerate the gingiva results in varying degrees of inflammation. Although for the most part such transient injuries undergo repair, they are needless sources of discomfort to the patient. Injudicious tooth separation and excessively vigorous condensing of gold foil restorations are sources of injury to the supporting tissues of the periodontium, which may be attended by acute symptoms such as pain and sensitivity to percussion.

Thermal injury artificially induced through reamed root canals produced necrosis in the surrounding periodontium and interrupted cementum formation in experimental animals.[4]

DENTAL PROBLEMS ASSOCIATED WITH MUSICAL WIND INSTRUMENTS

Wind instruments create forces on the teeth which may injure the periodontium and cause lossening and pathologic migration. With reed instruments such as the clarinet and saxophone, the mouthpiece is inserted between the teeth, causing excessive pressure against and displacement of the mandibular and maxillary incisors. It may also injure the lower lip by pressing it against the incisal edges of the mandibular teeth (Fig. 25–29). Brass instruments, which have an extraoral mouthpiece, produce lingually directed pressures through the lips to the maxillary and mandibular incisors.[40a]

Preventive and corrective measures include removable acrylic or metal splints over the facial surface and incisal edge of the anterior mandibular teeth, including the premolars, fixed splinting and elimination of sharp tooth edges.

RADIATION

Gingival ulceration, bleeding and suppuration, periodontitis, denudation of roots and bone, and loosening and loss of teeth have been noted following treatment with external and internal radiation in patients with malignancies of the oral cavity and adjacent regions.[5, 15, 54] Periodontal disease is a possible portal of entry for infection and the development of osteoradionecrosis following radiation therapy. Changes that vary in severity from edema and bleeding of the gingiva and widening of the periodontal ligament with disrupted deposition of cementum, to necrosis of the gingiva and periodontal ligament and resorption of alveolar bone, loosening and shedding of the teeth and the necrosis and sloughing of the oral mucosa, have been reported in experimental animals exposed to single and multiple head or total body roentgen radiation in individual doses of 10 r to 3000 r, to a total dosage of 11,000 r.[17, 19, 20, 31, 33, 49]

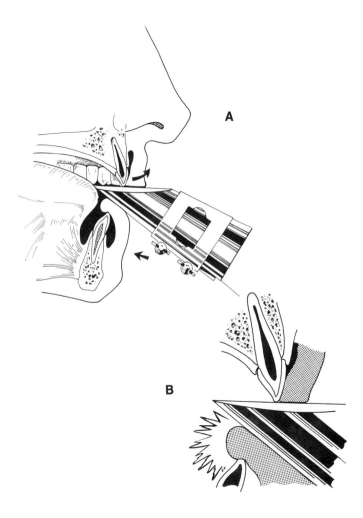

A

B

Figure 25–29 Trauma from Musical Instrument. *A*, Mouthpiece of single reed instrument (clarinet and saxophone) tends to displace maxillary incisors outward and push the mandibular incisors and mandible back. *B*, Pressure against the incisal edges may injure the lower lip. (From Porter, M. M.[40a])

REFERENCES

1. Anderson, W. S.: The Relationship of the Tongue-Thrust Syndrome to Maturation and Other Factors. Am. J. Orthodont., 49:264, 1963.
2. Arno, A., Schei, O., Lovdal, A., and Waerhaug, J.: Alveolar Bone Loss as a Function of Tobacco Consumption. Acta Odont. Scandinav., 17:3, 1959.
3. Arno, A., Waerhaug, J., Lovdal, A., and Schei, O.: Incidence of Gingivitis as Related to Sex, Occupation, Tobacco Consumption, Toothbrushing, and Age. Oral Surg., Oral Med. & Oral Path., 11:587, 1958.
4. Atrizadeh, F., and Zander, H. A.: Healing of the Periodontium after Thermal Injury. I.A.D.R., 48th General Meeting, 1970, 202, p. 99.
5. Aub, J. C., Evans, R. D., Hempelmann, L. H., and Martland, H. S.: The Late Effects of Internally-Deposited Radioactive Material in Man. Medicine (Baltimore), 31:221, 1952.
6. Baer, P. M., Kakehashi, S., Littleton, N. W., White, C. L., and Lieberman, J. E.: Alveolar Bone Loss and Occlusal Wear. Periodontics, 1:91, 1963.
7. Brandtzaeg, P.: The Significance of Oral Hygiene in the Prevention of Dental Diseases. Odont. T., 72:460, 1964.
8. Bruxism. Report of the 14th Congress of A.R.P.A. Internationale, Venice, Italy. Academy Review, 4:9, 1956.
9. Burwasser, P., and Hill, T. J.: The Effect of Hard and Soft Diets on the Gingival Tissues of Dogs. J. D. Res., 18:389, 1939.
10. Caloninius, P. E. B.: A Cytological Study on the Variation of Keratinization in the Normal Oral Mucosa of Young Males. J. West. Soc. Periodont., 10:69, 1962.
11. Carranza, F. A., and Carraro, J. J.: Lingual Pressure as Traumatizing Factor in Periodontics. Rev. A. Odont. Argent., 47:105, 1959.
12. Chaikin, B. S.: Anterior Periodontal Destruction Due to the Loss of One or More Unreplaced Molars. D. Items Int., 61:17, 1939.
13. Dechaume, M.: Importance du Sympathique, des Troubles de la Musculature Oro-Faciale et des Tics de Succion ou de Pulsion dans les Parodontopathies. Rev. Stomatol., 63:701, 1962.
14. Drum, N.: Classification of Parafunction. Deutsche Zahn. Zeit., 5:411, 1962.
15. Ellinger, F.: Effects of Ionizing Radiation on the Oral Cavity. Chapter 18 in: F. Ellinger (Ed.); Medical Radiation Biology. Springfield, Ill., Charles C Thomas, 1957.
16. Eschler, J.: Electrophysiologische and pathologische Untersuchungen des Kausystems. Forum Parodont., 5:1147, 1955.
17. Frandsen, A. M.: Periodontal Tissue Changes Induced in Young Rats by Roentgen Irradiation of the Molar Regions or the Head: Acta Odont. Scandinav., 20:393, 1962.
18. Frandsen, A. M., and Pindborg, J. J.: Tobacco and Gingivitis. III. Difference in the Action of Cigarette and Pipe Smoking. J. D. Res., 28:464, 1949.
19. Gowgiel, J. M.: Experimental Radio-osteonecrosis of the Jaws. J. D. Res., 39:176, 1960.
20. Greulich, R. C., and Ershoff, B. H.: Delayed Effects of Multiple Sublethal Doses of Total Body X-Irradiation on the Periodontium and Teeth of Mice. J. D. Res., 40:1211, 1961.
21. Hirschfeld, I.: Food Impaction. J.A.D.A., 17:1504, 1930.
22. Hirschfeld, I.: Individual Missing Tooth. J.A.D.A., 24:67, 1937.
23. Holden, S., Harris, J. E., and Ash, M. M., Jr.: Periodontal Disease in Nubian Children. I.A.D.R. Abstr., 48th General Meeting, 1970, 67, p. 65.
24. Ingle, J. I.: Occupational Bruxism and Its Relation to Periodontal Disease. J. Periodont., 23:7, 1952.
25. King, J. D., and Gimson, A. P.: Experimental Investigations of Paradontal Disease in the Ferret and Related Lesions in Man. Brit. D. J., 83:126, 1947.
26. Klingsberg, J., Cancellaro, L. A., and Butcher, E. O.: Effects of Air Drying on Rodent Oral Mucous Membrane: A Histologic Study of Simulated Mouth Breathing. J. Periodont., 32:38, 1961.
27. Kreshover, S. J.: The Effect of Tobacco on the Epithelial Tissues of Mice. J.A.D.A., 45:528, 1952.
28. Leof, M.: Clamping and Grinding Habits: Their Relation to Periodontal Disease. J.A.D.A., 31:184, 1944.
29. Lipke, D., and Posselt, U.: Parafunctions of the Masticatory System (Bruxism): Report of a Panel Discussion. J. West. Soc. Periodont., 8:133, 1960.
30. Lite, T., et al.: Gingival Pathosis in Mouth Breathers. A Clinical and Histopathologic Study and a Method of Treatment. Oral Surg., Oral Med. & Oral Path., 8:382, 1955.
31. Medak, H., and Burnett, G. W.: The Effect of X-ray Irradiation on the Oral Tissues of the Macacus Rhesus Monkey. Oral Surg., Oral Med. & Oral Path., 7:778, 1954.
32. Mehta, F. S., et al.: Relation of Betel Leaf Chewing to Periodontal Disease. J.A.D.A., 50:531, 1955.
33. Meyer, I., Shklar, G., and Turner, J.: A Comparison of the Effects of 200 KV Radiation and Cobalt-60 Radiation on the Jaws and Dental Structure of the White Rat. Oral Surg., Oral Med. & Oral Path., 15:1098, 1962.
34. Miller, J., and Hobson, P.: The Relationship Between Malocclusion, Oral Cleanliness, Gingival Conditions, and Dental Caries in School Children. Brit. D. J., 111:43, 1961.
35. Mühlmann, H. R., et al.: Okklusion und Artikulation im Atiologiekomplex Parodontaler Erkrankungen. Parodontologie, 11:20, 1957.
36. Nadler, S. C.: Bruxism, A Classification: Critical Review. J.A.D.A., 54:615, 1957.
37. Nadler, S. C.: The Importance of Bruxism. J. Oral Med., 23:142, 1968.
38. O'Leary, T. J., and Sosa, C. E.: Signs of Periodontal Breakdown in Patients with Malocclusion. J. Dent. Ed., 10:172, 1955.
39. Pindborg, J. J.: Tobacco and Gingivitis. II. Correlation between Consumption of Tobacco, Ulceromembranous Gingivitis and Calculus. J. D. Res., 28:461, 1949.
40. Pindborg, J. J.: Tobacco and Gingivitis. I. Statistical Examination of the Significance of Tobacco in the Development of Ulceromembranous Gingivitis and in the Formation of Calculus. J. D. Res., 26:261, 1947.
40a. Porter, M. M.: Dental Problems in Wind Instrument Playing. London, British Dental Association, 1968.
41. Poulton, D. R., and Aaronson, S. A.: The Relationship Between Occlusion and Periodontal Status. Am. J. Orthodont., 47:690, 1961.

42. Ramfjord, S. P.: Bruxism, A Clinical and Electromyographic Study. J.A.D.A., 62:21, 1961.

43. Ray, H. G., and Santos, H. A.: Consideration of Tongue-Thrusting as a Factor in Periodontal Disease. J. Periodont., 25:250, 1954.

44. Robinson, J., Reding, G., Zepelin, H., Smith, V., and Zimmerman, S.: Nocturnal Teeth-Grinding: A Reassessment for Dentistry. J.A.D.A., 78:1308, 1969.

45. Rosenzweig, K. A., and Langer, A.: Oral Disease in Yeshiva Students. J. D. Res., 40:993, 1961.

46. Ross, I. F.: The Effects of Tensional Clenching upon the Structures of the Neck. J. Periodont., 25:46, 1954.

47. Salley, J. J., and Kreshover, S. J.: Further Studies of the Effect of Tobacco on Oral Tissues. J. D. Res., 37:979, 1958.

48. Schour, I., and Sarnat, B. G.: Oral Manifestations of Occupational Origin. J.A.M.A., 120:1197, 1942.

49. Schüle, H., and Betzold, J.: Experimental Investigations on the Effect of X-ray Irradiation on Marginal Periodontal Tissues. Deutsche Zahn. Zschr., 24:140, 1969.

50. Sheppard, I. M.: Tongue Dynamics. D. Digest, 59:117, 1953.

51. Smoking and Noncancerous Oral Disease. The Health Consequences of Smoking, 1969 Supplement to the 1967 Public Health Service Review. U.S. Department of Health, Education and Welfare, Public Health Service.

52. Solomon, H., Priore, R., and Bross, I.: Cigarette Smoking and Periodontal Disease. J.A.D.A., 77:1081, 1968.

53. Sorrin, S.: Habit: An Etiologic Factor of Periodontal Disease. D. Digest, 41:290, 1935.

54. Stafne, E. C., and Bowing, H. H.: The Teeth and Their Supporting Structures in Patients Treated by Irradiation. Am. J. Orthodont., 33:567, 1947.

55. Straub, W. J.: Malfunction of the Tongue. Part II. The Abnormal Swallowing Habit: Its Causes, Effects, and Results in Relation to Orthodontic Treatment and Speech Therapy. Am. J. Orthodont., 47:596, 1961.

56. Summers, C. J., and Oberman, A.: Association of Oral Disease with 12 Selected Variables: I. Periodontal Disease. J. D. Res., 47:457, 1968.

57. Takahama, Y.: Bruxism. J. D. Res., 40:227, 1961.

58. Thaller, J. L.: The Use of the Cornell Index to Determine the Correlation between Bruxism and the Anxiety State: A Preliminary Report. J. Periodont., 31:138, 1960.

59. Thaller, J. L., Rosen, G., and Saltzman, S.: Study of the Relationship of Frustration and Anxiety to Bruxism. J. Periodont., 38:193, 1967.

60. Waerhaug, J.: Prevalence of Periodontal Disease in Ceylon. Association with Age, Sex, Oral Hygiene, Socioeconomic Factors, Vitamin Deficiencies, Malnutrition, Betel and Tobacco Consumption, and Ethnic Group. Final Report. Acta Odont. Scandinav., 25:205, 1967.

61. Wright, W. H.: Local Factors in Periodontal Disease. Periodontics, 1:163, 1963.

Chapter 26

NUTRITIONAL INFLUENCES IN THE ETIOLOGY OF PERIODONTAL DISEASE

The individual's nutritional status affects the condition of the periodontium, and injurious effects of local irritants and excessive occlusal forces may be aggravated by nutritional deficiencies. **However, no nutritional deficiencies of themselves cause gingivitis or periodontal pockets; local irritants are necessary to produce such changes.** Theoretically, there may be a "border zone" in which local irritants of insufficient severity to produce clinically detectable disease could cause gingival and periodontal disorders, if their effect upon the periodontium were aggravated by nutritional deficiencies. However, the extent to which the nutritional status may be altered before it affects the oral tissue is an individual matter, for which there are no measurements. Sometimes oral changes provide the first signs of the existence of nutritional deficiency.

Some nutritional deficiencies produce characteristic oral changes, some oral changes are common to several nutritional deficiencies, and the same deficiency may result in different oral changes in different patients. The problem of identifying oral

365

changes with specific deficiencies is complicated because multiple deficiencies occur together, and deficiency-induced oral changes are complicated by tissue injury caused by local irritating and traumatic factors.

PHYSICAL CHARACTER OF THE DIET

The physical character of the diet is an important factor in the etiology of gingival and periodontal disease. Soft diets, adequate in nutrients, may lead to accumulation of plaque and calculus and loosening of the teeth.[5, 11, 12, 24] Hard and fibrous foods provide surface cleansing action and stimulation which results in less plaque and gingivitis[7, 29] even if the diet is nutritionally inadequate.[14] They also provide the functional stimulation necessary for maintenance of the periodontal ligament and alveolar bone. An exception to the generally favorable observations regarding hard foods is the report of plaque reduction in animals after hard food was converted to a soft mixture by grinding and combining with 8 per cent vegetable oil.[26]

Local factors may induce conditioned nutritional deficiencies in the periodontium of patients with a satisfactory nutritional status. Degenerative changes in chronic inflammation and trauma from occlusion impair the capacity of the tissues to utilize available nutrients.

VITAMIN A DEFICIENCY

Deficiency of vitamin A results in keratinizing metaplasia of epithelium, increased susceptibility to infection,[10] disturbances in bone growth, shape and texture,[16] abnormalities in the central nervous system[33] and ocular manifestations—which include night blindness (nyctalopia), xerosis of the conjunctiva, xerosis of the cornea with subsequent corneal turbidity, ulceration and keratomalacia.[15]

Oral findings in experimental animals

The following changes have been reported in vitamin A deficient rats: widening of the periodontal ligament of the molars and incisors, degeneration of the principal fibers,[3] thickening of the cementum of the molars,[28] apical hypercementosis with imperfect root formation, retarded eruption and malposition of the teeth.[28] Hyperkeratosis of the oral epithelium produced by vitamin A deficiency in experimental animals is comparable to that resulting from prolonged administration of estrogen.[34] Alveolar bone changes in vitamin A deficient animals include increased density with fewer marrow spaces,[18] hypercalcification with retardation in the rate of bone deposition,[28] resorption with fibrosis,[4] atrophy with resorption (most pronounced in the furcation areas),[23] osteophytic formation,[3] osteoporosis and resorption of the crest of the alveolar bone, which may be the result of the deficiency or may occur secondary to gingival changes.[13]

Vitamin A deficiency and periodontal disease

Numerous studies in experimental animals suggest that vitamin A deficiency may predispose to periodontal disease.[2, 19, 20] Loss of neurotrophic stimulation as a result of peripheral nerve degeneration[13, 17, 22] and atrophy of the salivary glands[2] have been suggested as causative factors.

The gingiva shows epithelial hyperplasia and hyperkeratinization with proliferation of the epithelial attachment.[3, 13, 18] The life cycle of the epithelial cells is shortened as evidenced by early karyolysis.[7] Gingival hyperplasia with inflammatory infiltration and degeneration,[20] pocket formation[2, 3] and the formation of subgingival calculus[13] also occur.

Local irritation is necessary before abnormal epithelial tendencies associated with vitamin A deficiency are manifest in the gingival sulcus.[9] Pocket formation does not occur in vitamin A deficient animals in the absence of local irritation, but when local irritation is present, the pockets are deeper than in nondeficient animals and present associated epithelial hyperkeratosis. Repair of gingival wounds is retarded in vitamin A deficient animals,[8, 21] which are also subject to leukoplakia of the oral mucosa in areas other than the gingiva.[1]

In contrast with the abundance of evidence in experimental animals, there is little information regarding the effects of vitamin A deficiency upon the oral structures in humans. Low daily intake of vitamin A has been associated with periodontal disease.[25] Marshall-Day[6] reported a possible correlation between the incidence of periodontal disease and dermatologic lesions characteristic of vitamin A deficiency, and populations with a high incidence of periodontal disease tend to be deficient in vitamin A.[27]

Hypervitaminosis A

Large doses of vitamin A in young growing rats produce generalized bone resorptive activity and osteoporosis which result in multiple fractures. Developing dental tissues are not affected, but the alveolar bone shows marked resorption without repair.[32] Hypervitaminosis A may accelerate bone growth.[31] Furthermore, melanin-like pigmentation of the skin, scaling dermatosis, disturbed menstruation, itching, and exophthalmos have been identified with hypervitaminosis A in humans.[30]

REFERENCES

Physical Character of the Diet and Vitamin A

1. Abels, J. C., Rekers, P. E., Hayes, M., and Rhoads, C. P.: Relationship Between Dietary Deficiency and Occurrence of Papillary Atrophy of Tongue and Oral Leukoplakia. Cancer Res., 2:381, 1942.
2. Boyle, P. E.: Effect of Vitamin A Deficiency on the Periodontal Tissues. Am. J. Orthodont. & Oral Surg., 33:744, 1947.
3. Boyle, P. E., and Bessey, O. A.: The Effect of Acute Vitamin A Deficiency on the Molar Teeth and Paradontal Tissues, with a Comment on Deformed Incisor–Teeth in This Deficiency. J. D. Res., 20:236, 1941.
4. Burn, C. G., Orten, A. U., and Smith, A. H.: Changes in Structure of Developing Tooth in Rats Maintained on Diets Deficient in Vitamin A. Yale J. Biol. & Med., 13:817, 1941.
5. Burwasser, P., and Hill, T. J.: The Effect of Hard and Soft Diets on the Gingival Tissues of Dogs. J. D. Res., 18:389, 1939.
6. Day, C. D. M.: Nutritional Deficiencies and Dental Caries in Northern India. Brit. D. J., 76:143, 1944.
7. Egelberg, J.: Local Effect of Diet on Plaque Formation and Development of Gingivitis in Dogs. I. Effect of Hard and Soft Diets. Odont. Revy, 16:31, 1965.
8. Frandsen, A. M.: Periodontal Tissue Changes in Vitamin A Deficient Young Rats. Acta Odont. Scandinav., 21:19, 1963.
9. Glickman, I., and Stoller, M.: The Periodontal Tissues of the Albino Rat in Vitamin A Deficiency. J. D. Res., 27:758, 1948.
10. Green, H. N., and Mellanby, E.: Vitamin A as Anti-infective Agent. Brit. M. J., 2:691, 1928.
11. Haydak, M. H., Vivino, A. E., Bohfren, J. J., and Palmer, L. S.: A Clinical and Biochemical Study of Cow's Milk and Honey as an Essentially Exclusive Diet for Adult Humans. Am. J. M. Sc., 207:209, 1944.
12. Ivy, A. C., Morgan, J. E., and Farrel, J. I.: Effects of Total Gastrectomy. Surg., Gynec. & Obst., 53:602, 1931.
13. King, J. D.: Abnormalities in the Gingival and Subgingival Tissues due to Diets Deficient in Vitamin A and Carotene. Brit. D. J., 68:349, 1940.
14. King, J. D., and Glover, N. E.: The Relative Effects of Dietary Constituents and Other Factors Upon Calculus Formation and Gingival Disease in the Ferret. J. Path. & Bact., 57:353, 1945.
15. Kruse, H. D.: Medical Evaluation of Nutritional Status. IV. The Ocular Manifestations of Avitaminosis A, with Especial Consideration of the Detection of Early Changes by Biomicroscopy. Milbank Mem. Fund Quart., XIX:207, 1941.
16. Mellanby, E.: A Story of Nutritional Research. Baltimore, Williams & Wilkins Co., 1950.
17. Mellanby, E.: Xerophthalmia; Trigeminal Degeneration and Vitamin A Deficiency. J. Path. & Bact., 38:391, 1934.
18. Mellanby, H.: Effect of Maternal Dietary Deficiency of Vitamin A on Dental Tissues in Rats. J. D. Res., 20:489, 1941.
19. Mellanby, M.: Dental Research, with Special Reference to Parodontal Disease Produced Experimentally in Animals. D. Record, 59:227, 1939.
20. Mellanby, M.: Diet and the Teeth: An Experimental Study. Part I. Dental Structures in Dogs. Med. Res. Council (Brit.) Spec. Rep. Series No. 140, London, 1929.
21. Mellanby, M.: Diet and the Teeth: An Experimental Study. Part II. Diet and Dental Disease; B. Diet and Dental Structure in Animals Other than the Dog. Med. Res. Council (Brit.) Spec. Rep. Series No. 153, London, 1930.
22. Mellanby, M., and King, J. D.: Diet and the Nerve Supply to the Dental Tissues. Brit. D. J., 56:538, 1934.
23. Miglani, D. C.: The Effect of Vitamin A Deficiency on the Periodontal Structures of Rat Molars with Emphasis on Cementum Resorption. Oral Surg., Oral Med. & Oral Path., 12:1372, 1959.
24. Pelzer, R.: A Study of the Local Oral Effect of Diet on the Periodontal Tissues and the Gingival Capillary Structure. J.A.D.A., 27:13, 1940.
25. Radusch, D. F.: Nutritional Aspect of Periodontal Disease. Ann. Dent., 7:169, 1940.
26. Ramirez, J., and Stallard, R.: Diet: Its Role in the Accumulation of Local Etiologic Factors in Periodontal Disease. I.A.D.R. Abstr., 48th General Meeting, 1970, No. 342, p. 134.
27. Russell, A. L.: International Nutrition Surveys: A Summary of Preliminary Dental Findings. J. D. Res., 42:233, 1963.
28. Schour, I., Hoffman, M. M., and Smith, M. C.: Changes in Incisor Teeth of Albino Rats with Vitamin A Deficiency and Effects of Replacement Therapy. Am. J. Path., 17:529, 1941.
29. Strålfors, A., Thilander, H., and Bergenholtz, A.:

Caries and Periodontal Disease in Hamsters Fed Cereal Foods Varying in Sugar Content and Hardness. Arch. Oral Biol., *12*:1361, 1967.

30. Sulzberger, M. B., and Lazar, M. P.: Hypervitaminosis A. J.A.M.A., *146*:788, 1951.
31. Wolbach, S. B.: Vitamin A Deficiency and Excess in Relation to Skeletal Growth. Proc. Inst. Med. Chicago, *16*:118, 1946.
32. Wolbach, S. B., and Bessey, O. A.: Tissue Changes in Vitamin Deficiencies. Physiol. Rev., *22*:233, 1942.
33. Wolbach, S. B., and Bessey, O. A.: Vitamin A Deficiency and the Nervous System. Arch. Path., *32*:689, 1941.
34. Ziskin, D. E., Rosenstein, S. N., and Drucker, L.: Interrelation of Large Parenteral Doses of Estrogen and Vitamin A and Their Effect on the Oral Mucosa. Am. J. Orthodont. & Oral Surg., *29*:163, 1943.

VITAMIN B COMPLEX DEFICIENCY

The vitamin B complex includes the following substances: thiamine (vitamin B_1), riboflavin (vitamin B_2), nicotinic acid (niacin) or nicotinic acid amide (niacinamide), pantothenic acid, pyridoxine (vitamin B_6), biotin, para-aminobenzoic acid, inositol, choline, folic acid (folacin) and vitamin B_{12} (cyanocobalamin). Oral disease is rarely due to a deficiency in just one component of the B complex group. The deficiency is generally multiple. Oral changes common to deficiencies in the B complex group are gingivitis, glossitis, glossodynia, cheilosis, and inflammation of the entire oral mucosa. **The gingivitis in vitamin B deficiencies is nonspecific, caused by local irritation rather than by the deficiency, but it is subject to the modifying effect of the latter.**[1] Stomatitis and mild neuralgic disturbances with or without achlorhydria, and without anemia, have responded to B complex therapy.[28] An association has been hypothesized between vitamin B complex deficiency and herpetic-like oral vesicles based on the response of these lesions to vitamin B complex,[3, 10] or thiamine chloride therapy.[3]

Oral Findings Associated with Vitamin B Complex Deficiency

Thiamine (vitamin B_1)

The human manifestations of thiamine deficiency, called beriberi, are characterized by paralysis, cardiovascular symptoms (including edema) and loss of appetite. Frank beriberi is rare in the United States; however, less striking polyneuropathies do result from accompanying conditioning factors that interfere with absorption or utilization of thiamine. Many animals, including man, have microorganisms in their intestinal tracts that have the capacity to synthesize thiamine, thus complicating experimental inducement of deficiency of this vitamin.

The following oral disturbances have been attributed to thiamine deficiency: hypersensitivity of the oral mucosa;[26] minute vesicles (simulating herpes) on the buccal mucosa, under the tongue or on the palate; and erosion of the oral mucosa.[13] Glossitis could not be produced in humans by deprivation of thiamine.[38] Since thiamine is essential to bacterial and carbohydrate metabolism, it has been postulated that the activity of the oral flora is diminished in thiamine deficiency.[21]

Riboflavin (vitamin B_2)

The symptoms of riboflavin deficiency (ariboflavinosis) include glossitis, cheilosis, seborrheic dermatitis and a superficial vascularizing keratitis.[32, 33] The glossitis is characterized by a magenta discoloration and atrophy of the papillae. Disappearance of the papillae of the tongue varies, and depends upon the severity of the deficiency. In mild to moderate cases, the dorsum presents a patchy atrophy of the lingual papillae[1] and engorged fungiform papillae, which project as pebble-like elevations.[15] In severe deficiency, the entire dorsum is flat, having a dry and often fissured surface (Fig. 26–1). The margin of the tongue presents a scalloped appearance, caused by contiguous indentations that conform to the pattern of the interdental spaces of the dentition.

Cheilosis is one of the changes most frequently identified with riboflavin deficiency.[16, 17] According to Schour and Massler,[31] "The cheilosis begins as a tiny raw, red painful area at the commissure of the lips, at the mucocutaneous junction [Fig. 26–2]. The area becomes larger and is soon covered with an adherent white epithelial membrane. In severe cases, painful, multiple fissures develop. The lesion tends to spread to the lower lip, causing

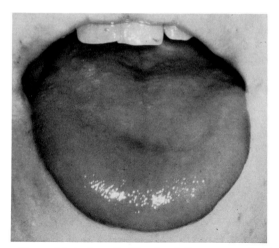

Figure 26-1 Smooth Discolored Tongue associated with riboflavin deficiency.

fissuring and cheilitis. It may also spread over the skin but characteristically spares the upper lip."

Riboflavin deficiency is not the only cause of cheilosis. Deficiencies of pyridoxine,[24] nicotinic acid,[14] the entire vitamin B complex,[15] calcium pantothenate[9] or iron may produce a comparable change. Loss of vertical dimension, together with drooling of saliva into the angles of the lips, may produce a condition similar to cheilosis which has been described as "pseudoriboflavinosis" and "pseudocheilosis."[7, 25] A lesion similar to cheilosis, termed "la perlèche," is attributed to bacterial and mycotic infection.[12] Riddle, Spies and Hudson[29] isolated *aureus* and *hemolyticus* from cheilotic lesions and concluded that in most angular lesions in riboflavin-deficient patients invasion by bacteria was a contributing factor.

Changes observed in riboflavin-deficient animals include severe lesions of the gingiva, periodontal tissues and oral mucosa (including noma),[4, 34] and retarded chondrogenic and osteogenic activity in the condylar growth center of the mandible.[23] Congenital malformation, including cleft palate and impaired mandibular development, results from prenatal riboflavin deficiency.[37] An association between alveolar bone loss[30] and riboflavin deficiency in humans has been suggested.

Nicotinic acid (niacin)

Nicotinic acid deficiency, or aniacinosis, results in *pellagra*, which is characterized

by dermatitis, gastrointestinal disturbances, neurological and mental disturbances (dermatitis, diarrhea and dementia),[18] glossitis, gingivitis and generalized stomatitis.[20]

ORAL CHANGES. Glossitis and stomatitis may be the earliest clinical signs of nicotinic acid deficiency.[27] In the acute form, there are hyperemia of the tongue, enlargement of the papillae and indentation of the margin, followed by atrophic changes and a resultant glazed surface. The tongue in acute nicotinic acid deficiency is "beefy-red" and **painful**, with "burning" (glossopyrosis)[22] (Fig. 26-3). In chronic nicotinic acid deficiency the tongue is thinned and fissured, with surface crevices, marginal serrations, and atrophy of the fungiform and filiform papillae. The gingiva may be involved in aniacinosis[19] with or without tongue changes. The most frequent finding is acute necrotizing ulcerative gingivitis, usually in areas of local irritation (Fig. 26-4).

Oral manifestations of vitamin **B** complex

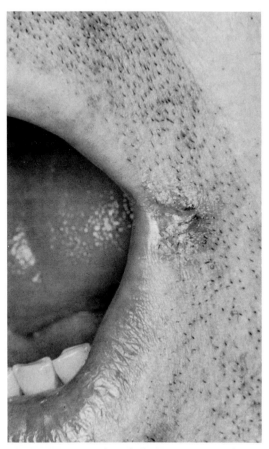

Figure 26-2 Angular Cheilosis in patient with conditioned vitamin B complex deficiency.

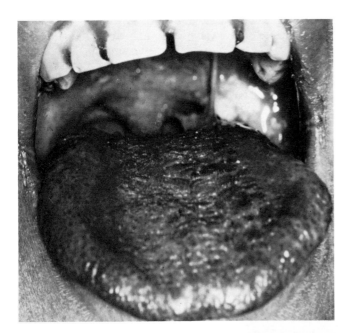

Figure 26-3 "Beefy," Crusted Tongue in Patient with Pellagra.

Figure 26-4 Ulceration of Buccal Mucosa in Patient with Nicotinic Acid Deficiency. Note sharp cusp of maxillary molar which initiated the irritation. (Courtesy Dr. David Weisberger.)

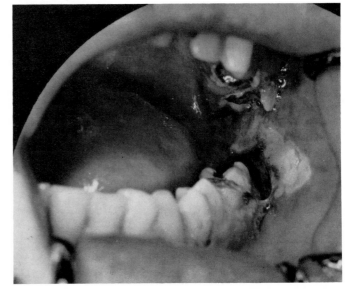

and nicotinic acid deficiencies in experimental animals include black tongue[1, 5, 8, 11] and gingival inflammation with destruction of the gingiva, periodontal ligament and alveolar bone.[2] Necrosis of the gingiva and other oral tissues, and leukopenia, are terminal features of nicotinic acid deficiency in experimental animals.

Pantothenic acid

Oral changes caused by pantothenic acid deficiency have been identified in animals but not in humans. These include[36, 40] angular cheilosis, hyperkeratosis with ulceration and necrosis of the gingiva and oral mucosa, proliferation of the basal layer of the oral epithelium, and resorption of the crest of the alveolar bone. Absence of an inflammatory response is a striking finding. Radiographically, narrowing of the periodontal ligament space, alveolar bone loss and rarefaction of bone may be observed.

Microscopically, the interdental papillae are necrotic, which in severe cases involves the

alveolar bone. There is very little inflammation. Diets deficient in the filtrate fraction of the vitamin B complex, which contains pantothenic acid plus other unknown elements, results in hyperkeratosis and degenerative changes with necrosis of the oral epithelium, reduction in height of the alveolar bone (with osteoporosis and replacement by adipose tissue), and malformation and resorption of the roots. Inflammatory changes are absent unless a deficiency in nicotinic acid is superimposed upon the filtrate fraction deficiency.

The oral mucosa and lips are glistening red, sometimes with ulceration. In the early stages salivary flow is increased and accompanied by drooling, but the dehydration which occurs as the disease progresses leads to reduced salivary flow and dryness.

Pyridoxine (vitamin B₆)

Anemia, cardiovascular disturbances, convulsions, retardation of growth,[39] and patchy atrophy of the dorsum of the tongue (similar to that observed in riboflavin deficiency) have been noted in experimental animals on diets deficient in pyridoxine.[1]

Humans with pyridoxine deficiency present angular cheilosis and glossitis with swelling, atrophy of the papilla, magenta discoloration and discomfort. When experimentally created in humans, the deficiency results in glossitis resembling that of nicotinic acid, reddening with small ulcerations of the mucosa and angular cheilosis.[35]

Folic acid (pteroylglutamic acid)

Folic acid deficiency results in macrocytic anemia with megaloblastic erythropoiesis, with oral changes and gastrointestinal lesions, diarrhea and intestinal malabsorption.[6]

ORAL CHANGES. Folic acid deficient animals present necrosis of the gingiva, periodontal ligament and alveolar bone without inflammation.[32a] The absence of inflammation is the result of deficiency-induced granulocytopenia.

In humans with sprue and other folic acid deficiency states there is generalized stomatitis, which may be accompanied by ulcerated glossitis, cheilitis and cheilosis. Ulcerative stomatitis is an early indication of a toxic effect of folic acid antagonists used in the treatment of leukemia.

In sprue, glossitis may be the presenting complaint; it usually occurs after the onset of steatorrhea. Swelling and redness at the tip and lateral margins are the initial disorders, accompanied in some cases by painful minute ulcers on the dorsum. Disappearance of the filiform and fungiform papillae is followed by the development of a smooth atrophic red tongue. Painful burning symptoms and increased salivation accompany the oral changes.

Vitamin B₁₂ (cyanocobalamin)

Vitamin B₁₂, the antipernicious anemia factor, is the only vitamin which contains cobalt. It is a patent catalyst and is involved in the synthesis of nucleic acid and folic acid metabolism. Pernicious anemia is the most severe form of vitamin B₁₂ deficiency. Other macrocytic anemias are thought to be mild forms of vitamin B₁₂ deficiency complicated by deficiency of folic acid. Oral changes in pernicious anemia are described in Chapter 28.

REFERENCES

Vitamin B Complex

1. Afonsky, D.: Oral Lesions in Niacin, Riboflavin, Pyridoxine, Folic Acid and Pantothenic Acid Deficiencies in Adult Dogs. Oral Surg., Oral Med. & Oral Path., 8:207, 315, 867, 1955.
2. Becks, H., Wainwright, W. W., and Morgan, A. F.: Comparative Study of Oral Changes in Dogs due to Deficiencies of Pantothenic Acid, Nicotinic Acid and Unknowns of B Vitamin Complex. Am. J. Orthodont. & Oral Surg., 29:183, 1943.
3. Burket, L. W., and Hickman, G. C.: Oral Herpes (Simplex) Manifestations; Treatment with Vitamin B Complex. J.A.D.A., 29:411, 1942.
4. Chapman, O. D., and Harris, A. E.: Oral Lesions Associated with Dietary Deficiencies in Monkeys. J. Infect. Dis., 69:7, 1941.
5. Denton, J.: A Study of Tissue Changes in Experimental Black Tongue of Dogs Compared with Similar Changes in Pellagra. Am. J. Path., 4:341, 1928.
6. Dreizen, S.: Oral Manifestations of Human Nutritional Anemias. Arch. Environ. Health, 5:66, 1962.
7. Ellenberg, M., and Pollack, H.: Pseudoariboflavinosis. J.A.M.A., 119:790, 1942.
8. Elvehjem, C. A., Madden, R. J., Strong, F. M., and Woolley, D. W.: Relation of Nicotinic Acid and Nicotinic Acid Amide to Canine Black Tongue. J. Am. Chem. Soc., 59:1767, 1937.

9. Field, H., Jr., Green, M. E., and Wilkinson, C. W.: Glossitis and Cheilosis Healed Following the Use of Calcium Pantothenate. Am. J. Digest. Dis., 12:246, 1945.

10. Gerstenberger, H. J.: Etiology and Treatment of Herpetic (Aphthous and Aphtho-Ulcerative) Stomatitis and Herpes Labialis. Am. J. Dis. Child., 26:309, 1923.

11. Goldberger, J., and Wheeler, G. A.: Experimental Black Tongue of Dog Compared with Similar Changes in Pellagra. Pub. Health Rep., 43:172, 1928.

12. Goodman, M. H.: Perlèche: A Consideration of Its Etiology and Pathology. Bull. Johns Hopkins Hosp., 51:263, 1932.

13. Govier, W. M., and Grieg, M. E.: Prevention of Oral Lesions in B_1 Avitaminotic Dogs. Science, 98:216, 1943.

14. Hon, H. S.: Riboflavin Deficiency Among Chinese. II. Cheilosis and Seborrheic Dermatitis. Chinese M. J., 59:314, 1941.

15. Jeghers, H.: Riboflavin Deficiency. IV. Oral Changes. Advances in Internal Medicine I. New York, Interscience Publishers Inc., 1942, p. 257.

16. Jolliffe, N., Fein, H. D., and Rosenblum, L. A.: Riboflavin Deficiency in Man. New England J. Med., 221:921, 1939.

17. Jones, H. E., Green, H. F., Armstrong, T. G., and Chadwick, V.: Stomatitis Due to Riboflavin Deficiency. Lancet, 1:721, 1944.

18. Kaufman, W.: Common Form of Niacinamide Deficiency Disease: Aniacinamidosis. New Haven, Yale University Press, 1943.

19. King, J. D.: Vincent's Disease Treated with Nicotinic Acid. Lancet, 2:32, 1940.

20. Kirkland, O.: Oral Manifestations of Pellagra. Internat. J. Orthodont., 22:1172, 1936.

21. Kneisner, A. H., Mann, A. W., and Spies, T. D.: Relationship of Dental Caries to Deficiencies of Vitamin B Group. J. D. Res. 21:259, 1942.

22. Kruse, H. D.: Lingual Manifestations of Aniacinosis with Especial Consideration of Detection of Early Changes by Biomicroscopy. Milbank Mem. Fund Quart., 20:262, 1942.

23. Levy, B. M.: The Effect of Riboflavin Deficiency on the Growth of the Mandibular Condyle of Mice. Oral Surg., Oral Med. & Oral Path., 2:89, 1949.

24. Machella, T. E.: Studies of B Vitamins in Human Subjects. III. Response of Cheilosis to Vitamin Therapy. Am. J. M. Sc., 203:114, 1942.

25. Mann, A. W., Dreizen, S., and Spies, T. D.: Further Studies in the Effect of the Correction of Mechanical Factors on Angular Cheilosis in Malnourished Edentulous Patients. Oral Surg., Oral Med. & Oral Path., 1:868, 1948.

26. Mann, A. W., Spies, T. D., and Springer, M.: Oral Manifestations of Vitamin B Complex Deficiencies. J. D. Res., 20:269, 1941.

27. Manson-Bahr, P., and Ransford, O. N.: Stomatitis of Vitamin B_2 Deficiency Treated with Nicotinic Acid. Lancet, 2:426, 1938.

28. Rhoads, C. P.: Conferences on Vitamin B Therapy. J.A.M.A., 113:297, 1939.

29. Riddle, J. W., Spies, T. D., and Hudson, N. P.: Note on the Interrelationship of Deficiency Disease and Resistance to Infection. Proc. Soc. Exper. Biol. & Med., 45:361, 1941.

30. Ross, J. A.: Some Observations on Dental Conditions in Possible Riboflavin Deficiency. Brit. J. Radiol., 17:247, 1944.

31. Schour, I., and Massler, M.: The Effects of Dietary Deficiencies Upon the Oral Structures. J.A.D.A., 32:714, 871, 1022, 1139, 1945.

32. Sebrell, W. H., and Butler, R. E.: Riboflavin Deficiency in Man. Pub. Health Rep., 53:2282, 1938; 54:2121, 1939.

32a. Shaw, J. H.: The Relation of Nutrition to Periodontal Disease. J. D. Res. (Suppl. 1), 41:264, 1962.

33. Sydenstricker, V. P.: Clinical Manifestations of Ariboflavinosis. Am. J. Pub. Health, 31:344, 1941.

34. Topping, N. H., and Fraser, H. F.: Mouth Lesions Associated with Dietary Deficiencies in Monkeys. Pub. Health Rep., 54:416, 1939.

35. Vilter, R. W., et al.: The Effect of Vitamin B_6 Deficiency Induced by Desoxypyridoxine in Human Beings. J. Lab. & Clin. Med., 42:335, 1953.

36. Wainwright, W. W., and Nelson, M.: Changes in Oral Mucosa Accompanying Acute Pantothenic Acid Deficiency in Young Rats. Am. J. Orthodont. & Oral Surg., 31:406, 1945.

37. Warkany, J., and Schraffenberger, E.: Congenital Malformations Induced in Rats by Maternal Nutritional Deficiency. VI. Preventive Factor. J. Nutrition, 27:477, 1944.

38. Williams, R. D., Masson, H. L., Wilder, R. M., and Smith, B. F.: Observations on Induced Thiamine Deficiency in Man. Arch. Int. Med., 66:785, 1940; 69:721, 1942.

39. Wolbach, S. B., and Bessey, O. A.: Tissue Changes in Vitamin Deficiencies. Physiol. Rev., 22:233, 1942.

40. Ziskin, D. E., Stein, G., Gross, P., and Runne, E.: Oral, Gingival and Periodontal Pathology Induced in Rats on a Low Pantothenic Acid Diet by Toxic Doses of Zinc Carbonate. Am. J. Orthodont. & Oral Surg. (Oral Surg. Sect.), 33:407, 1947.

VITAMIN C (ASCORBIC ACID) DEFICIENCY

Severe vitamin C deficiency in humans results in scurvy, a disease characterized by hemorrhagic diathesis and retardation of wound healing. The hemorrhages commonly occur in areas of trauma or marked function.[18] Clinical features of scurvy include fatigue, breathlessness, lethargy, loss of appetitie, sallow complexion, fleeting pains in joints and limbs, skin petechiae (particularly around hair follicles) epistaxis, ecchymosis (mainly in lower extremities), hemorrhage into muscles and deeper tissues (scurvy siderosis), hematuria, edema of the ankles and anemia.[22] Increased susceptibility to infection and impaired wound healing (see Chap. 36) are also features of vitamin C deficiency.

Vitamin C deficiency (scurvy) results in defective formation and maintenance of collagen,[13] mucopolysaccharide ground substance and intercellular cement substance in mesen-

chymal tissues.[33] **Its effect on bone is marked by retardation or cessation of osteoid formation, impaired osteoblastic function[25] and osteoporosis.[1, 9, 32] Vitamin C deficiency is also characterized by increased capillary permeability, susceptibility to traumatic hemorrhages, a hyporeactivity of the contractile elements of the peripheral blood vessels and sluggishness of blood flow.[18]**

Gingival and Periodontal Disease

Gingivitis

Gingivitis with enlarged hemorrhagic bluish red gingiva is described as the classic sign of vitamin C deficiency (see Chap. 7), **but gingivitis is not caused by vitamin C deficiency,** *per se.* Nor do all vitamin C deficient patients necessarily have gingivitis; it does not occur in the absence of local irritants. **If gingivitis is present in a vitamin C deficient patient it is caused by local irritants.** Vitamin C deficiency may aggravate the gingival response to local irritation and worsen the edema, enlargement and bleeding,[14] and the severity may be reduced by correcting the deficiency; but gingivitis will remain so long as local irritants are present.

The legendary association of severe gingival disease with scurvy led the presumption that vitamin C deficiency is an etiologic factor in gingivitis which is so common at all ages. Attempts to correlate the ascorbic acid level of the blood with the incidence and severity of gingivitis have produced mixed results. Some claim there is such a relationship,[2, 17, 31] but the majority disagree.[4, 5, 7, 8, 12, 20, 21, 23, 27]

Periodontal disease

It has been suggested that in humans alveolar bone loss results from ascorbic acid deficiency[3] and diets without citrus fruit juices,[28] but epidemiologic[24] and chemical[26] studies fail to identify vitamin C deficiency with the prevalence or severity of periodontal disease or tooth mobility.[19] In evaluating clinical studies dealing with ascorbic acid levels, it should be noted that it is the whole blood or leukocyte-platelet method of determination that is the reliable indicator.[5, 7, 23] Blood plasma levels fluctu-

ate with variations in intake; whole blood or leukocyte-platelet levels indicate the nutritional status of the tissues in regard to vitamin C.[6, 22]

Experimental evidence

Changes in the supporting periodontal tissues and gingiva in vitamin C deficiency have been documented extensively in experimental animals.[10, 15, 16, 30, 32] **Acute vitamin C deficiency results in edema and hemorrhage in the periodontal ligament, osteoporosis of alveolar bone, and tooth mobility; hemorrhage edema and degeneration of collagen fibers occur in the gingiva, but acute vitamin C deficiency does not cause or increase the incidence of gingivitis. Local irritation must be present for gingivitis to occur in experimental animals with acute vitamin C deficiency.[10, 11] The deficiency alters the response to irritation so that the gingiva are enlarged, edematous and hemorrhagic. Vitamin C deficiency also retards gingival healing.[29]**

Vitamin C deficiency does not cause periodontal pockets; local irritating factors are required for pocket formation to occur. However, when pocket formation does occur in vitamin C deficiency, it is of greater depth than that normally produced under comparable local conditions. The occurrence of pocket formation and destruction of underlying tissues in vitamin C deficiency is not attributable to the deficiency alone, but indicates the presence of a complicating local factor.

Acute vitamin C deficiency alters the response of the supporting periodontal tissues to the extent that the destructive effect of gingival inflammation upon the underlying periodontal membrane and alveolar bone is accentuated.[11] The exaggerated destruction results partly from inability to marshal a defensive delimiting reaction to the inflammation and partly from destructive tendencies caused by the deficiency itself. Factors contributing to the destruction of the periodontal tissues in vitamin C deficiency include inability to form a peripheral delimiting connective tissue barrier, reduction in inflammatory cells, diminished vascular response, inhibition of fibroblast formation, and differentiation to osteoblasts, impaired formation of collagen and mucopolysaccharide ground substance.

REFERENCES

Vitamin C

1. Albright, F., and Reifenstein, E. C., Jr.: Parathyroid Glands and Metabolic Bone Disease. Baltimore, Williams & Wilkins Co., 1948, p. 150.
2. Blockley, C. H., and Baenziger, P. E.: An Investigation into the Connection between the Vitamin C Content of the Blood and Periodontal Disturbances. Brit. D. J., 73:57, 1942.
3. Boyle, P. E.: Dietary Deficiencies as a Factor in the Etiology of Diffuse Alveolar Atrophy. J.A.D.A., 25:1436, 1938.
4. Burrill, D. Y.: Relationship of Blood Plasma Vitamin C Level to Gingival and Periodontal Disease. J. D. Res., 21:353, 1942.
5. Burrill, D. Y.: Oral Conditions in Experimental Vitamin C and B Deficiency. J.A.D.A., 33:594, 1946.
6. Butler, A. M., and Cushman, M.: Distribution of Ascorbic Acid in Blood and Its Nutritional Significance. J. Clin. Invest., 19:459, 1940.
7. Crandon, J. H., Lund, C. C., and Dill, D. B.: Experimental Human Scurvy. New England J. Med., 223:353, 1940.
8. Dalldorf, G., and Zall, G.: Tooth Growth in Experimental Scurvy. J. Exper. Med., 52:57, 1930.
9. Follis, R. H.: The Pathology of Nutritional Disease. Springfield, Ill., Charles C Thomas, 1948, p. 134.
10. Glickman, I.: Acute Vitamin C Deficiency and Periodontal Disease. I. The Periodontal Tissues of the Guinea Pig in Acute Vitamin C Deficiency. J. D. Res., 27:9, 1948.
11. Glickman, I.: Acute Vitamin C Deficiency and the Periodontal Tissues. II. The Effect of Acute Vitamin C Deficiency upon the Response of the Periodontal Tissues of the Guinea Pig to Artificially Induced Inflammation. J. D. Res., 27:201, 1948.
12. Glickman, I., and Dines, M. M.: Effect of Increased Ascorbic Acid Blood Levels on the Ascorbic Acid Level in Treated and Nontreated Gingiva. J. D. Res., 42:1152, 1963.
13. Gould, B. S.: Ascorbic Acid–Independent and Ascorbic Acid–Dependent Collagen-forming Mechanisms. Ann. New York Acad. Sc., 92:168, 1961.
14. Hodges, R. E., et al.: Experimental Scurvy in Man. Am. J. Clin. Nutrit., 22:535, 1969.
15. Hojer, J. A.: Studies in Scurvy. Acta Paediat. (Suppl.), 3:119, 1924.
16. Hojer, J. A., and Westin, G.: Jaws and Teeth in Scorbutic Guinea Pig. D. Cosmos, 67:1, 1925.
17. Keller, S. E., Ringsdorf, W. M., and Cheraskin, E.: Interplay of Local and Systemic Influences in the Periodontal Diseases. J. Periodont., 34:259, 1963.
18. Lee, R. E., and Lee, N. Z.: The Peripheral Vascular System and Its Reactions in Scurvy: An Experimental Study. Am. J. Physiol., 149:465, 1947.
19. O'Leary, T. J., Rudd, K. D., Crump, P. P., and Krause, R. E.: The Effect of Ascorbic Acid Supplementation on Tooth Mobility. J. Periodont.–Periodontics, 40:284, 1969.
20. Parfitt, G. J., and Hand, C. D.: Reduced Plasma Ascorbic Acid Levels and Gingival Health. J. Periodont., 34:347, 1963.
21. Perlitsh, M., Nielsen, A. G., and Stanmeyer, W. R.: Ascorbic Acid Plasma Levels and Gingival Health in Personnel Wintering Over in Antarctica. J. D. Res., 40:789, 1961.
22. Ralli, E. P., and Sherry, S.: Adult Scurvy and the Metabolism of Vitamin C. Medicine, 20:251, 1941.
23. Restarski, J. S., and Pijoan, M.: Gingivitis and Vitamin C. J.A.D.A., 31:1323, 1944.
24. Russell, A. L.: International Nutrition Surveys: A Summary of Preliminary Dental Findings. J. D. Res., 42:233, 1963.
25. Salter, W. T., and Aub, J. C.: Studies of Calcium and Phosphorus Metabolism. IX. Deposition of Calcium in Bone in Healing Scorbutus. Arch. Path., 11:380, 1931.
26. Shannon, I., and Gibson, W. A.: Intravenous Ascorbic Acid Loading in Subjects Classified as to Periodontal Status. J. D. Res., 44:355, 1965.
27. Spies, T. D.: Nutrition and Disease. Postgrad. Med., 17:2, 1955.
28. Thomas, A. E., Busby, M. C., Ringsdorf, W. M., and Cheraskin, E.: Ascorbic Acid and Alveolar Bone Loss. Oral Surg., Oral Med. & Oral Path., 15:555, 1962.
29. Turesky, S., and Glickman, I.: Histochemical Evaluation of Gingival Healing in Experimental Animals on Adequate and Vitamin C Deficient Diets. J. D. Res., 33:273, 1954.
30. Waerhaug, J.: The Role of Ascorbic Acid in Periodontal Tissue. J. D. Res., 39:1089, 1960.
31. Weisberger, D., Young, A. P., and Morse, F. W.: Study of Ascorbic Acid Blood Levels in Dental Patients. J. D. Res., 17:101, 1938.
32. Wolbach, S. B., and Bessey, O. A.: Tissue Changes in Vitamin Deficiencies. Physiol. Rev., 22:233, 1942.
33. Wolbach, S. B., and Howe, P. R.: Intercellular Substances in Experimental Scorbutus. Arch. Path., 1:1, 1926.

VITAMIN D (CALCIUM AND PHOSPHORUS) DEFICIENCIES

Vitamin D, a fat-soluble vitamin, is essential for the absorption of calcium from the gastrointestinal tract, and for the maintenance of the calcium-phosphorus balance and the formation of teeth and bones. The metabolism of calcium and phosphorus, and vitamin D, is interrelated. The effects of variations of the calcium, phosphorus and vitamin D intake upon the skeletal and dental structures are influenced by numerous other factors, such as parathyroid function, the presence of carbohydrate, fat and such inorganic elements as strontium and beryllium, and age. Deficiency in vitamin D and/or imbalance in the calcium-phosphorus intake result in *rickets* in the very young and *osteomalacia* in adults. Their effect upon the periodontal tissues of experimental animals has been described as follows:

Vitamin D deficiency with normal dietary calcium and phosphorus in young dogs is characterized by osteoporosis of alveolar bone;[5] osteoid formed at a normal rate, but remaining uncalcified; failure of osteoid to resorb, leading to its excessive accumulation; reduction in the width of the periodontal space; normal rate of cementum formation but defective calcification and some cementum resorption;[15] and distortion of the growth pattern of alveolar bone. In young rats the periodontium is unaltered in vitamin D deficiency, providing that the diet is adequate in minerals.[12]

In osteomalacic animals there is rapid, generalized severe osteoclastic resorption of alveolar bone, proliferation of fibroblasts which replace bone and marrow, and new bone formation around remnants of unresorbed bone trabeculae.[7] Radiographically there are generalized partial to complete disappearance of the lamina dura and reduced density of supporting bone, loss of trabeculae, increased radiolucence of trabecular interstices and increased prominence of remaining trabeculae. Microscopic and radiographic changes in the periodontium are almost identical with those in experimentally induced hyperparathyroidism.

In *vitamin D and calcium deficiency with normal dietary phosphorus* there are generalized bone resorption in the jaws, fibro-osteoid hemorrhage in the marrow spaces and destruction of the periodontal ligament.[5] The pattern is suggestive of changes in hyperparathyroidism.

Vitamin D and phosphorus deficiency with normal dietary calcium presents rachitic changes characterized by marked osteoid deposition.[11]

In *calcium and phosphorus deficiency with normal vitamin D* there is excessive bone resorption;[1, 5] resorption of alveolar bone and cementum occurs in adult animals on a calcium-deficient diet.[10]

In *phosphorus deficiency with normal dietary vitamin D and calcium,* jaw growth is disturbed, and tooth eruption and condylar growth retarded,[6, 14] accompanied by malocclusion.

Calcium deficiency in young rats produces osteoporosis and reduction in the number and diameter of periodontal fibers and increased cemental resorption.[12]

Hypervitaminosis D

Hypervitaminosis D in humans is characterized by nausea, vomiting, diarrhea, epigastric fullness, polyuria, polydipsia, albuminuria, impaired renal function, hypercalcemia or hyperphosphatemia. It may terminate fatally. In experimental animals, Follis[9] observed that excessive doses of vitamin D (125,000 units of vitamin D given daily for nine days) resulted in marked osteoblastic activity, and production of large quantities of osteoid about the trabeculae in the shafts of long bones. Baker[2] noted that guinea pigs maintained on hypervitaminotic D diets develop generalized osteoporosis and metastatic calcifications. Weinmann and Sicher[16] suggested that the bone destructive effect of hypervitaminosis D is a phenomenon secondary to renal damage which would create a condition of hyperparathyroidism.

Oral Findings. The periodontal findings in experimental hypervitaminosis D include osteosclerosis characterized by marked endosteal and periosteal bone formation (or deposition of an amorphous highly calcified material), osteoporosis and resorption of alveolar bone,[8] pathologic calcification in the periodontal ligament and gingiva, severe calculus formation, deposition of a cementum-like substance on the root surfaces (resulting in hypercementosis and the ankylosis of many teeth), and extensive periodontal disease.[3, 4] Calcification of periodontal ligament collagen has been produced in experimental animals by combining hypervitaminosis D with osteolathyrism, but not by the vitamin deficiency alone.[13]

REFERENCES

Vitamin D, Calcium and Phosphorus Deficiencies

1. Arnim, S. S., Clarke, M. F., Anderson, B. G., and Smith, A. H.: Dental Changes in Rats Consuming Diet Poor in Organic Salts. Yale J. Biol. & Med., 9:117, 1936.
2. Baker, S. L.: The General Pathology of Bone. In Shanks, S. C., and Kerley, P.: A Textbook of X-ray Diagnosis. 2nd ed. Philadelphia, W. B. Saunders Co., 1950, Vol. IV, Chaps. V, VI.
3. Becks, H.: Dangerous Effects of Vitamin D Overdosage on Dental and Paradental Structure. J.A.D.A., 29:1947, 1942.
4. Becks, H., Collins, D. A., and Freytog, R. M.:

Changes in Oral Structures of the Dogs Persisting after Chronic Overdoses of Vitamin D. Am. J. Ortho. & Oral Surg., 32:463, 1946.

5. Becks, H., and Weber, M.: Influence of Diet in Bone System with Special Reference to Alveolar Process and Labyrinthine Capsule. J.A.D.A., 18:197, 1931.

6. Burrill, D. Y.: The Effect of Low Phosphorus Intake on the Growth of the Jaws in Dogs. J.A.D.A., 30:513, 1943.

7. Dreizen, S., et al.: Studies on the Biology of the Periodontium of Marmosets. III. Periodontal Bone Changes in Marmosets with Osteomalacia and Hyperparathyroidism. Israel J. Med. Sc., 3:731, 1967.

8. Fahmy, H., Rodgers, W. E., Mitchell, D. F., and Brewer, H. E.: Effects of Hypervitaminosis D on the Periodontium of the Hamster. J. D. Res., 40:870, 1961.

9. Follis, R. H., Jr.: The Influence of Essential Nutrients and Hormones on Cartilage and Bone. Trans. Josiah Macy Jr. Foundation Conference on Metabolic Interrelations, 2:221, 1950.

10. Henrikson, P.: Periodontal Disease and Calcium Deficiency: An Experimental Study in the Dog. Acta Odont. Scandinav., 26:Suppl. 50:1, 1968.

11. MacCollum, E. V., Simmonds, N., Shipley, P. G., and Park, B. A.: The Production of Rickets by Diets Low in Phosphorus and Fat Soluble. A. J. Biol. Chem., 47:507, 1921.

12. Oliver, W. M.: The Effect of Deficiencies of Calcium, Vitamin D, or Calcium and Vitamin D and of Variations in the Source of Dietary Protein on the Supporting Tissues of the Rat Molar. J. Periodont. Res., 4:56, 1969.

13. Shoshan, S., Pisanti, S., and Sciaky, I.: The Effect of Hypervitaminosis D on the Periodontal Membrane Collagen in Lathyritic Rats. J. Periodont. Res., 2:121, 1967.

14. Weinmann, J. P.: Rachitic Changes of the Mandibular Condyle of the Rat. J. D. Res., 25:509, 1946.

15. Weinmann, J. P., and Schour, I.: Experimental Studies in Calcification. Am. J. Path., 21:821, 1047, 1945.

16. Weinmann, J. P., and Sicher, H.: Bone and Bones. St. Louis, C. V. Mosby Co., 1948, p. 147.

VITAMIN E, VITAMIN K AND VITAMIN P DEFICIENCIES

Vitamin E

No relationship has been demonstrated between deficiencies in vitamin E and oral disease.[5] Extirpation of the submaxillary and sublingual glands in vitamin E deficient animals results in gingival bleeding, loosening and exfoliation of the molars, and purulent discharge from the sockets.[2] In humans, a favorable response to vitamin E therapy has been reported in patients having severe periodontal disease, with a minimum of local irritating factors.[4]

Vitamin K

Vitamin K is necessary for the production of prothrombin in the liver; vitamin K deficiency results in a hemorrhagic tendency. It may cause excessive gingival bleeding after toothbrushing, or spontaneously. In humans it is synthesized by bacteria in the intestinal tract. Antibiotics and sulfa drugs which inhibit the bacterial action may interfere with vitamin K synthesis. Bile salts are important in the absorption of vitamin K; obstruction of the biliary tract may lead to hypoprothrombinemia. Vitamin K is used for the prevention and control of oral hemorrhage.

Vitamin P (citrin)

Vitamin P is involved in the maintenance of capillary integrity and the prevention of capillary fragility.[1, 6] It has been used therapeutically for the control of hemorrhage and in the treatment of blood dyscrasias.[7] Kreshover and Burket[3] suggested that the capillary fragility frequently encountered in patients with periodontal disease may be due in part to vitamin P deficiency. This is based on the finding of normal blood ascorbic acid levels in patients who manifested a high petechial count in capillary fragility testing. The use of citrin in the treatment of gingival disease is still in the experimental stage.

REFERENCES

Vitamin E, Vitamin K and Vitamin P Deficiencies

1. Bourne, G.: Vitamin P Deficiency in Guinea Pigs. Nature, 152:659, 1943.

2. Goldbach, H.: Success of Vitamin E Therapy in Periodontal Disease. Ztschr. f. Stom., 43:379, 1946.

3. Kreshover, S., and Burket, L.: cited in Burket, L.: Oral Medicine. Philadelphia, J. B. Lippincott Co., 1946, p. 411.

4. Lieb, H., and Mathis, H.: The Treatment of Periodontal Disease with Vitamin E. Ztschr. f. Stom., 47:358, 1950.

5. Nelson, M. A., and Chaudhry, A. P.: Effects of Tocopherol (Vitamin E) Deficient Diet on Some Oral, Para-Oral and Hematopoietic Tissues of the Rat. J. D. Res., 45:1072, 1966.

6. Rusznyák, S., and Szent-Györgyi, A.: Vitamin P: Flavonals as Vitamins. Nature, 138:27, 1936.

7. Scarborough, H.: Vitamin P. Biochem. J., 33:1400, 1939.

PROTEIN DEFICIENCY

Protein depletion results in hypoprotein-emia with many pathologic changes, including muscular atrophy, weakness, weight loss, anemia, leukopenia, edema, impaired lactation, decreased capacity to form antibodies, decreased resistance to infection, slow wound healing, lymphoid depletion, and reduced ability to form certain hormones and enzyme systems.[3] *Kwashiorkor*, a protein deficiency disease of children with a high mortality rate, is fairly widespread in malnourished populations.[12]

Oral Manifestations. Protein deprivation causes the following changes in the periodontium of experimental animals:[4, 6, 9] degeneration of the connective tissue of the gingiva and periodontal ligament, osteoporosis of alveolar bone, retardation in the deposition of cementum, delayed wound healing[13] (Fig. 26–5), and atrophy of the tongue epithelium.[15] Similar changes occur in the periosteum and bone in other areas. Osteoporosis results from reduced deposition of osteoid, reduction in number of osteoblasts, and retardation in the morphodifferentiation of connective tissue cells to form osteoblasts, rather than from increased osteoclasis. These observations are of interest in that they reveal loss of alveolar bone that is the result of the inhibition of normal bone-formative activity rather than the introduction of destructive factors.

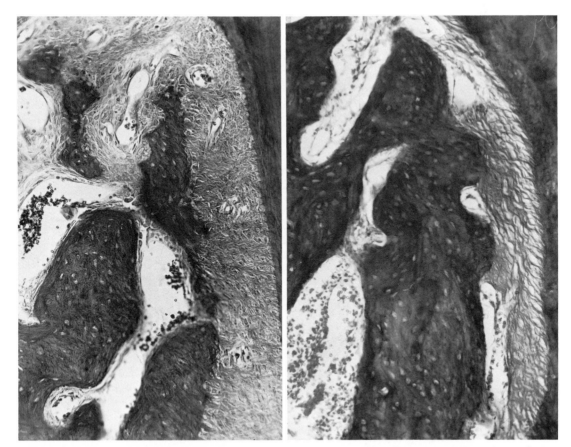

Figure 26–5 **The Effect of Protein Deprivation upon the Periodontium of the Albino Rat.** *Left,* **Control Animal.** Periodontal ligament and alveolar bone between the molar roots, showing dense collagen fibers. Note continuity of the collagen fibrils of the periodontal ligament with the matrix of the bone and polyhedral cells along the bone margin between the periodontal fibers. *Right,* **Protein Deprivation.** Periodontal ligament and alveolar bone between the molar roots. Note degeneration of the periodontal ligament marked by reduction in number and wavy outline of collagen fibrils. A clear-cut demarcation is seen between the bone matrix and the periodontal ligament (compare with control).

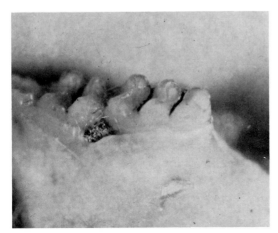

Fig. 26–6

Figure 26–6 Local Irritation Plus Starvation. Amalgam Inserted Interproximally to induce local irritation in experimental animal.

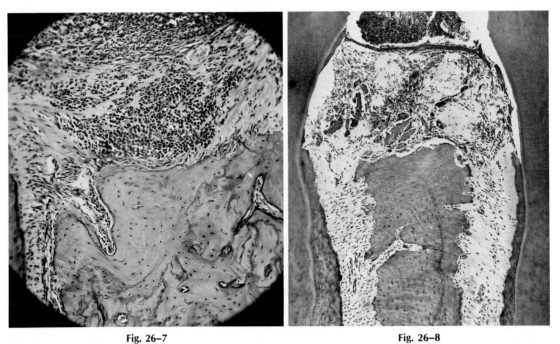

Fig. 26–7   Fig. 26–8

Figure 26–7 Margin of Alveolar Bone beneath area of artificially induced inflammation (Fig. 26–6) in albino rat on adequate diet. The bone surface in relation to the leukocytic infiltration presents lacunar resorption and an adjacent layer of osteoid lined with osteoblasts.

Figure 26–8 Interdental Bony Septum subjacent to artificially induced gingival inflammation in albino rat on starvation diet. The bone presents lacunar resorption without any evidence of new bone formation. (Compare with Fig. 26–7.)

Protein deficiency accentuates the destructive effects of local irritants[14] and occlusal trauma[11] upon the periodontal tissues, but the initiation of gingival inflammation and its severity depend upon the local irritants. Tryptophan deficiency in rats results in osteoporosis of alveolar bone.[1] A "pellagrous stomatitis" has been attributed to tryptophan deficiency in humans.[2]

Combined protein-vitamin deficiencies

Protein deficiency commonly produces anemia. However, protein deficiencies are always accompanied by those of hematopoietic vitamins and iron, and vitamin deficiencies include some degree of disturbed protein metabolism, so that anemia is often the result of combined protein-vitamin deficiency.[5] Such deficiency can produce macrocytic anemia with hematologic and oral changes identical with those of pernicious anemia (see Chap. 29). Several types of anemia occur in kwashiorkor, and the oral changes resemble those of pellagra, which is a mixed protein-vitamin deficiency state with severe oral manifestations.

STARVATION

The term "hunger osteopathy" connotes skeletal disturbances that occur in individuals in famine areas. Such disturbances are characterized by a reduction in the amount of normally calcified bone, and have been attributed to deficiencies in calcium, phosphorus, vitamin D and protein, and to associated hormonal dysfunction. In a study of controlled semi-starvation in young adults,[10] there were no changes in the oral cavity or skeletal system despite a 24 per cent loss of body weight.

Oral Changes. In experimental animals acute starvation results in osteoporosis of alveolar bone and other bones, reduction in the height of alveolar bone and accentuated bone loss associated with gingival inflammation[8] (Figs. 26–6 to 26–8). Furthermore, bone formation associated with extrusion of teeth following the extraction of functional antagonists is impaired by acute starvation.[7]

REFERENCES

Protein Deficiency

1. Bavetta, L. A., and Bernick, S.: Effect of Tryptophane Deficiency on Bones and Teeth of Rats. III. Effect of Age. Oral Surg., Oral Med. & Oral Path., 9:308, 1956.
2. Bean, W. B., Franklin, M., and Daum, K.: A Note on Tryptophane and Pellagrous Glossitis. J. Lab. & Clin. Med., 38:167, 1951.
3. Cannon, P. R.: Some Pathologic Consequences of Protein and Amino Acid Deficiencies. Springfield, Ill. Charles C Thomas Co., 1948.
4. Chawla, T. N., and Glickman, I.: Protein Deprivation and the Periodontal Structures of the Albino Rat. Oral Surg., Oral Med. & Oral Path., 4:578, 1951.
5. Dreizen, S.: Oral Manifestations of Human Nutritional Anemias. Arch. Environ. Health, 5:66, 1962.
6. Frandsen, A. M., et al.: The Effects of Various Levels of Dietary Protein on the Periodontal Tissues of Young Rats. J. Periodont., 24:135, 1953.
7. Glickman, I.: The Effect of Acute Starvation upon the Apposition of Alveolar Bone Associated with the Extraction of Functional Antagonists. J. D. Res., 24:155, 1945.
8. Glickman, I., Morse, A., and Robinson, L.: The Systemic Influence Upon Bone in Periodontoclasia. J.A.D.A., 31:1435, 1944.
9. Goldman, H. M.: Protein Deprivation in Rats. J. D. Res., 39:690, 1960.
10. Keys, A., et al.: The Biology of Human Starvation. Vol. 1, Chap. 12. Minneapolis, University of Minnesota Press, 1950.
11. Miller, S. C., Stahl, S. S., and Goldsmith, E. D.: The Effects of Vertical Occlusal Trauma on the Periodontium of Protein Deprived Young Adult Rats. J. Periodont., 28:87, 1957.
12. Scrimshaw, N. S., and Béhar, M.: Protein Malnutrition in Young Children. Science, 133:2039, 1961.
13. Stahl, S. S.: Effect of Protein Deprivation on Gingival Healing in Rats. I.A.D.R. Abs. of the 40th General Meeting, 1962, p. 9.
14. Stahl, S. S., Sandler, H. C., and Cahn, L.: The Effects of Protein Deprivation Upon the Oral Tissues of the Rat and Particularly upon the Periodontal Structures under Irritation. Oral Surg., Oral Med. & Oral Path., 8:760, 1955.
15. Stein, G., and Ziskin, D.: The Effect of Protein Free Diet on the Teeth and the Periodontium of the Albino Rat. J. D. Res., 28:529, 1949.

MINERAL DEFICIENCIES AND TOXICITIES

Iron

Pallor of the oral cavity and tongue are the most common and sometimes only oral manifestations of iron deficiency anemia.

The tongue may also be swollen with a blotchy or total atrophy of the papillary epithelium.[9, 24] Petechial hemorrhages in the mucosa and angular cheilosis occur in some cases.

Fluoride

Observations in populations using fluoride water supplies do not agree regarding the effects, if any, of ingested fluoride upon the condition of the periodontium (see Chap. 21). Findings in experimental animals vary, with some investigators reporting that fluoride increases periodontal disease,[26] and others that it decreases[8] or protects against it.[23] It has also been shown that fluoride reduces the severity of cortisone-induced alveolar bone resorption,[30] prevents adverse effects of hypervitaminosis D[13] and inhibits bone resorption in tissue culture.[15] Fluoride in the drinking water in levels used to prevent tooth decay presents no health hazards, although at much higher concentrations fluoride may affect the skeletal system adversely and produce spondylosis deformans characterized by progressive osteosclerosis, ossification of tendon and ligament insertions and spinal rigidity.[19] In experimental animals fluoride intoxication results in extensive periosteal bone deposition at sites of muscular insertion and generalized osteoporosis of the jaws.[4] Periodontal disease with loss of alveolar bone appeared to be associated with increased fluorine intake in South African natives.[1] Based upon increased bone density associated with high levels of ingested fluoride, as much as 100 mg. per day of sodium fluoride has been tried in the treatment of osteoporosis.[18]

Magnesium and molybdenum

Reduction in the rate of alveolar bone formation,[10] widening of the periodontal ligament,[10, 20] retarded tooth eruption and gingival enlargement with connective tissue hyperplasia have also been observed in magnesium-deficient animals.[6] Other changes include altered alveolar bone architecture (with the formation of a mosaic pattern[7]), increased resorption, fibrosis of the marrow, calculus formation, and loosening of the teeth. Molybdenum toxicity in experimental animals causes mandibular exostoses, cemental spurs,

hypercementosis, and disorganization of the odontoblastic layer.[25]

OSTEOLATHYRISM

Lathyrism is a disease of the nervous system in man and domestic animals caused by the ingestion of certain types of peas, such as *Lathyrus sativus*. It does not produce changes in the jaws or oral tissues. Animals fed diets rich in *Lathyrus odoratus* peas, or administered certain aminonitriles such as aminoacetonitrile, aminopropionitrile or methyleneaminonitrile develop osteolathyrism, a disease which bears no resemblance to lathyrism in humans.[28] Osteolathyrism is characterized by oral as well as systemic changes.

Exostoses occur on the jaws in areas of muscle attachment, and the condylar cartilage is enlarged. The fibroblasts of the periodontal ligament exhibit increased cytoplasmic basophilia and palisading, and the collagen fibers are fine, disoriented and embedded in amorphous eosinophilic material.[12, 22] Hydroxyproline activity and conversion of soluble collagen to the insoluble type are decreased according to some authors,[29] but in tissue culture studies with a lathyrogenic agent the synthesis and degradation of collagen are unaffected.[16] The alveolar bone is osteoporotic, and there are pronounced hypercementosis and loosening of teeth.[11] Mechanical force is an important contributing factor in the development of osteolathyritic changes in the jaws,[21] and systemic conditioning agents modify their severity.[14]

The electron microscope shows mottling of the bone matrix and disturbed development of osteoblasts.[3]

CALCIPHYLAXIS

Calciphylaxis is a condition of induced systemic hypersensitivity described by Selye,[27] in which tissues respond to appropriate challenging agents with precipitous, sometimes evanescent local calcification. Substances which predispose to calciphylaxis are known as sensitizers; agents which precipitate the calciphylaxis phenomenon are known as challengers. *Sensitizers* include dihydrotachysterol (DHT), vitamin D, parathormone, and sodium acetylsulfathiazole among many calcium salts and phosphates.

Challengers may be *direct* or *indirect.* Direct challengers include mechanical trauma and various chemical agents (salts of iron, chromium, aluminum, zinc, manganese, cesium) which cause calcification at the site of application and may elicit some form of systemic calciphylaxis when administered intravenously or intraperitoneally. Indirect challengers have little or no effect at the site of application and produce diverse systemic syndromes of calcification and sclerosis.

Prolonged administration of dihydrotachysterol (DHT) in rats produces a chronic intoxication syndrome with the following severe changes in the periodontium: osteosclerosis, pronounced osteoid formation, bulbous distortion in the shape of the bone, and degeneration of the marrow and the periodontal ligament. Intraperitoneal administration of ferric dextran (Fe-Dex) induced calciphylaxis which reduced the toxic effects of DHT upon the periodontium.[14a]

DISTURBANCES OF THE ACID-BASE BALANCE

The acid-base balance refers to the state of equilibrium that normally exists between the acid and base components of the tissues and fluids of the body. Acidosis is an abnormal state in which there is accumulation of acids or loss of alkali in the blood; it may be accompanied by changes in bone.[2] Acidosis from renal tubular insufficiency without glomerular insufficiency may result in osteomalacia in adults. Osteoporosis of the jaws has been described associated with acidosis in experimental animals.[5] Alkalosis is an abnormal state in which there is an accumulation of alkali or loss of acid. Retrograde changes in alveolar bone have been described in animals maintained on alkaline diets.[17]

REFERENCES

Mineral Deficiencies and Toxicities

1. Abrahams, L. C.: Masticatory Apparatus of the People of Calvinia and Namaqualand in the North-Western Cape of the Union of South Africa. J. D. A. South Africa, 1:5, 1946.
2. Albright, F., and Reifenstein, E. C.: The Parathyroid Glands and Metabolic Bone Disease. Baltimore, Williams & Wilkins, 1948, p. 241.
3. Amemiya, A.: Electron Microscopic Study of Periosteal Hyperostosis in Rats with Lathyrism Induced by Aminoacetonitrile. Bull. Tokyo Med. D. Univ., 13:319, 1966.
4. Bauer, W. H.: Experimental Chronic Fluorine Intoxication: Effects on Bones and Teeth. Am. J. Orthodont. & Oral Surg. (Oral Surg. Sect.), 31:700, 1945.
5. Bauer, W., and Haslhofer, L.: Veränderung der Kiefer und Zähne durch Zuckerverabreichung. Ztschr. f. Stomatol., 31:1359, 1933.
6. Becks, H., and Furuta, W. J.: Effect of Magnesium Deficient Diets on Oral and Dental Tissues. II. Changes in the Enamel Structure. J.A.D.A., 28:1083, 1941.
7. Becks, H., and Furuta, W. J.: The Effects of Magnesium Deficient Diets on Oral and Dental Tissues. III. Changes in Dentine and Pulp Tissue. Am. J. Ortho. & Oral Surg. (Oral Surg. Sect.), 28:1, 1942.
8. Costich, E. R., Hein, J. W., Hodge, H. C., and Shourie, K. L.: Reduction of Hamster Periodontal Disease by Sodium Fluoride and Sodium Monofluorophosphate in Drinking Water. J.A.D.A., 55:617, 1957.
9. Darby, W. J.: The Oral Manifestations of Iron Deficiency. J.A.M.A., 130:830, 1946.
10. Gagnon, J. A., Schour, I., and Patras, M. C.: Effect of Magnesium Deficiency on Dentin Apposition and Eruption in Incisor of Rat. Proc. Soc. Exper. Biol. & Med., 49:662, 1942.
11. Gardner, A. F.: Alterations in Mesenchymal and Ectodermal Tissues During Experimental Lathyrism. Apposition and Calcification of Cementum. Paradontol., 20:111, 1966.
12. Gardner, A. F.: Morphologic Study of Oral Connective Tissue in Lathyrism. J. D. Res., 39:24, 1960.
13. Gedalia, I., and Binderman, I.: Effect of Fluoride on Hypervitaminosis D in Rats. J. D. Res., 45:825, 1966.
14. Glickman, I., Selye, H., and Smulow, J. B.: Systemic Factors Which Influence the Manifestations of Osteolathyrism in the Periodontium. J. D. Res., 42:835, 1963.
14a. Glickman, I., Selye, H., and Smulow, J. B.: Reduction by Calciphylaxis of the Effects of Chronic Dihydrotachysterol Overdose upon the Periodontium. J. D. Res., 44:374, 1965.
15. Goldhaber, P.: The Inhibition of Bone Resorption in Tissue Culture by Nontoxic Concentrations of Sodium Fluoride. Israel J. Med. Sc., 3:617, 1967.
16. Golub, L., Stern, B., Glimcher, M., and Goldhaber, P.: The Effect of a Lathyrogenic Agent on the Synthesis and Degradation of Mouse Bone Collagen in Tissue Culture. Arch. Oral Biol., 13:1395, 1968.
17. Jones, M. R., and Simonton, F. V.: Mineral Metabolism in Relation to Alveolar Atrophy in Dogs. J.A.D.A., 15:881, 1928.
18. Jowsey, J., Schenk, R. K., and Reutter, F. W.: Some Results of the Effect of Fluoride on Bone Tissue in Osteoporosis. J. Clin. Endocrin. & Metab., 28:869, 1968.

19. Kemp, F. H., Murray, M. M., and Wilson, D. C.: Spondylosis Deformans in Relation to Fluorine and General Nutrition. Lancet, 243:93, 1942.

20. Klein, H., Orent, E. R., and McCollum, E. V.: Effects of Magnesium Deficiency on Teeth and Their Supporting Structures in Rats. Am. J. Physiol., 112:256, 1935.

21. Krikos, G., Beltran, R., and Cohen, A.: Significance of Mechanical Stress on the Development of Periodontal Lesions in Lathyritic Rats. J. D. Res., 44:600, 1965.

22. Krikos, G. A., Morris, A. L., Hammond, W. S., and McClure, H. H.: Oral Changes in Experimental Lathyrism (Odoratism). Oral Surg., Oral Med. & Oral Path., 11:309, 1958.

23. Likins, R. C., Pakis, G., and McClure, F. J.: Effect of Fluoride and Tetracycline on Alveolar Bone Resorption in the Rat. J. D. Res., 42:1532, 1963.

24. Monto, R. W., Rizek, R. A., and Fine, G.: Observations on the Exfoliative Cytology and Histology of the Oral Mucous Membranes in Iron Deficiency. Oral Surg., Oral Med. & Oral Path., 14:965, 1961.

25. Ostram, C. A., Van Reen, R., and Miller, C. W.: Changes in the Connective Tissue of Rats Fed Toxic Diets Containing Molybdenum Salts. J. D. Res., 40:520, 1961.

26. Ramseyer, W. F., Smith, C. A. H., and McCay, C. M.: Effect of Sodium Fluoride Administration on Body Changes in Old Rats. J. Geront., 12:14, 1957.

27. Selye, H.: Calciphylaxis. Chicago, University of Chicago Press, 1962.

28. Selye, H.: Lathyrism. Rev. Canad. de Biol., 16:3, 1957.

29. Smith, D. J.: Biochemical Aspects of Repair in Lathyrism. J. D. Res., 45:500, 1966.

30. Zipkin, I., Bernick, S., and Menczel, J.: A Morphological Study of the Effect of Fluoride on the Periodontium of the Hydrocortisone-Treated Rat. Periodontics, 3:111, 1965.

THE EFFECT OF NUTRITION UPON THE ORAL MICROORGANISMS

With increased interest in the role of microorganisms in the etiology of gingival and periodontal disease, attention has been directed to a relatively unexplored aspect of nutrition—namely, its effect upon the oral microorganisms. Although dietary intake is generally thought of in terms of sustaining the individual, it inadvertently is also the source of bacterial nutrients.

By its effect upon the oral bacteria the composition of the diet may influence the relative distribution of types of organisms, their metabolic activity and their pathogenic potential, which in turn affect the occurrence and severity of oral disease. Consideration of the role of nutrition upon the oral flora and of its possible implications in oral disease is in its early stages. Loesche and Gibbons present an excellent analysis of the information thus far available on this subject.[1]

It may be that oral changes considered to be the result of nutritional deficiencies upon the oral tissues could in part be first an effect upon the oral microorganisms, so that their products become increasingly injurious to the oral tissues. Carbohydrate content affects the bacterial composition and rate of dental plaque accumulation and the severity of experimentally induced periodontal disease;[2] the cariogenic potential of foods varies according to their utilization by acidogenic plaque bacteria.

REFERENCES

Nutrition and Oral Microorganisms

1. Loesche, W. J., and Gibbons, R. J.: Influence of Nutrition on the Ecology and Cariogenicity of the Oral Microflora. In Nizel, A. E.: The Science of Nutrition and its Application to Clinical Dentistry. Philadelphia, W. B. Saunders Company, 1966, p. 305.

2. Shaw, J. H., Krumins, I., and Gibbons, R. J.: Comparison of Sucrose, Lactose, Maltose and Glucose in the Causation of Experimental Oral Diseases. Arch. Oral Biol., 12:755, 1967.

Chapter 27

ENDOCRINOLOGIC INFLUENCES IN THE ETIOLOGY OF PERIODONTAL DISEASE

HORMONAL INFLUENCES ON THE PERIODONTIUM

Hormones are organic substances produced by the endocrine glands. They are secreted directly into the blood stream and exert an important physiologic influence upon the functions of certain cells and systems. The significance of hormonal disturbances in the causation of periodontal disease is presented here.

Hypothyroidism

The effects of hypothyroidism vary with the age at which it occurs. The basal metabolic rate is depressed and growth retarded.

Cretinism, juvenile myxedema and adult myxedema are the three clinical syndromes that result from hypothyroidism.

Cretinism is the manifestation of hypothyroidism that is either congenital or occurs shortly after birth. Delayed physical and mental development is characteristic of the disease. There is understature and disproportion; bone growth is retarded; craniofacial development is abnormal. The cranium is disproportionately large and the face is infantile and coarse; the jaws are small; the rate of tooth eruption is retarded.[62]

Juvenile myxedema occurs between the ages of six and twelve, and may be related to iodine deficiency or other injurious influences on the thyroid gland. Among the first symptoms are physical inactivity, mental dullness and inability to concentrate.[32] The body tissues have a pseudoedematous appearance. Oral changes may also give an early clue to the disorder. Tooth eruption is retarded, and the formation of the jaws is disturbed. The teeth are poorly formed; delayed formation of the dentin results in incompletely developed roots and patent pulp canals.

Hypothyroidism in the adult results in *myxedema*. The patient is easily fatigued, and usually gains weight in spite of lack of appetite. The characteristic nonpitting edema of subcutaneous tissues is seen. The basal metabolic rate and blood pressure are low, the pulse is slow, and the blood cholesterol is elevated.

Hypothyroidism and the periodontium

Aside from impaired development, no notable changes in the periodontal tissues have been attributed to cretinism. Chronic periodontal disease with severe bone loss has been described in patients with myxedema,[5, 29, 32, 37] with the suggestion that the latter condition contributes to the periodontal destruction. Degenerative changes in the gingiva have been reported in thyroidectomized animals.[3, 86]

In animals with thiouracil-induced hypothyroidism, apposition of alveolar bone is retarded[22] and the size of the haversian systems is reduced,[17] but there is no evidence of periodontal disease.[19] Animals with experimentally induced myxedema present hyperparakeratosis with some keratosis of the gingival epithelium, edema, and disorganization of the collagen bundles in the connective tissue, hydropic degeneration and fragmentation of the fibers of the periodontal ligament and osteoporosis of the alveolar bone.[55]

Hyperthyroidism

Hyperfunction of the gland is common in young and middle-aged adults. Among the symptoms are cardiovascular effects (increased pulse, hypertension, and cardiac enlargement), nervousness and emotional instability, loss of weight and exophthalmia. Infants with this disorder show increased growth and development in contrast to the hypothyroid condition, with early eruption of the teeth. The teeth and jaws are well formed and present no unusual irregularities. Alveolar bone appears somewhat rarefied and partially decalcified. In the adult, salivary flow is increased owing to sympathetic hyperstimulation, but there are no notable oral changes.[62]

Hyperthyroidism and the periodontium

Osteoporosis of the alveolar bone, lacunar resorption, increase in the size of the marrow spaces (with fibrosis of the marrow and an increase in the width and vascularity of the periodontal membrane) have been de-scribed in experimental animals fed thyroid extract over a period of one to sixteen weeks.[13] Thryoid feeding accentuates the osteoporosis of alveolar bone induced in animals by tryptophane deficiency.[4] Suppurative periodontal disease has been described in individuals with hyperthyroidism, without there having been established a cause and effect relationship between the hormonal disturbance and the oral condition.

Hypopituitarism

Hypopituitarism, a deficiency in the secretion of the anterior pituitary lobe, is marked by a retardation in the growth of all tissues. The earlier in life the condition occurs, the more severe the clinical changes. Hypopituitarism in children results in dwarfism. The pituitary dwarf is small, underdeveloped and usually well proportioned, although not always. Disproportion in growth is attributable to other endocrine glands affected by the hyposecretion of adrenotrophic, thyrotrophic and gonadotrophic hormones of the pituitary. The skeletal and genital systems are affected, but the nervous system is not involved; the patient is alert, and mentally exceeds the developmental age. The latter condition is in contradistinction to cretinism in which mental as well as physical development is affected.

In dwarfism, the cranium and face develop very slowly, resembling those of a child of a much earlier age. The face is relatively small compared with the cranium, and the sinuses are underdeveloped, especially the frontal. Retardation in development of the teeth and jaws has been noted by many observers. There is delayed resorption of the deciduous teeth and marked retardation in formation and eruption of the permanent teeth. The growth of the maxilla and mandible is arrested, with the mandible showing the greater degree of change. Retardation in the growth of the ramus resulting in failure in increase of the vertical height of the mandible, reduced intermaxillary space, crowding of the teeth and a tendency toward a distal relationship of the mandible have been attributed to hypopituitarism.

Hypopituitarism and the periodontium

The following is a summary of the microscopic changes observed in the periodontal tissues of experimental animals with artificially induced hypopituitarism:

Resorption of cementum in the molar bifurcation areas, reduced apposition of cementum, resorption of alveolar bone in animals with short postoperative life, with sclerosis and suggestion of mosaic pattern. The vascularity of the periodontal ligament is reduced and there is degeneration of the ligament with cystic degeneration and calcification of many of the epithelial rests. The epithelial attachment is often atrophic or absent. It has been suggested that the changes observed in these animals may not be specific for hypophysectomy, but may be attributable to an associated reduction in the blood supply, caused either by the hypophysectomy or resulting changes in other endocrine glands.[61, 65]

Hyperpituitarism

Hyperpituitarism, an increase in the secretion of the anterior lobe of the pituitary, results in giantism or acromegaly, depending upon the age at which it occurs. Hyperpituitarism before the age of six results in *giantism*, characterized by unusual height and disproportion. When hyperpituitarism occurs after the age of six, *juvenile acromegaly* is the result, with abnormal height, huge hands and feet, long face, and prognathic jaw.

In *adults*, hyperpituitarism results in *acromegaly*, which is characterized by a disproportionate overgrowth of the facial bones, with overdeveloped sinuses. The face is large with coarse features. The lips are greatly enlarged and localized areas of hyperpigmentation are often seen along the nasolabial folds. A marked overgrowth of the alveolar process causes an increase in size of the dental arch and consequently affects the spacing of the teeth. This may affect the periodontium by introducing the irritation of food impaction. Hypercementosis is another feature of the increased rate of growth.

Hypoparathyroidism

Hypoparathyroidism results from accidental removal of the glands in thyroidectomy or from deficiencies occurring early in life. There is a hypocalcemia and a resultant increased excitability of the nervous system. The condition is known as *parathyroid tetany*.

If the condition occurs in infancy, it causes enamel hypoplasia and disturbances in the calcification of dentin. The developing enamel and dentin show alternate irregular and accentuated zones of undercalcification and overcalcification. Dentin formed and calcified before the onset of the disease is not affected.

Hyperparathyroidism

Parathyroid hypersecretion produces generalized demineralization of the skeleton, the formation of bone cysts and giant cell tumors, increased osteoclasis, occasional osteoid formation and proliferation of the connective tissue in the marrow spaces and the haversian canals. The serum calcium is increased, serum phosphorus is decreased, and serum phosphatase may be normal or elevated.[81]

Hyperparathyroidism and the periodontium

Different investigators report the percentage of patients with hyperparathyroidism who present oral changes as 25,[76] 45[54] and 50[79] per cent.

The oral changes include malocclusion and tooth mobility, radiographic evidence of alveolar osteoporosis with closely meshed trabeculae, widening of the periodontal space, absence of the lamina dura and radiolucent cyst-like spaces.

Loss of lamina dura and giant cell tumors in the jaws are late signs of hyperparathyroid bone disease, which in itself is uncommon. Complete loss of the lamina dura does not occur often, and there is a danger of attaching too much diagnostic significance to it. Other diseases in which it may occur are *Paget's disease*, *fibrous dysplasia* and *osteomalacia*.

In hyperparathyroidism associated with renal insufficiency, Weinmann[81] **reported extensive**

resorption of lamellated bone and its replacement by immature coarse fibrillar spongy bone, and fibrosis of the bone marrow. In experimental animals,[82] *small doses* of parathormone induce a short period of osteoclasis followed by osteoblastic activity and osteosclerosis of the alveolar bone; *massive doses* lead to resorption of the bone and its replacement by connective tissue.

Diabetes

As far back as 1862, Seiffert described an association between diabetes mellitus and pathologic changes in the oral cavity. Despite a voluminous literature on the subject, opinions differ regarding the exact relationship of diabetes and oral disease. A variety of oral changes have been described in diabetic patients, such as dryness of the mouth; diffuse erythema of the oral mucosa; coated tongue and redness of the tongue, with marginal indentations and a tendency toward periodontal abscess formation; "diabetic periodontoclasia" and "diabetic stomatitis,"[83] enlarged gingiva, "sessile or pedunculated gingival polyps";[30] swollen, tender gingival papillae that bleed profusely; polypoid gingival proliferations and loosened teeth;[47, 56] and increased prevalence of periodontal disease,[68] with both vertical and horizontal bone destruction.[58]

Periodontal disease

Periodontal disease in diabetic patients follows no consistent pattern. Unusually severe gingival inflammation, deep periodontal pockets and periodontal abscesses often occur in patients with poor oral hygiene and calculus accumulation. In juvenile diabetic patients there is often extensive periodontal destruction, which is noteworthy because of their age. In many diabetic patients with periodontal disease, the gingival changes and bone loss are not unusual, although in others the severity of bone loss is impressive (Fig. 27–1).

The distribution and severity of local irritants and occlusal forces affect the severity of periodontal disease in diabetes. Diabetes does not cause gingivitis or periodontal pockets, but there are indications that it alters the response of the periodontal tissues to local irritants and occlusal forces, and that it hastens bone loss in periodontal disease and retards postsurgical healing of the periodontal tissues.

Studies in humans

Despite the generalized increased susceptibility to infection[53] and severe inflammation[46] in diabetes, some investigators[2, 11, 41, 49, 52, 80] recognize no relationship between diabetes and oral disease and maintain that when the two conditions exist together it is a coincidence rather than a specific cause and effect relationship. Others report increased severity of gingivitis[16] and periodontal disease, with increased tooth mobility not related to increased local irritants,[6, 19] and an associated increase in tooth loss.[18]

Microscopic changes described in the gingiva of diabetics include the following: hyperplasia with hyperkeratosis,[85] or a change from a stippled to smooth surface with diminished keratinization; intranuclear vacuolization in the epithelium; increased intensity of inflammation; fatty infiltration in the inflamed tissue;[20] an increase in calcified foreign bodies;[51] widening of the basement membrane of capillaries and precapillary arterioles[13, 34] but no osteosclerotic changes;[33] PAS fuchsinophilic thickening of small blood vessels,[42] and reduced staining of acid mucopolysaccharides. Oxygen consumption in the gingiva and oxidation of glucose are reduced.[14]

Arteriolar changes consisting of increased fuchsinophilia, thickened walls, narrowed lumen, medial degeneration and vacuolization have been reported in the gingiva of patients with diabetes and/or hypertensive cardiovascular disease.[78]

These microscopic changes are not unique or characteristic of diabetes, however, and the severity of the gingival inflammation is not correlated with the state of control of the diabetes.

Comparison of the salivary and blood sugar levels with the periodontal condition of diabetics revealed the following:

Salivary glucose levels (one hour after breakfast) were higher in diabetics but not to a degree which was diagnostic.[43] Salivary and blood sugar levels were correlated in nondiabetics, but only in diabetic females.[44] In diabetics and nondiabetics neither the salivary sugar nor the blood sugar was

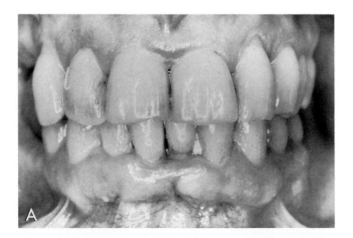

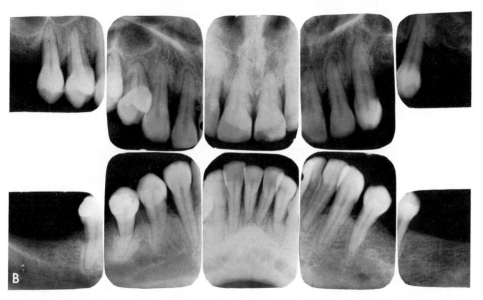

Figure 27–1   Diabetic Patient. *A,* Gingival inflammation and periodontal pockets in 34-year-old diabetic of long duration. *B,* Extensive generalized bone loss in patient shown in *A.* Failure to replace posterior teeth adds to the occlusal burden of the remaining dentition.

correlated with periodontal disease (periodontal index, Russell) or oral hygiene (oral hygiene index, Greene and Vermillion). Periodontal disease was more severe and the oral hygiene poorer in diabetics.[45]

Studies in animals

There have been many studies of the periodontium in animals with diabetes induced by injection of the drug alloxan. Some authors[15, 21] report that the prevalence, nature and severity of gingivitis are not affected by diabetes.

Osteoporosis and reduction in the height of alveolar bone (Fig. 27–2) occur in diabetic animals, with comparable osteoporosis in other bones. The periodontal ligament and cementum are not affected, but glycogen is depleted in the gingiva. Others report that gingival inflammation and bone destruction associated with local irritants are more severe in diabetic than in nondiabetic animals.[8, 9]

Generalized osteoporosis, resorption of the alveolar crest, and gingival inflammation and periodontal pocket formation associated with calculus have been described in Chinese hamsters with hereditary diabetes under

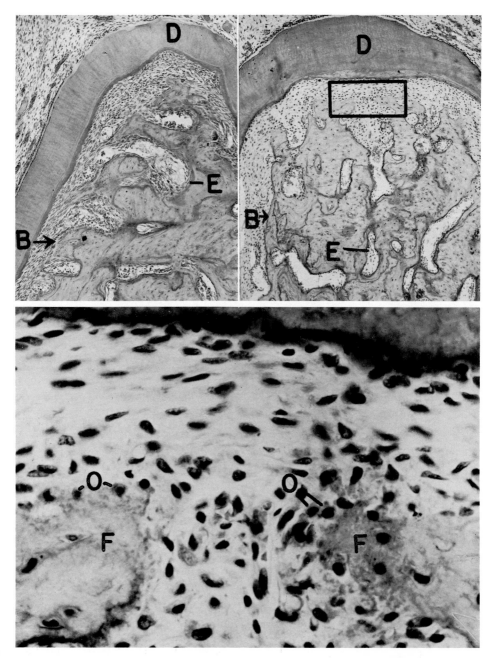

Figure 27–2 Changes in the Periodontium in Experimental Diabetes. *Top Left,* **Control Animal.** Bifurcation area of a mandibular molar (D) showing normal bone deposition adjacent to the periodontal ligament (B). The vessel channels and marrow spaces (E) are lined in part by newly formed bone and in part by resorption lacunae. *Top Right,* **Diabetic Animal.** Bone in bifurcation of a mandibular molar (D). Note absence of normal bone formation adjacent to the periodontal ligament (B) and along the vessel channels and marrow spaces (E). (Compare with control.) Bottom, High power study of the area enclosed within the rectangle above, showing fragmentation of the bone matrix (F) and release of the osteocytes (O).

insulin replacement therapy,[73] whereas no periodontal changes were observed in other animals with autosomal recessive diabetes.[67]

Periodontal injury produced by excessive occlusal forces[25] and periodontal atrophy from insufficient forces[35] are worsened in experimental diabetes, and postsurgical gingival healing is retarded.[25a]

The Gonads

Identification of several types of gingival disease with altered secretion of sex hormones (Chap. 12) has led to increased interest in hormonal effects upon the periodontal tissues and upon periodontal wound healing (Chap. 36).

Elevated levels of estrogen and progesterone increase gingival exudation in gingivitis-free and gingival diseased female animals, most likely because of hormone-induced increased permeability of gingival vessels.[38]

Progesterone alone produces dilatation of the gingival microvasculature which increases susceptibility to injury and exudation, but it does not affect the morphology of the gingival epithelium.[31] **Estrogen** injections counteract tendencies toward hyperkeratosis of gingival epithelium and fibrosis of vessel walls in castrated female animals.[60] Locally applied **progesterone, estrogen** and **gonadotrophin** appear to reduce the acute inflammatory response to chemical irritation.[39]

Ovariectomy results in osteoporosis of alveolar bone, reduced cementum formation and reduced fiber density and cellularity of the periodontal ligament[23] in young adult mice, but not in older animals;[50] and fibrosis of periodontal blood vessels.[59] There is also thinning and reduced cellular activity in the epithelium of the buccal mucosa, but not of the gingiva.[40] Gingival epithelium is atrophic in estrogen-deficient animals.[84]

Repeated injections of estrogen cause increased endosteal bone formation in the jaws[48, 74] and decreased polymerization of mucopolysaccharide protein complexes in the bone ground substance;[7] estrogen also stimulates bone formation and fibroplasia, which compensate for destructive changes in the periodontium induced by systemic administration of cortisone.[24]

Systemic administration of testosterone retards the downgrowth of sulcus epithelium over the cementum,[57] stimulates osteoblastic activity in aveolar bone, increases the cellularity of the periodontal ligament[71] and restores osteoblastic activity which is depressed by hypophysectomy.[72] Healing of oral wounds is accelerated by castration in males and is unaffected by ovariectomy.[12]

Corticosteroid Hormones

The systemic administration of cortisone in experimental animals results in osteoporosis of alveolar bone (Fig. 27–3), capillary dilatation and engorgement (with hemorrhage in the periodontal ligament and gingival connective tissue), degeneration and reduction in the number of collagen fibers of the periodontal ligament, and increased destruction of the periodontal tissues associated with inflammation caused by local irritation.[26] Loss of tooth-supporting bone has been noted in adrenalectomized animals.[1] Osteogenesis in alveolar bone which is reduced in adrenalectomized animals was restored by cortisone replacement,[70] but in another animal experiment there was no evidence that adrenalectomy, orchidectomy, or ovariectomy affected the initiation or progression of periodontal disease.[10]

In humans systemic administration of cortisone and ACTH appears to have no effect upon the incidence and severity of gingival and periodontal disease.[36]

THE GENERAL ADAPTATION SYNDROME AND THE DISEASES OF ADAPTATION

Many forms of stress such as trauma, cold, muscular fatigue, drug intoxication and nervous stimuli affect the body generally, and produce interrelated, nonspecific tissue changes. The composite of the systemic reactions that result from continued exposure to stress is termed the *general adaptation syndrome* (G.A.S.), which is described by Selye as the basis for the pathogenesis of many diseases previously considered to be of unrelated etiology.[63, 64] According to Selye, the general adaptation syndrome is a generalized group of physiologic mechanisms which represent an attempt by the body to resist the damaging effect of stress.

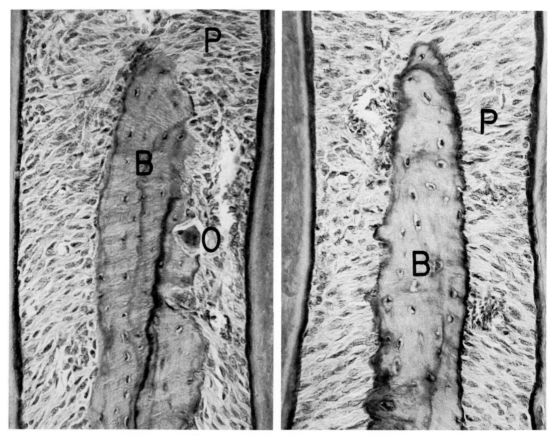

Figure 27–3   The Effects of Systemically Administered Cortisone upon the Periodontium. *Left,* **Control Animal, Interdental Septum.** There is a thin layer of newly formed osteoid bordered by a row of osteoblasts along one surface of the bone (B). The outer surface presents concavities of resorption with an occasional osteoclast (O). The periodontal ligament is shown at P. *Right,* **Cortisone-Injected Animal.** Note absence of normal osteoid and osteoblasts, and irregularly indented deeply staining bone margin (B). The connective tissue cells of the periodontal membrane (P) are reduced in number. The collagen fibers appear fibrin-like and fragmented.

Stress acts through the endocrine glands, particularly the anterior lobe of the pituitary and the adrenal cortex, to produce the morphologic and functional changes that comprise the general adaptation syndrome. Among these changes are enlargement of the adrenal cortex with increased secretion of adrenocorticoid hormones; involution of lymphatic organs; hyalinization and inflammatory changes in blood vessels with hypertension; gastrointestinal ulceration; and malignant nephrosclerosis. The "collagen" diseases of man are benefited by treatment with ACTH and cortisone, and they appear to be part of the general adaptation syndrome. Thus, the adaptive mechanism of the body in response to stress produces recognizable disease entities, referred to as the "diseases of adaptation."

The general adaptation syndrome de-velops in three stages: (1) the initial response, or "alarm reaction"; (2) the adaptation to stress—the "resistance stage"; and (3) a final stage marked by inability to maintain adaptation to the stress—the "exhaustion stage."

Stress and the periodontal tissues

The following observations have been reported in stressed experimental animals:

In the alarm reaction,[75] no significant changes; in the late stage of the stress syndrome, osteoporosis of alveolar bone,[28] epithelial sloughing, degeneration of the periodontal ligament and reduced osteoblastic activity;[51] in chronic stress, osteoporosis of alveolar bone, apical migration of the epithelial attachment and the formation of periodontal pockets.[69] Stress results in delayed healing of the connective tissue and bone in artificially induced gingival wounds but does not affect the epithelium.[77]

REFERENCES

1. Applebaum, E., and Seelig, A.: Histologic Changes in Jaws and Teeth of Rats Following Nephritis, Adrenalectomy, and Cortisone Treatment. Oral Surg., Oral Med. & Oral Path., 8:881, 1955.
2. Badanes, B. B.: Diabetes Acidosis and the Significance of Acid Mouth. D. Cosmos, 75:476, 1933.
3. Baume, L. J., and Becks, H.: The Effect of Thyroid Hormone in Dental and Parodental Structures. Paradentologie, 6:89, 1952.
4. Bavetta, L. A., Bernick, S., and Ershoff, B.: The Influence of Dietary Thyroid on the Bones and Periodontium of Rats on Total and Partial Tryptophan Deficiencies. J. D. Res., 36:13, 1957.
5. Becks, H.: Systemic Background of Paradentosis. J.A.D.A., 28:1447, 1941.
6. Belting, C. M., Hinicker, J. J., and Dummett, C. O.: Influence of Diabetes Mellitus on the Severity of Periodontal Disease. J. Periodont., 35:476, 1964.
7. Bernick, S., and Ershoff, B. H.: Histochemical Study of Bone in Estrogen-Treated Rats. J. D. Res., 42:981, 1963.
8. Bissada, N. F., and Schaffer, E. M.: Histopathological Changes in the Periodontium of Alloxan Diabetic Rats with and without Local Factors. Abst. No. 63, I.A.D.R. Abstracts, 1965.
9. Bissada, N. F., Schaffer, E. M., and Lazarow, A.: Effect of Alloxan Diabetes and Local Irritating Factors on the Periodontal Structures of the Rat. Periodontics, 4:233, 1966.
10. Boenheim, F.: Endocriner Status bei Paradentose. Zahnärztl. Rundsch., 37:1002, 1928.
11. Boenheim, F.: The Endocrine System in Periodontal Disease. In Miller, S. C.: Textbook of Periodontia. 2nd ed. Philadelphia, The Blakiston Co., 1943, p. 545.
12. Butcher, E. O., and Klingsburg, J.: Age, Gonadectomy and Wound Healing in the Palatal Mucosa. J. D. Res., 40:694, 1961.
13. Campbell, M. J. A.: An Electron Microscope Study of the Basement Membrane of the Small Vessels from the Gingival Tissue of the Diabetic and Nondiabetic Patient. J. D. Res., 46:1302, 1967.
14. Campbell, M. J. A.: The Oxygen Utilization and Glucose Oxidation Rate of Gingival Tissue from Non-Diabetic and Diabetic Patients. Arch. Oral Biol., 15:305, 1970.
15. Cohen, B., and Fosdick, L. S.: Chemical Studies in Periodontal Disease VI. The Glycogen Content of Gingival Tissues in Alloxan Diabetes. J. D. Res., 29:48, 1950.
16. Cohen, D. W., Friedman, L. A., Shapiro, J., and Kyle, G. C.: Studies on Periodontal Patterns in Diabetes Mellitus. J. Periodont. Res., Suppl., 4:35, 1969.
17. English, J. A.: Experimental Effects of Thiouracil and Selenium on the Teeth and Jaws of Dogs. J. D. Res., 28:172, 1949.
18. Fett, K. D., and Jutzi, E.: Die Bezahnung Bei Diabetikern in Abhängigkeit vom Lebensalter und der Diabetesdauer (Ger.). Deutsche Zahnärzt. Zeitschr., 20:121, 1965.
19. Fisher, R. L., and Mitchell, D. F.: Induced Hypothyroidism and the Periodontium of the Hamster. I.A.D.R. Abstracts of the 40th General Meeting, 1962, p. 67.
20. Gescheff, G.: Einige Lipoiduntersuchungen des Paradentiums bei Diabetes. 14 p. 8. Frankf. a. M. Verlagen [1931] Berlin.
21. Glickman, I.: The Periodontal Structures in Experimental Diabetes. New York J. D., 16:226, 1946.
22. Glickman, I., and Pruzansky, S.: Propyl-Thiouracil-Hypothyroidism in the Albino Rat. J. D. Res., 26:471, 1947.
23. Glickman, I., and Quintarelli, J.: Further Observations Regarding the Effects of Ovariectomy Upon the Tissues of the Periodontium. J. Periodont., 31:31, 1960.
24. Glickman, I., and Shklar, G.: The Steroid Hormones and Tissues of the Periodontium. Oral Surg., Oral Med. & Oral Path., 8:1179, 1955.
25. Glickman, I., Smulow, J., and Moreau, J.: Effect of Alloxan Diabetes Upon the Periodontal Response to Excessive Occlusal Forces. J. Periodont., 37:146, 1966.
25a. Glickman, I., Smulow, J. B., and Moreau, J.: Postsurgical Periodontal Healing in Alloxan Diabetes. J. Periodont., 38:93, 1967.
26. Glickman, I., Stone, I. C., and Chawla, T. N.: The Effect of Cortisone Acetate Upon the Periodontium of White Mice. J. Periodont., 24:161, 1953.
27. Goldman, H. M.: Experimental Hyperthyroidism in Guinea Pigs. Am. J. Orthodont. & Oral Surg., 29:665, 1943.
28. Gupta, O. P., Blechman, H., and Stahl, S. S.: The Effects of Stress on the Periodontal Tissues of Young Adult Male Rats and Hamsters. J. Periodont., 31:413, 1960.
29. Hirschfeld, I.: Discussion of "The Most Significant Findings of the California Stomatological Research Group in the Study of Pyorrhea" by F. V. Simonton. J. D. Res., 8:261, 1928.
30. Hirschfeld, I.: Periodontal Symptoms Associated With Diabetes. J. Periodont., 5:37, 1934.
31. Hugoson, A.: Gingival Inflammation and Female Sex Hormones. J. Periodont. Res., Supplement 5, 1970.
32. Hutton, J. H.: Relation of Endocrine Disorders to Dental Disease. J.A.D.A., 23:226, 1936.
33. Keene, J. J., Jr.: A Histochemical Evaluation for Small Vessel Calcification in Human Nondiabetic and Diabetic Gingival Biopsy Specimens, J. D. Res., 48:968, 1969 (Part II).
34. Keene, J. J., Jr.: Observations of Small Blood Vessels in Human Nondiabetic and Diabetic Gingiva. J. D. Res., 48:967, 1969 (Part II).
35. Komori, A.: Histological Studies of the Influence of Occlusal Function on the Periodontal Tissues of Alloxan Diabetic Rats. Bull. Tokyo Med. & D. University, 11:207, 1964.
36. Krohn, S.: The Effect of the Administration of Steroid Hormones on the Gingival Tissues. J. Periodont., 29:300, 1958.
37. Lewis, A. B.: Oral Manifestations of Endocrine Disturbances — Myxedema. D. Cosmos, 77:47, 1935.

38. Lindhe, J., Attström, R., and Björn, A.: Influence of Sex Hormones on Gingival Exudation in Gingivitis-Free Female Dogs. J. Periodont. Res., 3:273, 1968.

39. Lindhe, J., and Sonesson, B.: The Effect of Sex Hormones on Inflammation. II. Progestogen, Oestrogen, and Chorionic Gonadotropin. J. Periodont. Res., 2:7, 1967.

40. Litwack, D., Kennedy, J. E., and Zander, H. A.: Response of Oral Epithelia to Ovariectomy and Estrogen Replacement. Abstracts I.A.D.R. 48th General Meeting, 1970, No. 606, p. 200.

41. MacKenzie, R. S., and Millard, H. D.: Interrelated Effects of Diabetes, Arteriosclerosis and Calculus on Alveolar Bone Loss. J.A.D.A., 66:191, 1963.

42. McMullen, J., Gottsegen, R., and Camerini-Davalos, R.: PAS Fuchsinophilic Thickening of Small Blood Vessels in Diabetic Gingiva Due to Accumulation in the Periendothelial Area. J. Periodont., 5:61, 1967.

43. Mehrotra, K. K., and Chawla, T. N.: Quantitative Estimation of Salivary Glucose. J. Indian D. Assn., 40:243, 1968.

44. Mehrotra, K. K., Chawla, T. N., and Kumar, A.: Correlation of Salivary Sugar with Blood Sugar. J. Indian D. Assn., 40:265, 1968.

45. Mehrotra, K. K., Chawla, T. N., and Kumar, A.: Correlation of Salivary Sugar and Blood Sugar with Periodontal Health and Oral Hygiene Status Among Diabetics and Non-Diabetics. J. Indian D. Assn., 40:287, 1968.

46. Menkin, V.: Biochemical Factors in Inflammation and Diabetes Mellitus. Arch. Path., 34:182, 1942.

47. Niles, J. G.: Early Recognition of Diabetes Mellitus through Interstitial Alveolar Resorption. D. Cosmos, 74:161, 1932.

48. Nutlay, A. G., et al.: The Effect of Estrogen on the Gingiva and Alveolar Bone of Molars in Rats and Mice. J. D. Res., 33:115, 1954.

49. O'Leary, T. M., Shannon, I., and Prigmore, J. R.: Clinical and Systemic Findings in Periodontal Disease. J. Periodont., 33:243, 1962.

50. Piroshaw, N. A., and Glickman, I.: The Effect of Ovariectomy Upon the Tissues of the Periodontium and Skeletal Bones. Oral Surg., Oral Med. & Oral Path., 10:133, 1957.

51. Ray, H. G., and Orban, B.: The Gingival Structures in Diabetes Mellitus. J. Periodont., 21:85, 1950.

52. Reeve, C. M., and Winklemann, R. K.: Glycogen Storage in Gingival Epithelium of Diabetic and Non-Diabetic Patients. I.A.D.R. Abstracts of the 40th General Meeting, 1962, p. 31.

53. Richardson, R.: Influence of Diabetes on the Development of Antibacterial Properties in the Blood. J. Clin. Investigation, 12:1143, 1933.

54. Rosenberg, E. H., and Guralnick, W. C.: Hyperparathyroidism. Oral Surg., Oral Med. & Oral Path. 15:(Suppl. 2) 84, 1962.

55. Rosenberg, M. M., Goldman, H. M., and Garber, E.: The Effects of Experimental Thyrotoxicosis and Myxedema in the Periodontium of Rabbits. J. D. Res., 40:708, 1961.

56. Rudy, A., and Cohen, M. M.: The Oral Aspects of Diabetes Mellitus. New England J. Med., 219:503, 1938.

57. Rushton, M. A.: Epithelial Downgrowth: Effect of Methyl Testosterone. Brit. D. J., 93:27, 1952.

58. Rutledge, C. E.: Oral and Roentgenographic Aspects of the Teeth and Jaws of Juvenile Diabetics. J.A.D.A., 27:1740, 1940.

59. Schneider, H.: Changes in the Periodontium of the Rat Following Ovariectomy (Ger.). Paradont. Acad. Rev., 1:106, 1967.

60. Schneider, H., and Pose, G.: The Effect of Estrogen on Periodontal Conditions in Castrated Rats. Dtsch. Stomatol., 19:25, 1969.

61. Schour, I.: The Effect of Hypophysectomy on the Periodontal Tissues. J. Periodont., 5:15, 1934.

62. Schour, I., and Massler, M.: Endocrines and Dentistry. J.A.D.A., 30:595, 763, 943, 1943.

63. Selye, H.: The General Adaptation Syndrome and the Diseases of Adaptation. J. Clin. Endocrinol., 6:117, 1946.

64. Selye, H.: The Physiology and Pathology of Exposure to Stress. Acta Endocrinologica, Montreal, 1950.

65. Shapiro, S., and Shklar, G.: The Effect of Hypophysectomy on the Periodontium of the Albino Rat. J. Periodont., 33:364, 1962.

66. Shaw, J. H.: Endocrinopathies and the Periodontal Syndrome in the Rice Rat. J. D. Res., 45:977, 1966.

67. Sheehan, R., and Cohen, M.: The Periodontium of Diabetic Mice. Program and Abstracts, I.A.D.R. 48th General Meeting, Abst. No. 251, 1970, p. 111.

68. Sheppard, I. M.: Alveolar Resorption in Diabetes Mellitus. D. Cosmos, 78:1075, 1936.

69. Shklar, G.: Periodontal Disease in Experimental Animals Subjected to Chronic Cold Stress. J. Periodont., 37:377, 1966.

70. Shklar, G.: The Effect of Adrenalectomy and Cortisone Replacement on the Periodontium of the Rat. Periodontics, 3:239, 1965.

71. Shklar, G., Chauncey, H., and Peluso, D.: The Effect of Testosterone on the Periodontium of the Male Albino Rat. I.A.D.R. Abstracts of the 40th General Meeting, 1962, p. 68.

72. Shklar, G., Chauncey, H., and Shapiro, S.: The Effect of Testosterone on the Periodontium of Normal and Hypophysectomized Rats. J. Periodont., 38:203, 1967.

73. Shklar, G., Cohen, M. M., and Yerganian, G.: Disease in the Chinese Hamster with Hereditary Diabetes. J. Peridont., 33:14, 1962.

74. Shklar, G., and Glickman, I.: The Effect of Estrogenic Hormone on the Periodontium of White Mice. J. Periodont., 27:16, 1956.

75. Shklar, G., and Glickman, I.: The Periodontium and the Salivary Glands in the Alarm Reaction. J. D. Res., 32:773, 1953.

76. Silverman, S., Gordan, G., Grant, T., Steinbach, H., Eisenberg, E. and Manson, R.: The Dental Structures in Primary Hyperparathyroidism. Oral Surg., Oral Med. & Oral Path., 15:426, 1962.

77. Stahl, S. S.: Healing Gingival Injury in Normal and Systemically Stressed Young Adult Male Rats. J. Periodont., 32:63, 1961.

78. Stahl, S. S., Witrin, G. J., and Scoop, I. W.: Degenerative Vascular Changes Observed in Selected Gingival Specimens. Oral Surg., Oral Med. & Oral Path., 15:1495, 1962.

79. Strock, M. S.: The Mouth in Hyperparathyroidism. New England J. Med., 224:1019, 1941.

80. Ulrich, K.: Parodontopathy in Diabetes Mellitus. Deut. Zahnärtzl. Zschr., 4:221, 1962.

81. Weinmann, J. P.: Bone Changes in the Jaw

Caused By Renal Hyperparathyroidism. J. Periodont., *16*:94, 1945.

82. Weinmann, J. P., and Schour, I.: The Effect of Parathyroid Hormone on the Alveolar Bone and Teeth of the Normal and Rachitic Rat. Am. J. Path., *21*:857, 1945.

83. Williams, J. B.: Diabetic Periodontoclasia. J.A.D.A., *15*:523, 1928.

84. Ziskin, D. E., and Blackberg, S. N.: The Effect of Castration and Hypophysectomy on the Gingivae and Oral Mucous Membranes of Rhesus Monkeys. J. D. Res., *19*:381, 1940.

85. Ziskin, D. E., Loughlin, W. C., and Seigel, E. H.: Diabetes in Relation to Certain Oral and Systemic Problems. Part II. Am. J. Orthodont. & Oral Surg., (Oral Surg. Sect.), *30*:758, 1944.

86. Ziskin, R. D., and Stein, G.: The Gingiva and Oral Mucous Membranes of Monkeys in Experimental Hypothyroidism. J. D. Res., *21*:296, 1942.

Chapter 28

HEMATOLOGIC AND OTHER SYSTEMIC DISORDERS IN THE ETIOLOGY OF GINGIVAL AND PERIODONTAL DISEASE

HEMATOLOGIC DISORDERS IN THE ETIOLOGY OF GINGIVAL AND PERIODONTAL DISEASE

Oral changes are often the earliest indication of a hematologic disturbance but cannot be relied upon for the diagnosis of the patient's hematologic disorder. Oral findings suggest the existence of a blood disturbance; specific diagnosis requires complete physical examination and thorough hematologic study. Comparable oral changes occur in more than one form of blood dyscrasia, and secondary inflammatory changes produce a wide range of variation in the oral signs. For these reasons, gingival and periodontal disturbances associated with blood dyscrasias must be thought of in terms of fundamental interrelationships between the oral tissues and the blood and blood-forming organs, rather than as a simple association of dramatic oral changes with hematologic disease.

Abnormal bleeding from the gingiva, or other areas of the oral mucosa, that is difficult to control is an important clinical sign suggesting a hematologic disorder. Hemorrhagic tendencies occur in hematologic disorders whenever the normal hemostatic mechanism is disturbed[36] (Fig. 28–1).

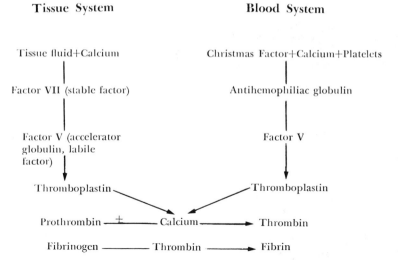

Figure 28–1 **Diagrammatic Representation of the Normal Hemostatic Mechanism** (after Robbins).

Gingival and Periodontal Disease in Leukemia

Oral manifestations occur with greatest frequency in acute and subacute monocytic leukemia, less frequently in acute and subacute lymphatic and myelogenous leukemia, and seldom in chronic leukemia.

In all forms of leukemia local irritation is the factor precipitating oral changes. Leukemic patients may be free of clinical periodontal changes in the absence of local irritants such as plaque, calculus, materia alba, food impaction, poorly contoured restorations, ill-fitting prosthesis or trauma.

Acute and subacute leukemia

Clinical changes that may occur in acute and subacute leukemia include a diffuse, cyanotic, bluish red discoloration of the entire gingival mucosa (whose surface becomes shiny), a diffuse edematous enlargement obliterating the details of the normal surface markings (see Chap. 8; Leukemic Gingival Enlargement), a rounding and tenseness of the gingival margin, blunting of the interdental papillae, and varying degrees of gingival inflammation with ulceration, necrosis and pseudomembrane formation (Figs. 28–2 and 28–3).

Microscopically, the gingiva presents a dense diffuse infiltration of predominantly immature leukocytes in the attached as well as the marginal gingiva (Fig. 28–4). Occasional

mitotic figures indicative of ectopic hematopoiesis may be seen. The normal connective tissue components of the gingiva are displaced by the leukemic cells (Fig. 28–5). The nature of the cells depends on the type of leukemia. The cellular accumulation is denser in the reticular connective tissue layer. In almost all cases, the papillary layer contains comparatively few leukocytes. The blood vessels are distended and contain predominantly leukemic cells. The red blood cells are reduced in number.

The epithelium presents a variety of changes. It may be thinned or hyperplastic. Degeneration associated with inter- and intracellular edema, and leukocytic infiltration with diminished surface keratinization, are common findings.

The microscopic picture of the marginal gingiva differs from that of the remainder of the gingiva in that it usually presents a notable inflammatory component in addition to the leukemic cells. Scattered foci of plasma cells and lymphocytes with edema and degeneration are common findings. The inner aspect of the marginal gingiva is usually ulcerated, and marginal necrosis with pseudomembrane formation may also be seen.

The periodontal ligament and alveolar bone may also be involved in acute and subacute leukemia.[3] The periodontal ligament may be infiltrated with mature and immature leukocytes. The marrow of the alveolar bone presents a variety of changes, such as localized areas of necrosis, thrombosis of blood vessels, infiltration with mature and immature leukocytes,

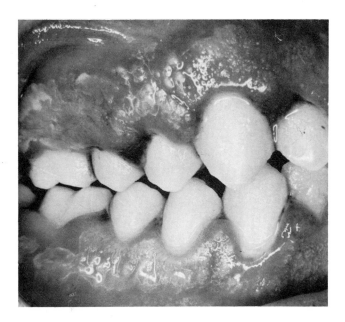

Figure 28–2   Acute Monocytic Leukemia. The gingiva is inflamed, edematous and discolored.

occasional red blood cells, and replacement of the fatty marrow by fibrous tissue.[7, 18, 38]

OTHER ORAL MUCOUS MEMBRANE CHANGES.   Areas of the oral mucous membrane other than the gingiva may be involved in acute or subacute leukemia. The site of involvement is generally an area subject to trauma, such as the buccal mucosa in relation to the line of occlusion or the palate. It appears as a *severe ulceration* or *abscess* that is resistant to treatment and spreads rapidly. Because of the difficulty of controlling the extension of infection and the severity of associated toxic complications, fatal termination is occasionally seen in such cases.

Chronic leukemia

In chronic leukemia there often are no clinical oral changes suggesting a hematologic disturbance. Tumor-like enlargement of the oral mucosa in response to local irritation,[9] generalized alveolar resorption, absence of the lamina dura, diffuse and irregular periodontal spaces, osteoporosis, subperiosteal elevation in the mental region, and analogous changes in other bones may occur in chronic leukemia.[3]

The microscopic changes in chronic leukemia may consist of replacement of the normal fatty marrow of the jaws by islands of mature lymphocytes (Fig. 28–6) or lymphocytic infil-tration of the marginal gingiva without dramatic clinical manifestations.

The gingival biopsy and leukemia

The existence of leukemia is sometimes revealed by a gingival biopsy taken to clarify the nature of a troublesome gingival condition. In such cases, the gingival findings must be corroborated by medical examination and hematologic study. The absence of leukemic involvement in a gingival biopsy does not rule out the possibility of leukemia. In chronic leukemia, the gingiva may simply present inflammatory changes with no suggestion of a hematologic disturbance. In patients with recognized leukemia, the gingival biopsy (Fig. 28–4) indicates the extent to which leukemic infiltration is responsible for the altered clinical appearance of the gingiva. Although such findings are of interest, their benefit to the patient is insufficient to warrant routine gingival biopsy in known leukemic patients.

Analysis of the relation of local irritation to gingival and periodontal changes in leukemia

In leukemia, the response to irritation is altered so that the cellular component of the inflammatory exudate differs both quantita-

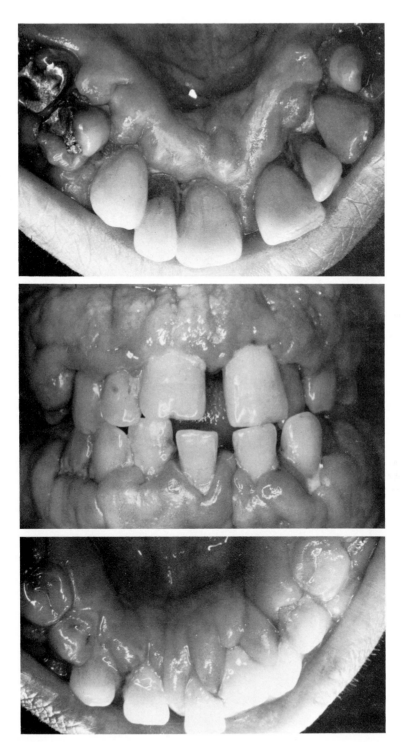

Figure 28–3   Gingival Enlargement in patient with myelocytic leukemia. *Top,* palatal view; *center,* labial view; *below,* lingual view of mandible.

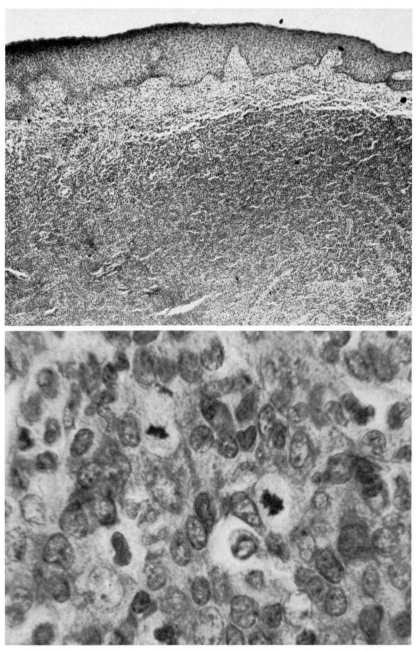

Figure 28–4 Gingival Biopsy of Patient with Acute Monocytic Leukemia. *Above,* Note dense diffuse cellular infiltration in the connective tissue and less cellular zone subjacent to the epithelium. The latter is a common microscopic finding. *Below,* Detailed study showing monocytic cells undergoing mitosis.

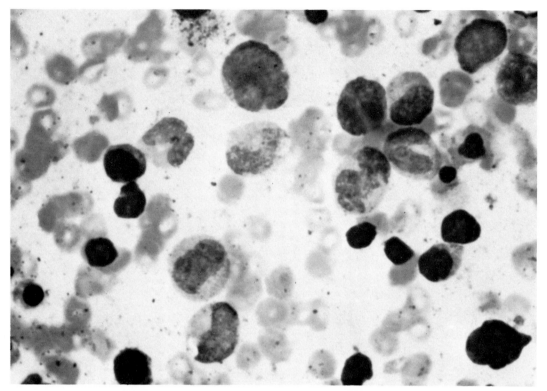

Figure 28–5   Bone Marrow Smear of Patient with Acute Monocytic Leukemia. The marrow is hyperplastic. There is a marked increase in granulopoiesis with a predominance of blast forms shown here. The cells are large, the nuclear chromatin is moderately thickened, and granules are notable in the cytoplasm. (Courtesy Dr. William Dameshek.)

tively and qualitatively from that which occurs in nonleukemic individuals. There is pronounced infiltration of immature leukemic cells, and a reduction in the red blood cells (in addition to the usual inflammatory cells). With the cellular infiltration there is degeneration of the gingiva.

The inflamed gingiva differs clinically from that of the nonleukemic individual. It is a peculiar bluish red in color, markedly sponge-like and friable, and bleeds persistently upon the slightest provocation, or even spontaneously. This markedly altered and degenerated tissue is extremely susceptible to bacterial infection. Because of the degenerated, anoxemic condition of the gingiva, the bacterial infection is so severe that acute gingival necrosis and pseudomembrane formation are comparatively common findings in acute and subacute leukemia. These oral changes produce associated disturbances that are a source of considerable difficulty to the patient, such as systemic toxic effects, loss of appetite, nausea, blood loss from persistent gingival bleeding and constant gnawing pain.

There is considerable variation in the gingival and periodontal changes observed in acute and subacute leukemia. The severity of the leukemia affects the extent of cellular infiltration of the gingiva and supporting periodontal structures. The local irritants and the severity of infection account for more striking clinical changes, such as gingival ulceration, necrosis and pseudomembrane formation, and gingival bleeding. These are the secondary changes superimposed upon the oral tissues altered by the blood disturbance. Differences in the degree of local irritation account for the variation in the oral changes seen in different patients. They also modify the oral picture at different times in the same patient. **By eliminating local irritants it is possible to alleviate severe oral changes in leukemia.**

In considering the relation of leukemia to gingival and periodontal disease, it is important to differentiate between (1) *primary changes*, those directly attributable to the hematologic disturbance; and (2) *secondary changes*, those superimposed upon the oral tissues by the almost omnipresent local

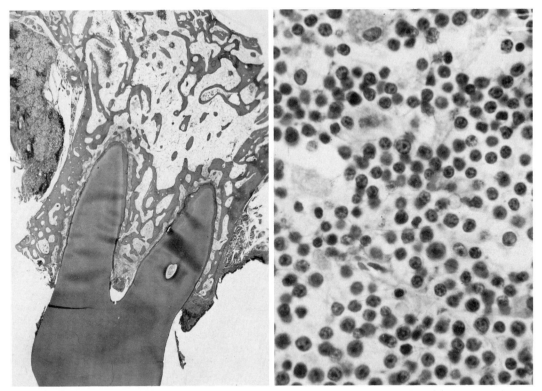

Figure 28–6   Chronic Lymphatic Leukemia. *Left*, Buccopalatal section through the maxilla (molar area) of a patient with chronic lymphatic leukemia, obtained at autopsy. *Right*, Detailed study of lymphocytes in the marrow of the maxilla.

factors, which induce a wide range of inflammatory changes.

Oral Changes in Anemia

Anemia refers to any deficiency in the quantity or quality of the blood as manifested by a reduction in the number of red blood cells and in the amount of hemoglobin. Anemia may be the result of blood loss, defective blood formation, or increased blood destruction. *Blood loss* may be acute, as in severe trauma, or chronic, as in gastrointestinal ulcer, or excessive, as in menstrual bleeding. *Defective blood formation* may be due to:

1. Deficiency of protein, iron or hematopoietically active vitamins, folic acid, vitamin B_{12}, pyridoxine, vitamin C and vitamin K.[13]

2. Depression of bone marrow activity by toxins, chemical substances such as the sulfonamides, physical agents such as roentgen rays, or mechanical interference such as neoplastic disease.

3. Unknown causes, as in "aplastic" anemia.

Increased blood destruction or hemolytic anemia may be due to infections or chemicals or to intrinsic causes.

The anemias are classified according to cellular morphology and hemoglobin content as (1) macrocytic hyperchromic (pernicious anemia), (2) microcytic hypochromic (iron deficiency anemia) and (3) normocytic normochromic anemia (hemolytic anemia; aplastic anemia).

Macrocytic hyperchromic anemia (pernicious or Addison's anemia)

Pernicious anemia is most frequently encountered in individuals past the age of 40. The sexes are equally affected. The disease, which has an insidious onset, is characterized by symptoms referable to the nervous, cardiovascular and gastrointestinal systems. The usual triad of symptoms includes a numbness and tingling of the extremities, weakness, and a sore tongue. Macrocytic hyperchromic anemia is characterized by a severe decrease in the number of erythrocytes (1,000,000 per cu. mm.) and elevated color index (1.5); a decreased hemoglobin value; a decreased platelet count (40,000); a decrease in the number of white blood cells; anisocytosis, poikilocytosis and polychromatophilia; and the presence of red cells containing nuclei or nuclear fragments.

ORAL CHANGES. Changes occur in the gingiva, the remainder of the oral mucosa, the lips and the tongue, which is involved in 75 per cent of the cases.[43] The earliest oral changes may be microscopic and consist of enlargement of epithelial cells with giant nuclei and nuclear pleomorphism.[6] The gingiva and mucosa are pale and yellowish and susceptible to ulceration. The tongue appears red, smooth and shiny owing to the uniform atrophy of the fungiform and filiform papillae. The tongue is sensitive to hot or spicy foods, and swallowing is painful. The patients complain that the tongue feels raw, and there are sensations of burning and numbness. Atrophy of the tongue may be a manifestation of deficiency of vitamin B complex.[21] *Marked pallor of the gingiva* is a striking finding in pernicious anemia, with a wide variety of inflammatory changes, depending upon the nature of the local irritation[16] (Figs. 28–7 and 28–8).

Pernicious anemia is cyclical, with intermittent symptom-free periods. Remissions may last for a short time or for years, but the glossitis of pernicious anemia persists during all but the most complete remissions. Exacerbation of the glossitis may be a signal of relapse.

Microcytic hypochromic anemia

This form of anemia is caused by a deficiency in iron and other substances concerned with hemoglobin production, occurs in chronic blood loss, and is associated with inadequate iron ingestion or absorption. It is seen more often in females. Weakness, fatigue and pallor are among the notable clinical features.

Microcytic hypochromic anemia is characterized by a moderate decrease in number of red blood cells (3,000,000), lowered color index (0.5), an increased platelet count (500,000), and a decreased hemoglobin.

ORAL CHANGES. Atrophy of alveolar bone and inflammation of the gingiva occur in animals with experimentally induced anemia.[20] Not all patients with hypochromic anemia present oral changes.[32] When involved, the most conspicuous change is pallor of the gingival mucosa and tongue, followed by erythema of the lateral

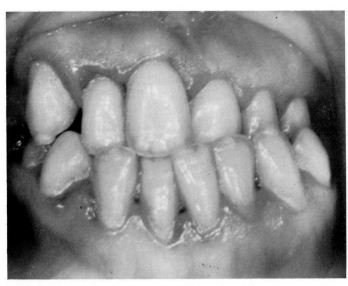
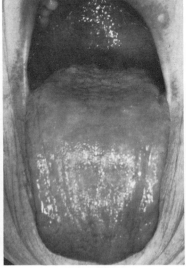

Fig. 28–7   Fig. 28–8

Figure 28–7   Diffuse Pallor of the Gingiva in Patient with Anemia. The discolored inflamed gingival margin stands out in sharp contrast to the adjacent pale attached gingiva.

Figure 28–8   Smooth Tongue in Patient with Pernicious Anemia.

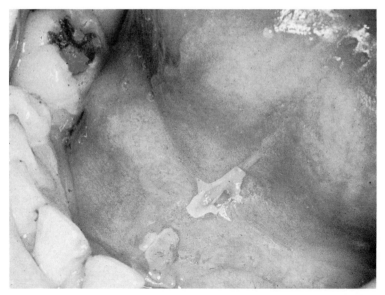

Figure 28–9 **Plummer-Vinson Syndrome** showing ulceration of the floor of the mouth at the base of the tongue.

border of the tongue with papillary atrophy and loss of muscle tone.[12, 17] Areas of gingival inflammation appear purplish red in contrast to the adjacent gingival pallor.

There is an initial erythema of the lateral border of the tongue, followed by pallor and papillary atrophy with loss of normal muscular tone.[12, 17] A correlation has been demonstrated between anemia and moderate to severe periodontal disease.[27] A syndrome consisting of glossitis, ulceration of the oral mucosa (Fig. 28–9) and oropharynx, and dysphagia, known as the *Plummer-Vinson syndrome,* may develop in patients with chronic anemia.

Sickle cell anemia

This is a hereditary and familial form of chronic hemolytic anemia and occurs almost exclusively in Negroes. It is characterized by pallor, jaundice, weakness, rheumatoid manifestations, leg ulcers and acute attacks of pain. The blood picture is distinguished by peculiar sickle-shaped and oat-shaped red corpuscles as well as signs of excessive blood destruction and active blood formation. Although not sex-linked, it occurs somewhat more frequently in females. Oral changes include generalized osteoporosis of the jaws, reported in about 80 per cent of the cases, with a peculiar stepladder align-

ment of the trabeculae of the interdental septa,[37] and pallor and yellowish discoloration of the oral mucosa.[31]

Normochromic normocytic anemia

In this group, the oral changes associated with *Cooley's anemia* are noteworthy. (See Chap. 20.)

Thrombocytopenic Purpura

In thrombocytopenic purpura there is spontaneous bleeding into the skin or from mucous membranes. Petechiae and hemorrhagic vesicles occur in the oral cavity, particularly in the palate and buccal mucosa. The gingiva is swollen, soft and friable. Bleeding occurs spontaneously or upon the slightest provocation and is difficult to control. Special note should be made of the fact that the gingival changes represent an abnormal response to local irritation; the severity of the gingival condition is dramatically alleviated by removal of the local irritants (Fig. 28–10).

Thrombocytopenic purpura may be idiopathic (e.g., of unknown etiology as in *Werlhof's disease*), or it may occur secondary to some known etiologic factor responsible for a reduction in the amount of functioning marrow and a resultant reduc-

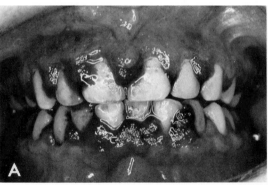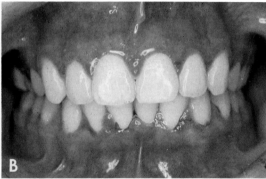

Figure 28–10 Thrombocytopenic Purpura. *A,* Hemorrhagic gingivitis in patient with thrombocytopenic purpura. *B,* Marked reduction in severity of gingival disease after removal of surface debris and careful scaling.

tion in the circulating platelets. The latter conditions include aplasia of the marrow; crowding out of the megakaryocytes in the marrow, as in leukemia for example; replacement of the marrow by tumor; destruction of the marrow by x-radiation or radium, or by drugs such as benzene, aminopyrine and the arsenicals.

Thrombocytopenic purpura is characterized by a low platelet count, a prolonged clot retraction and bleeding time, and by a normal or slightly prolonged clotting time.

Hemophilia

Hemophilia is an inherited sex-linked disease affecting only the male, and transmitted by the female. The afflicted male does not transmit the disease to his male offspring. The defect is passed to the female offspring, who exhibits no symptoms of the disease, but who transmits the defect to her son.

Hemophilia is characterized by prolonged hemorrhage from even slight wounds, and by spontaneous bleeding into the skin. Spontaneous bleeding from mucous membranes is not a feature of the disease.

The clotting time is markedly prolonged, but the bleeding time remains normal. The prolonged clotting time is due to a deficiency of serum protein antihemophiliac globulin (AHG; factor VIII), which presumably results from platelet resistance to disintegration. The normal bleeding time may be explained on the following basis:

When a hemophiliac person cuts himself,

the capillary, as it would normally, contracts with cessation of bleeding. When the capillary later expands, however, there is no clot present to plug the defect, and bleeding starts again.

Christmas Disease (Pseudohemophilia)

Christmas disease is characterized by abnormal bleeding tendencies that make it clinically indistinguishable from hemophilia. Another resemblance to hemophilia is that it is inherited by the male as a sex-linked recessive trait. It differs from hemophilia in that the hemostatic defect lies in the missing serum fraction, called plasma thromboplastin component (PTC), so named because it affects the production of thromboplastin, without which there is an abnormality in the clotting mechanism.

Mild Christmas disease may escape detection because the bleeding time, coagulation time and clot retraction time may be within normal limits. In patients with a history of abnormal bleeding, the prothrombin-consumption test or the thromboplastin-generation test may be necessary in order to rule out Christmas disease.[26]

Hereditary Hemorrhagic Telangiectasia

This comparatively rare vascular anomaly, sometimes known as *Rendu-Osler-Weber disease,* is characterized by multiple dilatations of capillaries and venules in the skin and mucous membrane, with a tendency toward hemorrhage. It appears to be transmitted in families as a simple dominant, affecting both sexes.[39]

The most common sites of the lesions, in order of involvement, are nasal mucosa, tongue, palate, lips, mucocutaneous junction and gingiva.[14] Lesions may occur, however, almost anywhere on the skin and mucous membranes of the body.

The telangiectases may be pinpoint in size or spider-like, with a central nodular pea-sized lesion. Although the condition may be present in childhood, the lesions increase in number as age advances.[40] The blood vessels do not attain their full size until about the age of 35, at which time the telangiectases appear bright-red, violaceous or purple. Epistaxis is a common symptom, and hemorrhage may occur wherever the lesions exist.

The *Sturge-Weber syndrome* is a congenital condition characterized by capillary angiomas (port-wine stain, nevus flammeus) on the face and on the meninges, with epileptiform symptoms. There are telangiectasis, vascular hyperplasia and enlargement of the gingiva with associated resorption of alveolar bone.

Infectious Mononucleosis

This is a benign infectious disease of unknown etiology. It usually occurs in children or young adults. The suspicion that it is communicable has not been well substantiated. It is characterized by sudden onset, headache, fever, muscular ache, sore throat, malaise, nausea, vomiting, swelling and tenderness of lymph nodes (particularly in the cervical area), occasional skin rash and lymphocytosis.

Soreness of the mouth and throat are often the patient's initial complaint. The oral findings include diffuse erythema of the entire mucosa with petechiae in some cases.[11] The marginal and interdental papillae are swollen and markedly reddened, and bleed on slightest provocation or even spontaneously.

After two to four weeks the systemic symptoms usually begin to subside, but the oral changes may persist.

The diagnosis of infectious mononucleosis is based upon the hematologic findings. Leukopenia is seen in the early stages, followed by a marked lymphocytosis. Characteristic of the blood picture are typical "monocytoid" lymphocytes, or Downey cells. The heterophile antibody test (Paul-Bunnell) is used as an aid in diagnosis. This is based on the agglutination of sheep red cells by the patient's serum. Agglutination with serum dilution of 1:64 or above is diagnostic.

Agranulocytosis (Granulocytopenia)

Agranulocytosis is an acute disease characterized by extreme luekopenia and neutropenia, and accompanied by ulceration of the oral mucosa, skin and gastrointestinal tract.

Drug idiosyncrasy is the most common cause of angranulocytosis, but in some instances its etiology cannot be explained. It has been reported following the administration of drugs such as aminopyrine,[25, 34] barbiturates and their derivatives, benzene ring derivatives,[28] sulfonamides,[30] gold salts or arsenicals. It generally occurs as an acute disease, but may reappear in cyclical episodes (cyclical neutropenia) that may be correlated with the onset of the menstrual period.[42] It may be periodic with recurring neutropenic cycles.[41]

The onset of the disease is accompanied by fever, malaise, general weakness and "sore throat." Ulceration in the oral cavity, oropharynx and throat is characteristic. The mucosa presents isolated necrotic patches that are black and gray and sharply demarcated from the adjacent uninvolved areas.[23, 29] **The absence of a notable inflammatory reaction because of lack of granulocytes is a striking feature.** The gingival margin may or may not be involved. Gingival hemorrhage, necrosis, increased salivation and fetid odor are accompanying clinical features.

Bauer[2] described the following microscopic changes in the periodontium: hemorrhage into the periodontal ligament with destruction of the principal fibers; osteoporosis of the cancellous bone with osteoclastic resorption; small fragments of necrotic bone in the hemorrhagic periodontal ligament; hemorrhage in the marrow adjacent to the teeth; areas in which the periodontal ligament is widened and consists of dense fibrous tissue with fibers parallel to the tooth surface, and the formation of new bone trabeculae. In cyclical neutropenia the gingival changes recur with recurrent exacerbation of the disease.[10]

Because infection is a common feature of agranulocytosis, differential diagnosis includes consideration of such conditions as acute necrotizing ulcerative gingivitis, diphtheria, noma and acute necrotizing inflammation of the tonsils. Definitive diagnosis depends upon the hematologic findings of pronounced leukopenia and almost complete absence of neutrophils.

Polycythemia

Polycythemia refers to an increase in the number of circulating red cells. It is to be distinguished from hemoconcentration ("relative" polycythemia), resulting from the loss of body fluid that accompanies persistent vomiting, diarrhea, or sweating. Polycythemia may be primary or secondary.

Primary polycythemia

Primary polycythemia is also known as polycythemia vera or rubra, or *Vaquez-Osler disease.* It is characterized by increased red cell production in the bone marrow, splenomegaly, and an increase in the red cell count ranging from 7 to 10 million per cubic millimeter. The total red cell volume, as well as the leukocyte and platelet counts, is also increased. The hemoglobin level is between 18 and 24 gm./100 cc., and the range of blood viscosity is 1.075 to 1.085, as compared with the normal range of 1.055 to 1.065.

Secondary polycythemia

Secondary polycythemia may occur as the result of a reduction in oxygen tension of

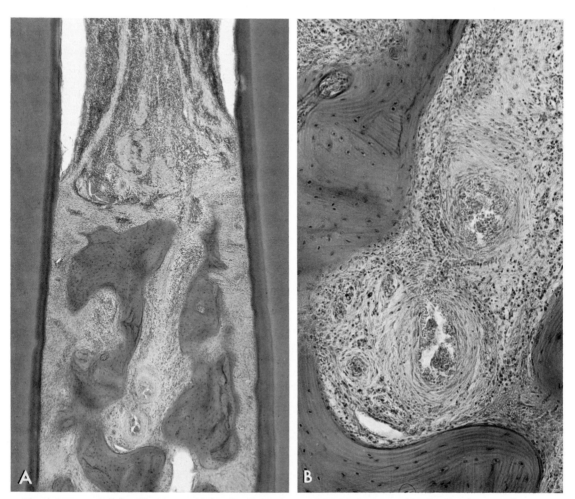

Figure 28–11   Vascular Changes in Aged Individual with Periodontal Disease. *A,* **Periodontitis,** showing inflammation extending from the gingiva into the interdental septum. *B,* Detailed view, showing arterioles with thickened walls in the marrow space of the interdental septum.

the inspired air, as in elevated altitudes. It may also be due to impaired transport of oxygen, or oxygenation of blood in the lungs, as in congenital or acquired heart disease and pulmonary disease. In secondary polycythemia, there is no increase in total red cell volume per kilogram of body weight, and the red cell count seldom exceeds 7 million per cubic millimeter of blood.

Polycythemia, either primary or secondary, is in most cases characterized by a reddish blue cyanotic discoloration of the skin, with comparable involvement of the oral and pharyngeal mucous membrane.[35, 43] Bright red diffuse discoloration of the gingiva and tongue[8] are sometimes seen with abnormal gingival bleeding.

Arteriosclerosis

In aged individuals arteriosclerotic changes characterized by intimal thickening, narrowing of the lumen, thickening of the media and hyalinization of the media and adventitia, with or without calcification, are common in vessels throughout the jaws as well as in areas of periodontal inflammation[33, 44] (Fig. 28–11). Periodontal disease and arteriosclerosis both increase with age, and it has been hypothesized that circulatory impairment induced by the vascular changes may increase the susceptibility to periodontal disease.[1]

In experimental animals partial ischemia of more than ten hours' duration, created by arteriolar occlusion, produces changes in the oxidative enzymes and acid phosphatase activity and in the glycogen and lipid content of the gingival epithelium.[22] Focal necrosis followed by ulceration occurs in the epithelium, with the epithelial attachment least affected.[24] DNA duplication is depressed. Changes typical of periodontal disease do not occur. Ischemia is followed by hyperemia, accompanied by metabolic changes and increased DNA synthesis in the epithelium plus epithelial proliferation and thickening—all considered to be part of the gingival response to arteriolar occlusion.

REFERENCES

1. Barrett, R., Cheraskin, E., and Ringsdorf, W., Jr.: Alveolar Bone Loss and Capillaropathy. J. Periodont–Periodontics, 40:131, 1969.

2. Bauer, W. H.: Agranulocytosis and the Supporting Dental Tissues. J. D. Res., 25:501, 1946.
3. Bender, I. B.: Bone Changes in Leukemia. Am. J. Orthodont. & Oral Surg., 30:556, 1944.
4. Bernick, S.: Age Changes in the Blood Supply to Human Teeth. J. D. Res., 46:544, 1967.
5. Bernick, S., Levy, B. M., and Patek, P. R.: Studies on the Biology of the Periodontium of Marmosets. VI. Arteriosclerotic Changes in the Blood Vessels of the Periodontium. J. Periodont.-Periodontics, 40:355, 1969.
6. Boen, S. T.: Changes in the Nuclei of Squamous Epithelial Cells in Pernicious Anemia. Acta Med. Scandinav., 159:425, 1957.
7. Burket, L. W.: A Histopathologic Explanation for the Oral Lesions in the Acute Leukemias. Am. J. Orthodont. & Oral Surg., 30:516, 1944.
8. Cecil, R. L., and Loeb, R. F.: Textbook of Medicine. 9th ed. Philadelphia, W. B. Saunders Co., 1955.
9. Chaundry, A. P., et al.: Unusual Oral Manifestations of Chronic Lymphatic Leukemia (Report of a Case). Oral Surg., Oral Med. & Oral Path., 15:446, 1962.
10. Cohen, D. W., and Morris, A. L.: Periodontal Manifestations of Cyclic Neutropenia. J. Periodont., 32:159, 1961.
11. Cottrell, J. E.: Infectious Mononucleosis. J. Periodont., 9:15, 1938.
12. Darby, W. J.: The Oral Manifestations of Iron Deficiency. J.A.M.A., 130:830, 1946.
13. Dreizen, S.: Oral Manifestations of Human Nutritional Anemias. Arch. Environ. Health, 5:66, 1962.
14. Durocher, R. T., Morris, A. L., and Burket, L. W.: Oral Manifestations of Hereditary Hemorrhagic Telangiectasia. Oral Surg., Oral Med. & Oral Path., 14:550, 1961.
15. El Mostehy, M. R., and Stallard, R. E.: The Sturge-Weber Syndrome: Its Periodontal Significance. J. Periodont.-Periodontics, 40:243, 1969.
16. Epstein, I. A.: Clinical Indications for the Use of Blood Examinations in the Practice of Periodontia. J. Periodont., 6:30, 1935.
17. Frantzell, A., et al.: Examination of the Tongue. Acta Med. Scandinav., 122:207, 1945.
18. Goldman, H. M.: Acute Aleukemic Leukemia. Am. J. Orthodont. & Oral Surg., 26:89, 1940.
19. Grant, D., and Bernick, S.: Arteriosclerosis in Periodontal Vessels of Aging Humans. J. Periodont., 41:170, 1970.
20. Hall, J. F., and Robinson, H. B. G.: Alveolar Atrophy in Anemic Dogs. J. D. Res., 16:345, 1937.
21. Hutter, A. M., Middleton, W. S., and Steenbock, H.: Vitamin B Deficiency and the Atrophic Tongue. J.A.M.A., 101:1305, 1933.
22. Itoiz, M. E., Litwack, D., Kennedy, J. E., and Zander, H. A.: Experimental Ischemia in Monkeys: III. Histochemical Analysis of Gingival Epithelium. J. D. Res. (Part 2), 48:895, 1969.
23. Kastlin, G.: Agranulocytic Angina. Am. J. Med. Sc., 173:799, 1927.
24. Kennedy, J. E., and Zander, H. A.: Experimental Ischemia in Monkeys: I. Effect of Ischemia on Gingival Epithelium. J. D. Res. (Part I), 48:696, 1969.
25. Kracke, R. R.: Granulopenia as Associated with Amidopyrine Administration. Report Made at Annual Session of A.M.A. June 1934.
26. Kramer, G., and Griffel, A.: Christmas Disease (Hemophilia B) in Periodontal Therapy. Oral Surg., Oral Med. & Oral Path., 15:1056, 1962.

27. Lainson, P., Brady, P., and Fraleigh, C.: Anemia, A Systemic Cause of Periodontal Disease. J. Periodont., 39:35, 1968.
28. Madison, F. W., and Squier, T. L.: Primary Granulocytopenia after Administration of Benzene Chain Derivatives. J.A.M.A., 102:755, 1934.
29. Mark, H. A.: Agranulocytic Angina. Its Oral Manifestations. J.A.D.A., 21:2119, 1934.
30. Meyer, A.: Agranulocytosis. Report of a Case Caused by Sulfadiazine. California and West Med. J., 61:54, 1944.
31. Mittleman, G., Bakke, B. F., and Scopp, I. W.: Alveolar Bone Changes in Sickle Cell Anemia. J. Periodont., 32:74, 1961.
32. Monto, R. W., Rizek, R., and Fine, G.: Observations on the Exfoliative Cytology and Histology of the Oral Mucous Membranes in Iron Deficiency. Oral Surg., Oral Med. & Oral Path., 14:965, 1961.
33. Quintarelli, G.: Histopathology of the Human Mandibular Artery and Arterioles in Periodontal Disease. Oral Surg., Oral Med. & Oral Path., 10: 1047, 1957.
34. Randall, C. L.: Granulocytopenia Following Barbiturates and Amidopyrine. J.A.M.A., 102:1137, 1934.
35. Reznikoff, P., Foot, N., and Bethea, J.: Etiological and Pathological Findings in Polycythemia Vera. Am. J. Med. Sc., 189:753, 1935.
36. Robbins, S. L.: Textbook of Pathology. 2nd ed. Philadelphia, W. B. Saunders Co., 1962, p. 156.
37. Robinson, I. B., and Sarnat, B. G.: Roentgen Studies of the Maxillae and Mandible in Sickle Cell Anemia. Radiol., 58:517, 1952.
38. Schonbauer, F.: Histological Findings in the Jaw in Septicemia and Leukemia. Zeit. f. Stomat., 27:804, 1929.
39. Schwartz, S., and Armstrong, B.: Familial Hereditary Hemorrhagic Telangiectasia in the Negro. New England J. Med., 239:434, 1948.
40. Scopp, I. W., and Quart, A.: Hereditary Hemorrhagic Telangiectasia Involving the Oral Cavity. Oral Surg., Oral Med. & Oral Path., 11:1138, 1958.
41. Telsey, B., Beube, F. E., Zegarelli, E. V., and Kutscher, A. H.: Oral Manifestations of Cyclical Neutropenia Associated with Hypergammaglobulinemia. Oral Surg., Oral Med. & Oral Path., 15: 540, 1962.
42. Thompson, W. P.: Observations on Possible Relation between Agranulocytosis and Menstruation with Further Studies on a Case of Cyclic Neutropenia. New England J. Med., 210:176, 1934.
43. Winter, L.: Blood Dyscrasias—Their Oral Manifestations. Am. J. Orth. & Oral Surg., 26:67, 1940.
44. Wirthlin, M. R., Jr., and Ratcliff, P. A.: Arteries, Atherosclerosis and Periodontics. J. Periodont.-Periodontics, 40:341, 1969.

OTHER SYSTEMIC DISORDERS

Metallic Intoxication

Ingestion of metals such as mercury, lead and bismuth in medicinal compounds and through industrial contact may result in oral manifestations owing to either (1) intoxication or (2) absorption without evidence of toxicity.

Bismuth intoxication[2]

Chronic bismuth intoxication is characterized by gastrointestinal disturbances, nausea, vomiting and jaundice, as well as an ulcerative gingivostomatitis, generally with pigmentation, accompanied by a metallic taste and burning sensation of the oral mucosa. The tongue may be sore and inflamed. Urticaria, exanthematous eruptions of different types, bullous and purpuric lesions as well as herpes zoster-like eruptions and pigmentation of the skin and mucous membranes are among the dermatologic lesions attributed to bismuth intoxication. Acute bismuth intoxication, which is less commonly seen, is accompanied by methemoglobin formation, cyanosis and dyspnea.

BISMUTH PIGMENTATION IN THE ORAL CAVITY. Bismuth pigmentation usually appears as a narrow blue-black discoloration of the gingival margin in areas of pre-existent gingival inflammation (see Chap. 6). Such pigmentation results from the precipitation of particles of bismuth sulfide associated with vascular changes in inflammation. It is not evidence of intoxication, but simply indicates the presence of bismuth in the blood stream. Bismuth pigmentation in the oral cavity also occurs in cases of intoxication. It assumes a linear form if the marginal gingiva is inflamed.

Lead intoxication[4]

The metal is slowly absorbed, and toxic symptoms are not particularly definitive when they do occur. There are pallor of the face and lips, gastrointestinal symptoms consisting of nausea, vomiting, loss of appetite and abdominal colic. Peripheral neuritis and psychological disorders and encephalitis have been reported. Among the oral signs are salivation, coated tongue, a peculiar sweetish taste, gingival pigmentation and ulceration. The pigmentation of the gingiva is linear (burtonian line), steel-gray and associated with local irritation. It may occur without toxic symptoms.

Mercury intoxication[1]

Mercury intoxication is characterized by headache, insomnia, cardiovascular symptoms, pronounced salivation (ptyalism) and metallic taste. Gingival pigmentation in linear form results from deposition of

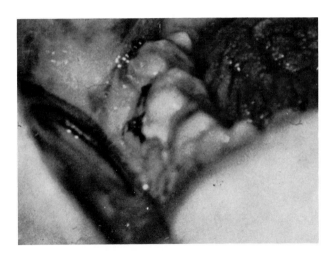

Figure 28–12   Ulceration of the Gingiva in Mercury Intoxication. Note linear pigmentation of the gingival margin adjacent to materia alba.

mercuric sulfide. The chemical also acts as an irritant which accentuates the pre-existent inflammation and commonly leads to notable ulceration of the gingiva and adjacent mucosa (Fig. 28–12) and destruction of the underlying bone. Mercurial pigmentation of the gingiva also occurs in areas of local irritation in patients without symptoms of intoxication.

Other Chemicals

Other chemicals such as *phosphorus*,[6] *arsenic*[3] and *chromium*[5] may cause necrosis of alveolar bone with loosening and exfoliation of the teeth. Inflammation and ulceration of the gingiva are usually associated with destruction of the underlying tissues. *Benzene*[6] intoxication is accompanied by gingival bleeding and ulceration with destruction of the underlying bone.

REFERENCES

Other Systemic Disorders

1. Akers, L. H.: Ulcerative Stomatitis following Therapeutic Use of Mercury and Bismuth. J.A.D.A., 23:781, 1936.
2. Higgins, W. H.: Systemic Poisoning with Bismuth. J.A.M.A., 66:648, 1916.
3. Hudson, E. H.: Purpura Hemorrhagica Caused by Gold and Arsenical Compounds with Report of 2 Cases. Lancet, 2:74, 1935.
4. Jones, R. R.: Symptoms in Early Stages of Industrial Plumbism. J.A.M.A., 104:195, 1935.
5. Lieberman, H.: Chrome Ulcerations of the Nose and Throat. New England J. Med., 225:132, 1941.
6. Schour, I., and Sarnat, B. G.: Oral Manifestations of Occupational Origin. J.A.M.A., 120:1197, 1942.

DEBILITATING DISEASES AND THE PERIODONTIUM

Debilitating diseases such as *syphilis, chronic nephritis* and *tuberculosis* may predispose to periodontal disease by impairing tissue resistance to local irritants and creating a tendency toward alveolar bone resorption.[23, 26] A type of membranous stomatitis has been described[4] associated with debilitation in uremia; and a sore dry mouth with edema, purulent inflammation and bleeding of the gingiva has been noted in primary renal disease.[31] The absence of periodontal disease in chronically ill patients has been presented as evidence that in individual cases systemic disease may exert no deleterious effect upon the periodontium.[25]

Difference of opinion exists regarding the relationship of tuberculosis to periodontal disease. Although an increased incidence of gingivitis and chronic destructive periodontal disease as well as alveolar bone changes, characterized by enlargement of the cancellous spaces, have been reported in tuberculous patients,[7, 21] these findings have not been corroborated in other studies.[13, 27] In patients with *leprosy* the chronic destructive periodontal disease has been described as nonspecific in nature and no *M. leprae* have been present in the gingiva.[28]

PSYCHOSOMATIC DISORDERS AND THE PERIODONTIUM

Harmful effects that result from psychic influences in the organic control of tissues are known as psychosomatic disorders.[14] There are two ways in which psychosomatic disorders may be induced in the oral cavity: (1) *through the development of habits which are injurious to the periodontium* and (2) *by the direct effect of the autonomic system upon the physiologic tissue balance.* Giddon[11] has presented an excellent review of experimental evidence which relates psychological factors to oral physiology.

Psychologically, the oral cavity is related directly or symbolically to the major human instincts and passions. In the infant, many oral drives find direct expression, as oral receptive and oral aggressive trends and oral eroticism.[24] In the adult, most of the instinctual drives are normally suppressed by education, and are satisfied in substitutive ways or are taken over by organs more appropriate than the mouth. **However, under conditions of mental and emotional duress, the mouth may subconsciously become an outlet for the gratification of basic drives in the adult.**

Gratification may be derived from neurotic habits, such as grinding or clenching of the teeth,[6, 9] nibbling on foreign objects, such as pencils or pipes, nail biting, or excessive use of tobacco, which are potentially injurious to the periodontium. Correlations have been reported between psychiatric and anxiety states and the occurrence of periodontal disease,[1, 3, 16, 17] and questioned by some.[2] Psychological factors in the etiology of acute necrotizing ulcerative gingivitis are discussed in Chapter 11.

It is necessary to correct local factors which may initiate harmful habits, but investigation of the psychic background is indicated in difficult cases. Saul[24] describes a case of sore throat, bleeding gums and ulceration of the buccal mucosa traced to mouth breathing and bruxism associated with oral-aggressive dreams. Psychoanalysis resulted in elimination of the underlying difficulty and habit and relief of the oral disease.

Disorders of psychosomatic origin may be produced in the oval cavity by the influence of the autonomic nervous system upon the somatic control of the tissues.[5] Alterations in the vascular supply caused by autonomic stimulation may adversely affect the health of the periodontium by impairing tissue nutrition.[22] Diminution in the secretion of saliva in emotional disorders may lead to xerostomia with painful symptoms. Weiss and English[30] outline the sequence of events whereby psychological disturbances affect tissue alterations as follows:

Psychological disturbance → Functional impairment → Cellular disease → Structural alteration

Autonomic influences upon the muscles of mastication may result in impairment of mandibular movement, which resembles organically induced temporomandibular joint disorders. In such cases, psychiatric management may suffice for the restoration of normal function of the mandible.

HEREDITY IN THE ETIOLOGY OF PERIODONTAL DISEASE

In experimental animals heredity appears to be a factor in calculus formation and periodontal disease.[18] Hypophosphatasia, an inherited disease characterized by rachitic-like skeletal changes, also presents premature loss of deciduous incisors and surrounding alveolar bone by ten months of age, and sometimes without the skeletal changes.[19]

In an investigation of blood types with a view toward the possibility of inheritance of predisposition, it was found that 49 per cent of patients with periodontal disease were of blood type A; the incidence of blood type A in patients without periodontal disease was 40 to 41.1 per cent.[20, 29] Gancotti[10] concluded that inherited tendency was a factor in 62 per cent of the cases of periodontal disease that he studied, whereas other investigators[8] found no indication that heredity affected gingival crevice depth or recession. Gorlin[12] has described numerous genetic disorders which result in oral mucous membrane changes. Heinrich[15] noted that periodontosis was more common in the pyknic type of individual than in the asthenic type.

REFERENCES

Debilitating Diseases and the Periodontium

1. Baker, E. G., Crook, G. H., and Schwabacher, E. D.: Personality Correlates of Periodontal Disease. J. D. Res., *40*:396, 1961.

2. Barry, J. R., and Dutkovic, T. R.: Oral Pathosis: Exploration of Psychological Correlates. J.A.D.A., 67:86, 1963.

3. Belting, C. M., and Gupta, O. P.: The Influence of Psychiatric Disturbances on the Severity of Periodontal Disease. J. Periodont., 32:219, 1961.

4. Bereston, E. S., and Herb, H.: Membranous Stomatitis with Debilitation and Uremia. Arch. Derm. & Syph., 44:562, 1941.

5. Biber, O.: Autonomic Symptoms in Psychoneurotics. Psychosomatic Med., 3:253, 1941.

6. Burstoen, M. S.: The Psychosomatic Aspects of Dental Problems. J.A.D.A., 33:862, 1946.

7. Cahn, L. R.: Observations in the Effect of Tuberculosis on the Teeth, Gums and Jaws. D. Cosmos, 67:479, 1925.

8. Ciancio, S., Hazen, S., and Cunat, J.: Periodontal Observations in Twins. J. Periodont. Res., 4:42, 1969.

9. Frohman, B. S.: Occlusal Neuroses. Psychoanalyt. Rev., 19:297, 1932.

10. Gancotti, M.: Hereditary Factors in Periodontal Diseases. Ann. Stomat. Roma, 5:117, 1956.

11. Giddon, D. B.: Psychophysiology of the Oral Cavity, J. D. Res., 45:1627, 1966.

12. Gorlin, R. J.: Genetic Disorders Affecting Mucous Membranes. Oral Surg., 28:512, 1969.

13. Gruber, I. E.: The Condition of the Teeth and the Attachment Apparatus in Tuberculosis. J. D. Res., 28:483, 1949.

14. Gupta, O. P.: Psychosomatic Factors in Periodontal Disease. Dent. Clin. North America, 1966, p. 11.

15. Heinrich, E.: Report on Sociologic and Constitutional Typologic Examinations on Paradentosis of 200 patients. Paradentium, 2:32, 1933.

16. Manhold, J. H.: Report of a Study on the Relationship of Personality Variables to Periodontal Conditions. J. Periodont., 24:248, 1953.

17. Miller, S. C., et al.: The Use of the Minnesota Multiplastic Personality Inventory as a Diagnostic Aid in Periodontal Disease. A Preliminary Report. J. Periodont., 27:44, 1956.

18. Moskow, B. S. Rennert, M. C., Wasserman, B. H., Khurana, H.: Interrelationship of Dietary Factors and Heredity in Periodontal Lesions in the Gerbil. Program and Abstracts, 48th General Meeting, I.A.D.R., 1970, p. 134.

19. Poland, C., III, Christian, J. C., and Bixler, D.: Hypophosphatasia: An Inherited Oral Disease. Program and Abstracts, 48th General Meeting, I.A.D.R., 1970, p. 228.

20. Polevitsky, K.: Blood Types in Pyorrhea Alveolaris. J. D. Res., 9:285, 1929.

21. Ramfjord, S.: Tuberculosis and Periodontal Disease, with Special Reference to the Collagen Fibers. J. D. Res., 31:5, 1952.

22. Ryan, E. J.: Psychobiologic Foundation in Dentistry. Springfield, Ill., Charles C Thomas, 1946, p. 27.

23. Sandler, H. C., and Stahl, S. S.: The Influence of Generalized Diseases on Clinical Manifestations of Periodontal Disease. J.A.D.A., 49:656, 1954.

24. Saul, L. J.: A Note on the Psychogenesis of Organic Symptoms. Psychoanalytic Quarterly, 4:476, 1935.

25. Scopp, I. W.: Healthy Periodontium in Chronically Ill Patients. J. Periodont., 28:147, 1957.

26. Stahl, S. S., et al.: The Influence of Systemic Diseases on Alveolar Bone. J.A.D.A., 45:277, 1952.

27. Tanchester, D., and Sorrin, S.: Dental Lesions in Relation to Pulmonary Tuberculosis. J. D. Res., 16:69, 1937.

28. Tochichara, Y.: Pyorrhea Alveolaris in Leprosy. Nippar No Shikai, 13:165, 1933.

29. Weber, R., and Pastern, W.: Uber die Frage der konstitutionellen Bereitschaft zur sog. Alveolar Pyorrhea (Alveolarpyorrhoe und Blutgruppen). Deutsch. Monatschr. f. Zahnheilkunde, 14:704, 1927.

30. Weiss, E., and English, O. S.: Psychosomatic Medicine. 2nd ed. Philadelphia, W. B. Saunders Co., 1949.

31. Weller, C. V.: Constitutional Factors in Periodontitis. J.A.D.A., 15:1081, 1928.

Chapter 29

THE SYSTEMIC CONDITION OF PATIENTS WITH PERIODONTAL DISEASE

Numerous clinical studies have been conducted to determine whether there are disorders that predispose to periodontal disease and also to determine the effect upon the patient of gingival and periodontal disease. The findings in such studies have been interpreted in the following ways:

1. There may be systemic disorders that predispose to periodontal disease.

2. Periodontal disease may predispose to certain systemic disorders.

3. There may be comparable factors that predispose patients to both periodontal disease and specific systemic disorders.

SYSTEMIC FINDINGS IN PERIODONTAL DISEASE

The following systemic aspects have been investigated in relation to periodontal disease. (Some studies differentiate be-

tween systemic findings in patients with periodontitis and those with periodontosis; others do not make this distinction.)

Metabolism

Patients with periodontitis present no characteristic metabolic pattern.[7-9] In periodontosis the metabolism has been reported as both lowered[12] and slightly elevated.[4, 6, 51] Opinions differ as to whether a correlation exists between the periodontal status and glucose tolerance levels.[37, 47]

Endocrine

Dysfunction of the parathyroid and pituitary glands, ovaries and thyroid (particularly hyperthyroidism),[5, 6] and abnormal serum calcium levels have been reported in periodontosis.[13] Hypothyroidism was observed in 43 out of 80 patients with periodontitis,[3] with and without other endocrine disorders (e.g., diabetes, hypogonadism and pituitary dysfunction). Disturbance in ovarian function[49] and reduced urinary estrogen levels[24] have been correlated with increasing severity of periodontal disease.

Blood chemistry

Elevated calcium,[50] lowered calcium with elevated phosphorus,[20] elevated serum glycoprotein,[15] uric acid, glucose, choles-

411

terol, citric acid, and bilirubin have been reported in the blood of patients with periodontosis.[25, 28, 46, 50] Serum glutamic oxaloacetic transaminase and serum glutamic pyruvic transaminase are not altered.[21]

In periodontitis, elevated blood calcium and lowered phosphorus,[2, 13, 19] elevated serum alkaline phosphatase,[34] and citric acid,[42] and lowered blood catalase[16] levels have been described. Some investigators suggest the possibility of a relationship between dietary inadequacy and deviations in blood chemistry in patients with periodontal disease.[22] Others note no significant changes in periodontal disease. The blood levels of calcium, glucose, cholesterol, ascorbic acid,[23, 45] sodium and potassium,[34] chloride, inorganic phosphate and urea nitrogen[31] are reported as unaltered. Serum total protein, albumin, globulin and uric acid show no significant relationship to periodontal status.[38, 39] The level of serum-free 17-hydroxycorticosterone is elevated in periodontal disease, but the significance of this finding has not been established. The glucose content of blood in the gingiva and the finger is the same in patients with periodontal disease,[25] but alkaline phosphatase in gingival blood is greater than in the general circulation.[32] C-reactive protein (CRP) (a nonspecific protein usually associated with diseases causing inflammation and tissue breakdown and not found in healthy individuals) was noted in patients with severe periodontal disease.[40]

Gastric chemistry

Gastric hyperacidity, hypoacidity and anacidity[8, 35] occur in patients with periodontal disease. The contention of Broderick,[10] that periodontal disease results from alkalosis and caries is caused by acidosis, has not been confirmed.

Hematologic aspects

Blood studies in patients with periodontal disease reveal the following: normal total and differential leukocyte count and low red blood count,[41] elevated counts, frequent secondary anemia of the hypochromic microcytic type,[18] decrease in hemoglobin values and a low erythrocyte count, as well as a relative lymphocytosis and a decrease in polymorphonuclear leukocytes.[27] Blood type A was noted in 49 per

cent of patients with periodontal disease in contrast with 40 to 41.1 per cent of patients without periodontal disease,[33, 48] but no significant relationship between blood grouping and periodontal disease,[1] or between arteriosclerosis and alveolar bone loss[26] has been established.

Comment

The preceding paragraphs reflect the rather unsettled status and sparseness of information regarding the systemic condition of patients with periodontal disease. It is difficult to evaluate many of the investigations because there is no uniformity in the criteria used to judge the periodontal disorders. The inadequacy of available information regarding the possible interrelation of systemic disorders and periodontal disease should not be misinterpreted as indicating an absence of such relationship. One must also guard against attributing too much significance to isolated, unconfirmed findings.

FOCAL INFECTION

According to the concept of focal infection, a primary site of infection in one part of the body may serve as the focus (Latin "hearth") from which infection emanates to other parts of the body. Interest in focal infection has fluctuated considerably from the initial enthusiasm stimulated by the original investigation of Rosenow in 1917. More recently, with the introduction of chemotherapy, attention has again been directed to the subject of focal infection.

In the early days of the focal infection concept, the oral cavity attracted attention because it harbored teeth with chronic apical disease. Physicians confronted with disease elsewhere in the body were drawn to the comparatively easily available "infected teeth." The persistence of disease in other areas of the body even after all the "infected" teeth had been removed, coupled with the revelation that not all pathologic apical lesions were necessarily infected, exerted a somewhat sobering influence upon the medical and dental professions in regard to the problem of focal infection.

TABLE 29-1 THE PERIODONTAL POCKET VS. PERIAPICAL DISEASE

Periodontal Pocket	Periapical Disease
1. Infection is always present.	1. Infection is not necessarily present in long-standing periapical lesions.[10]
2. The bacterial as well as mycotic organisms are of great variety and considerably more numerous as well as of greater pathogenic potentiality.	2. The bacterial organisms are not as varied, numerous nor of equal pathogenic significance.
3. Periodontal pockets are not circumscribed or walled off from the adjacent tissue.	3. Periapical areas are frequently well circumscribed within a fibrotic boundary.
4. Periodontal pockets are subject to constant mechanical stimulation in mastication which could drive bacteria into the blood stream.	4. Periapical areas are located centrally in the bone, in a comparatively undisturbed environment.
5. Periodontal pockets are more prevalent in adults in age groups likely to be subject to ailments requiring medical attention.	5. Less prevalent than periodontal pockets.

Periodontal disease and focal infection

Interest in the oral cavity as a possible source of focal infection has shifted recently from the periapical areas to the periodontal pocket.[44] Within the limitations which govern the concept of focal infection, **the periodontal pocket represents a greater potential menace than periapical disease for the reasons shown in Table 29-1.**

In patients with periodontal disease and a disturbance elsewhere in the body suspected of being of focal origin, **the responsibility for the decision regarding the fate of the teeth rests with the dentist.** It is reasonable to expect him to understand more about the periodontal tissues than other medical specialists. The physician, on the other hand, is in a position to inform the dentist regarding the likelihood of the patient's medical problem being caused by infection elsewhere in the body. It should be borne in mind that even in a patient with suppurative periodontal disease which the dentist might very well consider a potential focus of infection, there is no assurance that the patient's complaint is related to the oral condition.

BACTEREMIA IN GINGIVAL AND PERIODONTAL DISEASE*

The literature consistently points to disease of the gingiva as a source of bacteremia following mechanical manipulation of the teeth.[30, 36, 43] Murray and Moosnick[29] found

positive blood cultures in 55 per cent of the cases in which persons with varying degrees of dental caries and periodontal disease chewed paraffin cubes for 30 minutes. Fish and MacLean[17] reported positive blood cultures after tooth extractions in nine patients with periodontal disease. They assumed that luxation of the teeth in extraction caused alternate compression and stretching of the periodontal ligament and that streptococci were in this way pumped into the lymphatics and blood vessels. Okell and Elliott[30] reported 72 positive blood cultures following extraction in 100 patients with gingival disease. A significantly lower incidence of bacteremia was found in patients with no clinical periodontal disease. In addition, Elliott[14] found that where marked gingival disease was present, rocking of the teeth alone sufficed to produce bacteremia in 86 per cent of the patients. Bacteremia occurred more frequently associated with deep periodontal pockets. *Serratia viridans* was the organism most often seen. Burket and Burn[11] painted S. *marcescens* into the gingival sulcus prior to extraction and recovered it in postextraction blood cultures in 18 out of 90 cases.

REFERENCES

1. Barros, L., and Witkop, C. S. J.: Oral and Genetic Study of Chileans 1960—III Periodontal Disease and Nutritional Factors. Arch. Oral Biol., 8:195, 1963.
2. Becks, H.: Newer Aspects in Paradentosis. Ann. Int. Med., 6:65, 1932–3.
3. Becks, H.: Systemic Background of Paradentosis. J.A.D.A., 28:1447, 1941.
4. Biocca E., and Seppilli, A.: Human Infections Caused by Lactobacilli. J. Infect. Dis., 81:112, 1947.

---

*Bacteremia following periodontal treatment is discussed in Chapter 51.

5. Boenheim, F.: Endokriner Status bei Paradentose. Zahnärztl. Rundsch., 37:1326, 1928.

6. Boenheim, F.: Ist das endokrine Druesensystem bei Paradentose gestoert? Paradentium, 3:91, 1930.

7. Boenheim, F.: Pyorrhea Alveolaris as Systemic Disease. Brit. D. J., 53:12, 1932.

8. Boenheim, F.: Pathogenic Importance of the Endocrine Glands in Paradontal Disease. J. D. Res., 17:19, 1938.

9. Breuer, K.: Metabolic Studies in Disease of the Paradentium. Zschr. f. Stomat, 31:982, 1933.

10. Broderick, F. W.: Pyorrhea Alveolaris. London, John Bale Sons and Danielson, Ltd., 1931.

11. Burket, L. W., and Burn, G. G.: Bacteremia Following Dental Extraction. Demonstration of Source of Bacteria by Means of a Non-pathogen. J. D. Res., 16:521, 1937.

12. Chiuminatto, L.: Investigation of Metabolism in Paradentoses. Stomatologie, 27:269, 1929.

13. Citron, J.: Die Paradentose als Symptom von Endokrinen. Zeitschr. Clin. Med., 108:331, 1928.

14. Elliott, S. D.: Bacteremia and Oral Sepsis. Proc. Roy. Soc. Med., 32:747, 1939.

15. Engel, M. B., Laskin, D. M., and Gans, B. J.: Elevation of a Serum Glycoprotein in Periodontosis. J.A.D.A., 57:830, 1958.

16. Englander, H. R., et al.: The Relationship of Blood Catalase Activity and Periodontal Disease. J. Periodont., 26:233, 1955.

17. Fish, E. W., and MacLean, L.: Distribution of Oral Streptococci in the Tissues. Brit. D. J., 61:336, 1936.

18. Goldstein, H.: Systemic and Blood Picture in Several Hundred Periclasia-free and Periclasia-involved Individuals. J. D. Res., 16:320, 1937.

19. Grove, C. J., and Grove, C. T.: Blood Phosphorus Insufficiency in Pyorrhea. J. D. Res., 13:191, 1933.

20. Hawkins, H. F.: Nutritional Influences on Growth and Development. Int. J. Orth. & D. Children, 19:307, 1933.

21. Honjo, K., Nakamura, R., Tsunemitsu, A., and Matsumura, T.: Serum Transaminases in Periodontosis. J. Periodont., 35:247, 1964.

22. Karshan, M., et al.: Studies in Periodontal Disease. J. D. Res., 31:11, 1952.

23. Karshan, M., and Tenenbaum, B.: Blood Studies in Periodontoclasia. J. D. Res., 25:180, 1946.

24. Karshan, M., Tenenbaum, B., and Friedland, R.: Urinary Estrogen in Periodontosis. J. D. Res., 35:648, 1956.

25. Landgraf, E., et al.: Investigations of Uric Acid Blood Level in Periodontal Disease. Zeitschr. f. Stomat., 30:91, 1932.

26. Mackenzie, R. S., and Millard, H. D.: Interrelated Effects of Diabetes, Arteriosclerosis, and Calculus on Alveolar Bone Loss. J.A.D.A., 66:191, 1963.

27. Martin, D.: The Blood Associated with Pyorrhea Alveolaris. Austral. D. J., 9:488, 1937.

28. Morelli, G.: The Clinical and Therapeutic Evaluation of the Results Concerning Constitutional Factors in Cases of Paradentoses. Ann. Med., 41:648, 1935.

29. Murray, M., and Moosnick, F.: Incidence of Bacteremia in Patients with Dental Disease. J. Lab. & Clin. Med., 26:801, 1941.

30. Okell, C. C., and Elliott, S. D.: Bacteremia and Oral Sepsis. Lancet, 2:869, 1935.

31. O'Leary, T. J., Shannon, I. L., and Prigmore, J. R.: Clinical and Systemic Findings in Periodontal Disease. J. Periodont., 33:243, 1962.

32. Pelzer, R. H.: A Method for Plasma Phosphatase Determination for the Differentiation of Alveolar Crest Bone Types in Periodontal Disease. J. D. Res., 19:73, 1940.

33. Polevitsky, K.: Blood Types in Pyorrhea Alveolaris. J. D. Res., 9:285, 1929.

34. Rose, H. P., Kuna, A., and Kraft, E.: Systemic Manifestations of Periodontal Disease. J. Periodont., 34:253, 1963.

35. Sagal, Z.: Pyorrhea Alveolaris and Gastric Acidity. D. Cosmos, 68:1145, 1926.

36. Sand, R.: Periodontal Sepsis in Relationship to Systemic Disease. J.A.D.A., 28:710, 1941.

37. Shannon, I. L., and Gibson, W. A.: Oral Glucose Tolerance Responses in Healthy Young Adult Males Classified as to Caries Experience and Periodontal Status. Periodontics, 2:292, 1964.

38. Shannon, I. L., and Gibson, W. A.: Serum Total Protein, Albumin, and Globulin in Relation to Periodontal Status and Caries Experience. Oral Surg., Oral Med., & Oral Path., 18:399, 1964.

39. Shannon, I. L., Terry, J. M., and Chauncey, H. H.: Uric Acid and Total Protein in Serum and Parotid Fluid in Relation to Periodontal Status. J. D. Res., 45:1539, 1966.

40. Shklair, I., Loving, R., Leberman, O., and Rau, C.: C-Reactive Protein and Periodontal Disease. J. Periodont., 39:93, 1968.

41. Siegel, E.: Total Erythrocyte, Lymphocyte and Differential White Cell Counts of Blood in Chronic Periodontal Disease. J. D. Res., 24:270, 1945.

42. Simon, E., et al.: Citrate Content of Blood and Saliva in Relation to Periodontal Disease in Man. Arch. Oral Biol., 13:1243, 1968.

43. Stones, H. H.: Oral and Dental Diseases. Chronic Oral Sepsis and Relation to Systemic Diseases. Baltimore, Williams & Wilkins, 1948, Chap. XXXIII.

44. Storebecker, T. P.: Dental Infectious Foci and Diseases of the Nervous System. Acta Psychiat. Neurol. Scandinav., 36, Suppl. 157, 1961.

45. Tenenbaum, B., and Karshan, M.: Blood Studies in Periodontoclasia. J.A.D.A., 32:1372, 1945.

46. Tsunemitsu, A., et al.: Citric Acid Metabolism in Periodontosis. Arch. Oral Biol., 9:83, 1964.

47. Tuckman, M. A., et al.: The Relationship of Glucose Tolerance to Periodontal Status. J. Periodont., 41:513, 1970.

48. Weber, R., and Pastern, W.: Uber die Frage der Konstitutionellen Bereitschaft zur Sog. Alveolar Pyorrhoe (Alveolarpyorrhoe und Blutgruppen). Deutsch. Monatschr. F. Zahnheilkunde, 14:704, 1927.

49. Weiner, R., Karshan, M., and Tenenbaum, B.: Ovarian Function in Periodontosis. J. D. Res., 35:875, 1956.

50. Weinmann, J. P.: Study of Metabolism in Diffuse Atrophy. Zeitschr. f. Stomat., 25:822, 1927.

51. Weinmann, J. P.: Investigation of Metabolism in Diffuse Atrophy of the Alveolar Process. Zeitschr. f. Stomat., 28:1154, 1930.

Part IV
Classification of Gingival and Periodontal Disease

Chapter 30

CLASSIFICATION OF GINGIVAL AND PERIODONTAL DISEASE

Classification of gingival and periodontal disease provides a key for differentiating between various disease processes affecting the periodontium. To provide maximum assistance in diagnosis and treatment, the diseases have been classified here upon the basis of three criteria: (1) clinical features, (2) pathologic changes and (3) etiology.

Diseases of the periodontium are classified into two main groups: (1) gingival disease and (2) periodontal disease. Gingival diseases are those that appear clinically to be confined to the gingiva, whereas periodontal disease is destructive disease of the supporting periodontal tissues. Pathologic changes at the root apices are not customarily included under the term periodontal disease.

GINGIVAL DISEASE

The most common form of gingival disease is chronic inflammation, which usually spreads into the supporting tissues and initiates periodontal disease. Some forms of gingival disease remain confined to the gingiva.

Inflammation is a feature of all forms of gingival disease; however, the role of the inflammation varies. It may be the only disease process (*uncomplicated gingivitis*); it may be superimposed upon underlying systemically induced proliferative or degenerative gingival disease (*combined gingivitis*); or it may precipitate clinical disease in patients with systemic conditions that of themselves produce no clinically detectable gingival changes (*conditioned gingivitis*).

Classification

In the following classification (Table 30–1), diseases of the gingiva are grouped according to the role of inflammation.

416

TABLE 30–1 CLASSIFICATION OF GINGIVAL DISEASE

Type of Gingival Disease	Histopathology	Etiology
UNCOMPLICATED GINGIVITIS Chronic marginal gingivitis	**Chronic inflammation**	Local irritation (mechanical, chemical, bacterial)
Acute necrotizing ulcerative gingivitis	**Acute necrotizing inflammation with pseudomembrane formation**	Unknown—fusospirochetal bacterial complex suspected
Acute herpetic gingivostomatitis and other viral infections	**Acute inflammation with vesicle formation**	Herpes simplex and other viruses
Allergic gingivitis	**Acute inflammation with pronounced vascular response**	Various allergens (pollen, foods)
Nonspecific gingivitis	**Inflammation with or without ulceration**	Local irritation (chemical, mechanical, thermal)
Tuberculosis and syphilis	**Specific granulomatous inflammation**	Bacterial—*M. tuberculosis, T. pallidum*
Moniliasis (thrush) and other fungal infections	**Inflammation and ulceration with thick surface growth of fungi**	Mycotic—*Monilia albicans,* and other fungi
Pyostomatitis vegetans	**Hyperkeratosis and acanthosis of epithelium. Granulomatous inflammation with unruptured miliary abscesses**	Unknown
COMBINED GINGIVITIS Dermatoses affecting the gingiva (lichen planus, pemphigus, erythema multiforme, lupus erythematosus)	**Chronic inflammation with characteristic picture for different dermatoses**	Systemic (unknown) plus local irritation
Chronic desquamative gingivitis (gingivosis)	**Epithelial atrophy with desquamation, degeneration of the basement membrane and connective tissue ground substance and inflammation**	Systemic (unknown) plus local irritation
Chronic menopausal gingivostomatitis (senile atrophic gingivitis)	**Epithelial atrophy, degeneration of the basement membrane and connective tissue ground substance and inflammation**	Hormonal plus local irritation
Benign mucous membrane pemphigoid	**Chronic inflammation, epithelial degeneration, with sub-epithelial vesicle formation; histopathology varies**	Systemic (unknown) plus local irritation
CONDITIONED GINGIVITIS Gingivitis in pregnancy and puberty	**Inflammation plus exaggerated vascularity and edema**	
Gingivitis in vitamin C deficiency	**Inflammation plus collagen degeneration and interstitial hemorrhage**	Local irritation and systemic
Gingivitis in leukemia	**Inflammation plus diffuse infiltration of proliferating leukocytes**	

TABLE 30–1   CLASSIFICATION OF GINGIVAL DISEASE (*Continued*)

Type of Gingival Disease	Histopathology	Etiology
GINGIVAL ENLARGEMENT Inflammatory	**Chronic and acute inflammation**	Local irritation (chemical, microbial, thermal, mechanical)
Noninflammatory hyperplastic	**Noninflammatory hyperplasia of the epithelium and connective tissue**	Dilantin, hereditary, idiopathic
Combined	**Hyperplasia of epithelium and connective tissue plus superimposed inflammation**	Local irritation superimposed upon noninflammatory gingival enlargement
Conditioned	**Inflammation modified by systemic conditions**	Local irritation plus systemic conditioning—hormonal (pregnancy; puberty); leukemic; vitamin C deficiency
Neoplastic	**Tumor formation**	Etiology unknown
Developmental	**Chronic inflammation**	Location of gingiva on enamel in course of eruption plus local irritation

RECESSION
Gingival atrophy
	Denudation of cementum with migration of the epithelial attachment in the direction of the root apex	Physiologic (aging)
		Pathologic
		    Mechanical trauma (toothbrush, clasps)
		    Abnormal tooth position combined with mechanical trauma
		    Inflammation (associated with local irritation)
		    Disuse
		    Idiopathic

PERIODONTAL DISEASE

"Chronic destructive periodontal disease" is a nonspecific descriptive term that includes all forms of periodontal disease. It is customary to classify periodontal disease as one of three types: (1) *periodontitis* (*chronic suppurative periodontitis*)—destruction of the periodontium caused by local irritation; (2) *periodontosis*, noninflammatory degenerative disease ostensibly caused by systemic factors; and (3) *periodontal syndrome*—a combination of systemically caused degenerative changes and locally caused inflammation. Trauma from occlusion is often classified as a separate entity, *periodontal traumatism*,[31] distinct from other forms of periodontal disease.

Classification

The following classification is based upon the premise that trauma from occlusion, when present, is an integral part of periodontal disease rather than a separate disease process. It presents trauma from occlusion as a destructive change in the supporting periodontal tissues, sharing the responsibility for periodontal loss with inflammation (Table 30–2). This classification also makes allowance for the uncommon occurrence of trauma from occlusion as the sole pathologic process in periodontal disease.

Periodontitis

Periodontitis is the most common type of periodontal disease. It is referred to by such other terms as schmutzpyorrhea (Gottlieb) and paradentitis (Becks). Periodontitis results from extension of inflammation from the gingiva into the supporting periodontal tissues (Chaps. 14 and 15).

There are two types of periodontitis: *simple* (also referred to as *marginal periodontitis*), in which the destruction of periodontal tissues is caused by inflammation alone, and *compound*, in which the

TABLE 30–2 CLASSIFICATION OF PERIODONTAL DISEASE

Type	Histopathology	Etiology
PERIODONTITIS		
Simple periodontitis (marginal periodontitis)	Chronic inflammation of the gingiva; periodontal pockets; bone resorption; destruction of the periodontal ligament and tooth exfoliation.	Local irritation
Compound periodontitis	Chronic inflammation; resorption of alveolar bone and cementum; destruction of the periodontal ligament combined with vascular, degenerative and necrotic changes in the periodontal ligament; increased incidence of infrabony pockets and angular bone destruction.	Local irritation plus occlusal disharmony
PERIODONTOSIS		
Early periodontosis	Noninflammatory degeneration of the periodontal ligament, osteolysis(?), diminished formation of cementum(?).	Systemic(?)
Advanced periodontosis (periodontal syndrome)	Noninflammatory degeneration of the supporting periodontal tissues, complicated by inflammation and/or trauma from occlusion.	Systemic(?) plus local irritation and/or occlusal disharmony
TRAUMA FROM OCCLUSION	Degenerative and necrotic changes in the supporting periodontal tissues with tendency toward widening of the periodontal ligament and angular bone resorption.	Occlusal disharmony
PERIODONTAL ATROPHY		
Presenile atrophy	Reduction in the height of the periodontium.	Unknown
Disuse atrophy	Thinning of the periodontal ligament, thinning and reduction in the number of periodontal fibers, disruption of fiber bundle arrangement, thickened cementum, reduction in the height of alveolar bone.	Diminution or absence of occlusal forces

tissue destruction results from inflammation combined with trauma from occlusion. In individual patients the classification is determined by the predominant condition.

Simple periodontitis (marginal periodontitis)

CLINICAL FEATURES. Chronic inflammation of the gingiva, pocket formation—usually but not always with pus formation—bone loss, tooth mobility, pathologic migration and eventual tooth loss are the clinical features of simple periodontitis. It may be localized to a single tooth or group of teeth or generalized throughout the mouth, depending upon the distribution of the etiologic factors (Fig. 30–1).

Simple periodontitis progresses at a varied rate; its advanced stages are usually seen in late adulthood. It is noteworthy that pathologic migration occurs late in this disease, in contrast to periodontosis, in which pathologic migration is an early clinical sign.

Simple periodontitis is usually painless, but it may be accompanied by such symptoms as (1) sensitivity to thermal changes, food and tactile stimulation associated with denudation of the roots; (2) dull deep radiating pain during and after chewing, caused by the forceful wedging of food into periodontal pockets; (3) acute symptoms such as throbbing pain and sensitivity to percussion from periodontal abscess formation or superimposed acute necrotizing ulcerative gingivitis; (4) pulpal symptoms such as sensitivity to sweets, thermal changes or throbbing pain, which result from pulpitis associated with carious destruction of the root surfaces.

ETIOLOGY. Simple periodontitis is caused by a large variety of local irritants that cause gingival inflammation and extension of inflammation into the supporting periodontal tissues.

Compound periodontitis

CLINICAL FEATURES. The clinical features are the same as those of simple periodontitis with the following exceptions: there is a higher incidence of infrabony

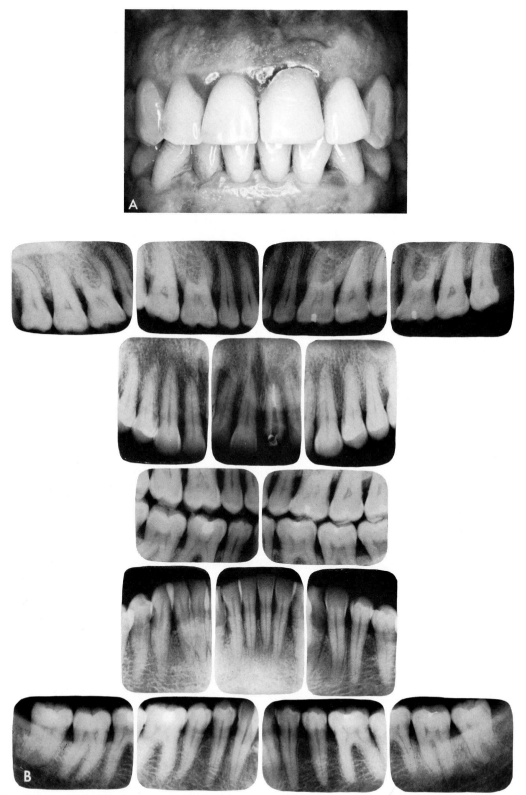

Figure 30–1 Simple Periodontitis in a 47-Year-Old Female. *A,* Clinical view showing generalized gingival inflammation and periodontal pocket formation. *B,* Radiographs showing generalized horizontal bone loss which varies in severity in different areas.

pockets,[10] and angular rather than horizontal bone loss (Fig. 30–2); widening of the periodontal ligament space is a more common finding; tooth mobility tends to be more severe, frequently with comparatively little gingival inflammation.

ETIOLOGY. Compound periodontitis is caused by the combined effects of local irritation plus trauma from occlusion. The degenerative changes in trauma from occlusion aggravate the destructive effects of inflammation.

Periodontosis

The term periodontosis designates chronic degenerative noninflammatory destruction of the periodontium originating in one or more of the periodontal tissues. It is characterized by early migration and loosening of the teeth in the presence or absence of secondary gingival inflammation and pocket formation. If permitted to run its course, it results in destruction of the periodontal tissues and loss of teeth. The condition is also referred to as *diffuse atrophy of the alveolar bone.*[15]

Clinical and microscopic features

Periodontosis affects both males and females and is seen most frequently in the period between puberty and the age of 30. In teenagers it is more prevalent in females. The maxillary and mandibular incisors and first molar areas are affected earliest and most severely and usually bilaterally,[26, 27] but with time the involvement becomes generalized (Fig. 30–3). Least destruction occurs in the mandibular premolar area.

THE THREE STAGES OF PERIODONTOSIS. Periodontosis develops in three stages with the following microscopic and clinical features (Orban and Weinmann):[33]

The first stage is characterized by degeneration and desmolysis of the principal fibers of the periodontal ligament (Figs. 30–4 and 30–5) and probable cessation of cementum formation. There is simultaneous resorption of the alveolar bone owing to (1) lack of functional stimulation from the tooth and (2) increased tissue pressure caused by edema and capillary proliferation.

Tooth migration is the earliest clinical sign and it occurs without detectable inflammatory involvement. The usual picture consists of labiodistal migration and extrusion and loosening of the maxillary incisors with diastema formation. Less frequently, distal migration of the mandibular incisors is seen. The rate of migration is affected by the occlusal relations of the anterior teeth and pressure from the tongue. Migration of posterior teeth in either a mesial or distal direction is occasionally seen.

The second stage is characterized by the rapid proliferation of the epithelial attachment along the root. Proliferation of the epithelial rests in the periodontal ligament may also occur.

The earliest signs of inflammatory involvement caused by local irritation are seen in the second stage. Clinically, both the first and second stages are of short duration and cannot be differentiated from each other.

The third stage is characterized by progressive gingival inflammation, trauma from occlusion, the development of deepened periodontal pockets and increased bone loss. The pockets are often of the infrabony type, but the presence of infrabony pockets is not necessarily evidence of the existence of periodontosis. This is the stage that is observed most frequently; it is referred to as advanced periodontosis or periodontal syndrome (Fig. 30–6). Periodontosis is a painless condition. In time, however, it may develop symptoms similar to those of periodontitis.

Radiographic features

Bone loss is initially confined to the mandibular and maxillary incisors and first molars. Destruction of the interdental septa is vertical, angular or arc-like rather than horizontal. Thickening of the periodontal space and absence or haziness of the lamina dura is observed in relation to many teeth. There may be generalized alteration in the trabecular pattern of the bone, characterized by less clearly defined trabecular markings and increased size of the cancellous spaces. As the disease progresses the bone destruction becomes generalized, obscuring the initial distribution of the bone loss.

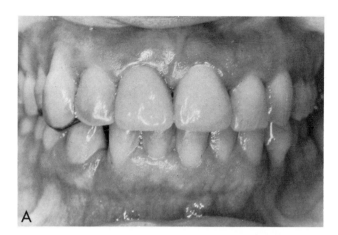

Figure 30–2 Compound Periodontitis in a 44-year-old Female. *A,* Generalized gingival inflammation with periodontal pocket formation. *B,* Generalized bone loss with angular destruction of the interdental septa caused by the combination of inflammation and trauma from occlusion.

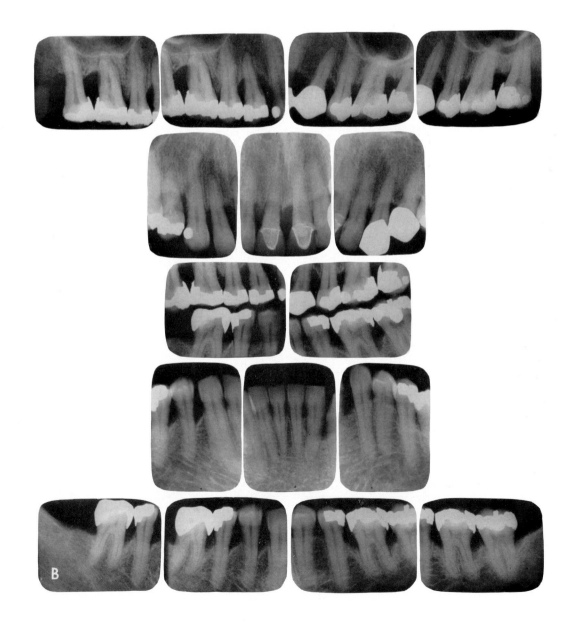

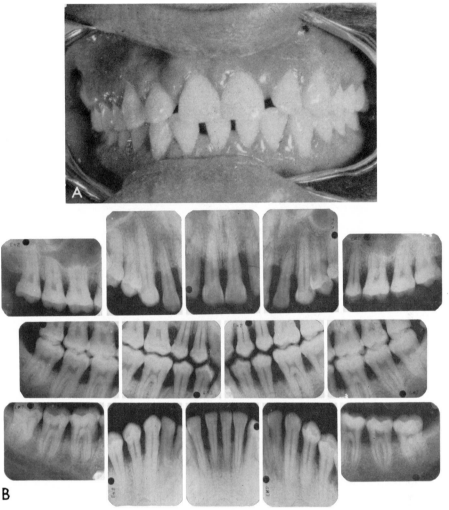

Figure 30–3 Periodontosis in a 24-year-old Male. *A,* Pathologic migration of the maxillary and mandibular anterior teeth. *B,* Generalized bone loss accentuated in the maxillary and mandibular anterior areas.

Etiology

The initial degeneration in periodontosis is considered to be of systemic etiology; the secondary inflammatory involvement is caused by local irritants; however, *the systemic origin of periodontosis has not been established.*[13]

Among systemic conditions suspected as potential causes of periodontosis are metabolic imbalance, inherited hormonal disturbances, debilitating disease, nutritional deficiency, diabetes, syphilis, hypertension, collagen disease and inherited inferiority of the dental organ.

Disturbance in physiologic continuous eruption is considered a contributing local etiologic factor. Trauma from occlusion may be responsible in part for the initial localization of the periodontal destruction to the anterior and molar regions and the angular rather than horizontal interdental bone destructive patterns.

Conditions resembling periodontosis have been described in experimental animals under various conditions such as excessively alkaline diets,[38] diets low in calcium and vitamin D,[5] protein depletion[11] and hyperthyroidism.[14]

Nature of the initial pathologic changes

Opinions differ regarding the nature of the initial pathologic changes in periodon-

Fig. 30–4

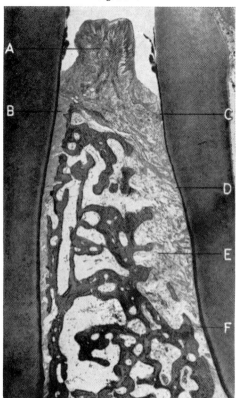

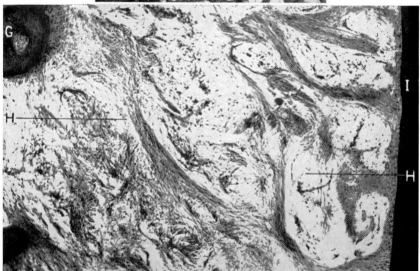

Fig. 30–5

Figure 30–4 Survey Mesiodistal Section Through the Interdental Space Between the Mandibular First Premolar *(left)* **and Second Premolar** *(right)* **from a Patient with Periodontosis.** *A,* Interdental papilla. *B,* Periodontal membrane of normal width on the distal side of the first premolar. *C,* Epithelial attachment. *D,* Epithelial island attached to the surface of the cementum. *E,* Widened periodontal space on the mesial side of the second premolar. *F,* Normal width of the portion of the periodontal membrane on the mesial side of the second premolar. (From Orban, B. and Weinmann, J. P., J. Periodont., *13*:41, 1946.)

Figure 30–5 Detailed study of area *(E)* in Figure 30–4 showing degeneration of the periodontal membrane at *(H).* The cementum is shown at *(I)* and the bone at *(G).*

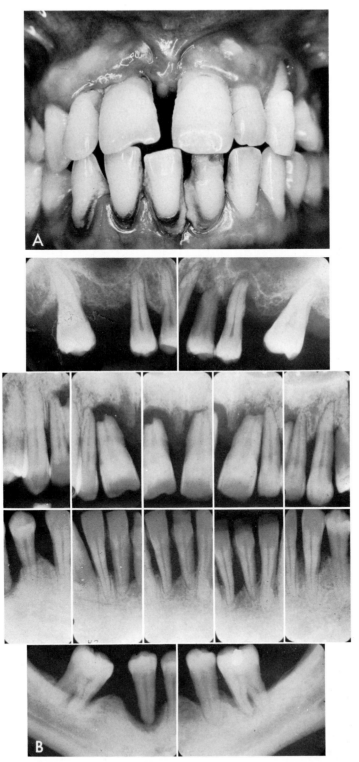

Figure 30–6 Advanced Periodontosis (Periodontal Syndrome) in a 28-year-old Female. *A*, Gingival inflammation, heavy calculus deposits, anterior open bite with diastema formation associated with tongue thrusting habit. *B*, Severe generalized bone destruction obscures the limitation of bone loss to the anterior and molar regions seen in early periodontosis.

tosis and the supporting tissue or tissues in which it occurs.

The prevalent opinion is that it starts as a noninflammatory degeneration of the principal fibers of the periodontal ligament[14, 15, 33, 37, 39] **which involves a single tooth, group of teeth, or the entire dentition. Other impressions of the initial changes in periodontosis include transformation of alveolar bone into fibrous connective tissue by a process of reversion,**[40] **deficiency in continuous deposition of cementum (described as deep cementopathia**[15, 17]**) followed by loss of attachment between tooth and bone and resorption of the adjacent bone.**[1] **The progressive loss of bone has been attributed to osteoclasis, pressure from edema and capillary proliferation and halisteresis. It is agreed that inflammation is secondary, starts in the gingiva, and is caused by local factors.**

The difference in opinion regarding the initial pathologic changes in periodontosis results in part from the fact that very few human jaws with the disease have thus far been studied. Periodontosis may be initiated by more than one type of pathologic change. The consensus regarding the pathology of periodontosis may be expressed as follows:

It originates as a degenerative change in one or more of the periodontal tissues which is followed by secondary inflammation and trauma from occlusion, which aggravate destruction of the periodontium and hasten tooth loss.

Papillon-Lefèvre syndrome

This is a rare condition, characterized by a combination of periodontosis and thickening of the epidermis of the hands and feet. It is described in Chapter 20.

Trauma from Occlusion

Because gingival inflammation is so common, trauma from occlusion seldom occurs without it. **When it is the sole pathological process it presents the following clinical features:** tooth mobility, pronounced periodontal space in the gingival region of the root (with an associated angular destruction of bone) and thickening of the periodontal ligament at the apex. Isolated teeth and

their antagonists are affected. There is no significant gingival inflammation, formation of periodontal pockets or pain.

Periodontal Atrophy

Atrophy is a decrease in the size of a tissue or organ or of its cellular elements after it has attained its normal mature size. Generalized reduction in the height of the alveolar bone, accompanied by recession of the gingiva without inflammation or trauma from occlusion occurs with increasing age and is termed *physiologic* or *senile atrophy.* Injurious local factors superimposed upon the underlying atrophy often cause additional bone loss. Atrophy of the periodontium in excess of the physiologic rate is a form of periodontal disease referred to as *presenile* or *disuse atrophy.*

Presenile atrophy

Presenile atrophy is premature reduction in the height of the periodontium that is uniform throughout the mouth and without apparent local cause (Fig. 30–7).

Disuse atrophy

Disuse atrophy results when the functional stimulation required for the maintenance of the periodontal tissues is markedly diminished or absent.

Disuse atrophy is characterized by thinning of the periodontal ligament, thinning and reduction in the number of periodontal fibers and disruption of the fiber bundle arrangement, thickened cementum and reduction in the height of the alveolar bone, and osteoporosis, which appears as a reduction in the number and thickness of the bone trabeculae.

Other Types of Periodontal Disease

Under the heading *periodontitis complex* Box[7] described a "systemic type" of periodontal disease, resembling periodontosis, characterized by the early appearance in the periodontal ligament of an inflammatory tissue change induced by occlusal trauma, termed *rarefying pericementitis fibrosa.* A noninflammatory *betel periodontosis* has been described as originating in the alveolar

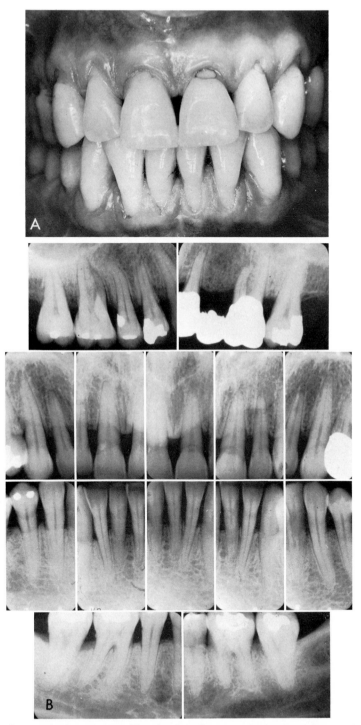

Figure 30–7 Presenile Atrophy in a 38-year-old Male. *A,* Reduction in the height of the periodontium and recession with slight gingival inflammation. *B,* Premature generalized bone loss.

TABLE 30-3 REPRESENTATIVE CLASSIFICATIONS OF GINGIVAL AND PERIODONTAL DISEASE

KANTOROWICZ, 1924[25]

Inflammatory disease
Paradentitis

Dystrophic disease with little inflammation
Presenile atrophy
Dystrophy from occlusal trauma
Dystrophy from lack of occlusion
Diffuse atrophy

SIMONTON, 1927[39]

Chemobacterial
Paradontitis

Systemic
Paradontitis
Diffuse atrophy

GOTTLIEB, 1928[16]

Inflammatory
Schmutzpyorrhea (poor oral hygiene)

Degenerative or atrophic
Diffuse alveolar atrophy (Systemic or metabolic causes)
Paradental pyorrhea

BECKS, 1929, 1931[3, 4]

Paradentitis
Simple
Secondary

Paradentosis
Presenile atrophy
Paradentosis due to trauma
Paradentosis due to lack of occlusion
Diffuse alveolar atrophy
Paradentosis secondary to paradontitis

Paradentoma

JACCARD, 1930, 1933[23, 24]

Inflammatory complex
Pure gingivitis
Preparadontal gingivitis
Inflammatory paradentosis

Osteopathic dystrophic complex
Dystrophic paradentosis
Presenile atrophy
Senile atrophy

ROY, 1935[36]

Alveolar pyorrhea, characterized by precocious senile alveolar resorption due to upset in general constitution of the individual
Pyorrhea with pockets
Common
Hyperemic } Gingivitis exists
Ischemic
Pyorrhea without pockets
Type with absence of local causes—no gingivitis
Juvenile atrophy—adolescent disease
Type with tooth movement due to laxity of paradentium—osteoporosis
Deformatory pyorrhea

ROBINSON, 1935[35]

Clinical types of paradentoses
Ortho pyorrhea—
Classic form of pyorrhea alveolaris
Hypertrophic pyorrhea
No alveolar crest resorption and seen in young people
Rubro pyorrhea
Uniform redness of the gingiva. Marked tooth attrition seen
Senile pyorrhea
A physiological alveolar resorption complicated by peridental inflammation

WESKI, 1937[41]

Paradentitis (Gingivitis)
Hypertrophic
Simple
Ulcerative

Paradentosis
Partial atrophic (true form of paradentosis)
Total atrophic (alveolar atrophy)

Paradentoma
Localized form
Epulis
Generalized form
Elephantiasis gingivae

THOMA AND GOLDMAN, 1937[40]

Inflammatory conditions
Gingivitis (may be of local or systemic origin)
Marginal. Hypertrophic. Ulcerative
Marginal paradentitis (poor oral hygiene)

Degenerative conditions
Paradontosis (bone resorption, in turn affecting other periodontal structures)

Atrophy
Gingival recession (faulty toothbrushing)
Presenile atrophy (normal physiologic process, recession of gingivae and resorption of alveolar crest)
Disuse atrophy
Decreased dental function or lack of function of jaws
Atrophy due to abnormal occlusal trauma

Syndrome of paradontitis and paradontosis

AMERICAN ACADEMY OF PERIODONTOLOGY, 1957[6]

Inflammation
Gingivitis
Periodontitis
Primary (simplex)
Secondary (complex)

Dystrophy
Occlusal traumatism
Periodontal disuse atrophy
Gingivosis
Periodontosis

HÄUPL AND LANG, 1927, 1940[18, 19]

Paradentitis
Marginal paradentitis
Etiology includes mechanical, thermal, chemical, infectious factors, as well as functional disturbances, tooth malformation, systemic disturbances, general resistance, etc.
Superficial marginal paradentitis
Epithelial changes
Regressive
Progressive
Formation of the pocket
Connective tissue changes
Subepithelial
Supra-alveolar
Changes in paradental bone
Marginal paradentitis profunda
Apical paradentitis

TABLE 30–3 REPRESENTATIVE CLASSIFICATIONS OF GINGIVAL AND PERIODONTAL DISEASE (Continued)

BOX, MCCALL, 1940, 1925[8, 29]	FISH, 1944[12]	HINE AND HINE, 1944[21]	ORBAN, 1942, 1949[31, 32]	HULIN, 1949[22]	HELD, 1949[20]
Gingivitis Acute Chronic **Periodontitis** Acute Chronic **Periodontitis simplex** (exogenous factors) **Periodontitis complex** or rarefying pericementitis fibrosa (endogenous factors)	**Gingivitis** Acute ulcerative Subacute marginal Chronic marginal Traumatic **Pyorrhea** Pyorrhea simplex (gradual deepening of sulcus) Pyorrhea profunda (deep pocket, pus formation, tooth mobility) Senile alveolar resorption **Neoplasia** Odontoclasma Cementoma Fibrous epulis	**Inflammation** **Gingivitis** Local—calculus, faulty restorations, poor contact areas, drugs Systemic—nutritional deficiencies, blood dyscrasias, etc. **Periodontitis simplex** (similar to gingivitis but more severe irritation) **Specific entities** Tuberculosis, syphilis Radiation **Atrophy or degeneration** Gingival recession Trauma Senile Disuse Idiopathic **Periodontitis complex** **Periodontitis** Systemic disturbances—Degeneration of connecting fibers in periodontal membrane Bone resorption **Hypertrophy** Gingival hypertrophy may accompany gingivitis Trauma Senile Disuse Idiopathic	**Inflammatory conditions** **Gingivitis** Localized to free margin of gingiva Swelling, shallow pockets Acute or chronic according to duration Ulcerative, purulent, etc. according to symptoms Local or systemic according to etiology Local (extrinsic). Infectious. Physical. Chemical Systemic (intrinsic). Dietary deficiency. Endocrine disturbance **Periodontitis** Inflammation extends to deeper supporting tissues. May be deep pockets, suppuration, abscess formation. Varying degrees of alveolar resorption Simplex—following gingivitis Complex—following periodontosis **Degenerative conditions** Gingivosis—systemic etiology Degeneration of connective tissue **Periodontosis** Degeneration of collagenous fibers of the periodontal membrane Irregular bone resorption Primarily systemic etiology—inherited inferiority of dental organ Early—no inflammation Late—deep pockets with periodontitis **Atrophic conditions** Periodontal atrophy—bone recession Precocious aging. Aging. Disuse—loss of normal function. Trauma—toothbrush, orthodontia *(Continued at right)* ORBAN (*Continued*) **Periodontal traumatism** Pressure necrosis and its consequences Primary—overstress, bruxism, etc. Secondary—loss of supporting tissue **Gingival hyperplasia** Overgrowth of gingiva in varying degrees Infectious—pyogenic granuloma. Endocrine dysfunction—pregnancy. Drugs—Dilantin. Idiopathic.	**Inflammatory processes** **Parodontitis** Exogenous gingivitis Tartar Bacteria Endogenous gingivitis Avitaminosis Intoxication **Degenerative processes** **Parodontosis** Precocious senile atrophy or Juvenile parodontosis Senile parodontosis Pyorrhetic parodontosis Traumatic paradontolysis **Parodontomes** Epulis Gingival elephantiasis	**True paradontopathia** Gingivitis Paradontolysis Paradontitis Periodontal atrophy **Symptomatic paradontopathia** (avitaminosis, blood dyscrasias etc.) **Enlargement conditions** Epulis Elephantiasis gingivae

TABLE 30–3 REPRESENTATIVE CLASSIFICATIONS OF GINGIVAL AND PERIODONTAL DISEASE (*Continued*)

PUCCI, 1950[34]	LYONS, 1951[28]	CARRANZA, 1959[9]		MILLER, 1950[30]
Marginal paradentitis	**Inflammatory**	Inflammatory	Superficial	**Gingivitis**
(benign)	**Gingivitis**	Periodontal		Acute, subacute, chronic exudative
Incipient	Acute	Syndrome	Deep	Hyperplastic, necrotizing, dietary, indo-
Hypertrophic	Simple	Traumatic	Compensated	lent (poor hygiene—filth pyorrhea)
Desquamative	Purulent	Periodontal		Endocrinopathic, allergic, hemopathic
Localized	Necrotizing	Syndrome	Uncompensated	**Periodontal abscess**
Advanced	Chronic	Combined	Compensated	Parodonta
Paradentosis (malignant)	Simple	Periodontal		Pericemental or gingival
Atrophic	Purulent	Syndrome	Uncompensated	Periapical
Constitutional	Necrotizing			**Alveoloclasia—bone resorption**
Horizontal alveolar atrophy with	Hyperplastic			Nutritional deficiency (alveoloclasia)
marginal paradentitis	Desquamative			Endocrinopathic (alveoloclasia)
Pure form	Pigmented			**Pericementoclasia**
Complicated form (vertical resorption)	**Periodontitis**			Pocket formation
Alveolar decalcification	Simplex—secondary to gingivitis			**Ulatrophia**
Physiologic alveolar atrophy	Complex—secondary to retrogressive			Ischemic or atrophic
Horizontal-precocious senile	disorders or trauma of the periodon-			Calcic
Accelerated passive eruption	tium			Afunctional
	Retrogressive			Traumatic
	Periodontosis			
	Atrophic periodontosis (periodontal			
	atrophy)			
	Senile			
	Presenile			
	Hyperfunctional periodontosis			
	Periodontosis gravis (systemic origin)			
	Deficiency disease			
	Endocrinopathies			
	Systemic toxicities			
	Blood dyscrasias			
	Metabolic diseases			
	Neoplastic			
	Benign			
	Fibroma			
	Elephantiasis gingivae			
	Malignant			

bone. The abrasive action of inveterate betel nut chewing[2] produces attrition and migration of the teeth, mostly the maxillary incisors, followed by spreading, loosening and extrusion of the maxillary incisors, which result from continued impact of the mandibular incisors. The molar teeth show signs of attrition but are not otherwise affected.

REVIEW OF OTHER CLASSIFICATIONS

Because of varied interpretations of the nature of gingival and periodontal disease their classification has been approached in many different ways. Representative classifications of gingival and periodontal disease are shown in Table 30–3.

REFERENCES

1. Baer, P., et al.: Advanced Periodontal Disease in an Adolescent. J. Periodont., *34*:533, 1963.
2. Balendra, W.: The Effect of Betel Chewing on the Dental and Oral Tissues and Its Possible Relationship to Buccal Carcinoma. Symposium on Oral Diseases in Tropical Countries. Brit. D. J., *87*:83, 1949.
3. Becks, H.: General Aspects in Pyorrhea Research. Pac. D. Gazette, *37*: 1929.
4. Becks, H.: Early Stage of Paradentosis. J.A.D.A., *18*:922, 1931.
5. Becks, H., and Fleming, W. C.: Is Osteodystrophic Type of Paradentosis, As Produced in Animals, Identical With One Form of Paradentosis in Man? J. D. Res., *15*:206, 1935.
6. Bernier, J. L.: Report of the Committee on Classification and Nomenclature. J. Periodont., *28*:56, 1957.
7. Box, H. K.: Studies in Periodontal Pathology. Bulletin No. 7. Canadian Dental Research Foundation, May, 1924.
8. Box, H. K.: Periodontal Studies. D. Items Int., *62*:915, 1940.
9. Carranza, F. A., and Carranza, F. A., Jr.: A Suggested Classification of Common Periodontal Disease. J. Periodont., *30*:140, 1959.
10. Carranza, F. A., and Erausquin, R.: First Periodontal Findings. Rev. Odont., *27*:485, 1939. Buenos Aires, Argentina.
11. Chawla, T. N., and Glickman, I.: Protein Deprivation and the Periodontal Structures of the Albino Rat. Oral Surg., Oral Med. & Oral Path., *4*:578, 1951.
12. Fish, E. W.: Paradental Disease. London, Eyre and Spottiswoode, 1944, p. 52.
13. Glickman, I.: Periodontosis. A Critical Evaluation. J.A.D.A., *44*:706, 1952.
14. Goldman, H. M.: Periodontosis in the Spider Monkey. A Preliminary Report. J. Periodont., *18*:34, 1947.
15. Gottlieb, B.: Etiology and Therapy of Alveolar Pyorrhea. Zschr. f. Stomatol., *18*:59, 1920.
16. Gottlieb, B.: Parodontal Pyorrhea and Alveolar Atrophy. J.A.D.A., *15*:2196, 1928.
17. Gottlieb, B.: The New Concept of Periodontoclasia. J. Periodont., *17*:7, 1946.
18. Häupl, K.: Basis of Histopathology of the Teeth and Their Supporting Structures. Leipzig, Johann Barth, 1940.
19. Häupl, K., and Lang, F. J.: Marginal Paradentitis. Berlin, H. Meusser, 1927.
20. Held, A. J.: Nomenclature and Classification of Diseases of the Dental Structures. Paradentologie, *3*:3, 85, 1949.
21. Hine, M. K., and Hine, C. L.: Classification of Periodontal Disturbances. J.A.D.A., *31*:1297, 1944.
22. Hulin, C.: Nomenclature and Classification. Paradentologie, *3*:82, 1949.
23. Jaccard, R.: Terminologie des Pyorrhees. Schwz. Mschr. f. Zahnhk., *40*:661, 1930.
24. Jaccard, R.: Necessity of an International Collaboration for Paradentosis Investigation. Schwz. Mschr. Zahnhk., *43*:196, 1933.
25. Kantorowicz, A.: Two Types of Pyorrhea. Klin. Zahnheilk., 1924.
26. Kaslick, R. S., and Chasens, A. I.: Periodontosis with Periodontitis: A Study Involving Young Adult Males. Part I. Review of the Literature and Incidence in a Military Population. Oral Surg., *25*:305, 1968.
27. Kaslick, R. S., and Chasens, A. I.: Periodontosis with Periodontitis: A Study Involving Young Adult Males. Part II. Clinical, Medical and Histopathologic Studies. Oral Surg., *25*:327, 1968.
28. Lyons, H.: Personal Communication, 1951.
28. McCall, J. O., and Box, H. K.: Chronic Periodontitis. J.A.D.A., *12*:1300, 1925.
30. Miller, S. C.: Oral Diagnosis and Treatment. 2nd ed. Philadelphia, Blakiston, 1950.
31. Orban, B.: Classification and Nomenclature of Periodontal Diseases. J. Periodont., *13*:88, 1942.
32. Orban, B.: Classification of Periodontal Disease. Paradentologie, *3*:159, 1949.
33. Orban, B., and Weinmann, J. P.: Diffuse Atrophy of the Alveolar Bone (Periodontosis). J. Periodont., *13*:31, 1942.
34. Pucci, F. M.: Periodontia. Montevideo, Uruguay, Barreiro y Ramos, 1950.
35. Robinson, H.: Pyorrhea, an Attempt to Differentiate Clinical Types with Suggestions for Nomenclature. Dent. Mag. & Oral Topics, *52(9)*:855, 1935.
36. Roy, M.: Alveolar Pyorrhea, Paris, Baillière et Fils, 1935.
37. Shroff, F. R.: The Behavior of Collagen Fibers in Some Types of Periodontal Disease. Oral Surg., Oral Med. & Oral Path., *6*:1202, 1953.
38. Simonton, F. V.: The Etiology of Paradontoclasia, Trans. 7th Int. Dent. Cong. II, 1646, 1926.
39. Simonton, F. V.: Parodontoclasia. Pac. D. Gazette, *35(4)*:251, 1927.
40. Thoma, K. H., and Goldman, H. M.: Classification and Histopathology of Parodontal Disease. J.A.D.A., *24*:1915, 1937.
41. Weski, O.: Paradentopathia and Paradentosis. Paradentium, *8*:169, 1937.

Chapter 31

THE "BONE FACTOR" CONCEPT OF PERIODONTAL DISEASE

The "bone factor" concept is a clinical guide for determining the diagnosis and prognosis of periodontal disease based upon the response of alveolar bone to local injurious factors.

BACKGROUND FOR THE "BONE FACTOR" CONCEPT

Normally, the height of alveolar bone is maintained by a physiologic equilibrium between bone formation and bone resorption. Local and systemic factors regulate this physiologic equilibrium, which reflects the condition of the bone throughout the body.[2-9] When there is a generalized skeletal tendency toward bone resorption, comparable changes occur in the alveolar bone that affect its response to inflammation and occlusal forces. *The systemic regulatory influence upon the response of alveolar bone is termed the "bone factor" in periodontal disease* (Fig. 31–1).

The fact that alveolar bone can be affected by systemic influences was recognized previous to the introduction of the "bone factor" concept. However, the experiments upon which the concept is based demonstrate (1) the manner in which different systemic influences alter the response of the alveolar bone to local irritation[7] and (2) the manner in which systemic influences cause destruction of the periodontal tissues in the absence of local destructive factors.

CLINICAL IMPLICATIONS OF THE "BONE FACTOR"

The individual "bone factor" affects the severity of bone loss associated with local destructive factors in periodontal disease.[8] The destructive effect of inflammation and trauma from occlusion varies with the status of the individual "bone factor." It is less severe in a healthy individual in the presence of a positive "bone factor," than when superimposed upon a systemically induced bone destructive tendency (negative "bone factor"). In the presence of a negative "bone factor" the normal adaptive capacity of alveolar bone to occlusal forces is altered so that a normal functional relationship becomes a local destructive force.[3]

Alveolar bone loss may occur in the absence of harmful local factors if the "bone factor" is sufficiently altered. Systemic disturbances that impair the bone-

432

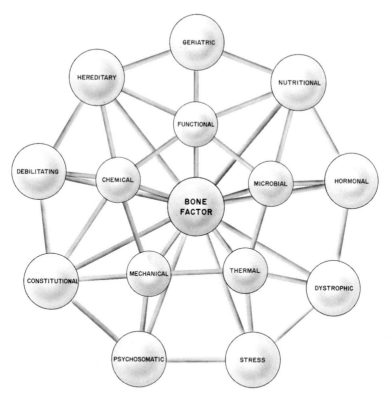

Figure 31–1   The "Bone Factor" Concept of the Nature of Periodontal Disease. The response of alveolar bone (*center circle*) to local etiologic agents in periodontal disease (*inner group*) is governed by interrelated systemic influences (*outer group*).

formative activity throughout the skeletal system result in loss of alveolar bone in the absence of local etiologic factors. Locally induced destruction aggravates the bone loss initiated by systemic disturbances.

The "bone factor" concept does not imply that alveolar bone is the tissue of origin in all cases of periodontal disease, or that it is the only periodontal tissue that may be affected by systemic disturbances, or that it is always affected by all systemic disorders.[10] The periodontal tissue in which destructive changes first appear is determined by the nature of the causative factors. It is as fallacious to assume that all cases of periodontal disease originate in the same tissue as it is to postulate that there is only a single condition, local or systemic, capable of inducing periodontal disease. However, *the crux of the problem of periodontal disease lies in the alveolar bone,* because in the final analysis it is the loss of alveolar bone that is responsible for tooth loss. Therefore, regardless of the

tissue in which periodontal disease originates, its clinical significance is ultimately gauged in terms of its effects upon the alveolar bone.

The "bone factor" concept differs from the traditional division of periodontal disease into "local" and "systemic" types. It envisions a systemic component in all cases of periodontal disease. It is the nature of the systemic component and not its presence or absence that influences the severity of periodontal destruction. If the systemic component is favorable, the destructive effect of local factors will be minimized; if it is unfavorable, the local destruction will be aggravated.

Individual cases of periodontal disease present various gradations in local and systemic etiology. Diagnosis entails the determination of the extent of systemic participation and whether it is favorable or harmful, rather than categorizing periodontal destruction into purely "local" and "systemic" types.

(Text continued on page 438.)

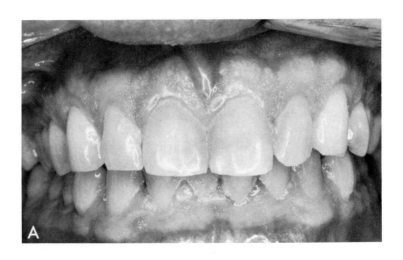

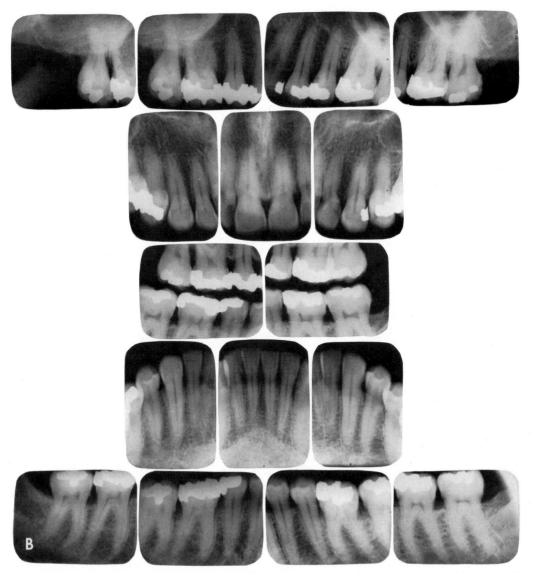

Figure 31-2   Positive "Bone Factor" in a 42-year-old Male. *A*, Gingival inflammation, poor oral hygiene and pronounced anterior overbite. *B*, The bone loss is slight considering the age of the patient and the unfavorable local factors. This is a patient with a positive "bone factor."

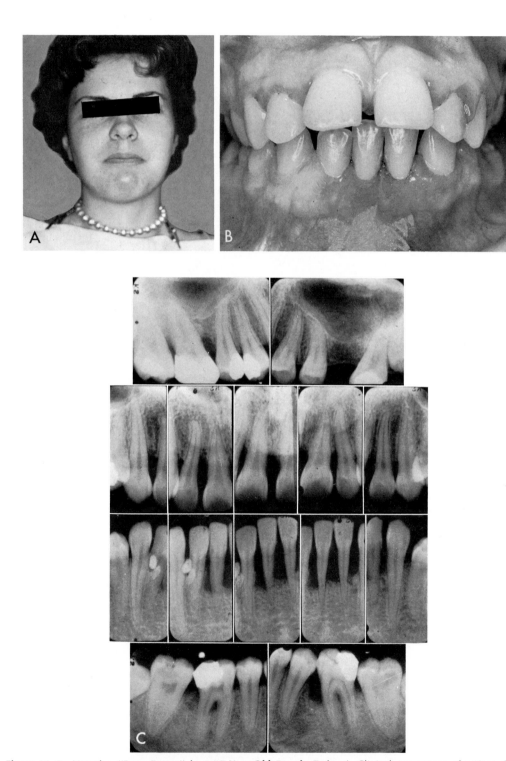

Figure 31–3 Negative "Bone Factor" in a 17-Year-Old Female Twin. *A,* Clinical appearance of patient. Compare with twin sister (Fig. 31–4, *A*). *B,* Gingival inflammation, periodontal pockets and pathologic migration. *C,* Severe bone destruction exceeds that which ordinarily occurs in 17-year-old patient with comparable local factors. This patient has a "negative bone factor." The distribution of bone loss in the anterior and first molar areas is considered typical of periodontosis. Note the bifurcation and trifurcation involvement of three remaining first molars.

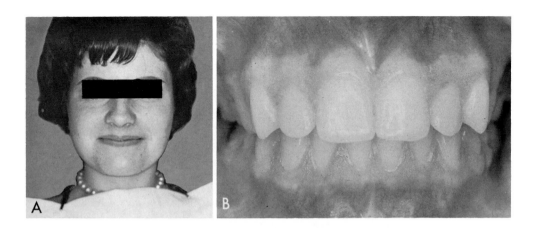

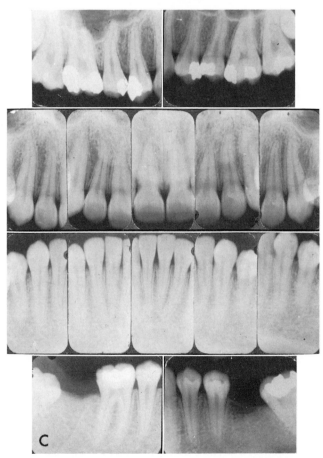

Figure 31–4   Positive Bone Factor. Twin sister of patient shown in 31–3, *A. A,* Clinical appearance. *B,* Excellent condition of gingiva. *C,* No bone loss despite missing mandibular first molar (*right*), tilted second molar and extruded maxillary first molar. Compare with the first molars in Figure 31–3, *C.*

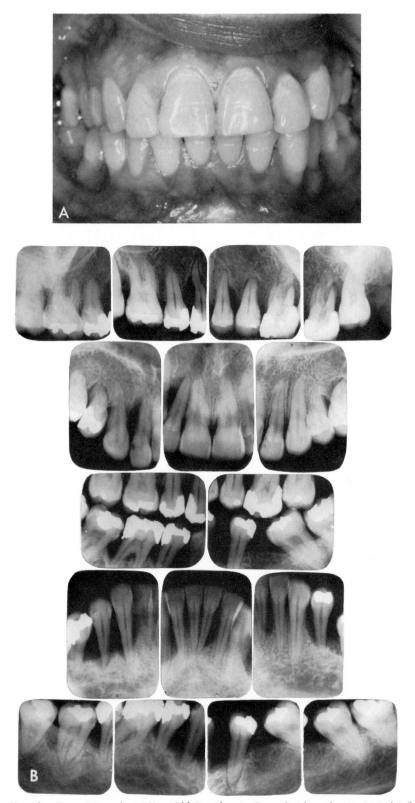

Figure 31–5 Negative Bone Factor in 34-Year-Old Female. *A,* Generalized moderate gingival inflammation with periodontal pocket formation. *B,* Bone loss more severe than ordinarily occurs in patient of this age with comparable local factors. The "bone factor" is therefore negative.

HOW THE "BONE FACTOR" IS APPLIED IN DETERMINING DIAGNOSIS AND PROGNOSIS

The clinical procedure whereby the "bone factor" concept is applied in the diagnosis and the determination of prognosis of periodontal disease is as follows:

1. *Determine the patient's age.*
2. *Evaluate the distribution, severity and duration of gingival inflammation and occlusal disharmonies, each of which is capable of inducing bone loss.*
3. *Determine the distribution, severity and rate of bone loss.*

The nature of the individual "bone factor" is determined from the above findings as follows:

A. A diagnosis of *"positive bone factor"* is made when the rate and severity of bone loss can be explained by the existing local factors (Fig. 31–2). It means that the systemic influences upon the alveolar bone are favorable so that new bone is constantly being formed in an effort to compensate for the increased resorption caused by the harmful local factors. Bone loss does occur, but it is maintained at a minimum. *In the presence of a positive bone factor, cessation of bone loss can be expected if the local factors are eliminated.*

B. The diagnosis of *"negative bone factor"* is made when the amount and rate of bone loss are in excess of that which clinical experience would lead one to expect at the patient's age in the presence of local factors of comparable severity and duration (Figs. 31–3 and 31–4). Since local factors are insufficient to account for the bone loss, factors other than those in the oral cavity must share the responsibility for it.

A diagnosis of "negative bone factor" does not mean that the patient has a bone disease or that the periodontal destruction necessarily originated in the alveolar bone. It means that prevailing systemic effects upon one or more of the tissues of the periodontium are such that the amount of bone loss caused by the local factors is accentuated. A diagnosis of "negative bone factor" is also made when alveolar bone loss occurs in the absence of local factors.

In patients with a "negative bone factor" the effectiveness of local treatment in arresting the bone destruction is limited by the extent to which systemic conditions are also responsible for it. However, *local treatment often suffices to retain the teeth in useful function for many years, even if systemic correction is not possible.*

Evaluation of the individual "bone factor" is predicated upon the history and findings at the time of examination. The "bone factor" is an expression of systemic influences and is not necessarily constant; it may be altered by changes in the individual systemic background.

COMPARISON OF THE DIAGNOSES "NEGATIVE BONE FACTOR" AND "PERIODONTOSIS"

The diagnoses "negative bone factor" and "periodontosis" have different implications. Patients with a "negative bone factor" may present features considered characteristic of periodontosis (Fig. 31–3, *C*), but many do not (Fig. 31–5). The connotation "periodontosis" implies the existence of a specific systemic type of periodontal disease considered to be a clinical entity, with characteristic features differentiating it from periodontitis. The term "negative bone factor" does not imply the presence of a specific type of periodontal disease. The clinical and radiographic features vary, depending upon the distribution and severity of local factors. Patients with a "negative bone factor" differ from those with a "positive bone factor" only in the response of alveolar bone to the local environment, and not because they represent different specific diseases.

REFERENCES

1. Chawla, T. N., and Glickman, I.: Protein Deprivation and the Periodontal Structures of the Albino Rat. Oral Surg., Oral Med. & Oral Path., 4:578, 1951.
2. Glickman, I.: The "Bone Factor" in Periodontoclasia. Bulletin Mass. Dental Soc., 20:14, 1944.
3. Glickman, I.: The Effect of Acute Starvation upon the Apposition of Alveolar Bone Associated with the Extraction of Functional Antagonists. J. D. Res., 24:155, 1945.
4. Glickman, I.: The Periodontal Structures in Experimental Diabetes. New York J. D., 16:226, 1946.
5. Glickman, I.: Acute Vitamin C Deficiency and Periodontal Disease. I. The Periodontal Tissues of the Guinea Pig in Acute Vitamin C Deficiency. J. D. Res., 27:9, 1948.

6. Glickman, I.: Acute Vitamin C Deficiency and Periodontal Disease. II. The Effect of Acute Vitamin C Deficiency Upon the Response of the Periodontal Tissues of the Guinea Pig to Artificially Induced Inflammation. J. D. Res., 27:201, 1948.

7. Glickman, I.: The Experimental Basis for the "Bone Factor" Concept in Periodontal Disease. J. Periodont., 20:7, 1951.

8. Glickman, I., Morse, A., and Robinson, L.: The Systemic Influence Upon Bone in Periodontoclasia. J.A.D.A., 31:1435, 1944.

9. Glickman, I., and Wood, H.: Bone Histology in Periodontal Disease. J. D. Res., 21:35, 1942.

10. King, J. D.: Abnormalities in the Gingival and Subgingival Tissues Due to Diets Deficient in Vitamin A and Carotene. Brit. D. J., 68:349, 1940.

Section Three · *The Prevention of Gingival and Periodontal Disease*

Chapter 32

PREVENTIVE PERIODONTICS

Increased awareness of the widespread prevalence of periodontal disease and the tooth loss it causes, plus the existence of a backlog of untreated disease which increases more rapidly than our ability to treat it, make it imperative that the emphasis in periodontics shift from treatment to prevention.[48] Emphasis on prevention does not detract from what can be accomplished by treatment, nor does it mean that the search for improved treatment methods should be relaxed. Treatment expertise will be necessary so long as people suffer from periodontal problems, but prevention represents a different approach. **Periodontal treatment starts with disease and aims to restore and preserve periodontal health even if it requires the most sophisticated techniques. Prevention starts with health and aims to preserve it by using the simplest, most universally applicable methods.** *Preventive periodontics is a cooperative program by the dentist, his ancillary personnel and the patient for the preservation of the natural dentition by preventing the onset, progress and recurrence of gingivitis and periodontal disease.*

443

GINGIVITIS AND PERIODONTAL DISEASE ARE PREVENTABLE

Most gingivitis, periodontal disease and tooth loss because of them can be prevented because they are caused by local factors which are accessible, correctable, and controllable. Local factors cause inflammation which is the predominant if not the sole pathologic process in gingivitis. Periodontal disease is an extension of gingivitis and is caused by the same local irritants plus trauma from occlusion. Trauma from occlusion is a co-destructive factor which contributes to the tissue breakdown in some cases of periodontitis.

Identifying local factors as the principal causes of periodontal disorders is not an oversimplification of the periodontal problem. Systemic influences affect the periodontal response to local irritants, but in the cases in which systemic etiology is suspected, it is usually difficult to establish what it is. The etiology of some forms of gingival disease is unknown, and severe periodontal disease occasionally occurs without apparent local cause, but such cases represent an extremely small segment of the total periodontal problem.

Neglect

Neglect is to blame for most if not all gingival and periodontal disease: neglect of the healthy mouth permits disease to occur; neglect of early disease permits it to destroy the tooth-supporting tissues; and neglect of the treated mouth permits disease to recur. Poor oral hygiene which permits plaque[8, 136] calculus and materia alba[53, 80] to accumulate overshadows all other local factors responsible for gingival disease. The status of the individual oral hygiene determines the prevalence and severity of gingivitis.[57, 65, 90, 118]

Most patients come for periodontal treatment in times of distress—either because of pain or the threat of losing their teeth—when they require the most time-consuming, complicated and often most costly treatment. More attention to preventing disease and treating it in its early stages would result in fewer problems from advanced and acute disease.

Dental Plaque

Dental plaque is the most important cause of oral disease.[*] It is the principal etiologic factor in gingivitis and dental caries. The products of plaque bacteria penetrate the gingiva and start gingivitis, which if untreated leads to periodontitis and tooth loss. Acid build-up in dental plaque initiates caries. Dental plaque is also important because it is the initial stage in the formation of dental calculus. After calculus is formed, it is the continuing deposit of new plaque on the surface, more than the inner calcified portion, which is responsible for perpetuating gingival inflammation. Another local irritant on the tooth surface which also contributes to gingivitis is materia alba, which is principally a concentration of bacteria and cellular debris.

Plaque Control

Plaque control is the prevention of the accumulation of dental plaque and other deposits on the teeth and adjacent gingival surfaces. **It is the most effective way of preventing gingivitis and is therefore a critical part of the many procedures involved in the prevention of periodontal disease. Plaque control is also the most effective way of preventing calculus formation.**

The most dependable way of controlling plaque thus far available is by mechanical cleansing with a toothbrush, dentifrice and other cleansing aids. Considerable progress has also been made in plaque control with chemical inhibitors (see page 467) in a mouthwash or in a dentifrice. However, for the total prevention of plaque accumulation all susceptible surfaces must be reached with some form of mechanical cleanser. It has not as yet been determined whether there is a minimal plaque level which the gingiva can tolerate, beyond which plaque accumulation need not be reduced, in order to prevent gingival and periodontal disease.

Preventive periodontics consists of many interrelated procedures, but plaque control is the keystone of the prevention of gingival and periodontal disease. It is basic to the practice of dentistry; without it oral health

---

[*]For a detailed discussion of dental plaque, calculus and material alba, see Chapter 22.

can neither be attained or preserved. **Every patient in every dental practice should be on a plaque control program.** For the patient with a healthy periodontium, plaque control means the preservation of health; for the patient with periodontal disease it means optimal post-treatment healing; and for the patient with treated periodontal disease plaque control means the prevention of recurrence of disease.

TOOTHBRUSHES AND OTHER ORAL HYGIENE AIDS

Toothbrushing removes plaque and materia alba,[35, 42, 76, 113, 138] and in so doing it reduces the onset and prevalence of gingivitis[19, 62, 83, 124] and retards the formation of calculus.[117, 142] Removal of plaque leads to resolution of gingival inflammation in its early stages,[25] and cessation of toothbrushing leads to its recurrence.[75, 87] For satisfactory results, toothbrushing requires the cleansing action of a dentifrice.[4, 40, 131]

The Kinds of Toothbrushes and Bristles

Toothbrushes vary in size, design, bristle hardness, length and arrangement (Fig. 32–1).[43] A toothbrush should clean efficiently and provide accessibility to all areas of the mouth. The choice is a matter of individual preference rather than a demonstrated superiority of any one type. Ease of manipulation by the patient is an important factor in brush selection. The effectiveness or potential injury from different types of brushes depends to a great degree upon how they are used.[22] The American Dental Association[2] refers to a range of acceptable brushes (brushing surface from 1.0 to 1.25 inches long and $5/16$ to $3/8$ inch wide, two to four rows, five to twelve tufts per row); but the design must fulfill the requirements of utility, efficiency and cleanliness.

Natural (hog bristle) and *nylon bristles* are equally satisfactory, but nylon bristles retain their firmness longer. Alternating between natural and nylon bristles is not recommended, because patients accustomed to the softness of an old natural bristle brush traumatize the gingiva when new nylon bristles are used with comparable vigor. The bristles may be grouped in separate tufts arranged in rows or evenly distributed throughout (multituft) (Fig. 32–1). The latter contain more bristles; both types are effective.[13] Rounded bristle-ends are assumed to be safer than flat-cut bristles with sharp ends, but this has been questioned,[59]

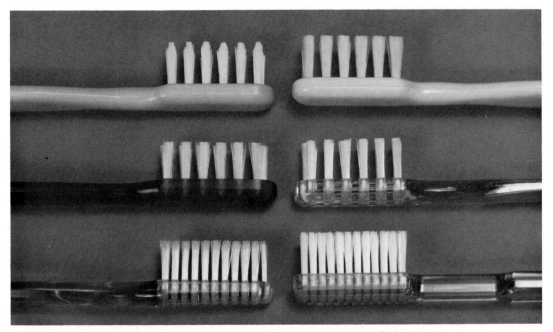

Figure 32–1   Types of Manual Brushes. Multituft types are in the bottom row.

and flat bristles round over slowly with use. The question of the most desirable **bristle hardness** is not settled. Bristle hardness is proportional to the square of the diameter and inversely proportional to the square of bristle length.[54] Bristle diameters in common use range from 0.007″ (soft), and 0.012″ (medium) to 0.014″ (hard). Soft bristle brushes of the type described by Bass (1948)[12] have been gaining acceptance. He recommended a straight handle, nylon bristles 0.007″ in diameter, 13/32″ long, with rounded ends, arranged in three rows of tufts, six evenly spaced tufts per row, with 80 to 86 filaments per tuft. For children, the brush is shorter, with softer (0.005″), shorter (11/32″) bristles.

Opinions regarding the merits of **hard and soft bristles** are based upon studies carried out under different conditions and are often inconclusive and not in agreement.[60] Medium bristles may cleanse better than soft bristles,[36] and are less likely to traumatize the gingiva or abrade the tooth substance and restorations. Soft bristles are more flexible, cleanse beneath the gingival margin (sulcal cleansing)[11] and reach more of the proximal tooth surface, but they may not completely remove heavy plaque deposits.[45] Soft bristles may cleanse better than hard[18] because of a "matting effect" by the combination of soft bristles and dentifrice. This increases tooth surface–dentifrice contact and adds to the cleansing action, but could also increase toothbrush abrasion.[54]

Dentifrices vary in abrasiveness (removal of root substance or restorative material).[1, 115] The manner in which the brush is used and the abrasiveness of the dentifrice affect the cleansing action and abrasion to a greater degree than the bristle hardness.[95]

Patients should be advised that toothbrushes must be replaced periodically, before the bristles become frayed. There is a tendency to use a brush "as long as it lasts," which often means after it no longer cleanses effectively and may be injurious to the gingiva.

Powered toothbrushes

There are many types of electric toothbrushes, some with an arcuate motion, or a back-and-forth reciprocal action, a combination of both, or a modified elliptical motion (Fig. 32–2). Regardless of the type, best results are obtained if the patient is instructed in its use.[7, 92] As a rule, patients who can develop the ability to use a toothbrush properly do equally well with a manual or electric brush. Less diligent brushers do better with an electric brush which compensates somewhat for their inadequacy. Electric brushes are more effective for handicapped individuals and for cleansing around orthodontic appliances.

Many researchers report that electrically powered toothbrushes are superior to manual brushes in terms of removing plaque, reducing plaque and calculus accumulation and improving gingival health,[76, 83, 93, 113, 117] but others claim that manual and powered brushes are equally effective.[8, 47, 101, 139] Electric brushes produce less abrasion of tooth substance and restorative materials than manual brushing,[96, 99] but the situation is reversed if the manual brush is used in a vertical rather than horizontal direction.[54]

Other Cleansing Aids

Teeth cannot be completely cleansed by toothbrushing and dentifrice alone, because bristles do not reach the entire proximal surface. Removal of interproximal plaque is essential because most gingival disease starts in the interdental papillae and the prevalence of gingivitis is highest there.[23, 69, 98, 119, 120, 125] For optimal plaque control toothbrushing should be supplemented with one or more other cleaning aids such as dental floss, interdental cleansers, oral irrigating devices, and mouthwashes. The supplemental aids required depend upon the individual rate of plaque formation, smoking habits, tooth alignment and special attention required for cleansing around orthodontic appliances and fixed prostheses.

TOOTHBRUSHING METHODS

There are many methods of toothbrushing.[58] **Except for overtly traumatic methods, thoroughness rather than technique is the important factor in determining the effectiveness of toothbrushing.** The needs of some patients are best served by combining selected features of different methods. Regardless of the technique you teach,

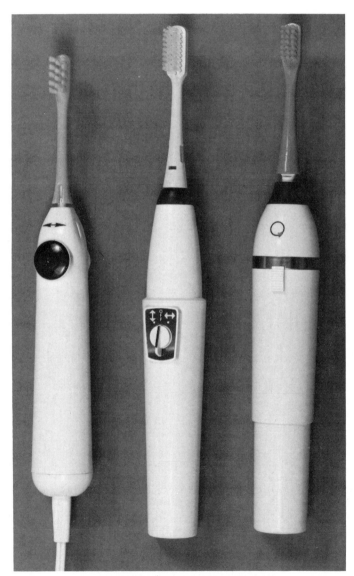

Figure 32–2   Types of Powered Brushes.

patients usually develop individualized modifications of it.

Several methods of toothbrushing are presented here, each of which if properly performed can accomplish the desired results. In all methods, the mouth should be divided into sections, starting with the maxillary right molar area and brushed in sequence until all accessible surfaces are cleaned. (Fig. 32–3).

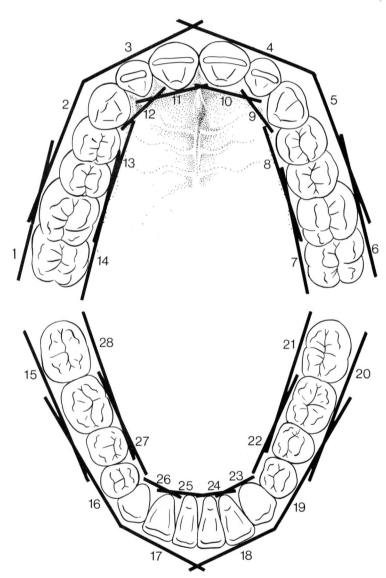

Figure 32–3   Toothbrush Positions for Systematic Cleansing.   Dark lines show toothbrush positions for coverage of the maxilla and mandible.

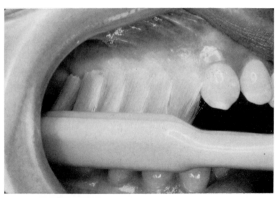

Figure 32–4

The Bass Method (Sulcal Cleansing)[10] with a Soft Brush

Maxillo-facial and facio-proximal surfaces

Starting with the facio-proximal surfaces in the right molar area, place the head of the brush parallel to the occlusal plane with the bristles at the tip behind the distal surface of the last molar (Figs. 32–4 and 32–5). Place the bristles at a 45° angle to the long axis of the teeth and force the bristle ends into the gingival sulci (Fig. 32–6) and over the gingival margin, making sure that the bristles extend as far as possible inter-proximally (Fig. 32–7). **Exert a gentle pressure in the long axis of the bristles** (Fig. 32–7, arrow), and activate the brush with a short back-and-forth vibratory motion, counting to ten without dislodging the tips of the bristles. This cleans behind the last molar, the marginal gingiva, within the gingival sulci and along the proximal tooth surfaces as far as the bristles reach.

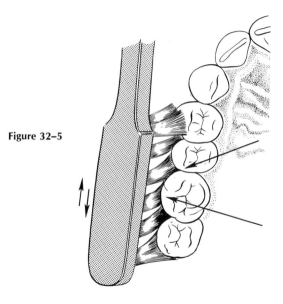

Figure 32–5

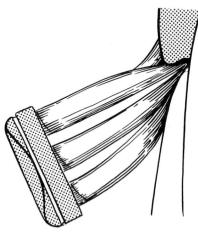

Figure 32–6

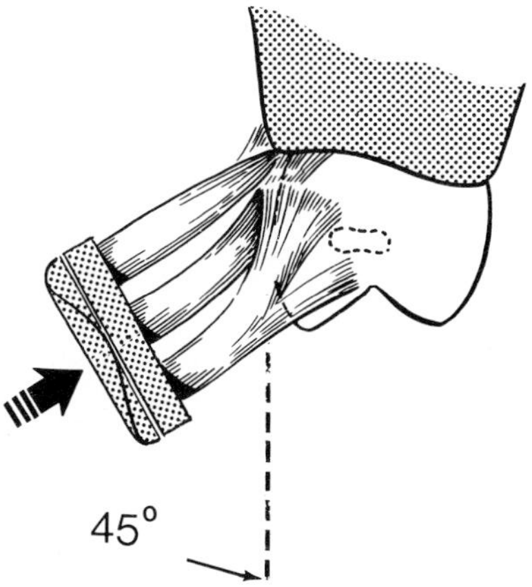

Figure 32–7

45°

COMMON ERRORS. The following errors in the use of the brush often result in unsatisfactory cleansing or soft tissue injury: (1) **The brush is inserted at an angle rather than parallel to the occlusal plane,** traumatizing the gingiva and the vestibular mucosa (Fig. 32–8). (2) The bristles are placed **on the attached gingiva rather than into the gingival sulcus** (Fig. 32–9). When the brush is activated, the gingival margin and tooth surfaces are neglected while the attached gingiva and alveolar mucosa are traumatized (Fig. 32–10). (3) **The bristles are pressed against the teeth rather than angulated into the gingival sulcus** (Fig. 32–11). Activating the brush cleanses the facial tooth surfaces but neglects other areas.

Lift the brush and move it anteriorly, and repeat the process in the premolar area (Fig. 32–12).

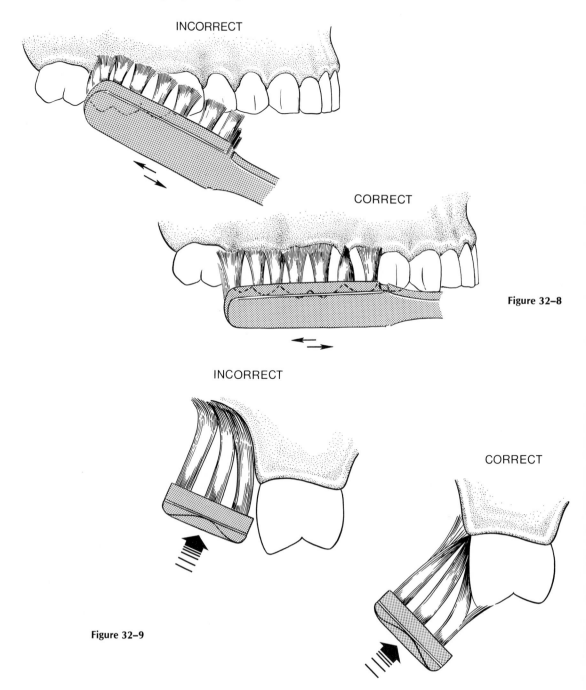

INCORRECT

CORRECT

Figure 32–8

INCORRECT

CORRECT

Figure 32–9

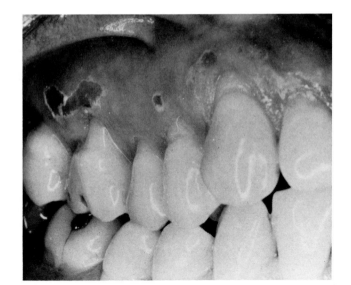

Figure 32–10   Scuffing of the Gingiva Produced by Improper Toothbrushing.

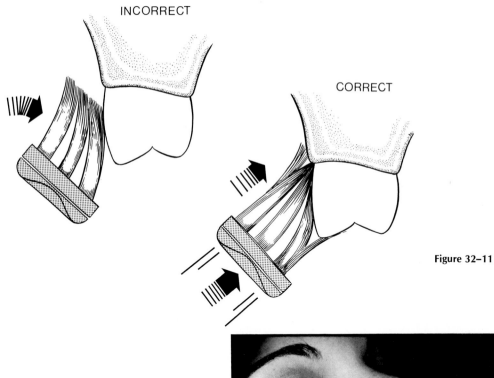

INCORRECT

CORRECT

Figure 32–11

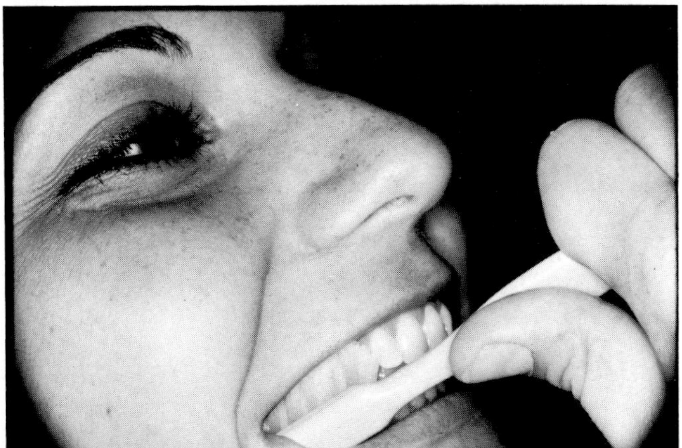

Figure 32–12

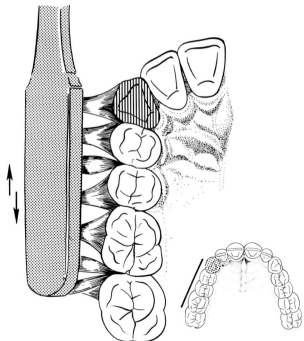

When the maxillary right canine is approached, **place the brush so that the last row of bristles is distal to the canine prominence—not over it** (Fig. 32–13). **Placing the brush across the canine prominence is incorrect** (Fig. 32–14). **It traumatizes the gingiva when pressure is applied to force the bristles into the mesial and distal interproximal spaces.** This could cause gingival recession at the canine prominence. Use the same precautions with the other canines. After the brush is activated, lift it and move it mesial to the canine prominence onto the maxillary incisors (Figs. 32–15 and 32–16).

Activate the brush, section by section, around the maxilla to the left molar area, making sure that the bristles reach behind the distal surface of the last molar.

Figure 32–13

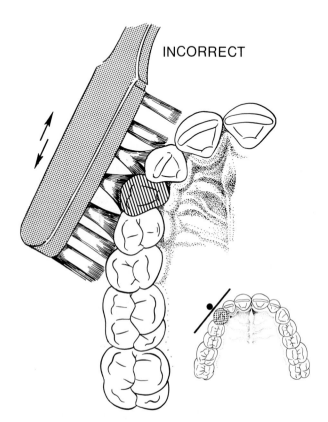

INCORRECT

Figure 32–14

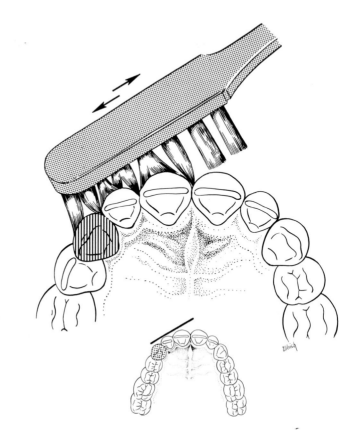

Figure 32–15

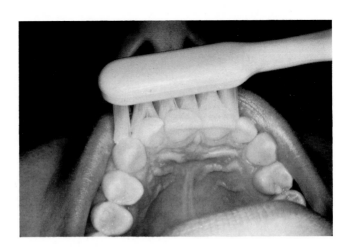

Figure 32–16

Maxillo-palatal and palato-proximal surfaces

Starting with the palatal and proximal surfaces in the maxillary left molar area, continue around the arch to the right molar area. Position the brush horizontally in the molar and premolar areas (Figs. 32–17 and 32–18). To reach the palatal surface of the anterior teeth, insert the brush vertically (Figs. 32–19 and 32–20). Press the end bristles into the gingival sulci and interproximally at about a 45° angle to the long axis of the teeth and activate the brush with repeated short strokes. If the shape of the arch permits, the brush is inserted horizontally between the canines with the bristles angulated into the gingival sulci of the anterior teeth (Fig. 32–21).

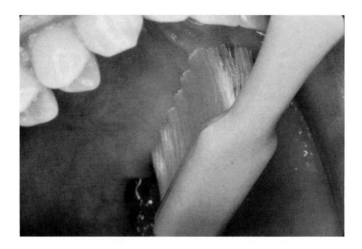

Figure 32–17

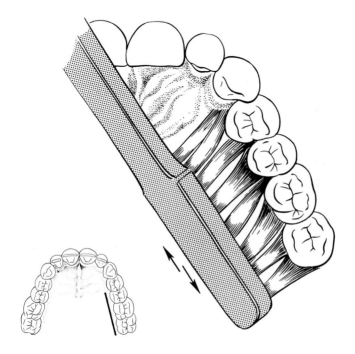

Figure 32–18

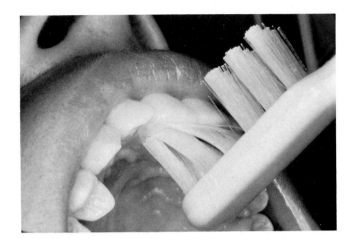

Figure 32–19

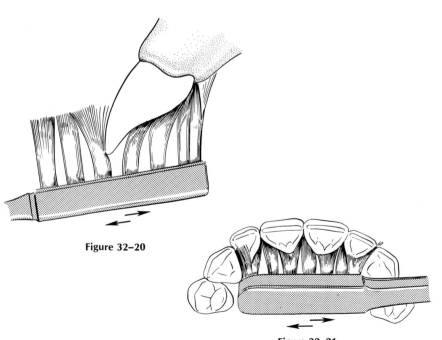

Figure 32–20

Figure 32–21

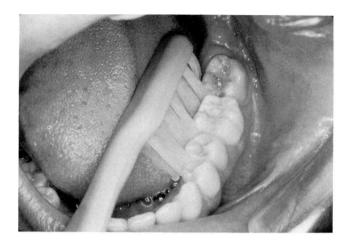

Figure 32–22

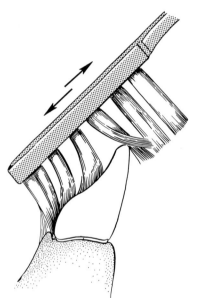

Figure 32–23

Mandibulo-facial, facio-proximal, lingual and linguo-proximal surfaces

After the maxilla is completed, continue on the facial and proximal surfaces of the mandible, section by section, from the distal of the right molar to the distal of the left molar. Then do the lingual and linguo-proximal surfaces, section by section, from the left to right molar areas (Fig. 32–22). In the mandibular anterior region the brush is inserted vertically, with the end bristles angulated into the gingival sulcus (Fig. 32–23). If space permits, the brush may be inserted horizontally between the canines with the bristles angulated into the sulci of the anterior teeth (Fig. 32–24).

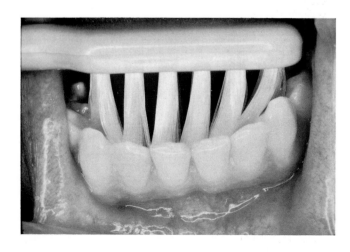

Figure 32–24

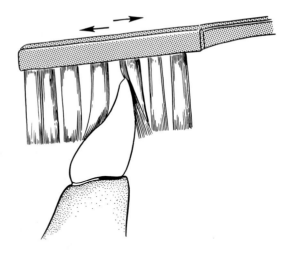

COMMON ERROR. The brush is placed on the incisal edge with the bristles on the lingual surface but not reaching into the gingival sulci (Fig. 32–25). When the brush is moved back and forth only the incisal edge and a portion of the lingual surface are cleaned.

INCORRECT

Figure 32–25

Occlusal surfaces

Press the bristles firmly on the occlusal surfaces with the ends deep into the pits and fissures (Fig. 32–26). Activate the brush with short back-and-forth strokes, counting to ten, advancing section by section until all the posterior teeth are cleaned.

COMMON ERROR. The brush is "scrubbed" across the teeth in long horizontal strokes instead of short back-and-forth movements.

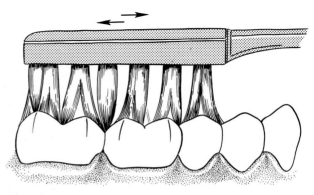

Figure 32–26

Stillman Method[130]

The brush is placed with the bristle ends resting partly on the gingiva and partly on the cervical portion of the teeth (Fig. 32–27). The bristles should be oblique to the long axis of the tooth and directed apically. Pressure is applied laterally against the gingival margin so as to produce a perceptible blanching. The brush is removed to permit the blood to return to the gingiva. Pressure is applied several times, and the brush given a slight rotary motion, with the bristle ends remaining in position.

The process is repeated on all the tooth surfaces, starting in the maxillary molar area and proceeding systematically around the mouth. To reach the lingual surfaces of the maxillary and mandibular anterior areas, the handle of the brush is parallel to the occlusal plane, with two or three tufts of bristles engaging the teeth and gingiva (Fig. 32–27).

The occlusal surfaces of the molars and premolars are cleaned with the bristles perpendicular to the occlusal plane and penetrating deeply into the sulci and interproximal embrasures.

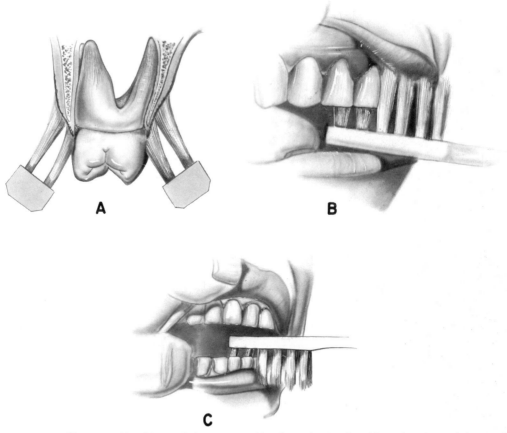

Figure 32–27 Stillman Toothbrushing Technique. *A,* Toothbrush on the facial and lingual surfaces of the maxillary posterior teeth. *B,* Toothbrush in maxillary anterior region. *C,* Toothbrush in mandibular anterior area.

Modified Stillman Method[61]

This is a combined vibratory action of the bristles with a stroking movement of the brush in the long axis of the teeth. The brush is placed at the mucogingival line, with the bristles pointed away from the crown and moved with a stroking motion along the attached gingiva, the gingival margin and tooth surface. The handle is rotated toward the crown and vibrated as the brush is moved.

Charters Method[34]

The brush is placed on the tooth at a 45° angle with the bristles pointed toward the crown (Fig. 32–28). The brush is then moved along the tooth surface until the sides of the bristles engage the gingival margin, preserving the 45° angle.

Twist the brush lightly, flexing the bristles so that the sides press on the gingival margin, the edges touch the tooth and some bristles extend interproximally. Without dislodging the bristles, rotate the head of the brush, maintaining the bent position of the bristles. The rotary action is continued while counting to ten. Move the brush to the adjacent area and repeat the procedure, continuing area by area on the entire facial surface, and then move to the lingual. Care should be taken to enter every embrasure.

To cleanse the occlusal surfaces, gently force the bristle tips into the pits and fisures and activate the brush with a rotary motion (not sweeping or sliding) without changing the position of the bristles. Repeat area by area until all chewing surfaces are cleansed.

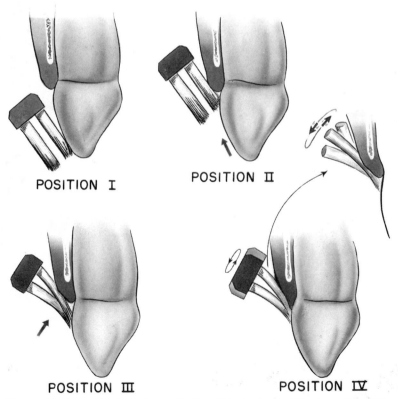

POSITION I

POSITION II

POSITION III

POSITION IV

Figure 32–28 Charters Toothbrushing Technique. *Position I,* Brush placed on the tooth with bristles angulated toward the crown. *Position II,* Brush moved so that bristles rest on the marginal gingiva. *Position III,* Bristles flexed against the tooth and gingiva. *Position IV,* Brush vibrated without changing the position of the bristle ends.

Fones Method

In the Fones method the brush is pressed firmly against the teeth and gingiva with the handle of the brush parallel to the line of occlusion and the bristles perpendicular to the facial tooth surfaces. The brush is then moved in a rotary motion with the jaws closed and the spherical pathway of the brush confined by the limits of the muco-buccal fold.

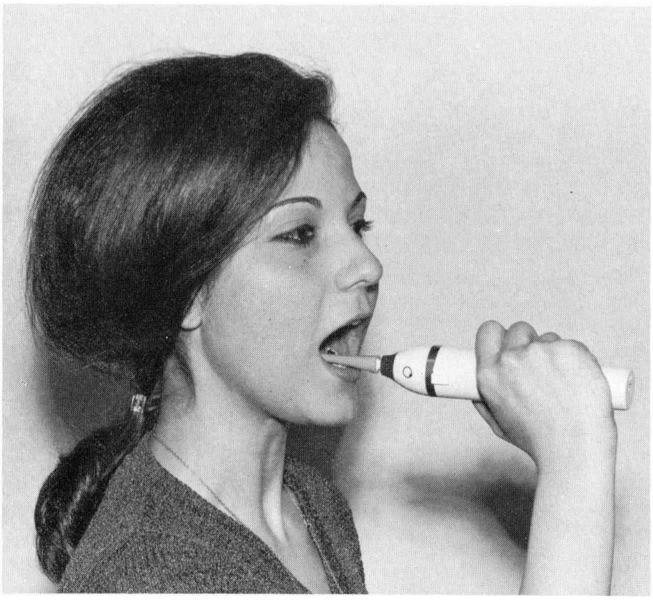

"Physiologic Method"[123]

Smith[123] and Bell[16] describe a method in which an effort is made to brush the gingiva in a manner comparable to the pathway of the food in mastication. This entails gentle sweeping motions, starting on the teeth and progressing over the gingival margin and attached gingival mucosa.

Methods of Toothbrushing with Powered Brushes

The mechanical action built into the brush affects the manner in which it is used. With the arcuate type (up and down) the brush moves from the crown to the marginal and attached gingiva and back. Brushes with a reciprocal motion (short back-and-forth strokes), or varied combinations of elliptical and reciprocal motions, can be used in a variety of ways: with the bristle ends in the gingival sulcus (Bass method) (Figs. 32–29 and 32–30), at the gingival margin with the bristles directed toward the crown (Charters method), or in a vertical, sweeping motion from the attached gingiva onto the crown (modified Stillman method).

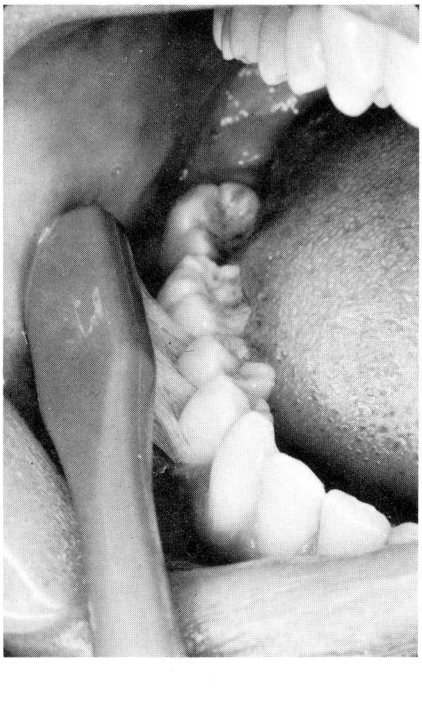

Figure 32–29. Use of a Powered Brush.

Figure 32–30 Powered Brush in Position Using the Bass Method.

HOW TO USE OTHER CLEANSING AIDS

Dental Floss

Dental floss is an effective way of cleansing proximal tooth surfaces.[46,104] Many prefer unwaxed high tenacity nylon (manufacturer's technical designation, 70–34/5 S3 Nylon 30 steam set)[11] but its superiority over waxed floss has not yet been demonstrated. There are several ways of using dental floss; the following is recommended: Cut a piece of floss about three feet long and wrap the ends around the middle finger of each hand. Pass the floss over the right thumb and left forefinger and insert it at the base of the gingival sulcus behind the distal surface of the last tooth on the right side of the maxilla. With a firm back-and-forth buccolingual motion move the floss occlusally to dislodge all soft surface accumulations. Repeat several times and move to the mesial interproximal space (Fig. 32–31).

Pass the floss gently through the contact area with a back-and-forth motion. Do not forcibly snap the floss past the contact area, because this will injure the gingiva. Place the floss at the base of the gingival sulcus on the mesioproximal surface. Cleanse the sulcus area and move the floss firmly along the tooth surface with a back-and-forth motion to the contact area. Move the floss over the interdental papilla to the base of the adjacent gingival sulcus and repeat the process on the disto-proximal surface.

The purpose of dental floss is to remove plaque, not to dislodge fibrous shreds of food wedged between the teeth and impacted into the gingiva. Chronic food impaction should be treated by correcting proximal contacts and "plunger" cusps. Removing impacted food with dental floss simply provides temporary relief and permits the condition to become worse.

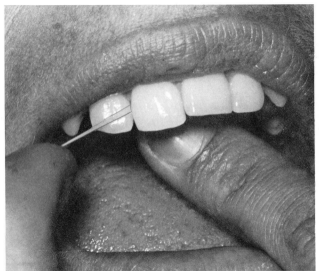

Figure 32–31 Dental Floss held with the right thumb and left index finger as it is moved past the contact area between the central and lateral incisors.

Rubber, Wooden and Plastic Interdental Cleansers (Interdental Tips)

There are various types of "tips" which are effective for cleansing proximal surfaces not accessible to the toothbrush. They are most useful when spaces have been created interdentally by the loss of gingival tissue. If the interdental papilla fills the space, the cleansing action of the tips is limited to the gingival sulcus on the proximal tooth surfaces. **The tip should not be forced be-** tween the intact interdental papilla and the teeth; this will create a space where none existed before.

Rubber tips are available at the end of the handle of some toothbrushes or in separate holders. When the gingiva fills the interdental space the rubber tip is used for cleansing the gingival sulcus along the proximal surfaces. The tip is placed at approximately a 45° angle to the tooth with the end in the sulcus and the side pressed against the tooth surface. The tip is then

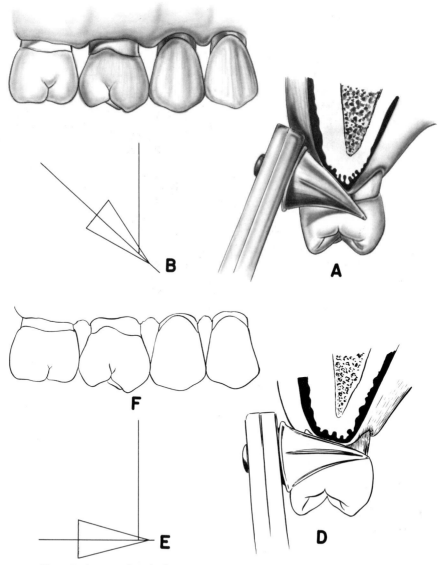

Figure 32–32 Rubber Tip for Interdental Cleansing. *Top,* **Correct Use.** *A,* Facio-lingual view of interdental space showing proper angulation of interdental tip. *B,* Diagrammatic illustration of proper tip angle. *C,* Gingival contour obtained by proper use of interdental cleanser in treated case of advanced periodontal disease. *Bottom,* **Incorrect Use.** *D,* Rubber tip inserted horizontally into interdental space instead of obliquely. *E,* Diagrammatic illustration of improper angulation of rubber tip (compare with *B*). *F,* Punched out interdental gingival craters produced by improper use of rubber tip.

moved along the tooth, following the base of the sulcus to the contact area. The procedure is repeated on the adjacent proximal surface, facially and lingually.

When there is space interdentally, the rubber tip is inserted at an angle of approximately 45° with the end pointed toward the occlusal surface and the lateral aspect resting against the interdental gingiva (Fig. 32–32, top). In this position the tip is more likely to create or preserve the normal tapered triangular contour of the interdental papilla. The tip is activated with a

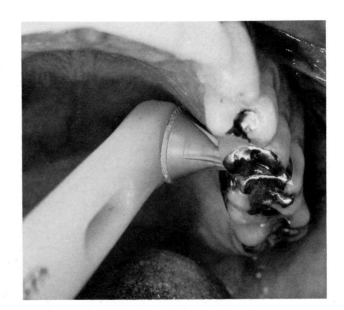

Figure 32–33 **Proper Angle for Insertion of Interdental Tip from the Palatal Side.**

rotary, lateral or vertical motion, cleansing the proximal tooth surfaces and at the time pressing against and cleansing the gingival surface. Each interdental space is treated from the facial and lingual sides (Fig. 32–33). Rubber tips are also useful for cleansing furcations.

Inflammation of the gingival papillae can be reduced by as much as 26.3 per cent by combining the rubber tip with toothbrushing as compared with 6.6 per cent reduction by toothbrushing alone,[50] and keratinization of the interdental gingiva can be increased.[49]

Common error

Patients tend to insert the rubber tip perpendicular to the long axis of the tooth (Fig. 32–32, bottom). This will increase gingival keratinization,[30] but will create flattened cupped-out interdental contours which are less desirable esthetically and functionally than the tapered contours produced by proper angulation of the rubber tip.

Other interdental cleansers (Fig. 32–34), such as wooden tips (Stimudents) and plastic tips (P/S, Polisher-Stimulator), the ends of toothpicks inserted in special holders (Char-stem, Perio-Aid) and pipe cleaners, are also useful for cleansing interdentally and in furcations, particularly in spaces too small for the rubber tip (Fig. 32–35). Interdental cleansers are also used for removing debris in the period immediately following periodontal therapy when the condition of the tissues does not permit vigorous brushing.

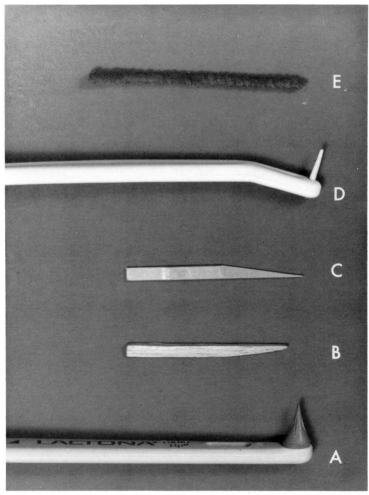

Figure 32–34   Interdental Cleansers. *A,* Rubber tip. *B,* Wooden tip (Stimudent). *C,* Plastic tip (P/S, Polisher-Stimulator). *D,* Toothpick in holder (Perio-Aid). *E,* Pipe cleaner.

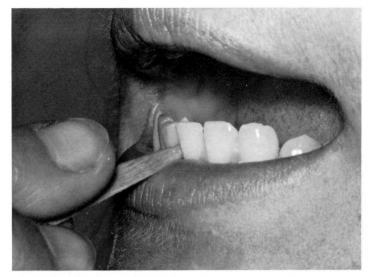

Figure 32–35 **Wooden Interdental Tip** inserted between the mandibular central incisors.

Oral Irrigating Devices

Oral irrigation devices, of which there are many types (Fig. 32–36), provide a steady or pulsating stream of water under pressure through a nozzle. The pressure is created by a built-in-pump or by attaching the device to the water faucet. Water irrigation is an effective oral hygiene aid which, when used in addition to toothbrushing, provides benefits beyond those attainable by toothbrushing alone. When used according to the manufacturer's instructions it causes no damage to soft or hard oral tissues or dental restorations.[74, 85] It does not detach plaque from the teeth but it retards the accumulation of plaque[63] and calculus[82] and reduces gingival inflammation and pocket depth.[74] It also increases gingival keratinization,[73] and clears bacteria from the oral cavity more effectively than toothbrushing and rinsing.[112, 137] Water irrigation reduces inflammation in the crestal region of periodontal pockets,[37] adds to the effectiveness of scaling in reducing gingival inflammation.[15] It is particularly helpful for cleansing around orthodontic appliances and fixed prostheses. Water irrigation does not create bacteremia in patients with healthy gingiva or gingivitis; some investigators find transient bacteremia following its use in periodontitis;[43a] others do not.[135] Bacteremia has also been reported following toothbrushing in 5 per cent of patients with periodontitis.[122a]

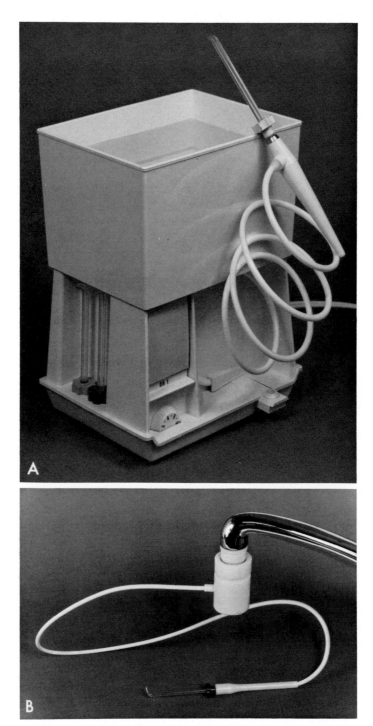

Figure 32–36 Oral Irrigation Devices. *A,* Type with built-in pump. *B,* Type which attaches to water faucet.

Mouthwashes

Mouthwashes may be used as an adjunct to, but not as a substitute for, toothbrushing and other cleansing aids. **Rinsing with a mouthwash alone is not enough to maintain good oral hygiene or gingival health.**[133] Mouthwashes are usually pleasant tasting, make the mouth feel clean and partially wash away loose food debris after eating,[144] but they do not dislodge dental plaque. Rinsing with water alone reduces the oral bacterial flora, and adding antimicrobial agents increases this effect.[94] However, the reduction is temporary,[109] and prolonged use of the same mouthwash appears to lessen its effectiveness.[3] **There is no evidence that nonspecific reduction in the oral microbial flora is beneficial.**

Gingival Massage

Despite the frequency with which gingival massage is mentioned in the periodontal literature, opinions differ as to whether it is beneficial or necessary for gingival health.[91] Massaging the gingiva with a toothbrush produces epithelial thickening and increased keratinization,[32,33,116,126,127] and increased mitotic activity in the epithelium and connective tissue.[20] Interdental cleansers also increase gingival keratinization.[30,49] It is generally assumed that epithelial thickening and increased keratinization are beneficial because they provide increased protection against bacteria and other local irritants, but this has not been proved. It is claimed that massage improves circulation, the supply of nutrients and oxygen to the tissues and the removal of waste products and tissue metabolism,[108] but the risk of gingival injury from unsupervised massage is also recognized. It is not clear whether the improved gingival health provided by toothbrushing and other oral hygiene procedures results from cleansing action alone, or whether there is a built-in massage effect which is also beneficial.

CHEMICAL PLAQUE AND CALCULUS INHIBITORS

Mechanical cleansing with toothbrush and supplemental aids is the most effective method for controlling plaque and calculus formation thus far available, but it is tedious and cannot be relaxed without risking new accumulations and the onset of gingival disease. There is a constant search for chemical aids which could prevent or significantly reduce plaque and calculus formation and lessen our dependence upon mechanical cleansing.[121] **Chemical preventives which would prevent plaque formation or its attachment to the tooth; destroy or remove the plaque before it calcifies; or alter the chemistry of the plaque so as to prevent calcification would also significantly reduce calculus formation.**

Many substances have been incorporated in toothpastes, mouthwashes, chewing gums and lozenges for the purpose of preventing plaque and calculus or to supplement mechanical cleansing in their control. Different degrees of effectiveness have been reported with such agents, but relatively few consumer products have thus far been developed. Some of the agents demonstrated capable of inhibiting the formation of plaque and/or calculus are ascoxal[107] (ascorbic acid, sodium percarbonate and copper sulfate), cetyl pyridinium chloride,[132] sodium rincinoleate,[122] water-soluble silicone,[39] urea,[17] victamine C, a cationic surface-active agent,[140,141] chlorhexidine gluconate (2 per cent),[86] enzymes such as dextranase (positive[68,81] and negative results[28]), mucinase,[4,40,77,128] mylase, prolase, β-glucuronidase, hyaluronidase alpha amylase, mannan depolymerase,[145] pectinase, β-amylase, chymotrypsin, peptidase papain,[97] proteolytic and amylolytic enzymes of bacterial and fungal origin;[55,105,110] acetates of zinc, manganese and copper[5] and antibiotics[88] such as vancomycin[100,103] (equivocal results), a macrolide antibiotic "CC10232"[143] and erythromycin.[84]

STEP-BY-STEP PROCEDURE FOR PLAQUE CONTROL INSTRUCTIONS

Plaque control serves three important purposes: (1) in the prevention of gingival and periodontal disease, (2) as a critical part of periodontal treatment, and (3) in the prevention of recurrence of disease in the treated mouth. In all these circumstances plaque control must be explained to the patient in a systematic manner. The following step-by-step procedure is suggested:

Step I. Patient Motivation

Before you teach a patient what to do, he must know why he is doing it. Instruction in proper oral hygiene techniques is not enough. The patient should understand what periodontal disease is, what its effects are, that he is susceptible to it and what he can do to protect himself.[38] **He must be motivated to want to keep his mouth clean for his own benefit and not to please his dentist.** It should be made crystal clear that the goal of plaque control is oral health and not simply the development of manual skills. Patients may become so involved in trying to imitate oral hygiene techniques that they lose sight of their purpose.

Step II. Patient Education

Most patients think of the toothbrush only in terms of cleansing the teeth;[79] its importance in the prevention of disease of the periodontium must be explained. **Toothbrushing is a most important patient-administered preventive and adjunctive therapeutic procedure. In no other field of medicine can the patient so effectively assist in preventing and reducing the severity of a disease as can be done in relation to gingivitis by toothbrushing, supplemented according to individual needs by interdental cleansing with dental floss, rubber and wooden interdental cleansers and water irrigation under pressure.** If a person maintained good oral hygiene from 5 to 50 years of age, he very likely could avoid the destructive effects of periodontal disease during this major period of his life.[53]

Patients must be made to understand that periodic scaling and cleansing of the teeth in the dental office are helpful preventive measures, but to be most effective they must be combined with the continuous protection against disease they themselves can provide by daily oral hygiene procedures at home. Explain that dental visits come two or three times a year, whereas adjunctive preventive dental care is available at home on a daily basis. Combining regular office visits with home oral hygiene significantly reduces gingivitis and loss of supporting periodontal tissues.[134] **Time spent in the dental office teaching the patient how to cleanse his teeth is a more valuable health** service than cleansing his teeth for him. **Ideally both should be provided.**

Demonstrate how to clean the teeth

With instruction and supervision patients can reduce the incidence of gingivitis far more effectively than with their usual oral hygiene habits.[52, 72, 134, 147] Chairside instruction in how to clean the teeth is more than a cursory demonstration in the use of a toothbrush and oral hygiene aids. It is a painstaking procedure which must be checked and rechecked on repeated visits until the patient demonstrates that he has developed the necessary proficiency.

First instruction visit

The patient reports for the first instruction visit with a new toothbrush and interdental cleanser which are kept in the office for use at future visits. Toothbrushing is first demonstrated on a cast, stressing the exact placement and activation of the bristles. This is followed by a demonstration in the patient's mouth while he observes with a hand mirror. The patient then uses the brush with the operator guiding and correcting him. The procedure is repeated with dental floss and interdental cleansers and water irrigation under pressure, according to the patient's needs. Teaching machines with film strips and slides should be used as adjuncts to person-to-person instruction—not as substitutes for it.

LOCATE THE PLAQUE. Small amounts of plaque are difficult to see, but heavier accumulations appear as gray-yellow or white (materia alba) material on the teeth. Disclosing stains in the form of solutions or chewable wafers[6] are used to locate the plaque and pellicle which would otherwise escape detection (Fig. 32–37, A and B). The disclosing solution (6 per cent tincture of basic fuchsin) is applied to the teeth with a pledget of cotton or a small spray or diluted in water as a mouthwash. The wafers (erythrosin or other dyes) are chewed and swished around the mouth for about one minute. Dental restorations do not take up the stain, but the oral mucous membrane and lips may retain it for one to two hours. Covering the lips lightly with vaseline before using the stain is helpful.

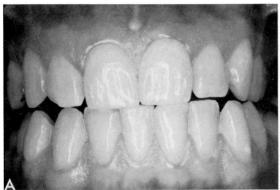

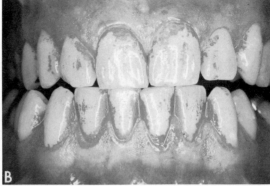

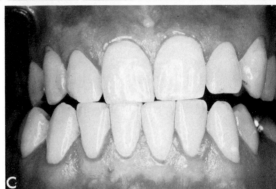

Figure 32–37 *A*, **Before Using Disclosing Solution.** Patient has gingivitis, but plaque is not apparent. *B*, **Stained with 6 per cent Tincture Basic Fuchsin.** The dark particulate material is dental plaque. *C*, **Restained with Basic Fuchsin after Thorough Cleansing.** The teeth appear free of plaque.

Show the patient the stained plaque. Small illuminated magnifying mirrors especially designed for this purpose will give him a close-up view (Fig. 32–38). Have the patient remove the stained plaque with his toothbrush; restain the teeth; then show him how to clean more effectively. **Stress the word "cleansing" rather than "toothbrushing."** Patients do better if they concentrate on cleansing the teeth rather than on learning a toothbrushing technique.

Even after vigorous brushing some stain usually remains on the proximal surfaces. Show the patient how to clean the proximal surface with dental floss and interdental cleansers, followed by water irrigation under pressure.

Restain the teeth with disclosing solution and repeat the instruction procedure until the patient can remove all the stainable material (Fig. 32–37, *C*).

The visit is terminated and the patient given the following instructions: **he is to clean his teeth at least twice a day, after meals, for a minimum of five minutes by the clock each time. Emphasize the words "by the clock."** Explain that it will take considerably longer than five minutes until he develops the necessary skills. Cleansing

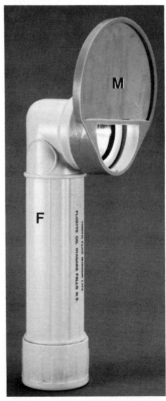

Figure 32–38 Magnifying mirror (M) (Floxite) Fits on Flashlight (F).

three times daily is only slightly more beneficial than twice a day,[127] but patients should cleanse after "bedtime" snacks. The patient is to return in one week.

Second and subsequent instruction visits

Stain the teeth with disclosing solution and have the patient demonstrate brushing and other cleansing procedures. What the patient does may bear little resemblance to what he was taught. Do not be discouraged — and do not say anything to discourage the patient. Make the necessary corrections, making sure that the patient understands what they are and why they are necessary. Explain that patients often develop their own variations of what they have been taught, with which they are comfortable and which accomplish the desired results so long as they are done thoroughly. Do not dismiss the patient until he demonstrates considerable improvement over his performance at the outset of the visit. Patience and repetition are the secrets of instruction in oral hygiene.

Schedule subsequent instruction visits, lengthening the intervals between them, until the patient attains the proficiency required to keep his mouth clean and healthy.

Plaque Control by Diet

Coarse fibrous foods

As part of the plaque control program patients should be advised to include hard fibrous foods in their diet, particularly at the end of meals. Although some investigators disagree,[18, 78] it is the consensus that hard fibrous foods reduce plaque accumulation and gingivitis on tooth surfaces exposed to their mechanical cleansing action during mastication.[6, 9, 27, 41, 129] Coarse fibrous foods also provide functional stimulation to the periodontal ligament and alveolar bone.

Soft diets lead to increased plaque accumulation and calculus formation, gingivitis and periodontal disease.[56, 64, 111] Animals fed soft diets enriched with vitamins and minerals develop severe periodontal disease with loosening of the teeth, which does not occur when the diet includes lengths of bone and adherent meat which require vigorous chewing.[70]

Limiting sucrose-containing foods

The fact that the ingestion of sucrose increases plaque formation is of great clinical importance. The polysaccharide dextran is a major component of the plaque matrix. It is a sticky substance which envelops the plaque bacteria and attaches the plaque to the tooth surface. The bacteria form the dextran from carbohydrates, particularly sucrose. Limiting the intake of sugar and sugar-sweetened foods assists in reducing plaque formation,[31] and patients should be instructed accordingly.

OTHER PROCEDURES IN PREVENTIVE PERIODONTICS

Critical though it is, plaque control by the patient is only one aspect of preventive periodontics. It must be combined with a regular program of other preventive procedures in the dental office. Prevention starts with the patient's history, particularly as related to the oral cavity and a thorough examination of the teeth, soft oral tissues and adjacent structures.

Education of patients to have periodic dental visits is in itself an important preventive measure. However, each visit must be a meaningful preventive service rather than simply a "cleansing" and checking for new cavities. It should consist of one or more of the following procedures, according to individual needs.

Oral Prophylaxis

As it is ordinarily used, the term *oral prophylaxis* refers to cleansing the teeth in the dental office, and consists of removing plaque, materia alba, calculus and stain and polishing the teeth. To provide the maximum benefit to the patient, oral prophylaxis should be more comprehensive and include the following:

1. Use disclosing solution or wafers to detect plaque.
2. Remove supra- and subgingival plaque and calculus and other surface accumulants.

3. Cleanse and polish the teeth. The teeth are cleansed and polished, using bristle wheels and rubber cups with a polishing paste (improved zirconium silicate[106]). Plaque is less likely to be deposited on smooth polished surfaces. Cleanse and polish the proximal tooth surfaces and pontics with dental floss and polishing paste. Flush the mouth with warm water to remove debris and restain with disclosing solution to check for unremoved plaque.

4. Apply topical caries-preventive agents, unless they were included in the polishing paste.

5. Check restorations and prostheses and correct overhanging margins and proximal contours of restorations. Cleanse removable prosthesis and check for proper fit, evidence of settling and gingival irritation in relation to clasps and tissue-borne sections.

6. Check for signs and symptoms of food impaction. Plunger cusps, abnormal proximal contacts and worn marginal ridges should be corrected to prevent or correct food impaction.

Check for Trauma from Occlusion

The most carefully adjusted dentitions undergo changes with time. Cuspal relationships of natural teeth and dental restorations which are modified by wear may lead to abnormal occlusal habits such as bruxing and clenching, damage the periodontium, or create muscle dysfunction and temporomandibular joint disorders. Periodontal signs of trauma from occlusion* include widening of the periodontal space, often accompanied by thickening of the lamina dura, tooth mobility in excess of that explainable by inflammation and reduced periodontal support, vertical and angular bone destruction, infrabony pockets, bifurcation and trifurcation involvement, and pathologic migration, particularly of the maxillary anterior teeth. Detection and correction of the responsible occlusal abnormalities plus elimination of local irritants which cause inflammation are essen-

---

*For a detailed discussion of the signs of trauma from occlusion, see Chapter 24.

tial for the prevention of progressive bone destruction and tooth loss.

Prophylactic occlusal adjustment in the absence of evidence of trauma from occlusion in anticipation of possible future damage is not recommended. Trauma from occlusion is the tissue injury produced by occlusal forces, not the forces themselves. Cuspal relationships that do not conform to an anatomic ideal are not necessarily injurious to the periodontium during function. The presence of "anatomically abnormal" occlusion without evidence of periodontal injury indicates that the periodontium had adapted to the existing occlusal forces. Interfering with a well-adapted functional relationship to create an anatomic ideal may precipitate the type of periodontal injury that the occlusal adjustment aims to prevent.

Radiographs should be taken at intervals determined by the nature of the patient's periodontal condition and caries experience.

One of the most important steps in a recall visit is the review of the patient's use of the toothbrush and other oral hygiene aids. This should be done in the mouth by the patient rather than on casts. Give it sufficient time, and if necessary have the patient report for another instruction session.

Prevention by Systemic Measures

Another approach to the prevention of gingival and periodontal disease is by systemic measures to (1) control or counteract local injurious agents such as bacteria and plaque and (2) improve the capacity of the periodontal tissues to resist them. Little has been accomplished in this phase of prevention, because systemic effects upon the periodontium are not as clearly defined as are the changes produced by local factors.

The systemic condition of the patient undoubtedly affects the metabolic processes responsible for the preservation of periodontal health. Although there are no systemic conditions which cause gingivitis or periodontal pockets, there is evidence that the injurious effects of local irritants and abnormal occlusal forces are aggravated by nutritional deficiency[102] or other systemic disorders.[51] It is possible that local irritants not severe enough to cause clinically detectable disease could produce periodontal disease if their effect were enhanced by systemically induced debility of the tissues. **What must be determined are the limits beyond which the systemic condition of the patient must change in order to significantly alter the periodontium or increase its susceptibility to disease.**

Systemic measures to prevent plaque or counteract its injurious effect

There are many interesting possibilities for development in this area. Systemically administered drugs that inhibit plaque and calculus formation would be a logical outgrowth of current research on topical anti-plaque and anti-calculus agents. In experimental animals, the rate of calculus formation has been changed by systemic measures,[14, 66] and plaque formation and gingival infection have been controlled by antibiotics in the diet.[67] There have been conflicting findings regarding the effectiveness of nutritional supplements in the prevention of periodontal disorders in humans. (See Chap. 57.)

The saliva and crevicular fluid[21, 26, 146] would be excellent vehicles for transporting systemically administered drugs to the periodontal area where they would be most effective. Antibiotics, immunoglobulins and antienzyme agents could be administered to counteract the noxious effects of plaque and bacteria and reinforce the capacity of the periodontium to resist them.

Other possibilities for preventive periodontics by systemic measures are vaccines to provide immunity against periodontal infection and catabolic hormones to reverse the aging of periodontal tissues and reduce their vulnerability to the cumulative effects of local irritants and changes in occlusion.

Dental Restorations in Preventive Periodontics

Dental restorations contribute significantly to the health of the periodontium, but they also introduce the risk of creating gingival and periodontal disease. **Man-made disease-producing conditions such as overhanging margins, incorrect contour and proximal contacts and traumatic occlusal relationships must be avoided.** The beneficial effects of dental restorations can be increased and the likelihood of causing periodontal irritation and injury reduced by attention to the details of construction described in Chapter 54.

Orthodontic Procedures in Preventive Periodontics

Orthodontic procedures are extremely important in the prevention of periodontal disease as well as in its treatment (see Chap. 56.) **The occlusion of the youngster casts the die for the condition of the periodontium in the adult.** Tooth irregularities and abnormal jaw relationships must be treated promptly because they initiate gingival and periodontal disorders which tend to worsen unless orthodontic correction is instituted.

PREVENTING THE MUTILATING EFFECTS OF PERIODONTAL DISEASE

The principal aim of preventive periodontics is to prevent the onset of disease, but if disease is already present, its purpose is to prevent further tissue destruction and tooth loss. Gingival and periodontal disease must be detected early and treated as soon as they are discovered. It is paradoxical that oral examinations performed carefully enough to use bite-wing radiographs to find pinpoint caries sometimes overlook gross gingival disease.

Gingival inflammation and periodontal pockets can be eliminated[89] and bone destruction arrested[114] by periodontal treatment. **It is simpler to treat slight gingivitis than severe gingivitis, to eliminate shallow pockets rather than deep pockets, and to prevent bone destruction and osseous defects rather than correct them.** Tooth loss by age 50 can often be prevented in a 30-year-old patient with periodontal disease by eliminating responsible local irritants and injurious occlusal relationships and by regular maintenance thereafter.

Interceptive Restorative Dentistry

Occlusal changes and loss of proximal contacts resulting from failure to replace missing molars are common causes of gingival and periodontal bone loss. Interceptive restorative dentistry refers to the use of simple dental restorations to correct conditions responsible for early periodontal breakdown (Fig. 32–39), in order to avoid heroic complicated restorative procedures to salvage dentitions mutilated by advanced periodontal disease.

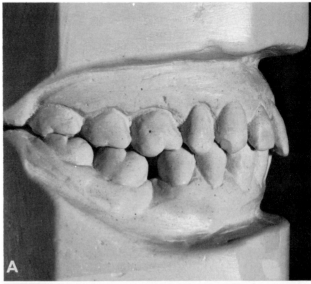
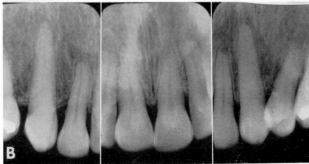
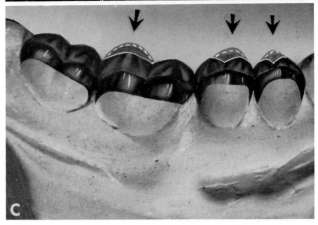

Figure 32–39   Interceptive Restorative Dentistry. *A,* Shift in tooth positions following failure to replace missing first molar in a 30-year-old patient. *B,* Early angular bone loss and widening of the periodontal ligament in the anterior maxilla resulting from trauma from occlusion secondary to disruption of the occlusion in the molar area. *C,* Interceptive restorative dentistry. Posterior abnormality corrected by restorations with proper occlusal and proximal relationships. The arrows indicate the old cuspal contours.

PREVENTION OF THE RECURRENCE OF DISEASE

The preservation of periodontal health after it has been attained requires as positive a program as the treatment of disease. It is a joint responsibility; the patient must adhere to the prescribed regimen of oral hygiene and periodic recall visits; the dentist must make each recall visit a meaningful preventive service.

PREVENTIVE PERIODONTICS – AT THE COMMUNITY LEVEL

To be effective, preventive periodontics must extend beyond the dental office into the community. Despite the fact that most gingival and periodontal diseases are preventable with methods equally or more effective than those for preventing dental caries,[71] periodontal disease remains the major cause of tooth loss in adults.* And the disease usually starts a long time before it necessitates tooth extraction.

By fifteen years of age, four out of every five persons have gingivitis, the initial stage of periodontal disease, and in 4 per cent of teenagers destructive periodontal disease is already present.[97] Judging from the high prevalence of periodontal disease, the preventive measures against it are not widely used. The public are either unaware of the importance of preventing periodontal disease or are disinterested and content to unnecessarily sacrifice their teeth to periodontal disease.

To overcome this situation, mass communication media such as the press, radio and television must be utilized to conduct psychological warfare on the public. The public must be educated regarding the nature and costly effects of periodontal disease and motivated to take advantage of available preventive methods, because it is in their best interest to do so.

As part of their professional responsibility to the community, the dentist and dental organizations must utilize every public forum for the following purposes:

Explain the damage wrought by periodontal disease in adults, but stress the fact that it starts in youngsters.

Dispel the notions that "pyorrhea is inevitable and incurable" and that "people are supposed to lose their teeth when they grow old."

Emphasize the facts that, unlike tooth decay, periodontal disease is usually painless; that regular dental examinations are required for its early detection; and that it should be treated as soon as it is detected.

Make it clear that effective periodontal treatment is available, and that the earlier treatment is instituted the more likely it is to succeed, but that prevention is the simplest, least time-consuming and most economical approach to the periodontal problem.

Stress the preventive value of good oral hygiene and regular dental care.

Explain that measures for preventing and treating gingival and periodontal disease must form the core of all group and community dental health plans, for patients of all ages, because the usefulness of all dental restorations depends upon the health of the tooth-supporting tissues.

REFERENCES

1. Abrasivity of Current Dentifrices. Report of the Council of Dental Therapeutics. J.A.D.A., *81*: 1177, 1970.
2. Accepted Dental Therapeutics. 3rd ed. Chicago, American Dental Association, 1969/70, p. 225.
3. Alderman, E. J., Jr., and Scallon, V. L.: An in Vivo Study of the Effect of Prolonged Use of a Specific Mouthwash on the Oral Flora. Chron. Omaha Dent. Soc., 28:284, 1965.
4. Aleece, A. A., and Forscher, B. K.: Calculus Reduction with a Mucinase Dentifrice. J. Periodont., 25:122, 1954.
5. Amdur, B., Brudevold, F., and Messer, A. C.: Observations on the Calcification of Salivary Sediment. I.A.D.R. Abstr., p. 18, 1962, No. 64.
6. Arnim, S. S.: The Use of Disclosing Agents for Measuring Tooth Cleanliness. J. Periodont., *34*:227, 1963.
7. Ash, M. M.: A Review of the Problems and Results of Studies on Manual and Power Toothbrushes. J. Periodont., *35*:202, 1964.
8. Ash, M. M., Gitlin, B. N., and Smith, W. A.: Correlation Between Plaque and Gingivitis. J. Periodont., *35*:424, 1964.
9. Baer, P. N., Stephan, R. M., and White, C. L.: Studies on Experimental Calculus Formation in the Rat. I. Effect of Age, Sex, Strain, High Carbohydrate, High Protein Diets. J. Periodont., *32*:190, 1961.
10. Bass, C. C.: An Effective Method of Personal Oral Hygiene, Part II. J. Louisiana St. Med. Soc., *106*:100, 1954.

---

*The epidemiology of gingival and periodontal disease is presented in Chapter 21.

11. Bass, C. C.: The Optimum Characteristics of Dental Floss for Personal Oral Hygiene. D. Items Int., 70:921, 1948.
12. Bass, C. C.: The Optimum Characteristics of Toothbrushes for Personal Oral Hygiene. D. Items Int., 70:696, 1948.
13. Bay, I., Kardel, K., and Skougaard, M. R.: Quantitative Evaluation of the Plaque-removing Ability of Different Types of Toothbrushes. J. Periodont., 38:526, 1967.
14. Becks, H., Wainwright, W. W., and Morgan, A. F.: Comparative Study of Oral Changes in Dogs Due to Deficiencies of Pantothenic Acid, Nicotinic Acid and Unknowns of the Vitamin B Complex. Am. J. Orth., 29:183, 1943.
15. Beget, B. C., and Bram, M.: Oral Irrigation and Inflammation. Forty-fifth General Meeting, International Association for Dental Research, Washington, D.C., March 1967, p. 36.
16. Bell, D. G.: Teaching Home Care to the Patient. J. Periodont., 19:140, 1948.
17. Belting, C. M., and Gordon, D. L.: In Vitro Effect of a Urea Containing Dentifrice on Dental Calculus Formation. II. J. Periodont., 37:26, 1966.
18. Bergenholtz, A., Hugoson, A., and Sohlberg, F.: An Evaluation of the Plaque-Removing Ability of Some Aids to Oral Hygiene. Svensk. Tandlak. T., 60:447, 1967.
19. Berman, C. L., Hosiosky, E. N., Kutscher, A. H., and Kelly, A.: Observations of the Effects of an Electric Toothbrush; Preliminary Report. J. Periodont., 33:195, 1962.
20. Bertolini, A.: Experimental Research on the Effects of Mechanical Gingival Massage. Paradontol., 9:144, 1955.
21. Bissada, N. F., Schaffer, E. M., and Haus, E.: Human Crevicular Fluid Flow: A 24 Hour Quantitative Study, I.A.D.R., Abstr. 1965, p. 72, No. 142.
22. Björn, H., and Lindhe, J.: On the Mechanics of Toothbrushing. Odont. Revy, 17:9, 1966.
23. Black, A. D.: Something of the Etiology and Early Pathology of the Diseases of the Periodontal Membrane with Suggestions as to Tooth Treatment. Cosmos 55:1219, 1913.
24. Brantzaeg, P.: The Significance of Oral Hygiene in the Prevention of Dental Diseases. Odont. T., 72:460, 1964.
25. Brandtzaeg, P., and Jamison, H. C.: The Effect of Controlled Cleansing of the Teeth on Periodontal Health and Oral Hygiene in Norwegian Army Recruits. J. Periodont., 35:308, 1964.
26. Brill, N., and Björn, H.: Passage of Tissue Fluid into Human Gingival Pockets. Acta Odont. Scandinav., 17:11, 1959.
27. Burwasser, P., and Hill, T. J.: The Effect of Hard and Soft Diets on the Gingival Tissues of Dogs. J. D. Res., 18:389, 1939.
28. Caldwell, R. C., et al.: The Effect of a Dextranase Mouthwash on Dental Plaque in Young Adults and Children. J.A.D.A., 82:124, 1971.
29. Cantor, M. T., and Stahl, S. S.: Interdental Col Tissue Responses to the Use of a Water Pressure Cleansing Device. J. Periodont.–Periodontics, 40:292, 1969.
30. Cantor, M. T., and Stahl, S. S.: The Effects of Various Interdental Stimulators upon the Keratinization of the Interdental Col. Periodontics, 3:243, 1965.

31. Carlsson, J., and Egelberg, J.: Effect of Diet on Early Plaque Formation in Man. Odont. Revy, 16:112, 1965.
32. Carter, S. B.: The Masticatory Mucosa and Its Response to Brushing; Findings in the Merion Rat, Meriones libycus, at Different Ages. Brit. D. J., 101:76, 1956.
33. Castenfelt, T.: Toothbrushing and Massage in Periodontal Disease. An Experimental Clinical Histologic Study. Stockholm, Nordisk Rotegravyr, 1952, P. 109.
34. Charters, W. J.: Eliminating Mouth Infections with the Toothbrush and Other Stimulating Instruments. D. Digest, 38:130, 1932.
35. Chilton, N. W., Didio, A., and Rothner, J. T.: Comparison of the Clinical Effectiveness of an Electric and a Standard Toothbrush in Normal Individuals. J.A.D.A., 64:777, 1962.
36. Conroy, C. W.: Comparison of Automatic and Hand Toothbrushes: Cleaning Effectiveness. J.A.D.A., 70:921, 1965.
37. Crumley, P. J., and Sumner, C. F.: Effectiveness of a Water Pressure Cleansing Device. Periodontics, 3:193, 1965.
38. Derbyshire, J. C.: Methods of Achieving Effective Hygiene of the Mouth. Dent. Clin. North America, March 1964, p. 231.
39. Draus, F. J., Leung, S. W., and Miklos, F.: Toward a Chemical Inhibitor of Calculus. D. Progress, 3:79, 1963.
40. Dudding, N. J., et al.: Patient Reactions to Brushing Teeth with Water, Dentifrice, or Salt and Soda. J. Periodont., 31:386, 1960.
41. Egelberg, J.: Local Effect of Diet on Plaque Formation and Development of Gingivitis in Dogs. I. Effect of Hard and Soft Diets. Odont. Revy, 16:31, 1965.
42. Elliott, J. R.: A Comparison of the Effectiveness of a Standard and an Electric Toothbrush. J. Periodont., 34:375, 1963.
43. Fanning, E. A., and Henning, F. R.: Toothbrush Design and Its Relation to Oral Health. Australian D. J., 12:464, 1967.
43a. Felix, J. A., Rosen, S., and App, G. R.: Detection of Bacteremia After the Use of an Oral Irrigation Device in Subjects With Periodontitis. J. Periodont., 42:785, 1971.
44. Fones, A. C.: Mouth Hygiene. 4th ed. Philadelphia, Lea and Febiger, 1934, p. 300.
45. Gilson, C. M., Charbeneau, G. T., and Hill, H. C.: A Comparison of Physical Properties of Several Soft Toothbrushes. J. Mich. Dent. Ass., 51:347, 1969.
46. Gjermo, P., and Flötra, L.: The Plaque Removing Effect of Dental Floss and Toothpicks: A Group Comparison Study. J. Periodont. Res., 4:170, 1969.
47. Glass, R. L.: A Clinical Study of Hand and Electric Toothbrushing. J. Periodont., 36:322, 1965.
48. Glickman, I.: Preventive Periodontics—A Blueprint for the Periodontal Health of the American Public. J. Periodont., 38:361, 1967.
49. Glickman, I., Petralis, R., and Marks, R.: The Effect of Powered Toothbrushing and Interdental Stimulation upon Microscopic Inflammation and Surface Keratinization of the Interdental Gingiva. J. Periodont., 36:108, 1965.
50. Glickman, I., Petralis, R., and Marks, R.: The Effect of Powered Toothbrushing plus Interdental

Stimulation upon the Severity of Gingivitis. J. Periodont., 35:519, 1964.

51. Glickman, I., Smulow, J. B., and Moreau, J.: Effect of Alloxan Diabetes upon the Periodontal Response to Excessive Occlusal Forces. I.A.D.R. Abstr., 1965, No. 65, p. 53.

52. Gravelle, H. R., Shackelford, M. F., and Lovett, J. T.: The Oral Hygiene of High School Students as Affected by Three Different Educational Programs. J. Pub. Health Dentistry, 27:91, 1967.

53. Greene, J. C.: Oral Hygiene and Periodontal Disease. Am. J. Pub. Health, 53:913, 1963.

54. Harrington, J. H., and Terry, I. A.: Automatic and Hand Toothbrushing Abrasion Studies. J.A.D.A., 68:343, 1964.

55. Harrisson, J. W. E., Salisbury, G. B., Abbott, D. D., and Packman, E. W.: Effect of Enzyme-Toothpastes upon Oral Hygiene. J. Periodont., 34:334, 1963.

56. Haydak, M. H., et al.: A Clinical and Biochemical Study of Cow's Milk and Honey as Essentially Exclusive Diet for Adult Humans. Am. J. M. Sc. 207:209, 1944.

57. Heylings, R. T.: A Study of the Prevalence and Severity of Gingivitis in Undergraduates at Leeds University. D. Practit. & D. Record 12:129, 1961.

58. Hine, M. K.: The Use of the Toothbrush in the Treatment of Periodontitis. J.A.D.A., 41:158, 1950.

59. Hine, M. K.: Toothbrush. Internat. D. J., 6:15, 1956.

60. Hiniker, J. J., and Forscher, B. K.: The Effect of Toothbrush Type on Gingival Health. J. Periodont., 25:40, 1954.

61. Hirshfeld, I.: The Toothbrush, Its Use and Abuse. D. Items Int., 3:833, 1931.

62. Hoover, D. R., and Lefkowitz, W.: Reduction of Gingivitis by Toothbrushing. J. Periodont., 36:193, 1965.

63. Hoover, D. R., Robinson, H. B. G., and Billingsley, A.: The Comparative Effectiveness of the Water-Pic in a Non-Instructed Population. J. Periodont., 39:43, 1968.

64. Ivy, A. C., Morgan, J. E., and Farrel, J. I.: Effects of Total Gastrectomy. Surg., Gynec. & Obst., 53:611, 1931.

65. James, P. M. C., Jackson, D., Slack, G. L., and Lawton, F. E.: Gingival Health and Dental Cleanliness in English School Children. Arch. Oral Biol., 3:57, 1960.

66. Kakehashi, S., Baer, P. N., and White, C.: Studies on Experimental Calculus Formation in the Rat. II. Effect of Calcium, Phosphate, Bicarbonate. J. Periodont., 33:186, 1962.

67. Keyes, P. H., and Jordan, H. V.: The Effect of Two Diets and an Antibiotic on Periodontal Disease in Hamsters. I.A.D.R. Abstr., 1965, No. 67, p. 53.

68. Keyes, P. H., et al.: Dispersion of Dextranous Bacterial Plaques on Human Teeth with Dextranase. J.A.D.A., 82:136, 1971.

69. King, J. D.: Gingival Disease in Dundee, D. Record, 65:9, 32, 55, 1945.

70. King, J. D., and Glover, R. E.: The Relative Effects of Dietary Constituents and Other Factors upon Calculus Formation and Gingival Disease in the Ferret. J. Path. & Bact., 57:353, 1945.

71. Knutson, J. W.: Recent Developments in the Prevention and Treatment of Periodontal Disease. J. South California D. A., 32:140, 1964.

72. Koch, G., and Lindhe, J.: The Effect of Supervised Oral Hygiene on the Gingiva of Children. The Effect of Toothbrushing. Odont. Revy, 16:327, 1965.

73. Krajewski, J., Giblin, J., and Gargiulo, A. W.: Evaluation of a Water Pressure Cleansing Device as an Adjunct to Periodontal Treatment. Periodontics, 2:76, 1964.

74. Lainson, P. A., Berquist, J. J., and Fraleigh, C. M.: Clinical Evaluation of Pulsar, A New Pulsating Water Pressure Cleansing Device. I.A.D.R. Abstracts, 48th General Meeting, 1970, No. 71, p. 66.

75. Larato, D., Stahl, S., Brown, R., Jr., and Witkin, G.: The Effect of a Prescribed Method of Toothbrushing on the Fluctuation of Marginal Gingivitis. J. Periodont–Periodontics, 40:142, 1969.

76. Lefkowitz, W., and Robinson, H. B. G.: Effectiveness of Automatic and Hand Brushes in Removing Dental Plaque and Debris. J.A.D.A., 65:351, 1962.

77. Leung, S. W., and Draus, F. J.: Effect of Certain Enzymes on Calculus Deposition (Abstr.). J. D. Res., 38:709, 1959.

78. Lindhe, J., and Wicén, P. O.: The Effects on the Gingivae of Chewing Fibrous Foods. J. Periodont. Res., 4:193, 1969.

79. Linn, E. L.: Oral Hygiene and Periodontal Disease: Implications for Dental Health Programs. J.A.D.A. 71:39, 1965.

80. Littleton, N. W.: Dental Caries and Periodontal Diseases among Ethiopian Civilians. Pub. Health Rep., 78:631, 1963.

81. Lobene, R. R.: A Clinical Study of the Effect of Dextranase on Human Dental Plaque J.A.D.A., 82:132, 1971.

82. Lobene, R. R.: The Effect of a Pulsed Water Pressure Cleaning Device on Oral Health. J. Periodont.–Periodontics, 40:667, 1969.

83. Lobene, R. R.: The Effect of an Automatic Toothbrush on Gingival Health. J. Periodont., 35:137, 1964.

84. Lobene, R. R., Brion, M., and Socransky, S. S.: Effect of Erythromycin on Dental Plaque and Plaque Forming Microorganisms of Man. J. Periodont.–Periodontics, 40:287, 1969.

85. Lobene, R. R., and Soparkar, P. M.: Effect of a Pulsed Water Pressure Cleansing Device on Oral Health, I.A.D.R. Abstr. No. 344, 1969, p. 126.

86. Löe, H., and Schiøtt, C. R.: The Effect of Mouthrinses and Topical Application of Chlorhexidine on the Development of Dental Plaque and Gingivitis in Man. J. Periodont. Res., 5:79, 1970.

87. Löe, H., Theilade, E., and Jensen, S. B.: Experimental Gingivitis in Man. J. Periodont., 36:177, 1965.

88. Löe, H., et al.: Experimental Gingivitis in Man: III. The Influences of Antibiotics on Gingival Plaque Development, J. Periodont. Res., 2:282, 1967.

89. Lövdal, A., Arno, A., Schei, O., and Waerhaug, J.: Combined Effect of Subgingival Scaling and Controlled Oral Hygiene on the Incidence of Gingivitis. Acta Odont. Scandinav., 19:537, 1961.

90. Lövdal, A., Schei, O., Waerhaug, J., and Arno, A.: Tooth Mobility and Alveolar Bone Resorption as a Function of Occlusal Stress and Oral Hygiene. Acta Odont. Scandinav., 17:61, 1959.

91. Lyons, H.: Fiction and Facts in Periodontology: An Appraisal. J.A.D.A., 39:513, 1949.

92. Manhold, B. S., Manhold, J. H., and Weisinger, E.: A Study of Total Oral Debris Clearance. J. New Jersey State D. Soc., 38:64, 1967.

93. Manhold, J. H.: Gingival Tissue Health with Hand and Power Brushing: A Retrospective with Corroborative Studies. J. Periodont., 38:23, 1967.

94. Manhold, J. H. Jr., Parker, L. A., and Manhold, B. S.: Efficacy of a Commercial Mouthwash: In Vivo Study. New York J. Den., 32:165, 1962.

95. Manly, R. S., and Brudevold, F.: Relative Abrasiveness of Natural and Synthetic Toothbrush Bristles on Cementum and Dentin. J.A.D.A., 55:779, 1957.

96. Manly, R. S., Wiren, J., Manly, P. J., and Keene, R. C.: A Method for Measurement of Abrasion of Dentin by Toothbrush and Dentifrice. J. D. Res., 44:533, 1965.

97. Marshall-Day, C. D., Stephens, R. G., and Quigley, L. F.: Periodontal Disease: Prevalence and Incidence. J. Periodont., 26:185, 1955.

98. Massler, M., Ludwick, W., and Schour, I.: Dental Caries and Gingivitis in Males 17–20 Years Old (at the Great Lakes Naval Training Center). J. D. Res., 31:195, 1952.

99. McConnell, D., and Conroy, C. W.: Comparisons of Abrasion Produced by a Simulated Manual Versus a Mechanical Toothbrush. J. D. Res., 46:1022, 1967.

100. McFall, W. T., Jr., et al.: Effect of Vancomycin on Inhibition of Bacterial Plaque. J. D. Res., 47: 1195, 1968.

101. McKendrick, A. J. W., Barbenel, L. M. H., and McHugh, W. D.: A Two Year Comparison of Hand and Electric Toothbrushes. J. Periodont. Res., 3:224, 1968.

102. Miller, S. C., Stahl, S. S., and Goldsmith, E. D.: The Effects of Vertical Occlusal Trauma on the Periodontium of Protein Deprived Young Adult Rats. J. Periodont., 28:87, 1957.

103. Mitchell, D. F., and Holmes, L. A.: Topical Antibiotic Control of Dentogingival Plaque. J. Periodont., 36:202, 1965.

104. Mohammed, C.: Dental Plaque Removed by Floss. J. New Jersey D. Soc., 36:419, 1965.

105. Mollé, W. H.: Efficacy of an Enzyme Toothpaste in the Retardation of Dental Plaque. J. Southern California D. A., 35:391, 1967.

106. Muhler, J. C., and Stookey, G. K.: The Development of an Improved $ZrSiO_4$ Prophylactic Paste. J. Periodont., 41:290, 1970.

107. Muller, E., et al.: The Effect of Two Oral Antiseptics on Early Calculus Formation. Helv. Odont. Acta., 6:42, 1962.

108. O'Rourke, J. T.: The Relation of the Physical Character of the Diet to the Health of the Periodontal Tissues. Am. J. Orth. & Oral Surg., 33:Sec. Oral Surg., 687, 1947.

109. Ostrolenk, M., and Weiss, W.: Effect of Mouthwashes on the Oral Flora. D. Abstr., 5:51, 1960.

110. Packman, E. W., Abbott, D. D., Salisbury, G. B., and Harrisson, J. W. E.: Effect of Enzyme Chewing Gums upon Oral Hygiene. J. Periodont., 34:255, 1963.

111. Pelzer, R. H.: A Study of the Local Oral Effect of Diet on the Periodontal Tissues and Gingival Capillary Structures. J.A.D.A., 27:13, 1940.

112. Phillips, J. E.: Effect of Water Irrigation on Oral Flora and Gingival Health. Masters Thesis, Graduate School, Marquette University, Milwaukee, Wisconsin, June, 1967.

113. Quigley, G. A., and Hein, J. W.: Comparative Cleansing Efficacy of Manual and Power Brushing. J.A.D.A., 65:26, 1962.

114. Rateitschak, K. H., Engelberger, A., and Marthaler, T. M.: Therapeutic Effect of Local Treatment on Periodontal Disease Assessed upon Evaluation of Different Diagnostic Criteria. 3. Radiographic Changes in Appearance of Bone. J. Periodont., 35:263, 1964.

115. Robinson, H. B. G.: Individualizing Dentifrices: The Dentist's Responsibility. J.A.D.A., 79:633, 1969.

116. Robinson, H. B. G. and Kitchin, P. C.: The Effect of Massage with the Toothbrush on Keratinization of the Gingivae. Oral Surg., Oral Med. & Oral Path., 1:1042, 1948.

117. Sanders, W. E., and Robinson, H. B. G.: Effect of Toothbrushing on Deposition of Calculus. J. Periodont., 33:386, 1962.

118. Schei, O., Waerhaug, J., Lövdal, A., and Arno, A.: Alveolar Bone Loss as Related to Oral Hygiene and Age. J. Periodont., 30:7, 1959.

119. Schour, I., and Massler, M.: Gingival Disease in Postwar Italy (1945). I. Prevalence of Gingivitis in Various Age Groups. J.A.D.A., 35:475, 1947.

120. Schour, I., and Massler, M.: Prevalence of Gingivitis in Young Adults. J. D. Res., 27:733, 1948 (abst.).

121. Schroeder, H. E.: Formation and Inhibition of Dental Calculus. Berne, Stuttgart, Vienna, Hans Huber Publishers, 1969.

122. Schroeder, H. E., Marthaler, T. M., and Mühlemann, H. R.: Effects of Some Potential Inhibitors on Early Calculus Formation. Helv. Odont. Acta, 6:6, 1962.

122a. Sconyers, J. R., Crawford, J. J., and Moriarty, J. D.: Study of Bacteremia Following Toothbrushing Using Sensitive Culture Methods. IADR Abtr., 1971, Abstr. No. 757.

123. Smith, T. S.: Anatomic and Physiologic Conditions Governing the Use of the Toothbrush. J.A.D.A., 27:874, 1940.

124. Smith, W. A., and Ash, M. M.: Effectiveness of an Electric Toothbrush. I.A.D.R., Abstr., 1963, No. 207, p. 86.

125. Stahl, S. S., and Goldman, H. M.: The Incidence of Gingivitis among a sample of Massachusetts School Children. Oral Surg., Oral Med. & Oral Path., 6:707, 1953.

126. Stahl, S. S., Wachtel, N., DeCastro, C., and Pelletier, G.: The Effect of Tooth Brushing on the Keratinization of the Gingiva. J. Periodont., 24: 20, 1953.

127. Stanmeyer, W. R.: A Measure of Tissue Response to Frequency of Toothbrushing. J. Periodont., 28:17, 1957.

128. Stewart, G. G.: Mucinase—A Possible Means of Reducing Calculus Formation. J. Periodont., 23:85, 1952.

129. Stewart, W. H., and Burnett, G. W.: The Relationship of Certain Dietary Factors to Calculuslike Formation in Albino Rats. J. Periodont., 31:7, 1960.

130. Stillman, P. R.: A Philosophy of the Treatment of Periodontal Disease. D. Digest, 38:314, 1932.

131. Strålfors, A., Thilander, H., and Bergenholtz, A.: Simultaneous Inhibition of Caries and Periodontal Disease in Hamsters by Disinfection,

Toothbrushing or Phosphate Addition. Arch. Oral Biol., *12*:1367, 1967.

132. Sturzenberger, O. P., and Leonard, G. J.: The Effect of a Mouthwash as Adjunct in Tooth Cleaning. J. Periodont–Periodontics, *40*:299, 1969.

133. Sumnicht, R. W.: Research in Preventive Dentistry. J.A.D.A., 79:1193, 1969.

134. Suomi, J. D., et al.: The Effect of Controlled Oral Hygiene Procedures on the Progression of Periodontal Disease in Adults: Results After Two Years. J. Periodont.–Periodontics, *40*:416, 1969.

135. Tamimi, H. A., Thomassen, P. R., and Moser, E. H., Jr.: Bacteremia Study Using a Water Irrigation Device. J. Periodont.–Periodontics, *40*:424, 1969.

136. Theilade, E., Wright, W. H., Jenson, S. B., and Löe, H.: Experimental Gingivitis in Man. II. A Longitudinal Clinical and Bacteriological Investigation. J. Periodont. Res., *1*:1, 1966.

137. Toto, P. D., Evans, C. L., and Sawinski, V. J.: Effects of Water Jet Rinse and Toothbrushing on Oral Hygiene. J. Periodont.–Periodontics, *40*:296, 1969.

138. Toto, P. D., and Farchione, A.: Clinical Evaluation of an Electrically Powered Toothbrush in Home Periodontal Therapy. J. Periodont., *32*:249, 1961.

139. Toto, P. D., Goljan, K. R., Evans, J. A., and Sawinski, V. J.: A Study on the Uninstructed Use of an Electric Brush. J.A.D.A., 72:904, 1966.

140. Turesky, S., Gilmore, N. D., and Glickman, I.: Calculus Inhibition by Topical Application of the Chloromethyl Analogue of Victamine C. J. Periodont., 38:142, 1967.

141. Turesky, S., Gilmore, N. D., and Glickman, I.: Reduced Plaque Formation by the Chloromethyl Analogue of Victamine C. J. Periodont., *41*:41, 1970.

142. Villa, P.: Degree of Calculus Inhibition by Habitual Toothbrushing. Helv. Odont. Acta, *12*:31, 1968.

143. Volpe, A. R., Kupczak, L. J., Brant, J. H., King, W. J., Kestenbaum, R. C., and Schlissel, H. J.: Antimicrobial Control of Bacterial Plaque and Calculus and the Effects of these Agents on Oral Flora. J. D. Res., *48*:832, 1969.

144. Wainwright, H. W., Bauer, F. K., and Thomas, P. B.: Removal of Radioactive Fat and Protein from the Mouth. J. D. Res., 38:392, 1959.

145. Wasserman, B. H., Mandel, I. D., and Levy, B. M.: In Vitro Calcification of Dental Calculus. J. Periodont., 29:144, 1958.

146. Weinstein, E., et al.: Studies of Gingival Fluid. I.A.D.R. Abstr., 1965, p. 72, No. 143.

147. Williford, J. W., Johns, C., Muhler, J. C., and Stookey, G. K.: Report of a Study Demonstrating Improved Oral Health Through Education. J. Dent. Child., *34*:183, 1967.

Section Four · The Treatment of Gingival and Periodontal Disease

PERIODONTAL TREATMENT consists of coordinated procedures for the purpose of creating a well-functioning dentition in a healthy periodontal environment.

It is a TOTAL TREATMENT which requires the interrelationship of the care of the periodontium with other phases of dentistry.

The concept of TOTAL TREATMENT is embodied in a MASTER PLAN which consists of the following:

I. THE SOFT TISSUE PHASE—Elimination of gingival inflammation and periodontal pockets and the factors that cause them.

II. THE FUNCTIONAL PHASE—Establishment of the optimal occlusal relationship for the entire dentition.

III. THE SYSTEMIC PHASE—Systemic adjuncts to local treatment and special precautions in patient management necessitated by systemic conditions.

IV. THE MAINTENANCE PHASE—Prevention of recurrence of disease in the treated patient.

Part I • *Diagnosis;*
Determination of the
Prognosis;
The Treatment Plan

DIAGNOSIS

Proper diagnosis is essential for intelligent treatment. In addition to recognizing the clinical and radiographic features of different diseases, diagnosis requires an understanding of the underlying disease processes and their etiology. **Our interest is in the patient who has the disease and not simply the disease itself.** Diagnosis must therefore include a general evaluation of the patient as well as consideration of the oral cavity.

Diagnosis must be systematic, and organized for specific purposes. It is not enough to assemble facts. The findings must be pieced together so that they provide a meaningful explanation of the patient's periodontal problem.

The diagnosis should provide answers to the following questions:

Which local factors are responsible for the gingival inflammation and periodontal pockets? Does the periodontium present evidence of trauma from occlusion? Are there occlusal relationships that account for the trauma from occlusion? Are the gingival and periodontal changes explainable by the local factors or do they suggest the possibility of contributing systemic etiology?

The following is a recommended sequence of procedures for the diagnosis of gingival and periodontal disease.

FIRST VISIT

Overall Appraisal of the Patient

From the first meeting, the operator should attempt an overall appraisal of the patient. This includes consideration of the patient's mental and emotional status, temperament, attitude and physiologic age. Observation of the patient as he enters the operating room and is seated in the chair may disclose gross manifestations of disease evidenced by the following:

Facies. Facial changes are associated with diseases such as hyperthyroidism, myasthenia gravis, acromegaly, myxedema, Paget's disease, parkinsonism, pernicious anemia, Bell's palsy and central facial paralysis. Facial expression is often indicative of anxiety, worry or depression.

Body Habitus. Marked obesity or wasting suggests the possibility of hormonal or nutritional disturbances or wasting disease such as malignancy or tuberculsosis.

Gait. Tertiary syphilis, Paget's disease and multiple sclerosis are frequently identified with abnormalities in gait.

Posture. Arthritis, tuberculosis of bone and Paget's disease.

Respiration. Dyspnea may indicate cardiac failure or pulmonary disease; wheezing respiration occurs in bronchial asthma.

Temperature. Elevated body temperature generally indicates infection.

Skin. Eruptions occur in the various dermatoses. Pigmentation is seen in Addison's disease, argyria and pellagra; pallor is seen in anemia or aortic insufficiency. Yellow dicoloration indicates jaundice, either obstructive, toxic or infectious. Cyanosis may be due to pulmonary or cardiac disease. Dryness is seen in cretinism and myxedema. Hemorrhage occurs in bleeding diatheses. Nevi, tumors, keloid or neurofibromatosis should be noted.

Eyes. Inflammation, exophthalmos or pupillary changes should be noted.

Nose. Purulent discharge indicates acute rhinitis or sinus infection. Deformities or obstruction of nasal passages may give rise to "mouth breathing."

Ears. Discharge is seen in acute and chronic infections.

Neck. Prominent neck veins may be associated with congestive heart failure or other disturbances of the cardiovascular system. Vigorous carotid pulsations may be indicative of hypertension. Masses in the neck may be due to lymphadenopathy, goiter or thyroid enlargement, cysts or tumors.

Submaxillary and Parotid Areas. Osteomyelitis, actinomycosis, obstruction of Wharton's duct and Ludwig's angina produce swelling in the submaxillary area. Epidemic parotitis, obstruction of Stensen's duct, Mikulicz's disease, or neoplasms may be responsible for swellings in these areas.

Systemic History

Most of the systemic history is obtained at the first visit and can be enlarged upon by pertinent questions at subsequent visits. The importance of the systemic history should be explained, because patients often omit information that they cannot relate to their dental problem. The systemic history will aid the operator in (1) **the diagnosis of oral manifestations of systemic disease,** (2) **the detection of systemic conditions that may be affecting the periodontal tissue response to local factors,** and (3) **the detection of systemic conditions that require special precautions and modifications in treatment procedures.** The systemic history should include reference to the following:

1. Is the patient under the care of a physician; if so, what is the nature and duration of the illness, and therapy? Special inquiry should be made regarding anti-

coagulants and corticosteroids—the dosage and duration of therapy.

2. History of rheumatic fever, rheumatic or congenital heart disease, hypertension, angina pectoris, myocardial infarction, nephritis, liver disease, diabetes, fainting spells.

3. Abnormal bleeding tendencies such as nose bleeds, prolonged bleeding from minor cuts, spontaneous ecchymoses, tendency toward excessive bruising and excessive menstrual bleeding.

4. Infectious disease, recent contact with infectious disease at home or at business, recent chest x-ray.

5. Possibility of occupational disease.

6. History of allergy—hay fever, asthma, sensitivity to foods, sensitivity to drugs such as aspirin, codeine, barbiturates, sulfonamides, antibiotics, procaine, laxatives or dental materials such as eugenol or acrylic resins.

7. Information regarding the onset of puberty and menopause and menstrual disorders or hysterectomy, pregnancies, miscarriages.

Dental History

Chief complaint

The following are some of the symptoms in patients with gingival and periodontal disease: "bleeding gums," "loose teeth," "spreading of the teeth with the appearance of spaces where none existed before," "foul taste in the mouth," "itchy feeling in the gums, relieved by digging with a toothpick." There may also be pain of varied types and duration, such as "constant dull gnawing pain," "dull pain after eating," "deep radiating pains in the jaws, especially on rainy days;" "acute throbbing pain," "sensitivity to percussion," "sensitivity to heat and cold," "burning sensation in the gums," "extreme sensitivity to inhaled air."

A preliminary oral examination is done to explore the source of the patient's chief complaint and determine whether *immediate emergency care* is required.

The dental history should also include reference to the following:

Visits to the dentist—frequency, date of last visit, nature of the treatment. "Oral prophylaxis" or "cleaning" by a dentist or hygienist—frequency and date of last one.

Toothbrushing—frequency, before or after meals, method, type of toothbrush and dentifrice, intervals at which brushes are replaced. Other methods for mouth care: mouthwashes, finger massage, interdental stimulation, water irrigation and dental floss.

Orthodontic treatment—duration and approximate time of termination.

Pain "in the teeth" or "in the gums." The manner in which it is provoked, its nature and duration and the manner in which it is relieved.

"Bleeding gums"—when first noted, whether it occurs spontaneously, upon brushing or eating, at night, with regular periodicity. Whether it is associated with the menstrual period or other specific factors. The duration of the bleeding and the manner in which it is stopped.

Bad taste in the mouth, areas of food impaction.

Tooth mobility—do the teeth feel "loose" or insecure? Is there difficulty in chewing?

History of previous "gum" trouble—the nature of the condition, previous treatment, duration, nature and approximate period of termination.

Habits—"grinding the teeth," "clenching the teeth" during the day or night— do the teeth or muscles feel "sore" in the morning? Other habits such as tobacco smoking or chewing, nail biting, biting on foreign objects.

Intra-oral radiographic survey

The radiographic survey should consist of a minimum of fourteen intra-oral films and posterior bite-wings.

Panoramic radiographs

Panoramic radiographs are a simple and convenient method of obtaining a survey view of the dental arch and surrounding structures (Fig. 33–1). They are helpful for the detection of developmental anomalies, pathologic lesions of the teeth and jaws and fractures, and for dental screening examinations of large groups. They provide an informative over-all radiographic picture of the distribution and severity of bone destruction in periodontal disease, but a com-

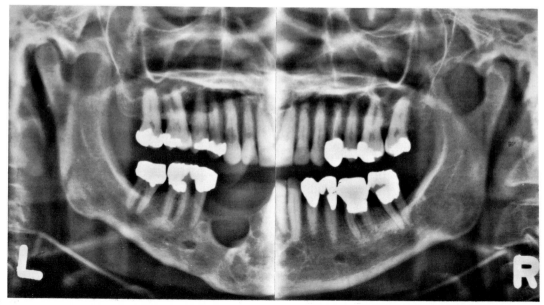

Figure 33–1 Panoramic Radiograph, showing temporomandibular joints, periodontal bone loss and "cystic" spaces in the jaw.

plete intra-oral series is required for definitive diagnosis and treatment planning.

Casts

Casts are extremely useful adjuncts in the oral examination. They indicate the position and inclinations of the teeth, proximal contact relationships, and food impaction areas. In addition, they provide a view of lingual cuspal relationships. They are important records of the dentition before it is altered by treatment. They also serve as "visual aids" in discussions with the patient and are useful for pre- and post-treatment comparisons as well as reference at check-up visits.

Clinical photographs

Kodachrome photographs are not essential but are useful for recording the appearance of the tissue before and after treatment. Photographs cannot always be relied upon for comparing subtle color changes in the gingiva; they do depict changes in gingival morphology.

If no emergency care is required, the patient is dismissed and instructed when to report for the second visit. Before this visit, a correlated examination is made of the radiographs and casts to relate the radiographic changes to unfavorable conditions represented on the casts. The casts are checked for evidence of abnormal wear, plunger cusps, uneven marginal ridges, malposed or extruded teeth, crossbite relationships or other conditions that could cause occlusal disharmony or food impaction. Such areas are marked on the casts, to be referred to in the detailed examination of the oral cavity to follow. The radiographs and casts are valuable diagnostic aids; however, it is the findings in the oral cavity that constitute the basis for diagnosis.

Nutritional status

Nutrition refers to the complex relationship between the individual total health status and the intake, digestion and utilization of nutrients. *Nutritional deficiency connotes an inadequacy in the nutritional status of the tissues.* Malnutrition or poor nutrition may result from excess food intake and improper nutrient balance as well as from an insufficiency of nutrients.

Nutritional deficiencies may be (1) *primary,* resulting from an overt insufficiency of nutrients; or (2) *secondary (conditioned),* resulting from bodily conditions which interfere with the ingestion, transport, cellular uptake or utilization of essential nutrients, in the presence of adequate food intake. Nutritional deficiencies usually develop in stages as follows: (1) *depletion of the tissue nutrient reserve,* (2) *biochemical tissue lesions,* (3) *morphologic and functional abnormalities which are expressed as* (4) *clinical signs and symptoms,* and finally (5) *tissue death.*

Diagnosis of nutritional deficiency

A nutritional diagnosis is based upon four sequential routes of inquiry: (1) medical and social history, and dietary history; (2) clinical examination; (3) laboratory tests; and (4) therapeutic trial.

MEDICAL AND SOCIAL HISTORY. Common complaints of patients with nutritional disorders include general weakness, chronic fatigue, failure of appetite, painful bleeding gums, sore lips, sore tongue and mouth, diarrhea, chronic nervousness, irritability, inability to concentrate, confusion, memory loss, dizziness, lethargy, photophobia, loss of manual dexterity, numbness, pain in the legs and skin rashes.

Attention should be given to conditions which could lead to secondary nutritional deficiencies such as the following:

Gastrointestinal disturbances which impair the digestion and absorption of nutrients. In diarrhea, hypermotility of the intestine does not permit sufficient time for water-soluble vitamins to be absorbed. Achlorhydria interferes with the absorption of calcium, phosphorus and iron. In diseases in which fat absorption is impaired, such as sprue, ulcerative colitis, dysentery and celiac disease, the absorption of the fat soluble vitamins (A, D, E, K) is inhibited. Excessive amounts of oxalic acid (found in spinach) or phytic acid (found in bran) will make minerals unavailable for utilization to the body. The daily use of mineral oil interferes with the absorption of carotene.

Interference with utilization of foods, which occurs as a feature of certain diseases such as diabetes, adrenal dysfunction, cirrhosis of the liver or thyroid disease.

Increased excretion, such as in polyuria of diabetes or in fever, which affects the nitrogen retention of the tissues as well as the water balance of the body. Lactation tends to reduce the thiamine level.

Factors which increase the nutritional requirements, such as hyperthyroidism, spurt growth periods, pregnancy, lactation, physical exertion or drug administration.

Factors which interfere with the ingestion of food, such as discomfort from caries and periodontal disease, absence of teeth, loss of appetite caused by infection, food allergy or nausea of pregnancy.

There is an important relationship between emotional status and appetite. Emotional problems often lead to overeating and obesity. "Breaking the smoking habit" frequently has a similar effect. Loss of appetite may result from bereavement or frustration. In alcoholics, diminished food intake may lead to nutritional deficiency.

DIETARY HISTORY. The dietary history should provide information regarding the patient's usual dietary practices and should include questions regarding the following:

Length of time the present diet has been followed.

History of any special diet, its type and duration. Therapeutic diets such as those prescribed in the treatment of ulcers, biliary disease and colitis, or "reducing diets" may be deficient in one or more essential nutrients.

Use of vitamins or other food supplements.

Regularity of meals.

Food likes, dislikes and idiosyncrasies.

Living conditions. Young individuals who live away from their families and prepare their own meals, and elderly individuals who live alone and find it difficult to obtain proper foods and prepare well-balanced meals often suffer from malnutrition.

Economic status and education. Inability to afford foods in necessary quantities and variety, and lack of knowledge regarding the requirement of a "good diet" are common causes of nutritional disorder.

After the desired information is obtained, the patient is given a "food diary," in which he is to record his daily food intake for at least five consecutive days which include a weekend.

EVALUATION OF THE DIET.[35a] The adequacy of the diet is evaluated by transposing the information in the dietary history into the basic four food groups: (1) *milk,* (2) *meat,* (3) *vegetable and fruit* and (4) *bread and cereal.* The *milk group* (milk, cheese) provides protein, calcium, riboflavin, vitamin A and other nutrients; the *meat group* (meat, fish, poultry, eggs, dried beans and peas)

TABLE 33–1 DIETARY EVALUATION CHART

Food Groups	Physical Form	1st Day	2nd Day	3rd Day	4th Day	5th Day	Average per Day	Recommended Intake	Difference
I. Milk	Liquid, soft	/ /		/	/	/ /	2	2 or more servings	OK
	Hard		/	/	/	/			
II. Meat	Soft, chopped	/	/ /	/		/ /	2	2 or more servings	OK
	Solid	/	/	/	/	/			
III. Vegetable and fruit	Juices, soft	/		/ /	/	/ /	2+	4 or more servings	−2
	Raw or slightly cooked	/		/	/	/ /			
IV. Bread and cereal	Soft, cooked	/ / / /	/ / /	/ / /	/ / /	/ / / /	5+	4 or more servings	+1
	Dry, crusty, toasted	/	/ /	/ /	/ /	/ /			

provides primarily protein, B complex vitamins and iron; the *vegetable and fruit group* provides most of the vitamins A and C as well as other minerals and vitamins; and the *bread and cereal group* furnishes B complex vitamins, iron, protein and carbohydrate. Foods which provide only calories such as sugar and sugar products should be kept to a minimum. The same is true of fats because they are usually contained in the milk and meat groups.

A chart such as that shown in Table 33–1 is helpful for evaluating the diet.[35] It separates the foods into different groups and also records their consistency so that inadequacies in coarse, hard foods which have a helpful cleansing effect upon the teeth and gingiva can be noted and corrected. A person who consumes less food than the amounts recommended in the evaluation chart is not necessarily nutritionally deficient. The recommendations represent amounts considered desirable for maintaining good nutrition in healthy patients, without bodily conditioning factors which interfere with food utilization. They represent goals to be strived for rather than requirements.

CLINICAL EXAMINATION. Certain signs and symptoms have been identified with different nutritional deficiencies.[51] However, many patients with nutritional disease do not exhibit classic signs of deficiency disorders, and different types of deficiency produce comparable clinical findings. Clinical findings are suggestive, but definitive diagnosis of nutritional deficiencies and their nature requires the combined information revealed by the history, clinical and laboratory findings and therapeutic trial. *Clinical findings* identified with specific nutritional deficiencies are presented in Table 33–2,[22] and the *oral manifestations of nutritional disorders* are described in detail in Chapter 26.

LABORATORY TESTS FOR NUTRITIONAL

DEFICIENCY. Blood, serum and urine tests reflect nutrient intake levels and absorption defects. The following are useful diagnostic aids: In the blood, *macrocytosis* may be the result of vitamin B_{12} and *folate deficiencies*, whereas a *microcytosis* may indicate lack of *iron* and *vitamin B_6. Hypochromia* is associated with *iron deficiency*. The *serum iron-binding capacity*, which normally is 300 to 450 μg./100 ml., is decreased to less than 18 per cent in *iron deficiency*.

A serum albumin value below 3.5 gm./100 ml. serum indicates *protein deficiency*. Serum *vitamin A levels* below 10 μg./100 ml. suggest deficiency of the vitamin. A serum carotene of 30 μg./100 ml. also indicates a vitamin A deficiency. Since *vitamin C* is not stored in the body, *serum ascorbic acid* levels reflect current intake. Serum values below 0.3 mg./100 ml. indicate inadequate intake; values below 0.01 mg./ml. are consistent with a diagnosis of *scurvy*. The normal serum level of *vitamin B_{12}* (cyancobolamine) should range between 7 and 15.9 mμg./ml. folate activity for *Lactobacillus casei*; below 7 mμg./ml. is subnormal.

Urinary creatinine is used as a reference unit in tests for several nutrients. Iodine intake is considered inadequate if its level in creatinine is less than 50 mg./gm. The N-methylnicotinamide content should be above 1.6 mg./gm. of creatinine. Riboflavin content below 80 μg./gm. of creatinine in adults and below 300 μg./gm. of creatine in children under six, and thiamine values less than 97 to 116 μg./gm. of creatine in adults and 120 μg./gm. of creatinine in children under six are considered indicative of inadequate intake.

TABLE 33–2 CLINICAL FINDINGS IDENTIFIED WITH NUTRITIONAL DEFICIENCIES*

System	Clinical Findings	Suggested Deficiency
General	Underweight	CHO, fat and protein
	Underheight	Protein, Ca, P, vitamins
	Pallor	Iron, folic acid, B_{12}, intrinsic factor
	Anorexia	Thiamine, niacin
	Weakness and fatigue	Calories, vitamin B complex
Skin	Dermatitis (pellagrous)	Niacin
	Intertrigo	Riboflavin
	Xerosis	Vitamin A
	Hyperkeratosis of hair follicle	Vitamin A
	Acne	Pyridoxine, vitamin A
Eyes	Nyctalopia or night blindness	Vitamin A
	Xerophthalmia	Vitamin A
	Photophobia	Riboflavin, vitamin A
	Bitot's spots	Vitamin A
	Vascular injection of conjunctiva and sclera	Riboflavin
Mouth	Angular cheilosis "Beefy red"	Riboflavin
	Scarlet red glossitis (pellagrous)	Niacin
	Lichen planus	B complex
	Leukoplakia	B complex
	Scorbutic gingivitis	Ascorbic acid
Skeletal	Rachitic deformities	Vitamin D, calcium and phosphorus
Neuromuscular	Muscle cramps (calf tenderness with or without edema)	Thiamine
	Paresthesia	Thiamine

*Comparable clinical findings may result from more than one type of deficiency.

SECOND VISIT

Oral Examination

Oral hygiene

The "cleanliness" of the oral cavity is appraised in terms of the extent of accumulated food debris, plaque, materia alba and tooth surface stains (Fig. 33–2). *Disclosing solution* (Chap. 32) *should be used routinely to detect plaque that would otherwise be unnoticed.*

Mouth odors

Halitosis, also termed "fetor ex ore" or "fetor oris," is foul or offensive odor emanating from the oral cavity.[30] Mouth odors may be of diagnostic significance; their origin may be either (a) local or (b) extra-oral or remote.

LOCAL SOURCES. Retention of odoriferous food particles on and between the teeth,[18] coated tongue, acute necrotizing ulcerative gingivitis, dehydration states, caries, artificial dentures, smoker's breath, healing surgical or extraction wounds. The fetid odor characteristic of acute necrotizing ulcerative gingivitis is easily identified. Chronic periodontal disease with pocket formation may also cause unpleasant mouth odor from accumulated debris and increased rate of putrefaction of the saliva.[3]

EXTRA-ORAL OR REMOTE SOURCES. These may include adjacent structures associated with rhinitis, sinusitis or ton-

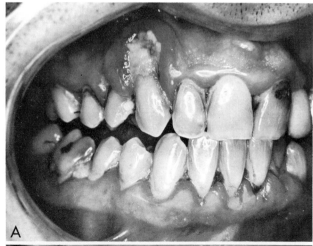

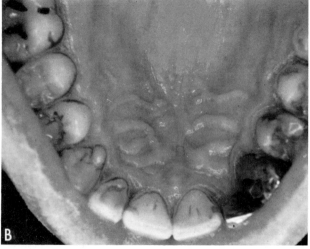

Figure 33–2 Poor Oral Hygiene. *A,* Gingival inflammation associated with plaque, materia alba and calculus in a patient with hemophilia. *B,* Palatal view of the same patient showing only slight gingivitis because the mechanical action of the tongue and food excursion reduces the accumulation of local irritants.

silitis; disease of the lungs and bronchi, such as chronic fetid bronchitis, bronchiectasis, lung abscesses, gangrene of the lung and pulmonary tuberculosis; odors excreted through the lungs from aromatic substances in the blood stream, such as metabolites from ingested foods or excretory products of cell metabolism. Of the latter group, alcoholic breath, acetone odor of diabetes and uremic breath in kidney dysfunction are examples.

Saliva

Ptyalism or excessive salivary secretion accompanies a variety of conditions such as the use of certain drugs (mercury, pilocarpine, iodides, bromides, phosphorus), acute necrotizing ulcerative gingivitis, various forms of stomatitis, Vincent's angina, irritation from smoking and psychic stimulation.

Decreased salivary secretion[9, 13] is seen in febrile diseases, chronic diseases such as chronic nephritis, uremia, diabetes mellitus, myxedema, neuropsychiatric disorders, lesions of the salivary glands, Plummer-Vinson and Sjögren syndromes and pernicious anemia. Xerostomia or "dry mouth" results from decreased salivary secretion and presents various clinical features such as generalized dryness and erythema with fissuring in extreme cases, and varying degrees of discomfort caused by a "burning" sensation.

Lips

Neoplasms, chancre, angular cheilosis, irritation from biting habits, indentations from occlusion and mucous cysts should be considered in the differential diagnosis of lesions of the lips.

Oral mucosa

A general survey of the color[9] and surface texture of the oral mucosa will indicate pathologic pigmentation, diffuse erythema associated with acute infection, diffuse erythema or bluish-red discoloration associated with vitamin B-complex deficiencies, smooth shiny atrophy with fissuring in senile or menopausal gingivostomatitis, patchy gray discoloration and desquamation associated with chronic desquamative gingivitis, and vesicles in pemphigus, erythema multiforme or benign mucous membrane pemphigoid (Fig. 33–3).

Cheek biting, irritating mouth washes, hot foods and topically applied drugs (Fig. 33–4) and ill-fitting dentures and denture clasps are common causes of painful ulceration. Leukoplakia, lichen planus, Koplik spots and inflammatory enlargement of the orifice of Stensen's duct are among other mucosal changes.

Floor of the mouth

Ranula, neoplasms and aphthae are often sources of pain.

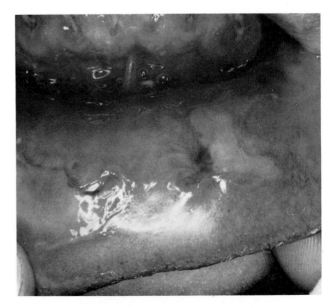

Figure 33–3   Vesicle in Benign Mucous Membrane Pemphigoid.

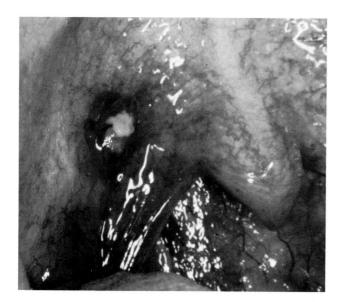

Figure 33–4   Aspirin Burn in the Oropharynx.

Tongue

The tongue should be examined for alterations in the color, size and nature of the papillae. Leukoplakia, lichen planus, erythema multiforme, pemphigus, pernicious anemia, vitamin B-complex deficiencies, Plummer-Vinson syndrome, syphilis and tuberculosis are among the systemic conditions in which the tongue may be involved. Other changes include erythema migrans (geographic tongue), moniliasis, congenital fissured tongue, median rhomboid glossitis and neoplasms. Tongue changes may be painless or accompanied by varying degrees of pain and burning. The operator should check carefully for local sources of irritation before seeking remote explanation of tongue problems. Rough spots on the teeth or margins of restorations, the incisal edges of irregularly aligned teeth, and calculus on the mandibular anterior teeth are common sources of irritation to the tongue.

BURNING TONGUE (OROLINGUAL PARESTHESIA, GLOSSOPYROSIS, GLOSSODYNIA). Burning and tingling tongue symptoms present a diagnostic and therapeutic problem. The tongue may appear normal or atrophic with or without dryness of the mouth (xerostomia) and atrophy and pain of the remainder of the oral mucosa. There are many possible causes of the tongue pain,[23] such as pernicious anemia, vitamin B complex deficiency, diabetes, hypothyroidism, post-menopausal syndrome, trigeminal neuralgia, mercurialism, use of tobacco and spices, antibiotic therapy, local mechanical irritation, electrogalvanic discharge between dental restorations constructed of different metals, and temporomandibular joint disturbances. Despite the numerous potential etiologic factors the tongue symptoms are often only explainable on a psychogenic basis.

Palate

Leukoplakia, "smoker's palate" with prominent inflamed mucous gland orifices, neoplasms and exostoses are commonly seen.

Oropharyngeal region

This is the site of pseudomembrane formation in Vincent's angina and diphtheria. Inflamed tonsils often cause radiating pain.

Examination of the Teeth

The teeth are examined for caries, developmental defects, anomalies of tooth form, wasting, hypersensitivity and proximal contact relationships.

Wasting disease of the teeth

Wasting is defined as any gradual loss of tooth substance characterized by the

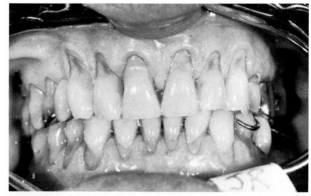

Figure 33–5 **Erosion** involving the enamel, cementum and dentin.

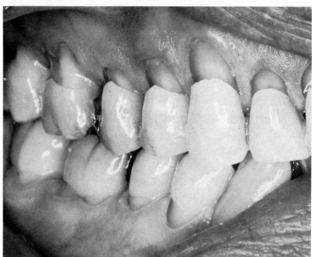

Figure 33–6 **Abrasion Attributed to Aggressive Toothbrushing.** Involvement of the roots is followed by undermining of the enamel.

formation of smooth polished surfaces without consideration of the possible mechanism of this loss. The forms of wasting are erosion, abrasion and attrition.

Erosion (cuneiform defect) is a sharply defined wedge-shaped depression in the cervical area of the facial tooth surface.[47] The long axis of the eroded area is perpendicular to the vertical axis of the tooth (Fig. 33–5). The surfaces are smooth, hard and polished. It generally affects a group of teeth. In the early stages, erosion may be confined to the enamel, but it generally extends to involve the underlying dentin as well as the cementum and dentin of the root.

The etiology of erosion is not known. Decalcification by acid beverages[31] or citrus fruits, and the combined effect of acid salivary secretion and friction are suggested causes. In patients with erosion the salivary pH, buffering capacity, calcium and phosphorus content have been reported as normal, with the mucin level elevated.[28]

Abrasion refers to the loss of tooth substance induced by mechanical wear other than that of mastication. Abrasion results in saucer-shaped or wedge-shaped indentations with a smooth shiny surface. Abrasion starts on exposed cementum surfaces rather than on the enamel, and extends to involve the dentin of the root. Continued exposure to the abrasive agent, combined with decalcification of the enamel by locally formed acids, may result in a loss of the enamel followed by the dentin of the crown (Fig. 33–6).

Toothbrushing[24] with an abrasive dentifrice or the action of clasps are common causes of abrasion. The former is by far the more prevalent. According to Manly,[26,27] the degree of tooth wear from toothbrushing depends upon the abrasive effect of the dentifrice and the angle of brushing. Horizontal brushing at right angles to the vertical axis of the teeth results in severest loss of tooth substance. Occasionally abrasion of the incisal edges occurs as a result of habits such as holding a bobby pin or tacks between the teeth.

Attrition. (See page 70.)

Hypersensitivity

Root surfaces exposed by gingival recession may be hypersensitive to thermal changes or tactile stimulation. Patients often direct the operator to the sensitive areas. They may be located by gentle exploration with a probe or cold air.

Proximal contact relations

Because there is a normal tendency toward mesial migration of the teeth, the location of the proximal contact area is important. Abnormal contact relationship may cause a shift in the median line between the central incisors, labial version of the maxillary canine, buccal or lingual displacement of the posterior teeth, and uneven relationship of the marginal ridges.

The location of proximal contact relations is of particular significance in the mandible. Since the mandibular arch is normally contained within the maxillary teeth, displacement of the mandibular teeth due to abnormally located proximal contact leads to a reduction in the circumference of the mandibular arch. This in turn results in increased overbite and loss of vertical dimension, often followed by food impaction, particularly on the lingual surfaces of the maxillary teeth. Proximal contacts are critical factors in the prevention of food impaction. They should be given careful attention when exploring the etiologic factors that contribute to the individual's periodontal problem.

Tooth mobility

All teeth have a slight degree of physiologic mobility. It varies in different teeth (highest in the central and lateral incisors) and at different times of the day.[36] It is highest upon arising in the morning and progressively decreases. The increased mobility in the morning is attributed to slight extrusion of the teeth because of limited occlusal contact during sleep. During the waking hours mobility is reduced by chewing and swallowing forces which intrude the teeth in the sockets.

Tooth mobility beyond the physiologic range (pathologic or abnormal mobility) is increased in periodontal disease as the result of the loss of supporting tissues, in inflammation and trauma from occlusion and in other conditions. (For a discussion of tooth mobility see Chap. 19.) Pathologic mobility is most common in the facio-lingual direction; it is less frequent mesio-distally, and vertical mobility occurs only in extreme cases.

Mobilometers or periodontometers are mechanical or electronic devices for the precise measurement of mobility.[34, 37, 39] They are not widely used despite the fact that standardization of the grading of mobility would be helpful in the diagnosis of periodontal disease and in evaluating the outcome of treatment. As a general rule mobility is graded clinically with a simple method such as the following:

The tooth is held firmly between the handles of two metal instruments, and an effort is made to move it in all directions; abnormal mobility most often occurs facio-lingually. Mobility is graded according to the ease and extent of tooth movement assessed by the individual therapist as follows:

Physiologic mobility.

Pathologic mobility, Grade 1 — slightly more than physiologic.

Pathologic mobility, Grade 2 — moderately more than physiologic.

Pathologic mobility, Grade 3 — severe mobility facio-lingually and/or mesio-distally combined with vertical displacement.

Sensitivity to percussion

Sensitivity to percussion is a feature of acute inflammation of the periodontal ligament. Gently percussing a tooth at different angles to the long axis often aids in localizing the site of the inflammatory involvement. Percussion also serves as a method of "sounding" for detecting teeth with reduced periodontal support.

Pathologic migration of the teeth

Alterations in tooth position should be carefully noted, particularly with a view toward abnormal occlusal forces, tongue thrusting or other habits that may be contributing factors. Pathologic migration of anterior teeth in young persons is often a sign of periodontosis.

The dentition with the jaws closed

Examination of the dentition with the jaws closed is not as revealing as examination of the jaws in function, but does indicate conditions of periodontal significance.

Irregularly aligned teeth, extruded teeth, improper proximal contact and areas of food impaction are all important sources of gingival irritation.

Overbite, *the projection of the maxillary teeth over the mandibular teeth in a vertical direction*, is a normal feature of the dentition. However, excessive overbite seen most frequently in the anterior region may cause impingement of the teeth upon the gingiva and food impaction, followed by gingival inflammation, enlargement and pocket formation (Fig. 33–7).

In open bite relationships, *abnormal vertical spaces exist between the maxillary and mandibular teeth.* The condition occurs most often in the anterior region, although posterior open bite is occasionally seen. Reduced mechanical cleaning by the passage of food may lead to accumulation of debris, calculus formation and extrusion of teeth.

In crossbite, *the normal relationship of the mandibular teeth to the maxillary teeth is reversed and the maxillary teeth are lingual to the mandibular teeth.* Crossbite may be bilateral, unilateral or may only

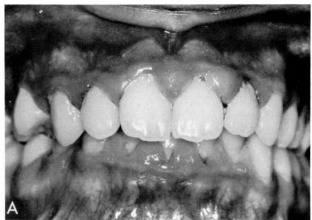

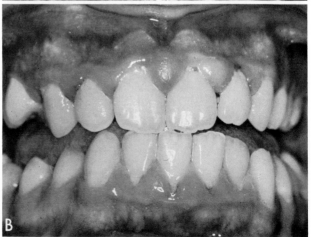

Figure 33–7 Excessive Anterior Overbite. *A,* Excessive anterior overbite with gingival inflammation and enlargement. *B,* Gingival enlargement in anterior region associated with overbite.

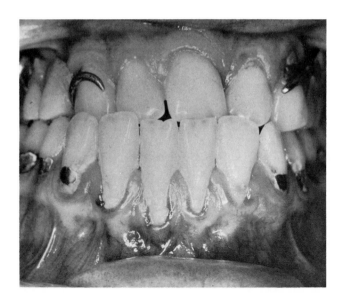

Figure 33–8 Crossbite Relationship with Associated Periodontal Disturbances.

affect a pair of antagonists. Trauma from occlusion, food impaction, spreading of the mandibular teeth and associated gingival and periodontal disturbances may be caused by crossbite (Fig. 33–8).

Examination of functional occlusal relationships

Examination of the functional occlusal relationships of the dentition is a critical part of the diagnostic procedure. Dentitions that appear normal when the jaws are closed may present marked functional abnormalities. Systematic procedures for the detection and correction of functional abnormalities are described in Chapter 53.

The temporomandibular joint

The clinical features, etiology (Chap. 52) and treatment (Chap. 53) of temporomandibular joint disorders are presented in later chapters.

Examination of the Periodontium

It is important to look for the earliest signs of gingival and periodontal disease. The examination should be systematic starting in the molar area in either the

maxilla or mandible and proceeding around the arch. This will avoid overemphasis of spectacular findings at the expense of other conditions which, though less striking, may be equally important.

Charts to record the periodontal and associated findings provide a guide for thorough examination and a record of the patient's condition (Fig. 33–9). They are also used for evaluating the response to treatment and for comparison at recall visits. However, excessively complicated mouth charting may lead to a frustrating maze of minutiae rather than clarification of the patient's problem.

Plaque and calculus

There are many methods of assessing plaque and calculus accumulation[11] (Chap. 21). For the detection of **subgingival calculus** each tooth surface is carefully checked to the level of the gingival attachment with a sharp No. 17 probe. Warm air may be used to deflect the gingiva and aid in visualization of the calculus. The amount of **supragingival calculus** may be measured with a calibrated periodontal probe.

The x-ray reveals heavy calculus deposits interproximally (Fig. 33–10) and sometimes on the facial and lingual surfaces, but cannot be relied upon for the thorough detection of calculus.

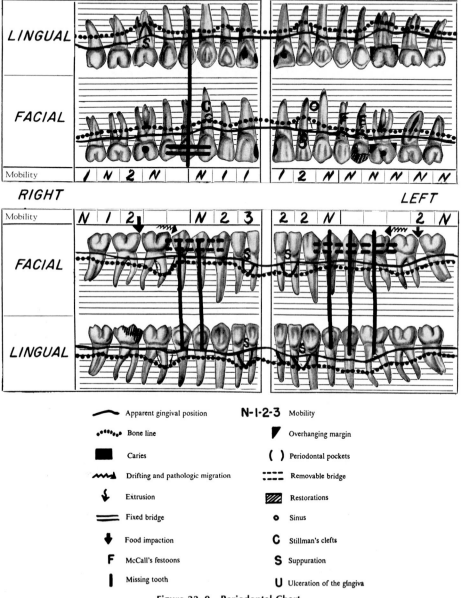

Apparent gingival position	N-1-2-3 Mobility
Bone line	Overhanging margin
Caries	( ) Periodontal pockets
Drifting and pathologic migration	Removable bridge
Extrusion	Restorations
Fixed bridge	o Sinus
Food impaction	C Stillman's clefts
F McCall's festoons	S Suppuration
I Missing tooth	U Ulceration of the gingiva

Figure 33–9 Periodontal Chart.

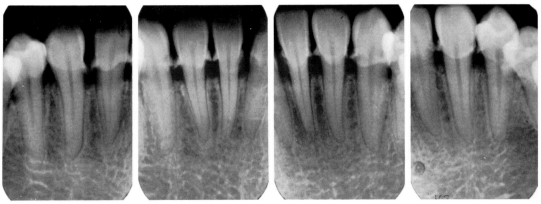

Figure 33–10   Calculus Appears Interproximally as Angular Spurs. The radiopaque image of calculus on the facial and lingual surfaces is superimposed on the teeth.

Gingiva

The gingiva must be dried before accurate observations can be made (Fig. 33–11). Light reflection from moist gingiva obscures detail. In addition to visual examination and exploration with instruments, firm but gentle palpation should be used for detecting pathologic alterations in normal resilience as well as for locating areas of pus formation.

Each of the following features of the gingiva should be considered: **color, size, contour, consistency, surface texture, position** and **ease of bleeding,** and **pain.** No deviation from the normal should be overlooked. The distribution of gingiva disease and acuteness or chronicity should also be noted.

The position of the gingiva warrants special mention. For accurate appraisal of recession, attention should be given to differentiating between the *apparent position* and the *actual position* of the gingival attachment on each tooth surface (Chap. 9).

Periodontal pockets

Examination for periodontal pockets should include consideration of the following: (1) presence and distribution on each tooth surface, (2) the type of pocket—whether it is suprabony or infrabony, simple, compound or complex; (3) pocket depth; (4) level of attachment on the root.

The only accurate method of detecting and evaluating periodontal pockets is care-

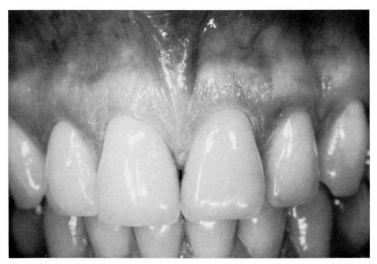

Figure 33–11   Normal Gingiva. Normal surface features are revealed by drying the gingiva.

ful exploration with a pocket probe or explorer. **Pockets are not detected or measured by radiographic examination.** The periodontal pocket is a soft tissue change. Radiographs indicate areas of bone loss where pockets may be suspected. They do not show whether pockets are present in these areas, nor do they reveal pocket depth or the location of the base of the pocket on the tooth surface.

Gutta percha points or calibrated silver points[20] are used with the x-ray to assist in determining the level of attachment of periodontal pockets and their relationship to the bone (Fig. 33–12). They may be used effectively for individual pockets, but their routine use throughout the mouth would be rather cumbersome. Clinical examination and probing are more direct and efficient.

In the examination for periodontal pockets, check each tooth surface. Probes calibrated in millimeters are available for measuring pocket depth. The probe should be inserted in line with the vertical axis of the tooth until the blunt end contacts the bottom of the pocket. The probe should not be forced into the underlying tissues. Calibrated pocket marking forceps (Fig. 33–13) may be used to locate the bottom of the pocket and mark it on the surface of the gingiva.

The level of attachment of the base of the pocket on the tooth surface is of greater diagnostic significance than the depth of the pocket. Pocket depth is simply the distance between the base of the pocket and the gingival margin. It may vary from time to time in untreated periodontal disease. For

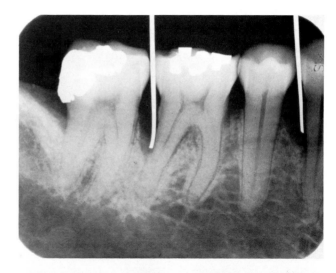

Figure 33–12 Blunted Silver Points Assist in Locating Base of Pockets.

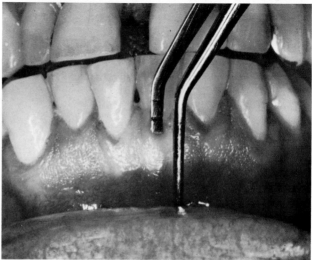

Figure 33–13 Calibrated Pocket Marking Forceps. The blunt calibrated end is inserted vertically into the pocket. The bottom of the pocket is marked on the outer surface by pressing the forceps together.

example, gingival bleeding caused by accidental mechanical irritation results in shrinkage of the pocket wall and some reduction in pocket depth. The level of attachment of the base of the pocket on the tooth surface affords a better indication of the severity of periodontal disease. **Shallow pockets attached at the level of the apical third of the roots connote more severe destruction than deep pockets attached in the coronal third of the roots.**

The level of attachment of the base of a periodontal pocket may vary on different surfaces of the same tooth and even on different areas of the same surface. Inserting the probe on all surfaces and in more than one area on individual surfaces reveals the depth and conformation of the pocket.

Suppuration

To determine whether pus is present in a periodontal pocket, the ball of the index finger is applied along the lateral aspect of the marginal gingiva and pressure is applied in a rolling motion toward the crown. Visual examination alone without digital pressure is not enough. Because the purulent exudate is formed on the inner pocket wall, the external appearance of the pocket may give no indication of its presence. Pus formation does not occur in all periodontal pockets, but digital pressure often reveals it in pockets where it is not suspected (Fig. 33–14).

Mucosa in relation to the root apices

Palpating the oral mucosa in the lateral and apical areas of the root is helpful in locating the origin of radiating pain which the patient cannot localize. Infection deep in the periodontal tissues and the early stages of periodontal abscess formation may also be detected by palpation.

Sinus formation

In children a sinus orifice along the lateral aspect of a root is usually the result of peri-

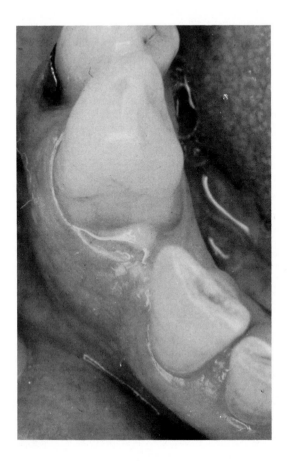

Figure 33–14 Pus Formation on the mesial surface of mandibular canine.

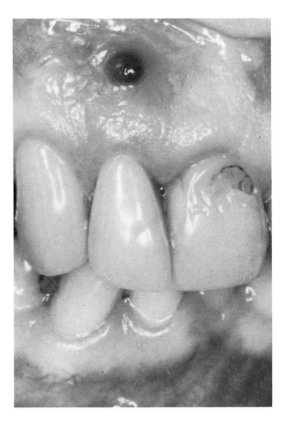

Figure 33–15 **Nodular Mass** at the orifice of a draining sinus.

apical infection of a deciduous tooth. In the permanent dentition it may be caused by a periodontal abscess as well as apical involvement. The orifice may be patent and draining or it may be closed and appear as a red nodular mass (Fig. 33–15). Exploration of such masses with a probe usually reveals a pinpoint orifice that communicates with an underlying sinus.

Alveolar bone loss

Alveolar bone levels are evaluated by clinical and radiographic examination. Probing is helpful for determining the height and contour of the facial and lingual bone obscured on the radiograph by the dense roots, and for determining the architecture of the interdental bone.

THE RADIOGRAPH IN THE DIAGNOSIS OF PERIODONTAL DISEASE

The x-ray is a valuable aid in the diagnosis of periodontal disease, the determination of

the prognosis and the evaluation of the outcome of treatment. **It is an adjunct to the clinical examination, not a substitute for it.** If a choice must be made, a more intelligent diagnosis can be made from the patient without the radiograph, than from radiographs without the patient.

The radiographic image results from the superimposition of tooth, bone and soft tissues in the pathway between the cone of the machine and the film. The x-ray reveals alterations in calcified tissue; it does not reveal current cellular activity, but shows the effects of past cellular experience upon the bone and roots. Changes in the soft tissues of the periodontium require special techniques which have not as yet attained routine clinical usage.

Normal interdental septa

Because the facial and lingual bony plates are obscured by the relatively dense root structure, radiographic evaluation of bone changes in periodontal disease is based upon the appearance of the interdental septa. The interdental septum normally presents a thin radiopaque border, adjacent to the periodontal ligament and at the crest, referred to as the *lamina dura* (Fig. 33–16). It appears radiographically as a continuous white line, but it is perforated by numerous small foramina containing blood vessels, lymphatics and nerves which pass between the periodontal ligament and the bone. Since the lamina dura represents the bone surface lining the tooth socket, the shape and position of the root and changes in the angulation of the x-ray beam produce considerable variations in its appearance.[29]

The width and shape of the interdental septum and the angle of the crest normally vary according to the convexity of the proximal tooth surfaces and the level of the cemento enamel junction of the approximating teeth.[46] The interdental space and the interdental septum between teeth with prominently convex proximal surfaces are wider anteroposteriorly than between teeth with relatively flat proximal surfaces. The faciolingual diameter of the bone is related to the width of the proximal root surface. The angulation of the crest of the interdental septum is generally parallel to a line between the cemento-enamel junction of the approximating teeth (Fig. 33–16). When there is a difference in the levels of the cemento-enamel junctions, the crest of the interdental bone is angulated rather than horizontal.

Distortion produced by variation in radiographic technique

Variations in x-ray technique produce artefacts which limit the diagnostic value of the radiograph. The bone level, the pattern of bone destruction, the width of the periodontal ligament space,[61] and the radiodensity, trabecular pattern and marginal contour of the interdental septum are modified by altering the exposure and development time, the type of film and the x-ray angulation.[38] Standardized reproducible techniques are required to obtain reliable radiographs for pre- and post-treatment comparisons.[40, 43] A grid calibrated in millimeters, superimposed upon the finished film, is helpful for comparing bone levels in radiographs taken under similar conditions[8] (Fig. 33–17).

The following are useful facts regarding the effects of angulation:

The long cone paralleling technique projects the most realistic image of the level of the alveolar bone[12] (Fig. 33–18). The bisection of the angle technique increases the projection and makes the bone margin appear closer to the crown; the level of the facial bone margin is distorted more than the lingual (Fig. 33–18). Shifting the cone mesially or distally without changing the horizontal plane projects the x-rays obliquely and changes the shape of the interdental bone, the width of the periodontal ligament

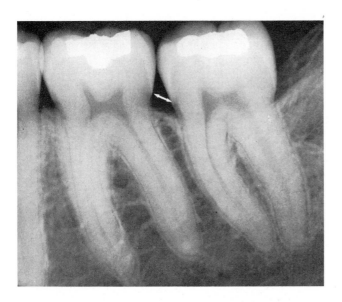

Figure 33–16 Crest of Interdental Septum Normally Parallel to a Line Drawn Between the Cemento-Enamel Junctions of Adjacent Teeth *(arrow).* Note also the radiopaque lamina dura around the roots and interdental septum.

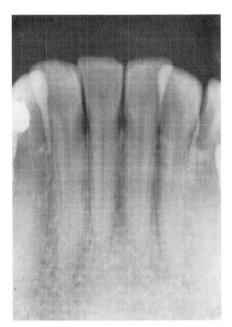

Figure 33–17   Radiograph with Superimposed Grid Calibrated in Millimeters.

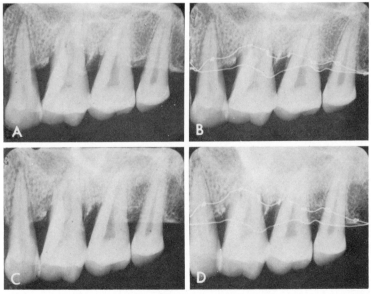

Figure 33–18   Long Cone Paralleling Technique and Bisection of the Angle Technique compared. (Courtesy of Dr. Benjamin Patur, Hartford, Conn.) *A*, Long cone technique. Radiograph of dried specimen. *B*, Long cone technique. Same specimen. The smooth wire is on the margin of the facial plate and the knotted wire is on the lingual plate to show their relative positions. *C*, Bisection of the angle technique. Same specimen. *D*, Bisection of the angle technique. Same specimen. Both bone margins are shifted toward the crown, the facial margin (*smooth wire*) more than the lingual margin (*knotted wire*) creating the illusion that the lingual bone margin has shifted apically.

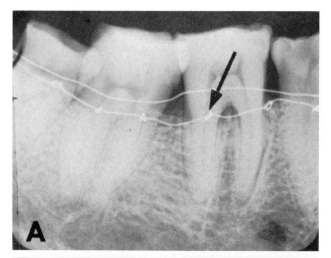

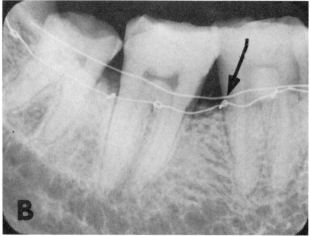

Figure 33–19 Distortion by Oblique Projection. *A,* **Long Cone Technique.** The smooth wire is on the facial bony plate, the knotted wire on the lingual. Note the knot (*arrow*) near the center of the distal root of the first molar, which shows bifurcation involvement. *B,* **Long Cone Technique. Cone Is Placed Distally Projecting the Rays Mesially and Obliquely.** The oblique projection shifts the image of all structures mesially. *The structures closest to the cone shift the most.* This creates the illusion that the knot (*arrow*) has moved distally. Note that the bifurcation involvement shown in *A* is obliterated in *B.*

space and the appearance of the lamina dura, and may distort the extent of furcation involvement (**Fig. 33–19**).

Bone destruction in periodontal disease

Because the radiograph does not reveal minor destructive changes in bone,[1,2,44] periodontal disease that produces even slight radiographic changes has progressed beyond its earliest stages. The earliest signs of periodontal disease must therefore be detected clinically. The radiographic image tends to be less severe than the actual bone loss.[59] The difference between the alveolar crest height and the radiographic appearance ranges from 0 to 1.6 mm.,[45] mostly accounted for by x-ray angulation.

The amount of bone loss

The x-ray is an indirect method for determining the amount of bone loss in periodontal disease. It indicates the amount of remaining bone rather than the amount lost. The amount of bone loss is estimated to be the difference between the physiologic bone level of the patient and the height of remaining bone. **To determine the amount of bone loss in periodontal disease it is necessary to (1) determine the age of the patient, (2) estimate the physiologic bone level at that age and (3) determine the difference between the physiologic bone level and the level of remaining bone indicated on the radiograph.** The same level of remaining bone indicates a different degree of bone loss in patients in different age groups (**Fig. 33–20**).

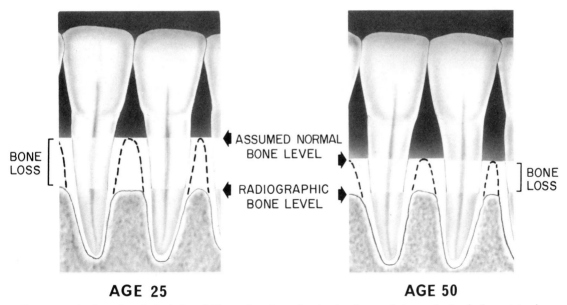

Figure 33–20   Bone Loss in Periodontal Disease is estimated to be the distance between the level of remaining bone and the bone level assumed to be normal for the patient's age. The same radiographic bone level represents greater bone loss in a 25-year-old patient than in a patient of age 50.

The distribution of bone loss

The distribution of bone loss is an important diagnostic sign. It points to the location of destructive local factors in different areas of the mouth, and in relation to differnet surfaces of the same tooth.

The pattern of bone destruction

In periodontal disease, the interdental septa undergo changes that affect the **lamina dura, the crestal radiodensity, the size and shape of the medullary spaces, and the height and contour of the bone.** The interdental septa may be reduced in height, with the crest horizontal and perpendicular to the long axis of the adjacent teeth (Fig. 33–21), or they may present angular or arcuate defects (Fig. 33–22). The former condition is called **horizontal bone loss,** and the latter, **angular or vertical bone loss or bone defects.**

Radiographs do not indicate the internal morphology or depth of crater-like interdental defects which appear as angular or vertical defects, nor do they reveal the extent of involvement on the facial and lingual surfaces. There are several reasons for this. Facial and lingual surface bone destruction is obscured by the dense root structure, and

bone destruction on the mesial and distal root surfaces may be partially hidden by a dense mylohyoid ridge (Fig. 33–23).

Dense cortical plates on the facial and lingual surfaces of the interdental septa obscure destruction which occurs in the intervening cancellous bone. This means that it is possible to have a deep crater in the bone between the facial and lingual plates without radiographic indication of its presence. In order for destruction of the interproximal cancellous bone to be recorded radiographically, the cortical bone must be involved. Reduction of only 0.5 or 1.0 mm. in the thickness of the cortical plate is sufficient to permit radiographic visualization of destruction of the inner cancellous trabeculae.[41]

Passing a probe through the gingiva to the bone helps determine the architecture of osseous defects produced by periodontal disease. It also aids in the location of dehiscences and fenestrations. Gutta percha packed around the teeth increases the usefulness of the radiograph for detecting the morpholoby of osseous craters and involvement of the facial and lingual surfaces (Fig. 33–24). However, surgical exposure and visual examination provide the most definitive information regarding the bone architecture produced by periodontal destruction.[42]

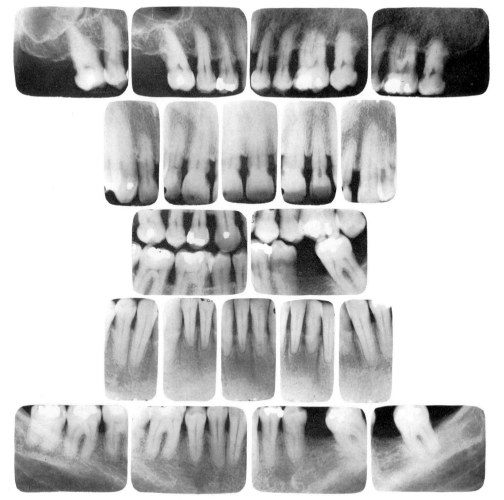

Figure 33-21 Complete Intraoral Series Showing Generalized Horizontal Bone Loss.

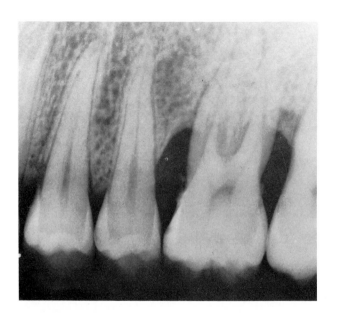

Figure 33-22 Angular Bone Loss on First Molar with Involvement of the Trifurcation.

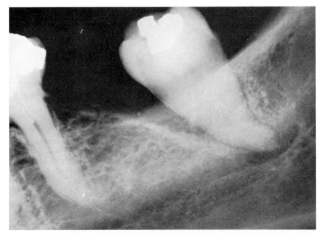

Figure 33–23 Angular Bone Loss on Mandibular Molar Partially Obscured by Dense Mylohyoid Ridge.

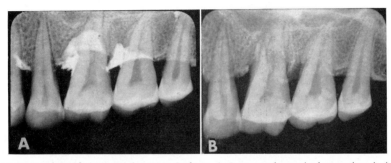

Figure 33–24 Gutta Percha Aids in Detecting Bone Defects. *A,* Gutta percha packed around teeth shows interproximal and facial and lingual bone loss. *B,* Same area without gutta percha gives little indication of the extent of bone involvement.

Radiographic changes in periodontitis

The following is the sequence of radiographic changes in periodontitis, and the tissue changes which produce them:

Fuzziness and a break in the continuity of the lamina dura at the mesial or distal aspect of the crest of the interdental septum are the earliest radiographic changes in periodontitis (Fig. 33–25, *A* and *B*).

These result from extension of inflammation from the gingiva into the bone and associated widening of the vessel channels, and a reduction in calcified tissue at the septal margin.

A wedge-shaped radiolucent area is formed at the mesial or distal aspect of the crest of the septal bone (Fig. 33–25, *B*). The apex of the area is pointed in the direction of the root.

This is produced by resorption of the bone of the lateral aspect of the interdental septum with an associated widening of the periodontal space.

The destructive process extends across the crest of the interdental septum and the height is reduced. Finger-like radiolucent projections extend from the crest into the septum (Fig. 33–25, *C*).

The radiolucent projections into the interdental septum are the result of the deeper extension of the inflammation into the bone. Inflammatory cells and fluid, proliferation of connective tissue cells, and increased osteoclasis cause increased bone resorption along the endosteal margins of the medullary spaces. The radiopaque projections, separating the radiolucent spaces, are the composite images of the partially eroded bone trabeculae.

The height of the interdental septum (Fig. 33–25, *D*) is progressively reduced by extension of inflammation and resorption of bone.

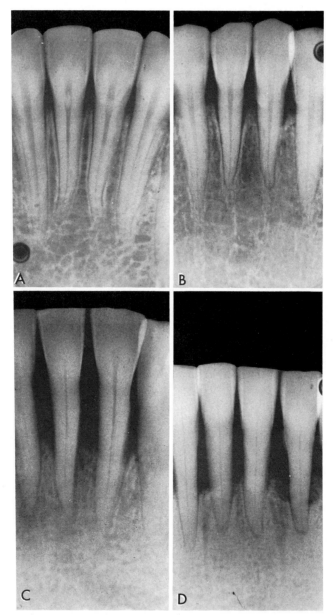

Figure 33–25   Radiographic Changes in Periodontitis. *A,* Normal appearance of interdental septa. *B,* Fuzziness and a break in the continuity of the lamina dura at the crest of the bone distal to the central incisor (*left*). There are wedge shaped radiolucent areas at the crests of the other interdental septa. *C,* Radiolucent projections from the crest into the interdental septum indicate extension of destructive processes. *D,* Severe bone loss.

When inflammation is the sole destructive factor in periodontal disease, the crest of the interdental septum is horizontal; when inflammation is combined with trauma from occlusion, the destruction is angular.

Radiographic changes in periodontosis

Periodontosis is characterized by a combination of the following radiographic features:

Loss of alveolar bone is localized in the early stages to a single tooth or group of teeth, and tends to become generalized as the disease progresses. The bone loss occurs initially in the maxillary and mandibular incisor and first molar areas, usually bilaterally (Fig. 33–26). The interdental septa present vertical, arc-like or angular destructive patterns. When the bone loss is generalized, it is least pronounced in the mandibular premolar areas.

A generalized alteration in the trabecular pattern of the alveolar bone consists of less clearly defined trabecular markings and increase in the size of the cancellous spaces.

The diagnosis of trauma from occlusion

Trauma from occlusion referes to *tissue injury* produced by occlusal forces—not to the occlusal forces themselves. The criterion that determines whether an occlusal force is injurious is whether it causes damage in the periodontal tissues; therefore the diagnosis of trauma from occlusion is made from the condition of the periodontal tissues. The periodontal findings are then used as a guide for locating the responsible occlusal relationships.

Periodontal findings that suggest the presence of trauma from occlusion are the following: excessive tooth mobility, particularly in teeth with radiographic evidence of widened periodontal space (Fig. 33–27), vertical and angular bone destruction (Figs. 33–23 and 33–28), infrabony pockets, and pathologic migration, especially of the anterior teeth.

Additional findings which suggest the presence of abnormal occlusal relationships are neuromuscular distrubances such as impaired function of the masticatory musculature, which in severe cases results

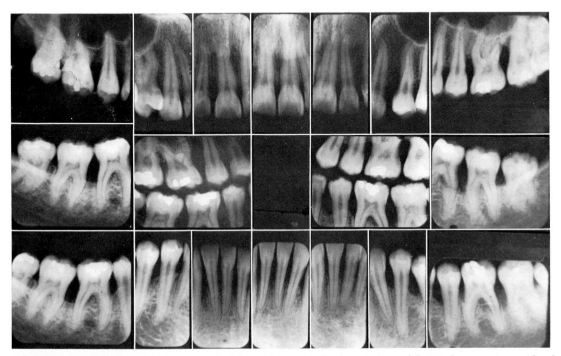

Figure 33–26 Periodontosis. The accentuated bone destruction in the anterior and first molar areas is considered characteristic of periodontosis.

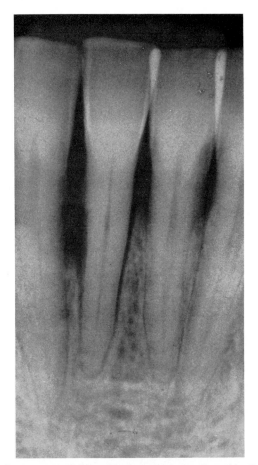

Figure 33–27 Widened Periodontal Space Caused by Trauma from Occlusion. Note the increased density of the surrounding bone caused by new bone formation in response to increased occlusal forces.

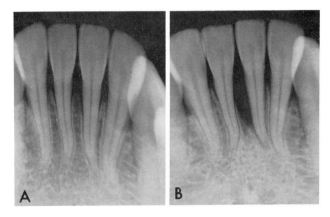

Figure 33–28 Angular Bone Loss Associated with Trauma from Occlusion. *A,* Thickening of periodontal space at crest of bone adjacent to central incisors. *B,* Six years later, angular bone destruction with formation of hemiseptum.

in muscle spasm and temporomandibular joint disorders.

Special mention should be made of pathologic migration of the anterior teeth as a sign of trauma from occlusion. Premature tooth contacts in the posterior region that deflect the mandible anteriorly contribute to destruction of the periodontium of the maxillary anterior teeth and pathologic migration (Figs. 33–29 and 33–30).

Additional radiographic criteria in the diagnosis of periodontal disease

A radiopaque horizontal line across the roots demarcates the portion of the root where the labial and/or lingual bony plate has been partially or completely destroyed from the remaining bone-supported portion (Fig. 33–31).

Vessel canals in the alveolar bone. Hirschfeld[20] described linear and circular radiolucent areas produced by interdental canals and their foramina respectively (Fig. 33–32). These canals indicate the course of the vascular supply of the bone and are normal radiographic findings. The radiographic image of the canals is frequently so prominent, particularly in the anterior region of the mandible, that they might be confused with radiolucence resulting from periodontal disease.

Differentiation between physiologic atrophy and chronic periodontal disease. In older persons it is sometimes necessary to determine whether the bone level is the result of physiological atrophy or if destructive periodontal disease is a contributory

factor. Clinical examination is the basic determinant. However, radiographically detectable alterations in the normal clearcut peripheral outline of the septa are corroborating evidence of periodontal disease.

SKELETAL DISTURBANCES MANIFESTED IN THE JAWS

Skeletal disturbances may produce changes in the jaws[5,15] that affect the interpretation of radiographs from the periodontal viewpoint. Included among the diseases in which destruction of tooth-supporting bone may occur are the following:

Osteitis fibrosa cystica (von Recklinghausen's disease of bone) causes a diffuse granular mottling, scattered "cyst-like" radiolucent areas throughout the jaws, and a generalized disappearance of the lamina dura.[48,55]

In *Paget's disease,* the radiographic appearance of the jaws varies. The normal trabecular pattern may be replaced by a hazy diffuse meshwork of closely knit, fine trabecular markings, with the lamina dura absent (Fig. 33–33), or there may be scattered radiolucent areas containing irregularly shaped radiopaque zones.[16]

Fibrous dysplasia may appear as a small radiolucent area at a root apex or as an extensive radiolucent area with irregularly arranged trabecular markings.[14] There may be enlargement of the cancellous spaces, with distortion of the normal trabecular pattern and obliteration of the lamina dura (Fig. 33–34).

In *Hand-Schüller-Christian* disease, the

(Text continued on page 515)

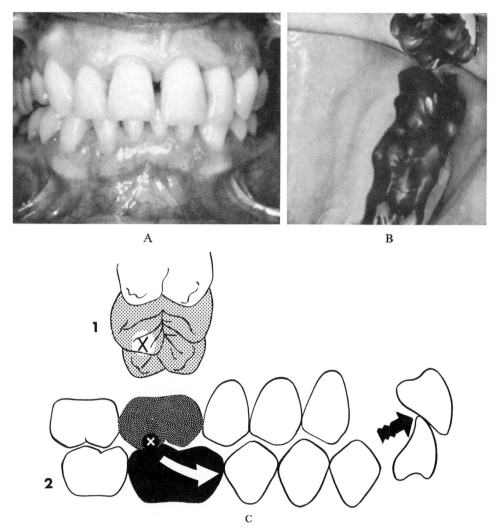

A

B

C

Figure 33–29   Pathologic Migration Associated with Trauma from Occlusion. *A,* Early pathologic migration of maxillary left central incisor. *B,* Mirror view of wax registration, showing prematurity on the mesiolingual incline of the maxillary molar which deflects the mandible anteriorly and traumatizes the maxillary incisors. *C,* Diagrammatic representation showing (1) Prematurity (X) on the maxillary molar and (2) anterior glide of the mandible (*arrow*) with impact against the maxillary incisors.

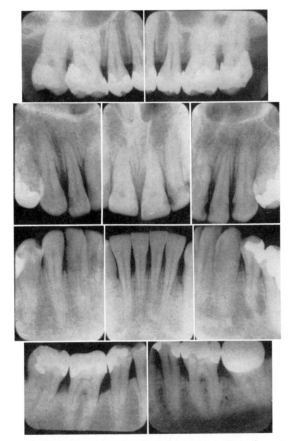

Figure 33–29 *Continued.* *D,* Radiographs of patient shown in *A.* Note the extensive bone destruction around the maxillary second molars and the maxillary and mandibular incisors.

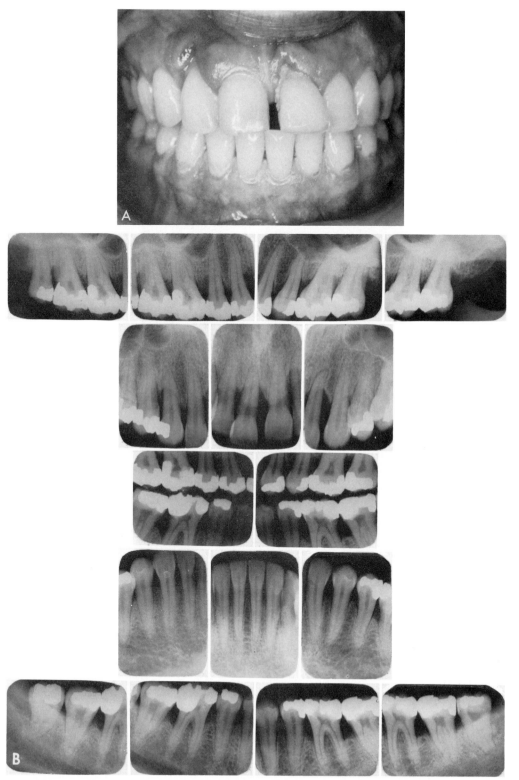

Figure 33–30   Periodontal Disease with Pathologic Migration of the Anterior Teeth. *A,* Periodontal inflammation and tissue loss, and pathologic migration in the anterior maxilla. *B,* Radiograph showing generalized bone loss and the angular pattern of bone destruction in the anterior maxilla.

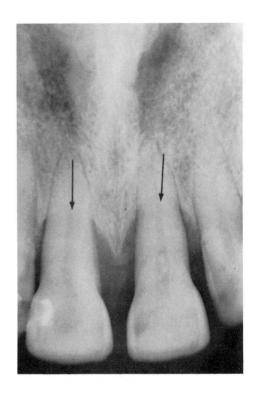

Figure 33–31 Horizontal Line across the roots of the central incisors (*arrows*). The area of the roots below the horizontal lines are partially or completely denuded of the facial and/or lingual bony plates.

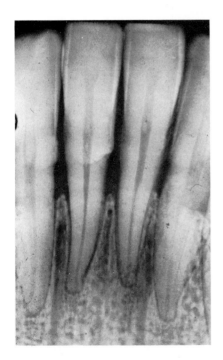

Figure 33–32 **Prominent Vessel Canals in the Mandible.**

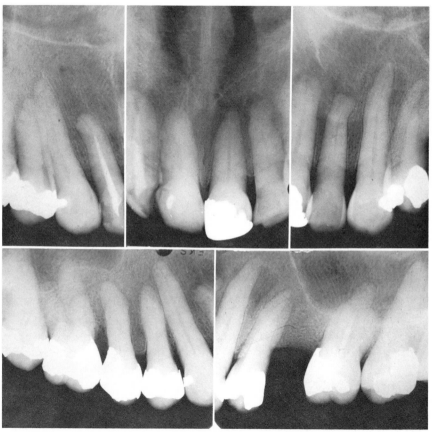

Figure 33–33   Altered Trabecular Pattern and Diminution in the Prominence of the Lamina Dura in Paget's Disease.

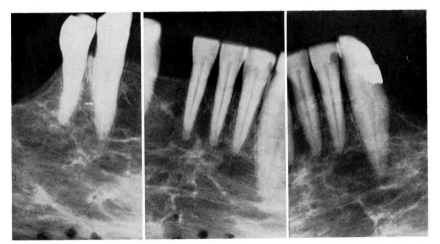

Figure 33–34   Osteoporosis and Altered Trabecular Arrangement in Fibrous Dysplasia.

radiographic appearance is that of single or multiple areas of radiolucency. Mobility of the teeth results from loss of bony support. *Letterer-Siwe disease and Gaucher's disease* may present comparable changes (Fig. 33–35).

Eosinophilic granuloma[49,56] appears as single or multiple radiolucent areas, which may be unrelated to the teeth or entail destruction of the tooth-supporting bone (Fig. 33–36).

Numerous radiolucent areas occur when the jaws are involved by *multiple myeloma.*

In *osteopetrosis* (marble-bone disease; Albers-Schönberg's disease),[10] the outlines of the roots may be obscured by diffuse

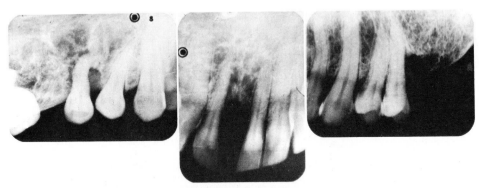

Figure 33–35   Osteoporosis in Gaucher's Disease.

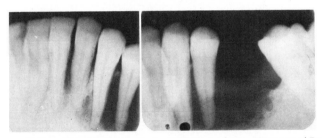

Figure 33–36   Bone Destruction Caused by Eosinophilic Granuloma. (Courtesy of Dr. Irving Salman).

radiopacity of the jaws. In less severe cases, the increased density is confined to the bone in relation to the nutrient canals and the lamina dura.

In *scleroderma* (Chap. 13) the periodontal ligament is uniformly widened at the expense of the surrounding alveolar bone (Fig. 33–37).

LABORATORY AIDS IN DIAGNOSIS

The Biopsy

The biopsy in the diagnosis of neoplasms

The diagnosis of neoplasms should be established by microscopic examination. If it is to serve the purpose for which it is intended, certain principles should govern the biopsy technique.

METHOD OF TAKING A BIOPSY. *Site of Biopsy.* 1. Where the lesion is small, it should be totally excised. The excision should be wide enough and deep enough to include a border of healthy tissue along the entire cut surface.

2. Where the size of the lesion is such that complete excision is not possible or feasible, *obtain a specimen representative of the lesion:*

a. *Select that portion of the lesion which demonstrates all of the pathologic changes noted clinically.* If this is not possible with one tissue section, select several areas.

b. *Take thin deep sections rather than broad shallow sections.* A small superficial tab of tissue may show nothing more than degenerative, inflammatory or necrotic changes.

c. *The section should include tissue at and beyond the lateral margins and base of the lesion.* In this way the transition from healthy to diseased tissue can be followed.

TECHNIQUE FOR OBTAINING TISSUE SPECIMEN. There are several biopsy techniques.

Incision. Incision can be performed with the scalpel or high frequency cutting current. Removal of the tissue with a sharp blade appears to be the method of choice. Electrosurgery may be used to advantage

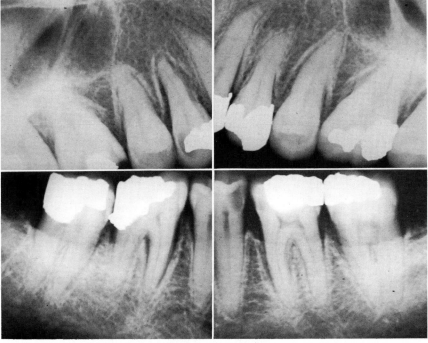

Figure 33–37 Scleroderma, showing typical uniform widening of the periodontal ligament and thickening of the lamina dura. (Courtesy of Drs. David F. Mitchell and Anand P. Chaudhry.)

in highly vascular tumors where bleeding may be a difficult complication.

Punch Biopsy. This method is of limited value in the oral cavity. Its greatest applicability is in the removal of small tissue specimens from inaccessible areas, such as the maxillary sinus and lateral or posterior pharyngeal walls.

Curettage. Tissue specimens are curetted from bony cavities and sinus tracts.

HANDLING OF THE TISSUE SPECIMEN.
1. The tissue should not be crushed or mutilated.

2. It should be placed in fixative immediately. Ten per cent formalin is an acceptable fixative. The volume of fixative should be approximately 20 times the volume of the tissue specimen. If the pathologist to whom you submit biopsy specimens prefers another fixative, it would be wise to keep on hand several small bottles containing this fixative.

If the specimen is too thick, only the peripheral portions of the tissue will be completely infiltrated and fixed, while the central area will undergo degenerative changes.

3. The specimen bottle should be properly labeled. Indicate whether the tissue specimen is soft tissue only, or whether it contains bone, and the time at which it was taken.

4. A brief history should accompany the specimen. This should include the name, age and sex of the patient, the location, a gross description of the lesion, its duration, the rate of growth or change in growth rate, and the method used in obtaining the specimen.

The biopsy in the diagnosis of gingival and mucosal disease

The gingival biopsy is important in the diagnosis of gingival disturbances. Microscopic study of gingival biopsies is often the only method of detecting local and systemic interrelationships that cannot be discerned by clinical examination. For example, amyloid is present in the gingiva in 78 per cent of patients with amyloidosis,[52] many of whom present no clinical gingival changes.

The amyloid is deposited extracellularly adjacent to the capillaries in the papillary layer immediately subjacent to the basal layer of the epithelium, and appears as amorphous hyalinized material which stains metachromatically with crystal violet.[32]

The presence of eosinophilic granuloma may be detected by gingival biopsy.[18] In addition to differentiating between different types of gingival enlargement, gingival biopsy is indispensable when the presence of diseases such as desquamative gingivitis, benign mucous membrane pemphigoid, pemphigus or lichen planus is suspected.

The marginal and attached gingiva should be included in the biopsy (Fig. 33–38). Inflammatory changes in the gingival margin tend to obscure any alterations that may be produced by a systemic disturbance. Inclusion of the attached gingiva, in which the effect of local irritants is less likely to be present, offers an opportunity to investigate tissue changes that may be produced by systemic disturbances.

Exfoliative Cytology

Exfoliative cytology is a diagnostic procedure consisting of the microscopic examination of cells obtained by scraping the surface of the suspected area, or by rinsing the oral cavity. The former is preferred. Its reliability for the diagnosis of cancer is 86 per cent, as compared with the close to 100 per cent reliability of an oral biopsy.[54] Cytology is not a substitute for biopsy but it is valuable if a biopsy cannot be done for some reason, and also in screening large groups of people for the presence of malig-

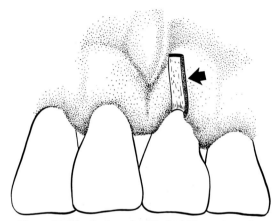

Figure 33–38 Rectangular Gingival Biopsy (*arrow*) **Includes Marginal and Attached Gingiva.**

nancy, provided it is used in conjunction with a careful oral examination. It is also helpful in the diagnosis of bullous and vesicular oral lesions.

To obtain a specimen, the entire surface of the abnormal mucosa is firmly scraped with the edge of a wooden tongue depressor. The material thus removed is spread directly on a glass slide and immediately fixed in 95 per cent alcohol and submitted for microscopic diagnosis.[50]

LABORATORY AIDS USED IN THE DIAGNOSIS OF SYSTEMIC DISEASE

When the nature and severity of gingival and periodontal disease cannot be explained by local causes, the possibility of contributing systemic factors must be explored. The dentist must understand the oral manifestations of systemic disease so that he can advise the physician regarding the type of systemic disturbance which may be involved in individual cases.

Numerous laboratory tests aid in the diagnosis of systemic diseases. The manner in which they are performed and the interpretation of findings are found in standard texts on the subject.[60] Those pertinent to the diagnosis of systemic disturbances often mainifested in the oral cavity are referred to briefly here.

The Hemogram

Blood smear

Examination of a stained blood smear reveals information regarding (1) the morphology, staining reaction and maturity of the red cells, (2) morphology and maturity of the various types of white cells, and (3) presence of parasites in the blood.

Red cell count

In males the average red cell count is 5.4 million per cubic millimeter with a range of 4.6 to 6.2. In females, the count is slightly lower with an average of 4.8 million per cubic millimeter, and a range of 4.2 to 5.4. A lowered red cell count or oligocythemia is present in pernicious anemia (1.5 to 2.5), hemolytic jaundice (1.5 to 3.0), iron

deficiency anemia (1.5 to 4.7), acute aplastic anemia (1.0 or less), chronic leukemia (average 4.2) and acute leukemia (1.0). An increased red cell count is seen in polycythemia (7.0 to 12.0).

Hemoglobin content

Total hemoglobin may be measured by the cyanmethemoglobin method. This is a spectrophotometric method and is the preferred technique.[6] Normal values of hemoglobulin vary with age and sex. The normal values for adult males is 16 ± 2.0 gm./100 ml., and for adult females is 14 ± 2.0 gm./100 ml. blood.[62]

White cell count

The normal number of leukocytes ranges from 5000 to 10,000 per cubic millimeter of blood, with an average of 7500.

The differential white cell count

Leukocytosis is the term applied to an increase in the number of white blood cells. Lymphocytic leukocytosis is an increase in the total white cell count with a predominance in the number of lymphocytes. It usually occurs in chronic inflammatory diseases, such as tuberculosis or syphilis, and in malaria, whooping cough and Hodgkin's disease. A neutrophilic leukocytosis is observed in a number of pathologic states: (a) in diseases caused by a pyogenic or pus-producing organism; (b) tissue necrosis, as for example, myocardial infarction; (c) acute massive hemorrhage; (d) malignant neoplasms; (e) gout; and (f) nephritis. An eosinophilic leukocytosis (eosinophilia) is seen in (a) parasitic dis-

TABLE 33–3 NORMAL VALUES FOR DIFFERENTIAL WHITE CELL COUNT

	Per Cent
Neutrophilic polymorphonuclear leukocytes	60–70
Segmented cells 52–67%; stab cells 3–5%; juveniles 0–1%, myelocytes 0%.	
Eosinophilic polymorphonuclear leukocytes	1–4
Basophilic polymorphonuclear leukocytes	0.25–0.50
Lymphocytes	25–28
Monocytes	2–6

eases caused by worms (helminthic infestations): (b) allergic diseases, such as asthma, hay fever and angioneurotic edema; (c) Hodgkin's disease; (d) periarteritis nodosa; and (e) skin diseases, such as pemphigus and psoriasis.

Leukemia represents an unrestrained growth of leukopoietic tissue resulting in the production of excessive numbers of immature white cells. Depending upon the cell type involved, myelogenous, lymphatic and monocytic leukemia can be distinguished. Leukemia may be either acute, subacute or chronic. During the course of leukemia, there may be periods when the white cell count is reduced instead of elevated. These periods are referred to as the aleukemic phases of leukemia (aleukemic leukemia), and are thought to be due to the inability of the white cells to leave the markedly hyperplastic marrow or lymphoid tissue. In the bone marrow, the hyperplastic leukopoietic tissue may encroach upon tissue that is forming red cells and blood platelets and cause anemia and thrombocytopenia, with all the complications associated with such deficiencies. Pallor, fatigue and weakness and tiny hemorrhages caused by anemia and platelet deficiency are often the presenting symptoms of leukemia.

A reduction in the white cell count below 5000 per cubic millimeter is termed leukopenia. The terms *leukopenia* and *granulopenia* are used interchangeably, because in most cases the granulocytes are the cells that are reduced in number. A leukopenia may be seen in a number of disease processes: bacterial infections, such as typhoid fever; viral diseases, such as measles; protozoal infections, malignant neoplasms, allergic diseases, aleukemic leukemia and agranulocytosis. *Agranulocytosis is a severe form of leukopenia in which the granulocytes may be completely absent from the blood, and the white cell count may be reduced to several hundred per cubic millimeter. In the absence of granulocytes, particularly the neutrophils, infections tend to run a rapid and often fatal course.

Erythrocyte sedimentation rate

The sedimentation rate is the rate at which red cells settle in shed blood. Increase in the sedimentation rate occurs in diseases characterized by widespread tissue injury and destruction, as in rheumatic fever, tuberculosis, arthritis, myocardial infarction and malignant neoplasms. The sedimentation rate is usually normal (Westergren method: 0–15 mm./hr. in men; 0–20 mm./hr. in women; 0–10 mm./hr. in children) or only slightly elevated in acute inflammations and infections of a very localized nature.

Laboratory Tests Employed in Exploring the Etiology of Spontaneous or Excessive Bleeding

COAGULATION TIME. The coagulation or clotting time is the time necessary for blood to clot after it has been removed and placed in a test tube or other container. For the determination of the clotting time, blood may either be obtained by skin puncture or venipuncture. The normal clotting time of blood obtained by skin puncture is 2 to 6 minutes. For blood obtained by vein puncture, the normal range is between 5 and 15 minutes. When siliconized tubes are used, the range is 19 to 60 minutes.

BLEEDING TIME. The bleeding time is the time necessary for a small cut to stop bleeding. In the *Duke* method for the determination of the bleeding time, a small cut is made in the ear lobe, and the blood is blotted with filter paper at 30 second intervals until bleeding ceases. The time interval between the first and the last drop is taken as the bleeding time. The normal range is 1 to 6 minutes, with the majority between 1 and 3 minutes. With the *Ivy* method, which entails the use of a cuff, the normal range is 1 to 9 minutes.

CLOT RETRACTION TIME AND CHARACTER OF THE CLOT. The clot retraction time is defined as the time it takes for a blood clot to retract from the wall of a test tube in which the blood is placed. Although the phenomenon of retractility is in some way related to the platelets, it is independent of the coagulation time. Usually the clot begins to retract within a few minutes to one hour after it is formed. Defective clots with prolonged retraction time are indicative of platelet deficiency.

THE PROTHROMBIN TIME. The prothrombin time is the time in seconds required for the formation of fibrin in oxalated plasma that has been recalcified after throm-

TABLE 33-4 CHARACTERISTICS OF THE VARIOUS HEMORRHAGIC DISEASES

Disease	Clotting Time	Clot Retraction Time	Bleeding Time	Platelet Count	Rumpel-Leede Test	Prothrombin Time
1. Idiopathic thrombocytopenic purpura	N	+	+	−	+	N
2. Hemophilia	+	N	N	N	N	N
3. Hereditary hemorrhagic telangiectasia	N	N	N	N	N	N
4. Pseudo-hemophilia	N	N	+	N	N	N
5. Secondary thrombocytopenic purpura	N	+	+	−	+	N
6. Anaphylactic purpura	N	N	±	N	+	N
7. Liver disease	+	N	±	N	N	+

N — normal
+ — prolonged
− — shortened

boplastin in excess has been added (Quick's method of determination). The normal prothrombin time is 12 to 14 seconds. The clotting mechanism will usually not be impaired until the prothrombin level has been reduced to approximately 20 per cent of normal.

CAPILLARY FRAGILITY TEST. The test most frequently employed in the determination of increased capillary fragility is the *Rumpel-Leede* test. A blood pressure cuff is placed on the upper arm and a pressure is maintained half way between systolic pressure for eight minutes. The appearance of more than 10 petechiae (tiny hemorrhages) in a circle 5 cm. in diameter below the bend of the elbow is indicative of increased capillary fragility.

The *characteristics of the various hemorrhagic diseases* are presented in Table 33-4.

BONE MARROW STUDIES. Aspiration biopsies are commonly employed in the investigation of blood dyscrasias. Such biopsies are usually taken from the sternum; the other sites are the ileum and spinous processes.

Patients with oral mucous membrane lesions of *suspected allergic origin* may be tested for sensitivity to a wide range of substances. The finding of eosinophilia is suggestive of allergy. A simple patch test for contact sensitivity has been devised for use in the oral cavity.[17] A small rubber suction cup lined with collodion is filled with cotton. The material to be tested is dropped on the cotton, and the cup is fastened to the oral mucosa with dental floss. An average contact time of 20 to 30 minutes is sufficient to elicit a severe localized tissue reaction in cases of sensitivity.

Exploration of Systemic Etiologic Factors in Patients with Excessive Bone Loss

In seeking for systemic disturbances in patients with severe and rapid alveolar bone loss, unexplained on the basis of local factors alone, the possibility of metabolic bone disease should be investigated.[53] The following are useful screening procedures:

1. RADIOGRAPHS OF THE SKULL AND SEVERAL LONG BONES.

2. DETERMINATION OF SERUM CALCIUM, SERUM PHOSPHORUS AND ALKALINE PHOSPHATASE. One must determine the serum calcium (normal values 9 to 11 mg./100 cc.), serum phosphorus (normal values 2.5 to 4.0 mg./100 cc. in adults; 3.5 to 6.0 mg./100 cc. in children) and alkaline phosphatase (normal values 1 to 5 Bodansky units per 100 cc. in adults; 5 to 12/100 cc. in children).

3. THYROID FUNCTION. The average basal metabolic rate of men between the ages of 27 and 50 is from 38 to 40 calories per square meter of body surface per hour, which is slightly above the normal for females of a comparable age group. A variation of ± 10 per cent is within normal range. A rise or decrease in the basal metabolic rate of 25 per cent or more is considered indicative of hyperthyroidism or hypothyroidism respectively.

The commonly used thyroid function test is the protein bound iodine (PBI). This test provides a valid estimate of total hormone bound to protein in peripheral blood in about 90 per cent of cases. The normal range for the PBI is 4.0 to 8.0 μg./100 ml. An increased PBI suggests hyperthyroidism; a decreased PBI suggests hypothyroidism.

Another thyroid function test is a radio-chemical method that measures displacement of I^{131}-labeled thyroxine from thyroxine-binding globulin (TBG) by thyroxine released from the patient's serum. This method is relatively unaffected by contamination and may be valuable in the presence of radiographic contrast media. However, diphenylhydantoin (Dilantin) may cause interference.

4. LABORATORY STUDIES FOR THE DETECTION OF DIABETES MELLITUS. *Fasting Blood Sugar Level.* The normal level of glucose in venous blood in the fasting state (8 to 14 hours after the last meal) is 60 to 100 mg./100 cc. This may normally rise to 160 mg./100 cc. after the ingestion of food. In untreated diabetes mellitus, the fasting blood sugar level may be between 200 and 280 mg./100 cc.

Postprandial Blood Sugar Level. Because the fasting blood glucose level may be normal in mild diabetics, the postprandial level taken two hours after eating is more reliable. Values between the 120 mg./100 cc. (normal) and 140 mg./100 cc. are suspicious. Patients with values above 140 mg./100 cc. are considered to be diabetic.

Glucose Tolerance Test. The glucose tolerance test provides an indication of the patient's capacity to regulate the blood sugar level following the ingestion of carbohydrate. It is the most reliable laboratory indication of the presence of diabetes. In the Standard Glucose Tolerance Test, the glucose level of the blood rises to a maximum (up to 160 mg./100 cc.) within the first hour after the ingestion of a test dose of glucose and returns to normal after two hours. In diabetic patients, the blood glucose rises above 180 mg./100 cc. and does not return to normal even after the two hour interval.

Urinary Glucose. Normally, a very small amount (0.5 to 1.5 gm. daily) of reducing substance is present in the urine, with glucose probably accounting for only a small fraction of this amount. The term glycosuria is applied to the presence of appreciable and abnormal amounts of glucose in urine. Glycosuria is associated with hyperglycemia in diabetes; however, negative urinary findings do not rule out the presence of the disease.

REFERENCES

1. Bender, I. B., and Seltzer, S.: Roentgenographic and Direct Observation of Experimental Lesions in Bone: I. J.A.D.A., 62:152, 1961.
2. Bender, I. B., and Seltzer, S.: Roentgenographic and Direct Observations of Experimental Lesions in Bone: II. J.A.D.A., 62:708, 1961.
3. Berg, M., Burrill, D. Y., and Fosdick, L. S.: Chemical Studies in Periodontal Disease. IV. Putrefactive Rate as Index of Periodontal Disease. J. D. Res., 26:67, 1947.
4. Björn, H., and Holmberg, K.: Radiographic Determination of Periodontal Bone Destruction in Epidemiological Research. Odont. Revy, 17:232, 1966.
5. Cahn, L.: The Jaws in Generalized Skeletal Disease. Ann. Toy. Coll. Surg. England, 8:115, 1951.
6. Cannar, R. K.: Proposal for the Distribution of a Certified Standard for Use in Hemoglobinometry. Am. J. Clin. Path., 25:376, 1955.
7. Easley, J.: Methods of Determining Alveolar Osseous Form. J. Periodont., 38:112, 1967.
8. Everett, F. G., and Fixott, H. C.: Use of an Incorporated Grid in the Diagnosis of Oral Roentgenograms. Oral Surg., 9:1061, 1963.
9. Faber, M.: Causes of Xerostomia. Acta Med. Scandinav., 113:69, 1943.
10. Fairbank, H. A. T.: Osteopetrosis. J. Bone & Joint Surg., 30:339, 1948.
11. Fischman, S. L., and Picozzi, A.: Review of the Literature: The methodology of Clinical Calculus Evaluation. J. Periodont- Periodontics, 40:607, 1969.
12. Fitzgerald, G. M.: Dental Radiography. IV. The Voltage Factor (k.p.). J.A.D.A., 41:19, 1950.
13. Furstenberg, A. C., and Crosby, E.: Disturbance of the Function of the Salivary Glands. Ann. Otol. Rhin. & Laryng., 54:243, 1945.
14. Glickman, I.: Fibrous Dysplasia in Alveolar Bone. Oral Surg., Oral Med. & Oral Path., 1:895, 1948.
15. Glickman, I.: The Oral Cavity; in S. L. Robbins: Textbook of Pathology. Philadelphia, W. B. Saunders Co., 1957, p. 711.
16. Glickman, I., and Glidden, S.: Paget's Disease of the Maxillae and Mandible. Clinical Analysis and Case Reports. J.A.D.A., 29:2144, 1942.
17. Goldman, L., and Goldman, B.: Contact Testing of the Buccal Mucous Membrane for Stomatitis Venenata. Arch. Dermat. & Syph., 50:79, 1944.
18. Grupe, H. E., and Orban, B.: Eosinophilic Granuloma Diagnosis by Gingival Biopsy. J. Periodont., 21:19, 1950.
19. Haggard, H. W., and Greenberg, L. A.: Breath Odors from Alliaceous Substances. J.A.M.A., 104:2160, 1935.
20. Hirschfeld, L.: A Calibrated Silver Point for Periodontal Diagnosis and Recording. J. Periodont., 24:94, 1953.

21. Hirschfeld, I.: Interdental Canals. J.A.D.A., *14*:617, 1927.

22. Jolliffe, N.: Clinical Signs of Malnutrition. Vitamin Methods. New York, Academic Press, 1951, Vol. II.

23. Karshan, M., Kutscher, A. H., Silver, H. G., Stein, G., and Ziskin, D. E.: Studies in the Etiology of Idiopathic Orolingual Paresthesias. Am. J. Digest Dis., *19*:341, 1952.

24. Kitchen, P. C.: The Prevalence of Tooth Root Exposure and the Relation of the Extent of Such Exposure to the Degree of Abrasion in Differing Age Classes. J. D. Res., *20*:565, 1941.

25. Kutscher, A. H.: Experiences with a Detailed Color Shade Guide for Use in the Study of the Oral Mucous Membranes in Health and Disease. Oral Surg., Oral Med. & Oral Path., *15*:408, 1962.

26. Manly, R. S.: Abrasion of Cementum and Dentin by Modern Dentifrices. J. D. Res., *20*:583, 1941.

27. Manly, R. S.: Factors Influencing Tests on the Abrasion of Dentin by Brushing with Dentifrices. J. D. Res., *23*:59, 1944.

28. Mannerberg, F.: Saliva Factors in Cases of Erosion. Odont. Revy, *14*:156, 1963.

29. Manson, J. D.: The Lamina Dura. Oral Surg., *16*: 432, 1963.

30. Massler, M., Emslie, R., and Bolden, T.: Fetor Ex Ore. Oral Surg., Oral Med. & Oral Path., *4*:110, 1951.

31. McCay, C. M., and Wills, L.: Erosion of Molar Teeth by Acid Beverages. J. Nutrition, *39*:313, 1949.

32. Meyer, I.: The Value of the Gingival Biopsy in the Diagnosis of Generalized Amyloidosis. J. Oral Surg., *8*:314, 1950.

33. Miller, W. D.: Experiments and Observations on the Wasting of Tooth Tissue Variously Designated as Erosion, Abrasion, Chemical Abrasion, Denudation, etc. D. Cosmos, *49*:1, 1907.

34. Muhlmann, H. R.: Tooth Mobility: A Review of Clinical Aspects and Research Findings. J. Periodont., *38*:686, 1967.

35. Nizel, A. E.: The Role of Diet and Nutrition in the Management of Gingival and Periodontal Disease; in The Science of Nutrition and Its Application in Clinical Dentistry, Philadelphia, W. B. Saunders Company, 1966.

35a. Nizel, A. E.: Nutrition in Preventive Dentistry: Science and Practice. Philadelphia, W. B. Saunders Company, 1972.

36. O'Leary, T. J.: Tooth Mobility. Dent. Clin. North America, *13*:567, 1969.

37. O'Leary, T. J., and Rudd, K. D.: An Instrument for Measuring Horizontal Tooth Mobility. USAF School of Aerospace Medicine TDR 63–58, August, 1963. Periodontics, *1*:249, 1963.

38. Parfitt, G. J.: An Investigation of the Normal Variations in Alveolar Bone Trabeculations. Oral Surg., Oral Med., & Oral Path., *15*:1453, 1962.

39. Parfitt, G. J.: The Dynamics of a Tooth in Function. J. Periodont., *32*:102, 1961.

40. Patur, B., and Glickman, I.: Roentgenographic Evaluation of Alveolar Bone Changes in Periodontal Disease. Dent. Clin. North America, March 1960, p. 47.

41. Pauls, V., and Trott, J. R.: A Radiological Study of Experimentally Produced Lesions in Bone. Practit., *16*:254, 1966.

42. Prichard, J. F.: Role of the Roentgenogram in the Diagnosis and Prognosis of Periodontal Disease. Oral Med. & Oral Path., *14*:182, 1961.

43. Puckett, J.: A Device for Comparing Roentgenograms of the Same Mouth. J. Periodont., *39*:38, 1968.

44. Ramadan, A. B. E., and Mitchell, D. F.: A Roentgenographic Study of Experimental Bone Destruction. Oral Surg., Oral Med. & Oral Path., *15*:934, 1962.

45. Regan, J. E., and Mitchell, D. F.: Roentgenographic and Dissection Measurements of Alveolar Crest Height. J.A.D.A., *66*:356, 1963.

46. Ritchey, B., and Orban, B.: The Crests of the Interdental Septa. J. Periodont., *24*:75, 1953.

47. Robinson, H. B. G.: Abrasion, Attrition and Erosion of Teeth. Health Center J., Ohio State Univ., *3*:21, 1949.

48. Rosenberg, E. H., and Guralnick, W. C.: Hyperparathyroidism. Oral Surg., Oral Med. & Oral Path., *15*:84, Suppl. 2, 1962.

49. Salman, I., and Darlington, C. G.: Eosinophilic Granuloma. Am. J. Orthodont. (Oral Surg. Sect.), *31*:89, 1945.

50. Sandler, H. C., Stahl, S. S., Cahn, L. R., and Freund, H. R.: Exfoliative Cytology for the Detection of Early Mouth Cancer. Oral Surg., Oral Med. & Oral Path., *13*:994, 1960.

51. Sanstead, H. H., Carte, J. P., and Darby, W. J.: How to Diagnose Nutritional Disorders in Daily Practice. Nutrition Today, *4*:20, 1969.

52. Selikoff, I., and Robitzek, E.: Gingival Biopsy for the Diagnosis of Generalized Amyloidosis. Am. J. Path., *23*:1099, 1947.

53. Sherwood, L. M., and Parris, E. E.: Physiologic and Pharmacologic Regulation of Bone Resorption. New England J. Med., *282*:909, 1970.

54. Shklar, G., Cataldo, E., and Meyer, I.: Reliability of Cytologic Smear in Diagnosis of Oral Cancer. A Controlled Study. Arch. Otolaryngol., *91*:158, 1970.

55. Silverman, S., Jr., Gordon, G., Grant, T., Steinback, H., Eisenberg, E., and Manson, R.: Dental Structures in Primary Hyperparathyroidism. Oral Surg., Oral Med. & Oral Path., *15*:426, 1962.

56. Sleeper, E.: Eosinophilic Granuloma of Bone. Oral Surg., Oral Med. & Oral Path., *4*:896, 1951.

57. Sponge, J. D.: Halitosis: A Review of Its Causes and Treatment. D. Practit. & D. Record, *14*:307, 1964.

58. Stallard, H.: Residual Food Odors of the Mouth. J.A.D.A., *14*:1689, 1927.

59. Theilade, J.: An Evaluation of the Reliability of Radiographs in the Measurement of Bone Loss in Periodontal Disease. J. Periodont., *31*:143, 1960.

60. Todd-Sanford Clinical Diagnosis by Laboratory Methods, Edited by Davidson, I., and Henry, J. B. 14th ed. Philadelphia, W. B. Saunders Company, 1969.

61. Van Der Linden, L. W. J., and Van Aken, J.: The Periodontal Ligament in the Roentgenogram. J. Periodont., *41*:243, 1970.

62. Wintrobe, M. M.: Clinical Hematology. 5th ed. Philadelphia, Lea & Febiger, 1961, p. 105.

Chapter 34

DETERMINATION OF THE PROGNOSIS

THE PATIENT AND THE PROGNOSIS

The prognosis is the prediction of the duration, course and termination of a disease and the likelihood of its response to treatment. It must be determined before the treatment is planned. The prognosis of gingival and periodontal disease is critically dependent upon the patient—his attitude, his desire to retain his natural teeth and his willingness and ability to maintain good oral hygiene. Without these, treatment will not succeed.

THE PROGNOSIS IN PATIENTS WITH GINGIVAL DISEASE

The prognosis of gingival disease depends upon the role of inflammation in the overall disease process. If inflammation is the only pathologic change the prognosis is favorable, provided all local irritants are eliminated, gingival contours conducive to the preservation of health are attained and the patient cooperates by providing good oral hygiene.

If inflammation is superimposed upon systemically caused tissue changes (such as in gingival enlargement associated with Dilantin therapy, or in patients with nutritional, hematologic or hormonal disorders) gingival health may be restored temporarily by local therapy alone, but the long-term prognosis depends upon control or correction of the contributing systemic factors.

THE PROGNOSIS IN PATIENTS WITH PERIODONTAL DISEASE

There are two aspects to the determination of the prognosis in patients with periodontal disease: *the overall prognosis* and the *prognosis of individual teeth.*

The Overall Prognosis

The overall prognosis is concerned with the dentition as a whole. It answers the questions, "Should treatment be undertaken?" and "Is it likely to succeed?" The

523

following factors are considered in determining the overall prognosis.

Assessment of the past bone response

The past response of the alveolar bone to local factors is a useful guide for predicting the bone response to treatment and the likelihood of arresting the bone-destructive process. Assessment of the past bone response entails consideration of severity and distribution of the periodontal bone loss in terms of the following: the patient's age; the distribution, severity and duration of local irritants such as plaque, calculus and food impaction; and occlusal abnormalities and habits.

If the amount of bone loss can be accounted for by the local factors, local treatment can be expected to arrest the bone destruction; the overall prognosis for the dentition is good (Fig. 34–1).

If the bone loss is more severe than one would ordinarily expect at the patient's age in the presence of local factors of comparable severity and duration, factors other than those in the oral cavity are contributing to the bone destruction. The overall prognosis is then poor, because of the difficulty generally encountered in determining the responsible systemic factors (Fig. 34–2). Local treatment can be relied upon to arrest bone destruction caused by the local factors, but unless the systemic etiologic factors are detected and corrected, bone loss may continue.

The prognosis is not necessarily hopeless without systemic therapy, provided the disease is detected early and sufficient bone remains to support the teeth. In such cases, local treatment often can retain the dentition in useful function for many years by eliminating local destructive factors and limiting the bone destruction to that caused by the systemic conditions.

Height of remaining bone

The next question is: "Assuming bone destruction can be arrested, is there enough bone remaining to support the teeth?" The answer is readily apparent in extreme conditions when there is so little bone loss that tooth support is not in jeopardy or when bone loss is severe and generalized and the remaining bone is obviously insufficient for proper tooth support. Most patients, however, do not fit into the extreme categories. The height of remaining bone lies somewhere in between, making the bone level alone inconclusive for determining the overall prognosis.

The patient's age

All other factors being equal, the prognosis is better in the older of two patients with comparable levels of remaining alveolar bone. The younger patient has suffered more bone destruction than the older patient because of the differences in the normal bone levels for their respective ages, and his condition represents a more rapid destructive process because of the shorter period in which the bone loss has occurred. The younger person would ordinarily be expected to have a greater bone-reparative capacity and better post-treatment prognosis. However, the fact that so much bone destruction has occurred in a relatively short period of time reflects unfavorably on the young patient's bone reparative capacity.

Number of remaining teeth

If the number and distribution of the teeth are inadequate for the support of satisfactory prosthesis, the overall prognosis is bad. The likelihood of maintaining periodontal health is diminished because of the inability to establish a satisfactory functional environment. Extensive fixed or removable prosthesis constructed on an insufficient number of natural teeth creates periodontal injury which is more likely to hasten the tooth loss than to provide a worthwhile health service.

Patient's systemic background

The patient's systemic background affects the overall prognosis in several ways.[4] In patients with extensive periodontal destruction that cannot be accounted for by local factors alone, it is reasonable to assume contributing systemic etiology. However, the detection of responsible systemic factors is usually difficult, so that the prognosis in such patients is usually poor. However, in patients with known systemic disorders

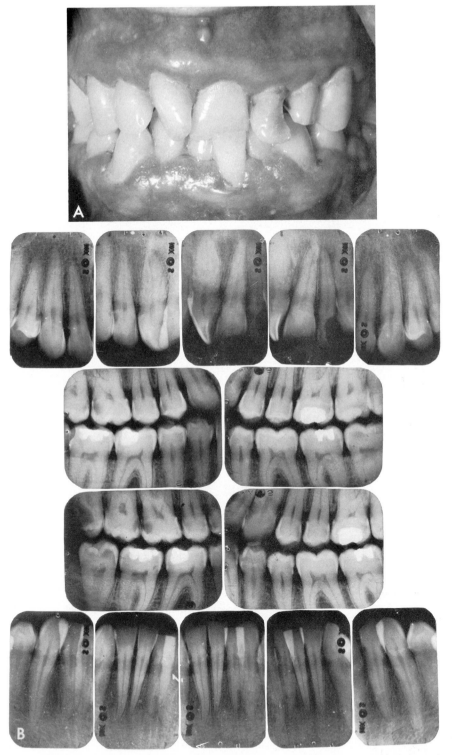

Figure 34–1 Good Bone Response, Overall Prognosis Favorable. *A,* Thirty-two-year-old male with generalized chronic marginal gingivitis and periodontal pocket formation, and excessive anterior overbite. *B,* Excellent bone picture despite unfavorable inflammatory and occlusal factors.

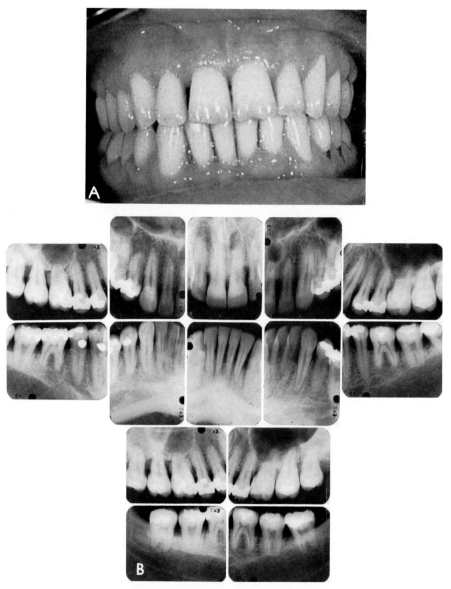

Figure 34–2 Poor Bone Response, Overall Prognosis Poor. *A,* Twenty-seven-year-old male with generalized chronic gingivitis and periodontal pocket formation. *B,* Bone destruction is in excess of that explainable by the local factors. The overall prognosis is poor.

that could affect the periodontium, such as diabetes, nutritional deficiency, hyperthyroidism and hyperparathyroidism, the prognosis of the periodontal condition benefits from their correction.

The prognosis must be guarded when surgical periodontal treatment is required but cannot be provided because of the patient's health. Incapacitating conditions

(such as Parkinson's disease) which prevent the patient from performing oral hygiene procedures also adversely affect the prognosis.

Gingival inflammation

Other factors being equal, the prognosis of periodontal disease is directly related to the severity of inflammation. In two patients with comparable bone destruction, the prognosis is better in the patient with the greater degree of inflammation. A larger component of the bone destruction is attributable to local irritation, and local treatment can be expected to be more effective in arresting the bone destruction.

Periodontal pockets

The location of the base of periodontal pockets is more important than pocket depth in deciding the overall prognosis. Because pocket depth and severity of bone loss are not necessarily related, a patient with deep pockets and little bone loss has a better prognosis than a patient with shallow pockets and severe bone destruction.

Malocclusion

Irregularly aligned teeth, malformation of the jaws and abnormal occlusal relationships are important factors in the etiology of periodontal disease. Correction by orthodontic or prosthetic means is essential if periodontal treatment is to succeed. **The overall prognosis is poor in patients with occlusal deformities which cannot be corrected.**

Tooth morphology

The prognosis is poor in patients with short tapered roots and relatively large crowns (Fig. 34–3). Because of the disproportionate crown-root ratio and the reduced root surface available for periodontal support,[1] the periodontium is more susceptible to injury by occlusal forces.

The prognosis of periodontosis (diffuse atrophy of alveolar bone)

In patients with periodontal disease diagnosed as periodontosis, systemic influences are considered responsible for the initiation and progress of the periodontal destruction. Local factors aggravate the systemically induced destructive changes. Ideally, treatment should include correction of the responsible systemic conditions, along with local measures, but the former are difficult to determine. However, **except in advanced cases of periodontosis in which the remaining bone is insufficient to support the teeth, the dentition can be retained in useful function by local treatment alone.**

The Prognosis of Individual Teeth

The prognosis of individual teeth is determined after the overall prognosis and is affected by it. For example, in a patient with a poor overall prognosis one would be disinclined to attempt to retain a tooth which is considered questionable because of local conditions. The following factors are considered in determining the prognosis of individual teeth:

Mobility

The principal causes of tooth mobility are loss of alveolar bone, inflammatory changes in the periodontal ligament and trauma from occlusion. (Tooth mobility is discussed in detail in Chapter 19.) Tooth mobility caused by inflammation and trauma from occlusion is correctable.[3] Tooth mobility resulting from loss of alveolar bone alone is not likely to be corrected. **The likelihood of restoring tooth stability is inversely proportional to the extent to which it is caused by loss of alveolar bone.**

Periodontal pockets

In suprabony pockets the location of the base of the pocket affects prognosis of individual teeth more than the pocket depth. **Proximity to frenum attachments and to the mucogingival line jeopardizes the prognosis unless corrective procedures are included in the treatment (Chap. 46.)**

PROXIMITY OF THE BASE OF THE POCKET TO THE APEX. The prognosis is adversely affected if the base of the pocket is close to the root apex even if there is no evidence of apical disease. **The incidence of degenerative pulp changes is increased in teeth affected by periodontal disease, usually without clinical symptoms or pulp necrosis.** The pulp changes are attributed to irritation from bacterial products through

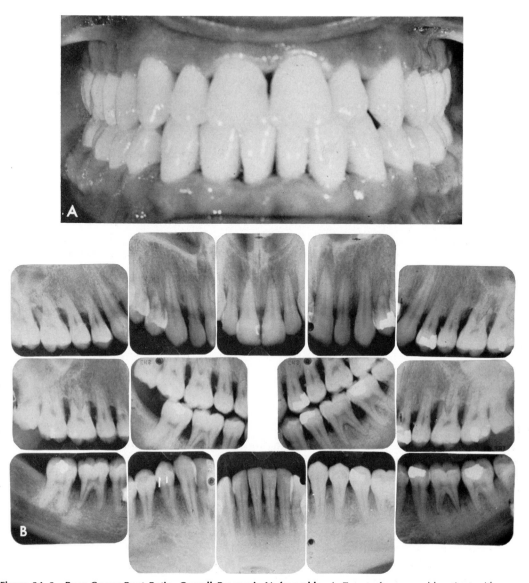

Figure 34–3 Poor Crown-Root Ratio, Overall Prognosis Unfavorable. *A,* Twenty-four-year-old patient with generalized gingivitis and periodontal pocket formation. *B,* Severity of bone destruction at this age indicates poor bone response. The contrast between the well formed crowns and relatively short tapered roots worsens the unfavorable prognosis.

the dentinal tubules of the exposed root surface wall of periodontal pockets and through lateral pulp canals. If the base of the pocket is close to the apex, injurious bacterial products may reach the pulp through the apical foramina. Root canal therapy is necessary in such cases to obtain optimal results from periodontal treatment.

When the periodontal pocket has extended to involve the apex the prognosis is generally poor. However, striking apical and lateral bone repair is sometimes obtained by combining endodontic and periodontal therapy (Chap. 45.)

Teeth adjacent to edentulous areas

Teeth that serve as abutments are subjected to increased functional demands. More rigid standards are required in evaluating the prognosis of teeth adjacent to edentulous areas.

Location of remaining bone in relation to the individual tooth surfaces

When greater bone loss has occurred on one surface of a tooth, the bone height on the less involved surfaces should be taken into consideration in determining the prognosis. Because of greater height of bone in relation to the latter surfaces, the center of rotation of the tooth will be nearer the crown (Fig. 34–4). The leverage upon the periodontium will therefore be more favorable than the bone loss on the most severely involved tooth surface suggests.

Relation to adjacent teeth

In dealing with a tooth with questionable prognosis, the chances of successful treatment should be weighed against the benefits that would accrue to the adjacent teeth if the tooth under consideration were extracted. **Heroic attempts to retain a hopelessly involved tooth jeopardizes the adjacent teeth.** Extraction of the questionable tooth is followed by partial restoration of the bone support of the adjacent teeth (Fig. 34–5).

Infrabony pockets

The likelihood of eliminating infrabony pockets depends upon several factors, critical among which are the contour of the osseous defects and the number of remaining bony walls (see Chapter 44, The Treatment of Infrabony Pockets).

Furcation involvement

The presence of bifurcation or trifurcation involvement does not indicate a hope-

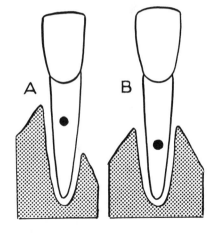

Figure 34–4 The Prognosis for Tooth *A* **Is Better Than That of Tooth** *B*, despite the fact that there is less bone on one of the surfaces. Because the center of rotation of tooth *A* is closer to the crown, the distribution of occlusal forces to the periodontium is more favorable than in *B*.

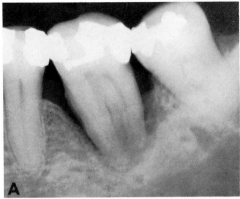
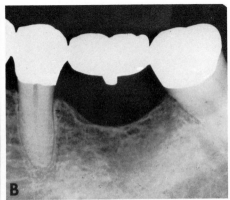

Figure 34–5 Extraction of Severely Involved Tooth to Preserve Bone on Adjacent Teeth. *A*, Extensive bone destruction around mandibular first molar. *B*, Eight and one-half years after extraction of first molar and replacement by prosthesis. Note the excellent bony support.

less prognosis (Chap. 45). The added support provided by multirooted teeth is an advantage over single-rooted teeth with comparable bone loss. However, infection through accessory canals in the furcation areas may lead to complicating pulpal changes.

Caries, nonvital teeth and tooth resorption

In teeth mutilated by extensive caries the feasibility of adequate restoration and endodontic therapy should be considered before undertaking periodontal treatment. Extensive idiopathic root resorption jeopardizes the stability of teeth and adversely affects the response to periodontal treatment. **The periodontal prognosis of treated nonvital teeth is not different from that of vital teeth.** Reattachment can occur to the cementum of nonvital or vital teeth. However, reattachment to exposed root dentin is not likely in nonvital teeth.[2] (For discussion of reattachment see Chapter 36.)

REFERENCES

1. Kay, S., Forscher, B. K., and Sackett, L. M.: Tooth Root Length-Volume Relationships. An Aid to Periodontal Prognosis. I. Anterior Teeth. Oral Surg., Oral Med. & Oral Path., 7:735, 1954.
2. Morris, M. L.: Healing of Human Periodontal Tissues Following Surgical Detachment and Expiration of Vital Pulps. J. Periodont., *31*: 23, 1960.
3. Morris, M. L.: The Diagnosis, Prognosis and Treatment of the Loose Tooth. Oral Surg., Oral Med. & Oral Path., 6:1037, 1953.
4. Schulte, W.: Limitations of Periodontal Therapy Due to Systemic Factors. Deutsche Zahnärzt. Zeitschr., 24:41, 1966.
5. Slatten, R. W.: An Evaluation of Factors Determining Prognosis in Inflammatory and Retrogressive Periodontal Disease. A. Series. J. Periodont., 25:30, 1954.

Chapter 35

THE TREATMENT PLAN

THE TREATMENT PLAN — NOT AN HEROIC ATTEMPT TO SALVAGE LOOSE TEETH

After the diagnosis and prognosis have been established, the treatment is planned. *The treatment plan is the blueprint for case management.* It includes all procedures required for the establishment and maintenance of oral health, such as decisions as to teeth to be retained or extracted, whether scaling and curettage or surgical techniques are to be used for pocket elimination, the need for mucogingival or reconstructive surgical procedures and occlusal correction, the type of restorations to be employed, which teeth are to be used for abutments, and the indications for splinting.

Unforeseen developments during treatment may necessitate modification of the initial treatment plan. However, **it is axiomatic that, except for emergencies, no treatment should be started until the treatment plan has been established.** Periodontal treatment requires long-range planning. **Its value to the patient is measured in years of healthful functioning** of the entire dentition, not by the number of teeth retained at the time of treatment. It is directed to establishing and maintaining the health of the periodontium throughout the mouth rather than to spectacular efforts to "tighten loose teeth."

The welfare of the dentition should not be jeopardized by an heroic attempt to retain questionable teeth. The periodontal condition of teeth we decide to retain is more important than their number. Teeth that can be retained with a minimum of doubt and a maximum margin of safety provide the basis for the total treatment plan. Teeth on the borderline of hopelessness do not contribute to the overall usefulness of the dentition, even if they can be saved in a somewhat precarious state. Such teeth become sources of recurrent annoyance to the patient and detract from the value of the greater service rendered by the establishment of periodontal health in the remainder of the oral cavity.

THE MASTER PLAN FOR TOTAL TREATMENT

The aim of the treatment plan is *total treatment* — that is, the *coordination of all treatment procedures for the purpose of creating a well-functioning dentition in a healthy periodontal environment.* The following "**master-plan**" which divides total treatment into four phases is prepared for each patient according to his needs.

1. The soft tissue phase

This entails elimination of gingival inflammation, periodontal pockets and the

531

factors which cause them; the establishment of gingival contour and mucogingival relationships conducive to the preservation of periodontal health; restoration of carious areas; correction of the margins of existing restorations; and recontouring proximal, facial and lingual surfaces and occlusal marginal ridges of existing restorations to provide proper proximal contact and food excursion pathways.

2. The functional phase

An optimal occlusal relationship is one that provides the functional stimulation necessary to preserve periodontal health. To obtain it may require occlusal adjustment; restorative, prosthetic and orthodontic procedures; splinting; and the correction of bruxism, clamping and clenching habits.

3. The systemic phase

Systemic conditions may necessitate special precautions in the course of periodontal treatment, affect the tissue response to treatment procedures or threaten the preservation of periodontal health after treatment is completed. Such situations should be taken care of in conjunction with the patient's physician. (For a discussion of systemic conditions which require special precautions, see Chapter 57.)

4. The maintenance phase

This entails all procedures for maintaining periodontal health after it has been attained. It consists of instruction in oral hygiene; recall of the patient at regular intervals according to his needs, to check on the condition of the periodontium, the status of the restorative dentistry and the need for further occlusal adjustment; and follow-up radiographs.

PLAQUE CONTROL IN PERIODONTAL TREATMENT

Plaque control is an integral part of periodontal treatment; no treatment, regardless of how expertly it is performed, can succeed without it. *Oral hygiene procedures performed by the patient to* *prevent the accumulation of dental plaque and food debris in the course of periodontal treatment are commonly referred to as "oral physiotherapy."* All local irritants must be removed in the treatment of periodontal disease. Irritation and infection from dental plaque are the most common causes of delayed healing. They cause inflammatory and degenerative changes that not only retard healing but may reverse it in the direction of recurrent disease.

Periodontal treatment is usually an entirely new experience for the patient. It is different from his previous dental experience in that he becomes an active participant in the treatment process. The patient must know what the dentist will do for him and what he will be expected to do for himself. The various oral hygiene procedures should be explained so that he understands their purpose and the effort they require. **It should also be emphasized that these procedures are to be continued after periodontal health has been attained in order to help prevent the recurrence of disease.**

When discussing the treatment plan, it is not enough simply to tell a patient that his cooperation will be required without explaining the effort it entails and the reasons for it. In his anxiety about his problem, the patient willingly promises to cooperate and often adds: "Doctor, I will do anything to save my teeth." Such assurance may be well intentioned, but it is not very meaningful when given without knowledge of the commitment involved.

Teaching plaque control as part of periodontal treatment

Teaching plaque control requires more chairside time with the patient than the total time required for the other periodontal treatment procedures. The step-by-step procedure for teaching plaque control is described on page 467. It may be started before or after the other treatment procedures are performed.

It is a good idea to start the overall treatment with plaque control. Placing the patient on a one-month oral hygiene regimen at the outset will help convince him of its high priority in the treatment program and will familiarize him with what he must

do to have a healthy mouth. It also gives the dentist an idea of what he can expect from the patient and provides an opportunity to demonstrate the benefits of plaque control in terms of improvement in the condition of the gingiva.

For all patients – those already started on a plaque control program and those who start after other treatment procedures are performed – there are certain special guidelines. After scaling and curettage or periodontal surgery, care should be taken not to injure the healing tissue. Cleansing should be started as soon as possible, but it should be confined initially to the gentle removal of superficial plaque and debris with a rubber tip or other interdental cleanser followed by light water irrigation. Brushing should be introduced as soon as the tissues permit, gradually developing the desired thoroughness.

In the early post-treatment days, the gingiva may bleed more when the teeth are cleaned than it did before treatment. **Unless there is pain, cleansing should be continued; the bleeding will subside as healing progresses.** Sometimes, sensitive root surfaces interfere with cleansing during the first two weeks. The sensitivity usually disappears gradually, but if it persists, it should be treated. (See The Treatment of Sensitive Roots, page 660.)

EXPLAINING THE TREATMENT PLAN TO THE PATIENT

The following are suggestions for explaining the treatment plan to the patient:

Be specific. Tell your patient: "You have gingivitis," or "You have periodontitis." Then, explain exactly what these conditions are, how they are treated and the future for the patient's mouth after treatment. **Avoid vague statements** such as: "You have trouble with your gums," or "Something should be done about your gums." Patients do not understand the significance of such statements and disregard them.

Start your discussion on a positive note. Talk about the teeth which can be retained and the long-term service they can be expected to render. Do not start your discussion with the statement: "The following teeth have to be extracted." This creates a negative impression which adds to the erroneous attitude of hopelessness the patient already may have regarding his mouth.

Make it clear that every effort will be made to retain as many teeth as possible, **but do not dwell on the patient's loose teeth.** Emphasize the fact that the important purpose of the treatment is to prevent the other teeth from becoming as severely diseased as the loose teeth.

Present the entire treatment plan as a unit. Avoid creating the impression that treatment consists of separate procedures, some or all of which may be selected by the patient. **Make it clear that dental restorations and prostheses contribute as much to the health of the gums as does the elimination of inflammation and periodontal pockets.** Do not speak in terms of "having the gums treated" and "then taking care of the necessary restorations later" as if these were unrelated treatments.

Patients frequently seek guidance from the dentist with such questions as: "Are my teeth worth treating?" "Would you have them treated if you were I?" "Why don't I just go along the way I am until the teeth really bother me, and then have them all extracted?"

If the condition is treatable, make it clear that the best results are obtained by prompt treatment. If the condition is not treatable, the teeth should be extracted. Explain that "doing nothing" or holding onto hopelessly diseased teeth as long as possible is inadvisable for the following reasons:

In periodontal disease, proper mastication of food is impaired because of looseness of the teeth and discomfort incurred by chewing. This leads to the "bolting" of food, which complicates the digestive process and may lead to gastrointestinal disturbances.

Exudate from periodontal pockets spoils the taste of food. In addition, the incorporation of purulent material into the food may irritate the mucosa of the stomach and lead to gastritis. Infection in the periodontal area is also a potential source of bacteremia.

Inability to chew properly leads to habits of food selection with preference for soft foods, which are for the most part carbohydrates.

It is not feasible to place restorations or

"bridges" on teeth with untreated periodontal disease, because the usefulness of the restoration is limited by the uncertain condition of the supporting structures.

Failure to eliminate periodontal disease not only results in loss of teeth already hopelessly involved, but also shortens the life span of other teeth which, with proper treatment, could serve as the foundation for a healthy, functioning dentition.

It is the dentist's responsibility to advise the patient of the importance of periodontal treatment. However, if treatment is to be successful, the patient must be sufficiently interested in retaining the natural teeth to provide the necessary oral hygiene. Individuals who are not particularly perturbed by the thought of losing their teeth are generally not good patients for periodontal treatment.

Part II • *The Soft Tissue Phase of Periodontal Treatment: Elimination of Gingival Inflammation and Periodontal Pockets and the Factors Which Cause Them*

Chapter 36

RATIONALE FOR PERIODONTAL TREATMENT

There are no forms of gingivitis or periodontal disease in which the removal of local irritants and prevention of their recurrence do not reduce the severity of the disease, lessen the rapidity of the destructive process and prolong the usefulness of the natural dentition.

The effectiveness of periodontal therapy is made possible by the remarkable healing capacity of the periodontal tissues (Fig. 36–1). Properly performed, periodontal treatment can be relied upon to accomplish the following: eliminate pain, eliminate gingival inflammation[46] and stop gingival bleeding, eliminate periodontal pockets and infection, stop pus formation, arrest the destruction of soft tissue and bone,[47] reduce abnormal tooth mobility,[16] establish optimal occlusal function, in some instances restore tissue destroyed by disease, re-establish physiologic gingival contour necessary for the preservation of periodontal health, prevent the recurrence of disease and reduce tooth loss[41] (Fig. 36–2).

LOCAL AND SYSTEMIC TREATMENT

Periodontal treatment consists principally of local procedures, because with infrequent exceptions gingival and periodontal diseases are caused by local factors, and local treatment suffices to achieve the desired results. When a systemic cause is suspected, it is generally difficult to determine its nature. Consequently, when systemic therapy is employed, it is usually as an adjunct to local measures and for specific purposes, such as the control of systemic complications from acute infections, chemotherapy to prevent harmful effects of post-treatment bacteremia, supportive nutritional therapy and the control of systemic diseases which aggravate the patient's periodontal condition or necessitate special precautions during treatment (Chap. 57).

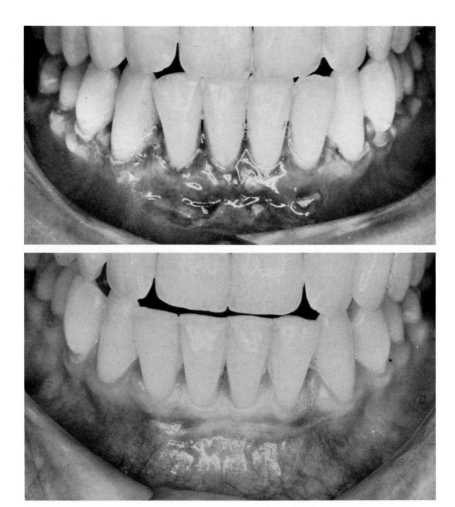

Figure 36-1 Excellent Healing Capacity of the Periodontium. *Above,* One week following periodontal surgery, after removal of periodontal dressing. *Below,* After seven months, showing healed tissues and restoration of physiologic gingival contour.

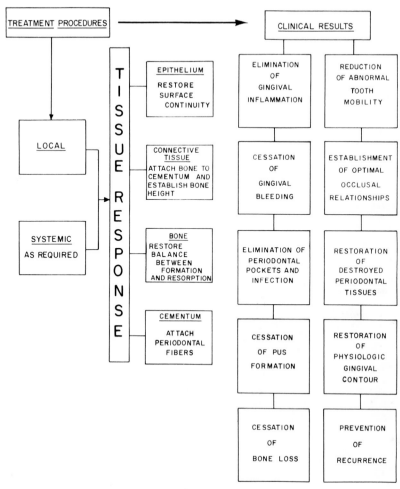

Figure 36–2 Tissue Response and Clinical Results Following Periodontal Treatment.

TWO LOCAL DESTRUCTIVE PROCESSES

The local etiologic factors in periodontal disease are numerous and varied, but in the final analysis they are divisible into two categories: (1) local irritants which cause gingival inflammation, such as plaque, cal-culus and food impaction; and (2) abnormal occlusal forces which cause trauma from occlusion, such as bruxing, clamping, or clenching (Fig. 36–3). To be effective, local treatment must eliminate inflammation and/or trauma from occlusion, as well as the factors which cause them, because these are the only local processes capable of pro-

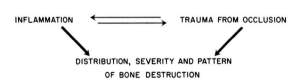

Figure 36–3 Local Etiologic Factors Divisible into Two Categories—Those Which Cause Inflammation and Those Which Cause Trauma from Occlusion.

ducing periodontal destruction. Periodontal destruction continues following treatment which eliminates inflammation-producing irritants and permits injurious occlusal relationships to persist, or treatment which creates optimal occlusal forces and disregards local irritants.

FACTORS WHICH AFFECT HEALING*

In the periodontium as elsewhere in the body, healing is affected by local and systemic factors.

Local factors

Systemic conditions which impair healing may reduce the effectiveness of local periodontal treatment and should be corrected prior to or along with local procedures. **However, it is the local factors such as contamination by microorganisms, irritation from plaque, food debris, and necrotic tissue remnants and trauma from occlusion which are the most common deterrents to healing following periodontal treatment.** Healing is also delayed by excessive tissue manipulation during treatment, trauma to the tissues and repetitive treatment procedures which disrupt the orderly cellular activity in the healing process. Topically applied cortisone and ionizing radiation retard healing.[42]

Healing is improved by local increase in temperature, debridement, the removal of degenerated and necrotic tissue, immobilization of the healing area and pressure on the wound. The cellular activity in healing entails an increase in oxygen consumption, but healing of the gingiva is not accelerated by artificially increasing the oxygen supply beyond the normal requirements.[19]

Systemic factors

The effects of systemic conditions upon healing have been extensively documented in animal experiments, but are less clearly defined in humans. Healing capacity diminishes with age.[10] Atherosclerotic vascular changes which are common in aging and the resultant reduction in blood circulation

may be responsible. Healing is delayed in diabetes and in patients with generalized infections and in other debilitating diseases.

The nutrient requirements of the healing tissues in minor wounds such as those created by periodontal surgical procedures are ordinarily satisfied by a well-balanced diet. Healing is retarded by insufficient food intake and by bodily conditions which interfere with the utilization of nutrients. Vitamin C deficiency[1, 15, 62] delays healing by depressing collagen formation and altering the integrity of capillary walls so that they are prone to rupture. Protein deficiency[58] also retards healing by reducing the supply of sulfur-containing amino acids such as cystine and methionine. Healing is also retarded by vitamin A deficiency, by a fat-rich diet and by overdose of vitamin D. The latter causes necrosis and calcification in the arterioles of the granulation tissue.

Healing is affected by hormones. Systemically administered glucocorticoids such as cortisone hinder repair by depressing the inflammatory reaction or by inhibiting the growth of fibroblasts and the production of collagen and formation of endothelial cells.[11] Systemic stress,[56] thyroidectomy, testosterone, ACTH and large doses of estrogen suppress the formation of granulation tissue and retard healing.[42] Progesterone increases and accelerates the vascularization of immature granulation tissue[30] and appears to increase susceptibility of gingiva to mechanical injury by producing dilation of marginal vessels.[24] Somatotropic hormone increases fibroplasia during gingival healing.[55]

Systemically administered antibiotics do not improve the epithelization of gingival wounds in experimental animals,*[59] nor do systemic antibiotics following gingivectomy in humans ("antibiotic umbrella") appear to prevent the occurrence of marked gingival inflammation.[60]

HEALING FOLLOWING PERIODONTAL TREATMENT

The basic healing processes are the same following all forms of periodontal therapy. They consist of the removal of degenerated tissue debris and the replacement of tis-

---

*For an excellent discussion of the subject of healing, the reader is referred to the presentation by Cameron.[11]

*For additional information regarding gingival healing the reader is referred to a comprehensive review by Stahl.[57]

sues destroyed by disease. **Regeneration and reattachment are aspects of periodontal healing which have a special bearing upon the results obtainable by treatment.**

Regeneration

Regeneration is the growth and differentiation of new cells and intercellular substances to form new tissues or parts. It consists of fibroplasia, endothelial proliferation, the deposition of interstitial ground substance and collagen, epithelial hyperplasia and the maturation of connective tissue.

Regeneration takes place by growth from the same type of tissue as that which has been destroyed, or from its precursor. In the periodontium, gingival epithelium is replaced by epithelium, and the underlying connective tissue and periodontal ligament are derived from connective tissue. **Bone and cementum are not replaced by existing bone or cementum, but from connective tissue, which is the precursor of both. Undifferentiated connective tissue cells develop into osteoblasts and cementoblasts which form bone and cementum.**

Regeneration of the periodontium is a continuous physiologic process. Under normal conditions new cells and tissues are constantly being formed to replace those which mature and die. This is termed "wear and tear repair." [27] It is manifested by mitotic activity in the epithelium of the gingiva [34] and the connective tissue of the periodontal ligament,[40] by the formation of new bone and by the continuous deposition of cementum.

Regeneration is also going on during active gingival and periodontal disease. Most gingival and periodontal diseases are chronic inflammatory processes and as such are healing lesions. Regeneration is part of the healing. However, local irritants, bacteria and bacterial products which perpetuate the disease process, and the inflammatory exudate they elicit are injurious to the regenerating cells and tissues and prevent the healing from proceeding to completion. In supporting periodontal tissues injured by abnormal occlusal forces (trauma from occlusion), the constantly present regenerative process attempts to repair the tissue damage.

By removing local irritants and periodontal pockets where bacteria accumulate and proliferate, periodontal treatment removes the obstacles to regeneration, and

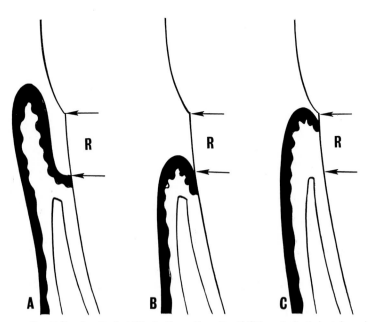

Figure 36–4 Regeneration Following Pocket Elimination—Two Possibilities. *A,* Periodontal pocket before treatment. The root surface (*R*) denuded by periodontal disease is marked by the arrows. *B,* One possibility. Normal sulcus re-established at the level of the base of the pre-existent pocket, the root (*R*) remains denuded. *C,* Another possibility is "reattachment." The periodontium is restored onto the root surface denuded by disease. New fibers and new cementum are formed on formerly denuded root (*R*) with a higher bone level and a healthy gingival sulcus attached closer to the crown.

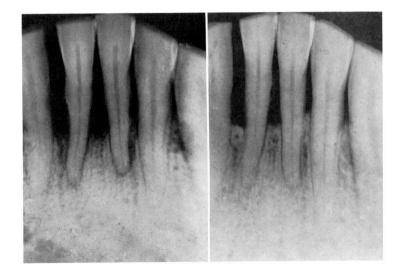

Figure 36–5 Bone Restored Following Periodontal Treatment. *Left,* Before treatment. *Right,* Five years later.

enables the patient to benefit from the inherent regenerative capacity of the tissues. There is a brief spurt in regenerative activity immediately following periodontal treatment, but there are no local treatment procedures which "promote" or "accelerate" regeneration.

Regeneration is a microscopic activity which differs in degree from clinically and/or radiographically detectable restoration of destroyed periodontal tissues. In most instances regeneration simply restores the continuity of the diseased marginal gingiva and re-establishes a normal gingival sulcus at the same level on the root as the base of the pre-existent periodontal pocket (Fig. 36–4). It arrests bone destruction without necessarily increasing bone height. Restoration of the destroyed periodontium to a degree which is clinically and/or radiographically detectable (Fig. 36–5) occurs less frequently, and is dependent upon the occurrence of reattachment.

Reattachment

To obtain clinically significant restoration of destroyed periodontium, reattachment must occur. *Reattachment is the re-embedding of new periodontal ligament fibers into new cementum and the attachment of gingival epithelium to tooth surface previously denuded by disease* (Fig. 36–4). The critical words in this definition are *"tooth surface previously denuded by disease."* Attachment of gingiva or periodontal ligament to areas of the tooth from which they may be re-

moved in the course of treatment or during the preparation of teeth for restorations represents *simple healing* of the periodontium, not reattachment. The term reattachment has unique usage in the periodontal field and refers specifically to the restoration of the marginal periodontium and not to repair of other areas of the root, such as that following traumatic tears in the cementum, tooth fractures or the treatment of periapical lesions.

Epithelial adaptation

"Epithelial adaptation" is different from reattachment. The former is close apposition of gingival epithelium to the tooth surface without complete obliteration of the pocket.[9, 28] The pocket space is too narrow to permit passage of a probe, but it does not prevent the entrance of bacteria and their products. This leads to inflammation of the inner pocket wall (Fig. 36–6), which escapes detection because of the deceptively healthy appearance of the external surface of the pocket. Spread of the inflammation into the supporting tissues with continued bone loss and periodontal abscess formation are potential sequelae.

Opinions differ regarding the extent and conditions under which reattachment is attainable by periodontal treatment.[29] It occurs more often following the treatment of infrabony pockets[12, 20, 21, 43, 65] than suprabony pockets,[29, 51, 54, 64] except in patients with one-wall infrabony defects (for the treatment of infrabony pockets, see Chapter

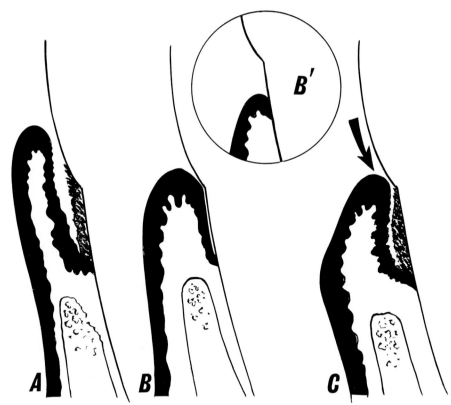

Figure 36–6 **"Epithelial Adaptation" Following Periodontal Treatment.** *A,* Periodontal pocket. *B,* After treatment. The pocket is *partially eliminated;* the remaining pocket is closely adapted to, but not attached to, the root. *C,* Seepage of bacteria and their products and other irritants between the pocket wall and tooth surface leads to recurrence of periodontal disease and continued bone loss. *B',* Result obtained had pocket been completely eliminated by initial treatment.

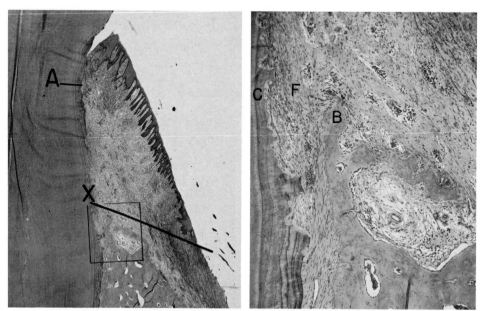

Figure 36–7 **Restoration of Periodontium in Animal Experiment (Glickman and Lazansky).** *Left,* Periodontium restored one month after gingiva and periodontal ligament were removed by incision at *X,* and the exposed cementum was scraped. The restored gingival sulcus is attached at *A. Right,* Detailed study of area within rectangle on left, showing regenerative capacity of tissues under experimental conditions. New cementum is deposited on irregularly indented cementum (*C*) which was exposed and scraped at time of operation. New fibers (*F*) are embedded in the cementum and in newly formed bone at *B.*

44). It has been demonstrated histologically following the treatment of infrabony pockets,[5, 14, 50] but with suprabony pockets both positive[8, 17, 33, 50] and negative microscopic findings[26, 36] have been reported. Reattachment has been observed histologically in experimental animals following healing of artificially created pockets,[25, 31, 32, 37, 44] and marginal wounds[2, 3, 4, 18, 25, 49] (Fig. 36–7), and following the surgical removal of inflamed gingiva.

FACTORS THAT AFFECT REATTACHMENT

The following factors affect the likelihood of attaining reattachment:

Removal of the epithelial attachment

Removal of the epithelial attachment in the treatment of deep suprabony and infrabony pockets increases the likelihood of obtaining reattachment. The post-treatment location of the epithelial attachment limits the height to which periodontal fibers become attached to the tooth. The level of attachment of the periodontal ligament in turn determines the maximum post-treatment height the bone can attain. **Leaving the epithelial attachment intact during periodontal treatment therefore automatically predetermines the post-treatment levels of the periodontal ligament and bone (Fig. 36–8).** Removal of the epithelial attach-

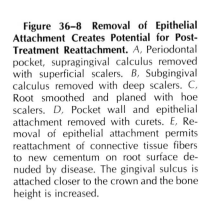

Figure 36–8 Removal of Epithelial Attachment Creates Potential for Post-Treatment Reattachment. *A,* Periodontal pocket, supragingival calculus removed with superficial scalers. *B,* Subgingival calculus removed with deep scalers. *C,* Root smoothed and planed with hoe scalers. *D,* Pocket wall and epithelial attachment removed with curets. *E,* Removal of epithelial attachment permits reattachment of connective tissue fibers to new cementum on root surface denuded by disease. The gingival sulcus is attached closer to the crown and the bone height is increased.

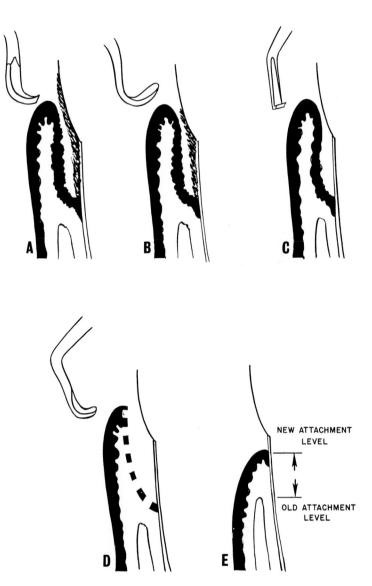

ment creates conditions in which connective tissue fibers could reattach to tooth surface coronal to the pretreatment level (Fig. 36–8), and creates the potential for increased bone height, and repair of infrabony defects.

When treating periodontal pockets, it cannot be determined by clinical examination whether or not the epithelial attachment has been completely removed. However, histologic studies indicate that it can be completely removed in every case treated by gingivectomy,[45, 63] but opinions differ regarding whether removal can be accomplished consistently by scaling and curettage. Some investigators report complete removal of the epithelial attachment,[39] the sulcal epithelium[6, 7, 38] and some of the underlying inflamed connective tissue following gingival curettage, whereas others observe in situ remnants of the epithelial attachment and sulcal epithelium.[48, 61, 64]

Thorough planing of the root surface

Changes in the tooth surface wall of periodontal pockets, such as degeneration of the remnants of Sharpey's fibers, accumulation of bacteria and their products, and disintegration of the cementum and dentin, interfere with reattachment. However, these obstacles can be eliminated by thorough root planing. Periodontally involved root surfaces produce cytotoxic effects on cells in tissue culture; nondiseased root surfaces do not.[23]

The clot

The clot forms the initial protective covering of the treated area. It is replaced by granulation tissue, which may extend up to the clot surface. The vascularity and bulk of the granulation tissue are reduced as it undergoes maturation to connective tissue. The height of the granulation tissue may affect the level at which the epithelium becomes attached to the root, because the proliferating epithelium is guided by the connective tissue surface along which it moves.

Other factors

Trauma from occlusion impairs post-treatment healing of the supporting periodontal tissues and reduces the likelihood of attain-ing reattachment. Widened periodontal spaces, angular bone defects and tooth mobility often result when trauma persists during healing.

Reattachment is more likely to occur when the destructive process has been rapid, such as following the treatment of pockets complicated by the formation of acute periodontal abscesses, and acute necrotizing ulcerative gingivitis.

The formation of new cementum and embedding of periodontal ligament fibers can occur on the cementum and dentin of vital teeth; in nonvital teeth it can occur on cementum but is not likely on exposed dentin.[35]

The likelihood of obtaining reattachment is increased by the elimination of infection and the correction of excessive tooth mobility.

GRANULATION TISSUE IN ACTIVE DISEASE AND POST-TREATMENT HEALING

The granulation tissue formed in post-treatment healing is the same type of tissue as that present in active chronic gingivitis and periodontal pockets. During active disease the granulation tissue does not mature to connective tissue because of the persistence of local irritation and inflammatory exudate. If all irritants are eliminated by scaling and curettage, without removing the granulation tissue, the inflammatory exudate is resorbed and maturation of the granulation tissue progresses. If periodontal pockets are treated by gingivectomy, the granulation tissue is removed to provide visibility and accessibility to the irritants on the root surface. New granulation tissue is formed early in healing and undergoes maturation, providing that all local irritants are removed. **From a clinical viewpoint, therefore, removal of granulation tissue in the treatment of periodontal pockets does not represent a sacrifice of tissue because it is replaced in the healing process.**

RECESSION AND POCKET ELIMINATION

The fact that more of the root surface is often visible after periodontal pockets are eliminated has led to the erroneous impres-

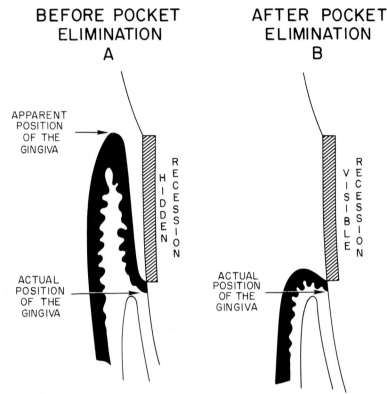

BEFORE POCKET
ELIMINATION
A

AFTER POCKET
ELIMINATION
B

APPARENT
POSITION
OF THE
GINGIVA

HIDDEN RECESSION

ACTUAL
POSITION
OF THE
GINGIVA

VISIBLE RECESSION

ACTUAL
POSITION
OF THE
GINGIVA

Figure 36–9 Amount of Recession is Determined by the Actual Position of the Gingiva, Not by the Apparent Position.
A, Before periodontal pocket is eliminated. Recession (**Hidden Recession**) is present, but it is covered by the disease pocket wall. *B,* After the periodontal pocket is eliminated, the recession which was present but hidden before treatment becomes visible (**Visible Recession**).

sion that periodontal treatment causes recession. This impression is based upon a misconception of what recession is. **The amount of recession depends upon the location of the epithelial attachment on the tooth surface, not the position of the crest of the gingiva.** *The former is the actual position of the gingiva; the latter is the apparent position* (Fig. 36–9).

Judging pre- and post-treatment recession by the location of the crest of the gingival margin is misleading. Recession is present before the periodontal pocket is treated, but the denuded root is hidden by the diseased pocket wall (Fig. 36–9). After the pocket is eliminated, the previously denuded root surface becomes exposed to view. **What happens is that hidden recession becomes visible recession** (Fig. 36–9).

Most often the amount of recession before and after the treatment of periodontal pockets is essentially the same. In some instances there may be more recession after treatment, and if reattachment occurs there is less. **However, in all instances the amount**

of recession is determined by the location of the epithelial attachment.

ESTABLISHMENT OF OPTIMAL OCCLUSAL RELATIONSHIPS

In addition to the elimination of periodontal pockets, treatment should include the establishment of a functional environment that fulfills the requirements of periodontal tissues. This is accomplished by one or more of the following: occlusal adjustment, restorative and orthodontic procedures, and the elimination of injurious habits. When the injurious occlusal forces are eliminated, the periodontium undergoes repair. To obtain the maximum benefits from occlusal correction, gingival inflammation should be eliminated first, because degenerative changes caused by the inflammation impair the reparative capacity of the periodontium. This sequence is modified in infrabony pockets where the pocket is treated and the occlusion is adjusted at the same time (Chap. 44).

REFERENCES

1. Barr, C. E.: Osteogenic Activity in Acute Ascorbic Acid Deficiency. J. Oral Therap., 4:5, 1967.
2. Beckwith, T. D., Fleming, W. C., and Williams, A.: Repair of the Tooth and Paradentium in the Guinea Pig, Rabbit and Cat. U. of Calif. Publications in Microbiology V–1, Nov. 1, 1943.
3. Beckwith, T. D., and Williams, A.: Regeneration of the Peridental Membrane in the Cat. Proc. Soc. Exp. Biol. & Med., 25:713, 1928.
4. Beckwith, T. D., Williams, A., and Fleming, W. C.: The Regeneration of the Rodent Peridental Membrane. Proc. Soc. Exp. Biol. & Med., 24:562, 1927.
5. Beube, F. E.: A Radiographic Histologic Study on Reattachment. J. Periodont., 23:158, 1952.
6. Beube, F. E.: Treatment Methods for Marginal Gingivitis and Periodontitis. Texas D. J., 71:427, 1953.
7. Blass, J. L., and Lite, T.: Gingival Healing Following Surgical Curettage: A Histopathologic Study. New York D. J., 25:127, 1959.
8. Box, H. K.: Studies in Periodontal Pathology. Canadian D. Res. Found. Bull. 7, May, 1924, p. 75.
9. Box, H. K.: Treatment of the Periodontal Pocket. Toronto, Univ. of Toronto Press, 1928, pp. 94, 105.
10. Butcher, E. O., and Klingsberg, J.: Age, Gonadectomy, and Wound Healing in the Palatal Mucosa. J. D. Res., 40:694, 1961.
11. Cameron, R.: Inflammation and Repair. Chapter 2 in Robbins, S. L.: Pathology. 3rd Ed. Philadelphia, W. B. Saunders Co., 1967.
12. Carranza, F. A.: A Technique for Treating Infrabony Pockets so as to Obtain Reattachment. D. Clin. North America, March 1960, p. 75.
13. Cheraskin, E., et al.: Resistance and Susceptibility to Oral Disease. II. A Study in Periodontometry and Carbohydrate Metabolism. Periodontics, 3: 296, 1965.
14. Cross, W. G.: Reattachment Following Curettage. A Histological Study. D. Practitioner, 7:38, 1956.
15. Dunphy, J. E.: On the Nature and Care of Wounds. Ann. Roy. Coll. Surg. Eng., 26:69, 1960.
16. Ferris, R. T.: Quantitative Evaluation of Tooth Mobility Following Initial Periodontal Therapy. J. Periodont., 37:190, 1966.
17. Fleming, W. E.: A Clinical and Microscopic Study of Periodontal Tissues Treated by Instrumentation. Pac. D. Gazette, 24:568, 1926.
18. Glickman, I., and Lazansky, J. P.: Repair of the Periodontium Following Gingivectomy in Experimental Animals. J. D. Res. (Abst.), 29:659, 1950.
19. Glickman, I., Turesky, S. S., and Manhold, J.: The Oxygen Consumption of Healing Gingiva. J. D. Res., 29:429, 1950.
20. Goldman, H. M.: Subgingival Curettage – A Rationale. J. Periodont., 19:54, 1948.
21. Gottlieb, B.: The New Concept of Periodontoclasia. J. Periodont., 17:7, 1946.
22. Gross, H.: Experiments on the Regenerative Capacity of the Gingiva in Dogs. Paradentium, 5:57, 1933.
23. Hatfield, C. G., and Baumhammers, A.: Cytotoxic Effects of Periodontally Involved Root Surfaces. I.A.D.R. Abstr. 48th General Meeting, 1970, p. 99, No. 203.
24. Hugoson, A.: Gingival Inflammation and Female Sex Hormones. J. Periodont. Res., Suppl. No. 5, 1970.
25. Jansen, M. T., Coppes, L., and Verdenius, H. H. W.: Healing of Periodontal Wounds in Dogs. J. Periodont., 26:292, 1955.
26. Kaplan, H., and Mann, J. B.: How Is Pyorrhea Cured? J.A.D.A., 29:1471, 1942.
27. Leblond, C. P., and Walker, B. E.: Renewal of Cell Populations, Physiol. Rev., 36:255, 1956.
28. Leonard, H. J.: Conservative Treatment of Periodontoclasia. J.A.D.A., 26:1308, 1939.
29. Leonard, H. J.: In Our Opinion – Reattachment. J. Periodont., Supp. to Jan., 1943, p. 5.
30. Lindhe, J., and Brånemark, P. I.: The Effect of Sex Hormones on Vascularization of a Granulation Tissue. J. Periodont. Res., 3:6, 1968.
31. Linghorne, W. J.: Studies in the Reattachment and Regeneration of the Supporting Structures of the Teeth. IV. Regeneration in Epithelialized Pockets Following the Organization of a Blood Clot. J. D. Res., 36:4, 1957.
32. Linghorne, W. J., and O'Connell, D. C.: Studies in the Reattachment and Regeneration of the Supporting Structures of the Teeth. III. Regeneration in Epithelialized Pockets. J. D. Res., 34:164, 1955.
33. McCall, J. O.: An Improved Method of Inducing Reattachment of the Gingival Tissues in Periodontoclasia. D. Items Int., 48:342, 1926.
34. Meyer, J., Marwah, A. S., and Weinmann, J. P.: Mitotic Rate of Gingival Epithelium in Two Age Groups. J. Invest. Derm., 27:237, 1956.
35. Morris, M. L.: Healing of Human Periodontal Tissues Following Surgical Detachment and Extirpation of Vital Pulps. J. Periodont., 31:23, 1960.
36. Morris, M. L.: Healing of Naturally Occurring Periodontal Pockets About Vital Human Teeth. J. Periodont., 26:285, 1955.
37. Morris, M. L.: The Reattachment of the Human Periodontal Tissue Following Surgical Detachment. J. Periodont., 25:64, 1954.
38. Morris, M. L.: The Removal of Pocket and Attachment Epithelium in Humans: A Histological Study. J. Periodont., 25:7, 1954.
39. Moskow, B. S.: The Response of the Gingival Sulcus to Instrumentation. A Histologic Investigation. II. Gingival Curettage. J. Periodont., 35:112, 1964.
40. Muhlemann, H. R., Zander, H., and Halberg, F.: Mitotic Activity in the Periodontal Tissues of the Rat Molar. J. D. Res., 33:459, 1954.
41. Oliver, R. C.: Tooth Mortality Following Periodontal Therapy. J. Periodont., 41:48, 1970 (Abstr.).
42. Perez-Tamayo, Ruy: Mechanisms of Disease and Introduction to Pathology. Philadelphia, W. B. Saunders Co., 1961, p. 105.
43. Prichard, J.: The Infrabony Technique as a Predictable Procedure. J. Periodont., 28:202, 1957.
44. Ramfjord, S. P.: Experimental Periodontal Reattachment in Rhesus Monkeys. J. Periodont., 22:67, 1951.
45. Ramfjord, S. P., and Costich, E. R.: Healing after Simple Gingivectomy. J. Periodont., 34:401, 1963.
46. Rateitschak, K.: The Therapeutic Effect of Local Treatment on Periodontal Disease Assessed upon Evaluation of Different Diagnostic Criteria. 2. Changes in Gingival Inflammation. J. Periodont., 35:155, 1964.
47. Rateitschak, K., et al.: The Therapeutic Effect of Local Treatment on Periodontal Disease Assessed upon Evaluation of Different Diagnostic Criteria.

3. Radiographic Changes in Appearance of Bone. J. Periodont., 35:263, 1964.

48. Sato, M.: Histopathological Study of the Healing Process after Surgical Treatment for Alveolar Pyorrhea. Bull. Tokyo Med. Dent. Univ., 1:71, 1960.

49. Schaffer, E. M., and Korn, N. A.: Comparison of Curettage and Gingivectomy in Dogs. (Abst.) I.A.D.R., 40:69, 1962.

50. Schaffer, E. M., and Zander, H.: Histological Evidence of Reattachment of Periodontal Pockets. Paradentologie, 7:101, 1953.

51. Shapiro, M.: Reattachment in Periodontal Disease. J. Periodont., 24:26, 1953.

52. Skillen, W. G., and Lundquist, G. R.: An Experimental Study of Peridental Membrane Reattachment in Healthy and Pathologic Tissues. J.A.D.A., 24:175, 1937.

53. Skillen, W. G., and Lundquist, G. R.: Experimental Gingival Injuries in Dogs. J. D. Res., 15:165, 1935.

54. Sorrin, S.: Bone Changes Induced by Periodontic Treatment. J. D. Res., 9:359, 1929.

55. Stahl, S. S.: Effect of Oral Somatotrophic Hormone Injections upon Gingival Wounds in Rats. J. D. Res., 38:725, 1959 (Abstr.).

56. Stahl, S. S.: Healing Gingival Injury in Normal and Systemically Stressed Young Adult Male Rats. J. Periodont., 32:63, 1961.

57. Stahl, S. S.: Healing of Gingival Tissues Following Various Therapeutic Regimens—a Review of Histologic Studies. J. Oral Therap. & Pharm., 2:145, 1965.

58. Stahl, S. S.: The Effect of a Protein-Free Diet on the Healing of Gingival Wounds in Rats. Arch. Oral Biol., 7:551, 1962.

59. Stahl, S. S.: The Influence of Antibiotics on the Healing of Gingival Wounds in Rats. I. Alveolar Bone and Soft Tissue. J. Periodont., 33:261, 1962.

60. Stahl, S. S., Soberman, A., and DeCesare, A.: Gingival Healing. V. The Effects of Antibiotics Administered During Early Stages of Repair. J. Periodont.-Periodontics, 40:521, 1969.

61. Stone, S., Ramfjord, S., and Waldron, J.: Scaling and Gingival Curettage. A Radioautographic Study. J. Periodont., 37:415, 1966.

62. Turesky, S. S., and Glickman, I.: Histochemical Evaluation of Gingival Healing in Experimental Animals on Adequate and Vitamin C Deficient Diets. J. D. Res., 33:273, 1954.

63. Waerhaug, J.: Depth of Incision in Gingivectomy. Oral Surg., Oral Med. & Oral Path., 8:707, 1955.

64. Waerhaug, J. Microscopic Demonstration of Tissue Reaction Incident to Removal of Subgingival Calculus. J. Periodont., 26:26, 1955.

65. Williams, C. H. M.: Rationalization of Periodontal Pocket Therapy. J. Periodont., 14:67, 1943.

Chapter 37

THE PERIODONTAL INSTRUMENTARIUM

Periodontal instruments are designed for specific purposes, such as the removal of calculus, planing the root surfaces, curettage of the gingiva or removal of diseased tissue. Upon first examination, the number of instruments available for similar purposes appears confusing. However, with experience one selects a relatively small set which fulfills all requirements. It is some-times necessary to reduce the size of instruments so that they fit into periodontal pockets without injuring the gingiva or tooth surfaces.[26, 33, 35]

CLASSIFICATION OF PERIODONTAL INSTRUMENTS

Periodontal instruments are classified according to the purposes they serve, as follows:

Periodontal probes and *pocket marking forceps* for location, measurement and marking of pockets, and determining their course on individual tooth surfaces.

Explorers, for location of deposits on the teeth.

Superficial (heavy) scalers, for removal of supragingival calculus.

Deep (fine) scalers, for removal of sub-gingival calculus.

Hoe scalers, for removal of subgingival calculus and planing root surfaces.

Curets for removal of the inner surface of the pocket wall and the epithelial attachment, and for smoothing root surfaces.

Ultrasonic instruments, for scaling and cleansing tooth surfaces and curetting the gingival wall of periodontal pockets.

Surgical periodontal instruments.

Cleansing and polishing instruments. Rubber cups, bristle brushes, portepolisher and dental tape for cleansing and polishing tooth surfaces.

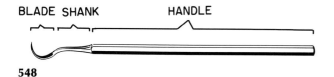

BLADE SHANK   HANDLE

Figure 37–1 The different sections of a typical periodontal instrument.

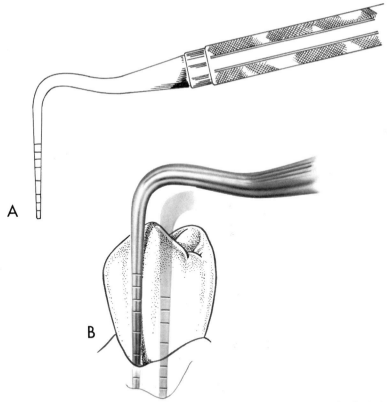

Figure 37–2 Glickman Periodontal Probe #26G. *A,* Calibrated blade offset from the shank. *B,* Pocket probed across the facial surface.

The wearing and cutting qualities of some types of steel used in periodontal instruments have been tested,[19, 20] but specifications vary with the manufacturers.

Each group of instruments has characteristic features; individual therapists often develop variations with which they operate most effectively. In the descriptions which follow, the first instrument or set in each group is the author's preference (the "G" series). The parts of each instrument, referred to as the "blade," "shank" and "handle," are shown in Figure 37–1.

Periodontal Probes

Periodontal probes are used to measure the depth of pockets and determine their conformation. The representative features are a tapered rod-like blade calibrated in 1

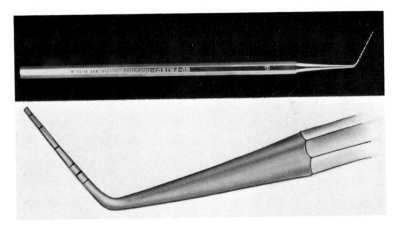

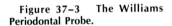

Figure 37–3 The Williams Periodontal Probe.

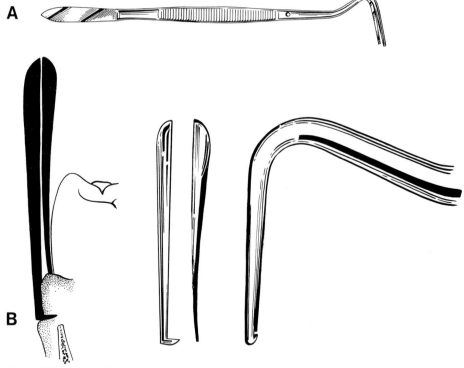

Figure 37–4   Glickman Periodontal Pocket Marker #27G and #28G (Hu-Friedy). *A,* The blade is joined to the shank with a goose-neck bend for accessibility to different tooth surfaces. *B,* Marker in periodontal pocket. The blunt end is slightly bowed to conform to the tooth.

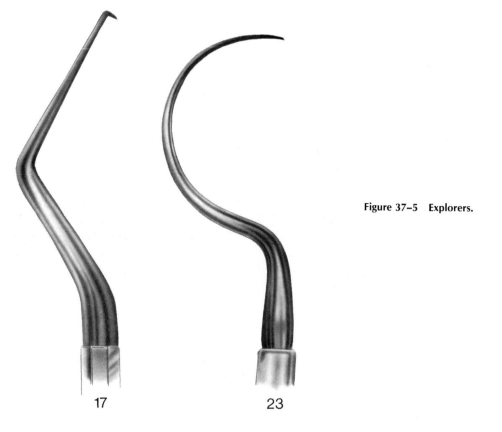

Figure 37–5   Explorers.

and 2 millimeter markings, and a blunt rounded tip. In some, a goose-neck bend joins the blade to the shank for better access to different tooth surfaces (Fig. 37–2, A) but there are many other types (Fig. 37–3). To measure a pocket, the probe is inserted with firm gentle pressure to the bottom of the pocket. **The blade should be aligned with the long axis of the tooth.** Several measurements are made to determine the course of the pocket on each surface (Fig. 37–2, B).

Periodontal Pocket Markers, #27G and #28G

This is a paired set of instruments shaped like cotton pliers (Fig. 37–4, A). One tip is sharp and bent at a right angle; the other is blunt and slightly bowed to conform to the tooth contour when it is inserted into the pocket. The blades are joined to the shank with a goose-neck bend to improve accessibility to different tooth surfaces.

To mark a pocket, the blunt tip is aligned in the long axis of the tooth and inserted to the bottom of the pocket (Fig. 37–4, B). The ends are pressed together, creating an ex-ternal bleeding point which corresponds to the bottom of the pocket. Multiple markings are used to trace the course of pockets on individual tooth surfaces.

Explorers

Of the many types of explorers the combined use of #23 and #17 is recommended. These are lightweight, delicate, highly tempered instruments; one of them is sickle-shaped (#23), and the other consists of a rod-like offset blade with a short right angle terminal bend (#17) (Fig. 37–5). Explorers are used to locate subgingival deposits before scaling and to check the smoothness of the root after treatment.

Superficial Scalers, #1G–#2G, #3G–#4G, #5G–#6G

This is a set of three double-ended scalers for removing supragingival deposits. #1G and #2G is a universal scaler with two blades in a straight line with the handle;

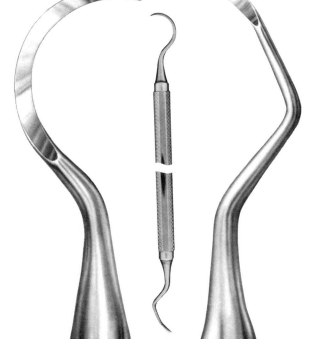

Figure 37–6 Universal Superficial Scaler #1G and #2G. One end is sickle-shaped with flatted sides; the other is trapezoidal.

1G   2G

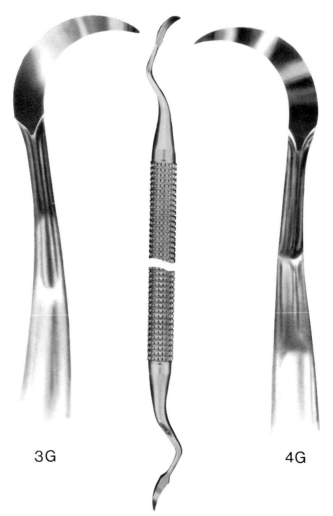

3G   4G

Figure 37–7   Superficial Scaler #3G and #4G.

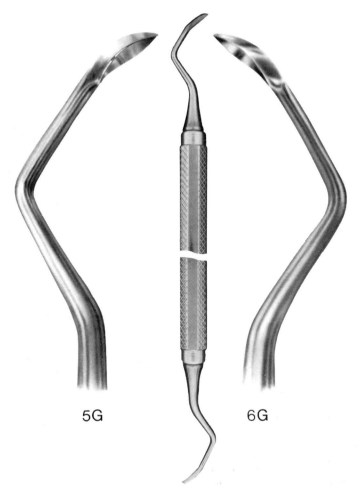

Figure 37–8 Superficial Scaler #5G and #6G.

#1G is sickle-shaped with flattened sides, and #2G is trapezoidal in cross section (Fig. 37–6). Instrument #3G and #4G has paired heavy sickle-shaped blades and angulated shanks. The inner surface is broad and tapers to a point. The end is rounded to preserve the effectiveness of the instrument when it is reduced by sharpening. Two cutting edges are formed by the junction of the inner and lateral surfaces (Fig. 37–7). The #5G–#6G is a finer superficial scaler with two small trapezoidal blades, each with two cutting edges (Fig. 37–8).

To avoid nicking the teeth these instruments are activated at an angle of slightly less than 90° with the tooth surface[35] (Fig. 37–9). The cutting edge engages the supragingival calculus at the level of the crest of the gingival margin, and the calculus is dislodged with a firm, steady motion toward the crown (Fig. 37–9). The procedure is systematically repeated until all visible calculus is removed.

JAQUETTE SUPERFICIAL SCALERS #1, #2 AND #3. Three instruments comprise the set. In #1 the blade and shank are in a straight line with the handle. Number 2 and #3 are paired with angulated shanks to facilitate accessibility to all tooth surfaces (Fig. 37–10). Instrument #1 is generally used in the anterior part of the mouth and #2 and #3 in the posterior part. The blade is triangular in cross section. The two lateral surfaces join the inner surface to form two working edges (Fig. 37–11). The inner surface tapers from a broad base at the shank to form a terminal point. These instruments are used with slightly less than a 90° angle of the blade to the tooth surface.

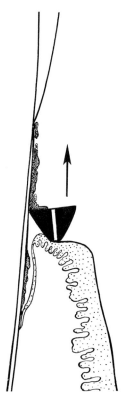

Figure 37–9 Removal of Supragingival Calculus with a #3G Superficial Scaler. The blade forms an angle of slightly less than 90° with the tooth surface.

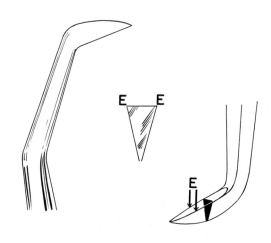

Figure 37–10 Jaquette Superficial Scalers #1, #2 and #3.

Figure 37–11 Jaquette Scaler, showing the blade in cross section and the cutting edges (E).

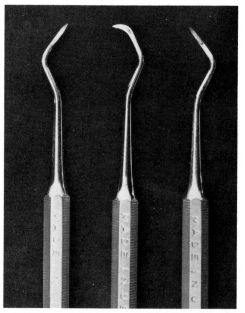

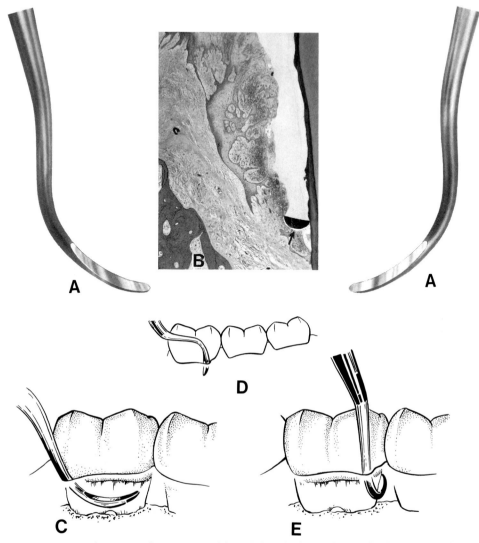

Figure 37–12 Deep Scaler #7G and #8G. *A,* Double-ended sickle shaped deep scaler for the removal of subgingival calculus. *B,* Cross section of the scaler blade against cemental wall of a deep periodontal pocket. *C,* Scaler in position at the base of a periodontal pocket on the buccal surface of a mandibular molar. *D,* Scaler inserted in pocket with the tip directed apically. *E,* Scaler in position at base of a periodontal pocket on the distal surface of mandibular molar.

Deep Scalers

DEEP SCALER, #7G–#8G. This instrument is used for the removal of deep deposits. It is finer than the superficial scalers and provides accessibility in deep pockets with a minimum of soft tissue trauma. The #7–#8 is a double-ended instrument (Fig. 37–12, *A*) with long, narrow, sickle-shaped blades. Each has an inner concave surface and an outer rounded surface. Two cutting edges are formed by the junction of the lateral borders of the inner and outer surfaces (Fig. 37–12, *A*). The inner surface be-

tween the cutting edges is flat. The outer and inner surfaces merge in a rounded flattened tip (Fig. 37–12, *A*). The angle of the blade to the shank provides accessibility to all areas of the mouth.

This instrument is used as follows:

(1) The blade is inserted to the depth of the pocket so that it forms an angle of slightly less than 90° with the tooth (Fig. 37–12, *B*. The subgingival calculus is engaged at its lowest border, close to the bottom of the pocket, and dislodged with a firm motion in the direction of the crown (Fig. 37–12, *C* and *E*).

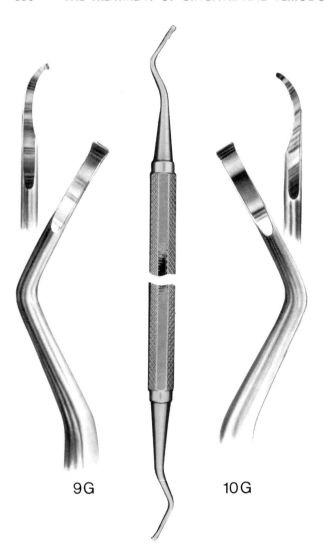

Figure 37–13 Deep Scaler #9G–#10G. Paired blades on a double-ended instrument.

9G   10G

(2) On the facial and lingual surfaces, the blade may be inserted into the pocket with the rounded tip pointed apically and the blade against the tooth surface (Fig. 37–12, *D*). The instrument is activated along the tooth surface.

The #7G–#8G scaler is best suited for removal of subgingival deposits, but it may also be used to smooth the root surface and remove the epithelial attachment from the tooth. The instrument cannot be used effectively if the blade is placed with the inner surface parallel to the tooth.

DEEP SCALER, #9G–#10G. This is a double-ended instrument with a small claw-shaped blade at each end (Fig. 37–13). The blade is slightly curved, with a straight cutting edge beveled at 45° and rounded at the

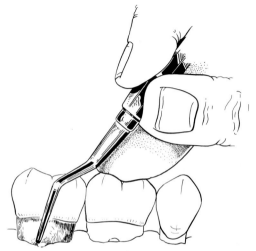

Figure 37–14 Deep Scaler #9G on the buccal aspect of the bifurcation of the mandibular second molar.

edges. This instrument is designed for deep scaling of posterior teeth, particularly in furcation areas (Fig. 37–14).

Hoe Scalers, #11G–#12G and #13G–#14G

Hoe scalers are used for planing and smoothing root surfaces, which entails removal of calculus remnants and softened cementum. The #11G–#12G and #13G–#14G hoes are double-ended instruments designed to provide accessibility to all root surfaces (Fig. 37–15, A). The blade is bent at a 99° angle; the cutting edge is formed by the junction of the flattened terminal surface with the inner aspect of the blade. The cutting edge is beveled at 45°. The blade is slightly bowed, so that it can maintain contact at two points on a convex surface. The back of the blade is rounded and the blade has been reduced to minimum thickness to permit access to the roots of deep pockets without interference from the adjacent tissues.

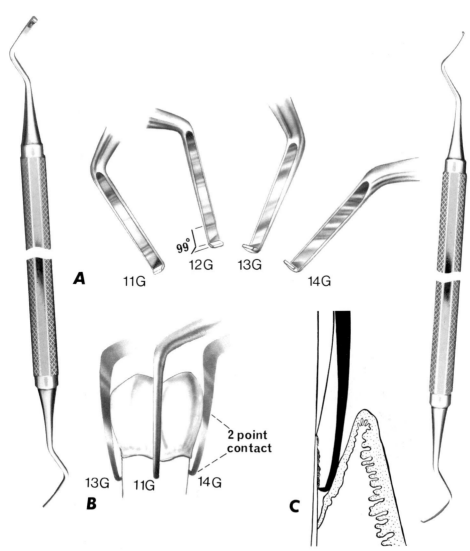

Figure 37–15 Hoe Scalers #11G–#12G and #13G–#14G. A, Double-ended hoe scalers with beveled cutting edge. B, Hoe scalers designed for different tooth surfaces, showing "two-point" contact. C, Hoe scaler in a periodontal pocket. The back of the blade is rounded for easier access. The instrument contacts the tooth at two points for stability.

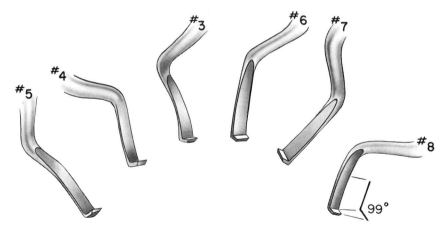

Figure 37–16   McCall's Hoe Scalers.

These instruments are used as follows:

1. The blade is inserted to the base of the periodontal pocket **so that it makes two-point contact with the tooth** (Fig. 37–15, *B* and *C*). This stabilizes the instrument and prevents nicking of the root.

2. The instrument is activated with a firm motion toward the crown, making every effort to preserve the two-point contact with the tooth.

McCalls' Hoe Scalers, #3, #4, #5, #6, #7 and #8.   This is a set of six hoe scalers designed to provide access to all tooth surfaces (Fig. 37–16). There is a different angular relationship between the shank and handle of each instrument.

Chisel Scalers #15G–#16G

The chisel scaler, designed for proximal surfaces of teeth too closely spaced to permit the use of other scalers, is usually used in the anterior part of the mouth (Fig. 37–17). The #15G–#16G is a double-ended instrument, with a curved and straight shank (Fig. 37–18); the blades are slightly curved with a straight cutting edge beveled at 45°.

The scaler is inserted from the facial surface. The slight curve of the blade makes it possible to stabilize it against the proximal surface, whereas the cutting edge engages the calculus without nicking the

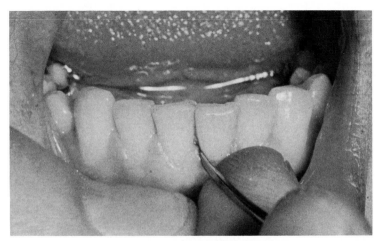

Figure 37–17   Chisel Scaler in Position.

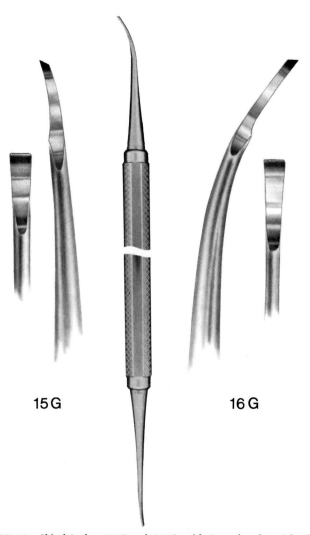

15 G   16 G

Figure 37–18 Chisel Scaler #15G and #16G, with Curved and Straight Shanks.

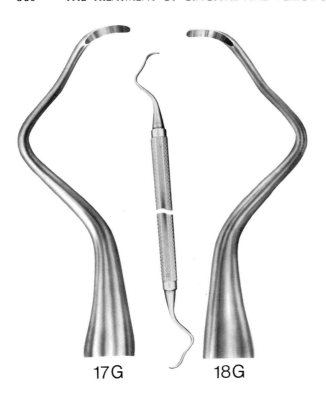

Figure 37-19 Universal Curet #17G and #18G.

17G   18G

tooth. The instrument is activated with a push motion, with the side of the blade held firmly against the root.

Curets

Curets are instruments with fine blades used primarily for the soft tissue wall of periodontal pockets, to remove the inner lining and epithelial attachment, and also for removing periodontal fibers from the walls of osseous defects associated with infrabony pockets. They are also used to remove calculus fragments, and smooth root surfaces.

UNIVERSAL CURET, #17G-#18G. The #17G-#18G universal curet has an angulated offset shank with a spoon-shaped blade (Fig. 37-19). The inner surface is flat and the outer surface is rounded, with two cutting edges formed where they meet.

The curet is used as follows:

The blade is inserted to the bottom of the pocket and the instrument is activated toward the crown with the cutting edge engaging the lining of the pocket wall (Fig. 37-20, A). **To prevent the pocket wall from moving away from the curet, gentle digital**

pressure is applied to the outer surface. The cutting edge on the other side of the blade may be used for smoothing the root surface.

To remove the epithelial attachment the curet is inserted with the blade pointed apically and the tip resting against the base of the pocket (Fig. 37-20, B). Slight vertical pressure is applied to push the tip into the attachment area, and the instrument is moved along the bottom of the pocket.

3. The curet may also be used for the partial removal of interdental gingival papillae (papillectomy). The blade is inserted at one side of the papilla and activated across it to remove the desired amount of tissue (Fig. 37-20, C and D).

GRACEY FINISHING CURETS. This is a widely used set of curets which are available as paired single instruments or as double-ended instruments. Three sets consisting of #3 and #4, #9 and #10, and #13 and #14 are adequate for most needs, but others are also available (Fig. 37-21, A). The instruments differ in the angulation of the shank to the handle. The blade is extremely fine and consists of a thin rounded bend, with two cutting edges formed by the junction of the outer and inner surfaces. The instrument is used for removing minute

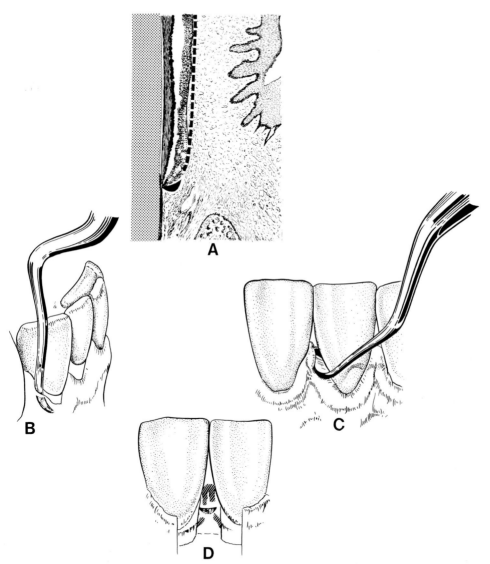

Figure 37–20 *A,* Cross section of the blade of a #17G universal curet at the base of a periodontal pocket. The blade starts beneath the epithelial attachment and moves along the broken line to remove the ulcerated inner pocket wall. *B,* Curet activated with the tip at the base of the pocket. *C,* Curet in a pocket on the mesial surface of a mandibular lateral incisor. *D,* Use of the curet to remove part of the interdental papilla. This is called papillectomy.

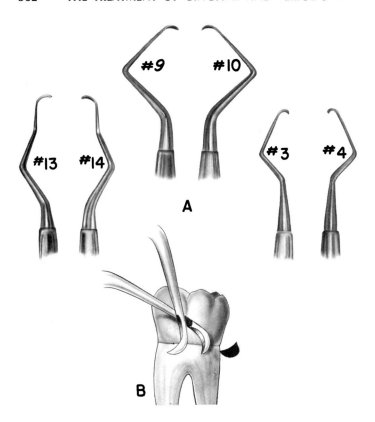

Figure 37–21 *A,* Gracey curets of different designs. *B,* Three different angles at which the Gracey curet may be applied to the tooth surfaces.

fragments of calculus and smoothing root surfaces as well as curettage of soft tissues. The design of the shank and size of the blade permit a wide range of movement on individual tooth surfaces (Fig. 37–21, *B*).

Files

Files were at one time popular, but they are no longer used very much for scaling and root planing, because they gouge and roughen root surfaces.[15] They are sometimes used for removing overhanging margins of dental restorations.

Surgical Instruments

Surgical hoe, #19G

This instrument has a flattened, fish-tail shaped blade with a pronounced convexity in its terminal portion (Fig. 37–22). The cutting edge is beveled with rounded edges and projects beyond the long axis of the

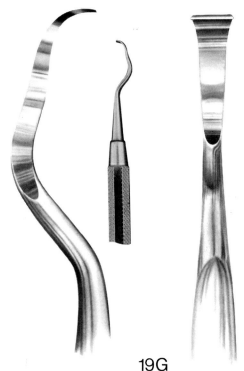

19G

Figure 37–22   Surgical Hoe #19G.

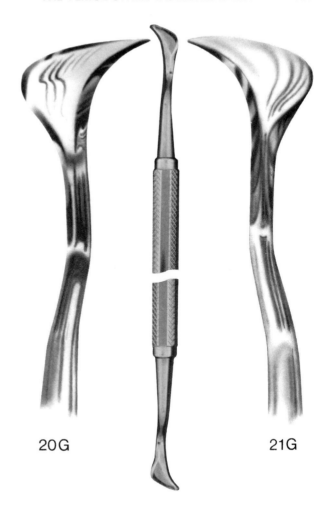

20G 21G

Figure 37–23 Periodontal Knives #20G and #21G. The tip of the blade is extended for interproximal access.

handle to preserve the effectiveness of the instrument when the blade is reduced by sharpening. The surgical hoe is generally used for detaching pocket walls after the gingivectomy incision, but it is also useful for smoothing root surfaces made accessible by any surgical procedure.

Periodontal knives, #20G and #21G

This is a double-ended instrument for gingivectomy and other periodontal surgery. It consists of a set of paired scaler-shaped blades attached to angulated shanks (Fig. 37–23). The entire periphery is a cutting edge, formed by the junction of the outer and inner surfaces. The tip of the blade is extended to provide access to proximal surfaces.

The interdent, #22G and #23G

This is a double-ended instrument designed especially for removing interdental tissue during gingivectomy. It is also useful for periodontal flaps and incising the inner wall of infrabony pockets. It consists of a pair of matched, elongated, slightly curved blades (Fig. 37–24). The cutting edges are tapered and form the periphery of the blade.

There are many other periodontal knives, of which the following are representative types: The Orban knives #1 and #2 are spear-shaped blades attached to the handle by an offset shank to provide accessibility to interproximal areas (Fig. 37–25). The blade has two cutting edges, formed by the junction of the rounded outer surface and the flat inner surface, and tapers to a sharp point.

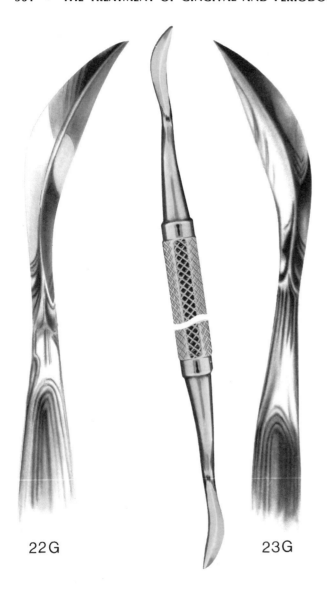

22G

23G

Figure 37–24 The Interdent #22G–#23G. Periodontal knives for gingivectomy (interdental tissue) and other surgical uses.

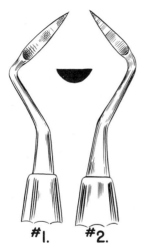

#1.   #2.

Figure 37–25   Orban Periodontal Knives, #1 and #2.

The Buck knives are spear shaped (Fig. 37–26), and the Monahan-Lewis knives have detachable blades (Fig. 37–27).

Kirkland surgical instruments

This is a complete set of instruments designed for the gingivectomy technique. Instruments #12K, #13K and #14K are especially adapted for removing diseased tissue following the gingivectomy incision and cleansing the root surfaces (Fig. 37–28). Numbers 2K, 3K, 4K, 5K, 7K, 8K, 9K, 17K, 18K, 19K, 20K, 21K and 22K, illus-

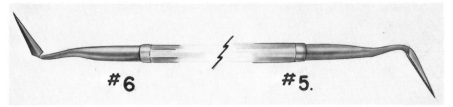

Figure 37–26　Buck Periodontal Knives.

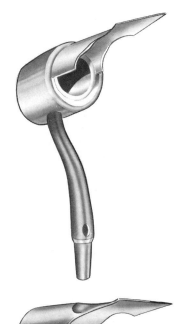

Figure 37–27　Monahan-Lewis Periodontal Knife with Detachable Blades.

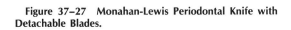

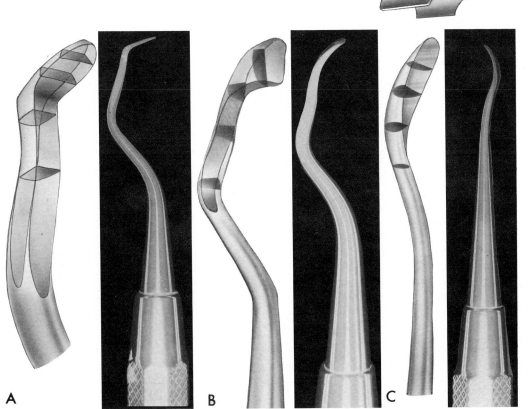

A　　　　　　　**B**　　　　　　　**C**

Figure 37–28　Kirkland Surgical Instruments. *A,* #12K. *B,* #13K. *C,* #14K.

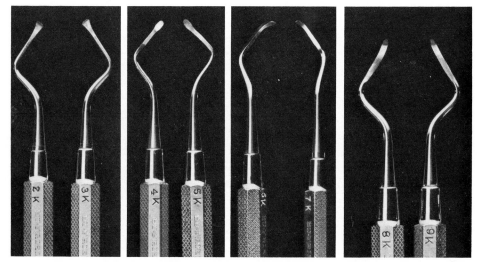

Figure 37–29 **Kirkland Surgical Instruments:** #2K and #3K; #4K and #5K; #6K and #7K; #8K and #9K.

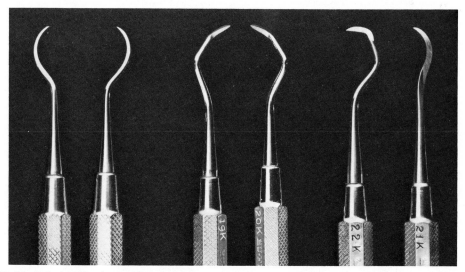

Figure 37–30 Paired Kirkland surgical instruments, #17K and #18K, #19K and #20K, and scalers #21K and #22K.

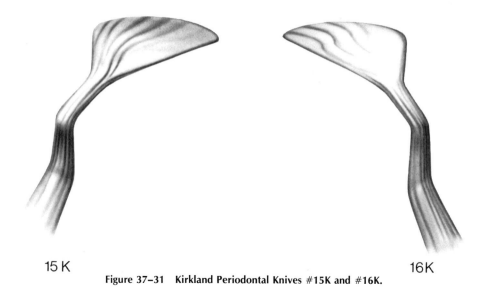

15 K   16K

Figure 37–31 Kirkland Periodontal Knives #15K and #16K.

trated in Figures 37–29 and 37–30, provide accessibility to all tooth surfaces for the removal of deposits and smoothing the roots.

The Kirkland periodontal knives #15K and #16K are paired instruments which consist of a thin flattened blade attached to the handle by an angulated shank. The outer edge is elliptical, and the inner edge is straight (Fig. 37–31).

Periosteal elevator, #24G

Periosteal elevators serve a variety of purposes in periodontal surgery. Greater versatility is provided by instruments with both rounded and straight blades (Fig. 37–32).

Scissors

Scissors are used in periodontal surgery for such purposes as removing tabs of tissue during gingivectomy, trimming the margins of flaps, enlarging incisions in periodontal abscesses and removing muscle attachments in mucogingival surgery. There are many types; the choice is a matter of individual preference. Illustrated in Figure 37–33 are the #25G with curved handle and curved beveled blade with serrations, and straight and curved scissors.

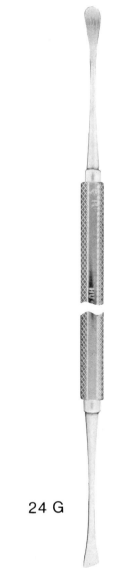

24 G

Figure 37–32 Periosteal Elevator #24G. Periosteal elevator with rounded and straight blades.

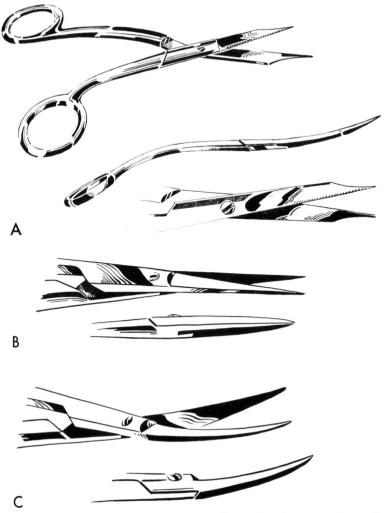

Figure 37–33 **Scissors.** *A,* #25G curved handle and curved bevelled blade with serrations. *B,* Straight scissors. *C,* Curved scissors.

Aspirators

Aspirators are indispensable in surgical periodontal procedures. Many types of aspirators and aspirator tips are available. The Frazier #3 tip is simple and efficient; its size and shape permit easy access to all areas (Fig. 37–34). It comes with a fitted stylet for removing entrapped tissue and debris.

Cleansing and Polishing Instruments

The rubber cup, portepolisher, bristle brush and dental tape are employed in the dental office for cleansing and polishing the tooth surfaces.

Rubber cups consist of a rubber shell with or without web-shaped conformations in the hollow interior. They are used in the handpiece with a special prophylaxis angle. There are many types of cleansing and polishing pastes, which should be kept moist to minimize frictional heat as the cup revolves. Aggressive use of the rubber cups may remove the layer of cementum which is very thin in the cervical area.

The *portepolisher* is a hand instrument constructed so as to hold a wooden point. The wooden point with a polishing paste is applied to the tooth with a firm burnishing action. The Ivory straight portepolisher with

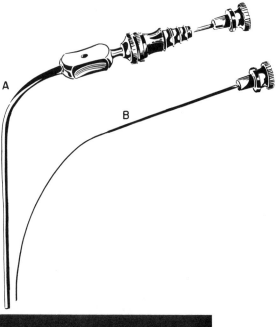

Figure 37–34 Frazier Aspirator Tip. *A,* Aspirator tip. *B,* Stylet for clearing the tip.

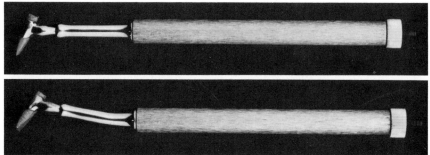

Figure 37–35 Portepolishers. *Above,* Straight type. *Below,* Angulated type.

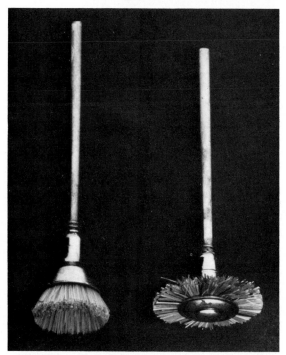

Figure 37–36 Bristle Brushes, Wheel and Cup Types.

the wood point set at an angle of 45° with the handle fulfills most needs (Fig. 37–35). A contra-angle portepolisher, angulated at 60°, for use in the posterior part of the mouth is also available (Fig. 37–35).

Bristle brushes are available in wheel and cup shapes (Fig. 37–36). The brush is used in the handpiece with a polishing paste. Because the bristles are very stiff, use of the brush should be confined to the crown to avoid injuring the cementum.

Dental tape with polishing paste is used for polishing proximal surfaces inaccessible to the other polishing instruments. The tape is passed interproximally, maintained at a plane at right angles to the long axis of the tooth, and activated in a firm labiolingual motion. Particular care is taken to avoid injury to the gingiva. The area should be cleansed with warm water to remove all remnants of paste.

569

Ultrasonic Instruments

Ultrasonic vibrations may be used for scaling, curettage and stain removal.[37] Their action is derived from physical vibrations of particles of matter, similar to sound waves, at frequencies above the range of human hearing which range from 20,000 to many million cycles per second.* In periodontal instrumentation, tipped instruments producing up to 29,000 vibrations per second are used.

Ultrasonic tips of different shapes are available for scaling, curettage, root planing and gingival surgery. All tips are made to operate in a wet field and have water outlets attached. The spray is directed at the end of the tip to dissipate the heat generated by the ultrasonic vibrations.

The instrument is used with a light touch and a limited number of strokes per unit area. Improper use may produce gouging and roughening of root surfaces. The tips work best against hard tooth surfaces but can also be used against gingival tissue. The gingiva can be made more rigid by injecting anesthetic solution directly into it.[4] When placed against a tooth or soft tissue surface the instrument mechanically debrides surface accumulations or necrotic tissue. The liquid sprayed on the vibrating tip reinforces the mechanical cleansing effect of the vibrations. The instrument should be kept away from bone to avoid the possibility of necrosis and sequestration. It should not be used on young growing tissues, and its use in the treatment of children is not recommended.[11]

When applied to the gingiva of experimental animals ultrasonic vibrations disrupt tissue continuity, lift off epithelium, dismember collagen bundles, and alter the morphology of fibroblast nuclei.[14] However, the simple application of ultrasonic vibration to the gingiva produces no clinically discernible morphologic changes, and use following gingivectomy does not appear to retard gingival healing.[12]

Ultrasonics is effective for removing calculus[5, 16, 22, 32] and debriding the epithelial lining of periodontal pockets.[14] It produces a narrow band of necrotic tissue (microcauterization) which strips off from the inner aspect of the pocket. The Morse type scaler and the rod-shaped instrument are used for this purpose. Some investigators find it as effective as manual instruments for curettage,[24] with less inflammation but more pronounced disruption of the uppermost periodontal fibers.[36] When debriding the gingival wall of periodontal pockets it tends to remove less of the underlying connective tissue than manual instrumentation but it does not smooth the root as well.[31] It tends to produce a stippled root with greater removal of tooth substance.[3] The volume and depth of tooth structure loss may be reduced by using a medium setting on the instrument and slight tactile force.[6]

There are reports that ultrasonic instrumentation roughens dentin surfaces[4] and causes more gouging and nicking of the roots than manual instruments,[1, 16] and that it is not as effective as manual instrumentation for root planing.[32] The roughness scores of teeth planed with ultrasonics have been reported as twice those of teeth planed with hand curets.[17]

Opinions differ regarding the effectiveness of ultrasonics for removing stains as compared with conventional methods of oral prophylaxis.[5, 16, 22] There is no significant difference in the incidence of bacteremia following subgingival procedures with manual and ultrasonic instruments.[2]

Electrosurgery

Electrosurgery refers to the use of high frequency electric currents for cutting or destroying tissue. There are two types of electrosurgical devices.* One consists of a spark-gap generator which produces a current characterized by surging peaks with intervals of highly reduced or damped-out energy; the other, most commonly used types, utilizes electronic circuitry to convert alternating electric current into high frequency radio current. Within this class are instruments which produce both *partially rectified* and *undamped fully rectified current* (multiple circuit units).[10] In *partially rectified currents, the alternating surging peaks are partially reduced or "damped"*

---

*"Cycles per second" are also referred to as Hertz or H$_z$.

*For an evaluation of dental electrosurgical devices, see the report prepared for the Council on Dental Materials and Devices of the American Dental Association (1969).[29]

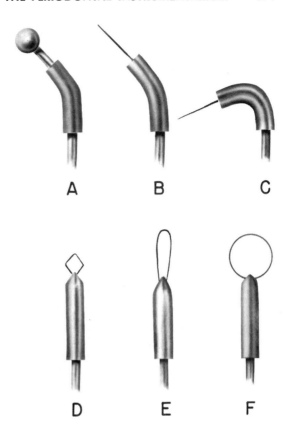

Figure 37–37 Electrodes Used in Electrosurgery. *A,* Ball; *B,* needle; *C,* bent needle; *D,* diamond; *E,* elliptical loop; *F,* spherical loop.

before peak cycles recur. This type of current is used for coagulation, desiccation and fulguration. *In fully rectified current the alternating cycles are filtered out, producing an undamped current* which is used for cutting tissue without coagulation.

The current is applied into the tissues through an electrode (active electrode); a conductive pad of flat metal or metallized rubber (passive electrode) in contact with the patient, but not necessarily in contact with the skin, is used to complete the circuit (biterminal circuit). Electrodes vary in design to serve specific purposes (Fig. 37–37). Most electrodes are single ended or monopolar and are used in a biterminal circuit, with the passive electrode in contact with the patient.

Desiccation is deep-penetrating cellular dehydration of tissue produced by a single electrode placed into tissue, using a highly damped high frequency alternating current. The small pointed electrode (Fig. 37–37) is commonly used for this purpose, without the pad.

Electrocoagulation is dehydration and coagulation of tissue and hemostasis, using a moderately or highly damped high frequency alternating current. A ball or loop type electrode is used with the conductive pad, usually for hemostasis or localized tissue destruction.

Fulguration is superficial dehydration and carbonization of tissue produced by placing a single electrode just above, not in contact with, the tissue surface. The current is a highly damped, high frequency alternating type, without the conductive plate. Fulguration may be used for destroying fistulous orifices, for eliminating tissue tabs and for hemostasis.

Electrosection ("cutting") is resecting tissue with fully rectified undamped high frequency biterminal current. The concentration of current causes molecular disintegration and volatilization of the tissues without coagulation and is considered self-limiting.

There are many uses for electrosurgery. **In restorative dentistry it is one of the methods of gingival retraction[23] to expose the margins of preparations.** It provides access to the tooth for finalizing the preparation and creates a gingival trough to accom-

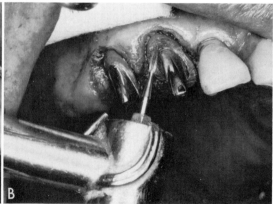

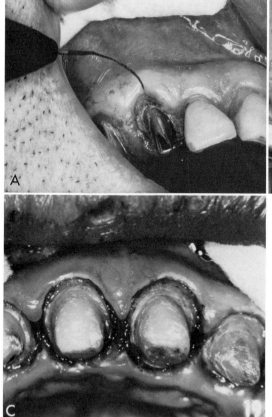

Figure 37–38 Gingival Retraction by Electrosurgery. *A,* Needle electrode removes inner surface of gingival margin which is covering the edge of the root. *B,* Access and visibility created for finalizing the preparation. *C,* Gingival trough provides space for impression material. (Courtesy of Dr. Mario Martignoni, Rome.)

modate impression material (Fig. 37–38). Gingival retraction is accomplished with the needle electrode carried along the inner surface of the gingival sulcus.

Electrosurgery is also used for **removing gingival tissue which covers the margins of carious lesions and interferes with cavity preparation.** A loop electrode is used for this purpose. The same procedure is used to remove tissue which interferes with the insertion of a rubber dam.[34]

In periodontics, electrosurgery is useful for a variety of purposes:

The removal of gingival enlargements and gingivoplasty[27] are performed with the needle electrode supplemented by the small ovoid loop or diamond-shaped electrodes for festooning (Fig. 37–39). A blended cutting and coagulating current is used. In all reshaping procedures the electrode is activated in a concise "paring" motion.

In the treatment of acute periodontal abscesses, the incision to establish drainage can be made with the needle electrode without exerting painful pressure. The incision will remain open because the edges are sealed by the current. After the acute symptoms subside, the regular procedure for the treatment of the periodontal abscess is followed (Chap. 48).

For hemostasis, the ball electrode is lightly touched to the bleeding surface with a coagulating current. Electrosurgery is very helpful for the control of isolated bleeding points. Bleeding areas located interproximally are reached with a thin, blade-shaped electrode.

Frenum and muscle attachments can be relocated to facilitate pocket elimination, using a loop electrode. For this purpose, the frenum or muscle is stretched and sectioned with the loop electrode and a coagulating current.

For cases of **acute pericoronitis,** drainage may be obtained by incising the flap with a bent needle electrode. A loop electrode is used to remove the flap after the acute symptoms subside.

Electrosurgery is a convenient and ef-

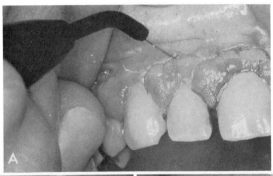

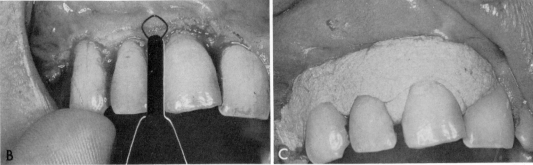

Figure 37–39 Gingival Resection and Gingivoplasty Using Electrosurgery. *A,* Gingival enlargement resected with needle electrode. *B,* Vertical interdental grooves created using diamond-shaped electrode. *C,* Periodontal pack in position.

fective method for cutting or eliminating tissue; it provides a clean operative field without hemorrhage.[28] However, **electrosurgery creates a risk of tissue damage and loss of periodontal support when it is used close to bone, which seriously limits its usefulness. It is valuable for superficial procedures such as the removal of gingival enlargement, gingivoplasty, relocating frenum and muscle attachments and incising periodontal abscesses and pericoronal flaps. It should not be used for procedures which involve proximity to the bone such as the treatment of infrabony pockets, flap operations or mucogingival surgery and some cases of gingival retraction.**

HEALING FOLLOWING ELECTROSURGERY. Some investigators report no significant differences in gingival healing following resection by electrosurgery and periodontal knives;[8, 18, 21] others find delayed healing, greater reduction in gingival height and more bone injury.[30] There appears to be little difference in the results obtained following **shallow** gingival resection with electrosurgery and periodontal knives. However, when used for **deep resections close to bone,** electrosurgery reportedly can produce gingival recession, bone necrosis and sequestration, loss of bone height, furcation exposure and tooth mobility which do not occur with the use of periodontal knives.[13]

Cryosurgery

Periodontal pockets have been eliminated by two freezing applications ($-35°$ C. to $-70°$ C.) with a cryostylet, without requiring anesthesia. A low-grade discomfort persists for two to three days after treatment. The initial gingival reaction to cryothermy is the formation of iceball-like lesions which after two days appear as surface vesicles. Healing is complete after two weeks.

REFERENCES

1. Allen, E. F., and Rhoads, R. H.: Effects of High Speed Periodontal Instruments on Tooth Surface. J. Periodont., *34:*352, 1963.
2. Bandt, C. L., et al.: Bacteremias from Ultrasonic and Hand Instrumentation. J. Periodont., *35:*214, 1964.

3. Belting, C. M.: Effects of High Speed Periodontal Instruments on the Root Surface During Subgingival Calculus Removal. J.A.D.A., 69:578, 1964.

4. Björn, H., and Lindhe, J.: The Influence of Periodontal Instruments on the Tooth Surface. Odont. Rev., 13:355, 1962.

5. Burman, L. R., Alderman, N. E., and Ewen, S. J.: Clinical Application of Ultrasonic Vibrations for Supragingival Calculus and Stain Removal. J. D. Med., 13:156, 1958.

6. Clark, S. M.: The Effect of Ultrasonic Instrumentation on Root Surfaces. J. Periodont., 39:135, 1968.

7. Clark, S. M.: The Ultrasonic Dental Unit: A Guide for the Clinical Application of Ultrasonics in Dentistry and in Dental Hygiene. J. Periodont.–Periodontics, 40:621, 1969.

8. Eisenmann, D., Malone, W. F., and Kusek, J.: Electron Microscopic Evaluation of Electrosurgery. Oral Sur., 29:660, 1970.

9. Everett, F. G., Foss, C. L., and Orban, B.: Study of Instruments for Scaling. Periodont., 16:61, 1962.

10. Ewen, S. J.: The Ultrasonic Wound—Some Microscopic Observation. J. Periodont., 32:315, 1961.

11. Ewen, S. J., and Glickstein, C.: Ultrasonic Therapy in Periodontics. Springfield, Ill., Charles C Thomas, 1968.

12. Frisch, J., et al.: Effect of Ultrasonic Instrumentation on Human Gingival Connective Tissue. Periodontics, 5:123, 1967.

13. Glickman, I., and Imber, L. R.: Comparison of Gingival Resection with Electrosurgery and Periodontal Knives—A Biometric and Histologic Study. J. Periodont., 41:142, 1970.

14. Goldman, H. M.: Histologic Assay of Healing Following Ultrasonic Curettage Versus Hand Instrument Curettage. Oral Surg., Oral Med. & Oral Path., 14:925, 1961.

15. Green, E., and Ramfjord, S. J.: Tooth Roughness after Subgingival Root Planing. J. Periodont., 37:44, 1966.

16. Johnson, W. N., and Wilson, J. R.: The Application of the Ultrasonic Dental Units to Scaling Procedures. J. Periodont., 28:264, 1957.

17. Kerrey, G. J.: Roughness of Root Surfaces after Use of Ultrasonic Instruments and Hand Curettes. J. Periodont., 38:340, 1967.

18. Klug, R. G.: Gingival Tissue Regeneration Following Electrical Retraction. J. Pros. Dent., 16:955, 1966.

19. Lindhe, J.: Evaluation of Periodontal Scalers. II. Wear Following Standardized or Diagonal Cutting Tests. Odont. Revy, 17:121, 1966.

20. Lindhe, J., and Jacobson, L.: Evaluation of Periodontal Scalers. I. Wear Following Clinical Use. Odont. Revy, 17:1, 1966.

21. Malone, W. F., Eisenmann, D., and Kusek, J.: Interceptive Periodontics with Electrosurgery. J. Pros. Dent., 22:555, 1969.

22. McCall, C. M., and Szmyd, L.: Clinical Evaluation of Ultrasonic Scaling. J.A.D.A., 61:559, 1960.

23. Miller, I. F., and Feinberg, E.: Electronic Surgery. New York J. Den., 32:172, 1962.

24. Nadler, H.: Removal of Crevicular Epithelium by Ultrasonic Curettes. J. Periodont., 33:220, 1962.

25. Odrich, R. B.: Cryotherapy of Periodontal Disease. Reported in Dental Abstracts, 12:107, 1967.

26. Orban, B., and Manella, V. B.: A Macroscopic and Microscopic Study of Instruments Designed for Root Planing. J. Periodont., 27:120, 1956.

27. Oringer, M. J.: Electrosurgery for Definitive Conservative Modern Periodontal Therapy. Dent. Clin. N. Amer., 13:53, 1969.

28. Oringer, M. J.: Electrosurgery in Dentistry. Philadelphia, W. B. Saunders Co., 1962.

29. Oringer, M. J.: Evaluation of Dental Electrosurgical Devices. J.A.D.A., 78:799, 1969.

30. Pope, J. W., Gargiulo, A. W., Staffileno, H., and Levy, S.: Effects of Electrosurgery on Wound Healing in Dogs. Periodontics, 6:30, 1968.

31. Sanderson, A. D.: Gingival Curettage by Hand and Ultrasonic Instruments—A Histologic Comparison. J. Periodont., 37:279, 1966.

32. Stende, G. W., and Schaffer, E. M.: A Comparison of Ultrasonic and Hand Scaling. J. Periodont., 32:312, 1961.

33. Waerhaug, J., et al.: The Dimension of Instruments for Removal of Subgingival Calculus. J. Periodont., 25:281, 1954.

34. Weisman, M. I.: Electrosurgery—An Adjunct in Rubber Dam Application in Endodontics. D. Digest, 75:193, 1969.

35. Wentz, F. M.: Therapeutic Root Planing. J. Periodont., 28:59, 1957.

36. Zach, L., and Cohen, G.: The Histology of the Response to Ultrasonic Curettage. J. D. Res., 40:751, 1961.

37. Zinner, D. D.: Recent Ultrasonic Dental Studies, Including Periodontia, Without the Use of an Abrasive. J. D. Res., 34:748, 1955 (abstract).

Chapter 38

GENERAL PRINCIPLES GOVERNING INSTRUMENTATION

Ensure Maximum Visibility, Accessibility and Illumination

Obtain Necessary Retraction

Hold the Instrument Securely and Stabilize the Hand for Operating

Instrument Grasp
Finger Rests

Be Certain the Instruments Are Sharp

Be Gentle and Careful

Maintain a Clean Field

Observe the Patient at All Times

Treat the Mouth in Orderly Sequence and Plan Each Treatment Visit

Comfort of the patient, operator and assistant is the first consideration for effective periodontal instrumentation. The following are additional fundamental requirements:

ENSURE MAXIMUM VISIBILITY, ACCESSIBILITY AND ILLUMINATION

Visibility is important for the detection of calculus and other deposits, destructive changes in the tooth surface and anomalies of tooth structure that require modification in instrumentation. In deep pockets, the cutting edge of the instrument is hidden so that thorough cleansing and planing of the root depend solely upon a keen tactile sense.

Accessibility facilitates thoroughness of instrumentation. The position of the patient and operator should be such as to provide maximum accessibility to the area of operation. Inadequate accessibility impedes thorough instrumentation, prematurely tires the operator and diminishes his effectiveness. It also inconveniences and tires the patient and diminishes patient cooperation.

Direct illumination is most desirable (Fig. 38–1). If it is not attainable, indirect illumination is obtained by using a mirror to

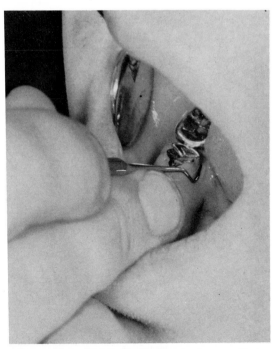

Figure 38–1 Direct Illumination in the mandibular right molar area.

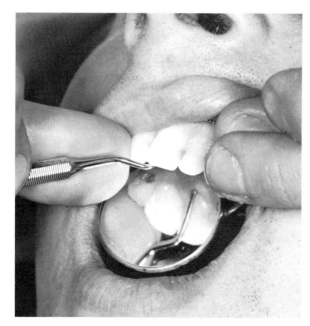

Figure 38–2 Indirect Illumination for operating upon the lingual surfaces of the maxillary anterior teeth with the operator behind the patient. The mirror reflects the light onto the field of operation.

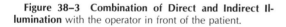

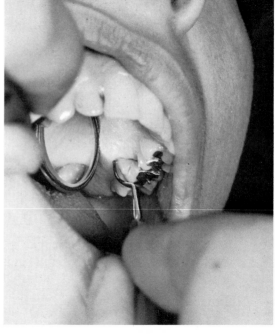

Figure 38–3 Combination of Direct and Indirect Illumination with the operator in front of the patient.

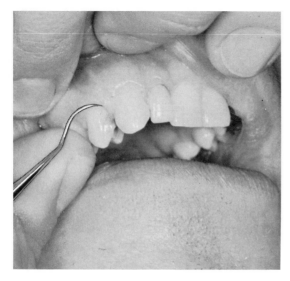

Figure 38–4 Retracting the Lip with the fingers of the nonoperating hand.

reflect the light to where it is needed (Fig. 38–2). Both are often used together (Fig. 38–3). The light source should be placed so that there is no glare in the patient's eyes.

OBTAIN NECESSARY RETRACTION

Retraction provides visibility, accessibility and illumination. The fingers, mirror, or both are used for retraction, depending upon the location of the area of operation.

The following illustrated methods are effective for retraction:

1. Use of the fingers of the nonoperating hand (Fig. 38–4).

2. Use of the mirror to deflect the cheek while the fingers of the nonoperating hand retract the lips and protect the angle of the mouth from irritation by the mirror handle (Fig. 38–5).

3. Use of the mirror to retract the tongue (Fig. 38–6).

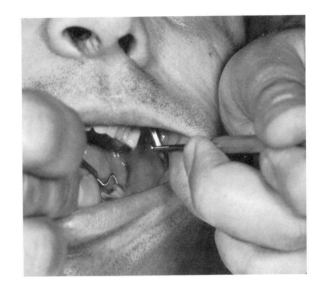

Figure 38–5 Retracting the Cheek with the mirror and the fingers of the nonoperating hand.

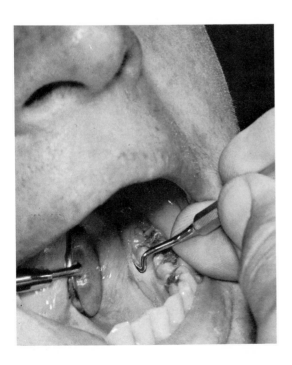

Figure 38–6 Retracting the Tongue with the mirror, and the cheek with the fingers.

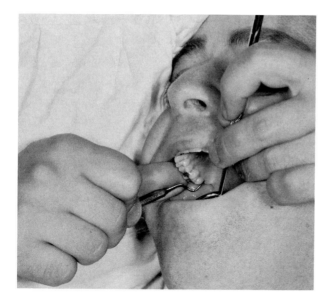

Figure 38–7 Retracting the Cheeks with the thumb of the operating hand and the fingers of the nonoperating hand.

4. Use of the fingers of the operating and nonoperating hands (Fig. 38–7).

5. Use of the mirror only to retract the lips and cheeks (Fig. 38–8).

6. Combinations of the above.

When retracting, care should be taken to avoid irritation to the angles of the mouth. In cold weather, softening the lips with petrolatum before operating is a helpful precaution against their cracking and bleeding.

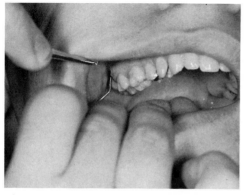

Figure 38–8 Retracting the Cheek with the mirror.

HOLD THE INSTRUMENT SECURELY AND STABILIZE THE HAND FOR OPERATING

Stability of the instrument and the hand is essential to control instrumentation and to avoid injury to the patient from sudden movement of the head. The two factors of major importance in providing stability are the *instrument grasp* and the *finger rests.*

Instrument grasp

The three methods for holding periodontal instruments in common usage are:

1. THE PEN GRASP (Fig. 38–9). The instrument is held between the thumb and second and third fingers, at the junction of the shank and handle of the instrument. The shank rests against the side of the pad of the third finger. The instrument is activated in a rolling motion by rotating the forearm and wrist with a steady finger rest as a fulcrum.

2. MODIFIED PEN GRASP (Fig. 38–10). The thumb and second finger engage the instrument at a point approximately one inch above the shank-handle junction. The shank rests against the side of the third finger opposite the ball of the finger, which

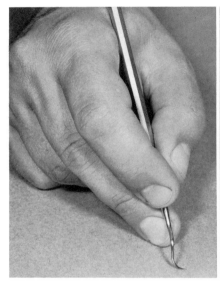

Figure 38–9   Pen Grasp.

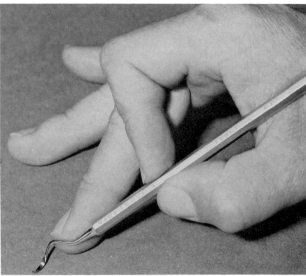

Figure 38–10   Modified Pen Grasp.

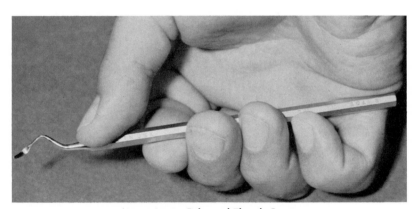

Figure 38–11   Palm and Thumb Grasp.

is used as a finger rest. In this grasp, the third finger is used not only as a finger rest and fulcrum but also to guide the direction of the instrument.

3. PALM AND THUMB GRASP (Fig. 38–11). The handle of the instrument is held in the cupped second, third and fourth fingers, with the ball of the thumb at the junction of the handle and the shank. The thumb acts as a fulcrum as the blade engages the tooth surface, and the handle of the instrument is activated by a coordinated movement of the forearm, wrist and cupped fingers.

Finger rests

The operating hand should be positioned to effectively activate the instrument and to provide sufficient control of the patient's jaws to prevent injury caused by sudden movement. The nonoperating hand and forearm are also helpful in controlling movement of the patient's head and in stabilizing the mandible.

It is important to obtain a firm finger rest. The finger rest serves to stabilize the instrument and the operating hand, to guide the instrument and to act as a fulcrum when the instrument is activated. The third finger is most commonly used as the finger rest. The finger rest may be on the teeth, gingiva, face, other fingers, or a combination of these. The following are the various locations and types of finger rests (Figs. 38–12 to 38–14):

1. THE THIRD FINGER ON THE TOOTH. The instrument is held in the *pen grasp*

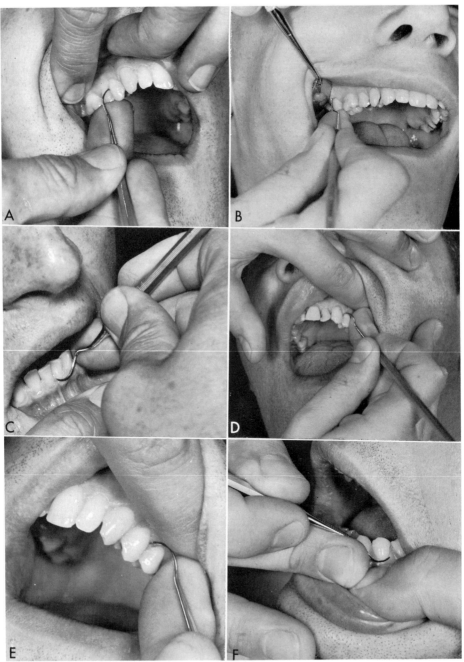

Figure 38–12 Finger Rests. *A,* Third finger rest on the occlusal surfaces of the teeth. *B,* Third finger rest on the occlusal surfaces of the teeth. *C,* Third finger rest on the facial surfaces of the teeth and gingiva. *D,* Third finger rest on finger and facial surfaces of the teeth. *E,* Detailed view of third finger rest on finger and facial surfaces of the teeth. *F,* Third finger rest on thumb.

with the shank resting against the third finger and the blade engaging the tooth surface (Fig. 38–12).

2. THE THIRD FINGER ON THE TOOTH. The instrument is held in the *modified pen*

grasp with the first and second fingers held high up on the handle and the shaft of the instrument resting against the side of the third finger (Fig. 38–12).

3. THE THIRD FINGER ON THE FACIAL

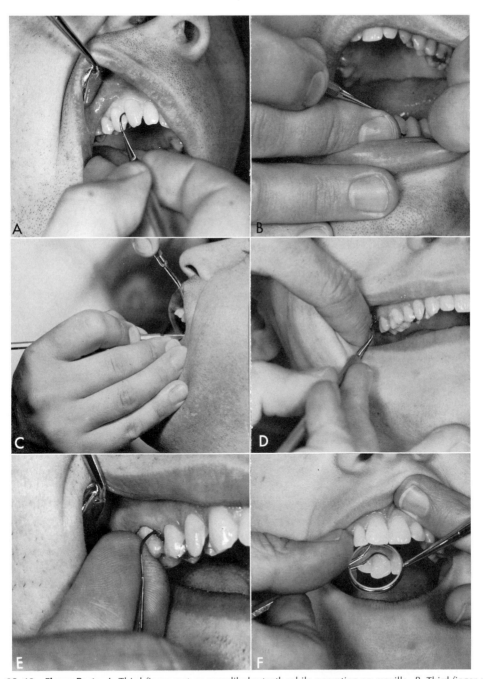

Figure 38–13 Finger Rests. *A,* Third finger rest on mandibular teeth while operating on maxilla. *B,* Third finger rest on teeth combined with fourth finger rest on chin. *C,* Finger rest on face. *D,* Fourth finger rest on face (operating hand), combined with additional stability and instrument guidance from finger of nonoperating hand. *E,* Thumb rest on posterior teeth. *F,* Thumb rest on anterior teeth.

Surface of the Teeth and the Gingiva. In some cases greater stability is obtained by resting the third finger on both the gingiva and the teeth (Fig. 38–12).

4. The Third Finger on Finger. The third finger rests upon the finger of the non-operating hand, which is being used for retraction (Fig. 38–12).

5. The Third Finger on the Incisal Edge of Occlusal Surface of the Mandibular Teeth. It is sometimes convenient to use this type of finger rest when operating on the maxilla (Fig. 38–13).

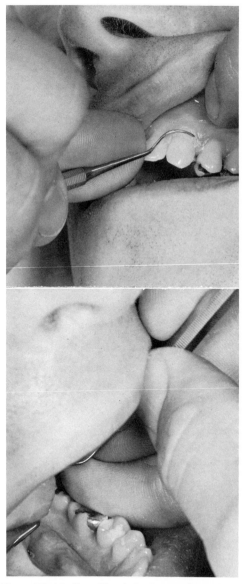

Figure 38–14 *Top,* **Thumb Rest on Incisors.** *Bottom,* **Fourth Finger Rest on Occlusal Surfaces** of the posterior teeth.

6. Auxiliary Finger Rests on the Face. When it is not possible to obtain a satisfactory rest position on the teeth or gingiva alone, the outer surface of the face is utilized to ensure stability (Fig. 38–13).

7. The Thumb on the Teeth. The palm and thumb grasp is used with the instrument pressing against the inner aspect of the ball of the thumb (Fig. 38–13).

8. The Fourth Finger on the Teeth. In operations in the mandibular molar area, stability is best obtained by resting the fourth finger on the occlusal surfaces while the instrument is guided by the second finger (Fig. 38–14).

BE CERTAIN THE INSTRUMENTS ARE SHARP

Instruments must be sharp to be effective. Successful treatment is not possible with dull instruments. Dull instruments inflict unnecessary trauma because of the excess force usually applied in an effort to compensate for their ineffectiveness. Instruments should be sharpened after each treatment visit. (See Chapter 40, Sharpening of Periodontal Instruments.)

BE GENTLE AND CAREFUL

Gentle, careful operating, in addition to being most considerate of the patient, is also the most effective way to operate. Tissue manipulation should be kept to a minimum; repetitive procedures interfere with the orderly cellular activity involved in healing.

Thoroughness is essential, but roughness must be avoided for the following reasons:

Roughness inflicts unnecessary pain in procedures carried out without anesthesia. It clutters the field of operation with excessive bleeding and debris and hinders the effectiveness of the operator. It produces excessive tissue injury and postoperative discomfort and delays healing.

It may cause gouging of the tooth surface and produce excessive postoperative sensitivity to touch and thermal changes.

It may force infected material into the deeper periodontal tissues and lead to serious postoperative infection.

MAINTAIN A CLEAN FIELD

During scaling and curettage, small gauze pads (2″ × 2″) and cotton rolls are extremely useful for isolating the field of operation and removing blood and debris. Bleeding is controlled by applying pressure with a pellet of cotton saturated with peroxide or with zinc chloride (8 per cent) or epinephrine (1:1000) in cases of pronounced bleeding. Deflecting the gingival margin with a gentle blast of warm air is helpful for checking the tooth surfaces during scaling and root planing. An aspirator is indispensable for obtaining the clean field required for periodontal surgery.

OBSERVE THE PATIENT AT ALL TIMES

It is essential to pay careful attention to the patient's reactions at all times. The facial expression indicates whether the patient is in pain; the onset of pallor and perspiration is a warning sign of patient weakness. Constant observation of the patient also helps the operator to anticipate sudden movements which might result in accidental trauma.

TREAT THE MOUTH IN ORDERLY SEQUENCE AND PLAN EACH TREATMENT VISIT

Treatment of the mouth should follow an orderly sequence, usually beginning with the maxillary right molar area, completing the maxilla, and then the mandible. Emergency care is given where necessary, after which the regular sequence is begun.

Have a detailed plan for each treatment visit. Prepare only the necessary instruments and arrange them in pairs in the order in which they are to be used. Consider the area to be treated in terms of tooth surfaces rather than in terms of single teeth. Use each instrument on all surfaces for which it is intended before putting it down. For example, one instrument may be used to scale all the proximal surfaces of the mandibular anterior teeth, followed by one for the facial surfaces and another one for the lingual surfaces. Scaling all surfaces of a single tooth with different instruments before proceeding to the next tooth entails many needless instrument changes.

Chapter 39

INSTRUMENTATION IN DIFFERENT AREAS OF THE MOUTH

Instrumentation in different areas of the mouth which affords maximum efficiency for the operator, and comfort for the patient is illustrated here in atlas form. More than one approach is presented for each area.

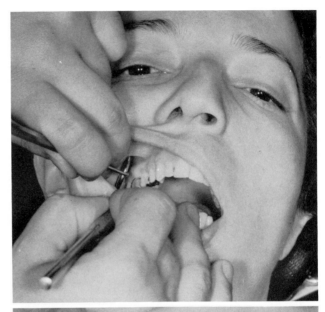

Figure 39–1 Maxillary Right Molar and Premolar Areas; Facial and Facioproximal Surfaces.

Illumination: Direct.
Visibility: Direct.
Instrument: Modified pen grasp.
Retraction: Mirror and fingers of nonoperating hand.
Finger Rest: Third and fourth fingers on occlusal surfaces of mandibular teeth and on face.

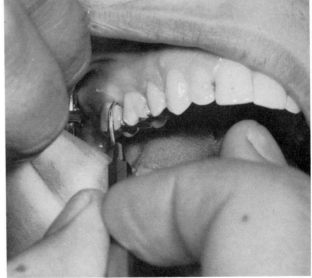

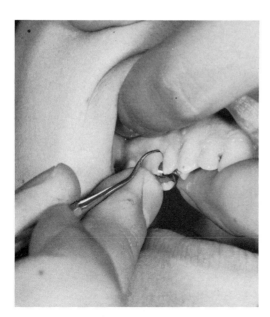

Figure 39–2 Maxillary Right Molar and Premolar Areas; Facial and Facioproximal Surfaces.

Illumination: Direct.
Visibility: Direct.
Instrument: Modified pen grasp.
Retraction: Fingers of nonoperating hand.
Finger Rest: Third finger on occlusal surfaces of molar or premolar teeth.

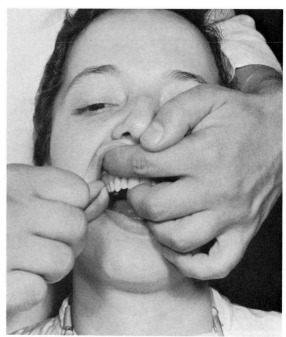

Figure 39–3 Maxillary Right Molar and Premolar Areas; Facial and Facioproximal Surfaces.

Illumination: Direct.
Visibility: Direct.
Instrument: Palm and thumb grasp.
Retraction: Thumb of operating hand and fingers of non-operating hand.
Finger Rest: Thumb on buccal surfaces of maxillary molar or premolar teeth.

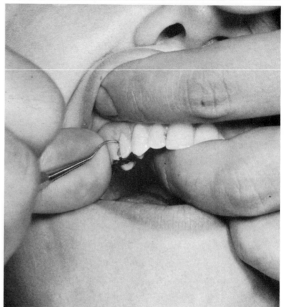

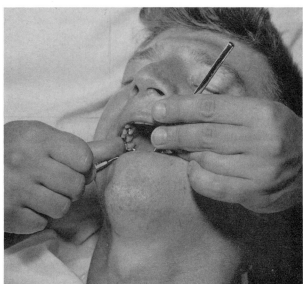

Figure 39–4 Maxillary Right Molar Premolar Areas; Lingual and Linguoproximal Surfaces.

Illumination: Direct and indirect.
Visibility: Indirect.
Instrument: Palm and thumb grasp.
Retraction: Thumb of operating hand; third and fourth fingers of nonoperating hand.
Finger Rest: Thumb on facial surfaces of maxillary molar and premolar teeth.

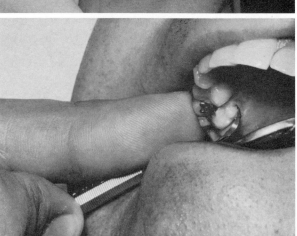

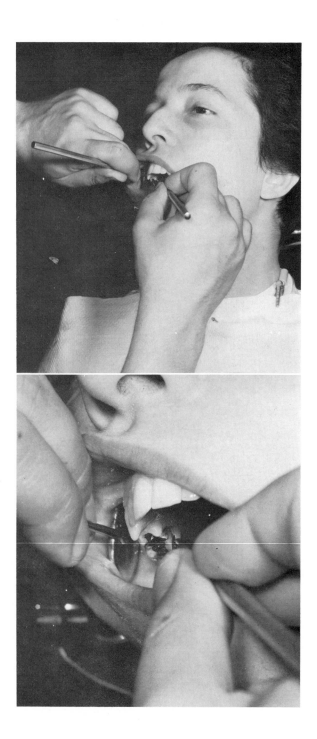

Figure 39–5 Maxillary Right Molar Area; Lingual and Linguoproximal Surfaces.

Illumination: Direct.
Visibility: Direct.
Instrument: Modified pen grasp.
Retraction: Fingers and mirror of nonoperating hand.
Finger Rest: Third finger on occlusal surfaces of mandibular teeth.

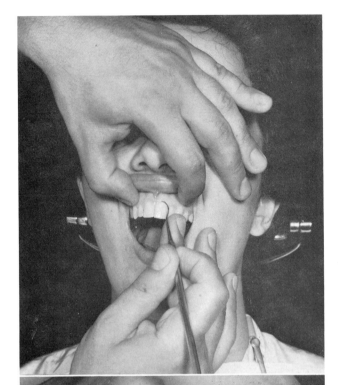

Figure 39–6   Maxillary Anterior Area; Facial and Facioproximal Surfaces.

Illumination: Direct.
Visibility: Direct.
Instrument: Modified pen grasp.
Retraction: Fingers of nonoperating hand.
Finger Rest: Third finger on incisal edges of maxillary teeth.

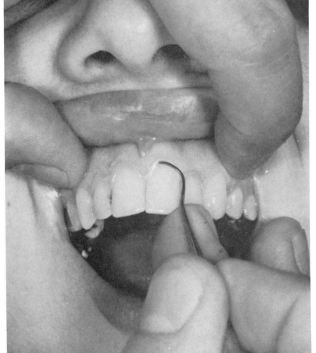

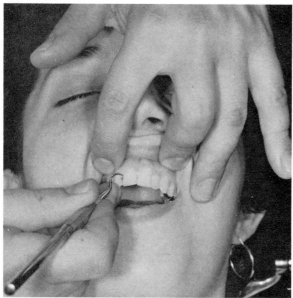

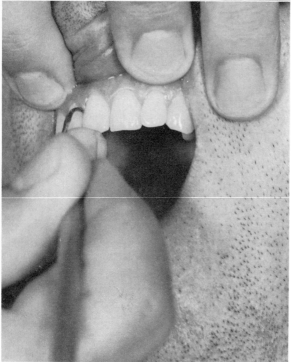

Figure 39–7   Maxillary Anterior Area; Facial and Facioproximal Surfaces.

Illumination: Direct.
Visibility: Direct.
Instrument: Modified pen grasp.
Retraction: Fingers of nonoperating hand.
Finger Rest: Third finger on incisal edges of maxillary anterior teeth.

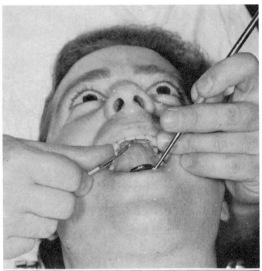

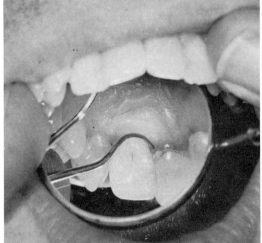

Figure 39–8 Maxillary Anterior Area; Lingual and Linguoproximal Surfaces.

Illumination: Indirect.
Visibility: Indirect.
Instrument: Palm and thumb grasp.
Retraction: Thumb of operating hand and fourth finger of nonoperating hand.
Finger Rest: Thumb on facial surfaces of anterior teeth.

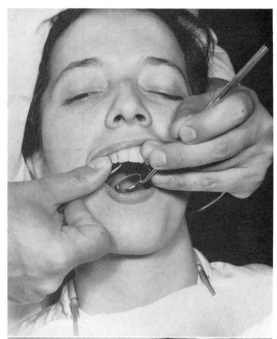

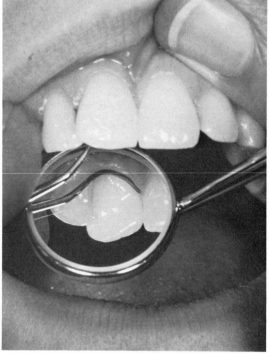

Figure 39–9 Maxillary Anterior Area; Lingual and Linguoproximal Surfaces.

Illumination: Indirect.
Visibility: Indirect.
Instrument: Palm and thumb grasp.
Retraction: Thumb of operating hand and fourth finger of nonoperating hand.
Finger Rest: Thumb on facial surfaces of maxillary premolars or anterior teeth.

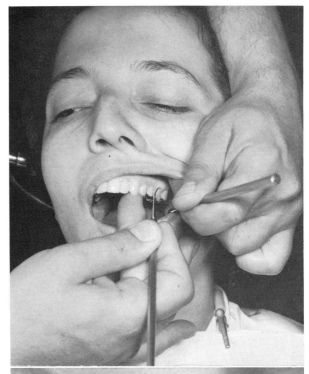

Figure 39–10 Maxillary Left Molar and Premolar Areas; Facial and Facioproximal Surfaces.

Illumination: Direct.
Visibility: Direct.
Instrument: Modified pen grasp.
Retraction: Mirror and second finger of non-operating hand.
Finger Rest: Third finger on occlusal surfaces of maxillary molars and premolars or incisal edges of anterior teeth.

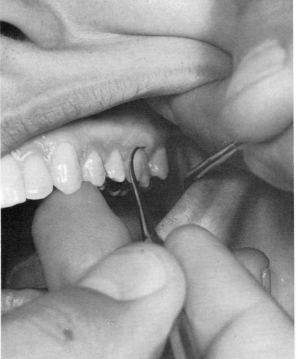

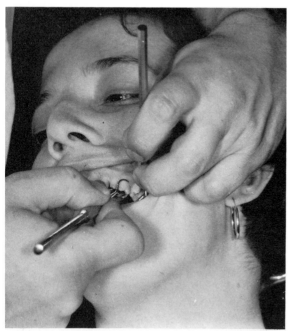

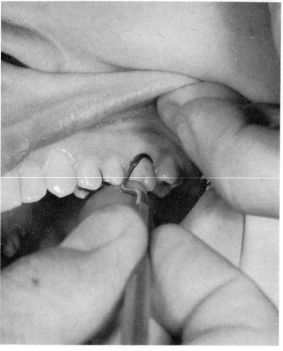

Figure 39–11 Maxillary Left Molar and Premolar Areas; Facial and Facioproximal Surfaces.

Illumination: Direct.
Visibility: Direct.
Instrument: Modified pen grasp.
Retraction: Mirror and third finger of non-operating hand.
Finger Rest: Third finger on occlusal surfaces of maxillary molar teeth.

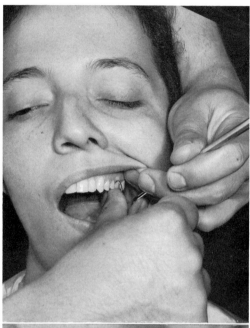

Figure 39–12 Maxillary Left Molar and Premolar Areas; Facial and Facioproximal Surfaces.

Illumination: Direct.
Visibility: Direct.
Instrument: Palm and thumb grasp.
Retraction: Mirror and third finger of nonoperating hand.
Finger Rest: Thumb on occlusal surfaces of maxillary molar or premolar teeth.

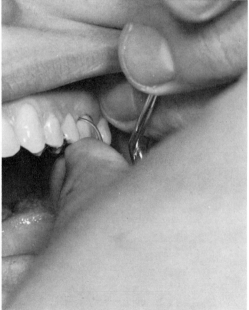

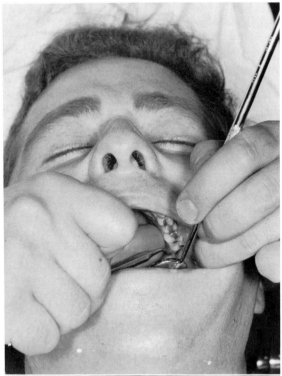

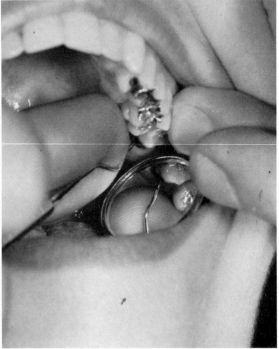

Figure 39–13 Maxillary Left Molar and Premolar Areas; Lingual and Linguoproximal Surfaces.

Illumination: Direct and indirect.
Visibility: Indirect.
Instrument: Palm and thumb grasp.
Retraction: Third and fourth fingers of nonoperating hand.
Finger Rest: Thumb on palatal surfaces of molar or premolar teeth.

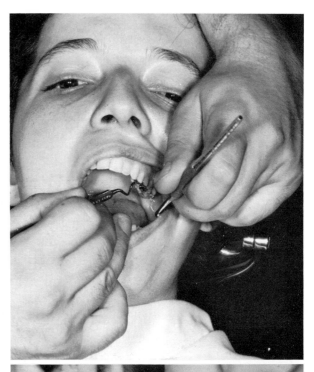

Figure 39–14 Maxillary Left Molar and Pre-molar Areas; Lingual and Linguoproximal Surfaces.

Illumination: Direct.
Visibility: Direct.
Instrument: Pen grasp.
Retraction: Fourth finger of operating hand and third finger of nonoperating hand.
Finger Rest: Third and fourth fingers of operating hand on incisal edges of mandibular anterior teeth.

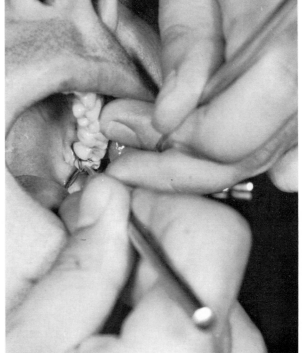

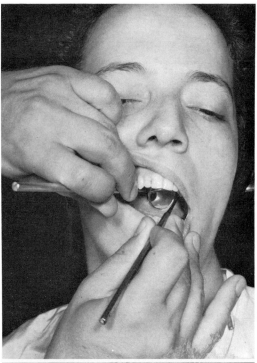

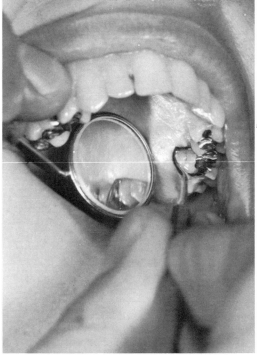

Figure 39–15 Maxillary Left Molar Area; Lingual and Linguoproximal Surfaces.

Illumination: Direct and indirect.
Visibility: Direct.
Instrument: Modified pen grasp.
Retraction: Fingers of nonoperating hand.
Finger Rest: Third fingers on occlusal surfaces of mandibular premolars and molars.

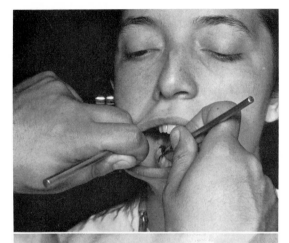

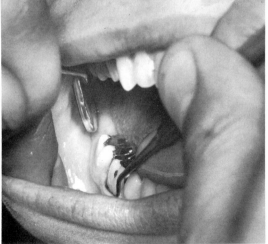

Figure 39–16 Mandibular Right Molar and Premolar Areas; Facial and Facioproximal Surfaces.

Illumination: Direct.
Visibility: Direct.
Instrument: Modified pen grasp.
Retraction: Mirror and third finger of nonoperating hand.
Finger Rest: Third finger on occlusal surfaces of premolars or incisal edges of mandibular anterior teeth.

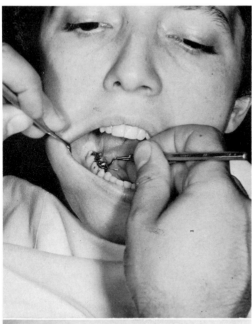

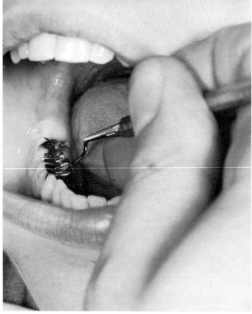

Figure 39–17 Mandibular Right Molar and Premolar Areas; Lingual and Linguoproximal Surfaces.

Illumination: Direct.
Visibility: Direct.
Instrument: Pen grasp.
Retraction: Mirror and fingers of operating hand.
Finger Rest: Third finger on incisal edges of anterior teeth or occlusal surfaces of premolars on other side.

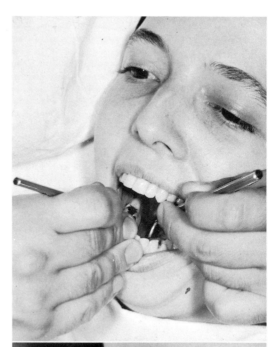

Figure 39–18 Mandibular Right Molar and Premolar Areas; Lingual and Linguoproximal Surfaces.

Illumination: Direct.
Visibility: Direct.
Instrument: Pen grasp.
Retraction: Mirror, third finger of operating hand and third finger of nonoperating hand.
Finger Rest: Third and fourth fingers of operatng hand on facial labial surfaces and incisal edges of anterior teeth.

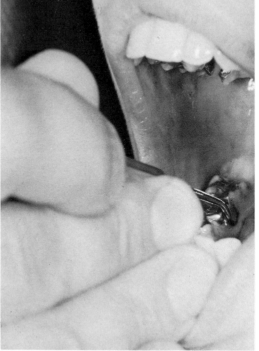

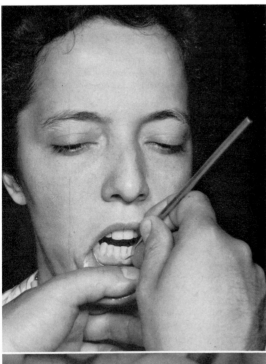

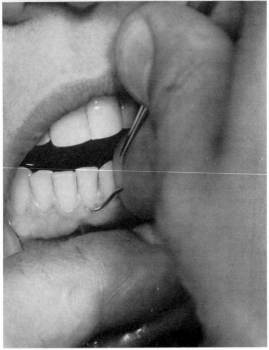

Figure 39–19 Mandibular Anterior Teeth; Facial and Facioproximal Surfaces.

Illumination: Direct.
Visibility: Direct.
Instrument: Modified pen grasp.
Retraction: Thumb of nonoperating hand.
Finger Rest: Third finger on facial surfaces of mandibular anterior teeth and gingiva.

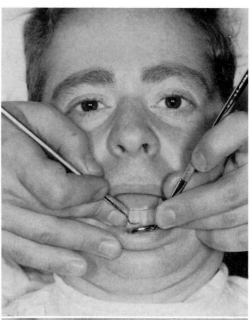

Figure 39–20 Mandibular Anterior Area; Facial and Facioproximal Surfaces.

Illumination: Direct.
Visibility: Indirect and direct.
Instrument: Pen grasp.
Retraction: Mirror and third finger of operating hand and fourth finger of nonoperating hand.
Finger Rest: Third finger on facial surfaces of mandibular anterior teeth.

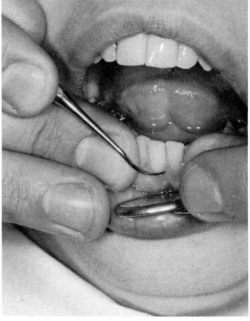

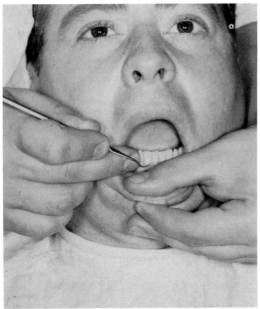

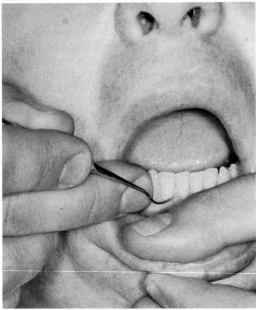

Figure 39–21 Mandibular Anterior Area; Facial and Facioproximal Surfaces.

Illumination: Direct.
Visibility: Direct.
Instrument: Pen grasp.
Retraction: Thumb and second finger of nonoperating hand.
Finger Rest: Third finger on facial surface of mandibular anterior teeth.

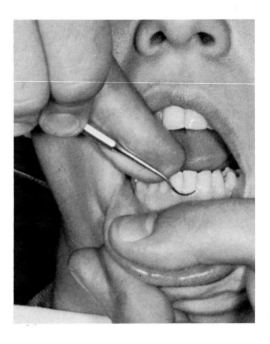

Figure 39–22 Mandibular Anterior Area; Facial and Facioproximal Surfaces.

Illumination: Direct.
Visibility: Direct.
Instrument: Palm and thumb grasp.
Retraction: Thumb and second finger of the nonoperating hand.
Finger Rest: Thumb on incisal edges of anterior teeth.

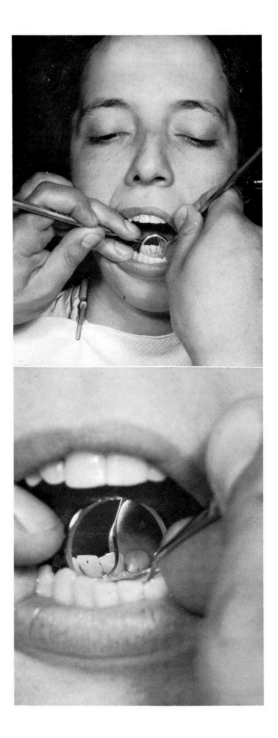

Figure 39–23 Mandibular Anterior Area; Lingual and Linguoproximal Surfaces.

Illumination: Indirect.
Visibility: Indirect.
Instrument: Pen grasp.
Retraction: Mirror and fingers of nonoperating hand. Fingers of operating hand.
Finger Rest: Third finger on incisal edges of mandibular anterior teeth.

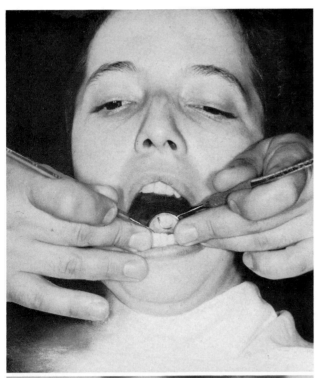

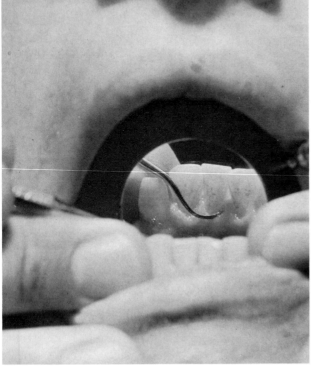

Figure 39–24 Mandibular Anterior Area; Lingual and Linguoproximal Surfaces.

Illumination: Indirect.
Visibility: Direct.
Instrument: Modified pen grasp.
Retraction: Mirror and third finger of operating hand and fourth finger of nonoperating hand.
Finger Rest: Third finger on facial surfaces of mandibular anterior teeth. Fourth finger on chin.

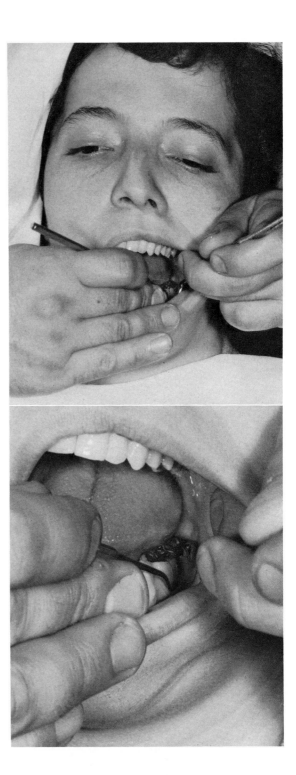

Figure 39–25 Mandibular Left Molar and Premolar Areas; Facial and Facioproximal Surfaces.

Illumination: Direct.
Visibility: Direct.
Instrument: Pen grasp.
Retraction: Mirror and third and fourth fingers of nonoperating hand and third finger of operating hand.
Finger Rest: Third finger on facial surfaces of mandibular premolars. Fourth and fifth fingers on chin.

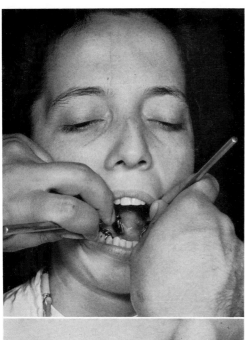

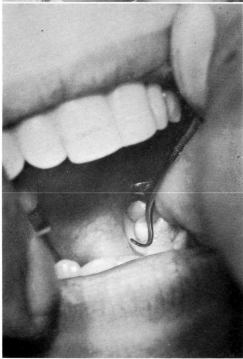

Figure 39–26 Mandibular Left Molar Area; Lingual and Linguoproximal Surfaces.

Illumination: Direct.
Visibility: Direct.
Instrument: Modified pen grasp.
Retraction: Mirror and fingers of nonoperating hand.
Finger Rest: Third finger on occlusal surfaces of mandibular teeth.

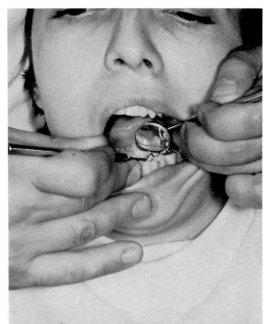

Figure 39–27 Mandibular Left Molar and Premolar Areas; Lingual and Linguoproximal Surfaces.

Illumination: Indirect.
Visibility: Direct.
Instrument: Modified pen grasp.
Retraction: Mirror and third and fourth fingers of operating hand.
Finger Rest: Third finger on facial surfaces and incisal edges of mandibular anterior teeth or facial surfaces of right premolars. Fourth finger on chin.

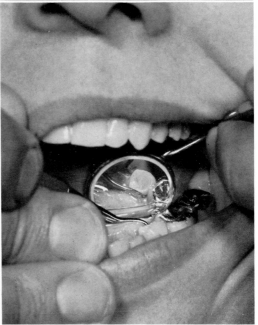

Chapter 40

SHARPENING OF PERIODONTAL INSTRUMENTS

To be effective, instruments must be sharp. An understanding of sharpening procedures is an essential prerequisite in the local treatment of periodontal disease. The principles governing sharpening and their application to periodontal instruments warrant detailed consideration.

The blade of each instrument has one or more cutting edges. Each cutting edge is formed by the junction of two surfaces of the blade. The cutting edge is the effective working portion of the instrument. When it is fine and smooth the instrument is sharp. When the cutting edge is blunt and rough the instrument is dull (Fig. 40–1). The sharpness of an instrument is checked by examining the edge in reflected light. In a dull instrument the edge presents a definite surface from which the light is reflected. As the instrument is sharpened, this surface is reduced until it appears as a fine line. Sharpening consists of cutting or grinding the surfaces which form the

edge of the blade until a fine thin linear cutting edge is restored. When the instrument is new, the surfaces forming the edge are set at a specific angle in accordance with the instrument design. The operator should familiarize himself with each instrument so that he understands the location and course of the cutting edges and the angles of the surfaces by which they are formed. **In sharpening, it is important to restore the cutting edge without distorting the original angles of the instrument.** Altering these angles impairs the effectiveness of the instrument to accomplish the purpose for which it was designed. *Honing is the final phase of sharpening;* it entails the use of a fine stone to attain a "finished" edge.

SHARPENING STONES

Sharpening is accomplished with stones which vary in grit or texture and design to meet different needs.

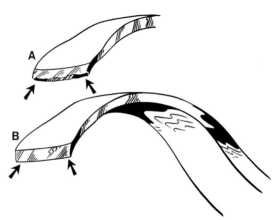

Figure 40–1 Creating a Sharp Cutting Edge. *A,* Dull cutting edge *(arrows). B,* Sharpened cutting edge *(arrows).*

Sharpening Stone Grit

Sharpening stones consist of masses of minute crystals, each of which is a sharp cutting point harder than steel. The coarseness or fineness, the hardness, the brittleness or toughness of these crystals determine the rate at which sharpening stones cut. Coarse stones cut comparatively rapidly.

The two most common grits used for sharpening dental instruments are the ruby stone, which is comparatively coarse and rapid cutting and is used for preliminary sharpening when an instrument is excessively dulled, and the Arkansas stone, which is a fine stone for the attainment of a finished edge.

Sharpening stones may be grouped according to method of use as follows:

MOUNTED STONES. Mounted stones are used in the hand piece. They are cylindrical in shape and may be obtained in varied sizes, in either the Arkansas or ruby grit (Fig. 40–2). Moyco ruby mounted cylindrical stones Nos. 5, 7, 8, 9, 11, 14 and 17 are well suited for sharpening most instruments.

UNMOUNTED STONES.

1. *Flat Stones.* These are rectangular stones of different sizes and grits which are either flat or have one surface grooved lengthwise with four different sized grooves (Fig. 40–3).

2. *Hand Stones.* These stones are held and activated by hand during sharpening. They may be cylindrical or of a special shape such as the number 309 carborundum stone which is tapered in the long axis and rectangular with rounded edges in cross section (Fig. 40–4).

PRINCIPLES OF SHARPENING

For proper sharpening, the following principles should be adhered to:

1. **Before starting to sharpen, establish the proper angle between the stone and the surface to be ground.** The plane of the surface being ground should be used as a guide.

2. Sharpening entails reducing the surface of the blade in relation to the dull edge; to accomplish this, **reduce the entire sur-**

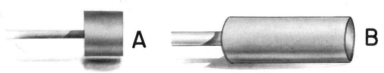

Figure 40–2 Mounted Sharpening Stones.

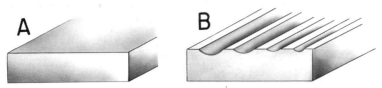

Figure 40–3 Flat Sharpening Stones. *A,* Without grooves. *B,* With grooves.

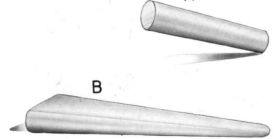

Figure 40–4 Hand Sharpening Stones. *A,* Cylindrical. *B,* Tapered.

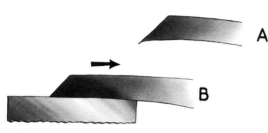

Figure 40–5 *A,* Wire edge extending from lower end of instrument after use of sharpening stone. *B,* Honing to remove the wire edge. Arrow indicates direction of instrument on stone.

face – do not create a new bevel at the cutting edge.

3. **Do not tilt the stone** so that it cuts unevenly across the surface being ground.

4. **Always lubricate the stone while sharpening.** This avoids unnecessary heat, which damages the edge temper, making the steel softer. With ruby stones, water is adequate, but for the Arkansas stones, oil should be used.

5. **Avoid excessive pressure.** This heats the edge, even though the stone is lubricated. A light touch is essential.

6. **Sharpen at the first sign of dullness.** The instrument will perform more satisfactorily and last longer.

7. The term "**wire edge**" is used to describe minute filamentous projections of metal which extend as a roughened ledge from the sharpened edge. Most sharpening techniques include the removal of the "wire edge" as a final stage. This is accomplished by gently honing the non-beveled surface of the blade adjacent to the cutting edge with a flat Arkansas stone (Fig. 40–5).

HOW TO SHARPEN INDIVIDUAL INSTRUMENTS

Sickle-shaped deep scalers

The two cutting edges to be sharpened are illustrated in Figure 40–6. The following methods may be used to sharpen these instruments:

1. USING A MOUNTED STONE. The instrument is held with a palm and thumb grasp, with the inner concave surface facing upward, and the tip toward the operator. The hand piece is held in the other hand with a palm and thumb grasp, the thumb resting firmly against the thumb of the hand holding the instrument, thus obtaining stabilization (Fig. 40–7). The stone, a Moyco No. 9 or 11, a water-lubricated ruby stone – or an Arkansas cylindrical stone which is oil-lubricated – may be used, depending upon the amount of grinding required. The stone is made to revolve slowly in the hand piece. The slowly re-

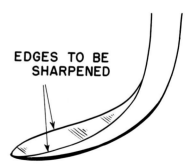

EDGES TO BE SHARPENED

Figure 40–6   Edges To Be Sharpened on the blade of a #7G or #8G deep scaler.

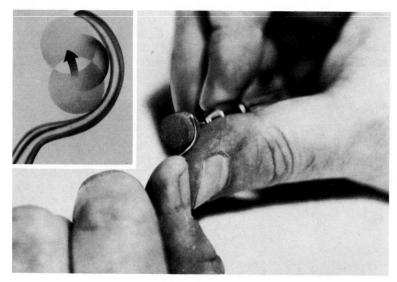

Figure 40–7   Proper Position of Fingers, Instrument and Stone for Sharpening with a Mounted Stone. *Inset,* The revolving stone is moved slowly from the junction of the blade and the shank to the tip.

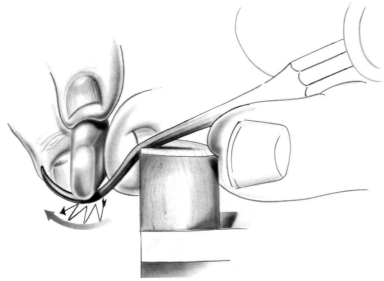

Figure 40–8 Sharpening a Scaler, Using a Tapered Hand Sharpening Stone. The instrument is stabilized in a wooden block held in a vise.

volving stone is placed against the inner surface at the junction of the blade and the shank, and then drawn slowly toward the tip, until it passes off the instrument. With the stone held correctly against the flat inner surface, both lateral edges will be sharpened simultaneously.

2. Using a Hand Stone. For optimal use of hand stones, the instrument should be stabilized while being sharpened, and the operator seated for controlled activation of the stone. Stabilization is obtained by holding the instrument in a notched depression at the edge of a small, wooden block held in a vise (Fig. 40–8). The instrument is placed so that the inner concave surface is upward and is parallel to the floor. The stone is placed on the inner surface of the blade at its junction with the shank and then moved back and forth in a sawing motion until it reaches the tip. The No. 309 carborundum stone is useful for this purpose. A cylindrical Arkansas stone, such as the Bates stone, which comes in two sizes (3/16 inch in diameter and 1/4 inch in diameter), may be used for finishing, following the No. 309 stone.

The outer surface is then honed slightly to remove the wire edge. To do this, the instrument is reversed in the sharpening block and rotated slightly so that the outer surface faces the operator. The stone is applied to the outer surface of the blade

and moved gently toward the cutting edge to remove filamentous wire projections.

The "wire edge" may also be removed with a grooved flat stone. The stone is held firmly on a flat surface with one hand, with long axis of the grooves directed away from the operator. The instrument is placed in a suitably sized groove with the tip in contact with the stone. The instrument is then pushed forward and upward against the stone so that the outer surface of the instrument is in contact with the side of the groove.

3. Recontouring the Blade. After being sharpened a number of times, the blade of scalers becomes thinned and flattened without a proportional narrowing of its width (Fig. 40–9). Proper shape is restored by grinding the outer aspect with a mounted stone (Fig. 40–10).

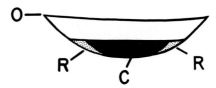

Figure 40–9 Reshaping Instrument after Repeated Sharpening. O, Cross section showing original shape of blade. R,C,R, Cross section showing blade reduced in size after repeated sharpening. R,R, Area removed to restore proper proportions to reduced blade. C, Cross section of recontoured blade.

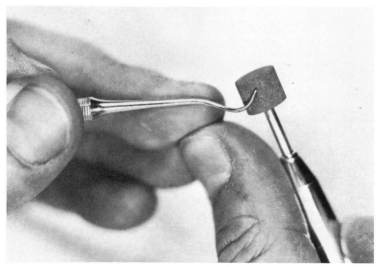

Figure 40–10 Position of fingers, instrument and stone when recontouring the outer surface of sickle-shaped scaler with a mounted stone.

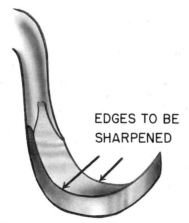

EDGES TO BE
SHARPENED

Figure 40–11 Cutting Edges To Be Sharpened on a sickle-shaped superficial scaler.

Sickle-shaped superficial scalers

The edges to be sharpened are shown in Figure 40–11. These instruments are sharpened in the same way as sickle-shaped deep scalers, with special care taken to preserve the angulation of the inner and lateral surfaces of the blade (Fig. 40–12).

Jaquette scalers

The edges to be sharpened are shown in Figure 40–13. The instrument is placed on a wooden block, with the inner aspect of the blade parallel to the floor (Fig. 40–8). A flat hand stone or the flat side of the No. 309 carborundum stone is moved back and forth across the inner surface.

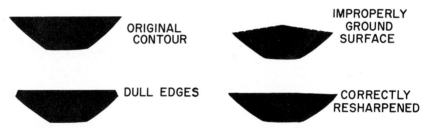

ORIGINAL
CONTOUR

IMPROPERLY
GROUND
SURFACE

DULL EDGES

CORRECTLY
RESHARPENED

Figure 40–12 Blade of a Sickle-Shaped Superficial Scaler, showing the contour when the instrument has dull edges and needs sharpening; the contour which results when the sharpening stone is not angulated properly; and the contour corrected by resharpening.

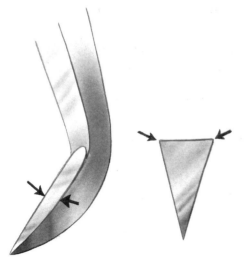

Figure 40–13 Jaquette Scaler, showing the cutting edges to be sharpened (*arrows*).

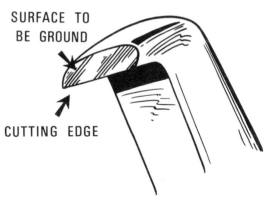

Figure 40–14 Blade of the #11G hoe scaler, showing the cutting edge to be sharpened and the surface to be ground.

Hoe scalers

The edge to be sharpened is shown in Figure 40–14. Hoes are sharpened with a flat stone. The instrument is placed with the bevel flat against the stone. One hand is used to control the angle at which the blade is held and the other supplies uniform downward pressure on the stone. Holding the wrists rigid, the blade is moved across the stone in a continuous "figure 8" pattern, with a swinging motion so that the upper part of the body as well as the arms participates in moving the instrument (Fig. 40–15).

The sharp corners of each end of the edge should be rounded to avoid laceration of the gingiva when this instrument is used. This is accomplished by holding the hoe in one hand with the blade facing the operator and rubbing the surface of a flat Arkansas stone across each corner in a rolling motion. To remove any wire edge that may be present, the undersurface of the blade is honed with the flat Arkansas stone.

The hoe scaler may also be sharpened using a straight stroke on a flat stone. The ball of the third finger against the side of the stone is used as a support and guide

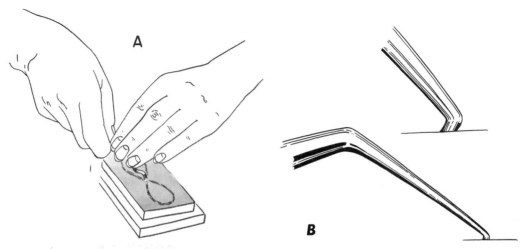

Figure 40–15 Sharpening Hoe Scaler. *A,* Using the "figure 8" technique on flat Arkansas stone. *B,* Placement of blade on stone so as to assure retention of proper angle.

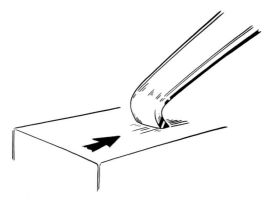

Figure 40–16 Sharpening Hoe Scaler on a flat stone. The instrument is moved in the direction of the arrow.

(Fig. 40–16). It should be noted that because of the bend in the blade, it is necessary to pull the instrument, instead of pushing it, in order to sharpen against the edge.

Chisel scalers

The edge to be sharpened is shown in Figure 40–17. This is best sharpened using a flat Arkansas stone. The stone is held firmly on a level surface with one hand. The other hand holds the instrument in a pencil grasp. The instrument is placed at the near end of the stone; the beveled surface flat against the stone. The ball of the third finger is used as a rest and **the instrument is pushed slowly forward without altering the stone-instrument angle.** The correct instrument-stone angle and incorrect angles are shown in Figure 40–17. To remove the wire edge, which remains following the sharpening of a chisel, the nonbeveled surface of the instrument is honed against a flat Arkansas stone.

The chisel scaler may also be sharpened using the "figure 8" technique described under hoe scalers (Fig. 40–15).

Curets

The edges to be sharpened are shown in Figure 40–18. These instruments are sharpened with the No. 7 Moyco mounted stone. The instrument is held in the hand with the palm and thumb grasp. The stone, rotating slowly in the hand piece, is moved along the length of the inner surface of the blade (Fig. 40–18) proceeding from the shank to the tip. The adjacent surfaces are

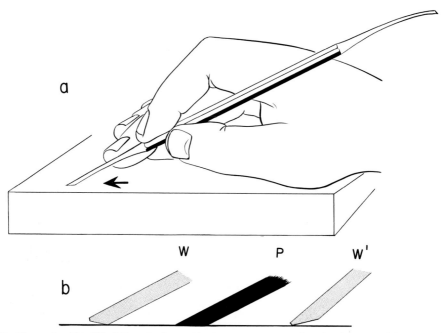

Figure 40–17 Sharpening The Chisel Type Scaler. a, The instrument is moved in the direction of the arrow. b, Proper angulation of the instrument on the stone is shown at P. Improper angulations are shown at W and W'.

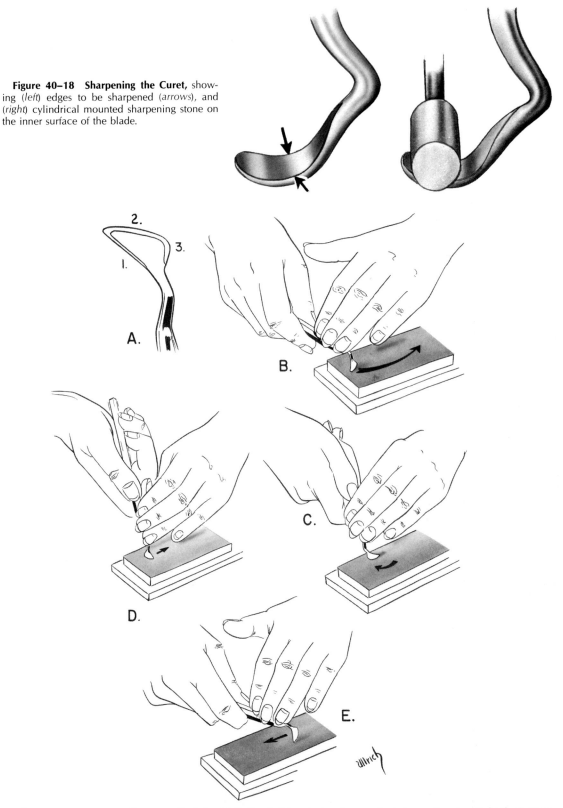

Figure 40–18 Sharpening the Curet, showing (*left*) edges to be sharpened (*arrows*), and (*right*) cylindrical mounted sharpening stone on the inner surface of the blade.

Figure 40–19 How to Sharpen a Periodontal Knife. *A,* Edges to be sharpened—1, inner; 2, outer; 3, back. *B,* Outer edge. Instrument stabilized on flat Arkansas stone and pushed from right to left (*arrow*). *C,* Other side of outer edge. Instrument reversed and returned across the stone (*arrow*). *D,* Inner edge. Instrument pushed in straight line (*arrow*). *E,* Other side of inner edge. Instrument reversed and returned across the stone (*arrow*).

honed with a flat, hand Arkansas stone to remove the wire edges. This instrument may also be sharpened with appropriately sized cylindrical hand stones.

Periodontal knives

Although they vary in length, most periodontal knives are sharpened either on a flat stone or with a rotating cylindrical stone. The #20G and #21G have three edges to be sharpened: the inner edge, the outer edge and the back edge (Fig. 40–19). They are sharpened on a flat Arkansas stone at least 6 inches long. The instrument is held in the right hand with the palm and thumb grasp and placed on the stone at an angle conforming to the bevel of the blade. The fingers of the left hand are then gently placed on the handle near the shank so as to stabilize the instrument on the stone. To sharpen the outer edge, the instrument is pushed across the stone from right to left, in a sweeping semicircular motion (Fig. 40–19). The blade is then reversed and the other side is pushed from left to right, in the same manner. To sharpen the inner and back edges, the above procedure is repeated, pushing the instrument across the stone in a straight line instead of in a semi-circle.

The periodontal knives may also be sharpened with a Moyco No. 9 ruby stone.

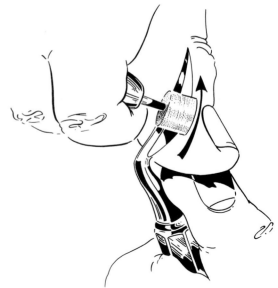

Figure 40–20 Sharpening a Periodontal Knife with a Mounted Stone. The handpiece is held in the right hand and the instrument in the left, and the rotating #9 ruby stone (Moyco) is moved along the blade in the direction of the arrow. The right thumb is stabilized on the thumb of the left hand.

The instrument is held in the left hand in the palm and thumb grasp, with the blade facing the operator (Fig. 40–20). The stone is placed flat against the surface of the blade, extending slightly beyond the edge. The slowly rotating stone is drawn along each surface, toward the tip, using the thumb of the right hand as a pivot.

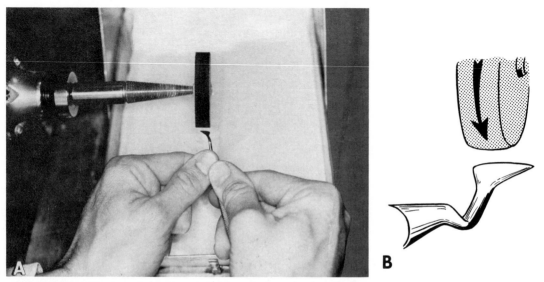

Figure 40–21 Renewing Sharpness with Hard Felt Wheel and Abrasive. *A*, Instrument in position. *B*, The direction of rotation is indicated by the arrow.

RENEWING SHARPNESS WITH A FELT WHEEL AND ABRASIVE

The sharpness of instruments can be renewed with a hard felt wheel and a metallic oxide abrasive. This is rapid and effective and prolongs the life of the instrument because it produces minimal wear. Cutting edges that have lost their original bevel or have become too blunt must first be sharpened with stones in order to benefit from the felt wheel.

Procedure

A metallic oxide compound such as chromium trioxide is applied to the rotating hard felt wheel mounted on a lathe. The instrument is held between the thumb and forefinger of both hands and applied with gentle pressure, as the wheel rotates at moderate speed *away from the cutting edge* (Fig. 40–21). **The hands are stabilized on the bench and the instrument is aligned** so as to preserve the original bevel of the cutting edge.

CARE OF THE SHARPENING STONES

With use, the surfaces of sharpening stones become blackened and clogged with metallic debris. Ruby stones or other water-lubricated stones may be cleansed with soap and water and a scrub brush. Arkansas and other oil stones are cleansed with gasoline.

The Arkansas stone should not be permitted to become dried. The surface should always be covered with a thin film of light oil when the stone is stored.

Ruby stones are sterilized in water. Arkansas stones are best sterilized by autoclaving or boiling in light oil.

To prevent grooving of a stone surface, an effort should be made to utilize the entire surface equally. Grooving of sharpening stone surfaces impairs the efficiency of the stone and the accuracy of the sharpening procedure. Unevenly worn or grooved stones may be reshaped with a Joe-Dandy disk.

Chapter 41

POCKET ELIMINATION

Pocket elimination consists of reducing the depth of periodontal pockets to that of a physiologic sulcus and restoring gingival health. It is important in the overall management of periodontal disease, but it is not the total treatment. Additional measures indicated by the requirements of the individual case must also be employed.

THE KEYSTONE OF PERIODONTAL TREATMENT

Elimination of the periodontal pocket **is the keystone of the overall periodontal treatment regimen** (Fig. 41–1). It is a critical factor in restoring periodontal health and arresting destruction of the supporting

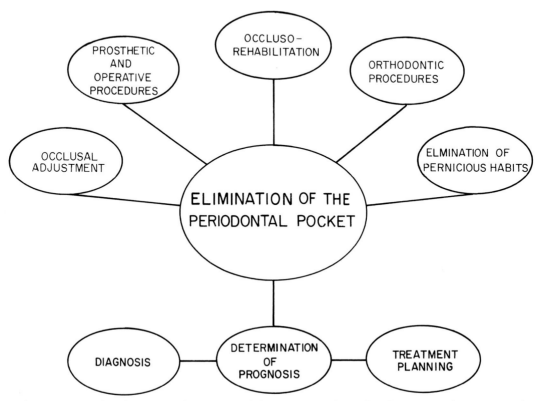

Figure 41–1 Pocket Elimination—the Keystone of the Treatment of Periodontal Disease, and a Basic Requirement for the Success of Associated Local Treatment Procedures.

periodontal tissues. Just as the removal of carious structure is essential before a restoration can be placed in a tooth, so too the successful outcome of all procedures involved in the total treatment of periodontal disease depends upon complete elimination of periodontal pockets (Fig. 41–1). Without pocket elimination the beneficial effects of occlusal adjustment and dental restorations upon the periodontium are diminished.

In the treatment of periodontal pockets, the goal is total elimination; partial reduction in pocket depth is a compromise which is not consistent with a healthy periodontium. Instead of trying to eliminate periodontal pockets, it is often possible to "maintain" them for years in what appears to be a healthy condition, with the pocket depth partially reduced or unchanged and without radiographic evidence of advancing bone loss.[1] This may be accomplished by regularly scheduled scaling and root planing and occasional gingival curettage, plus good patient oral hygiene. This temporizes the periodontal pocket with the ostensible advantage that preserving the pocket wall avoids exposure of root surface.

However, "pocket preservation" is not a substitute for pocket elimination in a treatment regimen aimed at the preservation of the periodontium. Persistent periodontal pockets are usually diseased, even though they appear healthy on the surface. The external appearance does not necessarily indicate the condition of the pocket wall. Pockets with severe inflammation and ulceration on the inside of the pocket wall often appear normal on the outer surface.

"Maintaining" periodontal pockets rather than eliminating them imposes the risk of tooth loss upon the patient. Spread of inflammation from periodontal pockets is a major cause of bone destruction in periodontal disease. The bone loss is progressive but not necessarily at a steady pace. There may be remissions and exacerbations, with periods of relative inactivity and even partial restoration of destroyed bone interspersed with periods of active bone destruction. (See Chapter 16, Bone Loss and Patterns of Bone Destruction in Periodontal Disease.) The timetable for the active bone destruction cannot be predicted, but the risk increases with the duration of periodontal pockets. Periodic radiographic check-ups in patients with persistent pockets can only reveal bone destruction after it has occurred. Eliminating periodontal pockets is the most effective way of arresting periodontal destruction caused by the spread of inflammation.

POCKET ELIMINATION – A TECHNICAL DISCIPLINE

An understanding of the underlying pathologic processes is helpful in the treatment of periodontal disease. However, pocket elimination per se is a technical procedure that must be mastered along with the many other techniques of general dentistry. The methods of pocket elimination are classified under two main headings: (1) *the scaling and curettage technique* and (2) *surgical techniques*, which include the *gingivectomy* and *flap operations*. The techniques, what they accomplish, and the factors governing their selection are presented in the next chapters.

RECURRENCE OF POCKET DEPTH

After treatment to eliminate periodontal pockets, some of the depth tends to return with time, regardless of whether the treatment is scaling and curettage or surgery.[2, 3] This occurs in patients with apparently good oral hygiene who are recalled at three-month intervals for maintenance prophylaxis and reinstruction in home care. The recurrence results from gingival inflammation caused principally by dental plaque. The pocket depth is produced by an increase in the height of the gingiva (gingival pocket) rather than by destruction of supporting periodontal tissues and apical shift in the epithelial attachment. The fact that some degree of pocket depth can return without loss of supporting tissues has led some to question whether elimination of pockets is essential for the maintenance of the periodontium.

OTHER PURPOSES SERVED BY POCKET ELIMINATION

In addition to arresting inflammation-induced bone resorption and restoring periodontal health, pocket elimination serves other purposes which are best illustrated by reviewing some of the potential complications of periodontal pockets:

Inflammation from periodontal pockets causes degeneration in the periodontal ligament which contributes to abnormal tooth mobility and impairs the capacity of the periodontium to withstand occlusal forces and support dental restorations and prostheses.

Periodontal pockets are sites of microbial concentration and potential sources of bacteremia, and provide conditions favorable for root caries and pulp disease.

Degenerative changes in the chronically inflamed pocket wall increase the susceptibility of the gingiva to superimposed acute necrotizing ulcerative gingivitis.

Periodontal pockets are sources of discomfort during mastication, interfere with the chewing required for the digestion of food, or lead to food selection habits which favor soft carbohydrates rather than fibrous protein foods.

The putrified contents of periodontal pockets spoil the taste of food and, in addition, contaminate it with material which may irritate the gastrointestinal tract.

REFERENCES

1. Oliver, R. C.: Quoted in Cohen, D. W.: Role of Periodontal Surgery. J. D. Res., 50:212, 1971.
2. Ramfjord, S. P.: Longitudinal Results Following Various Forms of Periodontal Treatment (Reported by M. Winslow). J. Periodont., 41:48, 1970.
3. Ramfjord, S. P., et al.: Subgingival Curettage Versus Surgical Elimination of Periodontal Pockets. J. Periodont., 39:167, 1968.

Chapter 42

THE SCALING AND CURETTAGE TECHNIQUE

The scaling and curettage technique is the basic, most commonly employed procedure for the elimination of periodontal pockets and the treatment of gingival disease. It consists of *scaling* to remove calculus, plaque and other deposits, *planing* the root to smooth it and remove necrotic tooth substance and *curetting* the inner surface of the gingival wall of periodontal pockets to separate away diseased soft tissue.

Scaling and curettage is performed in a confined area; it should be gentle and thorough and with minimum trauma to the infected tissues and the tooth surface.[9, 17] Each instrument should accomplish its purposes the first time it is used so that unnecessary repetition is avoided.

INDICATIONS

Scaling and curettage is the technique of choice for the following:

1. **Elimination of suprabony pockets in which the depth is such that the calculus on the root can be completely visualized by deflecting the pocket wall with a blast of warm air or a probe.** For scaling and curettage to succeed, the pocket wall must be edematous so that it can shrink to normal sulcus depth. **If the pocket wall is firm and fibrous, surgical treatment is required to eliminate the pocket regardless of the depth, because the fibrous pocket wall will not shrink sufficiently following scaling and curettage.**

2. **Most types of gingivitis, except gingival enlargement.**

3. **Scaling and curettage is also one of several techniques for the treatment of infrabony pockets.**

PRINCIPLES OF SCALING AND CURETTAGE

Scaling

Scaling removes dental plaque and calculus and stain and thereby eliminates factors provoking inflammation. Supragingival deposits are readily accessible for removal. The extent of subgingival calculus should be appraised before an effort is made to remove it. This entails sliding an instrument (explorer or fine scaler) gently along the calculus in the direction of the apex until the termination of the calculus on the root is felt. The distance between the edge of the calculus and plaque and the bottom of the pocket usually ranges from 0.2 to 1.0 mm., with the shorter distances and reduced accessibility in the deeper pockets. The operator should try to see the entire calculus mass by blowing warm air between the tooth and the gingival margin, or deflecting the gingiva with a probe or small pellet of cotton. The subgingival calculus is generally brown or chocolate-colored, or it may be lighter, approaching the color of the tooth and therefore escaping detection. It is often difficult to visualize the calculus in deep pockets because of the bulk of the soft tissue wall.

The complete removal of subgingival calculus requires the development of a delicate sense of touch. In the course of the scaling procedure, the smoothness of the root must be checked and rechecked, with a fine scaler or sharp explorer.[4]

It should be borne in mind that there is often a slight vertical groove on proximal root surfaces of the posterior teeth. Calculus lodged in these grooves gives the root a smooth contour and conveys the erroneous impression that the calculus is completely removed. Retained calculus prevents complete healing.

Root planing

It is not enough to remove the calculus; the root surface must also be planed until it is smooth. After the subgingival calculus has been completely removed, there may be areas in which the root feels somewhat softened (where the cementum has undergone necrotic changes). The softened material must be removed until firm tooth substance is reached. Removal of necrotic cementum may expose the dentin; although this is not the aim of treatment, there are circumstances in which it cannot be avoided.[18]

How to scale and plane

Scaling and planing consists of a "pull" motion, except on the proximal surfaces of closely spaced anterior teeth, where thin chisel scalers are used with a "push" motion (Chap. 37). In the "pull" motion, the instrument engages the apical border of the calculus and dislodges it with a firm movement in the direction of the crown (Fig. 42–1). Abrupt "sweeps" at the tooth result in "nicking" of the root surface which causes postoperative sensitivity.

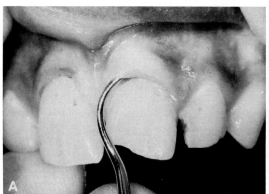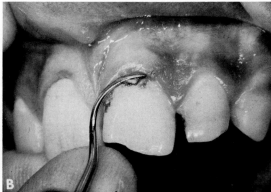

Figure 42–1   Removal of Subgingival Calculus. A, Deep scaler inserted below gingival margin. B, Flint-like subgingival calculus removed.

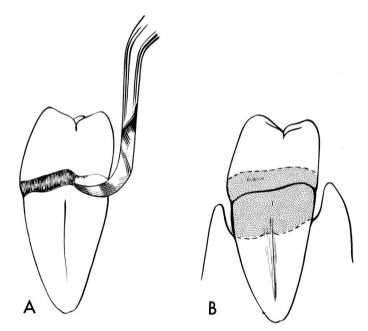

Figure 42–2 *A,* **Calculus Dislodged by Engaging the Lower Border with Cutting Edge of Scaler.** *B,* **The Instrumentation Zone** (shaded area) where scaling is confined for maximum efficiency.

The scaling motion is initiated in the **forearm** and transmitted from the wrist to the hand with slight flexing of the fingers. Rotation of the wrist is synchronized with the forearm. **The scaling motion is not initiated in the wrist or fingers, nor is it carried out independently without the use of the forearm.**

In the "push" scaling motion, the fingers activate the instrument. This method is used with the chisel scaler on the proximal surfaces of crowded anterior teeth. The instrument engages the lateral border of the calculus and the fingers provide a thrust motion, which dislodges the calculus. **To avoid forcing calculus into the supporting tissues,[12] do not push the instrument in an apical direction.**

The removal of calculus is not a whittling operation. The calculus is dislodged in its entirety, starting below its border; it is not "pared down" until the tooth surface is reached. After calculus is removed from one section of the tooth, the instrument is moved laterally to engage the adjacent deposits (Fig. 42–2).

Scaling is confined to a small area of the tooth on both sides of the cemento-enamel junction where the calculus and other deposits are located. This is the "instrumentation zone" (Fig. 42–2). Sweeping the instrument over the crown where it is not needed lengthens operating time, dulls the instrument and is contrary to the careful attention to detail required for effective instrumentation.

Curettage

Curettage consists of the removal of degenerated and necrotic tissue lining the gingival wall of periodontal pockets. The term curettage is sometimes used to designate smoothing of root surfaces; however, the author uses it only in connection with treatment of soft tissues. Smoothing of root surfaces is referred to as root planing. Curettage hastens healing by reducing the task of the body enzymes and phagocytes, which ordinarily remove tissue debris during healing. Also, by removing the epithelial lining of the periodontal pocket, curettage removes a barrier to reattachment of the periodontal ligament to the root surface. Some degree of irritation and trauma to the gingiva is unavoidable with scaling and curettage, even if it is performed with extreme care. The injurious effects are of microscopic proportion and generally do not significantly affect the healing. Overzealous scaling and curettage causes postoperative pain and retards healing.

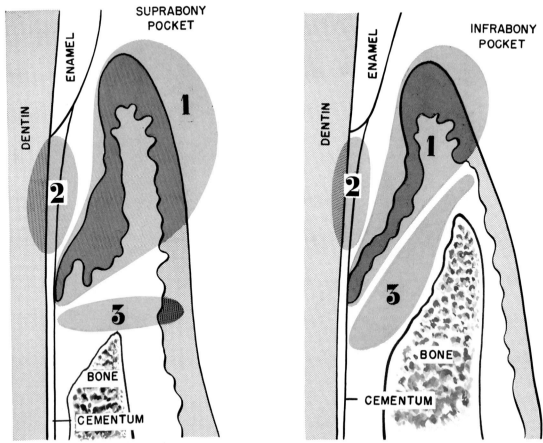

Figure 42–3   Critical Zones in Pocket Eradication. *Left,* Suprabony pocket; *right,* infrabony pocket. Zone 1: Soft tissue wall and epithelial attachment. Zone 2: Tooth surface. Zone 3: Connective tissue between the pocket wall and bone.

POCKET ELIMINATION BY SCALING AND CURETTAGE

In pocket elimination, just as in the preparation of a carious tooth for a restoration, it is necessary to have a plan of procedure before the operation is begun. As a guide to treatment, periodontal pockets may be subdivided into three critical zones (Fig. 42–3).

Critical Zones in Pocket Elimination

Zone 1. The soft tissue wall and epithelial attachment

The soft tissue wall of the pocket is inflamed and presents varying degrees of degeneration and ulceration with engorged blood vessels close to the surface, often separated from the contents of the pocket by only a thin layer of tissue debris. In this zone determine the following:

Whether the pocket wall extends in a straight line from the gingival margin or follows a tortuous course around the tooth.

The number of tooth surfaces involved by the pocket.

The location of the bottom of the pocket on the tooth surface, and the pocket depth.

The relationship of the pocket wall to the alveolar bone (Fig. 42–3). Is the entire pocket coronal to the crest of the bone (suprabony pocket), or is the bone lateral to the pocket wall (infrabony pocket)?

Zone 2. The tooth surface

Adherent to the tooth are calculus and other tooth surface deposits of varying amounts and texture. The superficial calculus is generally clay-like in consistency, obvious, and easily detached by well-directed instrumentation. However, deep in the pocket the calculus is hard, flint-like and tenaciously adherent to the surface. In the coronal portion of the root the cementum is extremely thin, and a ledge is often formed at the cemento-enamel junction, which must be taken into consideration when the tooth is scaled. The cementum surface may be softened by caries. It may be deformed by adherent cementicles.

The pocket itself contains bacteria, bacterial products, the products of food decomposition and calculus, all bathed in a slimy mucus medium. Pus may or may not be present.

In this zone determine the following:

1. The extent and location of deposits.

2. The condition of the tooth surface; the presence of softened, eroded areas.

3. The accessibility of the root surface to the necessary instrumentation.

Zone 3. The connective tissue between the pocket wall and the bone

In this zone, determine whether the connective tissue is soft and friable, or firm and bound to the bone. This is a significant consideration in the treatment of infrabony pockets (Chap. 44).

Elimination of Suprabony Pockets* by Scaling and Curettage

The following is a step-by-step procedure for eliminating suprabony pockets by scaling and curettage, with an explanation of what each step accomplishes.

Pocket elimination should be systematic, beginning in one section and proceeding in orderly sequence until the entire mouth is treated. Treatment is usually started in the right maxillary molar area, unless it is urgently needed in another section. The number of the teeth included at each visit varies with the skill of the operator, the type of patient and the severity of periodontal involvement.

---

*The use of scaling and curettage in the treatment of infrabony pockets is described in Chapter 44.

Step 1. Isolate and anesthetize the area

The field is isolated with cotton rolls or gauze pads and swabbed with a mild antiseptic such as Merthiolate or Metaphen. Throughout the scaling and curettage procedure the area is cleansed intermittently with pellets of cotton saturated with an equal mixture of warm water and 3 per cent peroxide. Strong antiseptics or escharotic drugs are not used because they may induce tissue injury and retard healing.

Topical or infiltration and block anesthesia are used according to the needs. Topical anesthetics are usually adequate for the elimination of shallow pockets, but for deep pockets more profound anesthesia by injection is advised. It is better to have slightly more anesthesia than not enough.

A fetish is sometimes made of not using any form of anesthetic for scaling and curettage. The removal of supragingival calculus does not require anesthesia, and experienced clinicians can perform subgingival scaling and curettage with a minimum of discomfort. The presence of anesthesia may foster abuse of the tissues. Judicious use of topical and injected anesthetics, however, is appreciated by the patient and precludes the likelihood of sacrificing thoroughness in an effort to avoid pain when anesthesia is not used.

Step 2. Remove the supragingival calculus

Remove the visible calculus and debris with superficial scalers. This will result in shrinkage of the gingiva because of bleeding elicited by even slight instrumentation.

Step 3. Remove the subgingival calculus

A deep scaler is inserted to the bottom of the pocket just beneath the lower border of the calculus and the calculus dislodged. The chisel type of scaler is used for proximal surfaces too close together to be reached with other types of scalers (Fig. 42–4, 1 and 2).

Step 4. Plane the tooth surface

Hoe scalers are then used to ensure removal of the deep deposits, removal of necrotic cementum and smoothing the root surface. Final smoothness is obtained with

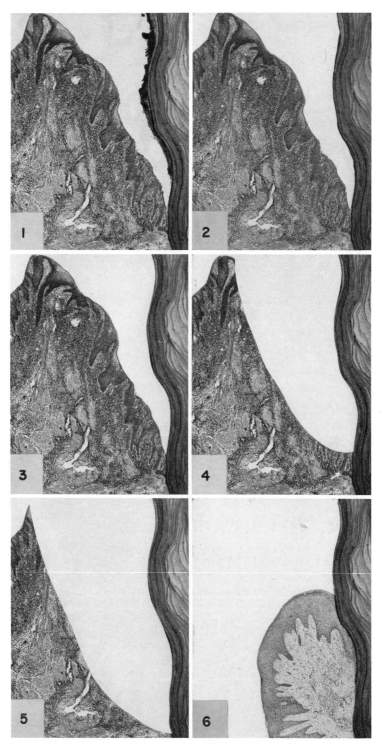

Figure 42–4   Diagrammatic Representation of the Anticipated Tissue Changes in Various Stages of Pocket Eradication Using Scaling and Curettage. *1,* The periodontal pocket with calculus on the root surface. *2,* Calculus removed. Note contour of the cementum. *3,* Root surface smoothed. *4,* Pocket wall curetted. Epithelial attachment (*arrow*) not disturbed. *5,* Alternate procedure to that shown in *4.* Pocket wall curetted. Epithelial attachment also removed. *6,* Pocket eradicated.

curettes (Fig. 42–4, 3), which produce significantly smoother surfaces than are obtainable with hoe scalers.[8]

The bacterial flora of the periodontal pocket is reduced after subgingival calculus is removed.[21, 22] The removal of necrotic cementum and dentin, in addition to removing local irritants, prepares the root so that new connective tissue may be deposited on its freshened surface. In the course of healing, new cementum is more likely to be deposited on a clean dentin surface than on necrotic cementum.

Step 5. Curette the soft tissue wall

Curettage is employed to remove the diseased inner lining of the pocket wall, including the epithelial attachment (Fig. 42–4, 4 and 5). If the epithelial attachment is permitted to remain, epithelium from the crest of the gingiva will proliferate along the curetted pocket wall to join it and prevent any possibility of reattachment of the connective tissue to the root surface.[11] Curettes are used for this purpose with cutting edges on two sides of the blade so that the root is smoothed in the same operation.

Removal of the inner pocket lining and the epithelial attachment is a two-stage procedure. The curette is inserted to engage the inner lining of the pocket wall and carried along the soft tissue to the crest of the gingiva. The pocket wall is supported by gentle finger pressure on the external surface. The curette is then placed under the cut edge of the epithelial attachment so as to undermine it. The epithelial attachment is separated away with a scooping motion of the curette to the tooth surface. Curettage removes degenerated tissue, proliferating epithelial buds and granulation tissue, which all go to form the inner aspect of the pocket wall, and creates a cut, bleeding connective tissue surface. The bleeding causes shrinkage in the height of the gingiva and reduction in pocket depth and facilitates healing by removing tissue debris.

Opinions differ regarding whether scaling and curettage consistently removes the pocket lining and epithelial attachment. Some report that scaling and root planing tear the lining epithelium, without removing it or the epithelial attachment,[13] but that both epithelial structures,[2, 3, 11] sometimes including underlying inflamed connective tissue,[14] are removed by curettage. Others report that the removal of lining epithelium and epithelial attachment is not complete.[19, 23, 25]

Step 6. Polish the tooth surface

Using a rubber polishing cup with Improved Zircate or a paste of fine pumice in water, the root surface and adjacent coronal surface are polished. The flexibility of the rubber cup permits access to the subgingival area without traumatizing the tissues. Brushes are not used for polishing the root surfaces at this stage because of the difficulty of avoiding soft tissue injury. After the root surfaces are polished, the field is cleansed with warm water and slight pressure is applied to adapt the gingiva to the tooth. The use of tissue varnish to cover the area is optional.

The patient is dismissed and advised to pursue his usual eating habits, but to be mindful that there may be some discomfort for a few days. He is to pay particular attention to keeping his teeth clean, gently at first, but gradually increasing the vigor of brushing, interdental cleansing and flossing, followed by water irrigation.

HEALING FOLLOWING SCALING AND CURETTAGE

Electromicroscopic studies reveal the following regarding roots which have been thoroughly scaled and planed:[20]

Immediately after treatment the surfaces are smooth; there may be some cracked and fragmented areas. In some sections the cementum is completely removed.

Pellicle and bacterial plaque are deposited on the surface within a few hours, followed by calcification of the root. Caries sometimes develops within seven days.

Within three to four weeks after exposure to the oral cavity a hypermineralized surface zone and a subsurface cuticle develop. These are produced by an interchange of minerals and organic components at the saliva-root interface. Remineralization occurs more frequently following scaling and root planing in periodontally diseased teeth than in periodontally healthy teeth.

Immediately after scaling and curettage

a blood clot fills the gingival sulcus. This is followed by a rapid proliferation of granulation tissue with a decrease in the number of small blood vessels as the tissue matures. Restoration and epithelization of the sulcus generally require from two to seven days,[10, 14, 15, 23] and restoration of the epithelial attachment occurs in animals as early as five days. Immature collagen fibers appear within 21 days post-treatment. Healthy gingival fibers inadvertently severed from the tooth by scaling, root planing and curettage,[16] and tears in the sulcular epithelium[13, 17] and epithelial attachment are repaired in the healing process.

Appearance of the gingiva after one week

The gingiva is reduced in height because of shrinkage and shift in the position of the gingival margin. The gingiva is also slightly redder than normal because of increased vascularity associated with healing. If the patient is not already on an instructed plaque control regimen, he is instructed at this visit, before the next area is treated.

Appearance of the gingiva after two weeks

At this time, with proper physiotherapy by the patient, the normal color, consistency, surface texture, and contour of the gingiva are attained and the gingival margin is well adapted to the tooth (Fig. 42–4, 6). Scaling and curettage removes irritants from the tooth surface; it must be accompanied by the elimination of all other forms of local irritation.

Sequelae of pocket elimination with the scaling and curettage technique

Healing is usually uneventful, but several types of complications may develop.

1. SENSITIVITY TO PERCUSSION. Inflammation of the periodontal ligament may develop within a day or two after treatment. The tooth is slightly extruded, sensitive to percussion and the patient complains of a throbbing pain. There may be localized lymphadenopathy. In such cases, antibiotics are administered systemically (Chap. 51) as a prophylactic measure. The involved tooth or its antagonist is ground slightly to relieve the occlusion. Using a topical anesthetic, the gingival margin is gently probed to stimulate bleeding and examined for any fragments of calculus that may be lodged in the tissues. The patient is instructed to avoid exertion and to rinse every hour with warm solution of a teaspoonful of salt in a glass of water. When the patient is seen after 24 hours, the condition is generally alleviated. The antibiotic therapy is continued for another 24 hours and rinsing reduced to three times a day.

2. BLEEDING. Bleeding may occur after two or three days. This results from inflammation around surface vessels, with rupture of the vessel walls. The area is generally partially covered with a small berry-like clot when the patient appears. To correct this condition, the clot is removed with a pellet of cotton saturated with peroxide, 3 per cent, and the bleeding point located. The surface is gently curetted and irritants are removed. Pressure is applied with either a gauze pad or a cotton pellet wedged interproximally for 20 minutes.

3. SENSITIVITY TO THERMAL CHANGES AND TACTILE STIMULATION. The patient may complain about sensitivity to cold and tactile stimulation. This is caused either by removal of cementum and exposure of the extremely sensitive granular layer of Tomes at the periphery of the root dentin,[5] or by exposure of root surface previously insulated from thermal changes by heavy calculus deposits.

Root sensitivity is treated with sodium fluoride desensitizing paste or other desensitizing agents (Chap. 51). Burnishing the clean root surface with a slightly warmed ball burnisher is frequently helpful in eliminating localized areas of sensitivity. Except in extreme cases, desensitization should not be undertaken the first week after treatment. It is advisable to postpone its use until shrinkage of the gingiva is complete and a well-developed epithelial covering is present. If the desensitizing agent is used the first week after treatment, gingival bleeding elicited in an effort to reach the denuded root surfaces diminishes the effectiveness of the desensitizing agent. There is also a tendency for post-treatment sensitivity to diminish spontaneously after two or three weeks have elapsed.

PACKING TECHNIQUES FOR POCKET ELIMINATION (BOX)

Box[6, 7] advocated a variation of the scaling and curettage technique for pocket eradication which included the use of periodontal packs. The packs consist of boracic acid, oil of peppermint, oxygen and other medicinals incorporated in a paraffin base, which is formed into sticks. The paraffin is heated and forced into the pocket areas by digital pressure or with a syringe designed for this purpose, where it remains for 24 to 48 hours. When it is removed, calculus exposed by shrinkage of the gingiva is removed by scaling.

A second application is made at this time or later, and repeated until gingival disease is eliminated. Individual packs may be changed daily or every other day, but may be left on longer. The period of treatment may be two or three weeks, at the end of which time excellent results are obtained. The effectiveness of the aforementioned procedure is enhanced if it is preceded by flushing the pockets with a special glycerin mixture (Mentho-Borate).

Advantages claimed for this technique include the following: It favors repair by covering the inflamed gingiva with a bland coating and separating it from the tooth. The pack also acts as a protective seal which prevents reinfection during healing. Mechanical pressure results in atrophy of the gingival margin and dilatation of the pocket which facilitates scaling with a minimum of trauma to the gingiva.

"CONSERVATIVE SURGICAL" TECHNIQUE (BARKANN)

Barkann[1] describes a modification of the scaling and curettage technique for pocket elimination which includes excision of the inner pocket wall and a phenol-camphor coagulating mixture. The following is the procedure:

Use a topical anesthetic and, after swabbing the pocket with an antiseptic, pack it with a cotton strand impregnated with a mixture of 25 per cent phenol and 75 per cent camphor. The strand remains in the pocket for an instant, and on its removal curetting is begun. The process of packing the strands and curetting is repeated, enlarging the pocket opening. As much coagulated tissue and pocket contents as possible are removed.

With a curved knife designed for this purpose, the papilla is excised with a semilunar incision and an internal bevel. With the sharp blade, the tissue walls within the pocket are scraped to create fresh bleeding surfaces. Special care must be exercised to retain the facial and lingual walls of the pocket, which form a trough for the retention of the blood clot through which regeneration of connective tissue proceeds.

After all extraneous matter has been removed, and the inner wall is bleeding freely, the pocket is packed with 1/4 inch gauze dressing, about 1 1/2 to 2 inches long, which has been moistened with sterile water and into which the phenol-camphor coagulating mixture has been incorporated. It is rarely necessary to pack a broad, hollow marginal pocket.

The following day the gauze is removed and the area is irrigated with normal saline solution and swabbed with an antiseptic. If very deep, the pocket is packed for another day with gauze saturated with an antiseptic such as Metaphen or Merthiolate. Plaque control is started as soon as the condition permits.

REFERENCES

1. Barkann, L.: A Conservative Surgical Technic for the Eradication of a Pyorrhea Pocket. J.A.D.A., 26:61, 1939.
2. Beube, F. E.: Treatment Methods for Marginal Gingivitis and Periodontitis. Texas D. J., 71:427, 1953.
3. Blass, J. L., and Lite, T.: Gingival Healing Following Surgical Curettage: A Histopathologic Study. New York D. J., 25:127, 1959.
4. Bodecker, C. F.: The Difficulty of Completely Removing Subgingival Calculus. J.A.D.A., 30:703, 1943.
5. Bodecker, C. F.: The Most Sensitive Areas of the Teeth and Their Operative Treatment. Trans. Seventh International Dental Congress I, 751, 1926.
6. Box, H. K.: Twelve Periodontal Studies. Toronto, University of Toronto Press, 1946, p. 138.
7. Cripps, S.: The Elimination of the Periodontal Pocket by Pressure Packing. Brit. D. J., 90:235, 1951.
8. Green, E., and Ramfjord, S. P.: Tooth Roughness after Subgingival Root Planing. J. Periodont., 37:396, 1966.
9. Hirschfeld, L.: Subgingival Curettage in Periodontal Treatment. J.A.D.A., 44:301, 1952.

10. Kon, S., et al.: Visualization of Microvascularization of the Healing Periodontal Wound. II. Curettage. J. Periodont.–Periodontics, *40*: 96, 1969.
11. Morris, M. L.: The Removal of the Pocket and Attachment Epithelium in Humans: A Histological Study. J. Periodont., *25*:7, 1954.
12. Moskow, B. S.: Calcifications in Gingival Biopsies. D. Progress, *1*:30, 1960.
13. Moskow, B. S.: The Response of the Gingival Sulcus to Instrumentation: A Histologic Investigation. I. The Scaling Procedure. J. Periodont., *33*:282, 1962.
14. Moskow, B. S.: The Response of the Gingival Sulcus to Instrumentation: A Histologic Investigation. II. Gingival Curettage. J. Periodont., *35*:112, 1964.
15. O'Bannon, J. Y.: The Gingival Tissues before and after Scaling the Teeth. J. Periodont., *35*:69, 1964.
16. Ramfjord, S., and Costich, E. R.: Healing after Simple Gingivectomy. J. Periodont., *34*: 401, 1963.
17. Ramfjord, S., and Kiester, G.: The Gingival Sulcus and the Periodontal Pocket Immediately Following Scaling of Teeth. J. Periodont., *25*:167, 1954.
18. Riffle, A. B.: The Cementum During Curettage. J. Periodont., *23*:170, 1952.
19. Sato, M.: Histopathological Study of the Healing Process after Surgical Treatment for Alveolar Pyorrhea. Bull. Tokyo Dent. College, *1*:71, 1960.
20. Selvig, K. A.: Biological Changes at the Tooth-Saliva Interface in Periodontal Disease. J. D. Res., *48*:846, 1969.
21. Simonton, F. V.: The Most Significant Findings of the California Stomatological Research Group in the Study of Pyorrhea. J. D. Res., *8*:235, 1928.
22. Steen, E.: The Occurrence of Bacteria in Gingival Pockets. Norske Tannlaegefore. Tid., *65*:230, 1955.
23. Stone, S., Ramfjord, S. P., and Waldron, J.: Scaling and Gingival Curettage. A Radiographic Study. J. Periodont., *37*:415, 1966.
24. Thebaud, J.: Some Microscopic Aspects of the Curetted Surface of the Cementum after the Subgingival Curettage. J. Canad. D. Assn., *17*:127, 1951.
25. Waerhaug, J.: Microscopic Demonstration of Tissue Reaction Incident to Removal of Subgingival Calculus. J. Periodont., *26*:26, 1955.

PERIODONTAL SURGERY

Many surgical periodontal procedures are described in the chapters which follow. The development of the use of surgery in periodontics,[1, 10] as its goals expanded from pocket elimination to the correction of disease-produced deformities and restoration of tissues destroyed by disease, is outlined below. This presentation should serve

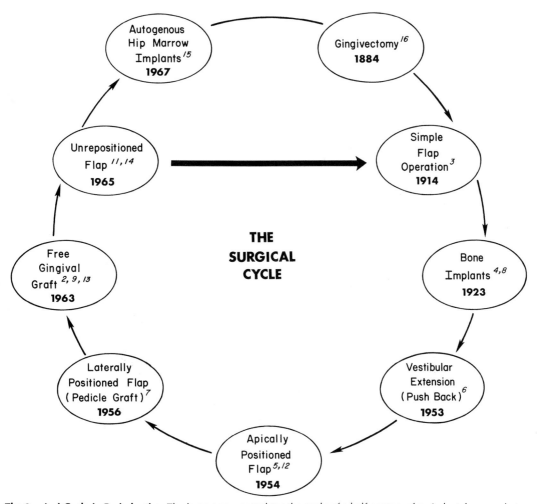

The Surgical Cycle in Periodontics. The large arrow completes the cycle of a half century of periodontal surgery between 1914 and 1965.

as an introduction to periodontal surgery and provide a background for evaluating current and future surgical techniques.

THE SURGICAL CYCLE

It is sometimes difficult to establish with certainty the originator of a technique or the exact date it was introduced, but it is apparent that techniques for surgery in periodontics have followed a cyclical trend (see figure on page 633). The start was with the gingivectomy in 1884,[16] followed by the simple flap procedure in 1914;[3] both operations were for eliminating periodontal pockets. In 1923, bone implants were tried for improving bone repair following periodontal surgery,[8] and although favorable results were reported,[4] the concept did not engender much enthusiasm at the time.

The vestibular extension (push-back) operation, in 1953,[6] broadened the scope of periodontal surgery to include the correction of mucogingival deformities. This stimulated an era of clinical experimentation with new procedures and modifications of older operations which had attracted little attention when first introduced.

The apically positioned flap, described in 1954,[5, 12] corrected mucogingival deformities without some of the pitfalls of earlier vestibular operations. It entailed less extensive surgery and, by covering the bone with a flap, it offered some protection against irreparable bone loss. The lateral sliding flap (pedicle graft), in 1956,[7] was aimed at covering isolated exposed roots, one of periodontics' enticing goals.

In the early 1960's,[2, 9, 13] the development of the free gingival graft enabled progressive clinicians to relocate gingiva to areas where it was more urgently needed. The unrepositioned flap appeared in 1965,[11] affording visibility and accessibility for pocket elimination, after which it was replaced to its presurgical location. This was similar to the simple flap operation which was introduced in 1914,[14] and completed the cycle of a half century of periodontal surgery (see figure).

During all this time, there had been a growing interest in obtaining "bone fill"

of osseous defects produced by periodontal disease. The challenge was approached by many techniques, used singly or in combination, such as sole dependence upon the natural reparative processes; reshaping the defects by osseous resection to make them more amenable to repair; and the use of implants of bovine anorganic bone, autogenous bone, dentin, cartilage and plaster of Paris. In 1967, autogenous hip marrow implants[15] were added to the continuing effort to improve bone repair following periodontal treatment.

REFERENCES TO THE LITERATURE

1. Beckham, L. C., Cederbaum, A. D., Levy, L., O'Connell, R., and Salkind, A.: A History of Periodontal Surgery and Suggested Changes in Terminology and Nomenclature. J. Periodont., 33:101, 1962.
2. Björn, H.: Free Transplantation of Gingiva Propria. Sveriges Tandlak-T., 22:684, 1963.
3. Cieszynski, A.: Bemerkungen zur Radikal—Chirurgischen Behandlung der sog. Pyorrhöe Alveolaries. Deutsch. Mschr. Zannheilk., 32:376, 1914.
4. Cross, W. G.: Bone Implants in Periodontal Disease. A Further Study. J. Periodont., 28:184, 1957.
5. Friedman, N.: Mucogingival Surgery: The Apically Repositioned Flap. J. Periodont., 33:328, 1962.
6. Goldman, H. M.: Periodontia. 3rd ed. St. Louis, C. V. Mosby Co., 1953, pp. 552–561.
7. Grupe, H. E., and Warren, R. F.: Repair of Gingival Defects by a Sliding Flap Operation. J. Periodont., 27:290, 1956.
8. Hegedüs, Z.: The Rebuilding of the Alveolar Process by Bone Transplantation. D. Cosmos, 65:736, 1923.
9. King, K., and Pennel, B. M.: Evaluation of Attempts to Increase the Width of Attached Gingiva. Presented before the Philadelphia Society of Periodontology, 1964.
10. Morris, M. L.: Surgical Procedures in Periodontia. New York J. Den., 17:303, 1947.
11. Morris, M. L.: The Unrepositioned Mucoperiosteal Flap. Periodontics, 3:147, 1965.
12. Nabers, C. L.: Repositioning the Attached Gingiva. J. Periodont., 25:38, 1954.
13. Nabers, J.: Free Gingival Grafts. Periodontics, 4:243, 1966.
14. Ratcliff, P. A.: Section on Periodontal Therapy—Review of Literature. In Proceedings of the World Workshop in Periodontics, 1966, University of Michigan Press, p. 307.
15. Schallhorn, R. G.: Eradication of Bifurcation Defects Utilizing Frozen Autogenous Hip Marrow Implants. Periodont. Abst., 15:101, 1967.
16. Stern, I. B., Everett, F. G., and Robicsek, K.: S. Robicsek—A Pioneer in the Surgical Treatment of Periodontal Disease. J. Periodont., 36:265, 1965.

Chapter 43

THE GINGIVECTOMY TECHNIQUE

In a limited literal sense, the term *gingivectomy* means excision of the gingiva. In reality, it is a *two-stage operation* consisting of *the removal of diseased gingiva and the scaling and planing of the root surface.*

Gingivectomy derives its effectiveness from the following:

1. **By removing the diseased pocket wall which obscures the tooth surface, it provides the visibility and accessibility that are essential for the complete removal of irritating surface deposits and thorough smoothing of the roots (Fig. 43–1).**

2. **By removing diseased tissue and local irritants, it creates a favorable environment for gingival healing and the restoration of physiologic gingival contour.**

As is often the case with treatment techniques in widespread use, many therapists claim to accomplish routinely with gingivectomy what others cannot, and

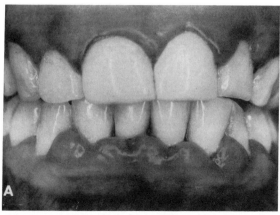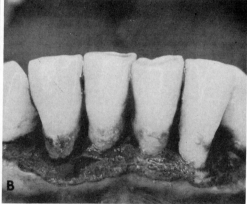

Figure 43–1 Visibility and Accessibility to Calculus. *A,* Gingival enlargement. *B,* Removal of diseased gingiva exposes calculus.

others cannot accomplish with it what many routinely do. When used for the purposes for which it is intended, gingivectomy is the most effective form of treatment available (Fig. 43–2). It will not succeed when more is expected of it than it can accomplish or when it is improperly performed.

WHEN TO USE GINGIVECTOMY

Gingivectomy is a definitive procedure for eliminating deep suprabony pockets[4, 13] (Fig. 43–2), suprabony pockets with firm fibrous walls, regardless of their depth, gingival enlargement (see Chap. 49), furcation involvement (see Chap. 45), periodontal abscesses (see Chap. 48), pericoronal flaps and some interdental gingival craters (see Chap. 50) and some infrabony pockets (see Chap. 44).

Pocket Elimination by Gingivectomy

The most common use for gingivectomy is the elimination of deep suprabony pockets in which the deposits on the root cannot be seen in their entirety when the pocket wall is deflected with a probe or blast of warm air. In pockets with a depth of more than 4 mm., calculus cannot be completely removed with any degree of predictability by hand scalers and/or ultrasonic scalers if the operator must rely solely upon tactile sensation.[11]

Gingivectomy is also used for the elimi-

nation of all suprabony pockets, regardless of their depth, if the pocket wall is fibrous and firm. Because fibrous gingival tissue does not shrink after scaling and curettage, some form of surgical treatment is necessary to eliminate the pocket.

Gingivectomy or Scaling and Curettage?

The scaling and curettage technique and gingivectomy are both effective for eliminating periodontal pockets. The question is not whether one should be used instead of the other, but when each should be used. To try to eliminate all pockets by scaling and curettage is erroneous, because it will not succeed; it is equally poor judgement to use gingivectomy for all periodontal pockets. A question frequently asked is: "How deep should a pocket be to require treatment by gingivectomy?" This cannot be answered in millimeters alone. In shallow or very deep pockets, the choice of treatment is apparent. However, in borderline cases, the decision depends upon the judgment and skill of the operator. **If there is any doubt that the pocket can be eliminated by scaling and curettage, the doubt indicates the need for gingivectomy and the patient should be given the benefit of the doubt.**

Pocket elimination should not be a matter of trial and error. Gingivectomy is not a last resort for treating pockets after scaling and curettage fails. Nor is scaling and curettage a preliminary treatment for

GINGIVECTOMY

Before   After

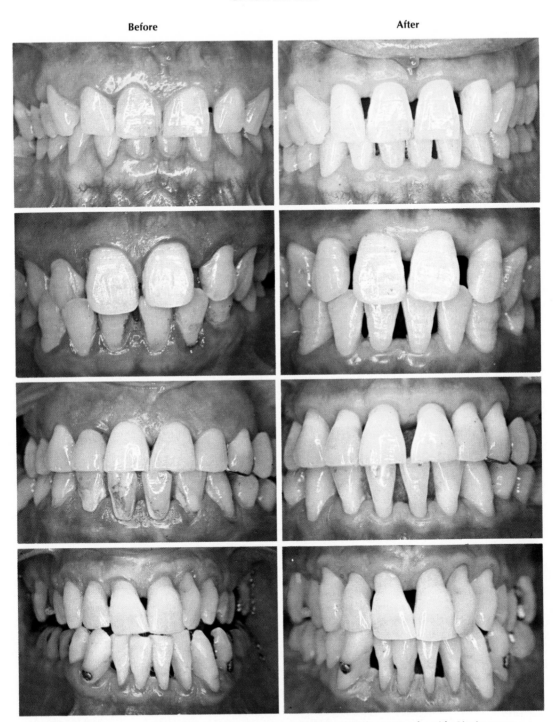

Figure 43–2 Results Obtained by Treating Suprabony Pockets of Different Depths with Gingivectomy.

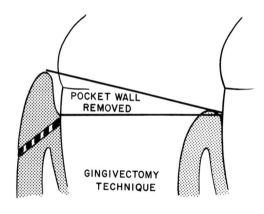

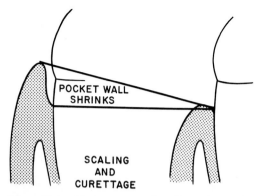

Figure 43–3 Gingivectomy and Scaling and Curettage Procedures produce the same esthetic result if pocket is completely eliminated.

pockets that require gingivectomy. The esthetic result is the same with both techniques if the pocket is completely eliminated (Fig. 43–3).

It should not be necessary to "try scaling and curettage first" to determine if the patient requires gingivectomy. **The therapist should develop the diagnostic acumen to decide upon the technique he is to use before treatment is begun so that the patient is not subjected to two operations to obtain a result which can be accomplished with one.** It is difficult for a patient to understand why the therapist has experimented with a doubtful procedure and withheld the technique he eventually uses with apparent success. Excessive scaling, in an unsuccessful effort to eliminate a pocket by scaling and curettage, causes excessive root sensitivity. "Heroic" scaling and curettage that fails also discourages the operator and undermines the patient's confidence in periodontal therapy.

Comparison of Results Obtained by Scaling and Curettage and Gingivectomy

Gingivectomy produces a greater reduction in pocket depth than does scaling and curettage. In patients with good oral hygiene and periodic post-treatment scaling, there is a gradual return of some pocket depth following both techniques, but to a lesser degree following gingivectomy.[31] The recurrence of pocket depth is greater on the facial and lingual surfaces than interproximally. It results from gingival height rather than apical migration of the epithelial attachment. Scaling and curettage of some deep pockets results in increased periodontal attachment (re-attachment); loss of attachment (recession) in gingivectomy-treated areas, reported in some studies,[7, 21, 29, 31, 40] is disputed in others.[8, 27, 28]

INITIAL PREPARATION BEFORE PERIODONTAL SURGERY

"Initial preparation" consists of preliminary procedures for the purpose of preparing the mouth for the overall periodontal treatment regimen which is to follow. It usually involves three or four visits, or more, depending upon the patient's condition. Initial preparation includes scaling and root planing, and the elimination of unfavorable local environmental factors such as overhanging restorations and areas of food impaction. Gross occlusal abnormalities are corrected and, if necessary, temporary splints and night guards are constructed to control excessive tooth mobility, reduce excessive occlusal forces and relieve parafunctional occlusal habits such as bruxism. Systemic conditions that may interfere with healing are also explored. The patient is instructed in a plaque control regimen which assists in the improvement of the periodontal condition and provides an opportunity to assess the effectiveness of the patient's cooperation in the treatment to follow.

Initial preparation is a preliminary, "less than complete" treatment. It improves the condition of the gingiva by reducing the severity of inflammation, and it lessens the extent of involvement. For example, the attached gingiva often undergoes degenerative changes secondary to the spread of inflammation from the gingival margin. Reducing the inflammation at its source also lessens its spread and results in improvement in the attached gingiva. The healing which occurs following initial preparation is also assumed to render the gingiva more suitable for surgical intervention.

Another purpose of initial preparation is to assist the therapist in determining what further treatment the patient requires. The tissue response is used as a guide to making a decision regarding the need for periodontal surgery and the most appropriate techniques to use.

The use of "initial preparation" is a matter of individual preference, depending upon the condition of the patient's mouth and the therapist's opinion of the benefits such preparation will provide.[15] It creates a cleaner mouth, reduces bleeding during surgery and improves the condition of the tissues upon which surgical procedures are to be performed.

However, there is no evidence that the tissue healing following initial preparation improves the results obtained by the treatment. Prescaling does not improve post-gingivectomy healing or gingival architecture.[1, 12, 36] Less bacteremia occurs during gingivectomies preceded by scaling, but the reduction is more than offset by the added bacteremia caused by the prescaling itself.[16, 20] Performing two procedures subjects the patient to a double risk. No other systemic blood changes ordinarily follow gingivectomy.[34]

Acute gingival disease must be eliminated before gingivectomy (Chap. 50), and the patient should be symptom-free for one month before the gingivectomy is performed.

A STEP-BY-STEP PROCEDURE FOR PERFORMING THE GINGIVECTOMY*

Premedication for the Apprehensive Patient

The apprehensive patient should be premedicated with Nembutal (100 mg.) or with other sedatives.

Anesthesia

Gingivectomy is a painless operation. The patient should be assured of this at the outset and should be thoroughly anesthetized, using local block and infiltration injections. Injection directly into the interdental papillae is not ordinarily required, but may be helpful.

Sequence of Treatments (Table 43–1)

A mouth with generalized pocket formation is treated in quadrants at weekly intervals. It is advisable to adopt a sequence for treating the quadrants in all patients, modifying it if there are urgent needs in a particular area. The author starts with the mandibular right quadrant. Because anesthesia is obtainable with fewer injections in the mandible and this area can be operated upon with the greatest facility, it simplifies the patient's first surgical visit. All periodontal conditions in the quadrant are treated, often by combining the gingivectomy with other surgical procedures (discussed in subsequent chapters).

The right maxilla is treated next, leaving the left side free for the patient to use for chewing. The left mandibular quadrant and the left maxillary quadrant are treated on successive weeks (Fig. 43–4).

---

*The gingivectomy technique described here is essentially that developed by Dr. Olin Kirkland with modifications by the author.

TABLE 43–1 SCHEDULE FOR GENERALIZED GINGIVECTOMY

First treatment visit	Operate right mandibular quadrant	
Second treatment visit	Remove pack from right mandibular quadrant; introduce plaque control by the patient	Operate right maxillary quadrant
Third treatment visit (Fig. 43–4, A, B)	Remove pack from the right maxillary quadrant; review plaque control	Operate left mandibular quadrant
Fourth treatment visit (Fig. 43–4, C)	Remove pack from the left mandibular quadrant; review plaque control	Operate left maxillary quadrant
Fifth treatment visit (Fig. 43–4, D)	Remove pack from the left maxillary quadrant; review plaque control	
Sixth and subsequent visits (Fig. 43–4, E)	Review plaque control and adjust occlusion if required	

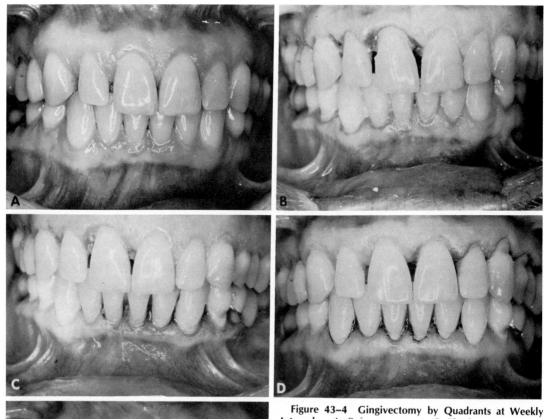

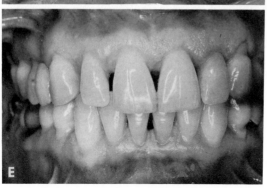

Figure 43–4 Gingivectomy by Quadrants at Weekly Intervals. *A,* Before treatment. *B,* Third treatment visit. The right mandibular and maxillary quadrants have been treated. The pack has just been removed from the right maxilla and the left mandibular quadrant is to be treated. Compare the right maxilla, at one week post-gingivectomy, with the right mandible, two weeks after operation.

C, Fourth treatment visit. Pack removed from mandibular left quadrant. To observe clinical changes in healing, compare the appearance of patient's right side with previous week (*B*).

D, Fifth treatment visit. Pack removed from maxillary left quadrant. Compare appearance of remainder of mouth with previous weeks (*B* and *C*).

E, After three months. Compare with *A.*

An aspirator is indispensable for performing the gingivectomy. It provides the clear view of each root surface, which is necessary for thorough removal of deposits and planing. Further, it permits accurate appraisal of the extent and pattern of soft tissue and bone involvement, and prevents seepage of blood into the floor of the mouth and oropharynx.

Mark the Pockets

The pockets on each surface are explored with a periodontal probe and marked with a #27G pocket marker. The instrument is held with the marking end in line with the vertical axis of the tooth. The straight end is inserted to the base of the pocket and the level marked by pressing the pliers together and producing a bleeding point on the outside surface (Fig. 43–5 and 43–6). The pockets are marked systematically, beginning on the distal surface of the last tooth, then on the facial surface, proceeding anteriorly to the midline. The procedure is repeated on the lingual surface. Each pocket is marked in several areas so as to outline its course on each surface.

Resect the Gingiva

The gingiva may be resected with periodontal knives, a scalpel or scissors. The removal of diseased gingiva is an important

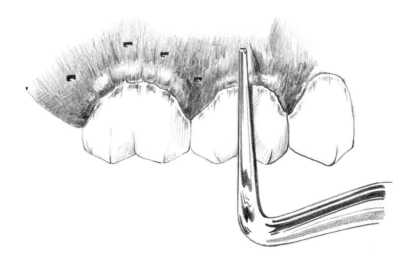

Figure 43–5 Pocket Marker #27G Makes Pin-Point Perforations which indicate pocket depth.

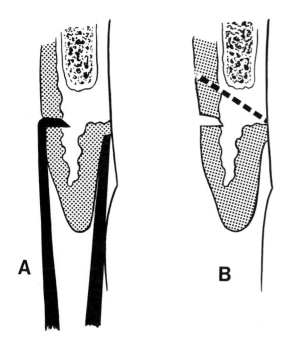

Figure 43–6 Marking the Depth of Suprabony Pocket. A, Pocket marker in position. B, Beveled incision extends apical to the perforation made by the pocket marker.

part of the gingivectomy, but the instrument with which it is done does not affect the outcome of treatment. The choice is based upon individual experience. The #20G and #21G periodontal knives are used by the author for incisions on the facial and lingual surfaces and distal to the terminal tooth in the arch. The interdental periodontal knives #22G and #23G are used for supplemental interdental incisions where necessary, and the Bard-Parker Blades #11 and #12 and scissors are used as auxiliary instruments.

Discontinuous and continuous incisions

Discontinuous or continuous incisions may be used, depending upon the operator's preference.

The *discontinuous incision* is started on the facial surface at the distal angle of the last tooth and carried forward, following the course of the pocket, and extending through the interdental gingiva to the distofacial angle of the next tooth (Fig. 43–7). The next incision is begun where the previous one crosses the interdental space, and is carried to the distofacial angle of the next tooth. Individual incisions are repeated until the midline is reached (Fig. 43–8).

The *continuous incision* is started on the facial surface of the last tooth and carried forward without interruption, following the course of the pockets, to the midline (Fig. 43–9). Frenum attachments in the paths of the incisions should be relocated (see Chap. 46) to avoid tension on the gingiva during healing.

After the incisions have been made on the facial surface, the procedure is repeated

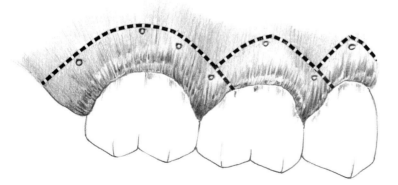

Figure 43–7 Discontinuous Incision apical to bottom of the pocket indicated by pinpoint markings.

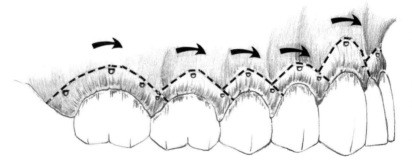

Figure 43–8 Quadrant Incised With Discontinuous Incision, which follows the outline of each pocket, apical to the pin-point markings.

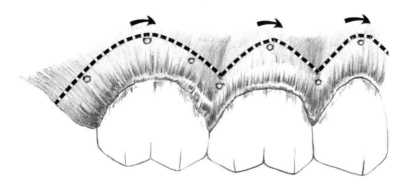

Figure 43–9 Continuous Incision begins on the molar and extends anteriorly without interruption.

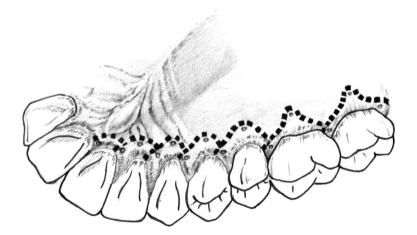

Figure 43–10   Discontinuous Incisions on the Palatal Surface follow the contours of deep periodontal pockets on the molars.

on the lingual surface (Fig. 43–10). To avoid the blood vessels and nerve of the incisive canal and also produce a better postoperative gingival contour, the incisions should be carried along the sides of the incisive papilla, not horizontally across it (Fig. 43–11).

The distal incision

After the facial and lingual incisions are completed, they are joined by an incision across the distal surface of the last erupted tooth. The distal incision is made with a #20G or #21G periodontal knife

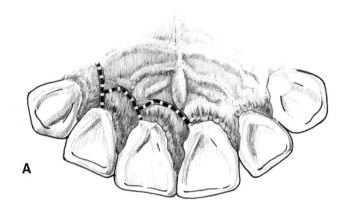

A

Figure 43–11   Incision Made Lateral to the Incisive Papilla. *A,* Discontinuous incision avoids cutting across incisive papilla. *B,* After pockets are removed.

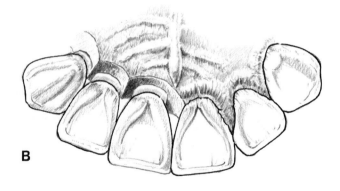

B

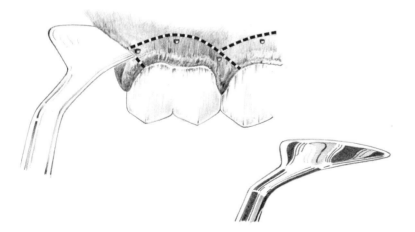

Figure 43–12 Beveled Distal Incision on the Maxilla with #20G periodontal knife.

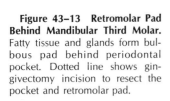

Figure 43–13 Retromolar Pad Behind Mandibular Third Molar. Fatty tissue and glands form bulbous pad behind periodontal pocket. Dotted line shows gingivectomy incision to resect the pocket and retromolar pad.

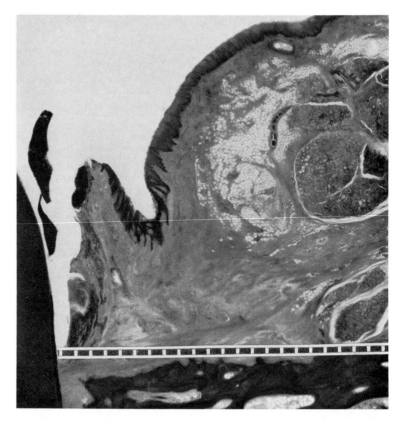

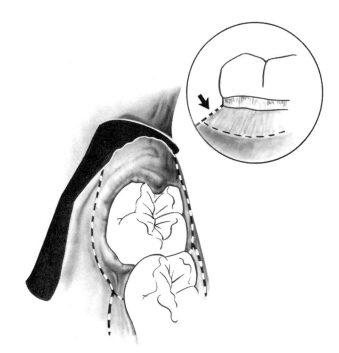

Figure 43–14 Distal Incision on the Mandible Joins the Facial and Lingual Incisions (*dotted lines*). *Inset,* The distal incision is beveled (*arrow*) to blend with the bevels on the facial and lingual surfaces.

inserted below the bottom of the pocket, and is beveled so that it blends with the facial and lingual incisions (Figs. 43–12, 43–13 and 43–14).

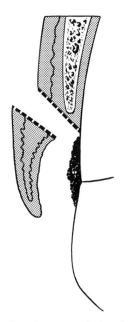

Figure 43–15 Complete removal of pocket wall assures exposure of calculus.

How to make the incision

The incision is made apical to the points marking the course of the pockets[2, 32, 40] between the base of the pocket and the crest of the bone. **It should be as close as possible to the bone without exposing it so as to remove the soft tissue coronal to the bone.** Removal of the soft tissue between the bottom of the pocket and the bone is important, because (1) it provides the greatest likelihood of removing the entire epithelial attachment; (2) it ensures the exposure of all root deposits at the bottom of the pocket (Fig. 43–15); and (3) it eliminates excessive fibrous tissue which interferes with the attainment of physiologic contour when the gingiva heals (Fig. 43–16). **This avoids the need for a second operation to reshape the gingiva after a gingivectomy is done.**

Exposure of bone is undesirable. Should it occur, healing usually presents no problem if the area is adequately covered by the periodontal pack.

The incision should be beveled at approximately 45 degrees to the tooth surface. This is most important where the pocket wall is enlarged and fibrous such

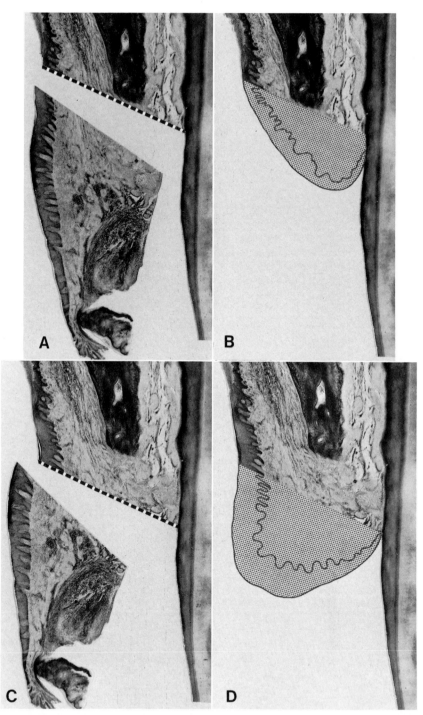

Figure 43-16 Incision Close to Bone Facilitates Healing Which Produces Physiologic Gingival Contour. *A,* Labial incision close beyond the pocket and close to the bone. *B,* Diagrammatic representation of healed gingiva with physiologic contour and normal sulcus. *C,* Incision is close to the bottom of the pocket but not deep enough. It leaves a remnant of epithelial attachment on the tooth and a wide band of inflamed fibrous connective tissue between the bottom of the pocket and the bone. *D,* Diagrammatic representation of bulbous gingiva and wide, deep sulcus formed on incompletely resected inflamed fibrous tissue.

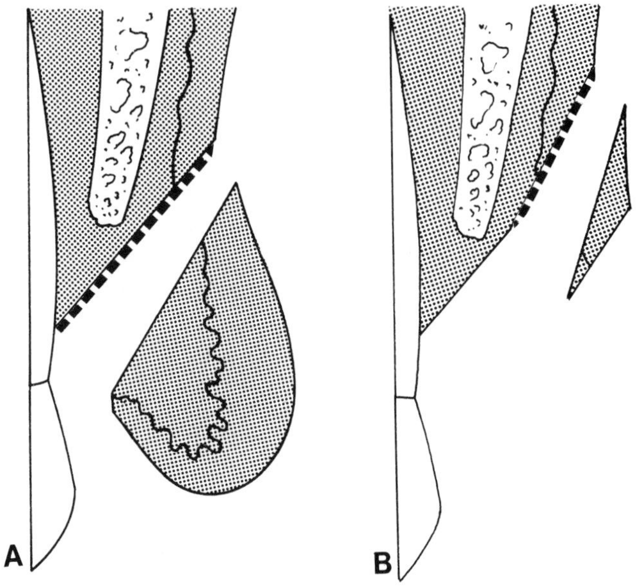

Figure 43–17 Beveled Incision for the Removal of Bulbous Fibrous Palatal Pocket. *A,* Bulbous gingiva on the palatal surface of maxillary first molar resected with a beveled incision. *B,* Corrective second incision sometimes required when proper contour cannot be obtained with single incision.

as on the palatal surface in the molar area (Fig. 43–17). Failure to bevel leaves a broad fibrous plateau which takes more time than ordinarily required to develop physiologic contour. In the interim, plaque and food accumulation may lead to recurrence of pockets.

The incision should recreate the normal festooned pattern of the gingiva as far as possible, but not if it means leaving part of the pocket wall intact. The diseased pocket wall must be completely removed even if it requires departure from the regular outline of normal gingiva.

The incision should pass completely through the soft tissue to the tooth (Fig. 43–18). Incomplete incisions make it difficult to detach the pocket wall, and leave adherent tissue tabs that must be removed with a scissors or periodontal knife.

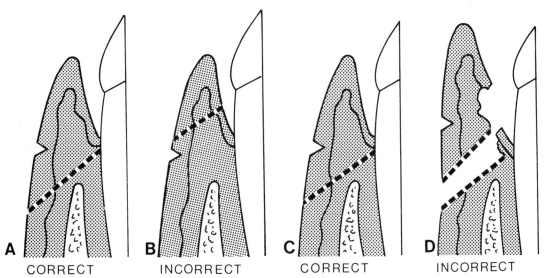

Figure 43–18 Correct and Incorrect Incisions. *A,* **Correct Incision** is apical to the bottom of the pocket, beveled and completely penetrates the soft tissue. The notch is made by the pocket marker at the level of the bottom of the pocket. *B,* **Incorrect Incision** is not deep enough, leaves part of pocket behind. *C,* **Correct Incision.** *D,* **Incorrect Incision** does not penetrate the soft tissues, leaves adherent tissue tab on the tooth.

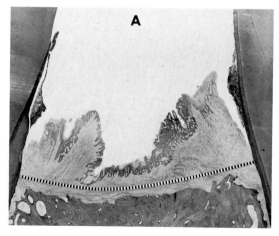

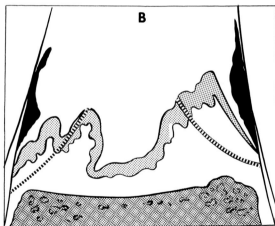

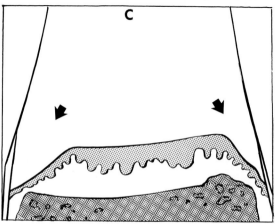

Figure 43–19 Incision Across Edentulous Space. *A,* Periodontal pockets adjacent to fibrous edentulous space. The proper incision is indicated by the dotted line. *B,* Incorrect incisions remove pockets separately, leaving fibrous mucosa intact. *C,* Troughs which result from improper incisions.

If in the course of the operation it becomes apparent that the incision is inadequate, it should be modified. The most common error is failure to make the incision close enough to the bone. Very often, deep calculus is revealed after the incision is corrected.

Teeth adjacent to edentulous areas

For pockets on teeth adjacent to an edentulous area, the usual incisions are made on the facial and lingual tooth sur-

faces. In addition, a single incision is made across the edentulous ridge apical to the pockets on the teeth and close to the bone (Fig. 43–19). Pockets adjacent to edentulous spaces should not be excised as separate units, as this creates gingival troughs (Fig. 43–19) that complicate subsequent prosthesis.

Remove the Marginal and Interdental Gingiva

Starting at the distal surface of the last erupted tooth, the gingival margin is de-

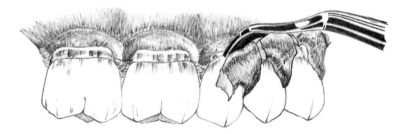

Figure 43–20 Detaching the Gingiva with a #19G Surgical Hoe. When the discontinuous incision is used, the marginal and interdental gingivae are removed as a unit.

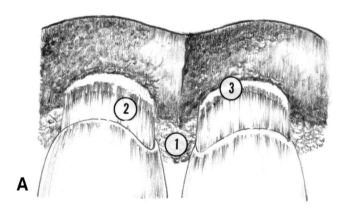

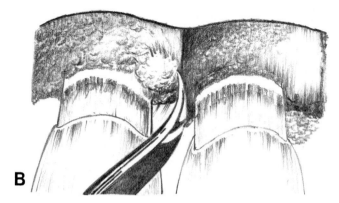

Figure 43–21 After the Pocket Wall Is Removed. *A,* Field of operation immediately after removing pocket wall. (1) Granulation tissue; (2) calculus and other root deposits; (3) clear space where bottom of the pocket was attached. *B,* Granulation tissue removed with curet to provide clear view of root surfaces. *C,* Root surfaces scaled and planed.

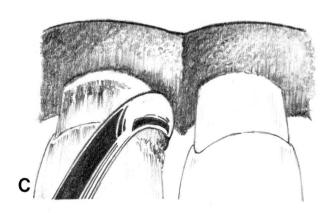

tached at the line of incision with the #19G surgical hoe and the #3G and #4G superficial scaler. The instrument is placed deep in the incision in contact with the tooth surface and moved coronally with a slow, firm motion (Fig. 43–20).

Appraise the Field of Operation

After the pocket wall is excised and the field is cleaned, the following features can be observed (Fig. 43–21, *A*).

1. Bead-like granulation tissue.
2. Calculus extending close to where the pocket was attached. **It is dark brown, slate-like in consistency, but some particles may be almost the same color as the root.**
3. A band-like light zone on the root where the base of the pocket was attached.

Other features that may be noted at this time are softening of the root surface, indentations produced by cellular resorption and cementum protuberances.

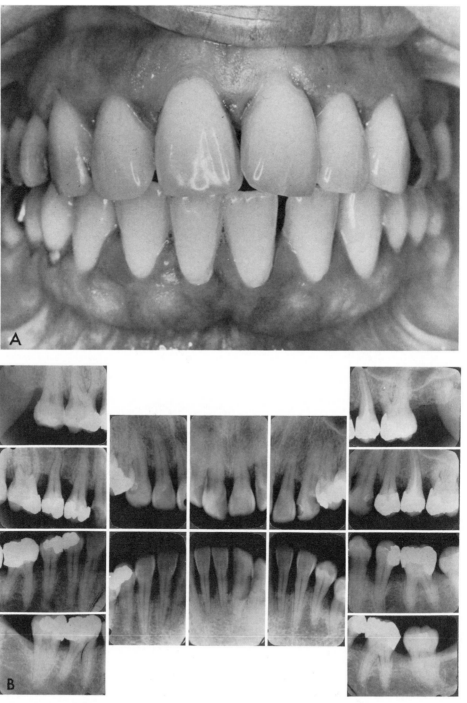

Figure 43–22 Bone Healing Following Gingivectomy. *A,* Generalized periodontal disease in 32-year-old patient. *B,* Extensive generalized bone loss. Patient has "negative bone factor." Note angular bone loss in mandibular incisor area.

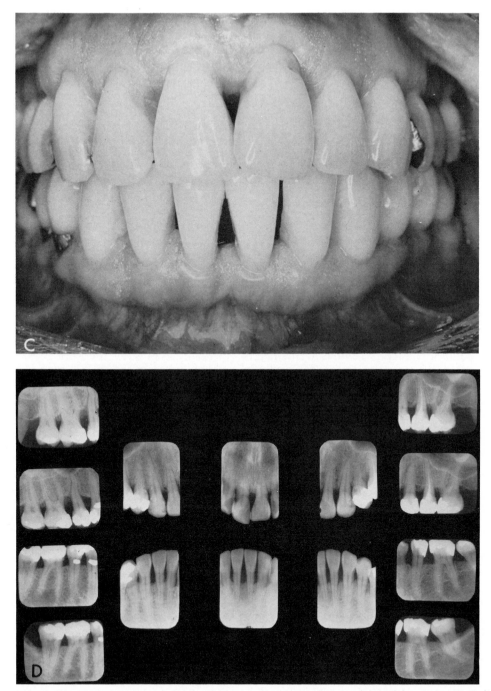

Figure 43–22 *Continued   C,* One year after gingivectomy showing excellent condition of the gingiva. *D,* Radiographs after one year showing generalized smoothing of the interdental margins and filling in of bony defect in mandibular incisor area (compare with *B*).

Remove the Granulation Tissue

The granulation tissue is removed before thorough scaling is attempted, so that hemorrhage from the granulation tissue will not obscure the scaling operation (Fig. 43–21, *B*).

Curets are used for this purpose. The curet is guided along the tooth surface and under the granulation tissue, separating it from the underlying bone. Removal of the granulation tissue will reveal either the surface of the underlying bone or a covering band of fibrous tissue.

Remove the Calculus and Necrotic Root Substance

The calculus and necrotic cementum are removed and the root surface is smoothed, using superficial and deep scalers and curets (Fig. 43–21, *C*).

The success of the gingivectomy depends in large measure upon the thoroughness with which the root is scaled and planed. This should be done immediately after the granulation tissue is removed and not postponed to a subsequent visit for the following reasons:

1. The roots are most visible and accessible after the granulation tissue is removed.

2. The gingiva cannot heal properly if root deposits are permitted to remain until the next visit when they will be obscured by inflamed gingiva.

3. Postponement introduces an unnecessary extra operation.

Management of the Alveolar Bone Margin

Bone is recontoured in the treatment of some types of infrabony pockets (Chap. 44) but in the treatment of suprabony pockets the bone should not be disturbed. The bone beneath periodontal pockets is viable tissue—it is neither infected nor necrotic. Filing or smoothing the bone to create an even, rounded margin is unnecessary and injurious, delays healing, and reduces the post-treatment bone height. Marginal defects are filled in and the bone margin rounded by the natural healing process (Fig. 43–22).

The trabeculae forming the "rough" bone margin under the pocket provide the scaffolding upon which new bone is deposited and into which new fibers are embedded for added tooth support. Removing these trabeculae reduces the potential height that can be attained by the bone during healing.

Filing the bone surface injures osteogenic cells lining the bone trabeculae and endosteal spaces, which form the new bone during healing. The injured cells become degenerated debris that must be removed by phagocytic and enzymatic activity before the constructive phase of healing can occur.

Filing the bone dislodges fragments, which undergo necrosis and act as irritants which prolong the exudative phase of inflammation and delay healing.

Pre-pack Hygiene

Before placing the periodontal pack each surface of every tooth is checked for calculus or soft tissue remnants, after which the area is washed several times with warm water and covered with a gauze sponge folded in a U shape. The patient is instructed to bite on the sponge, which remains in place until the bleeding stops. Persistent bleeding interferes with adaptation and setting of the periodontal pack. It usually can be traced to a bleeding point partially covered with clot. The clot is cleaned away with a pledget of cotton saturated with hydrogen peroxide. Pressure is then applied to the bleeding point with a pledget of cotton. If the bleeding is interproximal, the cotton is wedged between the teeth. In stubborn cases, the bleeding point is gently touched with an electrosurgery tip or electrocautery.

The Blood Clot

The cut surfaces should be covered by clot before the pack is applied. The clot protects the wound and provides a scaffolding for the new blood vessels and connective tissue cells formed in healing. The clot should not be too bulky. Excessive clot interferes with retention of the periodontal pack. It is also an excellent medium for bacterial growth and increases the possibility of infection and delays healing. This permits downgrowth of epithelium onto the root which limits the height of connective tissue attachment.[23]

The Periodontal Pack (Periodontal Dressing)

There are many types of periodontal packs, and new materials currently being investigated may soon become available for routine clinical use. Until then, the preference for use with gingivectomy is the Kirkland-Kaiser type. (For the composition of this and other types of periodontal packs, see Chapter 51.) It is easy to manipulate and apply, affords adequate working time before it sets, is firm enough to withstand mastication, is well tolerated by the tissues and is easily removed.

Preparation

The pack consists of a powder and liquid which are mixed on a wax paper pad with a wooden throat stick. The powder is grad-ually incorporated into the liquid until a thick paste is formed. More powder is kneaded into the paste with the fingers until it becomes a thick, not tacky, putty. **Proper consistency is important. The initial tendency is to make a mix which is too soft and, therefore, difficult to apply.** Tincture of green soap or orange solvent effectively removes the pack from the fingers.

How to apply the periodontal pack

The pack is rolled into two strips approximately the length of the treated quadrant. The end of one strip is bent into a hook shape and fitted around the distal surface of the last tooth, approaching it from the facial surface (Fig. 43–23). The remainder

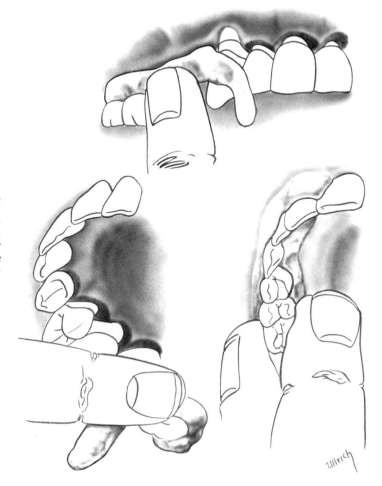

Figure 43–23   Inserting the Periodontal Pack. *A,* Strip of pack is hooked around last molar and pressed into place anteriorly. *B,* Lingual pack joined to the facial strip at the distal of the last molar and fitted into place anteriorly. *C,* Gentle pressure on facial and lingual surfaces joins pack interproximally.

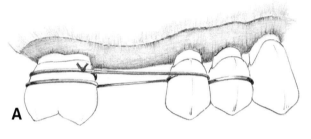

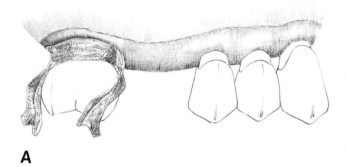

Figure 43–24   Dental Floss Loop Aids Retention of Pack Over Edentulous Area. *A,* Dental floss across edentulous space. *B,* Pack in place.

Figure 43–25   Pack Retained With Gauze Strip Around Isolated Tooth. *A,* Strip of 1/4" gauze loosely fitted to molar. *B,* Gauze embedded with pack is replaced on tooth, tightened and trimmed with scissors. *C,* Pack completed.

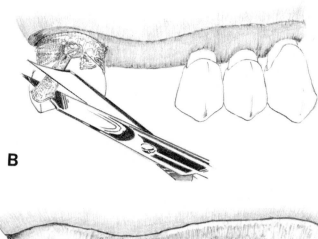

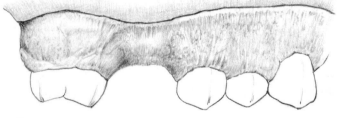

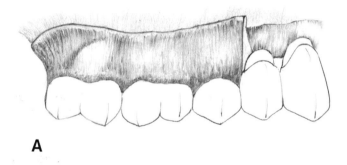

A

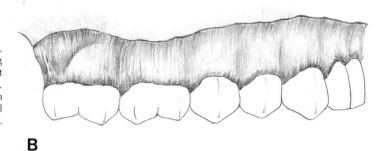

Figure 43–26 Pack in Place. *A,* Cross section showing pack extending just beyond the cut surface, without overextension onto uninvolved mucosa. *B,* Pack in place. *C,* Lingual pack in place, overextension onto palate will detach the pack and should be avoided.

B

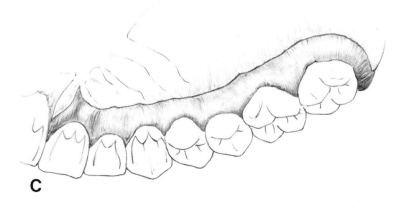

C

of the strip is brought forward along the facial surface to the midline, gently pressing it into place along the incised gingival margin and interproximally. The second strip of pack is applied from the lingual surface. It is joined to the pack at the distal surface of the last tooth, then brought forward along the cut gingival margin to the midline. The strips are joined interproximally by applying gentle pressure on the facial and lingual surfaces of the pack (Fig. 43–23).

For isolated teeth separated by edentulous spaces, the pack should be made continuous from tooth to tooth, covering the edentulous area. Joining the teeth with a loop of dental floss aids retention of the pack over the edentulous area (Fig. 43–24). When the edentulous space is long, isolated teeth may be packed separately to reduce the likelihood of displacement. To do this, a strip of one-fourth inch gauze is loosely fitted around the tooth. The gauze loop is removed, embedded with pack, replaced on the tooth and tightened (Fig. 43–25). The ends of the gauze are cut and pack is added.

The pack should completely cover the cut surface of the gingiva (Fig. 43–26), but overextension onto uninvolved mucosa

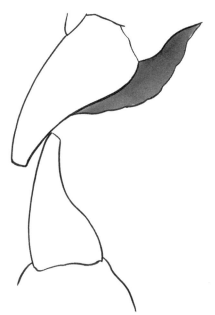

Figure 43–27 The Pack Should Not Interfere with the Occlusion.

should be avoided. **Excess pack irritates the mucobuccal fold and floor of the mouth, and interferes with the tongue.** Overextension also jeopardizes the remainder of the pack because it tends to break off, taking pack from the operated area with it. **Pack that interferes with the occlusion should be trimmed away before the patient is dismissed** (Fig. 43–27). Failure to do this causes discomfort and jeopardizes retention of the pack.

The operator should wait 15 minutes after the pack is applied before trimming it. This permits the lips, cheeks, and tongue to mold the pack while it is soft. Excess will be forced into areas where it is not needed and from which it can be easily removed.

The patient should not be dismissed until oozing of blood from beneath the pack has stopped.

Functions of the periodontal pack

There are no packs with any demonstrated curative properties. The value of the pack is indirect. It assists healing by protecting the tissue rather than by providing "healing factors." The pack serves the following functions:

1. Controls postoperative bleeding.
2. Minimizes the likelihood of postoperative infection and hemorrhage.
3. Provides some splinting of mobile teeth.
4. Facilitates healing by preventing surface trauma during mastication and irritation from plaque and food debris.

Additional facts regarding the periodontal pack

As a general rule, the pack is kept on for one week after gingivectomy. The one-week period is based upon the timetable of healing and clinical experience. It is not a rigid requirement; it may be extended, or the area may be repacked for an additional week.

If hemorrhage occurs through the pack at any time in the course of the week, the operator should remove the pack, locate the bleeding point and treat as indicated on page 657.

Fragments of the surface of the pack will come off during the week, but this presents no problem. If a portion of the pack is lost from the operated area and the patient is uncomfortable, it is usually best to repack the quadrant. Remove the remaining pack, wash the area with warm water and apply a topical anesthetic before replacing the pack, which is then to be retained for a week.

Patients may develop pain from an overextended margin which irritates the vestibule, floor of the mouth or tongue. The excess pack should be trimmed away, making sure that the new margin is not rough, before the patient is dismissed.

Patients report that the mouth feels unclean when the pack is on. Rinsing with a pleasant-tasting mouthwash diluted 1:3 with warm water, beginning on the second postoperative day, is helpful.

INSTRUCTIONS FOR THE PATIENT AFTER THE FIRST QUADRANT OF GINGIVECTOMY

After the pack is placed, the following printed instructions are given to the patient to be read before leaving the chair:

INSTRUCTIONS FOR

Mrs. Jane Smith

The operation which has been performed on your gums will help you keep your teeth. The following information has been prepared to answer questions you may have about how to take care of your mouth. Please read the instructions carefully—our patients have found them very helpful.

When the anesthesia wears off, you may have slight discomfort—not pain. Two 5-grain aspirin tablets will usually keep you comfortable. You may repeat every three hours if necessary.

We have placed a periodontal pack over your gums to protect them from irritation. The pack prevents pain, aids healing and enables you to carry on most of your usual activities in comfort. The pack will harden in a few hours, after which it can withstand most of the forces of chewing without breaking off. It may take a little while to become accustomed to it.

For your benefit the pack should remain in place as long as possible. **Do not remove it.** If particles of the pack chip off during the week do not be concerned as long as you do not have pain. If a piece of the pack breaks off and you are in pain, or if a rough edge irritates your tongue or cheek, please call the office. The problem can be easily remedied by replacing the pack. The pack will be removed at your next appointment.

For the first three hours after the operation avoid hot foods in order to permit the pack to harden. After this eat anything you can manage without chipping off the pack. Eggs, Jell-O, cereals, soups, milk, fish, hamburger or any semi-solid or finely minced foods are suggested. Avoid citrus fruits or fruit juices, highly spiced foods and alcoholic beverages. They will cause pain. Food supplements and/or vitamins are generally not necessary. We will prescribe them if needed.

Do not smoke—the heat and smoke will irritate your gums and delay healing. If at all possible, use this opportunity to give up smoking. Smokers have more gum disease than nonsmokers.

Rinsing is not part of the treatment, but it will help make your mouth feel refreshed. **Do not rinse today.** Beginning tomorrow, you may rinse as often as you wish with one of the popular, pleasant-flavored mouthwashes. Do not use it in concentrated form, dilute it—$1/3$ mouthwash to $2/3$ warm water.

Clean the parts of your mouth which have been treated on previous weeks using the methods in which you were instructed. The gums most likely will bleed more then they did before the operation. This is perfectly normal in the early stage of healing and will gradually subside. Do not stop cleaning because of it.

Follow your regular daily activities, but avoid excessive exertion of any type. Golf, tennis, skiing, bowling, swimming or sunbathing should be postponed for two days after the operation.

You may experience a slight feeling of weakness or chills during the first 24 hours. This should not be cause for alarm but should be reported at the next visit.

Swelling is not unusual, particularly in areas which required extensive surgical procedures. The swelling generally subsides in three or four days. If the swelling is painful or appears to become worse, please call the office.

There may be occasional blood stains in the saliva for the first four or five hours after the operation. This is not unusual and will correct itself. If there is considerable bleeding beyond this, take a piece of gauze, form it into the shape of a "**U**," hold it in the thumb and index finger, apply it to both sides of the pack and hold it under pressure for 20 minutes. Do not remove it during this period to examine it. If the bleeding does not stop at the end of 20 minutes, please contact the office. **Do not try to stop the bleeding by rinsing.**

If any other problems arise, please call the office.

THE PATIENT DURING THE FIRST POSTOPERATIVE WEEK

Properly performed, the gingivectomy presents no serious postoperative problems. Unfavorable sequelae are the exception rather than the rule; the following may arise in the first postoperative week:

1. PERSISTENT BLEEDING. The pack should be removed, the bleeding points located and the bleeding stopped either with pressure, electrosurgery or electro-

cautery. After the bleeding is stopped the pack is replaced.

2. SENSITIVITY TO PERCUSSION. Sensitivity to percussion may be caused by extension of inflammation into the periodontal ligament. The patient should be questioned regarding the progress of the symptoms. Progressively diminishing severity is a favorable sign. The pack should be removed and the gingiva checked for localized areas of infection or irritation which should be cleaned or incised to provide drainage. Particles of calculus that may have been overlooked should be removed. Relieving the occlusion is usually helpful.

Sensitivity to percussion may also be caused by excess pack which interferes with the occlusion. Removal of the excess usually corrects the condition.

3. SWELLING. Sometimes within the first two postoperative days patients report with a soft painless swelling of the cheek in the area of operation. There may be lymph node enlargement and the temperature may be slightly elevated. The area of operation itself is usually symptom-free. This type of involvement results from a localized inflammatory reaction to the operative procedure. It generally subsides by the fourth postoperative day, without necessitating removal of the pack. Penicillin, 250 mg. every four hours for 48 hours, is helpful as a prophylactic measure following the next operation.

4. FEELING OF WEAKNESS. Occasionally patients report having experienced a "washed-out" weakened feeling for about 24 hours after the operation. This repre-sents a systemic reaction to a transient bacteremia induced by the operative procedure. It is prevented by premedication with penicillin, 250 mg. every three hours, beginning 24 hours before the next operation and for a 24 hour postoperative period. Prophylactic chemotherapy is ordinarily not used except for patients with a history of rheumatic fever, cardiovascular disease, diabetes or prolonged corticosteroid therapy.

Removal of the Periodontal Pack and Return Visit Care

When the patient returns after one week, the pack is taken off by inserting a #19G surgical hoe along the margin and exerting gentle lateral pressure (Fig. 43–28). Pieces of pack retained interproximally and particles which adhere to the tooth surfaces are removed with scalers. Particles may be enmeshed in the cut surface and should be carefully picked off with fine cotton pliers. The entire area is syringed with warm water to remove superficial debris.

What to Look for at the Time of Pack Removal

The following are the usual findings when the pack is removed (Fig. 43–29):

The cut gingival surface is covered with a friable meshwork of new epithelium, which should not be disturbed.

The facial and lingual mucosa may be covered with a gray-yellow or white granu-

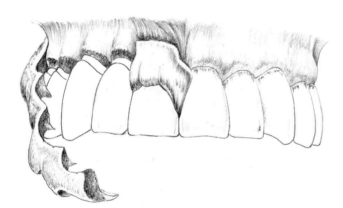

Figure 43–28 Removal of the Periodontal Pack.

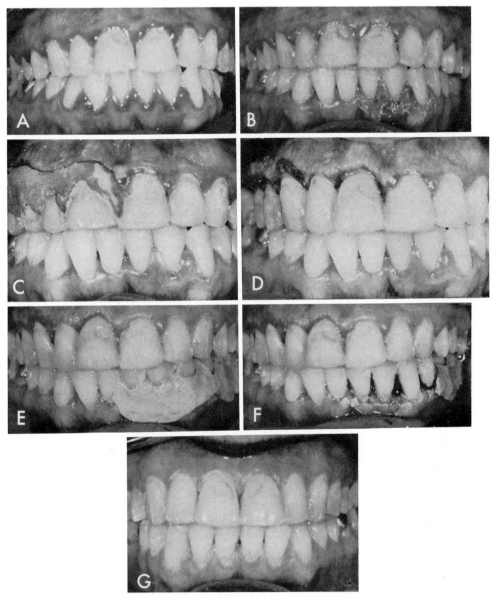

Figure 43–29 Appearance of the Gingiva Before, During and After Treatment by Gingivectomy. *A,* Generalized chronic marginal gingivitis with deep periodontal pockets. *B,* Two weeks after gingivectomy in the mandibular quadrant (*left*). Note excellent gingival contour in relation to the treated central, lateral and canine as compared with the inflammatory bulk of the gingiva in relation to the adjacent untreated anterior teeth. *C,* The patient returns one week after gingivectomy in the maxillary quadrant (*left*). The pack is still in position.

D, Immediately after the pack is removed; note the vascular appearance of the cut surface. *E,* The patient returns one week after gingivectomy in the mandibular quadrant (*right*). The pack is still in position. Note how the appearance of the gingiva in the maxilla (*left*) has changed as compared with the previous week (*D*). *F,* Immediately after the pack is removed from the mandible. The plaque-like material adherent to the gingiva is food debris which had seeped under the pack. *G,* Eighteen months after the generalized gingivectomy, note the excellent contour and position of the gingiva.

lar layer of food debris that has seeped under the pack. It is easily removed with a moist cotton pellet.

The root surfaces may be sensitive to a probe or thermal changes, and the teeth may be stained. There may be prominent bead-like remnants of calculus and granulation tissue.

Persistent granulation tissue

Red, bead-like protuberances of granulation tissue persist where calculus has not been completely removed. The granulation tissue is removed with a curet which exposes the calculus so that it can be removed and the root can be planed. Removal of the granulation tissue without removing the calculus will be followed by recurrence.

Calculus

Fragments of calculus delay healing. Each root surface should be rechecked visually and with a probe to be certain no calculus is present. Sometimes the color of the calculus is similar to that of the root. The grooves on proximal root surfaces and the furcations are areas in which calculus is likely to be overlooked.

After the pack is removed, the next quadrant is treated. It is usually not necessary to replace this pack. However, it is advisable to repack for an additional week for patients with (1) a low pain threshold who are particularly uncomfortable when the pack is removed, (2) unusually extensive periodontal involvement or (3) slow healing. Clinical judgment will help decide whether to repack the area or leave the initial pack on longer than one week.

Tooth mobility

Tooth mobility is increased immediately after gingivectomy,[6] but by the fourth week it diminishes beyond the pretreatment level.[39]

Final check on smoothness of the root surfaces

One week after the pack is removed from the final quadrant, all root surfaces are checked to see that they are smooth and firm. A rubber cup with fine pumice or Improved Zircate, and polishing strips are used for the final smoothing of the root at this time.

CARE OF THE MOUTH WHILE THE GINGIVECTOMY IS IN PROGRESS

Care of the mouth by the patient between the treatment of the first and final quadrants, as well as after the gingivectomy is completed, is extremely important. It begins after the pack is removed from the first quadrant. The patient either has been through a presurgical period of instructed plaque control or should be instructed at this time. (For a step-by-step procedure for plaque control, see Chapter 32.)

Vigorous brushing during the first week after the pack is removed is not feasible. However, the patient is informed that plaque and food accumulation will retard healing and he is advised **to try to keep the area as clean as possible** by the gentle use of interdental cleansers and dental floss and light water irrigation. Brushing is introduced when healing of the tissues permits; vigor of the overall hygiene regimen is increased as healing progresses. Patients should be told that there will most likely be more gingival bleeding than before the operation; that it is perfectly normal and will subside as healing progresses; and that it should not deter them from following their oral hygiene regimen.

Treatment of Sensitive Roots

When the pack is removed, there is a feeling of "emptiness" around the teeth because the patient has become accustomed to the pack. The roots may be sensitive to thermal changes and to touch. It is preferable to allow about two weeks to see if the sensitivity subsides. After this, sensitivity may be relieved by having the patient use the following solution:

Sodium fluoride 2% aqueous solution......8 ozs.
Color and flavor
Directions: Dip the toothbrush in a small amount of solution contained in a glass. Use the solution instead of a dentifrice. DO NOT SWALLOW.

The patient is usually comfortable by the time the solution is completely used. Areas of persistent sensitivity are treated with sodium fluoride paste or another desensitizing agent (Chap. 51). Elimination of sensitivity caused by root caries requires excavation and restoration.

HEALING FOLLOWING GINGIVECTOMY

The initial response after gingivectomy is the formation of a protective surface clot; the underlying tissue becomes acutely inflamed with some necrosis. The clot is replaced by granulation tissue. After 12 to 24 hours, epithelial cells at the margins of the wound show an increase in glycogen[36] and DNA synthesis and migrate over the granulation tissue to separate it from the contaminated surface layer of the clot. Epithelial activity at the margins reaches a peak in 24 to 36 hours,[9] and surface epithelization is generally complete after five to 14 days. During the first four weeks after gingivectomy, keratinization is less complete than prior to surgery; parakeratinization is most commonly seen.

In experimental animals, the surgically removed epithelial attachment is reconstructed on crown and root surfaces within two to three weeks.[17,18,22] Hemidesmosomes and basement lamina may be absent on the connective tissue side of the epithelial attachment. The outer surface of the gingival margin is healed by 14 days, but the epithelium of the gingival sulcus requires three to five weeks to heal.

In the initial 12 hours after gingivectomy, there is a slight reduction in cementoblasts and some loss of continuity of the osteoblastic layer on the outer aspect of the alveolar crest.[9] New bone formation occurs at the alveolar crest as early as the fourth day after gingivectomy,[29] and new cementoid appears at 10 to 15 days.[35]

By 24 hours, there is an increase in new connective tissue cells, mainly angioblasts, just beneath the surface layer of inflammation and necrosis; by the third day, numerous young fibroblasts are located in the area.[30] The highly vascular granulation tissue grows coronally, creating a new free gingival margin and sulcus.[26] Capillaries derived from blood vessels of the periodontal ligament migrate into the granulation tissue, and within two weeks they connect with gingival vessels.[41] Vasodilation and vascularity begin to decrease after the fourth day of healing and appear to be almost normal by the sixteenth day.[24] The connective tissue is still undergoing repair at the twenty-eighth day.

The flow of gingival fluid in humans is initially increased following gingivectomy and diminishes as healing progresses.[3,33] The maximum is reached after one week, coinciding with the time of maximum inflammation.

The tissue changes that occur in postgingivectomy healing are the same in all individuals, but the time required for complete healing varies considerably, depending upon the area of the cut surface and interference from local irritation and infection. Gingival healing is affected by age[19] but not by sex or socio-economic status.[36] In patients with physiologic melanosis, the pigmentation is diminished in the healed gingiva (Fig. 43–30).

Epithelization and re-formation of the epithelial attachment and re-establishment of the gingival and alveolar crest fiber system are slower in chemically created gingival wounds than in those produced by surgery.[38] Thirty-two days has been estimated as the average time required for complete repair of the epithelium following gingivectomy and 49 days for the connective tissue.[37]

The following time sequence for healing following gingivectomy in humans has also been reported:[5]

TWO DAYS. Clot formed. Bone covered by proliferating connective tissue from the sides of the wound. Numerous leukocytes and fibrin shreds present.

FOUR DAYS. A portion of the clot remains adjacent to the tooth surface. Underlying portion of the clot replaced by granulation tissue. Epithelium without rete pegs extends over part of the surface. Dense inflammatory infiltration.

SIX DAYS. Entire wound covered by fairly well differentiated stratified squamous epithelium. There is consolidation of the granulation tissue, some collagen formation. Inflammation present.

SIXTEEN DAYS. Epithelium appears mature with new rete pegs. Connective tissue very collagenous. Slight chronic inflammatory exudate still present.

TWENTY-ONE DAYS. Epithelial rete pegs well developed, some thickening of the stratum corneum, hyperplasia and

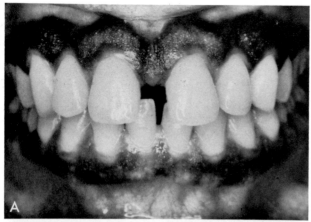

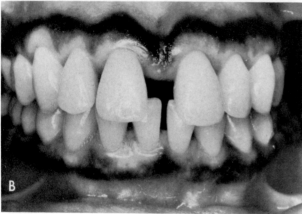

Figure 43–30 Physiologic Melanosis Diminished Following Gingivectomy. *A,* Before treatment—extensive physiologic pigmentation of the gingiva. *B,* One year after gingivectomy. Pigmentation is diminished; periodontal pockets are eliminated and physiologic gingival contour is restored.

spongiosis of the epithelium. Increased collagenization of the connective tissue. Gingiva clinically normal.

THE COMPLETE-MOUTH GINGIVECTOMY

Ordinarily, the gingivectomy is an office procedure performed in quadrants at weekly intervals. Under certain circumstances, however, it is in the best interest of the patient to treat the mouth (Figs. 43–31 and 43–32) in one operation with the patient hospitalized. Periodontal surgical procedures which may be required in addition to the gingivectomy are done at the same time.

Indications

PATIENT PROTECTION. There are patients with systemic conditions that are not severe enough to contraindicate elective surgery but that may require special precautionary measures, best provided in

a hospital. This group includes patients with cardiovascular disease, diabetes, hyperthyroidism, those undergoing prolonged steroid therapy, and those with a history of rheumatic fever or abnormal bleeding tendencies.

The purpose of hospitalization is to protect patients by anticipating their special needs—not to perform periodontal surgery when it is contraindicated by the patients' general condition. There are patients for whom elective surgery is contraindicated regardless of whether it is performed in the dental office or the hospital. When consultation with the patients' physician leads to this decision, palliative periodontal therapy, in the form of scaling and curettage if permissible, is the necessary compromise.

THE APPREHENSIVE PATIENT. Gentleness, understanding and preoperative sedation usually suffice to calm the fears of most patients. For some patients, however, the prospect of a series of surgical procedures is sufficient stress to trigger disturbances

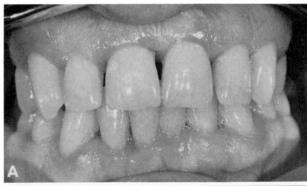

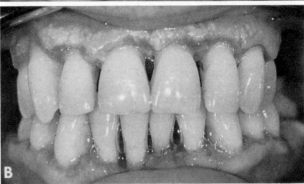

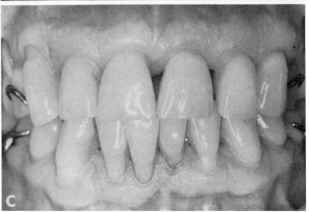

Figure 43–31 Complete-Mouth Gingivectomy. *A,* Generalized periodontal disease with fibrotic periodontal pockets. *B,* One week after operation. Note that the outline of the incision is irregular so as to follow the depth of individual pockets. *C,* after seven months. Physiologic contours restored by gingival healing. Note slight stain and calculus at recall visit.

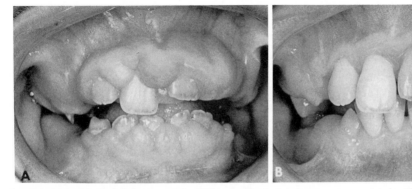

Figure 43–32 Gingival Enlargement in Child. *A,* Gingival enlargement associated with Dilantin therapy treated by complete-mouth gingivectomy. *B,* After healing.

that jeopardize the well-being of the patient and hamper treatment. Explaining that the treatment at the hospital will be performed painlessly, and that it will be preceded by a depth of sedation that is not practical for ambulatory patients visiting a dental office, are important steps toward allaying their fears. The thought of completing the necessary surgical procedures in one session rather than in repeated visits is an added comfort to the patient, because it eliminates the prospect of repeated anxiety in anticipation of each treatment.

With the complete-mouth gingivectomy, there is less stress for the patient. It is performed after a night's rest in the hospital and under ample sedation rather than after coming from the street into the dental office (sometimes after rushing to be on time for the appointment). The patient is returned to his room after the gingivectomy for a check of his physical condition and for a restful postoperative sleep, instead of leaving the dental office and making the trip home.

EXTENSIVE MUCOGINGIVAL SURGERY. For patients who require extensive mucogingival procedures (see Chap. 46), the fact that the operation is performed under the sterile conditions of the operating room reduces the risk of complicating infections and delayed healing.

When extensive adjunctive mucogingival surgery is performed, the immediate postoperative period spent in the hospital is particularly beneficial. Nursing care for administering cold compresses is prescribed for the first four hours, and other assistance is given, so that emergencies such as hemorrhage or shock, although extremely rare, can be dealt with promptly.

PATIENT CONVENIENCE. For patients whose occupation entails considerable contact with the public, the gingivectomy performed in quadrants at weekly intervals sometimes presents a special problem. It means that for a period of a month, some area of the mouth will be covered by the periodontal pack. With the complete-mouth technique, the pack is ordinarily retained for only one week. Patients find this a very acceptable alternative to a month of involvement with the pack. For a variety of other reasons, patients may desire to attend to their surgical needs in one session under optimal conditions.

Hospital admission and pregingivectomy medical examination

If, after consideration of all factors, the complete-mouth gingivectomy is selected as the procedure of choice, a hospital appointment is made. The days immediately preceding and during the menstrual period are avoided because there may be excessive postoperative bleeding at that time.

The length of the hospital stay is 48 hours. The patient enters early in the afternoon preceding the morning of the operation, to allow time for a physical examination, hemogram and other laboratory procedures, and medical consultations.

Preparations are made for special precautionary measures that may be required before, during or after the gingivectomy. For example, diabetics who consider themselves to be "under control" sometimes require a short period of dietary supervision and regulation of insulin before surgery. The medical examination occasionally reveals disease of which the patient is not aware as well as conditions which the patient felt were not relevant to his dental problem and were thus omitted from the case history taken in the dentist's office.

Premedication and anesthesia

PREMEDICATION. Many combinations of drugs may be used for sedation. The following has been found to be effective.

The **night before gingivectomy, before retiring: Seconal 100 mg.; one hour before gingivectomy: Nembutal, intramuscular; one half hour before anesthesia: scopolamine, 0.4 mg., and morphine sulfate, 10 mg.** Patients with a history of rheumatic fever, cardiovascular disease, diabetes or prolonged corticosteroid therapy are premedicated with antibiotics.

ANESTHESIA. Local or general anesthesia may be used. Local anesthesia is our method of choice, except for especially apprehensive patients. It permits unhampered movement of the head which is necessary for optimal visibility and accesibility to the various root surfaces.

The following injections are used for the mandible: bilateral mandibular and long buccal injections; for the maxilla: bilateral anterior palatine nerve injections at the posterior palatine foramen and the nasopalatine nerve injection in the incisive foramen, plus buccal infiltration in the molar, premolar and anterior regions. Injection directly into the interdental papillae is not ordinarily required; it may be used in areas in which sensitivity persists.

The operation

The gingivectomy is performed on the operating table with the patient's back elevated at an angle of approximately 30 degrees and the head at the level of the operator's elbows. The assistant responsible for the aspirator stands on the side of the table opposite the operator.

The mandible is usually treated first. The technique is the same as that employed when the gingivectomy is done in quadrants, along with other necessary periodontal surgery. The periodontal pack is applied after bleeding stops.

Postoperative instructions at the hospital

The patient is returned to his room; the following postoperative instructions are entered in the record:

Cold semi-solid foods only
Demerol, 50 mg. every four hours if necessary
Discharge tomorrow (date) morning
Periodontal pack is to remain in place, to be removed at the doctor's office

If mucogingival surgery was performed:

Cold compresses to the appropriate area, on and off, at 15 minute intervals for four hours.

The patient is discharged from the hospital the morning following the operation, with an appointment for a week later at the dentist's office.

Instructions for the patient following complete-mouth gingivectomy

The patient is given a printed booklet containing the following instructions:

INSTRUCTIONS FOR

Mr. Alan Jones

The operation which has been performed on your gums will help you keep your teeth.

The following information has been prepared to answer questions you may have about how to take care of your mouth. Please read the instructions carefully—our patients have found them very helpful.

We have placed a periodontal pack over your gums to protect them from irritation. The pack prevents pain, aids healing and enables you to carry on most of your usual activities in comfort.

For your benefit the pack should remain in place as long as possible. **Do not remove it.** If particles of the pack chip off during the week, do not be concerned as long as you do not have pain. If a piece of the pack breaks off and you are in pain, or if a rough edge irritates your tongue or cheek, please call the office. The problem can be easily remedied.

Eat anything you can manage without chipping off the pack. Eggs, Jell-O, cereals, soups, milk, fish, and hamburger or any semi-solid or finely minced foods are suggested. **Avoid citrus fruits or fruit juices, highly spiced foods and alcoholic beverages. They will cause pain.** You may supplement your diet with a multivitamin preparation for the next two weeks.

Do not smoke—the heat and smoke will irritate your gums and delay healing. If at all possible, use this opportunity to give up smoking. Smokers have more gum disease than nonsmokers.

Rinsing is not part of the treatment, but it will help make your mouth feel refreshed. At home you may rinse gently as often as you wish with one of the popular mouthwashes. Do not use it in concentrated form; dilute it—$1/3$ mouthwash to $2/3$ warm water.

Cleanse the surface of the pack with a soft tooth brush moistened with water, without a dentifrice. A water irrigation device used at low pressure with room temperature water, is also helpful.

Please remain at home the day you return from the hospital. After this you may follow your regular daily activities, avoiding excessive exertion of any type. Golf, tennis, skiing, bowling, swimming or sunbathing should be postponed for four days after the operation.

For the first two days you will be unaccustomed to having the pack in your mouth and it may be uncomfortable. Should you have pain take two aspirin tablets, 5 grains every three hours. If the pain is not relieved, please call the office.

Swelling is not unusual, particularly in areas which required extensive surgical procedures. The swelling generally subsides in three or four days. If the swelling is painful or appears to become worse, please call the office.

There may be occasional blood stains in the saliva for the first four or five hours after the operation. This is not unusual and will correct itself. If there is considerable bleeding beyond this, take a piece of gauze, form it into the shape of a "**U**," hold it in the thumb and index finger, apply it to both sides of the pack and hold it under pressure for 20 minutes. Do not remove it during this period to examine it. If the bleeding does not stop at the end of 20 minutes, please contact the office. **Do not try to stop the bleeding by rinsing.**

If other problems arise, please call the office.

First postoperative office visit

The patient is seen at the office one week after the operation. The pack is usually removed and the patient is instructed in plaque control. If surgical procedures were performed in addition to the gingivectomy, the area may be repacked or the initial pack may remain for another week.

GINGIVECTOMY BY CHEMOSURGERY (ORBAN)

There is a gingivectomy technique in which the gingiva is removed with chemicals rather than with a knife.[25] It entails the use of a 5 per cent paraformaldehyde (tri-oxymethylene) paste consisting of the following:

The powder:
Zinc oxide............................ 70.0 gm.
Zinc acetate......................... 1.0 gm.
Zinc stearate........................ 1.0 gm.
Rosin................................. 28.0 gm.
Paraformaldehyde................. 5.0 gm.
The liquid:
Eugenol.............................. 85.0 cc.
Cottonseed oil..................... 15.0 cc.

When used properly, the paste is effective. Undesirable side effects are (1) periodontal abscess formation if it is packed so

tightly that it prevents drainage of exudate from the pocket, and (2) tissue necrosis if it is used in deep infrabony pockets. The following is the suggested step-by-step procedure for performing a chemosurgical gingivectomy:

1. Mix the powder and liquid on a waxed paper slab to a creamy consistency and add a few cotton fibers.
2. Place the mixture on the tooth at the gingival margin and carry into the pocket with a thin spatula (a few fibers of dry cotton on the surface of the mix will prevent it from adhering to the spatula).
3. Spatulate the remainder of the mixture on the slab and add to the softer mix which has been placed in the pockets.
4. After the mix hardens, cover with cavity varnish.
5. Remove the mix after two days (no harmful effects result from permitting it to remain longer).
6. Repeat several times, if necessary, until all excess tissues are removed.
7. Cauterize granulating wound surface with silver nitrate (concentrated), 10 per cent zinc chloride, or 20 per cent trichloroacetic acid to prevent excessive granulation.
8. After the necrotic tissue has sloughed off, treat the gingival margin with 30 per cent Superoxol. (Neutralize the acidity of the Superoxol by adding 1 drop of 5 per cent bicarbonate of soda solution to 10 drops or less of Superoxol.)
9. Absorb the Superoxol in cotton fibers and carry to the gingival tissue on a flat instrument. Repeat until the tissue blanches. The whiteness will disappear in 15 to 20 minutes.
10. Repeat the Superoxol twice a week for five weeks.
11. Apply silver nitrate or other agents mentioned above whenever granulation tends to overgrow.
12. Remove all calculus and polish tooth surfaces.
13. Adjust the occlusion, administer systemic therapy where indicated and check the patient every three to six months.

GINGIVOPLASTY

Gingival and periodontal disease often produce deformities in the gingiva which

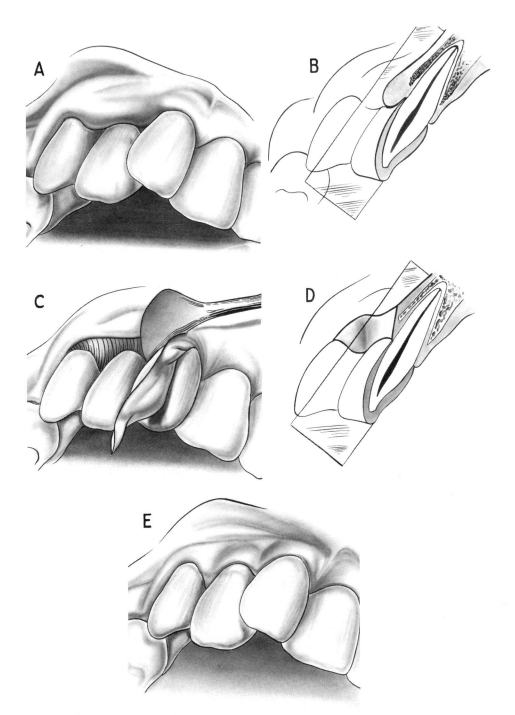

Figure 43–33   Reshaping the Gingiva With Proper Gingivectomy Incision. *A,* Fibrous chronic inflammatory gingival enlargement in relation to malposed anterior teeth. *B,* Diagram showing the relationship of the enlarged gingiva to the tooth. *C,* Removal of the gingiva with a fan-like incision. This resects the gingival margin and tapers the gingiva to desirable contour. The root surfaces are then thoroughly scaled and smoothed and periodontal pack is placed for a period of one week. *D,* Diagram showing the angle at which the gingiva is trimmed. *E,* After healing. The gingival disease is eliminated and physiologic contour is restored.

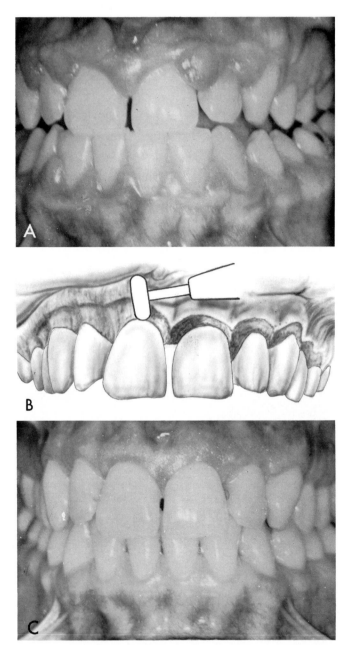

Figure 43–34 Properly Contoured Gingivectomy Incision produces same gingival architecture as improperly contoured gingivectomy incision followed by later gingivoplasty. *A,* Gingival enlargement. *B,* Patient's left side; maxilla and mandible treated by gingivectomy. Right side treated by gingivectomy followed by gingivoplasty with rotary diamond stones. *C,* After two months, the gingival contour is the same on both sides. In the early postoperative period healing was slower in the gingivoplasty quadrants.

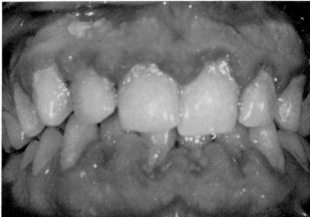

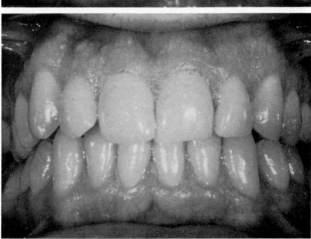

Figure 43–35 Attainment of Desired Gingival Contour by Properly Beveling the Gingivectomy Incision. Before treatment (*above*). Pronounced gingival enlargement consisting of a combination of edematous and fibrous tissue. After treatment (*below*). Gingival contour attained by properly beveling the incision in the regular gingivectomy technique.

interfere with normal food excursion, collect irritating plaque and food debris, and prolong and aggravate the disease process. Gingival clefts and craters, shelf-like interdental papillae caused by acute necrotizing ulcerative gingivitis and gingival enlargement are examples of such deformities. *Artificially reshaping the gingiva to create physiologic gingival contours is termed gingivoplasty.*[14] It is usually performed as a second operation on healed gingiva in which abnormalities persist after previous treatment.

Most deformities of the gingiva can be corrected by the gingivectomy technique described earlier in this chapter without requiring a follow-up gingivoplasty, providing that the gingivectomy is properly performed. This means that the incision must be deep enough to remove extraneous fibrous tissue between the bottom of the pocket and the bone, and the incision must be properly beveled (Fig. 43–33).

Indications

Gingivoplasty is required as an adjunctive procedure when gingival recontouring is not included in the initial treatment or when healing unexpectedly results in gingival abnormalities. Gingivoplasty may be done with a periodontal knife, scalpel, rotary coarse diamond stones[10] (Fig. 43–34) or electrosurgery. It consists of procedures that resemble those performed in festooning artificial dentures—namely, tapering the gingival margin, creating an escalloped marginal outline, thinning the attached gingiva and creating vertical interdental grooves and shaping the interdental papillae to provide sluiceways for the passage of food.

Comment

It is the natural tendency for gingival healing to produce physiologic gingival contours (Fig. 43–35), not gingival abnormalities, providing that local conditions do not interfere with the healing process. This means that, in addition to surgery, irregularly aligned teeth, excessive anterior overbite with impingement upon the maxillary and mandibular gingivae, improperly contoured restorations and areas of food impaction must be corrected. Effective oral hygiene is also essential for the attainment and maintenance of physiologic gingival contours.

REFERENCES

1. Ambrose, J. A., and Detamore, R. J.: Correlation of Histologic and Clinical Findings in Periodontal Treatment. Effect of Scaling on Reduction of Gingival Inflammation Prior to Surgery. J. Periodont., 31:238, 1960.
2. Ariaudo, A. A.: Symposium on the Surgical Approach to the Periodontal Problem. Procedure for Gingivectomy. J. Periodont., 28:62, 1957.
3. Arnold, R., et al.: Alterations in Crevicular Fluid Flow During Healing Following Gingival Surgery. J. Periodont. Res., 1:303, 1966.
4. Benjamin, E. M.: The Quantitative Comparison of Subgingival Curettage and Gingivectomy in the Treatment of Periodontitis Simplex. J. Periodont., 27:144, 1956.
5. Bernier, J., and Kaplan, H.: The Repair of Gingival Tissue After Surgical Intervention. J.A.D.A., 35:697, 1947.
6. Burch, J., et al.: Tooth Mobility Following Gingivectomy. A Study of Gingival Support of the Teeth. Periodontics, 6:90, 1968.
7. Burgett, F. G., et al.: Variation of Pocket Depth and Attachment Level with Periodontal Therapy. I.A.D.R. Abstr., 48th General Meeting, No. 69, 1970.
8. Donnenfeld, O. W., and Glickman, I.: A Biometric Study of the Effects of Gingivectomy. J. Periodont., 37:447, 1966.
9. Engler, W. O., Ramfjord, S., and Hiniker, J. J.: Healing Following Simple Gingivectomy. A Tritiated Thymidine Radioautographic Study. I. Epithelialization. J. Periodont., 37:298, 1966.
10. Fox, L.: Rotating Abrasives in the Management of Periodontal Soft and Hard Tissues. Oral Surg., Oral Med. & Oral Path., 8:1134, 1955.
11. Frisch, J., Levin, M. P., and Bhaskar, S. N.: Calculus Removal: Effectiveness of Scaling. J. S. Calif. D. Assn., 38:36, 1970.
12. Glickman, I.: The Effect of Prescaling Upon Healing Following Periodontal Surgery—A Clinical and Histologic Study. J. D. Med., 16:19, 1961.
13. Glickman, I.: The Results Obtained with the Unembellished Gingivectomy Technic in a Clinical Study in Humans. J. Periodont., 27:247, 1956.
14. Goldman, H. M.: The Development of Physiologic Gingival Contours by Gingivoplasty. Oral Surg., Oral Med. & Oral Path., 3:879, 1950.
15. Gottsegen, R.: Should the Teeth Be Scaled Prior to Surgery? J. Periodont., 32:301, 1961.
16. Gutverg, M., and Haberman, S.: Studies on Bacteremia Following Oral Surgery: Some Prophylactic Approaches to Bacteremia and the Results of Tissue Examination of Excised Gingiva. J. Periodont., 33:105, 1962.
17. Henning, F.: Epithelial Mitotic Activity After Gingivectomy. Relationship to Reattachment. J. Periodont. Res., 4:319, 1969.
18. Henning, F.: Healing of Gingivectomy Wounds in the Rat: Reestablishment of the Epithelial Seal. J. Periodont., 39:265, 1968.
19. Holm-Pedersen, P., and Löe, H.: Wound Healing in the Gingiva of Young and Aged Individuals. J. Periodont. Res., 2:245, 1967.
20. Korn, N. A., and Schaffer, E. M.: A Comparison of the Postoperative Bacteremias Induced Following Different Periodontal Procedures. J. Periodont., 33:226, 1962.
21. Korn, N. A., Schaffer, E. M., and McHugh, R. B.: An Experimental Assessment of Gingivectomy and Soft Tissue Curettage in Dogs. J. Periodont., 36:96, 1965.
22. Listgarten, M. A.: Electron Microscopic Features of the Newly Formed Epithelial Attachment After Gingival Surgery. J. Periodont. Res., 2:46, 1967.
23. Morris, M. L.: Healing of Human Periodontal Tissues Following Surgical Detachment from Vital Teeth: The Position of the Epithelial Attachment. J. Periodont., 32:108, 1961.
24. Novaes, A. B., et al.: Visualization of the Microvascularization of the Healing Periodontal Wound. III. Gingivectomy. J. Periodont. – Periodontics, 40:359, 1969.
25. Orban, B.: New Methods in Periodontal Treatment. Bur, 42:116, 1942.
26. Persson, P. A.: The Healing Process in the Marginal Periodontium after Gingivectomy with Special Regard to the Regeneration of Epithelium (an Experimental Study on Dogs). Odont. T., 67:593, 1959.
27. Prandi, E. C., Blitzer, B., and Carranza, F. A., Jr.: Evaluación Biométrica de la Técinca de Gingivectomia en Humanos. Rev. Assoc. Odont. Argent., 57:84, 1969.
28. Prince, J. P.: Gingival Position and Contour Following Gingivectomy. Paradontologie and Academy Review, 2:153, 1968.
29. Ramfjord, S., and Costich, E. R.: Healing After Simple Gingivectomy. J. Periodont., 34:401, 1963.
30. Ramfjord, S. P., et al.: A Radiographic Study of Healing Following Simple Gingivectomy. II. The Connective Tissue. J. Periodont., 37:179, 1966.
31. Ramfjord, S. P., et al.: Subgingival Curettage versus Surgical Elimination of Periodontal Pockets. J. Periodont., 39:167, 1968.
32. Ritchey, B., and Orban, B.: The Periodontal Pocket. J. Periodont., 23:199, 1952.
33. Sandalli, P., and Wade, A. B.: Alterations in Crevicular Fluid Flow During Healing Following Gingivectomy and Flap Procedures. J. Periodont. Res., 4:314, 1969.
34. Scopp, I. W., and Cantor, M. T.: Hematologic Analysis After Gingivectomy. J.A.D.A., 70:1422, 1965.
35. Stahl, S. S.: Soft Tissue Healing Following

Experimental Gingival Wounding in Female Rats of Various Ages. Periodontics, 1:142, 1963.

36. Stahl, S. S., et al.: Gingival Healing. II. Clinical and Histologic Repair Sequences Following Gingivectomy. J. Periodont., 39:109, 1968.

37. Stanton, G., Levy, M., and Stahl, S. S.: Collagen Restoration in Healing Human Gingiva. J. D. Res., 48:27, 1969.

38. Tonna, E., and Stahl, S.: A Polarized Light Microscopic Study of Rat Periodontal Ligament Following Surgical and Chemical Gingival Trauma. Helv. Odont. Acta, 11:90, 1967.

39. von Majewsky, I., and Sponholz, H.: Ergibnesse nach parodontal therapeutischen Massnahmen unter besonderer Berucksichtigung der Zahnbeweglichkeitssusung mit dem Makroperiodontometer nach Muhlemann. Zahnarztl. Rundschau, 75:57, 1966.

40. Waerhaug, J.: Depth of Incision in Gingivectomy. Oral Surg., Oral Med. & Oral Path., 8:707, 1955.

41. Watanabe, Y., and Suzuki, S.: An Experimental Study in Capillary Vascularization in the Periodontal Tissue Following Gingivectomy or Flap Operation. J. D. Res., 42:758, 1963.

Chapter 44

TREATMENT OF INFRABONY POCKETS

The infrabony pocket differs from the suprabony pocket in that it is situated in an osseous defect with its base apical to the margin of the alveolar bone rather than coronal to it. **The aims of treatment are elimination of the pocket, reattachment of the periodontal ligament to the root surface and filling in of the osseous defect.**

The periodontal pocket and the osseous

defect are interrelated; successful treatment requires that both be eliminated; the persistence of one leads to the recurrence of the other. Treatment consists of (1) the elimination of inflammation and local irritants and conditions which lead to their accumulation; and (2) the correction of factors which share the responsibility with inflammation for the formation of infrabony pockets, namely trauma from occlusion and, in some instances, food impaction.

FOUR CRITICAL AREAS IN THE TREATMENT OF INFRABONY POCKETS

There are four critical areas basic to all techniques for treating infrabony pockets and their associated osseous defects (Fig. 44–1, *A*): (1) the soft tissue pocket wall, (2) the root surface, (3) the periodontal fibers covering the bone surface and (4) the walls of the osseous defect.

1. Management of the soft tissue pocket wall

The soft tissue wall consists of the epithelial lining of the pocket, the epithelial attachment and the adjacent granulation tissue. The epithelial structures must be removed to make it possible for new connective tissue fibers to reattach to the tooth surface (Fig. 44–1, *B*). If the epithelial attachment is permitted to remain, it will be joined by proliferating epithelium from the adjacent gingiva and form an epithelial barrier between the healing connective tissue and the tooth. This will recreate the pocket, obstruct the connective tissue from reaching the root and prevent filling in of the osseous defect (Fig. 44–2).

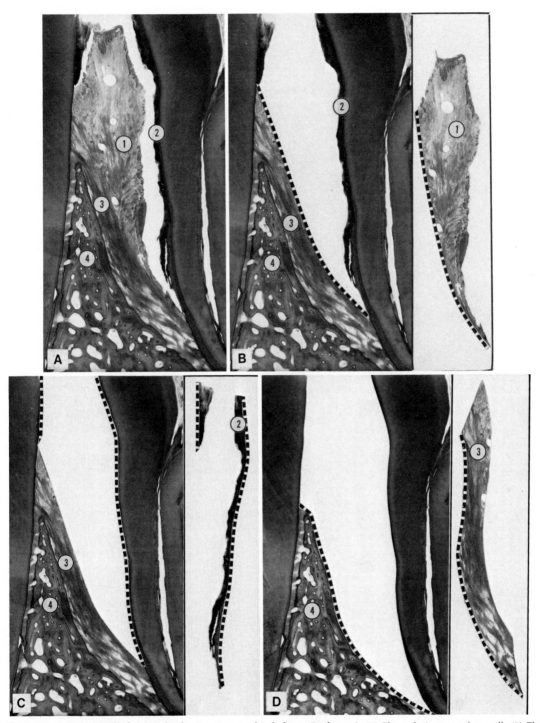

Figure 44–1   Four Critical Areas in the Treatment of Infrabony Pockets. *A,* (1) The soft tissue pocket wall. (2) The root surface. (3) The periodontal fibers which cover the bone surface. (4) The walls of the osseous defect. *B,* The inner lining of the pocket wall (1) is removed. *C,* The calculus (2) is removed and the roots are planed. *D,* The periodontal ligament fibers (3) are removed from the bone, leaving the scarified walls of the osseous defect (4).

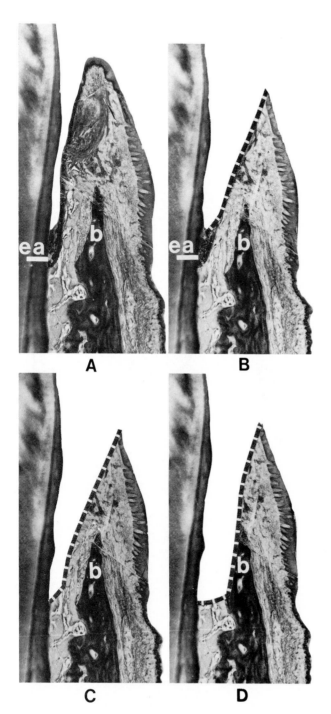

Figure 44–2 Removal of the Epithelial Attachment in the Treatment of Infrabony Pockets (A Composite Illustration). *A,* Infrabony pocket on the facial surface, showing the relationship of the epithelial attachment (ea) at the bottom of the pocket to the bone (b). *B,* Incomplete removal of pocket lining (*dotted line*) leaves the epithelial attachment on the tooth. *C,* Complete removal of the epithelial attachment (*dotted line*) creates the possibility of reattachment of new periodontal ligament fibers. *D,* Removal of periodontal ligament fibers from the bone surface (*dotted line*) facilitates migration of osteogenic cells from the bone into the defect.

2. Management of the root surface

The root surface should be prepared for the deposition of new cementum and the embedding of new periodontal ligament fibers. It must be meticulously scaled and planed to remove all deposits, softened tooth structure and adherent remnants of the epithelial attachment (Fig. 44–1, C).

3. Management of periodontal fibers covering the bone surface

In infrabony pockets, periodontal ligament fibers extend in an angular course over the surfaces of the osseous defects. One of the effects of abnormal occlusal forces upon the periodontium is to alter the alignment of the transseptal fibers (interproximally) and the alveolar crest fibers (facially and lingually). When infrabony pockets are formed, the walls of the angular (vertical) bone defects are covered with these fibers, and both the bone surface and fibers are aligned perpendicular to the direction of the injurious force.

The fibers must be removed to permit the flow of blood and osteogenic cells into the osseous defect (Fig. 44–1, D). Intact fibers must be firmly curetted from the bone surface. When inflamed, the fibers undergo degeneration and are partially or completely replaced by granulation tissue which is more easily removed.

4. Management of the walls of the osseous defect

The walls of the osseous defect should be curetted to form a clean surface with multiple small bleeding points. In some long-standing pockets, condensation of bone has produced a comparatively dense cortical wall. If necessary, perforations may be made in the bone surface with a small round bur[23] to facilitate passage of blood and osteogenic cells from the bone into the osseous defect.

MANAGEMENT OF OSSEOUS DEFECTS

Osseous defects characteristically are associated with infrabony pockets, but they also may occur with suprabony pockets. There are two ways defects may be corrected: (1) by repair of the defect, that is, by filling in with new bone and reattachment of new periodontal fibers to the root, or (2) by remodeling the defect, that is, trimming the walls of the defect to eliminate it, or to make it more amenable to bone repair. The former is the more desirable; it occurs often and in response to different treatment techniques, but not consistently enough to be predictable.[26,38] The healing process fills in the osseous defect and restores smooth physiologic bone contours (Fig. 44–3). Nature reduces sharp bony margins, eliminates abrupt inconsistencies between the bone levels interdentally and on the roots and reduces the facial and lingual walls of interdental craters, along with filling in the depressed craters with new bone. The likelihood of obtaining "bone fill" depends in large measure upon the architecture and the number of bony walls in the defect.[28] Broad, shallow defects are less likely to be filled in with bone than narrow deep ones, except where the space between the tooth and bone is too narrow to permit the necessary instrumentation.

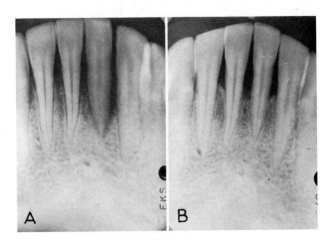

Figure 44–3 Correction of Osseous Defect by Natural Healing Processes. *A,* Before treatment — note angular defect on the distal surface of central incisor. *B,* One year after treatment, showing repair of defect. (Courtesy of Dr. H. Schwartz, Boston.)

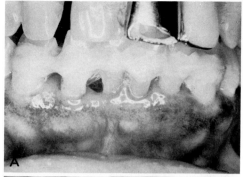

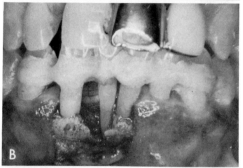

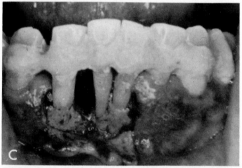

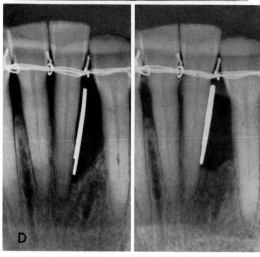

Figure 44–4 Flap Operation Followed by Repair of Two and One-Half Wall Infrabony Defect. (Part of a clinical experiment. Patur and Glickman.[26]) *A,* Mandibular teeth splinted with wire ligature covered with acrylic. *B,* Before treatment, flap reveals two and one-half wall osseous defect. It consists of a lingual wall, proximal wall and one-half wall on the facial surface.

C, Eight and one-half months after treatment without artificially reshaping the bone. Bone defect filled and bone recontoured by the natural healing process. *D, Left,* Before treatment. Bone defect with silver point at base of pocket. *Right,* After eight and one-half months bone defect repaired. Clinical measurements indicate 3.5 mm. increase in bone height and 4.5 mm. soft tissue reattachment.

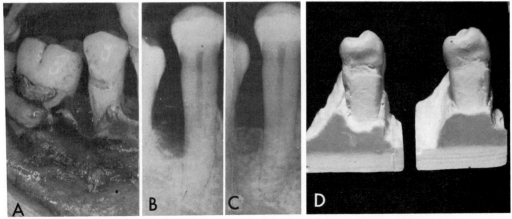

Figure 44–5   Repair of Two-Wall Osseous Infrabony Defect Following Flap Operation. *A,* Flap reveals two-wall defect on distal surface of second premolar. It consists of a lingual wall and a proximal wall. *B,* Before treatment. Radiographs of defect shown in *A. C,* Seven and one-half months after treatment without osseous surgery. The bone is repaired, there is a 4 mm. increase in bone height and 4.5 mm. soft tissue reattachment. (Bone repair occurred despite fact that proximal contact was not restored because of conditions of clinical experiment in which this case was treated.)

D, Models from impressions taken of the bone distal to the premolar before treatment and after seven and one-half months. Note that the crater has been filled in and recontoured by natural healing process.

The prognosis is best in three-wall osseous defects;* two- and two-and-one-half-wall defects also undergo satisfactory repair but less consistently (Figs 44–4 and 44–5). One-wall osseous defects tend to persist after treatment. There may be a slight reduction in the height of the osseous wall and an increased radiopacity of the inner surface, but the pocket generally recurs.

Except in cases of one-wall defects, infrabony pockets are treated with the objective of obtaining optimal repair by natural healing processes. The following techniques are used for this purpose.

TECHNIQUES FOR TREATING INFRABONY POCKETS AND OSSEOUS DEFECTS

Diagnosis

The initial step is an assessment of the depth and course of the pocket, the morphology and dimensions of the osseous defect, and tooth mobility. Each tooth surface is carefully probed to determine the level at which the pocket is attached. The radio-

graph is helpful in estimating the severity of bone destruction but is of limited value in determining the morphology and dimensions of the osseous defect. Piercing the surface of the gingiva with a sharp instrument provides some impressions regarding the contours of the underlying bone but not the definitive information obtainable after surgical exposure.

Diagnosis includes an evaluation of the likely etiologic factors. This should include checking the occlusion, parafunctional occlusal habits, alignment of the teeth, anatomy of the surrounding bone and food impaction areas. The flap operation is the treatment of choice, but the scaling and curettage technique and gingivectomy are also used. Best results are often obtained by a combination of techniques.

The flap operation (See Fig. 44–6, shown on the following page)

ISOLATE THE AREA.   After the area is anesthetized, it is isolated with gauze packs, dried, and painted with antiseptic solution.

PROBE THE COURSE OF THE POCKET AND BONY DEFECT.   The course of the pocket is explored with a pocket probe to determine where to locate the initial incisions. The dimension of the defect can be approximated by passing an instrument through the gingiva to the underlying bone surface.

---

*Sometimes referred to as "intrabony"[29] rather than infrabony to emphasize that the defect is entirely "within bone."

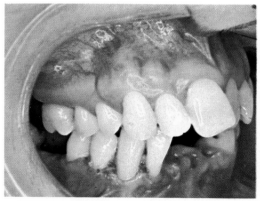

A, Before treatment.

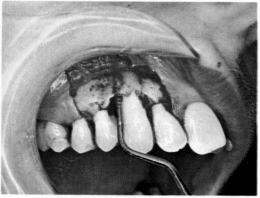

B, Deep three wall infrabony defect with measuring probe inserted.

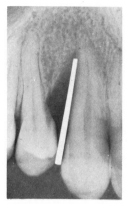

C, Radiograph before treatment indicates angular osseous defect. Gutta percha point extends to base of pocket.

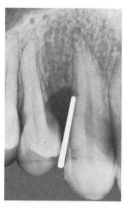

D, Nine months after treatment. Radiograph indicates repair of osseous defect. Gutta percha point shows new level of sulcus.

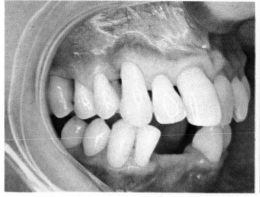

E, Nine months after treatment. Gingiva healed with physiologic contour.

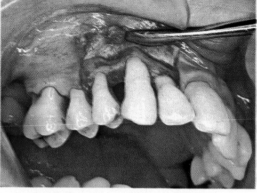

F, Elevation of flap confirms radiographic appearance of repaired bone defect and reattachment of periodontium to tooth.

Figure 44–6 Flap Operation for Infrabony Pocket.

REFLECT A FLAP. Vertical incisions are made on each side of the involved area on the facial or lingual surfaces or both, depending upon the requirement to obtain access. The incisions should extend from the gingival margin into the alveolar mucosa and should be spaced sufficiently apart to expose the entire infrabony defect without stretching the tissues, and deep enough to permit elevation of a muco-periosteal flap (Fig. 44–7, A and B).

REMOVE THE POCKET WALL AND GRAN-ULATION TISSUE. After the vertical in-cisions are made and before the flap is elevated, an internal incision is made along the gingival margin to separate the soft tissue wall of the pocket from the flap. Elevate a mucoperiosteal flap; then curet the adherent pocket wall from the tooth surface. The osseous defect will be partially filled with granulation tissue which is removed with a curet. This will expose the deposits on the root and facilitate thorough exploration of the dimensions and morphol-ogy of the defect (Fig. 44–7, B).

TREAT THE ROOT. Remove all deposits, softened root substance and adherent tabs of tissue, and smooth the root surface. Be sure to reach the root at the base of the defect.

REMOVE FIBERS FROM THE BONE SURFACE. Collagen fibers covering the bone should be curetted away to permit unobstructed bleeding into the defect. If necessary, perforate the bone surface with a small, round bur to facilitate bleeding.

REPLACE THE FLAP. After a clot is formed, replace the flap, suture it firmly over the bone and roots and cover with periodontal pack. Remove the pack and sutures after one week. Repacking is usually not necessary (Fig. 44–7, C).

The gingivectomy

After the area is anesthetized, the course of the pocket is marked and the gingivec-tomy is performed as follows:

FIRST INCISION. With periodontal knives, or the Bard-Parker scalpel, #11 or #12, the pocket wall above the bone is resected and removed, exposing the orifice of the osseous defect (Fig. 44–8, A).

SECOND INCISION. With the interdent periodontal knives #22G and #23G the inner pocket wall is resected from the bone (Fig. 44–8, B).

REMOVE THE GRANULATION TISSUE. Insert a curet along the root surface to the bottom of the pocket, move it laterally to undermine the soft granulation tissue and remove it. This will expose the deposits on the root and provide an opportunity to

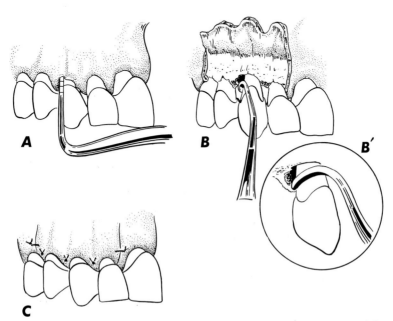

Figure 44–7 Infrabony Pocket Treated by Flap Operation. A, Periodontal probe in deep infrabony pocket on distal surface of the maxillary right canine. B, Area exposed by elevating a simple flap. Root surface scaled and smoothed after granulation tissue is removed. B', Blade of scaler in position on root surface. C, Flap returned and sutured in position.

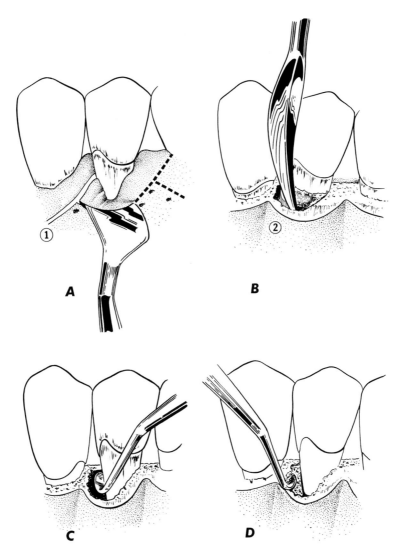

Figure 44–8 Gingivectomy Technique for Eliminating Infrabony Pocket. *A,* First incision (1) resects pocket wall above markings made by pocket marker. *B,* After removal of the pockets, a second incision (2) is made to resect the inner pocket wall. The interdent periodontal knife #22G–23G, shown here, or a #12 Bard-Parker blade is used for the purpose. *C,* After the inner pocket wall is removed, the root surface is scaled and planed. *D,* Granulation tissue and periodontal fibers covering the bone are removed with a curet, exposing the walls of the osseous defect.

evaluate the dimensions and architecture of the bone defect.

SCALE AND PLANE THE ROOT. Scale and plane the root to remove all deposits and necrotic tooth substance and smooth the root (Fig. 44–8, *C*). Pay particular attention to the area at the base of the pocket to assure removal of all soft tissue in the area of the epithelial attachment.

REMOVE THE FIBROUS COVERING OF THE BONE. Intact fibrous tissue is removed from the bone surface with the cutting edge of the curet (Fig. 44–8, *D*). This will expose a bleeding bone surface. If necessary, make several small perfora-

tions in the bone surface with a small round bur to facilitate bleeding into the defect.

PLACE A PERIODONTAL PACK. Cleanse the area with warm water to remove fragments of calculus and soft tissue. After bleeding stops, cover the area with a periodontal pack, without displacing the clot. The pack is removed after one week and the area is cleansed.

The scaling and curettage technique

Scaling and curettage are essential features of all methods for treating infrabony pockets.[37] However, in selected cases it is possible to treat effectively by scaling and curettage alone.

The area is anesthetized, and the pocket is probed and marked on the facial and lingual surfaces. Starting at the base of the defect and moving coronally along the bony wall, the epithelial lining and connective tissue of the pocket are curetted and removed with curets. The root is scaled and smoothed, making a special effort to remove all soft tissue remnants in the area of the epithelial attachment. The bony walls of the defect are curetted to remove fibrous covering in order to facilitate bleeding from the bone into the defect.

CORRECTION OF ASSOCIATED ETIOLOGIC FACTORS

Adjusting the occlusion in the treatment of infrabony pockets

The correction of trauma from occlusion is especially important in the treatment of infrabony pockets. Occlusal forces are important in the etiology of infrabony pockets and also affect the outcome of treatment.[41] Of itself, trauma from occlusion does not cause periodontal pockets. However, when combined with local irritation, trauma from occlusion modifies the supporting periodontal tissues and the pathway of gingival inflammation in such a way as to lead to the formation of infrabony pockets and osseous defects (Chap. 24).

The bony walls and the covering periodontal ligament fibers are often aligned perpendicular to the injurious occlusal forces. The periodontal ligament fibers on the bone surface are removed during treatment. The successful repair of the osseous defect depends upon reattachment of new periodontal ligament fibers formed in the healing process. Since the alignment of the fibers is functionally oriented, the new fibers will be attached at the same angular pattern as the old one, and preclude the repair of the osseous defect, unless the abnormal occlusal forces are corrected.

The occlusion is adjusted at the time the pocket is treated or before. Occlusal correction involves the entire dentition, and not simply the affected area.* Grinding

confined to the involved teeth and their antagonists to "relieve the bite" is inadequate. The involved teeth are often secondarily traumatized because of a shift in the occlusion caused by occlusal prematurities in other areas of the dentition. Orthodontic correction is necessary in the treatment of infrabony pockets around irregularly aligned teeth and teeth which have undergone pathologic migration. This will improve the functional forces upon the periodontium and restore proper proximal contacts.[48]

Repeatedly reducing the occlusal surfaces of the affected teeth to permit accelerated eruption reportedly improves the repair of osseous defects in periodontosis.[11]

Treatment splints

To prevent injury from occlusal forces, mobile teeth should be splinted previous to or at the time of treatment. Mobility deflects occlusal forces away from the vertical axis of the teeth, converting vertical forces into potentially injurious lateral forces which interfere with healing. The occlusion should be adjusted before the splint is applied, and the splint should conform to the corrected occlusion.

Food impaction

Food impaction is often an etiologic and complicating factor, and should be eliminated. Contours and margins of restorations should be checked and all other local irritants and conditions leading to their accumulation should be eliminated.

TRANSPLANTS IN THE TREATMENT OF OSSEOUS DEFECTS*

Background Information

In an effort to induce bone growth and increase the likelihood of obtaining "bone fill" and reattachment, autogenous, homog-

---

*Occlusal adjustment is described in Chapter 53.

*Transplants are tissues taken from one location in the body for grafting to another location of the same or a different individual. Implants are materials from any source which are grafted into the body.

enous and heterogenous (allograft) bone implants, bone derivatives (anorganic bone),[14] osseous coagulum[31] and bone marrow[17, 39, 40, 44] have been used in artificially created[19, 25, 47] and naturally occurring osseous defects.[4,5,9,12,15,20,21,2 3,24,33,43] Cartilage,[38] cementum and dentin particles[36,42] and plaster of Paris[3] have also been used.[1,30] Whole teeth have been implanted in extraction wounds created by extracting teeth with osseous defects.[2]

The most commonly used implant materials are autogenous bone obtained from the patient's jaw and hip bone marrow. The subject of osseous grafts has been reviewed in several articles.[22,27,45] In successful cases, the bone graft serves as a source of osteoblasts and as an inductor upon connective tissue cells to develop into osteoblasts. The bone graft is resorbed and replaced by new bone; cancellous bone resorbs more rapidly than cortical bone and is more likely to provide osteogenic cells.[6,18] The few healing studies that have been reported thus far show that the implant is partially resorbed and remodeled. There is some bone formation around it, and the part that remains is nonvital.[27,34]

Red bone marrow, when transplanted from its original site to the jaws, has the capacity to differentiate into osteoblasts.[10,32,46] Combining it with autogenous bone seems to enhance the osteogenic potential of the marrow implant.[5]

Clinical Procedures

Autogenous bone transplants in the treatment of osseous defects (Nabers and O'Leary)[23]

STEP 1: INITIAL PREPARATION. The area is scaled and curetted, the occlusion is adjusted and the patient is instructed in plaque control.

STEP 2: PREPARATION OF THE IMPLANT SITE. A mucoperiosteal flap is elevated (Fig. 44–9, A); granulation tissue is removed from the defect, and the osseous walls are curetted to remove covering periodontal fibers. If the bony walls are dense, multiple perforations are made with a small round bur to facilitate vascularization of the graft. The root surfaces are thoroughly scaled and planed (Fig. 44–9, B and C).

STEP 3: OBTAINING THE IMPLANT. Cancellous bone from the patient's jaw is used for the implant. Sources of the bone are healing extraction wounds (Fig. 44–9, D), edentulous ridges, bone removed during osteoplasty and ostectomy, bone trephined from within the jaw without damaging the roots (Fig. 44–10) and newly formed bone in wounds specially created for this purpose.[15] The bone may be transferred directly to the defect or placed in a dappen dish with isotonic saline solution.

STEP 4: INSERTING THE BONE. After the defect is cleansed with pellets of cotton, particles of bone are loosely packed into it until the defect is filled to a rounded surface contour (Fig. 44–9, E).

The flaps are replaced and sutured, making sure that the bone is completely covered (Fig. 44–9, F), and that the area is covered with periodontal pack. The sutures and pack are removed after one week, and the area is repacked for two or three additional weekly intervals (Fig. 44–9, G). Antibiotics are prescribed for the evening before surgery and for a 48-hour postoperative period.

Autogenous hip bone marrow transplants in the treatment of osseous defects (Schallhorn, Hiatt and Boyce)[40]

Bone repair of one-, two- and three-wall infrabony defects and furcations, and increase in the height of crestal bone, have been reported following the implantation of autogenous marrow and cancellous bone obtained from the iliac crest. Root resorption is an infrequent but not serious complication (two in a series of 182 areas). The following is the implantation procedure:

STEP 1: INITIAL PREPARATION. The area is scaled and curetted, gross occlusal abnormalities are corrected and the patient is instructed in plaque control (Fig. 44–11, A and B).

STEP 2: PREPARATION OF THE IMPLANT SITE. To preserve as much tissue as possible to cover the implant, a full or partial thickness flap is reflected without an internal bevel incision at the margin. Soft tissue curettage is performed before the flap is elevated.

After the area is exposed, granulation tissue is removed and the roots are scaled

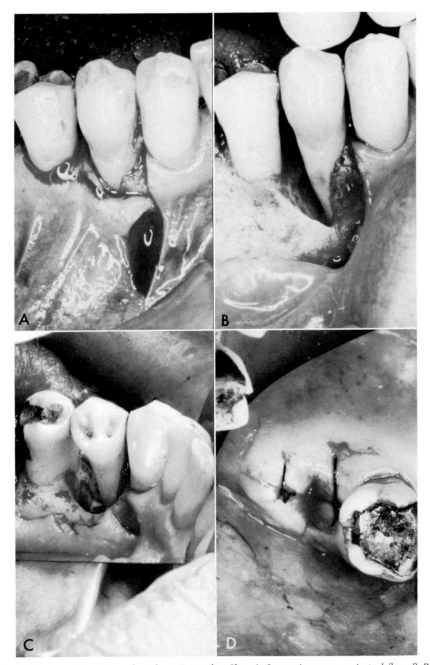

Figure 44–9 Autogenous Bone Transplant from Extraction Site. *A,* Separating mucoperiosteal flap. *B,* Buccal view of angular defect on the distal surface of the first premolar. *C,* Elevating lingual mucoperiosteal flap and view of angular defect. *D,* Bone obtained from six week old extraction site.

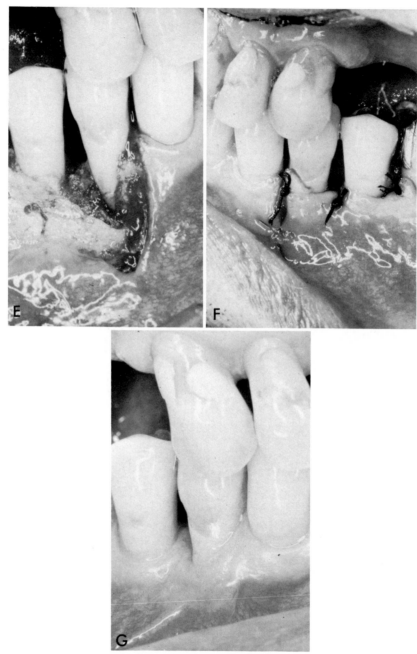

Figure 44–9 *Continued*   *E,* Defect filled with bone implant. *F,* Flap replaced and sutured. *G,* Two and one-half months after treatment. Note excellent gingival contour. (Courtesy of Edward S. Cohen, D.M.D.)

and planed (Fig. 44–11, C and D). The cortical bone in the walls of the osseous defect is perforated with a small round bur in several areas, to permit vascularization of the implant.

STEP 3: OBTAINING THE IMPLANT. Cores of marrow and cancellous bone (an outpatient procedure) are removed from the posterior iliac crest and spine and placed in one of several solutions, depending on the mode of storage. The biopsy site is covered with a bandage.

If the biopsy is to be used immediately, it is carried to the dental office in a nutrient media (minimum essential media) where it can remain for up to three hours. Implants to be used for from three hours to one week after removal are stored in vials containing 5 to 15 per cent glycerol in a refrigerator at 4° C. The vials are removed at 37° C. before the implant is used. For longer periods (months) the biopsies are stored in 25 per cent glycerol in a minimum essential medium stored in a low temperature freezer (−79° C.).[40]

STEP 4: PLACING OF THE IMPLANT. The cores of marrow and cancellous bone are placed snugly into the defect, which is overfilled if possible (Fig. 44–11, E). The flaps are returned over the area and sutured, covered with dry foil and periodontal pack. The pack is changed weekly for two to five weeks. Antibiotics are used prophylactically, beginning the evening before surgery and for a 48-hour postoperative period. Healing is usually uneventful, with normal gingival contours restored within two months (Fig. 44–11, F).

Bone swaging in the treatment of osseous defects (Ewen)[12]

Swaging adjacent bone is another approach to obtaining repair of osseous defects. The technique varies with the location of the defect.[35] In essence it consists of separating a section of bone and forcefully pushing it to fill the space in the defect.

For defects adjacent to edentulous space, the following procedure is used:

STEP 1: PREPARE THE RECIPIENT SITE. Mucoperiosteal flaps are elevated, granulation tissue is removed from the defect and the roots are scaled and smoothed.

STEP 2: TRANSFERRING THE BONE. The dimension of the required bone transfer is determined, and it is separated from the bone bordering the defect with a thin linear bur cut (Fig. 44–12). A thin, blunted surgical chisel is inserted into the cut, and with a mallet the bone is pushed into the defect (Fig. 44–12).

The flaps are returned over the area, sutured and covered with periodontal pack. Sutures and pack are removed in a week, and the pack is replaced for another week if necessary.

Interdental craters are filled by forcefully collapsing the facial and lingual walls inward.

Osseous coagulum transplants in the treatment of osseous defects (Robinson)[31]

Though not on an entirely predictable basis, repair of osseous defects and early furcation involvement has been obtained with implants of an osseous coagulum of bone dust and blood,[31] using the following technique:

STEP 1: PREPARING THE RECIPIENT SITE. After presurgical scaling and some occlusal adjustment, the defect is exposed by elevating a mucoperiosteal flap with an internal bevel. Root deposits and granulation tissue are removed, the root is planed and the bony wall of the defect is perforated with a small round bur or stainless steel cowhorn explorer.

STEP 2: OBTAINING THE IMPLANT. Sources of the implant material include the lingual ridge on the mandible, exostoses, edentulous ridges, the bone distal to a terminal tooth, bone removed by osteoplasty or ostectomy and the lingual surface of the mandible or maxilla at least 5 mm. from the roots. Bone is removed with a carbide bur, #6 or #8, at speeds between 5000 and 30,000 r.p.m. The coagulum formed by mixture of the bone particles and blood is placed in an autoclaved dappen dish.

STEP 3: PLACING THE IMPLANT. The coagulum is placed in the defect a little at a time, starting at the bottom and packing and drying with gauze until there is a considerable excess. The flap is replaced over the coagulum, sutured, compressed with wet gauze for three minutes and covered with dry tin foil adapted to the teeth, followed by a periodontal pack, and covered again with foil. Erythromycin, 250 mg. four times

(Text continued on page 690)

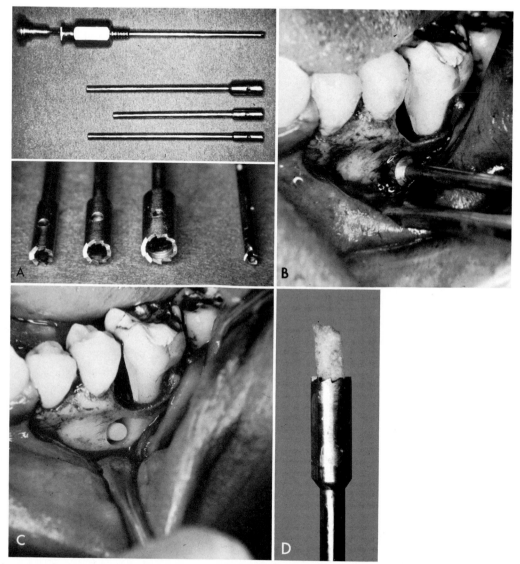

Figure 44–10 Autogenous Bone Transplant Obtained With Trephine. *A,* Trephines. *Top,* Manual trephine. *Center,* Different-sized power trephines #2, #4 and #6. *Bottom,* Orifices of trephines. *B,* Mucoperiosteal flap elevated, showing osseous defect on the mesial surface of the first molar. Trephine inserted into bone distal to the second molar. *C,* Bone separated by trephine. *D,* Bone transplant; the cancellous portion is used, the cortical layer is removed.

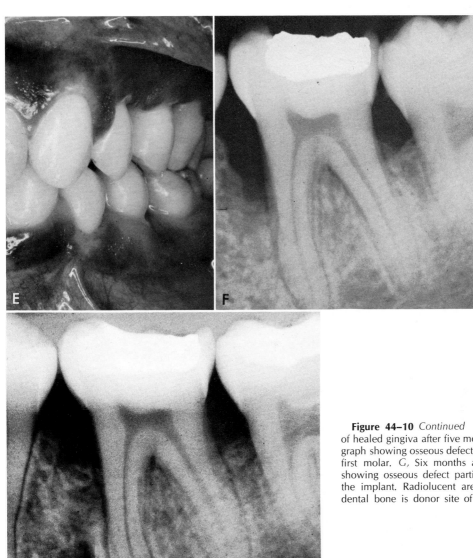

Figure 44–10 *Continued   E,* Appearance of healed gingiva after five months. *F,* Radiograph showing osseous defect on mandibular first molar. *G,* Six months after treatment, showing osseous defect partially filled with the implant. Radiolucent area in the interdental bone is donor site of the transplant.

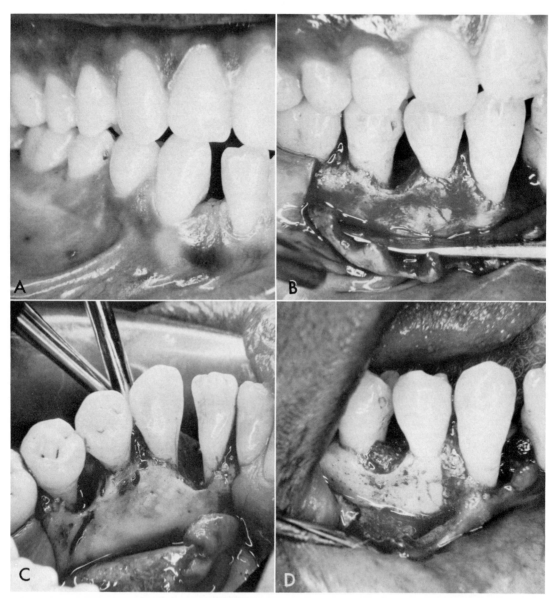

Figure 44–11 Autogenous Hip Marrow Implant. *A,* Before treatment. *B,* Mucoperiosteal flap reveals osseous defect on the second premolar. *C,* Lingual view of infrabony defect revealed by periosteal flap. (Note the defect between the canine and lateral.) *D,* Hip marrow implant in premolar osseous defect.

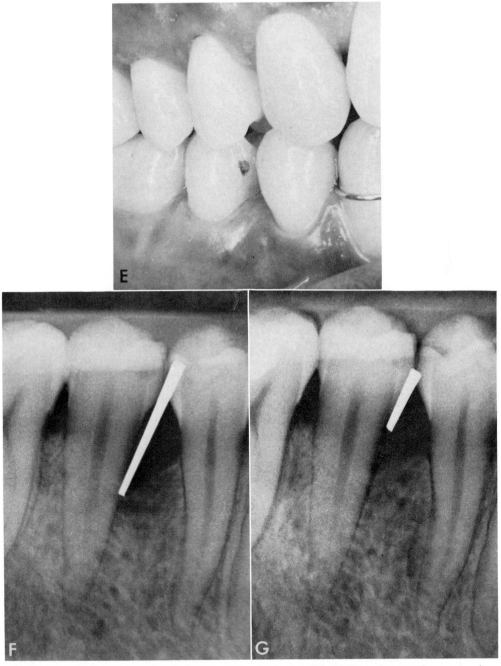

Figure 44–11 *Continued* E, Seven months after treatment. F, Osseous defect before treatment. The gutta percha point is at the base of the pocket. G, Seven months after treatment. The bone is repaired. The gutta percha point is at the base of the healed sulcus which is now attached higher on the root. (Courtesy of Edward S. Cohen, D.M.D.)

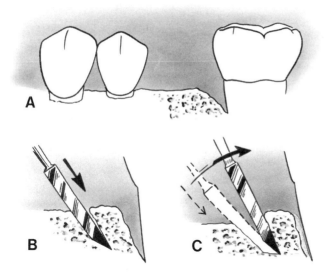

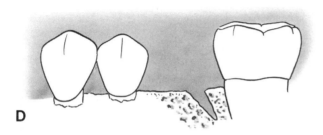

Figure 44–12 **Bone Swaging to Fill Infra-bony Defect.** *A,* Infrabony defect of the mesial of the mandibular molar. *B,* Chisel separate section *(arrow).* *C,* Bone swaged into infrabony defect *(arrow).* *D,* Infrabony defect filled with bone.

daily, is prescribed for three days beginning the evening before surgery, and the sutures and pack are removed after a week, followed by plaque control (Fig. 44–13).

Corrective remodeling of osseous defects

If, at approximately nine months after treatment, bone defects are not sufficiently repaired so that periodontal health can be maintained by vigorous plaque control and periodic maintenance scaling, they can be eliminated by removing the osseous walls and recontouring. This is done by re-entering the area and using rotary diamond stones, chisels or rongeurs. (See the section on Osseous Surgery in Chapter 46.)

Experienced clinicians sometimes anticipate the results and include bone remodeling as part of the initial treatment to avoid subjecting the patient to a second corrective operation. This is often the procedure in the combined type of defect with three

walls in the apical portion, and one, two or two and one-half walls coronally (Fig. 44–14). The coronal portion of the walls is reduced until only a three-wall defect, with the best prognosis for post-treatment "bone fill," remains.

One-wall infrabony defects

To eliminate one-wall infrabony defects on the facial or lingual surface, the margin of the bone is reduced to the level of the base of the defect and then rounded[7, 8, 13] (Fig. 44–15). Interproximally, one-wall defects often produce a hemiseptum formed by the remnant of the interdental bone. In the treatment of this condition, the bone is reduced to the level of the defect, and facial and lingual surfaces are thinned and tapered toward the crown. In one-wall defects adjacent to edentulous spaces, the edentulous ridge is reduced to the level of the osseous defect (Fig. 44–16).

Artificial remodeling of bone is not re-

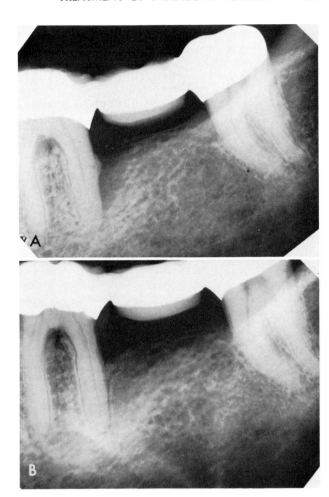

Figure 44–13 Bony Defect on Distal Root of First Molar Treated With Osseous Coagulum Transplant. *A,* Before treatment. *B,* One year after treatment. (Courtesy of Dr. R. Earl Robinson, San Mateo, California.)

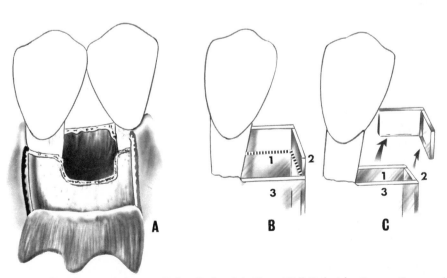

Figure 44–14 Combined Type of Osseous Defect Reduced to Three-Wall Defect by Osseous Surgery. *A,* Reflected flap reveals infrabony osseous defect. *B,* There are three osseous walls in the apical half of the defect (1, lingual; 2, distal; 3, facial) and only two walls in the coronal half (1, lingual; 2, distal). *C,* The two walls in the coronal half are removed, leaving the three-wall defect in the apical half.

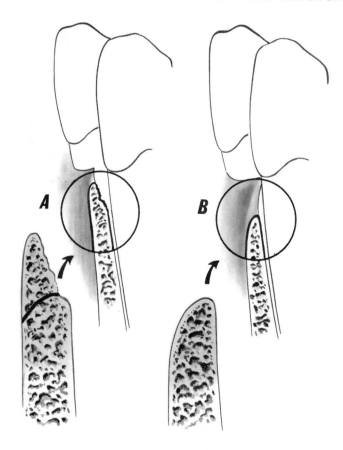

Figure 44–15 Bone Recontoured to Correct One Wall Infrabony Defect. *A,* Angular defect in the facial bone on a premolar is shown in the circle and in enlarged view. The dark line shows the level to which the bone is reduced to correct the defect. *B,* Recontoured bone shown in the circle and in enlarged view.

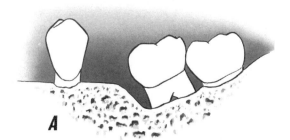

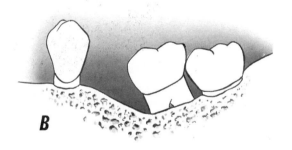

Figure 44–16 Reduction of One Wall Infrabony Angular Defect. *A,* Angular bone defect mesial to tilted molar. *B,* Defect reduced by "ramping" angular bone.

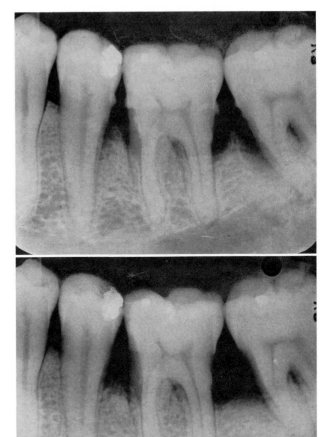

Figure 44–17 Infrabony Pockets on Mesial and Distal Surfaces of Same Interdental Septum. *Above,* Before treatment. One wall osseous defects on proximal surfaces of molars and premolar. *Below,* Seven months after treatment of infrabony pockets without artificially remodelling the osseous defects are corrected by natural healing.

quired when one-wall infrabony defects are "back to back" on the same interdental septum. Treatment of the pockets without altering the bone is generally followed by resorption of the intervening bony septum which also eliminates the one-wall defects on both sides of it (Fig. 44–17).

REFERENCES

1. Alderman, N. E.: Sterile Plaster of Paris as an Implant in the Infrabony Environment: A Preliminary Study. J. Periodont.–Periodontics, *40*:11, 1969.
2. Baer, P., and Gamble, J.: Autogenous Dental Transplants as a Method of Treating the Osseous Defect in Periodontosis. An in-Progress Report of Four Cases. Oral Surg., *22*:405, 1966.
3. Bahn, S. L.: Plaster: A Bone Substitute. Oral Surg., *21*:672, 1966.
4. Beube, F. E.: A Study on Reattachment of the Supporting Structures of the Teeth. J. Periodont., *18*:55, 1947.
5. Beube, F. E., and Silvers, H. F.: Influences of Devitalized Heterogenous Bone Powder on Regeneration of Alveolar and Maxillary Bone of Dogs. J. D. Res., *14*:15, 1934.
6. Burwell, R. G.: Studies in the Transplantation of Bone. VII. The Fresh Composite Homograft–Autograft of Cancellous Bone. J. Bone & Joint Surg., *46-B*:110, 1964.
7. Carranza, F. A.: When and Why the Elimination of Bone Is Necessary in the Treatment of Periodontal Disease. Anales del Ateneo del Instituto Municipal de Odontologia (Buenos Aires), *3*:311, 1941.
8. Carranza, F. A., and Carranza, F. A., Jr.: The Management of the Alveolar Bone in the Treatment of the Periodontal Pocket. J. Periodont., *27*:29, 1956.
9. Cross, W. G.: The Use of Bone Implants in the Treatment of Periodontal Pockets. Dent. Clin. North America, March, 1960, p. 107.
10. Cushing, M.: Autogenous Red Marrow Grafts: Their Potential for Induction of Osteogenesis. J. Periodont.–Periodontics, *40*:492, 1969.
11. Everett, F., and Baer, P.: A Preliminary Report on the Treatment of the Osseous Defect in Periodontosis. J. Periodont., *35*:63, 1964.
12. Ewen, S. J.: Bone Swaging. J. Periodont., *36*:57, 1965.

13. Fröhlich, von E.: Grundsätzliche Fragen der chirurgische Behandlung der marginalen Parodontitis. Deutsche Zahnartzl. Zschr., 8:523, 1953.

14. Gurkan, S., and Melek, S.: Anorganic Bone Implantation in Infrabony Periodontal Pockets. Internat. D. J., 13:703, 1963.

15. Halliday, D. G.: The Grafting of Newly Formed Autogenous Bone in the Treatment of Osseous Defects. J. Periodont.–Periodontics, 40:511, 1969.

16. Hegedüs, Z.: The Rebuilding of the Alveolar Process by Bone Transplantation. D. Cosmos, 65:736, 1923.

17. Hiatt, W. H.: The Induction of New Bone and Cementum Formation. III. Utilizing Bone and Marrow Allografts in Dogs. J. Periodont., 41:596, 1970.

18. Holmstrand, K.: Biophysical Investigations of Bone Transplants and Bone Implants. Acta Orth. Scandinav., Suppl. No. 26, 1957.

19. Hurt, W. C.: Freeze-Dried Bone Homografts in Periodontal Lesions in Dogs. J. Periodont., 39:89, 1968.

20. Kromer, H.: Implantation of Bone Homografts in Periodontal Pockets. Dent. Clin. North America, July, 1962, p. 471.

21. Melcher, A. H.: The Use of Heterogenous Anorganic Bone in Periodontal Bone Grafting: A Preliminary Report. J. D. Assn. S. Afr., 13:80, 1958.

22. Nabers, C. L.: What Is The Place of Bone Grafts in Periodontal Therapy? J. Western Soc. Periodont., 15:149, 1967.

23. Nabers, C. L., and O'Leary, T. J.: Autogenous Bone Transplants in the Treatment of Osseous Defects. J. Periodont., 36:5, 1965.

24. Older, L. B.: The Use of Heterogenous Bovine Bone Implants in the Treatment of Periodontal Pockets. J. Periodont., 38:539, 1967.

25. Patterson, R., Collings, K., and Zimmermann, E.: Autogenous Implants in the Alveolar Process of the Dog with Induced Periodontitis. Periodontics, 5:19, 1967.

26. Patur, B., and Glickman, I.: Clinical and Roentgenographic Evaluation of the Post-Treatment Healing of Infrabony Pockets. J. Periodont., 33:164, 1962.

27. Pfeifer, J. S.: The Present Status of Bone Grafts in Periodontal Therapy. Dent. Clin. North America, 13:193, 1969.

28. Prichard, J.: A Technique for Treating Infrabony Pockets Based on Alveolar Process Morphology. Dent. Clin. North America, March 1960, p. 85.

29. Prichard, J. F.: The Etiology, Diagnosis and Treatment of the Infrabony Defect. J. Periodont., 38:455, 1967.

30. Ray, R., and Sabet, T.: Bone Grafts: Cellular Survival Versus Induction. J. Bone & Joint Surg., 45A:377, 1963.

31. Robinson, R. E.: Osseous Coagulum for Bone Induction. J. Periodont.–Periodontics, 40:503, 1969.

32. Rosenbaum, J. H., and McFall, W. T., Jr.: A Histological Evaluation of Autogenous Marrow Transplants in Rat Maxilla. I.A.D.R. Abst., 1970, p. 103, No. 220.

33. Rosenberg, M. M.: Reentry of an Osseous Defect Treated by a Bone Implant After a Long Duration. J. Periodont., 42:360, 1971.

34. Ross, S. E., and Cohen, D. W.: The Fate of a Free Osseous Tissue Autograft: A Clinical and Histologic Case Report. Periodontics, 6:145, 1968.

35. Ross, S. E., Malamed, E. H., and Amsterdam, M.: The Contiguous Autogenous Transplant—Its Rationale, Indications and Technique. Periodontics, 4:246, 1966.

36. Schaffer, E. M.: Cementum and Dentine Implants in a Dog and a Rhesus Monkey. J. Periodont., 28:125, 1957.

37. Schaffer, E. M.: Subgingival Curettage. J. Periodont., 28:60, 1957.

38. Schaffer, E. M., and Packer, M. W.: Bone Regeneration: Cartilage and Tooth Grafts in Periodontal Pockets. Dent. Clin. North America, July, 1962, p. 459.

39. Schallhorn, R. G.: Eradication of Bifurcation Defects Utilizing Frozen Autogenous Hip Marrow Implants. Periodont. Abstr., 15:101, 1967.

40. Schallhorn, R. G., Hiatt, W. H., and Boyce, W.: Iliac Transplants in Periodontal Therapy. J. Periodont., 41:566, 1970.

41. Schärer, P., Butler, J. H., and Zander, H. A.: Healing of Bony Pockets in Connection with Occlusal Dysfunctioning. Schweiz. Mschr. Zahnheilk., 79:244, 1969.

42. Scopp, I. W., Kassouny, D. Y., and Register, A. A.: Human Bone Induction by Allogenic Dentin Matrix. I.A.D.R. Abst., 1970, p. 100, No. 205.

43. Scopp, I. W., Morgan, F. H., Dooner, J. J., Fredrics, H. J., and Heyman, R. A.: Bovine Bone (Boplant) Implants for Infrabony Oral Lesions. Periodontics, 4:169, 1966.

44. Seibert, J. S.: Reconstructive Periodontal Surgery: Case Report. J. Periodont., 41:113, 1970.

45. Shellow, R. A., and Ratcliff, P. A.: The Problems of Attaining New Alveolar Bone After Periodontal Surgery. J. Western Soc. Periodont., 15:154, 1967.

46. Sullivan, H. C., Vito, A. A., Meltzei, A. M., and Rabinowitz, J. L.: Evaluation of the Use of Hemopoietic Marrow in Intrabony Periodontal Defects., I.A.D.R. Abst., 1971, p. 171, No. 474.

47. Yuktanandana, I.: Bone Graft in the Treatment of Infrabony Periodontal Pocket in Dogs. A Histological Investigation. J. Periodont., 30:17, 1959.

48. Zamet, J.: Combined Periodontal Surgery and Orthodontic Movement in the Treatment of an Isolated Palatal Infrabony Pocket. D. Pract. (Bristol), 17:314, 1967.

Chapter 45

TREATMENT OF FURCATION INVOLVEMENT; AND COMBINED PERIODONTAL-ENDODONTIC THERAPY

The prognosis of teeth with furcation involvement is governed by the same factors that determine the prognosis of single-rooted teeth with comparable periodontal destruction, **but multirooted teeth have the advantage of added stability provided by the extra root anchorage.** The principles governing the treatment of furcations are the same as those applicable to periodontal disease in general, with certain special procedural considerations which are presented here.

CLASSIFICATION OF FURCATION INVOLVEMENT

The following classification of furcation involvement, based upon severity of destruction, provides one of the criteria for treatment in individual cases; the types of pockets and the presence or absence of osseous defects are additional important diagnostic considerations.

Grade I involvement (incipient)

Involvement of the periodontal ligament in the furcation without gross or radiographic evidence of bone loss (Fig. 45–1).

695

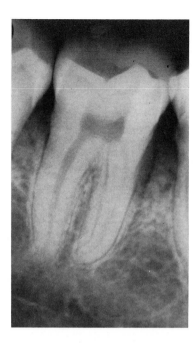

Figure 45–1   Grade I Bifurcation Involvement (Incipient). No marked radiographic change in the bifurcation area.

Grade II involvement

In these cases (Fig. 45–2), bone is destroyed on one or more aspects of the furcation, **but a portion of the alveolar bone and periodontal ligament remains intact.** The intact periodontal structures permit only partial penetration of the furcation with a blunt probe.

Grade III involvement

In these cases (Fig. 45–2), the furcation may be occluded by gingiva, but the bone has been destroyed to such a degree as to permit the complete passage of a probe faciolingually or mesiodistally.

Grade IV involvement

The periodontium has been destroyed to such a degree that the furcation is open and exposed and permits unobstructed passage of a probe (Fig. 45–2).

TREATMENT OF FURCATION INVOLVEMENT

Furcations are treated by scaling and curettage, gingivectomy or the simple flap operation, depending upon the severity of involvement and the architecture of the destructive process. Suprabony pockets without osseous deformities are treated by scaling and curettage or gingivectomy; furcations with infrabony pockets and osseous defects are treated with the flap operation. Furcation involvement may be confined to a single tooth, but very often several teeth are affected. The furcations are treated as they are encountered in the systematic care of the mouth.

Treatment of grade I involvement (with suprabony pockets)

Early furcation involvement usually presents suprabony pockets which are treated by scaling and curettage or gingivectomy, depending upon pocket depth and fibrosity of the pocket walls. Since the destructive process is in its incipient stages, it is not necessary to enter the furcation in the treatment process. Elimination of the pocket is followed by resolution of inflammation and repair of the periodontal ligament and adjacent bone margin.

Treatment of grade II involvement (with suprabony pockets)

Under local anesthesia, each tooth surface is probed down to the bone to deter-

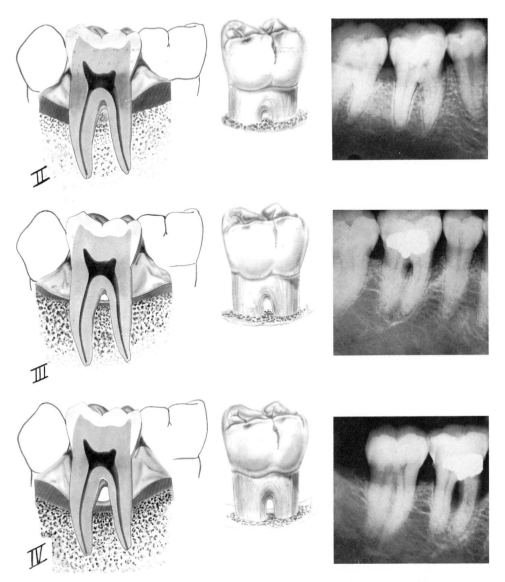

Figure 45–2 *II,* **Grade II Bifurcation Involvement.** Radiograph reveals a small area of radiolucence. A remnant of bony wall is still present in the bifurcation area. *III,* **Grade III Bifurcation Involvement.** Radiograph reveals distinct triangular area of radiolucence. A probe can be passed buccolingually through the bifurcation. *IV,* **Grade IV Bifurcation Involvement.** Radiograph reveals pronounced bone loss. There is obvious clinical exposure of the bifurcation area.

mine the pattern of periodontal destruction. One aspect of the furcation is intact in grade II involvement; treatment is from the most extensively involved side and is usually gingivectomy. Pinpoint markings are made on the gingiva at the base of the pockets on all surfaces (Fig. 45–3).

A gingivectomy incision is made through the pinpoint markings, conforming to the outline of the underlying bone margin (Fig. 45–3, *A*). The incision is made with periodontal knives or a Bard-Parker scalpel

#12 and is beveled at approximately a 45 degree angle to the tooth (Fig. 45–3, *B*). The resected gingiva is detached, exposing underlying bead-like granulation tissue which is removed with curets. The root is scaled and planed.

The area is cleaned with warm water, and strips of periodontal pack are placed on the facial and lingual surfaces and pressed together so that they join interproximally for retention (Fig. 45–3, *D*). The pack is removed after one week.

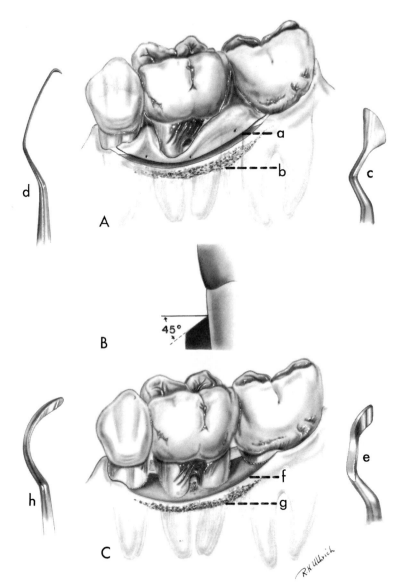

Figure 45–3 Gingivectomy Technique for the Treatment of Bifurcation Involvement. *A,* (a) Line of incision for removing the gingiva. (b) The level of the underlying bone. *B,* The gingiva is cut at a 45° angle to the tooth. *C,* Appearance of the area after the diseased gingiva is removed. (f) The cut surface. (g) The level of the underlying bone.

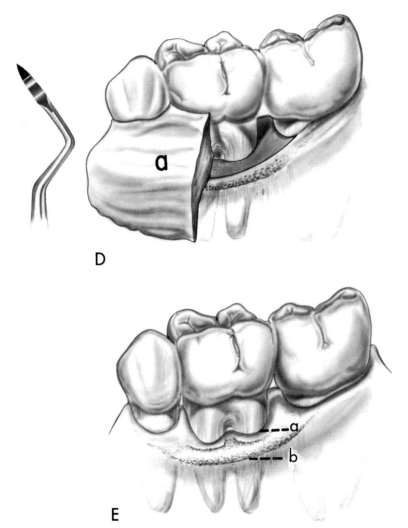

D

E

Figure 45–3 *Continued   D,* The pack (a) in position. Part of the field is uncovered to show the relationship of the pack to the furcation. This part is also covered with pack. *E,* The healed lesion showing the contour of the gingiva (a) and the level of the bone (b). **Compare with Treated Cases shown in Figure 45–4.**

When the pack is removed, the area is cleaned and the roots checked for small particles of calculus and smoothness. The patient is instructed in plaque control (if this has not been done earlier in the course of treatment), with particular emphasis upon cleansing the furcation. Interdental cleansers such as rubbertips, Stimudents and Perio-aids should be applied to the tooth at an acute angle (see Chap. 32) to avoid the crater-like gingival conformation which results when they are inserted perpendicular to the tooth.

Treatment of grade III and grade IV involvement (with suprabony pockets)

In these conditions, interradicular tissue destruction permits a probe to pass freely through the furcation. The gingiva is resected just coronal to the bone to provide visibility and access from all directions so that the involved root surfaces may be throughly planed and smoothed without disturbing the bone. The periodontal pack is placed for one week except when patient comfort requires repacking for an additional week.

POST-TREATMENT GINGIVAL CONTOUR

Removal of all root deposits, planing of all exposed root surfaces and fastidious patient care are essential for obtaining optimal post-treatment gingival contour in the furcation areas (Fig. 45–4). Bulging of the gingival margin and recurrence of pockets invariably can be traced to calculus or roughness of the root or inadequate plaque control. In the treatment of early bifurcation involvement, the buccal groove is sometimes eliminated by reshaping the tooth (**odontoplasty**) to reduce post-treatment accumulation of irritating plaque and debris.[4]

TREATMENT OF FURCATION INVOLVEMENT COMPLICATED BY PERIODONTAL ABSCESS

When furcation involvement is complicated by periodontal abscess formation, the abscess is eradicated as part of the treatment of the furcation (Fig. 45–5).

TREATMENT OF FURCATION INVOLVEMENT COMBINED WITH INFRABONY POCKETS AND OSSEOUS DEFECTS

When infrabony pockets and osseous defects are part of the clinical picture of furcation involvement, the treatment of choice is the simple flap operation and adjunctive procedures usually used for these conditions as described in Chapter 44.

To preserve as much bony support as possible in the furcation area, these lesions are treated without removing bone from the osseous defects (Fig. 45–6). The aim of this approach is to obtain bone repair and recontouring by the natural healing processes (Fig. 45–7). Autogenous bone and hip marrow implants may also be used to obtain bone repair in the osseous defect. If bone repair is not obtained after nine months to one year, the osseous defects may be eliminated by reshaping the bone.

Successful results have been reported in the treatment of furcations with implants consisting of plastic and bone.[6] To make the implant, 1 gram of a mixture by weight of 20 per cent grated anorganic bone and 80 per cent polymethacrylate is mixed with 0.5 cc. autopolymerizing monomer (liquid). The furcation is exposed by elevating a flap; the area is cleansed and the roots are scaled and smoothed. The implant is inserted with an amalgam carrier and packed with amalgam pluggers. After the defect is filled, excesses are removed and the plastic surface is contoured. The flap is replaced and sutured, and covered with periodontal pack for ten days.

Occlusal adjustment in the treatment of furcations with infrabony pockets and osseous defects

Furcation involvement is not of itself indicative of the presence of trauma from occlusion; inflammation may be the only responsible destructive factor. **However, of all the areas of the periodontium, the**
(Text continued on page 704.)

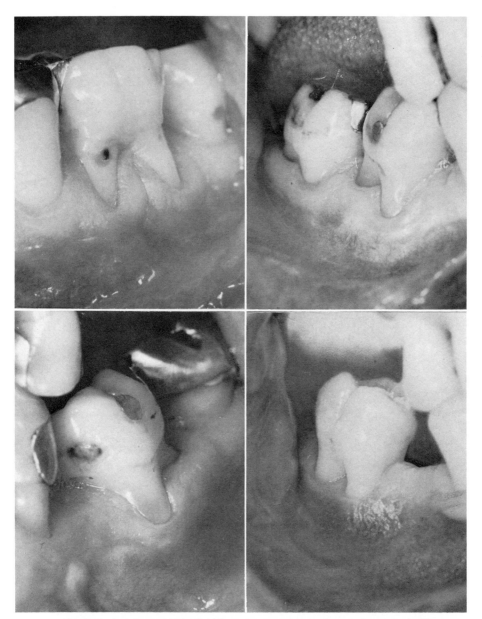

Figure 45–4   Optimal Gingival Contour Obtained by Treatment of Furcation Involvement of Different Severity.

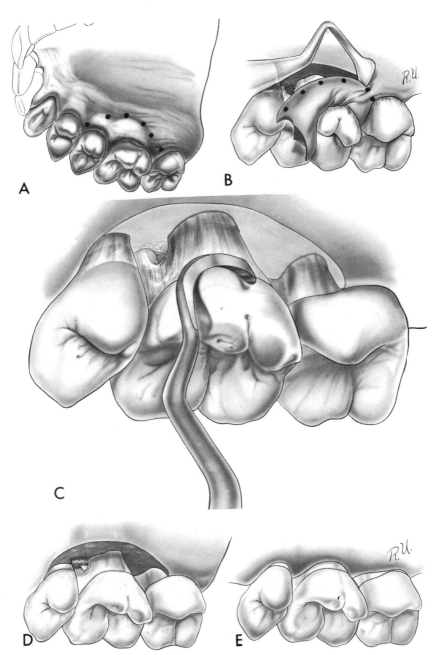

Figure 45–5 Gingivectomy for the Treatment of Furcation Involvement Complicated by Periodontal Abscess. *A,* Periodontal abscess outlined by pinpoint markings. *B,* Abscess excised apical to the markings. *C,* After the calculus is removed, the roots are smoothed with a curet. Note the exposed tricurcation. *D,* Furcation cleansed before inserting periodontal pack. *E,* Area healed.

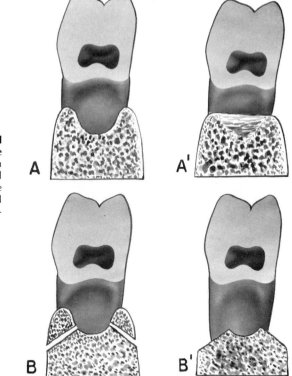

Figure 45–6 Potential Benefit of Retaining Facial and Lingual Bone in the Treatment of Osseous Defects in the Furcation Area. *A,* Faciolingual view showing crater in bifurcation of mandibular molar *A',* Undisturbed facial and lingual plates provide scaffolding for filling in of the defect by healing process. *B,* When the facial and lingual plates are artificially reshaped the potential height obtainable by healing is reduced (*B'*).

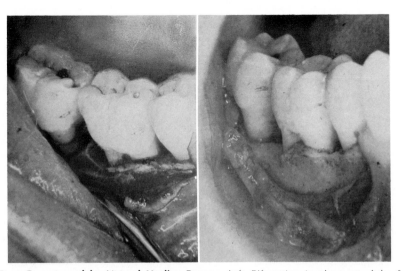

Figure 45–7 Bone Recontoured by Natural Healing Process. *Left,* Bifurcation involvement of the first and second molars with crater-like interdental bony defect and bony shelf. *Right,* One year after treatment without reshaping the bone, the area was re-entered to examine the bone. Note that the buccal ledge has been recontoured and the interdental defect has been eliminated by the natural healing process.

furcation is most susceptible to injury from excessive occlusal forces. When furcation involvement is complicated by infrabony pockets and osseous defects, or if the tooth is excessively mobile, checking the occlusion and adjusting it, if necessary, are essential. If the treated teeth are used as abutments for restorations, every effort should be made to align the occlusal forces in the vertical axis of the teeth in order to attain optimal bone repair (Fig. 45–8).

ROOT RESECTION AND HEMISECTION IN THE MANAGEMENT OF FURCATION INVOLVEMENT (HEMISECTION)

Under special circumstances, a root may be resected or a tooth may be sectioned in half **(hemisection)**, to preserve teeth with furcation involvement.[1,7] These are not routine forms of treatment, but are resorted to if it is not possible to obtain success by the regular methods.

Root resection and hemisection should be restricted to firm teeth. The prognosis is best when the bone destruction is concentrated around one root or the roots are well supported.

Root resection

This procedure may be used on any root of a multirooted maxillary tooth, but the mesiobuccal or distobuccal root of the maxillary molars is the most suitable.

Technique for root resection

This procedure consists of filling the root canals, resecting the root and placing a restoration in the severed root canal (Fig. 45–9).

STEP 1. Endodontic therapy is performed first, with the involved root only partially filled. In this way, the patient is spared the discomfort that may occur if the root is resected and there is a time lapse before endodontic therapy.

STEP 2. Under local anesthesia, probe

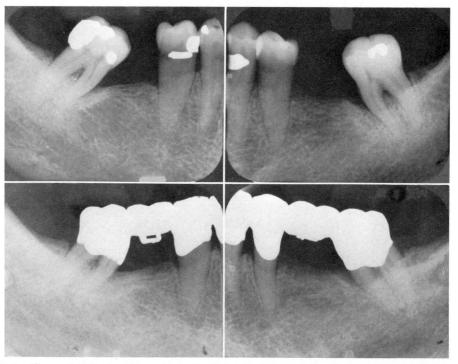

Figure 45–8 Alignment of Occlusal Forces in the Vertical Axis of the Teeth to Obtain Optimal Bone Repair of Furcation Involvement. *Above,* Furcation involvement of mandibular molars with angular osseous defects on the mesial surface. *Below,* Eight years after treatment. The teeth have been reshaped with crowns to direct the occlusal forces toward the vertical axis. Note the improvement in the appearance of the bone. (Restorations by Dr. R. Sheldon Stein, Boston, Mass.)

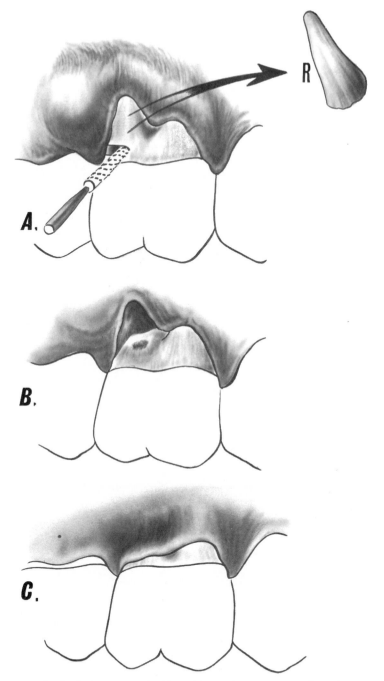

Figure 45–9 Root Resection in the Treatment of Trifurcation Involvement. A, Distobuccal root resected and removed (R). B, Tooth surface smoothed, showing the root canal which was filled before the resection. C, After healing.

the area to determine the extent and outline of alveolar bone destruction around the root to be removed (Fig. 45–10, A).

STEP 3. Make vertical or oblique incisions in the gingiva and mucosa mesial and distal to the involved tooth, and ele-

vate a mucoperiosteal flap (Fig. 45–10, B, and C).

STEP 4. With a contra-angle handpiece and a cross-cut bur, sever the root where it joins the tooth (Fig. 45–10, D). Remove the root (Fig. 45–10, E).

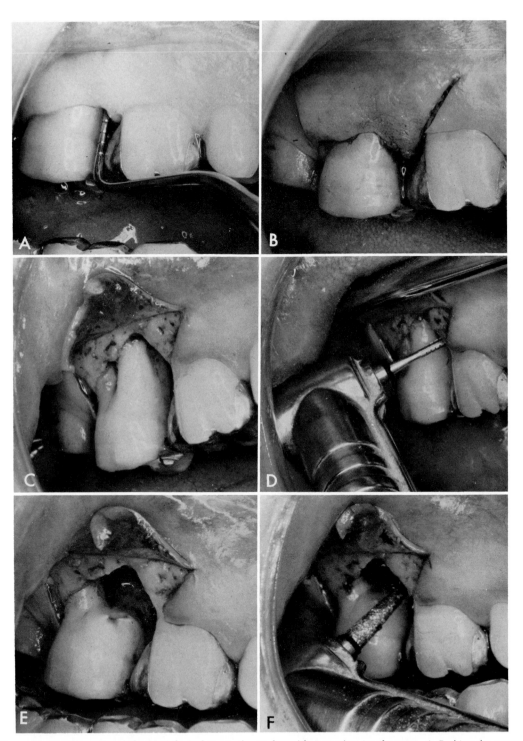

Figure 45–10   Resection of the Mesiobuccal Root of a Molar with Furcation Involvement. *A,* Probing the extent of periodontal destruction. *B,* Incisions for a flap. *C,* Mucoperiosteal flap elevated, revealing extensive bone loss and osseous defect on mesiobuccal root. *D,* Root resected with cross-cut bur. *E,* Root removed; sharp stump remains. *F,* Sharp stump smoothed and tooth contoured to prevent food entrapment.

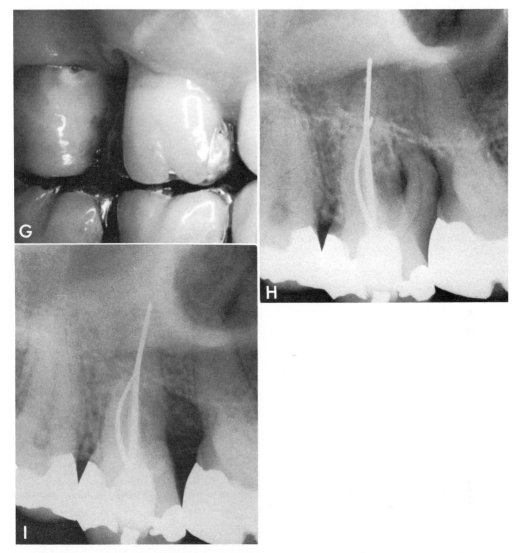

Figure 45–10 *Continued* *G,* Area healed, showing excellent gingival contour where root was removed. *H,* Before treatment. Radiograph shows extensive bone loss around mesiobuccal root. *I,* Nine months after treatment, showing bone repair where root was removed.

STEP 5. With a stone or diamond point, **smooth the resected root stump** and **contour the tooth to permit unimpaired passage of food** (Fig. 45–10, *F*). Insert a pinpoint restoration in the severed root canal.

STEP 6. Scale and plane root surfaces which become visible and more accessible when the root is removed. This is a most critical part of the treatment.

STEP 7. Clean the area, replace the flap, suture and cover with periodontal pack. Remove the pack and suture after one week. Physiologic gingival contour is usually restored by two months (Fig. 45–10, *G*), and bone repair is detectable radiographically by nine months (Figs. 45–10, *H* and *I*).

Hemisection

Hemisection involves the same technique as that used for root resection, except that half the crown is removed along with one of the roots of a mandibular molar. The retained mesial or distal half serves as a useful abutment for a dental restoration (Fig. 45–11).

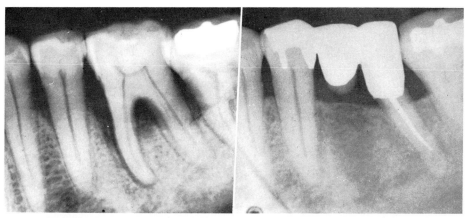

Figure 45–11 Hemisection. *Left,* Bifurcation involvement of first molar. *Right,* Two years and three months after resection of the mesial half of the first molar. (Courtesy of Dr. John Cane, Philipsburg, N.J.)

COMBINED PERIODONTAL-ENDODONTIC THERAPY

Periodontics and endodontics are separate specialties, but the periodontium is not similarly divided into periodontal and periapical halves; the periodontium is a continuous unit. As inflammation spreads from the gingiva into the alveolar bone and periodontal ligament, it may reach the pulp through the root apices or accessory pulp canals near the apex or in the furcation. Periapical destruction caused by pulpal infection may spread along the root and cause a retrograde periodontitis,[8] or inflammation in the pulp may spread through accessory canals and cause inflammation and periodontal destruction in the furcation.[9] There are, therefore, many occasions when the survival of a tooth depends upon combined periodontal and endodontic approaches to treatment.[5]

Indications

Combined periodontal-endodontic therapy is indicated when there is continuity of destruction between the gingival margin and the periapical region. The diagnosis is made by probing the periodontal pocket to the root apex; radiographs with gutta percha points are helpful diagnostic aids (Fig. 45–12). The pulp in such cases is usually nonvital.

Combined periodontal-endodontic therapy is also sometimes indicated for **teeth with periodontal destruction which extends close to but does not reach the periapical** area. Such teeth often resist repeated attempts at periodontal treatment. The pulp usually responds to vitalometer and other tests. However, repair of the periodontal lesion is strikingly improved after endodontic therapy.

The prognosis of combined periodontal-endodontic therapy depends upon the degree of mobility and the severity and distribution of bone loss. Best results are obtained on firm teeth with bone loss con-

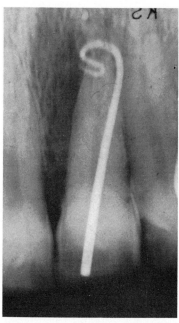

Figure 45–12 Gutta Percha Point Indicates that Periodontal Pocket Extends to the Apex of Maxillary Central Incisor.

fined to one root surface or one root of a multirooted tooth. **Since occlusion provides the stimulation required for a healthy periodontium and post-treatment healing of the periodontium is adversely affected by injurious occlusal forces, the prognosis is improved by consideration of the occlusion and correction when necessary.**

Sequence of combined treatment

The types of periodontal and endodontic therapy vary in individual cases; properly performed, they produce gratifying results (Fig. 45–13). Since the healing responses of the periodontium to both forms of therapy are interrelated, they should be performed together. If they are done at different times, there is no rule regarding which should be first. Treating the periodontal pocket first might be beneficial to periapical healing by shutting off bacterial flow from the oral cavity. Treating the root canal first could force toxic bacterial products and chemical irritants through the dentinal tubules which injure the cementum[2] and interfere with the outcome of periodontal treatment. Re-

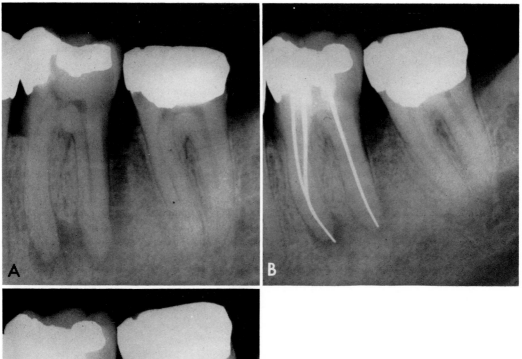

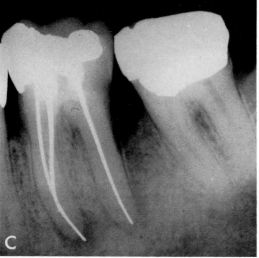

Figure 45–13 Combined Periodontal-Endodontic Therapy. *A,* Before treatment, showing vertical radiolucent zone from the margin to the periapical region of the distal root of the first molar and a radiolucent area on the mesial root. *B,* One year after combined periodontal-endodontic treatment, showing considerable improvement. *C,* Three years after treatment, showing further improvement.

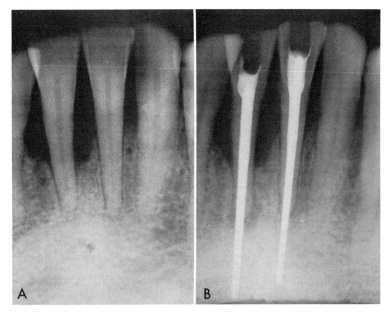

Figure 45–14 Endodontic Endosseous Implants. *A,* Before. *B,* After. (Courtesy of Dr. Robert L. Kittredge, Boston.)

lief of pain often governs the sequence of treatment in these cases.

ENDODONTIC ENDOSSEOUS IMPLANTS

Endodontic endosseous implants are used as adjuncts to periodontal therapy, to stabilize periodontally involved teeth.[3] The implant consists of a metal post embedded in the bone beyond the apex (approximately 10 mm.) of an endodontically treated tooth (Fig. 45–14). It improves the crown-root ratio by adding to the length of bone-supported root structure.

The implants are employed when replacement of a single periodontally involved tooth would require using adjacent teeth which ordinarily would not need restorations, or which are not suitable as abutments; and to preserve teeth which are the only remaining potential abutments for prostheses, particularly in the mandible. Contraindications are proximity of the root apex to the maxillary sinuses, floor of the nose, mandibular canal and mental foramen, and debilitating systemic disease.

The results with endodontic endosseous implants are not predictable, but when successful they provide valuable service to the patient (Fig. 45–14).

REFERENCES

1. Amen, C. R.: Hemisection and Root Amputation. Periodontics, *4*:197, 1966.
2. Erausquin, J., and Muruzabál, M.: Necrosis of Cementum Induced by Root Canal Treatments in the Molar Teeth of Rats. Arch. Oral Biol., *12*:1123, 1967.
3. Frank, A. L.: Improvement of the Crown-Root Ratio by Endodontic Endosseous Implants. J.A.D.A., *74*:451, 1967.
4. Goldman, H. M.: Therapy of the Incipient Bifurcation Involvement. J. Periodont., *29*:112, 1958.
5. Hiatt, W. H.: Periodontic Pocket Elimination by Combined Endodontic–Periodontic Therapy. Periodontics, *1*:152, 1963.
6. Hodosh, M., and Shklar, G.: A New Method of Treating Teeth with Furcation Involvement. R. I. Dent. J., *2*:19, 1969.
7. Messinger, T. F., and Orban, B.: Elimination of Periodontal Pockets by Root Amputation. J. Periodont., *25*:213, 1954.
8. Simring, M., and Goldberg, M.: The Pulpal Pocket Approach: Retrograde Periodontitis. J. Periodont., *35*:22, 1964.
9. Winter, G. B., and Kramer, I. R. H.: Changes in Periodontal Membrane and Bone Following Experimental Pulpal Injury in Deciduous Molar Teeth in Kittens. Arch. Oral Biol., *10*:279, 1965.

Chapter 46

MUCOGINGIVAL AND RECONSTRUCTIVE SURGERY

Mucogingival surgery consists of plastic surgical procedures for the correction of gingivo–mucous membrane relationships which complicate periodontal disease and may interfere with the success of periodontal treatment. The term "reconstructive

711

periodontal surgery" refers to plastic surgical procedures which are undertaken to restore destroyed or diseased periodontal tissues. The terms overlap somewhat, because many operations fit into both categories.

MUCOGINGIVAL SURGERY

In the first half of this century, periodontal surgery was confined to eliminating disease and arresting tissue destruction; more recently, there has been considerable clinical experimentation with mucogingival and reconstructive procedures to correct disease-induced deformities and restore destroyed tissue. In the attempt to broaden the scope of periodontal therapy and increase the longevity of the natural dentition, operations have often been performed before the research was done to determine their usefulness and limitations. When such information became available, some operations were discarded and others were refined. **Before surgical procedures are per-** formed on a patient, there should be acceptable evidence that the operation is likely to solve his problem, and the extent to which it is experimental should be made clear to the patient.[110]

Indications for Mucogingival Surgery

Mucogingival surgery is performed as an adjunct to regular pocket elimination procedures for the following purposes:

1. **To relocate frena and muscle attachments which encroach upon periodontal pockets and pull them away from the tooth surface.** Tension from such attachments (a) distends the gingival sulcus and fosters the accumulation of irritants which lead to gingivitis and pocket formation, and (b) aggravates the progress of periodontal pockets and causes their recurrence after treatment (Fig. 46–1). The problem is more common on the facial surface, but it occasionally occurs on the lingual surface (Fig. 46–2).

2. **To widen the zone of attached gingiva**

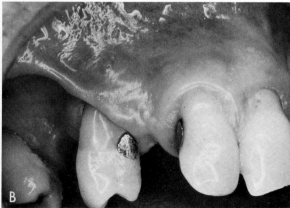

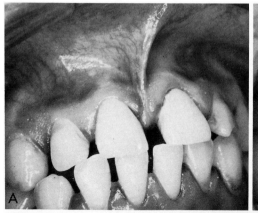

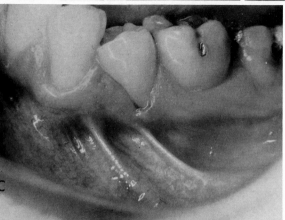

Figure 46–1 High Frenum Attachments. *A,* Frenum between maxillary central incisors. *B,* Frenum on the mesial surface of the maxillary second premolar. *C,* Frenum attached to pocket wall on mandibular first premolar.

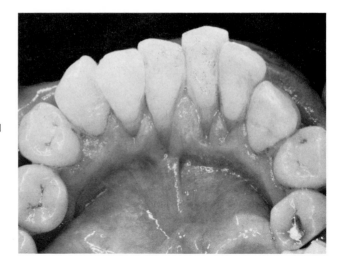

Figure 46–2 Frenum attached to pocket wall on lingual surface of incisor.

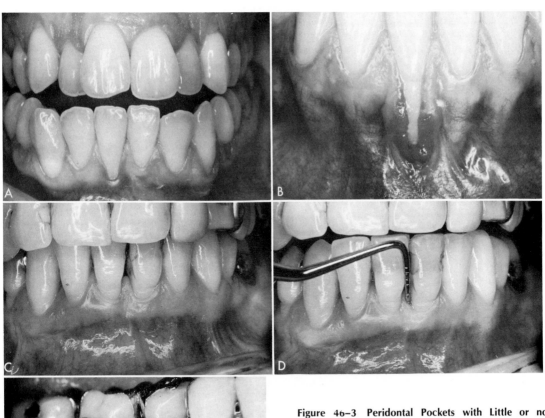

Figure 46–3 Peridontal Pockets with Little or no Attached Gingiva. A, Pocket on mandibular incisor extends into alveolar mucosa. B, Pocket on mandibular incisor extends into alveolar mucosa. Note pronounced inflammation. C, Periodontal pockets in mandibular area. D, Probe indicates 4 mm. pocket on the mesial surface of the central incisor reaches to the mucogingival line. E, Extreme exposure of the mesiobuccal root of the mandibular first molar.

or create a new zone of attached gingiva when periodontal pockets extend close to or beyond the mucogingival junction (Fig. 46–3), **or into the alveolar mucosa** (Fig. 46–3). This is the most common purpose for which mucogingival surgery is performed. The procedure is based upon the premise that a minimum width of attached gingiva is required to support the gingival fibers which brace the marginal gingiva and prevent it from being deflected from the tooth during mastication.

The width of the attached gingiva varies in different individuals and on different teeth. It is generally greatest in the incisor region (3.5 to 4.5 mm. in the maxilla and 3.3 to 3.9 mm. in the mandible) and less in the posterior segments, with the least width in the first premolar area (1.9 mm. in the maxilla and 1.8 mm. in the mandible).[1] No minimum width of attached gingiva has been established as a standard necessary for gingival health; even as little as 1 mm. may create no problems in a patient with excellent oral hygiene.[13]

The following are useful guides for determining whether mucogingival surgery is required for correction of the attached gingiva:

If the base of periodontal pockets is apical to the mucogingival line, some attached gingiva must be created to separate the healed gingival sulcus from the alveolar mucosa and prevent pockets from recurring.

The tension test

If the base of periodontal pockets is close to the mucogingival line, the functional adequacy of the post-treatment attached gingiva can be predicted by the following test. Retract the cheeks and lips laterally with the fingers. If such tension pulls the marginal gingiva from the teeth, the attached gingiva is too narrow and should be widened along with the treatment of the pockets.

3. **To deepen the oral vestibule.** The principal reason for deepening the oral vestibule is to create space for a widened zone of attached gingiva or for relocation of frena. The deepened vestibule will also provide space for unimpaired food excursion and lessen food retention at the gingival margin; it may also facilitate improved

toothbrushing, but this has not been substantiated.[7, 109]

4. **To cover denuded root surfaces.** Root surfaces denuded by gingival disease and recession are functional and esthetic problems. Gingiva may be transplanted onto exposed roots by plastic operations and may become so adherent to the root that it does not permit the entrance of a periodontal probe. Reattachment involves the formation of new cementum and the embedding of new connective fibers into the root. Some reattachment (3.5 mm.)[104, 105] on exposed roots has been reported in artificially created defects in experimental animals,[119] and in isolated clinical studies in humans,[101] but the likelihood of obtaining it is not predictable.

Factors Which Affect the Outcome of Mucogingival Surgery

Anatomic structures

The structures involved in mucogingival surgery are (Figs. 46–4 and 46–5) the marginal and attached gingiva, mucogingival line (junction), alveolar mucosa, periodontal ligament, cementum, alveolar bone and alveolar periosteum, regional blood vessels, lymphatics and nerves, muscle and frenum attachments and fornix of the oral vestibule. The reader is referred to Chapters 1 to 4 for a review of these structures, except for muscle and frenum attachments and the mental nerve, which are discussed here.

MUSCLE ATTACHMENTS. Tension from high muscle attachments interferes with mucogingival surgery by postoperative reduction in vestibular depth and width of attached gingiva. To prevent this, muscle attachments in the operative field must be separated from the bone (Fig. 46–6). The following muscles may be encountered in mucogingival operations:

1. The mentalis: Originates on the facial surface of the alveolar process in the incisive fossa and is inserted into the skin of the chin (Fig. 46–7).

2. The incisivus labii inferioris: Originates on the alveolar process close to the border in the mandibular lateral incisor area and passes to the lower lip (Fig. 46–7).

3. The depressor labii inferioris: Origin-

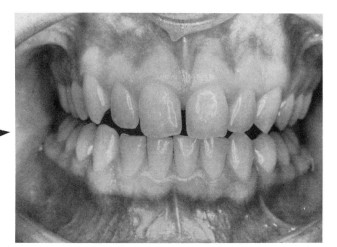

Figure 46–4 Normal Relationship of the Marginal and Attached Gingiva to the Mucogingival Line which demarcates the gingiva from the alveolar mucosa. Also shown are the oral vestibule, the vestibular fornix and frena attachments in the incisor and premolar areas. ▶

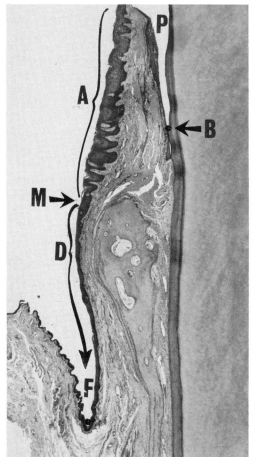

Figure 46–5 Mucogingival Area. Periodontal pocket (P) encroaches upon the mucogingival line (M). The bottom of the pocket is at B. Part of the attached gingiva (A) forms the wall of the pocket. Also note the alveolar mucosa (D), and vestibular fornix (F).

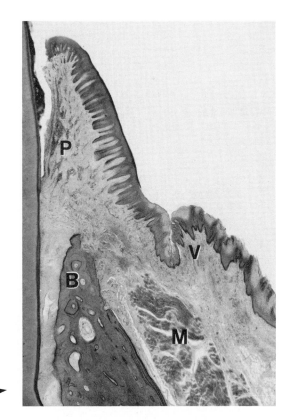

Figure 46–6 Muscle Attachment (M) close to vestibular fornix (V) and crest of the facial bone (B) in an autopsied ▶ jaw with periodontal disease. P, Periodontal pocket.

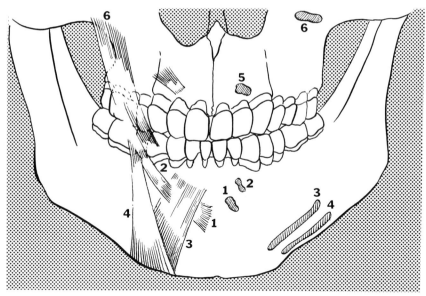

Figure 46–7 Muscle Attachments Which May be Encountered in Mucogingival Surgery. The origin of the muscle is shown on the right; the insertion on the left. 1. Mentalis. 2. Incisivus labii inferioris. 3. Depressor labii inferioris. 4. Depressor anguli oris (triangularis). 5. Incisivus labii superioris. 6. Levator anguli oris (caninus).

ates on the oblique line of the mandible between the symphysis and the mental foramen and passes upward and medially into the lower lip, where it blends with the orbicularis oris and fibers of the opposite side (Fig. 46–7).

4. The depressor anguli oris (triangularis): Originates on the oblique line of the mandible to be inserted into the angle of the mouth.

5. The incisivus labii superioris: Originates from the alveolar process close to the border in the maxillary lateral incisor area and passes to the upper lip (Fig. 46–7).

6. Levator anguli oris (caninus): Arises from the canine fossa below the infraorbital foramen and inserts into the angle of the mouth (Fig. 46–7).

THE MENTAL NERVE. Trauma to the nerve can produce uncomfortable paresthesia of the lip which recovers slowly. Familiarity with the location and appear-

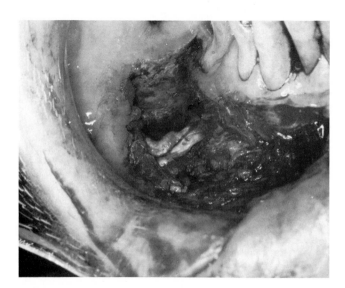

Figure 46–8 Mental Nerve. Emerging From the Foramen in the Premolar Area.

ance of the mental nerve reduces the likelihood of injuring it. The mental nerve emerges from the mental foramen located apical to the first and second mandibular premolars and usually divides into three branches (Figs. 46–8, 46–9 and 46–10).

One turns forward and downward to the skin of the chin. The other two course anteriorly and upward to supply the skin and mucous membrane of the lower lip and the mucosa of the labial alveolar surface.

Other Factors Which Affect the Outcome of Mucogingival Surgery

Irregularity of teeth

Abnormal tooth alignment is an important cause of gingival deformities that require corrective surgery and is an important factor in determining the outcome of treatment. The location of the gingival margin, the width of the attached gingiva and alveolar bone height and thickness are all affected by tooth alignment. On teeth which are tilted or rotated labially, the labial bony plate is thinner and located further apically than

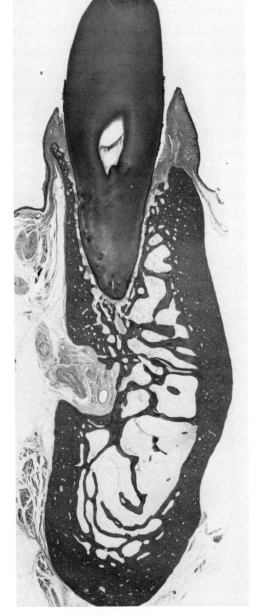

Figure 46–9 Mental Nerve and Blood Vessels in Mental Foramen. Note the relationship of the mental foramen to the apex of the second premolar and the oral vestibule.

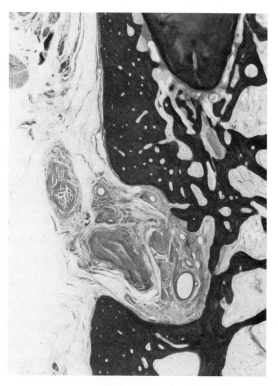

Figure 46–10 Detailed View of Mental Nerve and Blood Vessels in the Mental Foramen. Note Relationship to Premolar Root.

on the adjacent teeth, and the gingiva is receded so that the root is exposed.[122] On the lingual surface of such teeth, the gingiva is bulbous and the bone margins are closer to the cemento-enamel junction. The level of gingival attachment on root surfaces and the width of attached gingiva following mucogingival surgery are affected as much, or more, by tooth alignment as by variations in treatment procedures (Fig. 46–11).

Orthodontic correction is indicated when mucogingival surgery is performed on malposed teeth in an attempt to widen the attached gingiva or to restore the gingiva over denuded roots. If orthodontic treatment is not feasible, the prominent tooth should be ground to within the borders of the alveolar bone with special care taken to avoid pulp injury.

Roots covered with thin bony plates comprise a hazard in mucogingival surgery. Even the simplest type of flap (partial thickness) creates the risk of bone resorption on the periosteal surface.[48] Resorption in amounts that ordinarily are not significant may cause loss of bone height when the bony plate is thin or tapered at the crest.

Occlusion

The occlusion should be adjusted prior to or along with mucogingival surgery, because occlusion affects the post-treatment contour of the bone. Excessive or in-

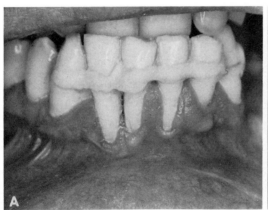
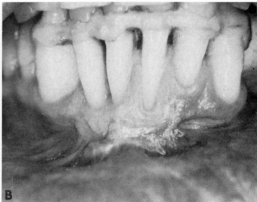
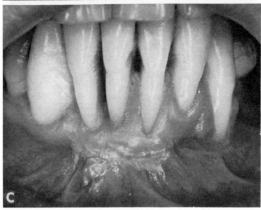

Figure 46–11 Gingival Recession and Narrow Band of Attached Gingiva Persist Around Labially Positioned Roots After Mucogingival Surgery. *A,* Before treatment, showing gingival recession with narrow band of attached gingiva around labially prominent teeth. *B,* Three months after mucogingival surgery. The attached gingiva around the central and lateral incisors has been widened. *C,* Five months after surgery. Recession is increased and the attached gingiva is narrowed around the prominent roots. Compare the patient's left canines in *B* and *C.*

sufficient occlusal forces interfere with healing of the supporting periodontal tissues[88] and produce thinning of the gingival half and bulging of the apical portion of the labial plate.[44] Loose teeth should be stabilized by splinting, because excessive tooth mobility may lead to abnormal occlusal forces. Gingival healing and the location of the gingival sulcus do not appear to be affected by occlusal forces.

The mucogingival line (junction)

Normally, the mucogingival line in the incisor and canine areas is located approximately 3 mm. apical to the crest of the alveolar bone on the radicular surfaces and 5 mm. interdentally.[100] In periodontal disease and on malposed disease-free teeth, the bone is located further apically and may extend beyond the mucogingival line.

The distance between the mucogingival line and the cemento-enamel junction before and after periodontal surgery is not necessarily constant. After inflammation is eliminated, there is a tendency for the tissue to contract and draw the mucogingival line in the direction of the crown.[33]

Instruments for Mucogingival Surgery

The following is a representative selection of instruments which are used in addition to those ordinarily required for the different pocket elimination techniques; the choice is a matter of individual preference: Bard-Parker scalpels, blades #11, #12 and #15, bone chisels, fine thumb forceps, locking needle holder (small), mosquito hemostats, periosteal elevator, scissors, sutures 4-0 and 5-0, tissue nippers, and tissue retractors.

Suturing Techniques

There are many types of sutures, suture needles and materials;[32,62] the following methods, using a ⅜ circle reverse cutting needle and 4-0 black braided silk, fill most needs in periodontal surgery:

1. INTERDENTAL LIGATION (Fig. 42–12). This technique is used to join facial and lingual flaps; each interdental space is sutured separately. The needle is inserted through the facial aspect of the facial flap through the interdental space to penetrate the lingual flap from its inner surface (Fig. 46–12, A and B). It is then reversed through the same interdental space, passing over the lingual flap and the facial flaps (Fig. 46–12, C) and tied on the facial side (Fig. 46–12, D).

2. SLING LIGATION (Fig. 46–13). This technique can be used for a flap on one surface of a tooth, involving two interdental spaces. The needle is passed from the lingual side, through one of the interdental spaces, beneath the contact point to pierce the facial flap from its inner aspect and emerge on the facial side (Fig. 46–13, B). The needle is returned through the same interdental space, the thread passing over the facial flap and then looping around the lingual surface of the tooth (Fig. 46–13, C and D). It is then passed through the other interdental space to pierce the facial flap from its inner aspect (Fig. 46–13, B and D). The needle is reversed through the same interdental space, the thread passing over the facial papilla and the needle emerging on the lingual side (Fig. 46–13, E) where the tie is made. The suture is started on the facial side for a lingual flap.

3. VERTICAL MATTRESS SUTURE (Fig. 46–14). This suture is used when there is a flap on the facial or lingual surface and another procedure such as gingivectomy on the other. The suture is started in the attached gingiva of the flap, and a vertical "bite" is taken with the needle beneath the interdental papilla (Fig. 46–14, A and B). The needle is then passed through the interdental space, around the lingual surface of the tooth and through the next interdental space to emerge on the facial surface. A vertical "bite" is taken with the needle on the facial surface of the flap beneath the interdental papilla (Fig. 46–14, C and D). The needle is then reversed through the same interdental space (Fig. 46–14, E), around the lingual surface and through the other interdental space onto the facial surface (Fig. 46–14, F), where a tie is made (Fig. 46–14, G).

4. CONTINUOUS SLING SUTURE – TYPE I (Fig. 46–15). This is used when there is a flap involving many teeth on one surface with another procedure such as gingivec-

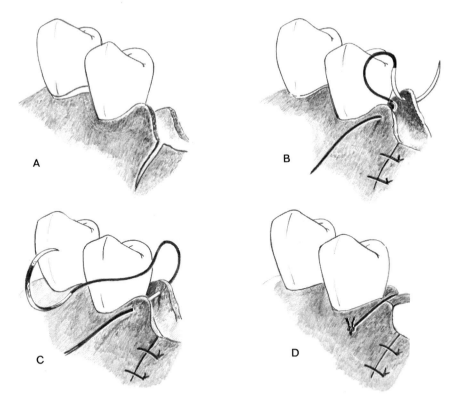

Figure 46–12 **Interdental Ligation.** *A,* Facial and lingual flaps to be sutured. *B,* The vertical incision is closed by simple, interrupted sutures. To suture interdentally, the needle is inserted through the facial aspect of the facial papilla and through the lingual papilla from its inner side. *C,* The needle is reversed through the same interdental space. *D,* A tie is made on the facial side.

tomy on the other surface. The suture closely adapts the flap to the bone and fixes it at the desired level in relation to the bony crest. When suturing a flap on the facial surface the needle is passed through the corners of the flap distal to the last tooth and tied at the end to hold it there (Fig. 46–15, *A*). The thread is looped around the distal surface of the tooth and onto the lingual, and the needle is passed through the interdental space to emerge on the facial surface. The needle is then reversed, pierces the facial flap from its external aspect and is returned through the same interdental space (Fig. 46–15, *B*). The thread is hooked around the lingual surface of the adjacent tooth, and the previous procedure is repeated until the next to last tooth in the group is reached (Fig. 46–15, *B*).

The lingual loop on this tooth is left loose. The needle is then passed through the interdental space to the facial surface. It pierces the flap from the external aspect and is returned through the same inter-dental space to the lingual surface. A tie is made with the loose loop of thread that was left on the lingual surface (Fig. 46–15, *C* and *D*).

5. CONTINUOUS SLING SUTURE – TYPE II (Fig. 46–16). This is another type of suture which can be used when there is a flap involving many teeth on one surface with another procedure such as gingivectomy on the other surface. For a flap on the facial surface, the needle is started from the lingual side and engages the outer surface of the distogingival corner of the flap. The needle is passed through the flap, leaving a long end on the lingual side which is to be used later for a tie (Fig. 46–16, *A*). The thread is looped around the distal and lingual surfaces of the last tooth, and the needle is passed through the interdental space to the facial side. It engages the facial flap from its outer aspect, penetrates it and passes back through the same interdental space. This process is continued until the entire flap is sutured (Fig. 46–16, *B*). The

(Text continued on page 725.)

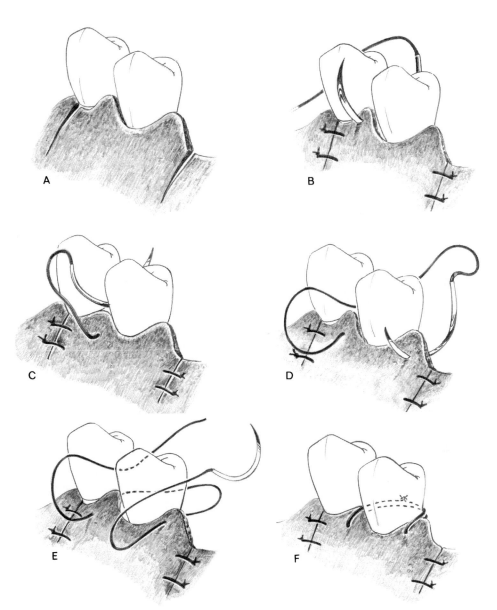

Figure 46–13   Sling Ligation. *A,* Tooth with a flap on the facial surface and a gingivectomy on the lingual. *B,* The vertical incisions are closed by simple, interrupted sutures. The needle is passed through the interdental space from the lingual to the facial side and pierces the flap from its inner aspect. *C,* The needle is returned over the edge of the flap through the same interdental space to the lingual side. *D,* The thread is looped around the lingual surface of the tooth, and the needle is passed through the adjoining interdental space from the lingual side to pierce the flap from its inner aspect. *E,* The needle is reversed through the same interdental space to the lingual side. (Dotted lines show thread on the lingual surface.) *F,* A tie is made on the lingual surface of the tooth (shown in dotted lines).

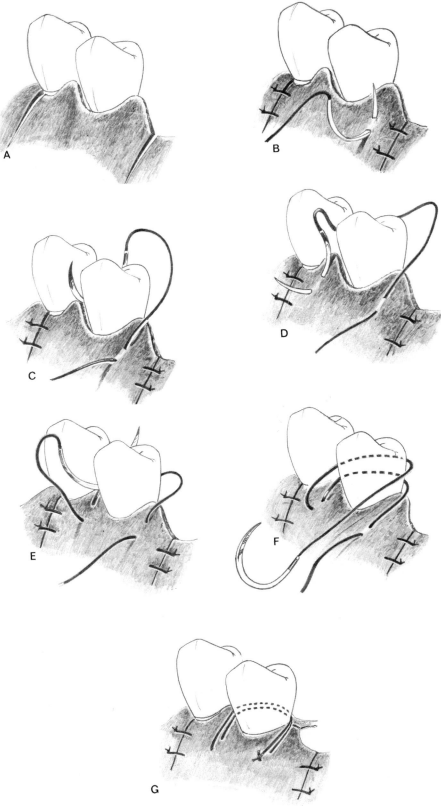

Figure 46–14   *See opposite page for legend.*

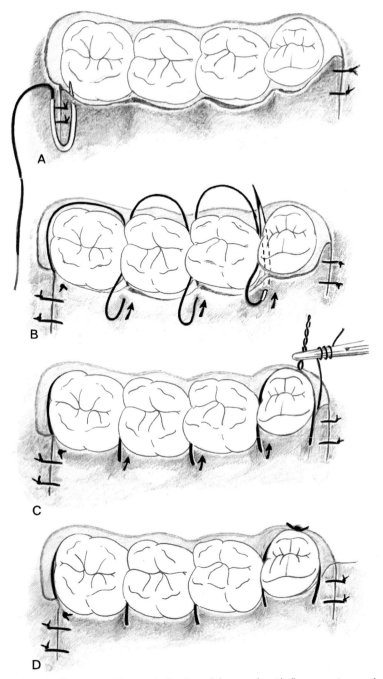

Figure 46–15 Continuous Sling Suture, Type I. *A,* Section of the mouth with flap operation on the facial surface and gingivectomy on the lingual. Vertical incisions are closed with interrupted sutures. The needle is inverted into the disto-gingival corner of the flap for an initial tie. *B,* The needle is being returned to the lingual side of the interdental space, after penetrating the flap from its outer aspect. *C,* Loose loop of thread left on the lingual surface of the premolar is twisted and tied with the other end of the suture. *D,* Tie is made on the lingual surface of the premolar.

Figure 46–14 Vertical Mattress Suture. *A,* Tooth with a facial flap and a lingual gingivectomy. *B,* Vertical incisions are closed by simple, interrupted sutures. Mattress suture is started in the flap by taking a vertical "bite" with the needle. *C,* The needle is then passed through the first interdental space, around the lingual surface of the tooth and through the adjoining interdental space in the direction of the facial surface. *D,* A vertical "bite" is taken with the needle through the external surface of the flap. *E,* The needle is reversed through the second interdental space. *F,* The thread is carried around the lingual surface and the needle is passed through the first interdental space to emerge on the facial side. Dotted lines represent the thread on the lingual surface. *G,* A tie is made on the facial side.

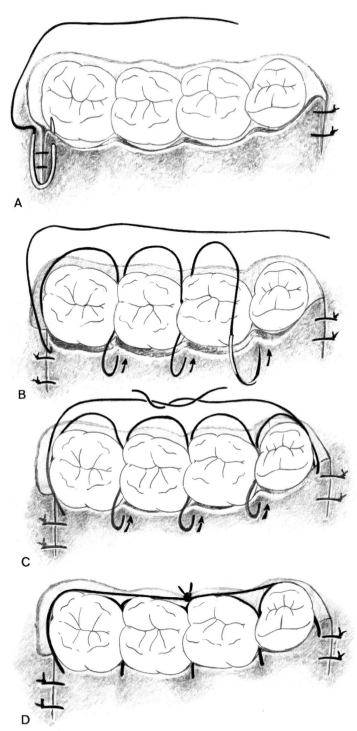

Figure 46–16 Continuous Sling Suture, Type II. *A,* Section of the mouth with flap on the facial surface and gingivectomy on the lingual. The two vertical incisions are closed with interrupted sutures. The needle has been passed from the lingual surface to the external surface of the facial flap and through the distogingival corner of it. One end of the thread is left on the lingual side. *B,* The thread passes around the distal and lingual surfaces and the needle is passed through the interdental space to the facial side. It engages the facial flap from its outer aspect and is passed back through the same interdental space to the lingual. *C,* Suturing is completed on the mesial aspect of the second premolar and the suture is tied with the end of the thread initially left on the lingual side. *D,* Lingual tie is completed.

needle is carried through the final interdental space onto the lingual surface, where a tie is made with the long end of the suture initially left there (Figs. 46–16, C and D).

Periodontal Flaps and Grafts

Periodontal flaps

A periodontal flap is a section of gingiva and/or mucosa surgically separated from the underlying tissues to provide visibility and accessibility necessary for treatment. **There are two basic types: the simple flap (unrepositioned flap), which is replaced to its presurgical location at the end of the operation; and the positioned (repositioned) flap, which is placed in a new location at the end of the operation. The flaps originally used in periodontics were the simple type, and their purpose was to eliminate periodontal pockets.**[26] **In recent years, the objectives of the flap have been expanded beyond pocket elimination to include the correction of mucogingival defects and the restoration of tissues destroyed by disease. Positioned flaps are used for these purposes** (Fig. 46–17).

THE SIMPLE FLAP OPERATION FOR ELIMINATING PERIODONTAL POCKETS. There are many variations[112, 124, 125] of the flap operation for eliminating periodontal pockets; The Neumann[67] and Widman[115] techniques utilized most of the representative procedures which are described below:

Step 1. Internal incision to remove inner aspect of pocket wall.

Step 2. Retraction of the flap consisting of gingiva, mucosa and alveolar periosteum, exposing the bone from the gingival margin to the apices of the teeth (Fig. 46–18).

Step 3. Removal of granulation tissue and calculus and smoothing of the root surfaces.

Step 4. Trimming the margin of the alveolar bone.

Step 5. Suturing of the flap in its original position (Fig. 46–18).

The simple flap operation was very popular at one time, but it fell out of favor as a technique for eliminating suprabony pockets. There was a high proportion of relapses.[110] The healed flap margin did not reattach to the tooth, and it formed bulbous contours which retained irritating debris. It remains one of the preferred methods for the treatment of infrabony pockets, because it provides excellent visibility and access to the osseous defects.

POSITIONED FLAPS FOR POCKET ELIMINATION, CORRECTION OF MUCOGINGIVAL DEFECTS AND THE RESTORATION OF TISSUE DESTROYED BY DISEASE. The many types of positioned flaps which are relocated from their original site for the combined purposes of pocket elimination, correction of mucogingival defects and the restoration of tissue destroyed by disease are described in detail in this chapter.

Positioned flaps may be relocated in three directions: apically, laterally or coronally. *A full thickness (mucoperiosteal) flap consists of the surface epithelium and connective tissue plus the periosteum of the underlying bone; a partial thickness (split thickness or mucosal) flap consists of epithelium and a thin layer of the underlying connective tissue.*[102, 103]

Grafts

Grafts are tissues transferred from one site to replace damaged structures in another. Gingiva, oral mucosa, bone and bone marrow are the tissues usually used as grafts. *The area from which a graft is obtained is called the donor site. Grafts which remain attached to the donor site by a base or "pedicle" are known as pedicle grafts.* The graft is transferred to the recipient site by sliding (transposition) or by rotating it on its base (rotation). The terms "pedicle graft" and "positioned flap" are interchangeable because they refer to the same procedure. *A free graft refers to tissues completely removed from one location and transferred to another without retaining connection with the donor site,* i.e., "free gingival graft." Grafts are classified according to source as follows: *Autologous grafts (autografts) are tissues obtained from the same individual; homologous grafts (homografts) are obtained from different individuals of the same species; and heterologous (heterografts) are obtained from another species.*

Grafts are classified according to structure as follows: *A mucoperiosteal (full thickness)*

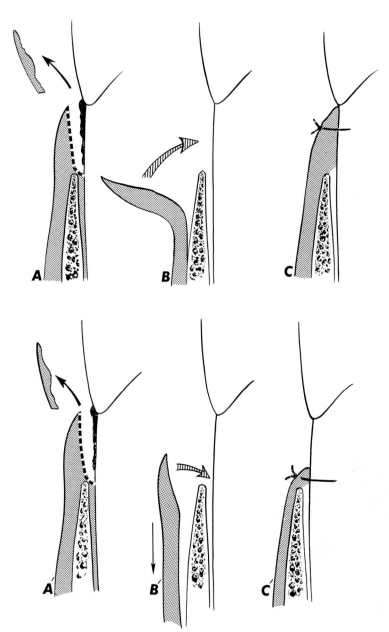

Figure 46–17   Difference Between a Simple Flap (*A, B, C*) **and an Apically Positioned Flap** (*A', B', C'*). *A,* **Simple Flap;** internal bevel incision removes inner pocket wall (*arrow*). *B,* Simple flap elevated, tooth cleaned and smoothed and flap returned to original location (*arrow*). *C,* Flap sutured. *A',* **Apically Positioned Flap;** internal bevel incision removes inner pocket wall (*arrow*). *B',* Flap elevated, tooth cleaned and smoothed, flap moved apically (*vertical arrow*) and positioned at the level of the bone crest (*arrow*). *C',* Apically positioned flap sutured at the crest of the bone.

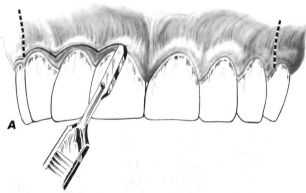

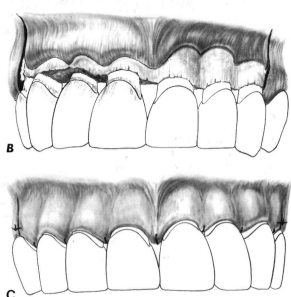

Figure 46–18 Simple Flap Operation for Elimination of Periodontal Pockets. *A,* Vertical incisions outline flap. Inner pocket wall resected with internal bevel incision. *B,* Inner pocket wall removed, full thickness flap elevated, teeth on the left side scaled and smoothed and bone margin trimmed. *C,* Flap returned to presurgical position and sutured.

graft consists of surface epithelium and connective tissue plus the periosteum of the underlying bone; a mucosal (partial thickness) graft consists of epithelium and a thin layer of underlying connective tissue.[102, 103]

MUCOGINGIVAL OPERATIONS

The following are representative procedures for correcting mucogingival defects designated by terms used by the American Academy of Periodontology* and by other terms in common usage. The description of each operation is followed by its accomplishments and limitations as revealed by

---

*Current Procedural Terminology for Periodontics. 2nd ed. American Academy of Periodontology, 1969.

studies in humans and experimental animals. In some instances, the reported findings are inconclusive or conflicting. This is to be expected for many reasons, such as subtle differences in the way the same operation is performed by different clinicians; the difficulty of obtaining histologic material to corroborate what appear to be obvious clinical results; differences between postoperative healing of artificially created and naturally occurring periodontal lesions; differences in tissue response among animal species, between animals and humans and among different individuals; differences in oral hygiene among humans; and the **difference between pre- and post-treatment impressions gathered from clinical observations and photographs, rather than facts based upon measurements subjected to statistical analysis.**

Frenectomy or Frenotomy (Repositioning Frenum Attachment)

A frenum is a fold of mucous membrane, usually with enclosed muscle fibers, that attaches the lips and cheeks to the alveolar mucosa and/or gingiva and underlying periosteum. A frenum becomes a problem if its attachment is too close to the marginal gingiva. It may then pull upon a healthy gingival margin and invite the accumulation of irritants; it may deflect the wall of a periodontal pocket and aggravate its severity; or it may interfere with post-treatment healing, prevent close adaptation of the gingiva and lead to pocket formation, or interfere with proper toothbrushing.

Purposes

The terms "frenectomy" and "frenotomy" represent operations that differ in degree. *Frenectomy is complete removal of the frenum, including its attachment to underlying bone, such as may be required in the correction of an abnormal diastema between maxillary central incisors. Frenotomy is partial removal of the frenum.* Both are used, but the latter generally suffices for periodontal purposes, namely to relocate the frenum attachment so as to create the zone of attached gingiva between the gingival margin and the frenum. Frenectomy or frenotomy is usually performed in conjunction with other periodontal treatment procedures, but occasionally is done as a separate operation.

Frenum problems occur most often on the facial surface between the maxillary and mandibular central incisors and in the canine and premolar areas,[111] and, less frequently, on the lingual surface of the mandible.

Procedure

If the vestibule is deep enough, the operation is confined to frenum, but it is often necessary to deepen the vestibule to provide space for the repositioned frenum. This is accomplished as follows:

1. Anesthetize the area.
2. Engage the frenum with a hemostat inserted to the depth of the vestibule (Fig. 46–19, *A* and *B*).
3. Incise along the upper surface of the hemostat, extending beyond the tip (Fig. 46–19, *C*).
4. Make a similar incision along the under surface of the hemostat (Fig. 46–19, *D*).
5. Remove the triangular resected portion of frenum with the hemostat (Fig. 46–19, *E*). This exposes the underlying brushlike fibrous attachment to the bone.
6. Make a horizontal incision, separating the fibers, and bluntly dissect to the bone.
7. If the vestibule is shallow, deepen it by extending the dissection laterally for a distance of three teeth in each direction (Fig. 46–19, *F*).
8. Clean the field of operation and pack with gauze sponges until bleeding stops.
9. Insert the periodontal pack. First pack the marginal area, as is ordinarily done following gingivectomy. Then, using the marginal pack as a stable base, add thin strips on the edge to the depth of the incision (Fig. 46–19, *G*).
10. Remove the pack after two weeks and repack twice at weekly intervals. One month from the time of operation is usually required for the formation of an intact mucosa with the frenum attached in its new position (Fig. 46–19, *H*).

In patients with a deep oral vestibule, it may not be necessary to extend the depth in order to relocate the frenum (Fig. 46–20).

High frenum attachments on the lingual surface are uncommon. To correct these without involving the structures in the floor of the mouth, approximately 2 mm. of the attachment is separated from the mucosa with a periodontal knife at weekly intervals until the desired level is reached. The area is covered with periodontal pack in the intervals between treatments.

Vestibuloplasty (Vestibular Extension Procedures)

Procedures used to alter the form of the oral vestibule are referred to as vestibuloplasty. Their principal purpose is to increase vestibular depth to provide space for an increased zone of attached gingiva.[47] The increased depth may also facilitate improved oral hygiene and gingival health.[7, 109]

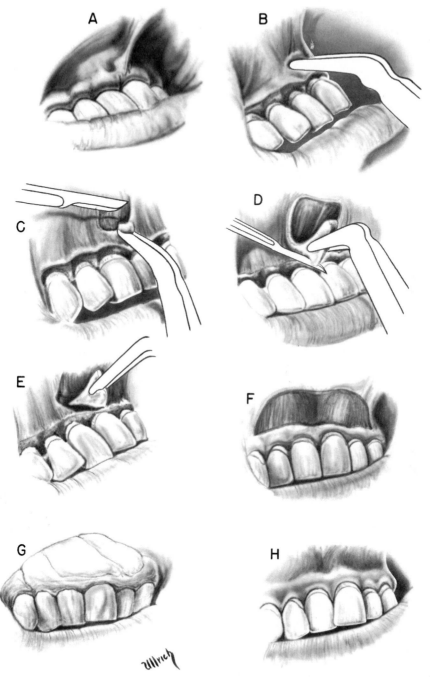

Figure 46-19 Repositioning the Frenum Attachment. *A,* Frenum attached close to periodontal pocket. *B,* After pockets are resected the frenum is engaged with hemostat. *C,* Incision along upper margin of hemostat. *D,* Incision along lower margin of hemostat. *E,* Resected portion of frenum removed. *F,* Vestibular trough deepened in the midline and lateral areas. *G,* Periodontal pack in position. *H,* Periodontal pockets eliminated and frenum attachment in raised position.

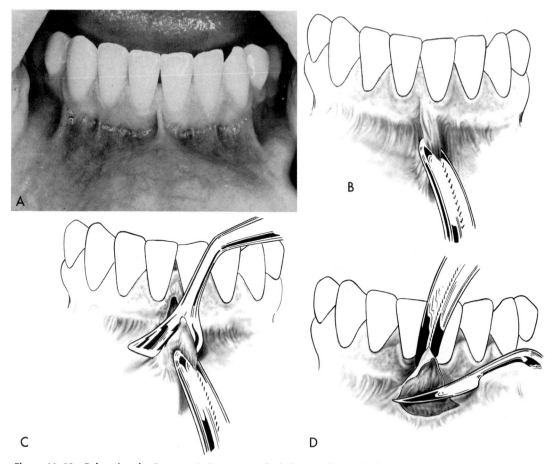

Figure 46–20 Relocating the Frenum. *A,* Frenum attached close to the gingival margin. *B,* Hemostat engages frenum. *C,* Incision along the upper border of the hemostat. *D,* Incision along the lower border of the hemostat removes a wedge-shaped section of the frenum.

Vestibular extension using a partial thickness (mucosal) flap (mucosal stripping or separation)[55, 83, 86]

This operation consists of reflecting a partial thickness flap and deepening the vestibular fornix for the purposes of increasing the width of the attached gingiva and relocating frenum attachments (Fig. 46–21).

PROCEDURE. *Step 1.* Make a gingivectomy incision slightly apical to the base of the pockets, even if this entails incising into the alveolar mucosa (Fig. 46–21, *A*). Resect the pockets; remove the calculus and plane the root surfaces.

Step 2. Make vertical incisions from the gingival margin into the fornix of the vestibule, outlining the area where increased depth is desired.

Step 3. Place a #15 Bard-Parker blade flat against the gingiva with the point directed apically and insert it into the mucogingival junction at one end of the operative field (Fig. 46–21, *B*). Move it along the mucogingival junction, separating a flap consisting of epithelium and a thin layer of underlying connective tissue. Hold the edge of the flap with fine tissue forceps and dissect it away from the underlying tissue, deepening the oral vestibule in the process.

When the desired depth is reached (approximately twice that of the desired zone of attached gingiva), apply slight lateral pressure against the cheeks and lips, drawing the flap apically until the edge of the flap is at the newly established vestibular depth (Figs. 46–21, *C* and 46–22).

As alternative procedures, the mucosal separation may be started from the line of gingivectomy incision (Figs. 46–21, *D* and

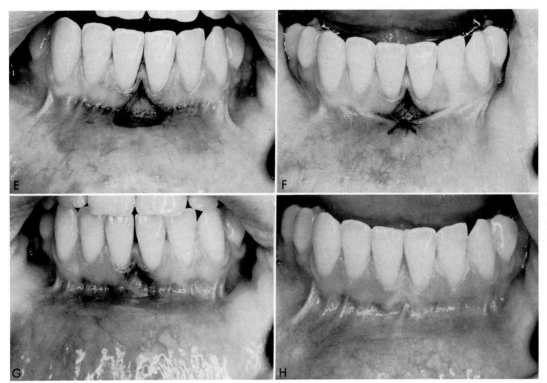

Figure 46–20 *Continued E,* After removal of the frenum. *F,* Mucosa sutured in position. *G,* After one week, periodontal pack and suture removed. *H,* After six months, frenum relocated at the mucogingival line.

E, or directly from the gingival margin (Fig. 46–23).

Step 4. Cleanse the periosteum. Remove muscle and frenum attachments and soft tissue from the periosteum to provide a smooth, firm base for the granulation tissue which covers the wound and will finally form the widened band of attached gingiva. Special effort should be made to remove the muscle attachments to minimize post-treatment loss of vestibular depth.

The edge of the flap may be sutured to the periosteum at the base of the operative field, but this is not necessary. Control the bleeding with a 2″ × 2″ gauze pad under pressure. When a clot forms, the flap adheres to the underlying tissue at the base of the fornix.

Step 5. Insert the periodontal pack. Remove excess clot and insert the periodontal pack* in two stages. First, place the pack over the cut gingival margin as is

ordinarily done for gingivectomy (Fig. 46–24). This provides a firm base for stabilizing the pack which is to cover the remainder of the operative field. Second, take a strip of pack which is wide enough to reach the base of the fornix and add it to the marginal pack so that it forms an apron-like protection for the entire area (Fig. 46–24). Exert gentle pressure on the lip and cheek so as to mold the pack into position.

Overpacking is a common cause of post-operative problems. Patients should remain in the chair after the pack is inserted to permit the lips, cheeks and tongue to mold the pack while it is soft. Excess pack which interferes with the occlusion should be removed. Biting into excess pack after it hardens loosens the remainder of the pack and causes irritation and inflammation of the wound. This in turn causes delayed healing, post-treatment bleeding and excessive granulation tissue which may result in increased resorption along the bone surface.

Pack insertion may be modified in many

---

*The Kirkland-Kaiser pack used by the author and other types of packs available for mucogingival surgery are described in Chapter 51.

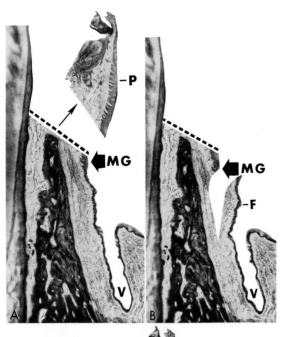

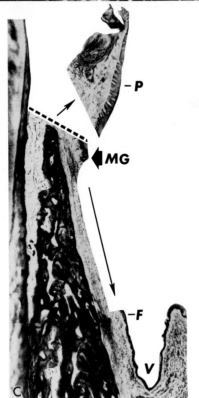

Figure 46–21 Mucosal Stripping. *A,* Pocket (P) resected by gingivectomy incision. MG, Mucogingival junction. V, Vestibular fornix. *B,* Periodontal pocket is removed; tooth is scaled and planed. Incision made at the mucogingival junction (MG) separates away partial thickness flap (F), leaving periosteum and layer of connective tissue on the bone. *C,* Partial thickness flap moved apically along the bone, increasing the depth of the oral vestibule (V).

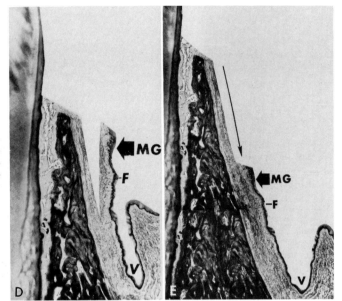

Figure 46–21 *Continued D,* **Variation of the operation,** when little or no attached gingiva remains after gingivectomy. The incision separating the partial thickness flap (F) is made at the cut edge of the gingiva. *E,* Partial thickness flap (F) moved apically. Note that the oral vestibule is deepened (V).

ways, such as by covering the exposed bone with Telfa (a form of surgical dressing) in an effort to lessen postoperative pain; and by using acrylic stents, dental floss or soft stainless steel wire loops around the teeth to aid pack retention, or chrome cobalt tissue tacks to stabilize the flap during the first postoperative week.[90] However, the method described above is effective and without undesirable complications if the pack is well adapted interproximally and not overextended.

After the pack is inserted, place an ice-bag on the face. Have the patient hold it there during the 15-minute period before you trim away the excess pack. **This is extremely helpful following extensive mucogingival procedures because it reduces postoperative swelling, discoloration and discomfort.**

Give the patient two 5-grain tablets of aspirin with instructions to repeat at three-hour intervals, if necessary. A prescription for stronger analgesics is given to the patient to be filled, if required. A.S.A. and codeine, gr. 1/4, two tablets every four hours, or Darvon Compound 65, one capsule every four hours, are effective. **Keep a carbon copy of all prescriptions in the patient's record.**

Explain the postoperative instructions to the patient, and provide a typewritten or printed copy such as the following for review at home:

Postoperative Instructions Following Mucogingival Surgery:

For_____

1. Use an ice pack "on and off" at ten-minute intervals for three hours after the operation.
2. Take two 5-grain tablets of aspirin every three hours, if necessary. If pain persists, fill the prescription and use as directed.
3. Clean your mouth as usual in the un-operated areas. Modify your cleansing procedures in the operated area to avoid disturbing the periodontal pack. After the first day, you may rinse with a pleasant-tasting mouthwash diluted one to three in a glass of water. Water irrigation under medium pressure is useful for cleansing food debris from the pack.
4. For the first three or four days, there will be some discomfort which can usually be managed with aspirin, and some swelling. Small pieces of pack may break off, but this usually presents no problem. If large sections fall off, please call the office.

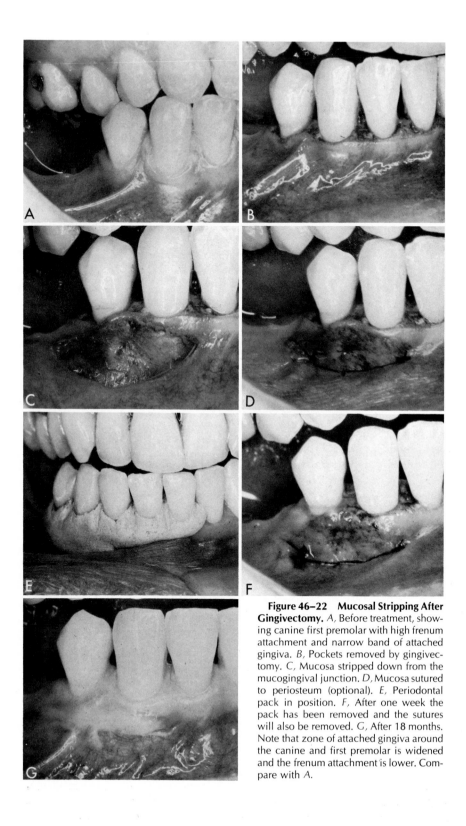

Figure 46–22 Mucosal Stripping After Gingivectomy. *A,* Before treatment, showing canine first premolar with high frenum attachment and narrow band of attached gingiva. *B,* Pockets removed by gingivectomy. *C,* Mucosa stripped down from the mucogingival junction. *D,* Mucosa sutured to periosteum (optional). *E,* Periodontal pack in position. *F,* After one week the pack has been removed and the sutures will also be removed. *G,* After 18 months. Note that zone of attached gingiva around the canine and first premolar is widened and the frenum attachment is lower. Compare with *A.*

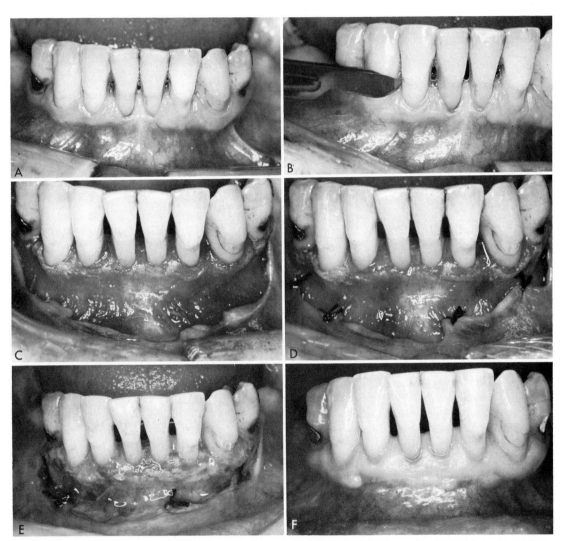

Figure 46–23   Mucosal Stripping with Internal Bevel. *A,* Before treatment, showing periodontal pockets, exposed roots and narrow band of attached gingiva. *B,* Inner surface of periodontal pockets resected with internal bevel. *C,* Mucosa has been separated away, leaving the bone covered with periosteum. The inner pocket walls have been removed from the teeth, and the roots are scaled. *D,* The mucosa is sutured to the periosteum (optional). *E,* After one week, the periodontal pack has been removed. The sutures will also be removed. *F,* After eight months, the pockets are eliminated and there is a widened zone of attached gingiva. (Compare with *A.*)

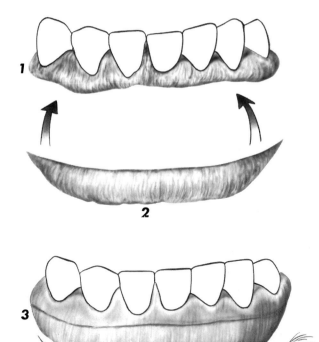

Figure 46–24 Method of Inserting Periodontal Pack in Two Stages. 1, Pack applied at margin as ordinarily done following gingivectomy. 2, Apron-shaped section which conforms to the shape of the vestibule to be added to the marginal section. 3, Apron-shaped section in position.

Step 6. Remove the pack after two weeks, cleanse the area and repack two more times at weekly intervals, after which the area is usually sufficiently healed for the pack to be discontinued.

POSTOPERATIVE COURSE. Patients sometimes develop painful ulceration at the edge of the pack. To relieve this, flush the area with warm water, dry and apply topical anesthetic. Remove pieces of pack which adhere to the tissues. Smooth the margin of the pack and, if necessary, add new pack to it. Line the edge of the pack with Orabase, which forms a soothing, protective cushion and usually makes the patient comfortable. Instruct the patient to reapply the Orabase at home at four-hour intervals, if necessary. Emphasize the importance of removing food debris after meals.

Paresthesia. Slight numbness of the lip sometimes persists after vestibular extension operations in the mandible, occasionally with a slight drooping of the lip and drooling. Such complications usually disappear within one to three weeks and the patient should be reassured of this. However, special precautions must be taken to avoid injury to the mental nerve which could produce similar, but more severe, problems that last six months to a year.

ACCOMPLISHMENTS OF VESTIBULAR EXTENSION WITH A PARTIAL THICKNESS FLAP (MUCOSAL STRIPPING). The depth of the fornix and the zone of attached gingiva are increased by this operation, but the increases diminish as healing progresses.[10-12, 25] The long-term expectancy is retention of a little less than half the initial extension in most regions, with slightly more in the canine areas and less in the molars.[56] The shrinkage of vestibular depth may stop or reverse itself,[7] but not consistently or to a significant degree.[56]

THE NEW ZONE OF ATTACHED GINGIVA. The new surface of the attached gingiva is initially smooth and shiny; the normal stippling develops in six to nine months.

Microscopically, the gingiva initially appears as a connective tissue scar similar to attached

gingiva but differing from it in that its epithelial rete pegs are short and broad, and the connective tissue is arranged in horizontal bundles without differentiation into a vertical papillary layer. With time, the tissues develop microscopic features that are indistinguishable from those of normal attached gingiva.[57]

There may be a thin, horizontal scar at the junction of the attached gingiva and alveolar mucosa where the margin of the flap joins with the new tissue covering the bone. Eighteen or 24 months are sometimes required for the scar to disappear.

Vestibular extension using a full thickness (mucoperiosteal) flap

This operation[45, 114] is the same as the one described above, except that the bone is denuded and the alveolar periosteum is included in the flap. It was one of the earliest mucogingival procedures, but was discontinued because of the tissue loss it produced.[22, 113, 120]

Vestibular extension using a combined full thickness and partial thickness flap[4, 68]

This procedure is based upon the hypothesis that the level to which the bone is denuded of periosteum determines the post-treatment width of the attached gingiva. The coronal portion of the flap includes the periosteum; the apical portion is partial thickness.

PROCEDURE (Fig. 46–25). *Step 1.* Short vertical incisions are made from the gingival margin to the bone at the anterior and posterior borders of the operative field.

Step 2. Periodontal pockets are eliminated by gingivectomy.

Step 3. A mucoperiosteal flap is elevated, exposing approximately 4 mm. of bone. The vertical incisions are extended apically without penetrating the periosteum.

Step 4. The flap is continued, leaving the periosteum on the bone. The result is a single flap with the marginal area of the facial plate denuded of periosteum; the apical portion remains covered.

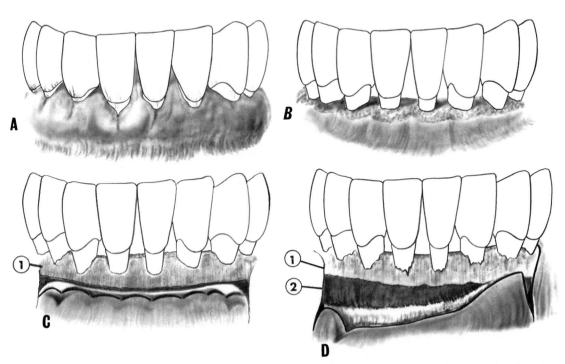

Figure 46–25 Combined Full Thickness and Partial Thickness Flap. *A,* Before operation, deep periodontal pockets extend into the alveolar mucosa. *B,* Periodontal pockets removed by gingivectomy. *C,* Full thickness section of flap is elevated (1); the periosteum is removed from the margin of the bone. *D,* Partial thickness section of flap is elevated (2). The periosteum is left on the bone.

Step 5. The bone is contoured, if desired; the flap is sutured in position, and the area is covered with a periodontal pack.

ACCOMPLISHMENTS. The attached gingiva is increased, but not necessarily to the same degree as that to which the bone was denuded.[66] A full thickness flap in the marginal zone also increases the risk of reducing the height of the labial plate.

Edlan-Mejchar operation for vestibular deepening[36, 109]

This technique produces statistically significant vestibular deepening (4.72 mm.) in the mandibular area, which reportedly persists in patients observed for periods of up to five years. It is recommended as a method of creating an environment for achieving and maintaining gingival health in patients without periodontal pockets but with little or no gingiva remaining around the mandibular anterior teeth.

PROCEDURE. *Step 1: Outline the Operative Field* (Fig. 46–26, A). Starting at the junction of the gingival margin and attached gingiva, make a vertical incision at each end of the operative field, extending approximately 12 mm. from the alveolar margin into the vestibule. Join the vertical incisions with a horizontal incision.

Step 2: Reflect a Flap (Fig. 46–26, B). Separate a mucosal flap and elevate it to expose the periosteum of the bone.

Step 3: Separate the Periosteum from the Bone (Fig. 46–26, C). Starting at the crest of the facial bone, just under the elevated flap separate the periosteum and attached muscle fibers from the bone and transpose them to the lip.

Step 4: Replace the Mucosal Flap (Fig. 46–26, D). Fold the mucosal flap down over the bone and suture it to the inner surface of the periosteum. The fornix of the vestibule is now formed by the junction of the mucosal flap and the transposed periosteum.

Step 5: Suture the Periosteum (Fig. 46–26, E). The upper edge of the periosteum is sutured to the mucosa of the lip or vestibule where the horizontal initial incision was made. According to Edlan and Mejchar, the periosteum is covered with epithelium within seven to ten days and the mucous membrane attaches to the bone in two to three weeks.

Fenestration procedure[29, 83, 85, 86] (periosteal separation with periosteal retention)

This operation is designed to widen the zone of attached gingiva with a minimum loss of bone height. It utilizes a partial thickness flap, except in a rectangular area at the base of the operative field, where the periosteum is elevated and the bone is exposed (Fig. 46–27). This is the area of fenestration. Its purpose is to create a scar which is firmly bound to the bone and will prevent separation from the bone and narrowing of the width of the attached zone.

PROCEDURE. *Step 1: Eliminate the Periodontal Pockets.* With a #15 Bard-Parker blade, make a shallow, vertical incision from the gingival margin to the vestibular fornix at each end of the operative field. With a gingivectomy incision, resect the periodontal pockets; remove the calculus and plane the root surfaces (Fig. 46–27, A).

Step 2: Elevate a Partial Thickness Flap. A partial thickness flap consists of epithelium and a thin underlying layer of connective tissue. The periosteum is left intact as a protective covering for the bone. To start the flap, hold a #15 Bard-Parker blade flat against the facial surface and insert it on the field (Fig. 46–27, B). Make a shallow incision along the mucogingival line.

Hold the corners of the mucosa with fine forceps and insert the Bard-Parker blade midway between the epithelial surface and the periosteum. Slowly incise across the operative field, gently separating a partial thickness flap with the forceps. If the periodontal pockets extend into the aveolar mucosa and no attached gingiva remains after they are resected, the flap is started from the cut mucosal surface (Figs. 46–27, E and F, and 46–28).

Extend the dissection apically, reflecting the flap and deepening the vestibular fornix as you progress (Fig. 46–27, C). The fornix should be deepened to a level approximately twice the desired width of the new attached gingiva. With a scissors remove irregularities in the flap margin. Slide the flap apically until the edge is at the newly created level of the vestibule.

Step 3: Cleanse the Periosteum. At this stage, there is a wide area of bone covered by periosteum and a thin layer of connective tissue. With a scissors, remove

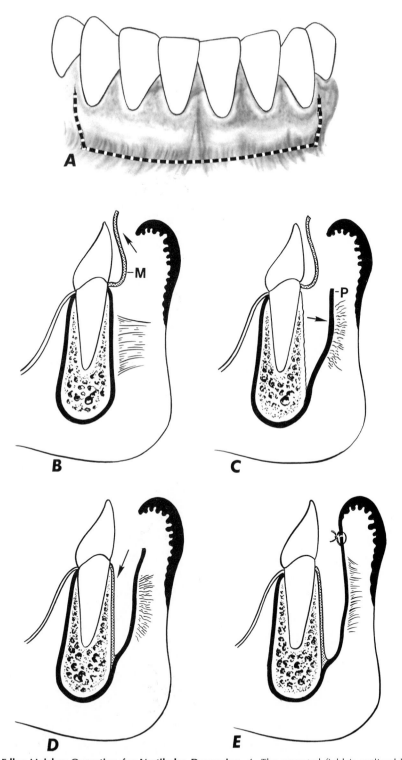

Figure 46–26   Edlan-Mejchar Operation for Vestibular Deepening. *A,* The operated field is outlined by two vertical incisions from the junction of the marginal and attached gingiva to approximately 12 mm. from the alveolar margin into the vestibule. The vertical incisions are joined by a horizontal incision. *B,* A mucosal flap (M) is elevated, exposing the periosteum of the bone. *C,* The periosteum (P) is separated from the bone, starting from the line of attachment of the mucosal flap; the periosteum, including muscle attachments, is transposed to the lip. *D,* The mucosal flap is folded down over the bone (*arrow*) and sutured to the inner surface of the periosteum. *E,* The periosteum is transposed to the lip and sutured where the initial horizontal incision was made.

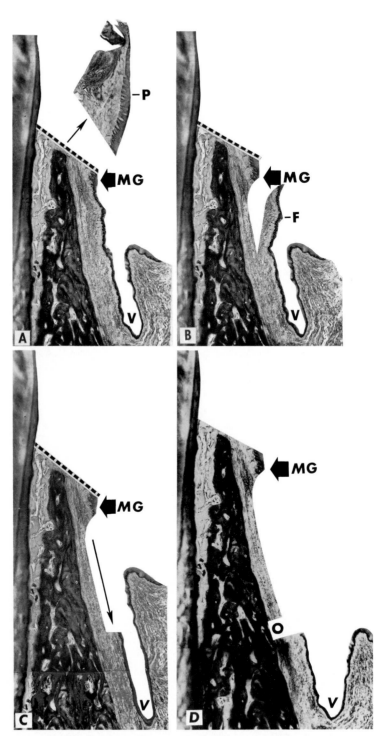

Figure 46–27 **Fenestration.** *A,* Periodontal pocket (P) resected with gingivectomy incision. MG, Mucogingival junction. V, Vestibular fornix. *B,* Incision at mucogingival junction separates partial thickness flap, (F), leaving periosteum and layer of connective tissue on the bone. *C,* Partial thickness flap moved apically, deepening the oral vestibule (V). *D,* Fenestration (O) cut through the periosteum, leaving the bone exposed.

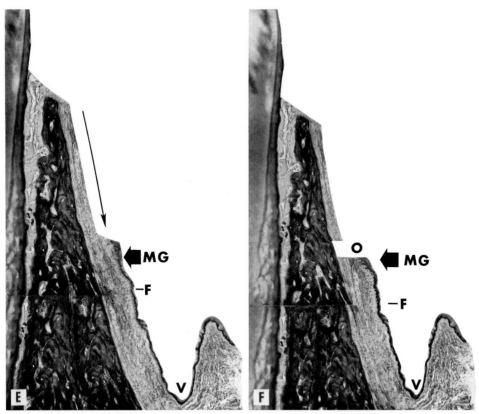

Figure 46–27 *Continued* *E,* Variation of operation when little or no attached gingiva remains following gingivectomy. Partial thickness flap is separated at the cut gingival margin and moved apically (F), deepening the oral vestibule (V) in the process. *F,* Fenestration (O) cut through the periosteum, exposing the bone.

all muscle fibers and soft tissue from the periosteum until the surface is smooth and firm.

Step 4: Fenestration. At the deepest level in the vestibule, make an incision through the periosteum to the labial plate along the length of the operative field. Bluntly dissect the periosteum and overlying tissue from the bone (a fenestration) across the operative field (Fig. 46–27, *D*). The margin of the flap may be sutured to the periosteum at the lower border of the fenestrated area, but this is not necessary.

Apply pressure with 2″ × 2″ gauze pads until the bleeding stops; remove excess clot; then insert a periodontal pack (Fig. 46–28). Replace the pack after two weeks and twice again at weekly intervals. If sutures are used, remove them after one week.

ACCOMPLISHMENTS OF THE FENESTRATION OPERATION. The fenestration produces an increase in the width of attached gingiva and in vestibular depth approximately one half of that created at the time of operation.

A scar forms in the fenestration area which ultimately develops microscopic features resembling those of attached gingiva.[75,85] The scar is initially firmly attached to the underlying bone[21] and prevents narrowing of the new zone of attached gingiva (Fig. 46–28, *G*). The binding effect lasts about four weeks;[3] by three months the width of attached gingiva is reduced by approximately 28 per cent[81] and remains that way for approximately a year, after which the width is usually further reduced. **Post-treatment shrinkage of the attached gingiva is anticipated at the time of operation by providing space for twice the desired width of attached gingiva.**

The tendency of repositioned muscle attachments to return to their original position is an important limiting factor in vestibular extension operations. The most lasting results are obtained when minimal invasion of musculature is required in

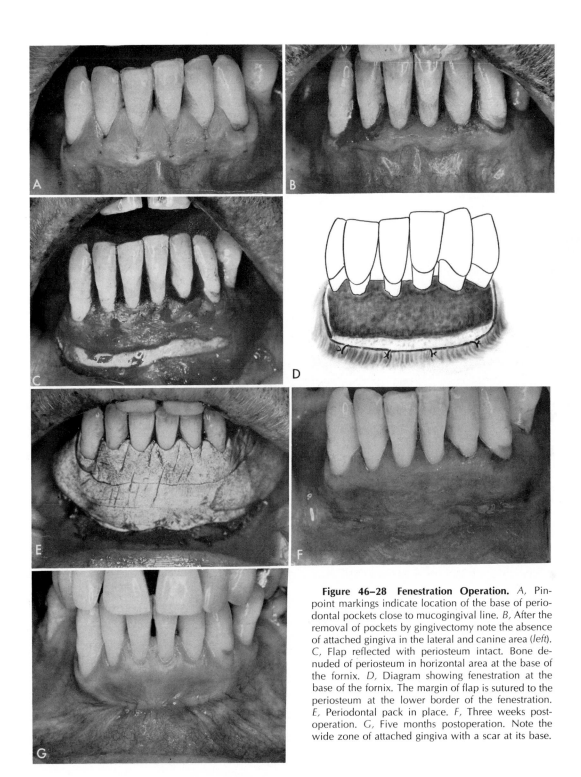

Figure 46–28 Fenestration Operation. *A,* Pinpoint markings indicate location of the base of periodontal pockets close to mucogingival line. *B,* After the removal of pockets by gingivectomy note the absence of attached gingiva in the lateral and canine area (*left*). *C,* Flap reflected with periosteum intact. Bone denuded of periosteum in horizontal area at the base of the fornix. *D,* Diagram showing fenestration at the base of the fornix. The margin of flap is sutured to the periosteum at the lower border of the fenestration. *E,* Periodontal pack in place. *F,* Three weeks postoperation. *G,* Five months postoperation. Note the wide zone of attached gingiva with a scar at its base.

order to create increased space for attached gingiva.[75] Muscle attachments encountered in the course of deepening the vestibule must be removed to reduce the likelihood of their return. Contraction of the scar also tends to reduce post-treatment vestibular depth.[95]

The Apically Positioned Flap[4, 5, 37, 39, 65, 66, 116]

Positioned flaps are used to correct mucogingival deformities without some of the limitations of vestibular extension operations, and with less extensive surgical interference. This operation utilizes the apically positioned flap, partial thickness or full thickness, for the combined purposes of pocket elimination, widening the zone of attached gingiva, deepening the oral vestibule and relocating frena apically. The partial thickness (mucosal) flap is generally used to avoid exposing bone and the accompanying risks of bone resorption and aggravation of bone dehis-

cences and fenestrations.[87, 96] The full thickness (mucoperiosteal) flap is indicated when accessibility to the bone is desired for recontouring purposes.

The apically positioned partial thickness flap

There are three distinguishing features of this operation: (1) the internal (reverse) bevel incision for removing the inner aspect of periodontal pockets (Fig. 46–29), (2) the partial thickness flap and (3) the location of the flap (Figs. 46–30, 46–31 and 46–32).

Step 1: Vertical Incisions. Make a vertical incision from the gingival margin into the fornix of the vestibule at each end of the operative field. The incisions should be placed at the distofacial angle of the terminal teeth rather than interproximally to avoid unequal shrinkage and notching of the interdental papillae. The incision should penetrate to the periosteum, but not through it.

Step 2: The Internal Bevel Incision.

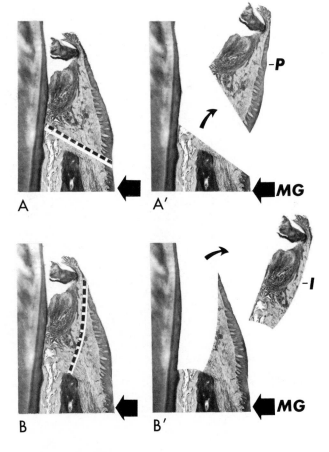

Figure 46–29 Comparison of Gingivectomy Incision and Internal Bevel Incision (Reverse Bevel). *A* and *A'*, Gingivectomy incision. Periodontal pocket (P) is removed, leaving small zone of attached gingiva above the mucogingival junction (MG). *B* and *B'*, Internal incision. Inner wall (I) of periodontal pocket removed, leaving outer pocket wall plus attached gingiva above the mucogingival junction (MG).

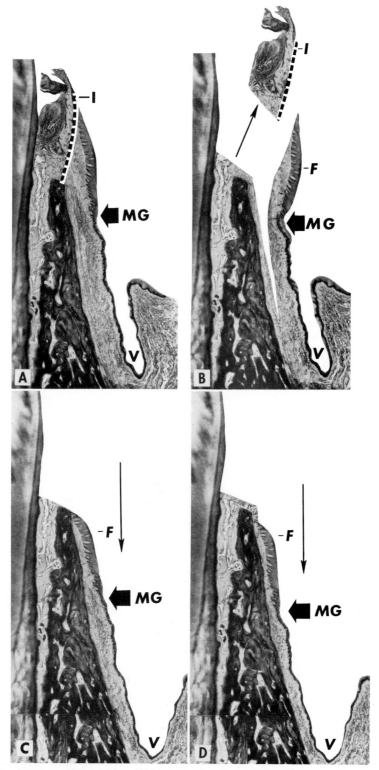

Figure 46–30 Apically Positioned Partial Thickness Flap. *A,* Internal incision (I) separates inner wall of periodontal pocket. MG, Mucogingival junction. V, Vestibular fornix. *B,* Partial thickness flap (F) separated away, leaving periosteum and layer of connective tissue on the bone. Inner wall of periodontal pocket (I) is removed and the tooth scaled and planed. *C,* Partial thickness flap (F) positioned apically with the edge of the flap at the crest of the bone. Note that the vestibular fornix is also moved apically. *D,* Partial thickness flap (F) positioned apically with the edge of the flap several millimeters below the crest of the bone.

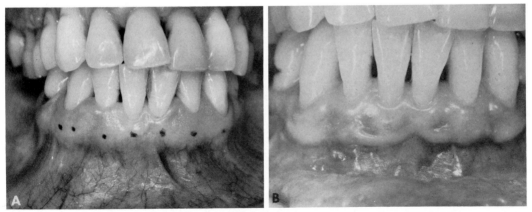

Figure 46–31 Deep Periodontal Pockets Encroach Upon Mucogingival Line. *A,* Marks inserted to show location of the base of deep periodontal pockets in relation to the mucogingival line. *B,* Two months after apically repositioned flap operation. The attached gingiva is ruffled because the flap was not separated deep enough in the fornix.

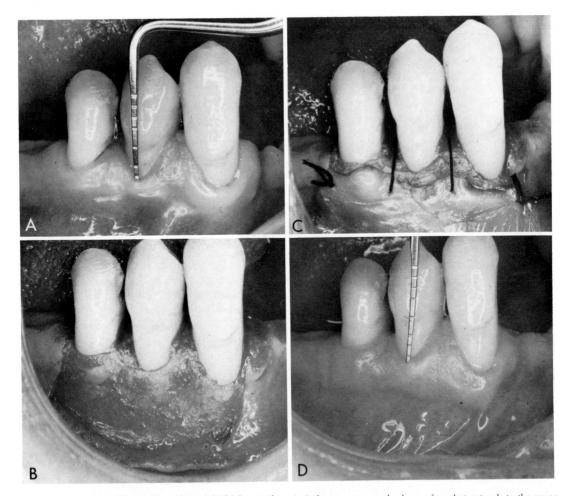

Figure 46–32 Apically Positioned Partial Thickness Flap. *A,* Before treatment, the base of pocket extends to the mucogingival line. *B,* Mucosal flap separated from the periosteum, teeth scaled and smoothed. *C,* Flap replaced below the crest of the bone. *D,* Eight months after treatment. Note the shallow sulcus and widened zone of attached gingiva. Compare with *A.*

With a Bard-Parker blade or the #22G or #23G periodontal knives, make an incision on the inside of the periodontal pockets from the tip of the gingival margin to the crest of the labial plate (Fig. 46-30,A). This incision differs from the gingivectomy incision in that it removes the diseased inner aspect of the pocket and retains the outer gingival wall. The outer gingival wall is important in this operation, because it contributes to the increased width of the attached gingiva. To avoid bulky gingival contours, the internal bevel should thin the pocket wall at the same time that it removes the diseased inner portion.

Step 3. Insert a #15 Bard-Parker blade into the internal incision, and separate the outer wall of the periodontal pockets. Continue with the blade under the attached gingiva, separating a flap consisting of epithelium and a thin layer of underlying connective tissue from the periosteum (Fig. 46-30, B). Progressively dissect the flap toward the fornix of the vestibule.

Be sure to separate the flap far enough into the fornix to provide space for the flap to be positioned apically without "buckling." If the space is inadequate, the healed gingiva will have a "ruffled" surface which requires several months to become smooth (Fig. 46-31).

Step 4. Remove the inner wall of the periodontal pockets from the teeth; scale the root surfaces free of all deposits and smooth.

Step 5. Position the flap apically. Trim the edge of the flap to conform to the contour of the bone margin and place it on the labial plate. The edge of the flap may be located in three possible positions in relation to the bone: (1) **Slightly coronal to the crest of the bone,** in an attempt to preserve the attachment of supracrestal fibers. This location may also result in thick gingival margins and interdental papillae with deep sulci, and create the risk of recurrent pockets. (2) **At the level of the crest of the labial plate** (Fig. 46-30, C). This provides satisfactory gingival contour, provided the flap is adequately thinned. (3) **Two millimeters short of the crest** (Fig. 46-30, D). This position produces the most desirable gingival contour and the same post-treatment level of gingival attachment as is obtained by placing the flap at the crest of the bone.[42] New tissue will cover the crest of the bone to produce a firm, tapered gingival margin. Placing the flap short of the crest increases the risk of a slight reduction in bone height,[31] but this is compensated for by the advantages of a well-formed gingival margin.

Step 6. Secure the flap. Remove excess clot; be sure the flap rests firmly on the underlying tissue and suture it with interrupted suspensory and lateral sutures with 4-0 silk.

Step 7. Protect the flap. Apply a gauze sponge until bleeding stops, and cover the area with periodontal pack. Remove the pack and sutures after one week. Repacking is not usually necessary.

ACCOMPLISHMENTS. This operation produces an increase in the width of attached gingiva and relocates the fornix of the vestibule and frena apically. It results in less postoperative discomfort and heals more rapidly than vestibular extension procedures.[54] The width of the attached gingiva is increased by approximately half the pretreatment depth of the pockets.[35] The post-treatment width can be estimated before the operation by using the following formula:

$$\text{Estimated post-treatment width of attached gingiva} = \frac{\text{Pretreatment depth of pockets}}{2} + \text{Pretreatment width of attached gingiva}$$

This is applicable if the flap is positioned at the crest. Since the pocket wall contributes to the increase in attached gingiva, the operation is best suited for patients with deep pockets who require additional attached gingiva. The final width of attached gingiva may be increased by placing the flap further apically from the crest (Figs. 46-32 and 46-33).

The apically positioned full thickness flap

This is the same operation as the apically positioned partial thickness flap, except that it employs a full thickness (mucoperiosteal) flap (Fig. 46-34). It is used when the bone is to be recontoured as part of the

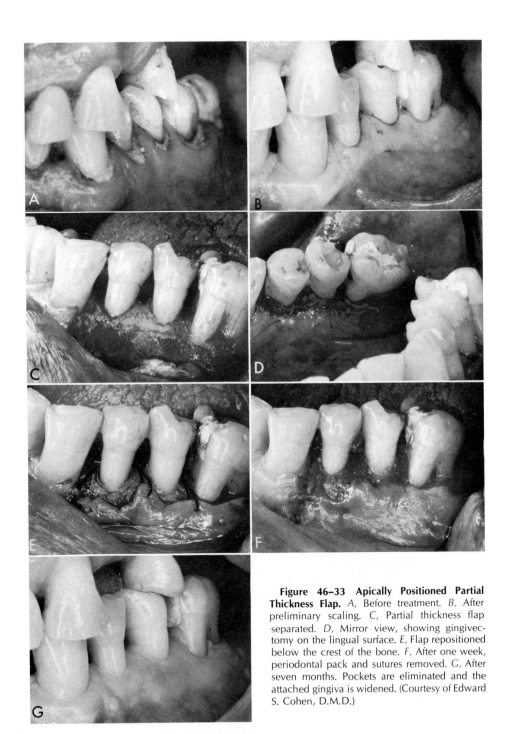

Figure 46–33 Apically Positioned Partial Thickness Flap. *A,* Before treatment. *B,* After preliminary scaling. *C,* Partial thickness flap separated. *D,* Mirror view, showing gingivectomy on the lingual surface. *E,* Flap repositioned below the crest of the bone. *F,* After one week, periodontal pack and sutures removed. *G,* After seven months. Pockets are eliminated and the attached gingiva is widened. (Courtesy of Edward S. Cohen, D.M.D.)

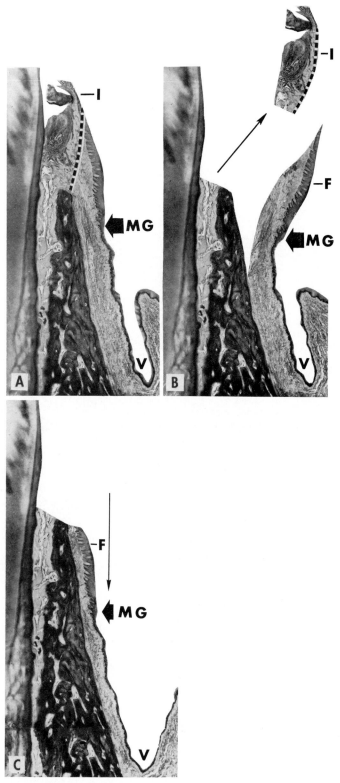

Figure 46–34 Full Thickness (Mucoperiosteal) Apically Positioned Flap. *A,* Internal incision (I) separating inner wall of periodontal pocket. MG, Mucogingival junction. V, Vestibular fornix. *B,* Full thickness flap (F), including periosteum, is separated from the bone. Inner wall of periodontal pocket removed. Tooth scaled and smoothed. *C,* Flap positioned apically on the bone with the edge of the flap at the bony crest.

total operation. It should not be used when bone dehiscence or fenestration is suspected, which is more likely on labially prominent teeth.[87]

The procedure is the same as that described above for the apically positioned flap, except that in Step 3 the periosteum is included when the flap is elevated, leaving the bone exposed (Fig. 46–35).

Comparison of results obtained with partial thickness (mucosal) and full thickness (mucoperiosteal) apically positioned flaps

Both operations eliminate periodontal pockets and correct mucogingival deformities with some limiting side effects. They are not indicated for pocket elimina-

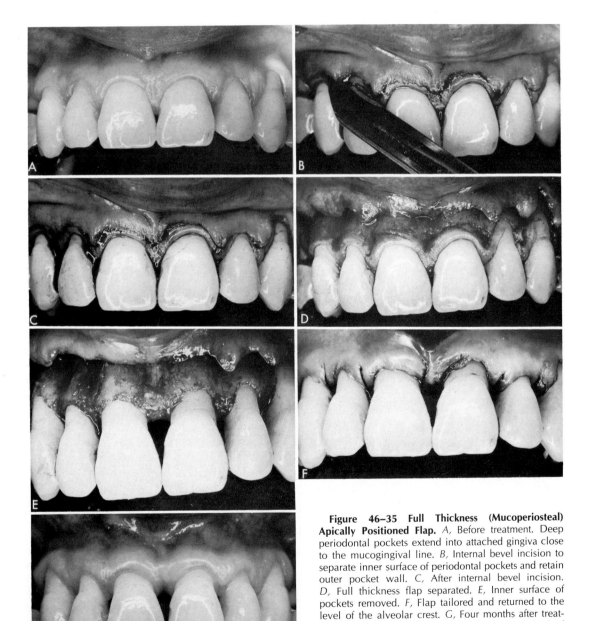

Figure 46–35 Full Thickness (Mucoperiosteal) Apically Positioned Flap. A, Before treatment. Deep periodontal pockets extend into attached gingiva close to the mucogingival line. B, Internal bevel incision to separate inner surface of periodontal pockets and retain outer pocket wall. C, After internal bevel incision. D, Full thickness flap separated. E, Inner surface of pockets removed. F, Flap tailored and returned to the level of the alveolar crest. G, Four months after treatment. Pockets eliminated with healthy zone of attached gingiva.

tion alone, because they result in bone loss and gingival recession not encountered following gingivectomy,[23, 35] without necessarily producing equally satisfactory gingival contours (Fig. 46–36).

Elevating any type of flap results in inflammation and bone resorption and introduces the risk of thinning of bone and loss in bone height,[43, 99, 106, 118] particularly over the roots; some of the damaged tissue undergoes repair. Full thickness flaps produce more bone loss and gingival recession than the partial thickness type,[22, 30, 35, 71, 78, 82, 98, 106, 113, 117, 120] and healing is slower.[18] Mucoperiosteal flaps may create a deeper vestibule, but the gain in width of attached gingiva at the apical end is more than offset by the added gingival recession.[24] Some hold different opinions regarding the relative merits of these flaps[79, 121] and note that they may heal at the same rate[8] or that full thick-

ness flaps heal more rapidly, with less vascular congestion or tissue necrosis.[107]

Laterally (Horizontally) Positioned Flap–Pedicle Graft[50]

Purpose

The purpose of this operation is to cover root surfaces denuded by a gingival defect or periodontal disease and widen the zone of attached gingiva.

Procedure

Step 1: Prepare the Recipient Site. Make a rectangular incision, resecting the periodontal pockets or gingival margin around the exposed root (Figs. 46–37, *A* and Fig. 46–38). The incision should extend to the periosteum and include a border of 2 to 3

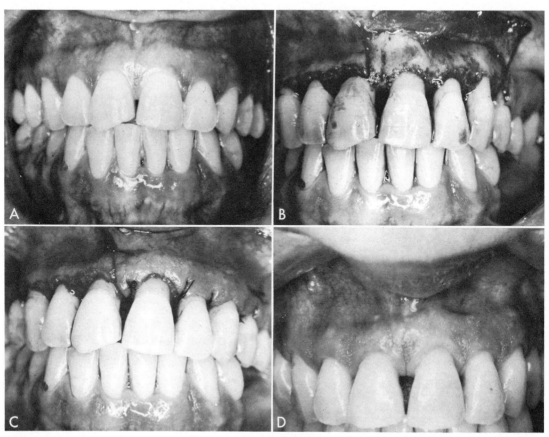

Figure 46–36 Comparison of Gingivectomy and Apically Positioned Full Thickness Flap. *A,* Before treatment. *B,* Gingivectomy on patient's right, full thickness apically positioned flap on the left. *C,* Flap sutured at the crest of the alveolar bone. *D,* Nine months after treatment. The gingival contour is better on the patient's right (gingivectomy side).

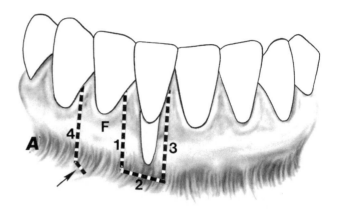

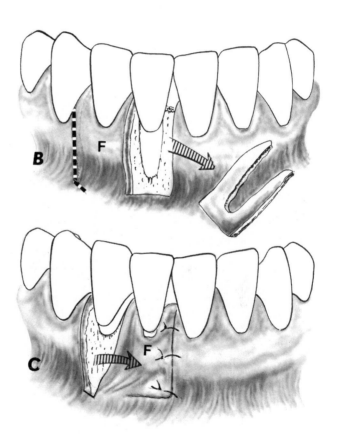

Figure 46–37 Laterally Positioned Flap. *A,* Incisions (1,2,3) made around gingival defect on central incisor. A vertical incision (4) at the distal of the lateral outlines the flap (F) to be positioned. A small angular releasing incision (*arrow*) relieves tension when flap is moved. *B,* Diseased gingival tissue removed from around central incisor (*arrow*), including the periosteum. Tooth scaled and smoothed. *C,* Flap (F), including periosteum, is transferred from the lateral incisor onto the central.

mm. of bone mesial and distal to the root to provide a connective tissue base to which the flap can attach. The rectangle should extend apically for a sufficient distance into the alveolar mucosa to provide space for the zone of attached gingiva.

Remove the resected soft tissue without disturbing the narrow zone of periosteum around the root, and scale and smooth the root surface (Fig. 46–37, *B*).

Step 2: Prepare the Flap. The donor site should be periodontally healthy, with a satisfactory width of attached gingiva and minimal loss of bone, and without dehiscences or fenestrations. Malposed or rotated teeth should be avoided. Inflammation should be eliminated before the flap operation is undertaken. A full thickness or partial thickness flap may be used, but the latter is preferable because it offers

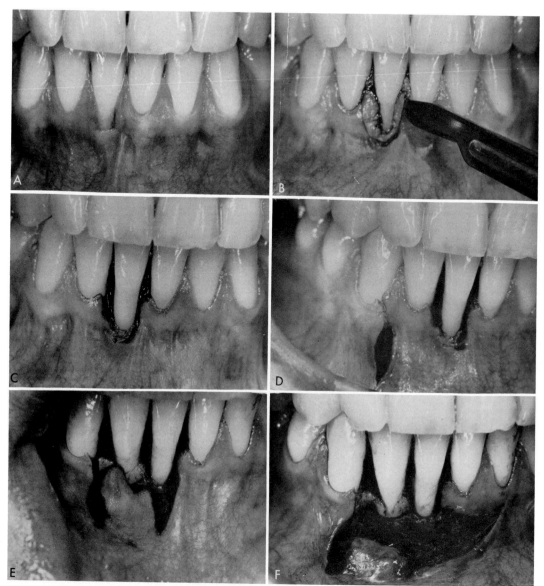

Figure 46–38 Horizontally Repositioned Flap Combined With Relocation of Frenum Attachment. *A,* Gingival defect on central incisor. *B,* Defect incised. *C,* Gingiva removed and tooth scaled and planed. *D,* Vertical incision on canine for sliding flap. *E,* Sliding flap detached. Note high frenum attachment between the central incisors. *F,* Frenum detached and resected to level of vestibular fornix.

the advantage of more rapid healing in the donor site[8] and reduces the risk of loss of facial bone height, particularly if the bone is thin or dehiscence or fenestration is suspected. However, if the gingiva is thin, partial thickness may not be sufficient for flap survival.

With a #15 Bard-Parker blade, make a vertical incision from the gingival margin to outline a flap adjacent to the recipient site. Incise to the periosteum of the bone and extend the incision into the oral mucosa to the level of the base of the recipient site (Fig. 46–37, *B*). The flap should be sufficiently wider than the recipient site to cover the root and provide a broad margin for attachment to the connective tissue border around the root. The interdental papilla at the distal end of the flap or a major portion of it should be included to secure the flap in the interproximal space between the donor and recipient teeth.

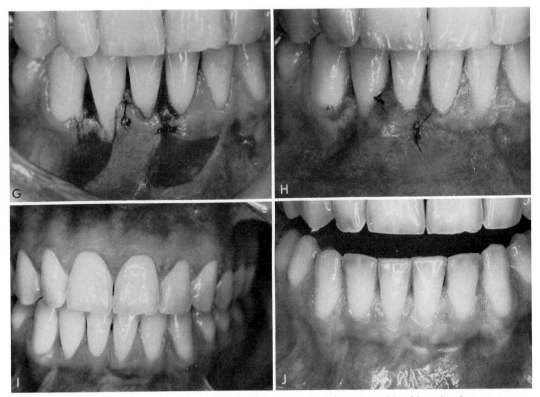

Figure 46–38 Continued G, Sliding flap repositioned laterally on central incisor and fixed lateral and suspensory suture. H, One week postoperation, sutures to be removed. I, Five weeks after operation. J, Seven years after treatment. Note the preservation of gingival position and contour.

Make a vertical incision along the gingival margin and interdental papilla. Insert a #15 Bard-Parker blade into the incision and, directing the blade apically, separate away a flap consisting of epithelium and a thin layer of connective tissue, leaving the periosteum on the bone. Hold the edge of the flap with a tissue forceps, and continue the dissection to the desired depth in the oral vestibule. Tailor the margin of the flap to conform to the recipient site, and thin it if necessary so that it will not be bulbous.

It is sometimes necessary to make a *releasing incision* to avoid tension on the base of the flap which impairs the circulation when the flap is moved. To do this, make an oblique incision into the alveolar mucosa at the distal corner of the flap, pointing in the direction of the recipient site (Fig. 46–37, B).

Step 3: Transfer the Flap. Slide the flap laterally onto the adjacent root, making sure that it lies flat and firm without excess tension on the base. Fix the flap with interrupted sutures to the adjacent gingiva and alveolar mucosa. A suspensory suture may be made around the involved tooth to prevent the flap from slipping apically (Fig. 46–37, C).

Step 4: Protect the Flap and Donor Site. Cover the operative field with a soft periodontal pack, extending it interdentally and onto the lingual surface to secure it. Remove the pack and sutures after one week, and repack twice at weekly intervals.

Variations

There are many variations in the incisions for this operation. A common one is the use of converging oblique incisions over the recipient site and a vertical or oblique incision at the distal end of the donor site (Fig. 46–39) so that the transposed flap is slightly wider at its base. In another modification, the marginal attachment in the donor site is preserved to reduce the likelihood of recession and mar-

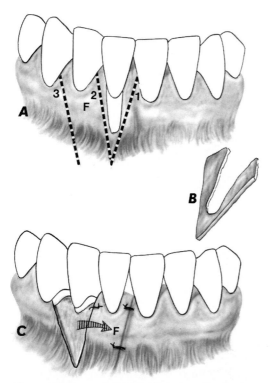

Figure 46–39 Lateral Sliding Flap Using Oblique Incisions. A, Oblique incisions (1 and 2) to remove gingiva around exposed incisor root. Parallel incision (3) to outline flap (F) which is transferred onto root. B, Gingiva removed from around root. C, Partial thickness flap (F) transferred onto incisor root and sutured.

the root remains partially covered. Better results are obtained with narrow, long gingival defects than with broad, shallow ones.

The extent to which the flap "reattaches" to the root with the formation of new cementum and the embedding of new connective tissue fibers has not been settled. Reattachment has been reported on artificially denuded roots in experimental animals,[119] and in some clinical studies in humans,[101, 104, 105] but it does not occur consistently enough to be predictable.

In the donor site, there is uneventful repair and restoration of gingival health and contours, with some loss of radicular bone (0.5 mm.) and recession (1.5 mm.) reported with full thickness flaps.

Double Laterally Positioned Flaps

The laterally repositioned flap is most often used on single teeth. However, when two adjacent roots are exposed, twin flaps are used to correct the condition. The procedure is the same as that for a single lateral flap, except that there are two teeth in the recipient site and there are two donor sites, one on each side of the involved area. The results are the same as those following laterally positioned flaps on single teeth.

ginal bone resorption, but this requires a donor site with a wide zone of attached gingiva.[49]

Accomplishments

Attainment of a functionally satisfactory zone of attached gingiva in the recipient site is not a problem (Figs. 46–38 and 46–40). Some cellular degeneration and necrosis is associated with the transfer of the flap, but this is followed by repair. The morphologic features of the transplanted tissues do not change.[91-93]

Coverage of the exposed root surface is a less definitive matter. The flap attaches to the connective tissue bordering the root and bridges over the formerly denuded root surface. It appears to be attached and may adhere so firmly to the root as to resist insertion of a periodontal probe.[2] There is some shrinkage of the flap with time, but

Double Papillae Positioned Flaps[27, 52]

The purposes of this operation are to restore the zone of attached gingiva and to attempt to cover roots denuded by isolated gingival defects with a flap formed by joining two interdental papillae. It is recommended when the areas bordering the gingival defect are unsatisfactory for a laterally positioned flap because of insufficient attached gingiva or deep periodontal pockets. These problems are overcome by utilizing the contiguous halves of the adjacent interdental papillae. The interdental papillae provide a zone of attached gingiva which is usually wider than on the radicular surface and also reduce the risk of loss in radicular bone height because the bone is thicker interdentally than on the roots.

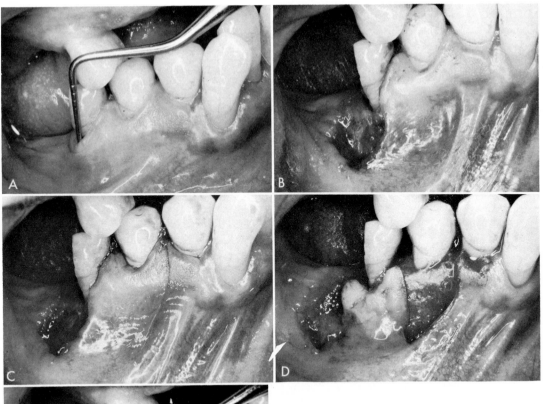

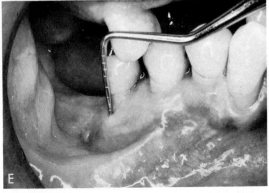

Figure 46–40 Partial Thickness Lateral Sliding Flap. *A,* Before treatment. Periodontal pocket on second premolar extends into the alveolar mucosa. *B,* Second premolar—V-shaped recipient site prepared to receive the flap. *C,* Flap outlined on the first premolar. *D,* Partial thickness flap transferred to second premolar. *E,* Seven months after treatment, showing shallow gingival sulcus and widened zone of attached gingiva. Compare with *A.* (Courtesy of Edward S. Cohen, D.M.D.)

Procedure

Step 1: Prepare the Recipient Site. With periodontal knives or a #15 Bard-Parker blade, make a V-shaped incision and re-section the diseased gingiva around the involved root. Scale and smooth the root surfaces (Fig. 46–41, *A* and *B*).

Step 2: Prepare the Flaps. With a #15 Bard-Parker blade, start at the gingival margin lateral to the mesial and distal interdental papillae and make a slightly oblique incision into the oral vestibule to the level of the V-shaped incision on the involved root. This will outline the flaps,

each of which consists of part of the inter-dental papillae on both sides of the root (Fig. 46–41, *B*). Each flap is broader at its base than at the gingival margin. Make a horizontal incision across the tip of each interdental papilla. Separate a partial thick-ness flap on each side of the root by inserting a #15 Bard-Parker blade into the oblique incision beneath the alveolar mucosa and moving it to the tip of the inter-dental papilla. Thin the edge of the flap to avoid a bulky gingival margin after healing.

Step 3: Transfer and Secure the Flaps. Move the flaps together until they meet

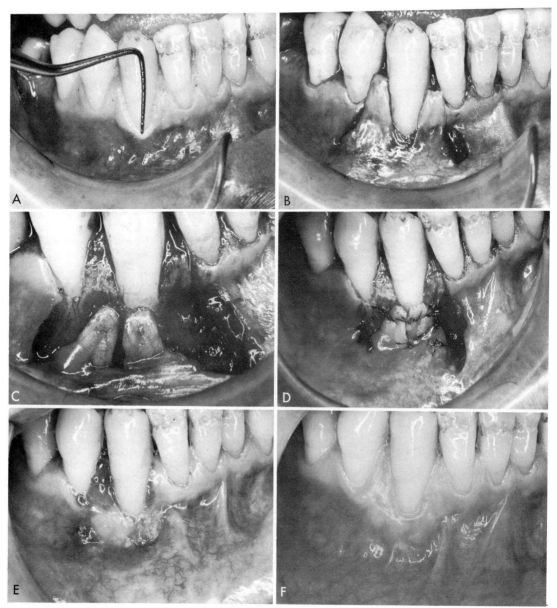

Figure 46–41 Double Papillae Flap. *A,* Before treatment. Narrow band of attached gingiva on the canine. *B,* Mesial and distal papillae separated. *C,* Papillae transferred to the canine. *D,* Papillae placed on bony plate and sutured to the periosteum. *E,* After one week. *F,* After seven months. Note the widened zone of attached gingiva. Compare with *A.* (Courtesy of Edward S. Cohen, D.M.D.)

over the root surface (Fig. 46–41, *C*). The outer epithelium of one section is sometimes removed so that the flaps can be overlapped with two connective tissue surfaces in contact. Suture the flaps together on the bone with interrupted sutures secured to the periosteum to prevent the flaps from slipping apically (Fig. 46–41, *D*). A suspensory suture through the margin of the joined flaps and around the neck of the tooth may also be used for this purpose.

Step 4: Protect the Flaps. Cover the operative field with a soft periodontal dressing for one week. Remove the sutures and repack for another week (Fig. 46–41, *E* and *F*).

Sliding Partial Thickness Flap from an Edentulous Area (Pedicle Graft)

The purpose of this operation is to restore attached gingiva on teeth adjacent to edentulous spaces with denuded roots and a small vestibular fornix, often complicated by tension from a frenum.[28] A partial thickness flap of masticatory mucosa from the adjacent edentulous ridge is used.

Procedure

Step 1: Prepare the Recipient Site. With a #15 Bard-Parker blade, make a V-shaped incision from the gingival margin mesial

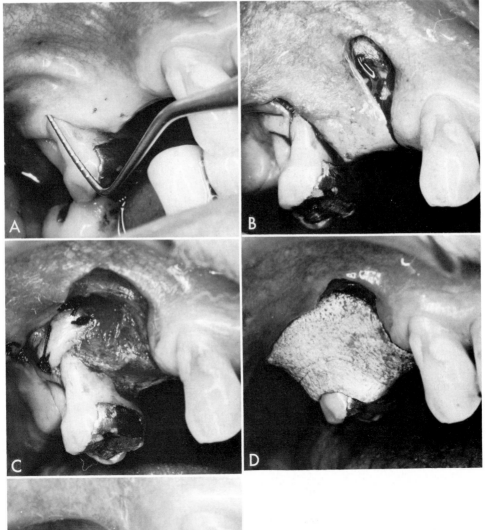

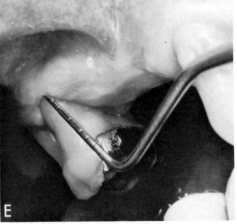

Figure 46–42 Laterally Positioned Flap From Edentulous Area. *A,* Before treatment. Note absence of attached gingiva on the mesiobuccal root of the molar. *B,* Wedge-shaped recipient site prepared over mesiobuccal root and partial thickness flap outlined in edentulous area. *C,* Flap transferred to bone over mesiobuccal root and sutured. *D,* Periodontal pack in position. *E,* After eight months. Note the zone of attached gingiva on the mesiobuccal root. Compare with *A.* (Courtesy of Edward S. Cohen, D.M.D.)

and distal to the involved tooth into the alveolar mucosa apical to the root apex or apices (Fig. 46–42, *A* and *B*); include frenum attachments in the resected area. Elevate the tip of the tissue wedge outlined by the incision with a tissue forceps, and dissect away the wedge of tissue with a #15 Bard-Parker blade. Leave the periosteum and covering connective tissue on the bone, except in areas where bone is to be recontoured. Remove the loose strands or clumps of tissue from the connective tissue surface to provide a firm base for the transferred flap.

Step 2: Scale and Smooth the Root Surfaces.

Step 3: Prepare the Flap. Make an incision along the crest of the edentulous ridge from the proximal tooth surface for a distance equal to or slightly longer than the width of the recipient site. From the end of the incision make a vertical incision from the crest of the ridge into the alveolar mucosa to the level of the base of the wedge-shaped recipient site, outlining a flap which is wider at the base (Fig. 46–42, *B*). Insert a periodontal knife into the incision at the crest of the ridge, and separate away a partial thickness flap of masticatory mucosa, leaving the periosteum on the bone, and continue the separation into the alveolar mucosa.

If the mucogingival junction is high on the edentulous ridge and the buccal masticatory mucosa is narrow, masticatory mucosa from the lingual surface is included in the graft. The initial incision is made on the lingual surface close to, but not at, the mucogingival junction.

Step 4: Transfer the Flap. To facilitate free movement of the flap without stretching or twisting the pedicle and interfering with the circulation, a short, oblique releasing incision may be made at the base in the direction the flap is to be moved. Check the recipient site to be sure bleeding has stopped and remove excessive clot from the surface.

Move the flap laterally and place it firmly on the recipient surface with the free end of the flap at the margin of the bone. Suture one margin of the flap to the adjacent cut tissue surface and the other to the periosteum (Fig. 46–42, *C*). A suspensory suture may be made through the free margin of the flap around the tooth to prevent the flap from slipping apically. Cover the area with a periodontal pack which is removed with the sutures after one week (Fig. 46–37, *D*). Repack two more times at weekly intervals (Fig. 46–37, *E*).

Coronally Positioned Pedicle Graft (Kalmi, Moscor, Goranov[59])

Of historical interest is an operation developed in an effort to improve the esthetics in patients with teeth denuded by advanced periodontal disease. It consists of covering denuded roots of maxillary anterior teeth by sliding pedicle flaps from adjacent uninvolved gingiva and alveolar mucosa as follows (Fig. 46–43):

Periodontal pockets are resected by gingivectomy, and the roots are scaled and smoothed. A mucoperiosteal flap as wide as the exposed root surface and outlined by a horizontal incision across the anterior maxilla is elevated from the bone (Fig. 46–43, *A* and *B*). The flap is divided in two by a midline V-shaped incision at the frenum, and the two flaps are moved onto the roots and sutured. Reattachment of the flaps to the exposed roots has been reported in experimental animals,[54] but not in humans.[74]

Coronally Positioned Flap[51]

The purposes of this operation are to eliminate periodontal pockets and to attempt to obtain reattachment of the gingiva to root surface previously denuded by disease.

Procedure

The inner wall of the periodontal pockets is separated from the outer wall, and a mucoperiosteal flap is laid back, exposing the diseased area. The inner walls of the pockets are removed, and the tooth surfaces are scaled free of deposits and smoothed.

The flap is returned and sutured in place at a level **coronal to the pretreatment position**. The area is covered with periodontal pack, which is removed with sutures after one week. The pack is repeated for an additional week if necessary.

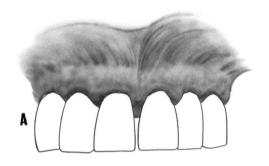

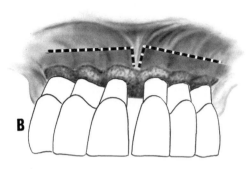

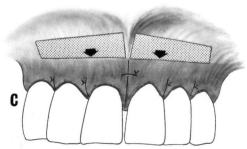

Figure 46–43 Coronally Positioned Pedicle Flap. *A,* Patient with deep periodontal pockets. *B,* Periodontal pockets removed and roots scaled and planed. Mucoperiosteal flaps are outlined by horizontal and vertical incisions indicated by dotted lines. *C,* Flaps drawn down over the root surfaces as indicated by arrows and joined and sutured in position over the roots. The bone in the stippled areas is denuded.

The Unrepositioned Flap[63]

The purposes of this procedure are to eliminate disease from periodontal pockets and to attempt to obtain gingival reattachment to previously denuded root surfaces. It is similar to the simple flap in that it utilizes mucogingival flaps which are sutured to their presurgical location at the end of the operation.

Procedure

Step 1: Resect the Inner Pocket Wall. Under local anesthesia, mark the bottom of the periodontal pockets and make a vertical incision from the gingival margin to the vestibular fornix at each end of the field of operation on the facial and lingual surfaces. Separate the inner aspect of the periodontal pockets from the outer pocket wall by inserting a #15 Bard-Parker blade from the margin of the pockets to the crest of the underlying bone.

Step 2: Elevate the Flaps. With a periosteal elevator, lay back the facial and lingual mucoperiosteal flaps from the outer wall of the periodontal pockets to the vestibular fornix.

Step 3: Remove the Inner Pocket Wall from the Root. Remove the adherent inner walls of the periodontal pockets from the roots, making a special effort to remove the entire epithelial attachment.

Step 4: Scale and Smooth the Tooth Surfaces.

Step 5. Replace the flaps on the teeth and bone and suture in firm apposition with the root surfaces. The area is covered with periodontal pack, which is removed with the sutures after one week.

The Management of Bulbous Tuberosities and Retromolar Pads (Distal Wedge Operation[84] and Linear Distal Incision Operation[16])

The treatment of periodontal pockets on the distal surface of terminal molars is frequently complicated by the presence of bulbous fibrous tissue over the maxillary tuberosity or prominent retromolar pads in the mandible. The most direct approach to pocket elimination in such cases is to resect the bulbous tissue and the pocket wall with a gingivectomy incision (Fig. 46–44). To assure complete removal of the bulbous tissue, the incision is started on the distal surface of the tuberosity and carried forward to the distal surface of the tooth apical to the base of the pocket.

When there is little attached gingiva or an

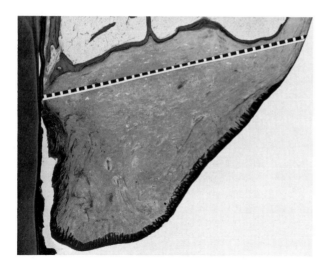

Figure 46–44 Removal of Bulbous Fibrous Tissue Over Maxillary Tuberosity With Gingivectomy Incision.

infrabony pocket with an osseous defect, it is desirable to reduce the bulbous tissue rather than remove it, for the following reasons: to produce attached gingiva, to provide access to the osseous defect and to preserve mucosa for protection of the healing wound. Reduction of bulbous tuberosity pads or retromolar pads entails removing the central core of tissue responsible for the bulk and preserving the mucosal walls to serve as covering flaps.

Operation

Operations for this purpose were described by Robinson[84] and Braden.[16] They may be modified according to individual requirements. The following is a representative procedure:

Step 1. A triangular wedge is cut in the bulbous tuberosity or retromolar pad, extending from the distal surface of the tooth (the base of the triangle) to the distal border of the soft tissue and from the external surface to the periosteum. The facial and lingual incisions should be extended anteriorly for a short distance on the tooth to provide accessibility to the entire distal surface (Fig. 46–45, A) and for additional periodontal surgery, if necessary.

Step 2. Deflect the facial and lingual walls of the fibrous pad and, with a periodontal knife, resect the central core of tissue at its base, including the periosteum if recontouring of bone is intended (Fig. 46–45, A).

Step 3. With reverse bevel incisions,

undermine the walls of the flaps to the width of the underlying bone. Remove the resected tissue, leaving twin buccal and palatal flaps (Fig. 46–45, B). Separate the flaps and the periosteum from the buccal and lingual surfaces of the tuberosity to increase visibility and accessibility to the bone (Fig. 46–45, C). If necessary, make an oblique releasing incision at the distal end of each flap to avoid tension on the tissues (Fig. 46–45, D).

Step 4. Scale and smooth the root surface. If an osseous defect is present, curette the inner walls to remove intact fibers which interfere with vascularization and healing.

Step 5. Cleanse the area with warm water. Apply pressure with 2″ × 2″ gauze pads until a clot is formed and remove the excess. Adapt the buccal and lingual flaps over the bone, trimming the edges to avoid overlapping and suture for one week (Fig. 46–45, E).

Palatal Flaps

Osseous defects are frequently corrected more effectively and with less tissue loss when approached from the palate than from the buccal surface. Palatal flaps are used for osseous correction and for the reduction of bulbous fibrous tissue.

The palatal flap operation consists of resecting the inner aspect of the periodontal pockets with an internal bevel from the tip of the gingival margin to a point

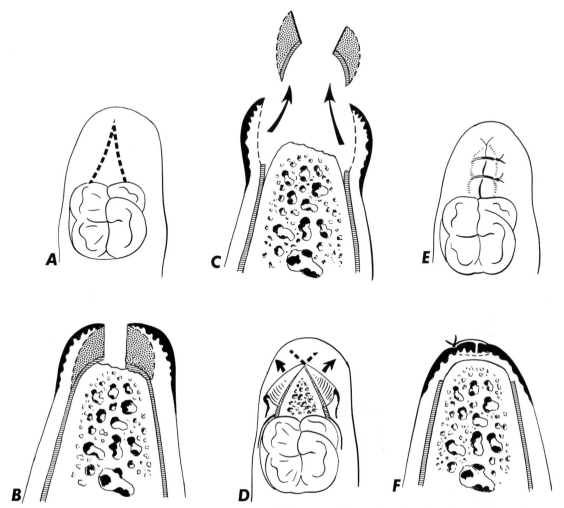

Figure 46–45 Distal Wedge Operation for Reduction of Fibrous Maxillary Tuberosity Pad and Treatment of Osseous Defect. *A,* Distal wedge outlined by triangular incisions. *B,* Section of bulbous fibrous tissue removed, including the periosteum over osseous defect. Additional tissue to be removed is shown in dotted areas. *C,* Fibrous pads removed, including the periosteum (*lined area*), exposing osseous defect and creating thin palatal and buccal flaps. *D,* Releasing incisions (*dotted lines*) provide greater access to underlying bone. Flap extended onto the buccal and palatal surfaces of the molar. *E,* Flaps replaced and sutured after tooth is scaled and smoothed and bone is contoured. *F,* Cross section showing buccal and palatal flaps sutured and bone contoured.

slightly apical to the crest of the palatal bone (Fig. 46–46, *A*). A periodontal knife is inserted into the incision, and a full thickness flap is separated from the bone to provide access for bone corrective procedures (Fig. 46–46, *A*, *B* and *C*). The inner aspect of the pockets is removed; the roots are scaled and smoothed, and the osseous defects are corrected. The flap is replaced and sutured (Fig. 46–46, *E*) and covered with periodontal pack. The sutures and pack are removed in a week, and the area is replaced for an additional week or more if necessary.

Free Gingival Autografts[9,64,77,94]

Free gingival grafts are used to create a widened zone of attached gingiva and to deepen the vestibular fornix to provide space for it. They have also been tried for covering denuded roots.

Procedure

Step 1: Eliminate the Pockets. With a gingivectomy incision, resect the periodontal pockets and scale and smooth the root surfaces.

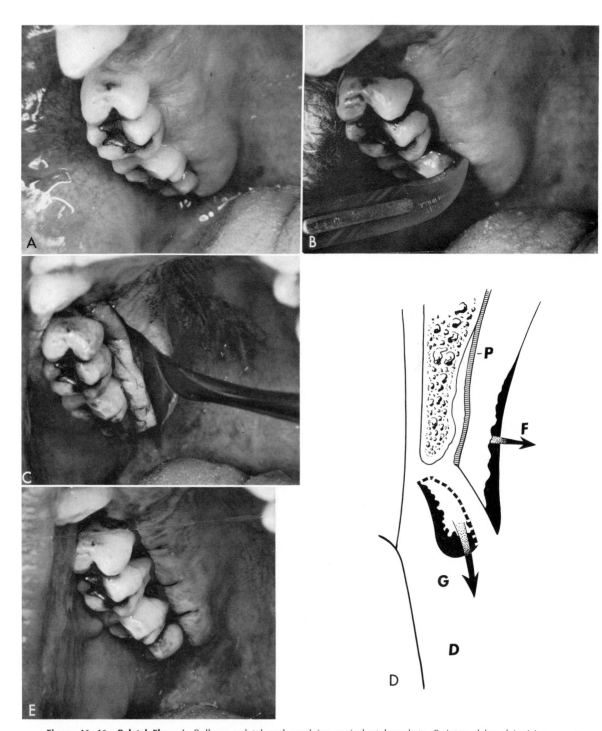

Figure 46–46   Palatal Flap. *A,* Bulbous palatal pad overlying periodontal pockets. *B,* Internal bevel incision resects inner pocket wall and thins palatal gingiva. *C,* Palatal tissue separated from inner pocket wall along line of incision. *D,* Inner pocket wall (G) removed. Flap (F) including periosteum (P), is elevated from bulbous bone. *E,* Bone is contoured, teeth are scaled and planed and thinned palatal tissue is sutured.

Step 2: Prepare the Recipient Site. The purpose of this step is to prepare a firm connective tissue bed to receive the graft. With a #15 Bard-Parker blade outline the recipient site with two vertical incisions from the cut gingival margin into the alveolar mucosa (Fig. 46–47, *A* and *B*). Extend the incisions to approximately twice the desired width of the attached gingiva, allowing for 50 per cent contrac-

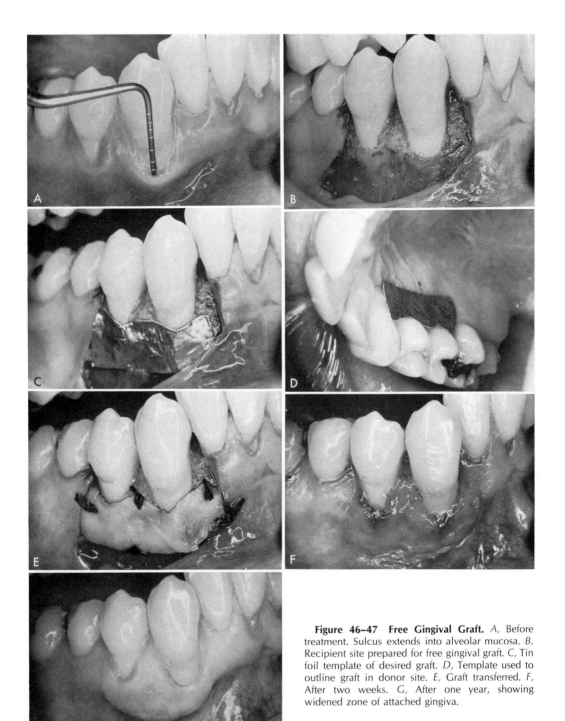

Figure 46–47 Free Gingival Graft. *A,* Before treatment. Sulcus extends into alveolar mucosa. *B,* Recipient site prepared for free gingival graft. *C,* Tin foil template of desired graft. *D,* Template used to outline graft in donor site. *E,* Graft transferred. *F,* After two weeks. *G,* After one year, showing widened zone of attached gingiva.

tion of the graft when healing is complete. The amount of contraction depends upon the extent to which the recipient site penetrates the muscle attachments. The deeper the recipient site, the greater is the tendency for the muscles to elevate the graft and reduce the final width of the attached gingiva. The periosteum along the apical border of the graft is sometimes penetrated in an effort to prevent postoperative narrowing of the attached gingiva.[17]

Insert a #15 Bard-Parker blade along the cut gingival margin, and separate a flap consisting of epithelium and underlying connective tissue without disturbing the periosteum. Extend the flap to the depth of the vertical incisions. Make a horizontal incision to resect and remove the flap. If a narrow band of attached gingiva remains after the pockets are eliminated, it should be left intact and the recipient site started by inserting the blade at the mucogingival junction, instead of at the cut gingival margin.

Prepare the recipient bed for the graft by removing extraneous soft tissue with a curved scissors #25G or tissue nippers, leaving a firm connective tissue surface. Control the bleeding with a 2" × 2" sponge and pressure, and protect the area with a sponge moistened with saline. Make a template of tinfoil or wax template of the recipient site to be used as a pattern for the graft (Fig. 46–47, C and D).

Step 3: Obtain the Graft from Donor Site. A partial thickness graft is used; the sites from which it is obtained are, in order of preference, attached gingiva, masticatory mucosa from an edentulous ridge, and palatal mucosa. The graft should consist of epithelium and a thin layer, approximately 3 mm., of underlying connective tissue. Proper thickness is important for survival of the graft. It should be thin enough to permit ready diffusion of nutritive fluid from the recipient site, which is essential in the immediate post-transplant period. A graft which is too thin may shrivel and expose the recipient site.[77] If it is too thick, its peripheral layer is jeopardized because of the excessive tissue which separates it from new circulation and nutrients.[40]

Place the template over the donor site, and make a shallow incision around it with a #15 Bard-Parker blade. Insert the blade

to the desired thickness at one edge of the graft. Elevate the edge and hold it with a tissue forceps. Continue to separate the graft with the blade, lifting it gently as separation progresses to provide visibility. Placing sutures at the margins of the graft helps control it during separation and transfer and simplifies placement and suturing to the recipient site.[6]

After the graft is separated, remove loose tissue tabs from the undersurface. Thin the edge to avoid bulbous marginal and interdental contours. Special precaution must be taken with grafts from the palate. The submucosa in the posterior region is thick and fatty and should be trimmed so that it will not interfere with vascularization. Grafts tend to re-establish their original epithelial structure so that mucous glands may occur in grafts obtained from the palate.

Step 4: Transfer and Immobilize the Graft. Remove the sponge from the recipient site, reapply with pressure if necessary until bleeding is stopped. Clean away excess clot. A thick clot interferes with vascularization of the graft;[72] it is also an excellent medium for bacteria and increases the risk of infection.

Position the graft and adapt it firmly to the recipient site. Space between the graft and the underlying tissue (dead space) will retard vascularization and jeopardize the graft. Suture the graft at the lateral borders and to the periosteum to secure it in position (Fig. 46–47, E). Before suturing is complete, elevate the unsutured portion and cleanse the recipient bed beneath it with an aspirator to remove clot or loose tissue fragments. Press the graft back into position and complete the sutures. Be sure the graft is immobilized, because movement interferes with healing. Avoid excessive tension which will warp the graft and may pull it away from the underlying surface.

Respect for tissue is essential for success. Use every precaution to avoid injury to the graft. Use tissue forceps delicately to avoid crushing it. Use a minimum number of sutures to avoid unnecessary tissue penetration. The graft can survive some injury, but abuse may damage it beyond recovery.

Cover with periodontal pack for one week when the sutures are removed (Fig. 46–47, F). Repack for another week.

Step 5: Protect the Donor Site. Cover the donor site with periodontal pack for one week and repeat if necessary. Retention of the pack on the donor site is sometimes a problem. If facial or buccal attached gingiva was used, the pack may be retained by locking it through the interproximal spaces onto the lingual surface. If there are no open interdental spaces, the pack can be covered by a plastic stent wired to the teeth. A modified Hawley retainer is useful to cover the pack on the palate and over edentulous ridges.

The fate of the graft

The success of the graft depends upon survival of the connective tissue (Fig. 46–47, G). Sloughing of the epithelium occurs in most cases, but the extent to which the connective tissue withstands the transfer to the new location determines the fate of the graft. Fibrous organization of the interface between the graft and the recipient bed occurs within two to several days.[97]

The graft is initially maintained by a diffusion of fluid from the host bed, adjacent gingiva and alveolar mucosa.[40] The fluid is a transudate from the host vessels and provides nutrition and hydration essential for the initial survival of the transplanted tissues. During the first day, the connective tissue becomes edematous and disorganized and undergoes degeneration and lysis of some of its elements. As healing progresses, the edema is resolved and degenerated connective tissue is replaced by new granulation tissue.

Revascularization of the graft starts by the second[15] or third day.[58] Capillaries from the recipient bed and from periodontal ligament included in the recipient site proliferate into the graft to form a network of new capillaries and anastomose with pre-existing vessels.[58] Many of the graft vessels degenerate and are replaced by new ones, and some participate in the new circulation. The central section of the surface is the last to vascularize, and is complete by the tenth day.

The epithelium undergoes degeneration and sloughing, with complete necrosis occurring in some areas.[72] It is replaced by new epithelium from the borders of the recipient site. A thin layer of new epithelium is present by the fourth day, with rete pegs developing by the seventh day. In skin grafts the basement membrane remains in situ, disengaged from the overlying epithelium and attached to the underlying connective tissue. New epithelial cells migrate over the basal membrane and appear to be guided by it. The plasma membrane of the cells thickens and forms hemidesmosomes that attach to the basement membrane, and the regenerating epithelium synthesizes new basement membrane.[41]

Microscopically, healing of a graft of intermediate thickness (0.75 mm.) is complete by ten and one half weeks; thicker grafts (1.75 mm.) may require 16 weeks or longer.[46]

The gross appearance of the graft reflects the tissue changes within it. At the time of transplant, the graft vessels empty and the graft is pale. The pallor changes to an ischemic gray-white during the first two days, until vascularization begins and pink color appears. The plasmatic circulation accumulates and causes softening and swelling of the graft, which is reduced when the edema is removed by the new blood vessels from the recipient site. Loss of epithelium leaves the graft smooth and shiny. New epithelium creates a thin, gray, veil-like surface which develops normal features as the epithelium matures.

Functional intergration of the graft occurs by the seventeenth day, but the graft is morphologically distinguishable from surrounding tissue for months. It may eventually blend with adjacent tissues, but more often, although it is pink, firm and healthy, it tends to be somewhat bulbous (Figs. 46–48 and 46–49). This ordinarily presents no problem, but if it traps irritating plaque or is esthetically unacceptable, thinning of the graft may be necessary.

Thinning bulbous grafts

Paring down the surface will not reduce the bulbous condition, because the surface epithelium tends to proliferate again. The graft should be thinned as follows:

Step 1. With a #15 Bard-Parker blade, make vertical incisions along the lateral border of the graft to the gingival margin. If the graft does not extend to the gingival margin, make the incisions along three of the borders.

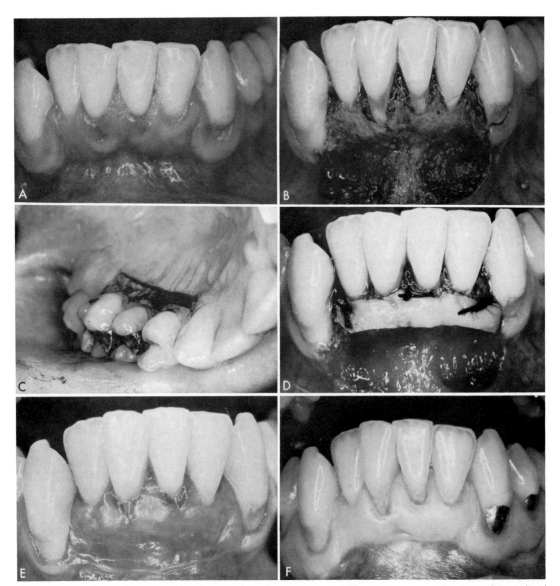

Figure 46–48 Free Gingival Graft (same patient as Fig. 46–47). *A,* Before treatment—pockets extend into alveolar mucosa. *B,* Recipient site prepared for graft. *C,* Graft obtained from the palate. *D,* Graft sutured in position. *E,* After two weeks. *F,* After one year. Note the widened zone of attached gingiva.

Step 2.   Elevate the graft from the underlying periosteum, and thin it by removing tissue from the undersurface.

Step 3.   Replace the graft and suture.

Accomplishments of free gingival grafts

Free gingival grafts effectively widen the attached gingiva and deepen the oral vestibule. Compared with other operations for the same purposes, they entail involvement of an additional operative site (the donor site). Some feel that grafts protect the underlying bone,[108] in that they cause less osteoclastic activity and stimulate osteoblastic activity and thickening of the bone.[15] If this were so, it would be advantageous to use grafts for widening attached gingiva when the facial bone is thin.

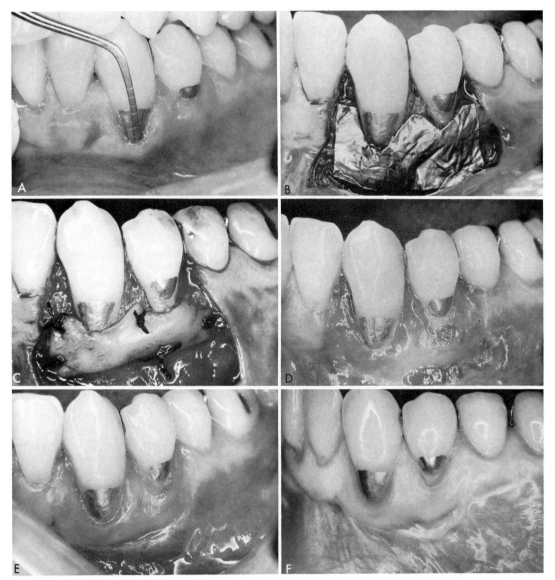

Figure 46–49 **Free Gingival Graft** (same patient as Figs. 46–47 and 46–48). *A,* Before treatment—periodontal pocket in the canine extends into the alveolar mucosa. *B,* Recipient site prepared and template made for desired graft. *C,* Graft sutured in place. *D,* After two weeks. *E,* After nine weeks. *F,* After one year. Note the widened zone of healthy attached gingiva. Compare with *A.*

Free gingival grafts and denuded roots

Roots denuded by gingival defects are unattractive and are commonly the sites of plaque accumulation and persistent gingival disease. The incentive for experimenting with procedures which offer promise of restoring the gingiva on denuded roots is great. Grafts placed over exposed roots generally shrink, re-exposing part of the root, but covering a portion of it, particularly when the gingival defect is long and narrow.

Since the vascular bed is required for preservation of a free gingival graft, it cannot be expected to correct extensive root exposure.[53, 97] However, if the gingival defect is narrow, collateral circulation from the connective tissue around the margins of the recipient site aids survival of the graft over the root.[102] The graft may be firmly adherent and resist separation from the tooth by a periodontal probe,[64] but the extent to which it is reattached to the root by new fibers embedded into new cementum has not been established. Reattachment of free gingival grafts has been reported on artificially exposed roots in animals,[73] but the results in humans are as yet inconclusive.[101, 103]

OSSEOUS SURGERY

The term osseous surgery refers to surgical procedures performed on bone for the purposes of reshaping or restoring it. Osseous surgery is concerned with the correction of bony defects produced by periodontal disease or anatomic deformity or a combination of both. They are most often associated with infrabony pockets, but may also occur beneath the suprabony type. The defects include interproximal craters or angular defects, facial and lingual angular defects, thick bony ledges and irregularities in the level of interproximal and radicular bone and exostoses. (For a description of osseous defects and their formation, see Chapter 16.)

The procedures in osseous surgery fit into two categories: (1) bone resection and reshaping to correct osseous defects and create physiologic osseous contours, and (2) implant procedures to stimulate bone growth and restore tissue destroyed by disease.

Correction of Osseous Defects by Bone Resection and Remodeling

The procedures used for this purpose are designated by such terms as "osseous resection,"[69, 89] "plastic remodeling,"[20] "osteoplasty" and "osteoectomy."[38] *Osteoplasty refers to reshaping the bone without removing tooth-supporting bone. Osteoectomy includes removal of tooth-supporting bone.* There is considerable difference of opinion regarding the wisdom of artificially remodeling bone in the treatment of periodontal disease. It is a severe form of therapy which involves more than just the mechanical reshaping of a structure; biologic processes involved in the bone response may produce more severe alterations

in bone morphology than the therapist intended.

The need for reshaping bone to an idealized form is based upon the assumption that if defects are permitted to persist following periodontal treatment, they will cause deformity of the overlying gingiva followed by retention of irritating plaque and debris and recurrence of pockets. **However, in healing, following periodontal surgery the gingiva does not necessarily follow the contour of the underlying bone.** The morphology of the interdental gingiva depends more upon the shape and contour of the proximal tooth surfaces than upon the shape of the underlying bone.[123] On the facial and lingual surfaces, the level of attachment and contour of the gingiva are often unrelated to the height or shape of the underlying radicular bone.[43]

Osteoplasty and osteoectomy are used in association with pocket elimination procedures and mucogingival operations. Most bone defects under suprabony pockets are remodeled by osteoclastic and osteoblastic activity in normal post-treatment healing (Fig. 46–50). Osseous defects associated with infrabony pockets are a more serious problem, but every effort should be made to obtain natural remodeling and filling in of the defects before resorting to bone resection. Removing facial and lingual bone and soft tissue to the level of interproximal craters in an attempt to eliminate interproximal pockets may result in undesirable reductions in the level of gingival attachment.[80] (For the treatment of infrabony pockets, see Chapter 44.)

When used with mucoperiosteal periodontal flaps, bone recontouring by grinding increases the post-treatment loss in bone height.[34] Slight reshaping with chisels is reportedly followed by complete restoration of bone in experimental animals.[18] The post-treatment contour of the facial bone under periodontal flaps is also affected by the occlusion.[44]

Grinding with stones causes bone degeneration and necrosis on the bone surface where tissue viability is required for healing. It retards healing because of the additional time required for the cellular and enzymatic removal of the injured tissue before the reconstruction phase of repair occurs. New bone can form in vascular spaces adjacent to necrotic zones produced

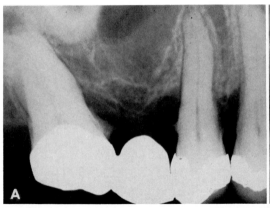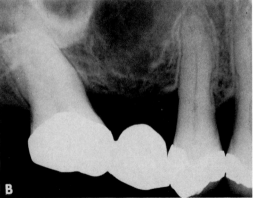

Figure 46–50 Angular Bone Defects Repaired by Healing Without Osseous Surgery. *A,* Angular bone defects under bridge. *B,* Three years after pocket elimination and occlusal adjustment. (Dr. Carl Stoner, New London, Conn.)

by grinding; it is more likely to occur in areas cut with high-speed rather than low-speed rotary instruments.[14] The thickness of the bone affects the results produced by grinding. Interdental septa may retain the shapes artificially created for them,[61] but grinding thin radicular bone produces bone necrosis which, despite attempts at repair, results in loss of bone and unpredictable morphology.[60] Reducing the crest of thick cancellous facial bone by osteoectomy and osteoplasty is followed by repair and restoration of presurgical levels, but further reduction of height occurs if the bone is thin.[76]

Despite the risk it entails, there are instances in which recontouring of the bone is required. In patients with exostoses, when it can be anticipated that the bone deformity will interfere with the attainment of satisfactory post-treatment oral hygiene and gingival health, the bone is reshaped when the pockets are eliminated (Fig. 46–51). In other situations, the bone should not be artificially remodeled until other treatment procedures combined with conscientious patient cooperation fail to achieve the desired results.

Techniques for remodeling bone

The bone is most often remodeled with coarse mounted diamond stones (Fig. 46–52), but bone files, rongeurs, chisels or large round burs may be used. With diamond stones or burs, the area is bathed in a stream of warm water to minimize injury from frictional heat.

Correction of exostoses

Make a vertical incision from the gingival margin to the mucobuccal fold mesial and distal to the involved area, and raise a gingival flap, including the periosteum of the bone (Fig. 46–53). With a coarse rotating diamond stone, under a stream of water, reduce the bulk of the bone and reshape it in conformity with the prominence of the roots, create interdental grooves, taper the interproximal bone inward toward the crest, and eliminate marginal irregularities. Remove all tissue debris, replace the flap, suture and cover with periodontal pack.

The pack is removed after one week and repeated at weekly intervals until the patient is comfortable.

Correction of interdental craters

Interdental craters may be corrected by reducing the facial or lingual wall or both to the base of the crater and tapering the bone inward and toward the crown. To preserve the facial bone in the anterior maxilla[19] (Fig. 46–54) and avoid bone loss and denudation of the buccal roots of the maxillary molars, the major correction is done on the lingual surface[70] (Fig. 46–55). The lingual wall of the crater is reduced and the bone is ramped and tapered toward the tooth.

Correction of thick bony ledges

Persistent, thick, shelf-like marginal ledges which interfere with the main-
(Text continued on page 777.)

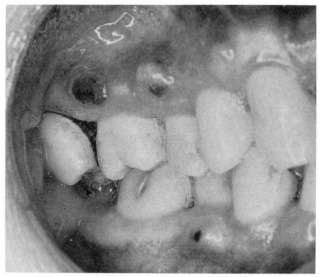

Figure 46–51 Patient with Exostoses on Maxilla and Mandible. Note the scuffing caused by toothbrushing.

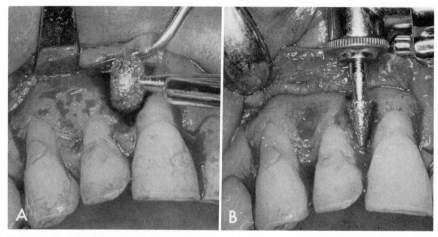

Figure 46–52 Bone Contoured with Diamond Stone. *A,* Round stone used to reduce prominence of labial bone. *B,* Tapered stone used to create interdental sluiceways.

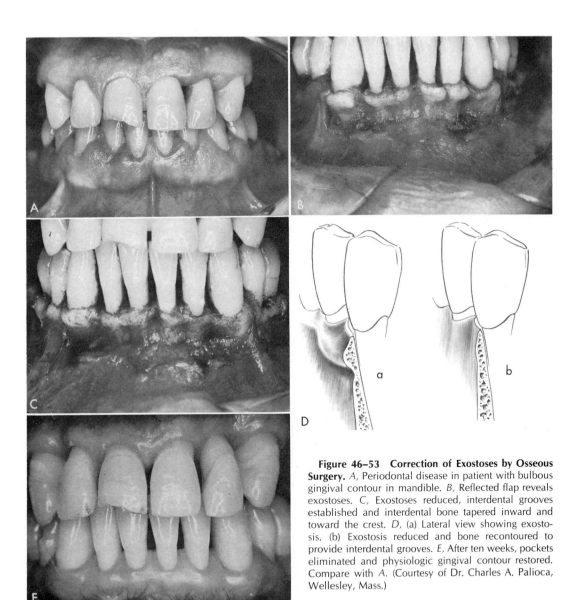

Figure 46–53   Correction of Exostoses by Osseous Surgery. *A,* Periodontal disease in patient with bulbous gingival contour in mandible. *B,* Reflected flap reveals exostoses. *C,* Exostoses reduced, interdental grooves established and interdental bone tapered inward and toward the crest. *D,* (a) Lateral view showing exostosis. (b) Exostosis reduced and bone recontoured to provide interdental grooves. *E,* After ten weeks, pockets eliminated and physiologic gingival contour restored. Compare with *A.* (Courtesy of Dr. Charles A. Palioca, Wellesley, Mass.)

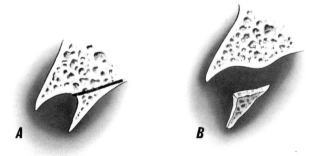

Figure 46–54   Palatal Approach to Correction of Interdental Crater. *A,* Interdental crater between maxillary incisors. Bone correction is indicated by black line. *B,* Corrected bone contour attained by bone removal. (After Carranza.)

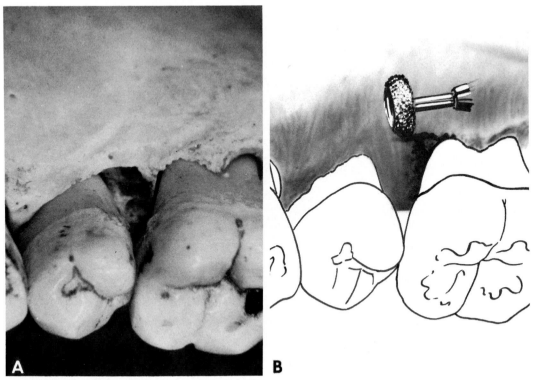

Figure 46–55   Interdental Defect Reduced by Palatal Approach. *A,* Palatal view of osseous defect on the distal surface of maxillary second premolar. *B,* Palatal wall of crater reduced and tapered with diamond stone.

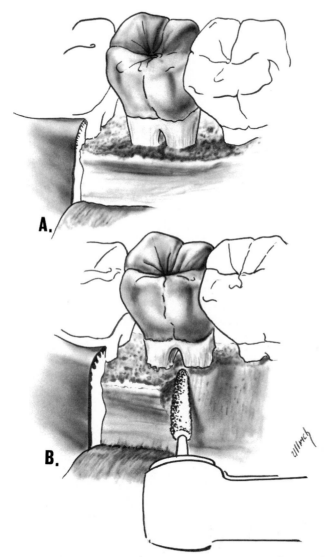

Figure 46–56   A. Remodeling of Bulky Bony Margins. *A,* Bony ledge interferes with proper healing of bifurcation area. *B,* Bone reshaped and tapered with diamond stone to eliminate shelf-like margin.

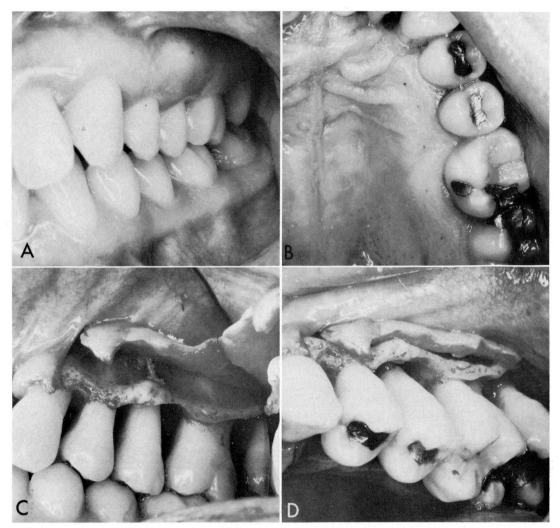

Figure 46–57 Osteoplasty for Reduction of Bulbous Bone Undermined by Craters. *A,* Before treatment. Note the bulbous contour in the premolar area. *B,* Before treatment. Bottom of pockets marked on the palate. *C,* Elevation of full thickness flap reveals irregular bulbous bony ledge. *D,* Craters under bulbous bony ledge.

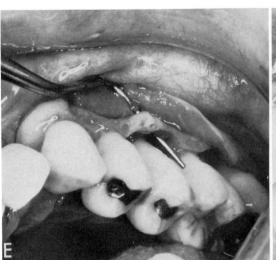

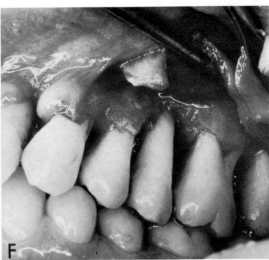

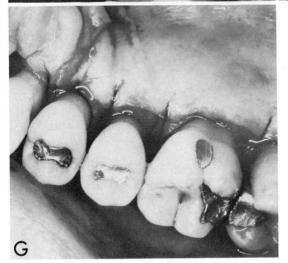

Figure 46–57 *Continued* *E,* Probe demonstrates dehiscence in the bone. *F,* Bony ledge and craters removed by osseous surgery. *G,* Palatal flap sutured to flap on the facial surface. (Courtesy of Edward S. Cohen, D.M.D.)

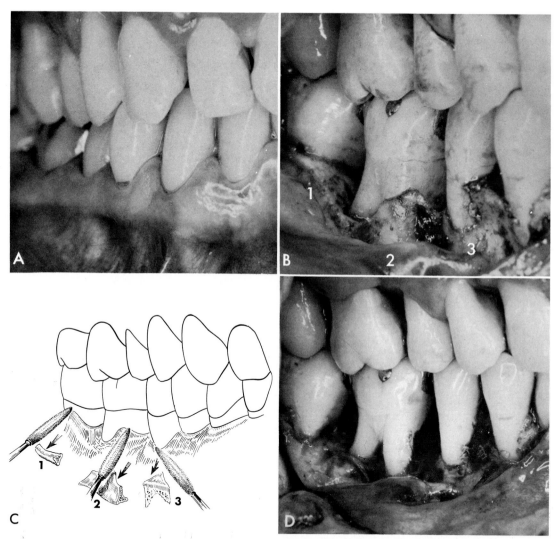

Figure 46–58   Bone Recontoured by Osteoplasty. *A,* Patient with deep periodontal pockets and bone loss. *B,* Elevation of full thickness flap reveals broad osseous plateau (1) and bone irregularities (2 and 3). *C,* Osseous deformities (1, 2 and 3) recontoured by osteoplasty. *D,* After correction of osseous deformities. (*A, B* and *D* courtesy of Edward S. Cohen, D.M.D.)

tenance of gingival health in furcations are thinned and tapered inwardly (Fig. 46–56). Crater-like defects which undermine bulbous marginal bone are caused by removing the overlying bony ledge (Fig. 46–57). Abrupt irregularities in the bone margin are reduced in order to create continuity between the interdental and radicular bone (Fig. 46–58).

Implant Procedures to Stimulate Bone Growth and Restore Tissue Destroyed by Disease

See Chapter 44, section on Transplants in the Treatment of Osseous Defects.

REFERENCES

1. Ainamo, J., and Löe, H.: Anatomical Characteristics of Gingiva. A Clinical and Microscopic Study of the Free and Attached Gingiva. J. Periodont. 37:5, 1966.
2. Albano, E. A., Caffesse, R. G., and Carranza, F. A., Jr.: A Biometric Analysis of Laterally Displaced Pedicle Flaps. Rev. Asoc. Odontol. Argent., 57:351, 1969.
3. Allen, D. L., and Shell, J. H.: Clinical and Radiographic Evaluation of a Periosteal Separation Procedure. J. Periodont., 39:290, 1968.
4. Ariaudo, A. A., and Tyrrell, H. A.: Elimination of Pockets Extending to or Beyond Mucogingival Junction. Dent. Clin. North America, March 1960, p. 67.
5. Arnold, N. R., and Hatchett, C. M., Jr.: A Comparative Investigation of Two Mucogingival Surgical Methods. J. Periodont., 33:129, 1962.
6. Becker, N. G.: A Free Gingival Graft Utilizing a Pre-suturing Techinque. Periodontics, 5:194, 1967.
7. Bergenholtz, A., and Hugoson, A.: Vestibular Sulcus Extension Surgery in Cases with Periodontal Disease. J. Periodont. Res., 2:221, 1967.
8. Bhaskar, S. N., et al.: Healing Under Four Types of Mucogingival Flaps. Programs and Abstracts, I.A.D.R., 48th General Meeting, 1970, p. 100, Abst. #207.
9. Björn, H.: Free Transplantation of Gingiva Propria. Sveriges Tandlak. T., 22:684, 1963.
10. Bohannan, H. M.: Studies in the Alteration of Vestibular Depth. I. Complete Denudation. J. Periodont., 33:120, 1962.
11. Bohannan, H. M.: Studies in the Alteration of Vestibular Depth: II. Periosteum Retention. J. Periodont., 33:354, 1962.
12. Bohannan, H. M.: Studies in the Alteration of Vestibular Depth: III. Vestibular Incision. J. Periodont., 34:209, 1963.
13. Bowers, G. M.: A Study of the Width of Attached Gingiva. J. Periodont., 34:201, 1963.
14. Boyne, P. J.: Histologic Response of Bone to Sectioning by High-Speed Rotary Instruments. J. D. Res., 45:270, 1966.
15. Brackett, R. C., and Gargiullo, A. W.: Free Gingival Grafts in Humans. J. Periodont., 41:581, 1970.
16. Braden, B. E.: Deep Distal Pockets Adjacent to Terminal Teeth. Dent. Clin. North America, 13:161, 1969.
17. Bressman, E., and Chasens, A. I.: Free Gingival Graft with Periosteal Fenestration. J. Periodont., 39:298, 1968.
18. Caffesse, R. G., Ramfjord, S. P., and Nasjleti, C.: Reverse Bevel Periodontal Flaps in Monkeys. J. Periodont., 39:219, 1968.
19. Carranza, F. A.: When and Why the Elimination of Bone Is Necessary in the Treatment of Periodontal Disease. Anales Del Atoneo del Instituto Municipal de Odontologica (Buenos Aires), 3:311, 1941.
20. Carranza, F. A., and Carranza, F. A., Jr.: The Management of the Alveolar Bone in the Treatment of the Periodontal Pocket. J. Periodont., 27:29, 1956.
21. Carranza, F. A., Carraro, J. J., Dotto, C. A., and Cabrini, R. L.: Effect of Periosteal Fenestration in Gingival Extension Operations. J. Periodont., 37:335, 1966.
22. Carranza, F. A., Jr., and Carraro, J. J.: Effect of Removal of Periosteum on Postoperative Result of Mucogingival Surgery. J. Periodont., 34:223, 1963.
23. Carranza, F. A., Jr., and Carraro, J. J.: Mucogingival Techniques in Periodontal Surgery. J. Periodont., 41:294, 1970.
24. Carraro, J. J., Carranza, F. A., Jr., Albano, E. A., and Joly, G.: Effect of Bone Denudation in Mucogingival Surgery in Humans. J. Periodont., 35:463, 1964.
25. Chacker, F. M., and Cohen, D. W.: Regeneration of Gingival Tissues in Non-Human Primates. J. D. Res., 39:743, 1960.
26. Cieszyknsi, A.: Bemerkungen zur Radikal-Chirugischek. Behandlung der Sog. Pyorrhoe Alveolaries. Deutsch Mschr. Zahneilk. 32:376, 1914. A Work on Special Dental Pathology. Chicago, C. V. Black Medico-Dental Publication Company, 1915, p. 64.
27. Cohen, D. W., and Ross, S. E.: The Double Papillae Repositioned Flap in Periodontal Therapy. J. Periodont., 39:65, 1968.
28. Corn, H.: Edentulous Area Pedicle Grafts in Mucogingival Surgery. Periodontics, 2:229, 1964.
29. Corn, H.: Periosteal Separation—Its Clinical Significance. J. Periodont., 33:140, 1962.
30. Costich, E. R., and Ramfjord, S. P.: Healing After Exposure of Periosteum and Labial Bone in Periodontal Surgery. J. D. Res., 43:791 (Suppl.), 1964 (Abst.).
31. Costich, E. R., and Ramfjord, S. P.: Healing After Partial Denudation of the Alveolar Process. J. Periodont., 39:127, 1968.
32. Dahlberg, W. H.: Incisions and Suturing: Some Basic Considerations About Each in Periodontal Flap Surgery. Dent. Clin. North America, 13:149, 1969.

33. Donnenfeld, O. W., and Glickman, I.: A Biometric Study of the Effects of Gingivectomy. J. Periodont., 37:447, 1966.
34. Donnenfeld, O. W., Hoag, P. M., and Weissman, D. P.: A Clinical Study in the Effects of Osteoplasty. J. Periodont., 41:131, 1970.
35. Donnenfeld, O. W., Marks, R., and Glickman, I.: The Apically Repositioned Flap: A Clinical Study. J. Periodont., 35:381, 1964.
36. Edlan, A., and Mejchar, B.: Plastic Surgery of the Vestibulum in Periodontal Therapy. Internat. D. J., 13:593, 1963.
37. Friedman, N.: Mucogingival Surgery: The Apically Repositioned Flap. J. Periodont., 33: 328, 1962.
38. Friedman, N.: Periodontal Osseous Surgery: Osteoplasty and Osteoectomy. J. Periodont., 26:257, 1955.
39. Friedman, N., and Levine, H. L.: Mucogingival Surgery: Current Status. J. Periodont., 35:5, 1964.
40. Gargiulo, A. W., and Arrocha, R.: Histo-clinical Evaluation of Free Gingival Grafts. Periodontics, 5:285, 1967.
41. Giacomatti, L., and Parakkal, P. F.: Skin Transplantation: Orientation of Epithelial Cells by the Basement Membrane. Nature, 223:514, 1969.
42. Glickman, I., Smulow, J. B., Ellinger, H. A., and Foulke, C. N.: Healing of Apically Positioned Mucosal Flaps and Free Gingival Grafts. I.A.D.R. Abst., #468, 1971, p. 169.
43. Glickman, I., Smulow, J. B., O'Brien, T., and Tannen, R.: Healing of the Periodontium Following Mucogingival Surgery. Oral Surg., Oral Med. & Oral Path., 16:530, 1963.
44. Glickman, I., Smulow, J., Vogel, G., and Passamonti, G.: The Effect of Occlusal Forces on Healing Following Mucogingival Surgery. J. Periodont., 37:319, 1966.
45. Goldman, H. M.: Periodontia. 3rd ed. St. Louis, C. V. Mosby Co., 1953, pp. 552–561.
46. Gordon, H. P., Sullivan, H. C., and Atkins, J. H.: Free Autogenous Gingival Grafts. II. Supplemental Findings—Histology of the Graft Site. Periodontics, 6:130, 1968.
47. Gottsegen, R.: Frenum Position and Vestibule Depth in Relation to Gingival Health. Oral Surg., Oral Med. & Oral Path., 7:1069, 1954.
48. Grant, D. A.: Experimental Periodontal Surgery: Sequestration of Alveolar Bone. J. Periodont., 38:409, 1967.
49. Grupe, H. E.: Modified Technique for the Sliding Flap Operation. J. Periodont., 37:491, 1966.
50. Grupe, H. E., and Warren, R. F., Jr.: Repair of Gingival Defects by a Sliding Flap Operation. J. Periodont., 27:92, 1956.
51. Harvey, P. M.: Management of Advanced Periodontitis. Part I. Preliminary Report of a Method of Surgical Reconstruction. New Zeal. D. J., 61:180, 1965.
52. Hattler, A. B.: Mucogingival Surgery—Utilization of Interdental Gingiva as Attached Gingiva by Surgical Displacement. Periodontics, 5:126, 1967.
53. Hawley, C. E., and Staffileno, H.: Clinical Evaluation of Free Gingival Grafts in Periodontal Surgery. J. Periodont., 41:105, 1970.
54. Helburn, R. L., Cohen, D. W., and Chacker, F. M.: Healing of Repositioned Mucogingival Flaps in Monkeys. I.A.D.R. Abstracts, 41:116, 1963.
55. Hileman, A. C.: Surgical Repositioning of Vestibule and Frenums in Periodontal Disease. J.A.D.A., 55:676, 1957.
56. Hilming, F., and Jervoe, P.: Surgical Extension of Vestibular Depth on the Results in Various Regions of the Mouth in Periodontal Patients. Tandlaegebladet, 74:329, 1970.
57. Ivancie, G. P.: Experimental and Histological Investigation of Gingival Regeneration in Vestibular Surgery. J. Periodont., 28:259, 1957.
58. Janson, W. A., et al.: Development of the Blood Supply to Split-Thickness Free Gingival Autografts. J. Periodont.—Periodontics, 40:707, 1969.
59. Kalmi, J., Moscor, M., and Goranov, Z.: The Solution of the Aesthetic Problem in the Treatment of Periodontal Disease of Anterior Teeth: Gingivoplastic Operation. Paradentologie, 3:53, 1949.
60. Lobene, R., and Glickman, I.: The Response of Alveolar Bone to Grinding with Rotary Diamond Stones. J. Periodont., 34:105, 1963.
61. Matherson, D. G., and Zander, H. A.: An Evaluation of Osseous Surgery in Monkeys. I.A.D.R. Abst., #325, 1963, p. 116.
62. Morris, M.: Suturing Techniques in Periodontal Surgery. Periodontics, 3:84, 1965.
63. Morris, M.: The Unrepositioned Muco-periosteal Flap. Periodontics, 3:147, 1965.
64. Nabers, J.: Free Gingival Grafts. Periodontics, 4:243, 1966.
65. Nabers, C. L.: Repositioning the Attached Gingiva. J. Periodont., 25:38, 1954.
66. Nabers, C. L.: When Is Gingival Repositioning an Indicated Procedure? J. Western Soc. Periodont., 5:4, 1957.
67. Neumann, R.: Radical Surgical Treatment of Alveolar Pyorrhea. Viertelj. f. Zahnheilk., 2: 113, 1921.
68. Ochsenbein, C.: Newer Concepts of Mucogingival Surgery. J. Periodont., 31:175, 1960.
69. Ochsenbein, C.: Osseous Resection in Periodontal Surgery. J. Periodont., 29:15, 1958.
70. Ochsenbein, C., and Bohannan, H. M.: The Palatal Approach to Osseous Surgery. I. Rationale. J. Periodont., 34:60, 1963.
71. Ochstein, A. J., Hansen, N. M., and Swenson, H.: A Comparative Study of Cyanoacrylate and Other Periodontal Dressings on Gingival Surgical Wound Healing. J. Periodont.–Periodontics, 40:515, 1969.
72. Oliver, R. C., Löe, H., and Karring, T.: Microscopic Evaluation of the Healing and Revascularization of Free Gingival Grafts. J. Periodont. 3:84, 1968.
73. Oliver, R. C., and Woofter, C., Healing and Revascularization of Free Mucosal Grafts over Roots. I.A.D.R. Abst., #469, 1971, p. 170.
74. Patur, B., and Glickman, I.: Gingival Pedicle Flaps for Covering Root Surfaces Denuded by Chronic Destructive Periodontal Disease—A Clinical Experiment. J. Periodont., 29:50, 1958.
75. Pennel, B., King, K. O., Higgason, J. D., Towner, J. D., Fritz, B. D., and Sadler, J. F.: Retention of Periodontium in Mucogingival Surgery. J. Periodont., 36:39, 1965.
76. Pennel, B. M., King, K. O., Wilderman, M. H., and Barron, J. M.: Repair of the Alveolar Process Following Osseous Surgery. J. Periodont., 38: 426, 1967.

77. Pennel, B. M., Tabor, J. C., King, K. O., Towner, J. D., Fritz, B. D., and Higgason, J. D.: Free Masticatory Mucosa Graft. J. Periodont.–Periodontics, 40:162, 1969.

78. Pfeifer, J. S.: The Reaction of Alveolar Bone to Flap Procedures in Man. Periodontics, 3:135, 1965.

79. Ramfjord, S. P., and Costich, E. R.: Healing After Exposure of Periosteum on the Alveolar Process. J. Periodont., 39:199, 1968.

80. Ramfjord, S. P., Nissle, R. R., Schick, R. A., and Cooper, H., Jr.: Subgingival Curettage Versus Surgical Elimination of Periodontal Pockets. J. Periodont., 39:167, 1968.

81. Redondo, V. F., Bristailante, A., and Carranza, F. A., Jr.: Evaluacion Biometrica de la Tecnica de Extension Gingival con Fenetracion Periosticuar. Rev. Asoc. Odontol. Argent, 56:346, 1968.

82. Redondo, V. F., and Carranza, F. A., Jr.: Estudio Biometrico de la Tecnica de Colgajo Desplazado Apicalmente. Rev. Asoc. Odontol. Argent. (in press).

83. Robinson, R. E.: Periosteal Fenestration in Mucogingival Surgery. J. West. Soc. Periodont., 9:107, 1961.

84. Robinson, R. E.: The Distal Wedge Operation. Periodontics, 4:256, 1966.

85. Robinson, R. E., and Agnew, R. G.: Periosteal Fenestration at the Mucogingival Line. J. Periodont., 34:503, 1963.

86. Rosenberg, M. M.: Vestibular Alterations in Periodontics. J. Periodont., 31:231, 1960.

87. Roth, H.: Some Speculations as to Predictable Fenestrations Prior to Mucogingival Surgery. Periodontics, 3:29, 1965.

88. Schärer, P., Butler, J., and Zander, H.: Healing of Bony Pockets in Connection with Occlusal Dysfunctioning. Schweiz. Mschr. Zahnheilk. 79:244, 1969; Periodont. Abstr., 17:66, 1969.

89. Schluger, S.: Osseous Resection: A Basic Principle in Periodontal Surgery. Oral Surg., Oral Med. & Oral Path., 2:316, 1949.

90. Seibert, J. S.: Technique for the Stabilization of Soft Tissue Flap Employing Chrome-Cobalt Alloy Tissue Tacks. J. Periodont., 32:283, 1961.

91. Simaan, G.: Histology Study of the So-Called Attached Gingiva Following the Deepening of the Vestibulum by the Mucosal Flap Technique. Czas. Stomat. 69:91, 1969; Periodont. Abstr., 17:116, 1969.

92. Smith, R. M.: A Study of the Intertransplantation of Alveolar Mucosa. Oral Surg., 29:328, 1970.

93. Smith, R. M.: A Study of the Intertransplantation of Gingiva. Oral Surg., 29:169, 1970.

94. Snyder, A. J.: A Technic for Free Autogenous Gingival Grafts. J. Periodont., 40:702, 1970.

95. Spengler, D. E., and Hayward, J. R.: Study of Sulcus Extension Wound Healing in Dogs. J. Oral Surg., 22:413, 1964.

96. Staffileno, H.: Palatal Flap Surgery: Mucosal Flap (Split Thickness) and Its Advantages Over the Mucoperiosteal Flap. J. Periodont.–Periodontics, 40:547, 1969.

97. Staffileno, H., and Levy, S.: Histologic and Clinical Study of Mucosal (Gingival) Transplants in Dogs. J. Periodont.–Periodontics, 40:311, 1969.

98. Staffileno, H., Levy, S., and Gargiulo, A.: Histologic Study of Cellular Mobilization and Repair Following a Periosteal Retention Operation via Split Thickness Mucogingival Flap Surgery. J. Periodont., 37:117, 1966.

99. Staffileno, H., Wentz, F., and Orban, B.: Histological Study of Healing of Split Thickness Flap Surgery in Dogs. J. Periodont., 33:56, 1962.

100. Strahan, J. D.: The Relation of the Mucogingival Junction to the Alveolar Bone Margin. D. Practit. & D. Rec., 14:72, 1963.

101. Sugarman, E. F.: A Clinical and Histological Study of the Attachment of Grafted Tissue to Bone and Teeth. J. Periodont.–Periodontics, 40:381, 1969.

102. Sullivan, H. C., and Atkins, J. H.: Free Autogenous Gingival Grafts. I. Principles of Successful Grafting. Periodontics, 6:5, 1968.

103. Sullivan, H. C., and Atkins, J. H.: The Role of Free Gingival Grafts in Periodontal Therapy. Dent. Clin. North America, 13:133, 1969.

104. Sullivan, H. C., Carman, D., and Dinner, D.: Histological Evaluation of Laterally Positioned Flap. I.A.D.R. Abst. #467, 1971, p. 169.

105. Sullivan, H. C., Dinner, D., and Carman, D.: Clinical Evaluation of the Laterally Positioned Flap. I.A.D.R. Abst. #466, 1971, p. 169.

106. Tavtigian, R.: The Height of the Facial Radicular Alveolar Crest Following Apically Positioned Flap Operations. J. Periodont., 41:412, 1970.

107. Tisot, R. J., and Sullivan, H. C.: Evaluation of the Survival of Partial Thickness and Full Thickness Flaps. I.A.D.R. Abst. #470, 1971, p. 170.

108. Vande Voorde, H. E.: Gingival Grafting and Gingival Repositioning. J.A.D.A., 79:1415, 1969.

109. Wade, A. B.: Vestibular Deepening by the Technique of Edlan and Mejchar. J. Periodont., Res., 4:300, 1969.

110. Waerhaug, J.: Review of Cohen: "Role of Periodontal Surgery." J. D. Res., 50:219, 1971.

111. Waltzer, R. E., and Halik, F. J.: Repositioning of the Frenum in Periodontal Involvement. J. Oklahoma D. A., 43:10, 37, 1954.

112. Ward, A. W.: The Surgical Eradication of Pyorrhea. J.A.D.A., 15:2146, 1928.

113. West, T. L., and Bloom, A.: A Histologic Study of Wound Healing Following Mucogingival Surgery. J. D. Res., 40:675, 1961.

114. Whinston, G. J.: Frenotomy and Mucobuccal Fold Resection Utilized in Periodontal Therapy. New York D. J., 22:495, 1956.

115. Widman, L.: Antwort auf Neumanns "Erwiderung Über die Prioritätsfrage Betreffs der Radikal-Chirurgischen Behandlung der Sogenannten Alveolarpyorrhoe." Viert. f. Zahn., 39:186, 1923.

116. Widman, L.: E. Paradencio, su Patologia de Tratamiento, by Pucci, F. M. Barreiro y Ramos, Montevideo, 1951, p. 523.

117. Wilderman, M. N.: Exposure of Bone in Periodontal Surgery. Dent. Clin. North America, March, 1964, p. 23.

118. Wilderman, M. N.: Repair After a Periosteal Retention Procedure. J. Periodont., 34:487, 1963.

119. Wilderman, M. N., and Wentz, F. M.: Repair of a Dentogingival Defect with a Pedicle Flap. J. Periodont., 36:218, 1965.

120. Wilderman, M. N., Wentz, F. M., and Orban, B. J.: Histogenesis of Repair After Mucogingival Surgery. J. Periodont., 31:283, 1960.

121. Wood, D. L., and Hoag, P. L.: Alveolar Crest Reduction Following Full and Partial Thickness Flaps. Joint Meeting of the American and Canadian Academies of Periodontology, Montreal, September 16-19, 1970.

122. Woofter, C.: The Prevalance and Etiology of Gingival Recession. Periodont. Abstr., *17*:45, 1969.

123. Zander, H. A., and Matherson, D. G.: The Effect of Osseous Surgery on Interdental Tissue Morphology in Monkeys. I.A.D.R. Abst., #326, 1963, p. 117.

124. Zemsky, J. L.: Surgical Treatment of Periodontal Diseases with the Author's Open-View Operation for Advanced Cases of Dental Periclasia. D. Cosmos, 68:465, 1926.

125. Zentler, A.: Suppurative Gingivitis with Alveolar Involvement. A New Surgical Procedure. J.A.M.A., *71*:1530, 1918.

Chapter 47

TREATMENT OF UNCOMPLICATED CHRONIC GINGIVITIS

Uncomplicated chronic gingivitis is the most common disease of the gingiva. It affects the interdental and marginal gingiva. **It should be detected in its earliest stages and treated as soon as it is detected** (Figs. 47–1 and 47–2). Usually painless, it is the most common cause of gingival bleeding. Failure to treat it invites destruction of the underlying periodontal tissues and premature tooth loss.

Separation of the treatment of chronic gingivitis from the scaling and curettage technique for eliminating periodontal pockets (Chap. 42) is somewhat artificial, because both conditions usually occur together. However, chronic gingivitis is the initial stage in pocket formation and should be treated before pockets develop.

Chronic gingivitis is always caused by local irritation. Systemic conditions may aggravate the inflammation caused by local irritants and should be appropriately dealt with (Chap. 57), but **no systemic conditions of themselves cause chronic gingivitis.**

TREATMENT

Treatment should be preceded by careful examination to detect all sources of local irritation, such as dental plaque, calculus, food impaction, overhanging or improperly contoured restorations, or irritating removable prostheses. The teeth should be stained with disclosing solution to detect plaque,

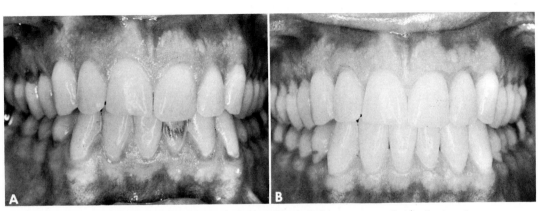

Figure 47–1 Slight Chronic Marginal Gingivitis. *A,* Before treatment. *B,* After treatment.

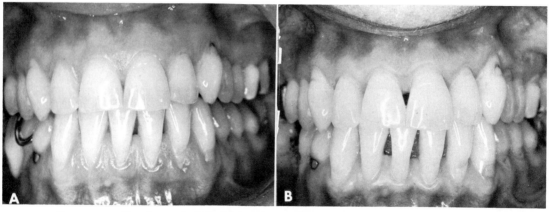

Figure 47–2 Chronic Marginal Gingivitis and Recession. A, Before treatment. B, After treatment.

and carefully probed with the #17 or #21 explorers to locate small particles of calculus.

Step 1. Treatment of uncomplicated gingivitis is started by explaining the importance of plaque control and teaching the patient how to achieve it. **This gives the patient a realistic perspective regarding the treatment of gingivitis: that it includes something he must do for himself, as well as something the dentist does for him.** It also provides an opportunity to demonstrate that plaque control really benefits his gums. After the patient is instructed in plaque control, he is given an appointment for the next visit.

Step 2. The condition of the gums is reviewed with the patient, and improvement is pointed out to him. The teeth are stained with disclosing solution and plaque control is reviewed, with the patient demonstrating the various procedures he used.

The teeth are scaled to remove all deposits, and all tooth surfaces are polished with a paste of fine pumice or Improved Zircate.

Polishing is an important preventive measure against the recurrence of gingivitis. Plaque, the most important cause of gingivitis and the initial stage in the formation of calculus, tends to form more readily on rough surfaces.

Other sources of local irritation referred to earlier should be eliminated.

Step 3. The gingivae are examined and plaque control is reviewed. Special attention is given to areas of persistent inflammation, which usually entails rescaling and emphasis on patient technique for cleansing the area.

These procedures are repeated at subsequent visits until the gingivae are healthy. The patient is then placed on "recall," **with a careful explanation of the reasons for periodic visits and the importance of the care he gives his mouth in the intervening periods.**

CAUSES OF FAILURE

Treatment of chronic gingivitis should present no problems. However, if disease persists, the following are the most likely causes:

1. Failure to remove minute particles of calculus, often just beneath the cemento-enamel junction.

2. Failure to polish the tooth surfaces after deposits are removed.

3. Failure to eliminate sources of irritation other than deposits on the teeth. Food impaction is one of the frequently overlooked factors.

4. Inadequate plaque control because of one or more of the following: (a) insufficient patient instruction, (b) premature dismissal of the patient before he demonstrates competence in plaque control or (c) lack of patient cooperation.

5. A tendency to seek remote systemic etiology for persistent gingivitis caused by overlooked local irritants.

6. Dependence upon vitamins, mouthwashes and topical application of drugs, particularly hormones, antibiotics and oxidizing agents. **Except for topical anesthetics, drugs serve no significant purpose in the treatment of chronic gingivitis.**

Chapter 48

TREATMENT OF THE PERIODONTAL ABSCESS

The most effective way to treat periodontal abscesses is with surgical procedures which provide the necessary visibility and access to the responsible local irritants. There are two types of periodontal abscesses: (1) abscesses deep in the supporting tissues, which are usually treated with the simple (unrepositioned) flap operation; and (2) abscesses contained in the walls of periodontal pockets, which are usually treated by gingivectomy.

SIMPLE FLAP OPERATION FOR THE PERIODONTAL ABSCESS DEEP IN THE SUPPORTING TISSUES

The abscess may be either acute or chronic. If it is acute, preliminary measures are instituted, following which the condition is treated as a chronic lesion.

Treatment for the Acute Periodontal Abscess

Day one

After the diagnosis is established, the patient's temperature is taken and the general systemic reaction is evaluated. The abscess is isolated with gauze sponges and dried and swabbed with an antiseptic solution, followed by a topical anesthetic. After waiting two or three minutes for the anesthetic to become effective, the abscess is palpated gently to locate the most fluctuant area.

With the Bard-Parker #12 blade, a vertical incision is made through the most fluctuant part of the lesion, extending from the mucogingival fold to the gingival margin (Fig. 48–1). If the swelling is on the lingual surface, the incision is started just apical to the swelling and extended through the gingival margin. The blade should penetrate to firm tissue to be sure to reach deep purulent areas. After the initial extravasation of blood and pus, irrigate with warm water and gently spread the incision to facilitate draining.

If the tooth is extruded, it should be ground slightly to avoid contact with its antagonists. Stabilize the tooth with the index finger to reduce vibration and discomfort. It is often preferable to relieve the teeth in the opposing jaw to avoid discomfort.

After drainage stops, the area is dried and painted with an antiseptic. Patients without systemic complications are instructed to rinse hourly with a solution of a teaspoonful of salt in a glass of warm water, and to return

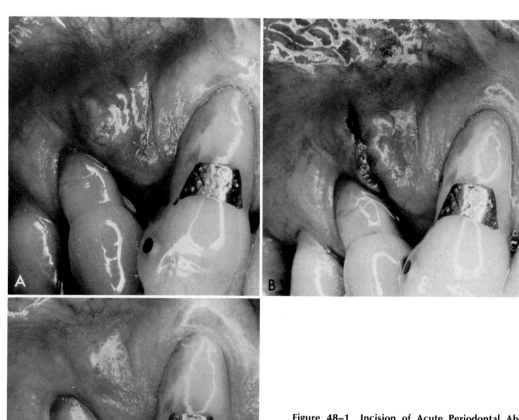

Figure 48–1 Incision of Acute Periodontal Abscess. *A,* Fluctuant acute periodontal abscess. *B,* Abscess incised. *C,* After acute signs subside.

the next day. Penicillin or other antibiotics (see Chap. 51, Page 815) are prescribed for patients with elevated temperatures, in addition to the rinses. The patient is also instructed to avoid exertion and is put on a copious fluid diet. If necessary, bed rest is recommended. Analgesics are prescribed for pain.

Day two

The next day, the swelling is generally markedly reduced or absent, and the symptoms have subsided. If acute symptoms persist, the patient is instructed to continue the regimen prescribed the previous day, and return in 24 hours. The symptoms invariably disappear by then and the lesion is ready for usual treatment for a chronic periodontal abscess (Fig. 48–2).

Chronic Periodontal Abscess

The area is isolated with gauze, dried and painted with antiseptic, facially and lingually, and injected to ensure adequate anesthesia.

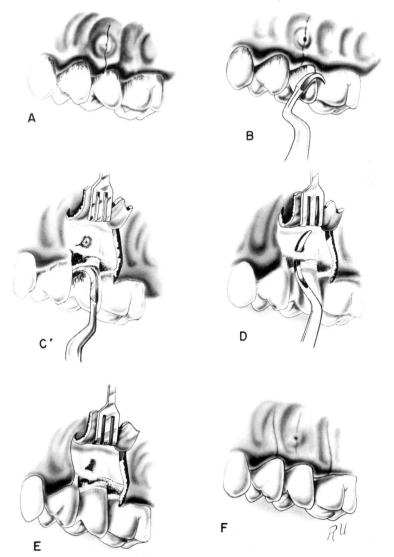

Figure 48–2 Incision of Acute Periodontal Abscess Followed by Flap Operation. *A,* Vertical incision of acute periodontal abscess deep in the supporting periodontal tissues. *B,* Superficial calculus removed. *C,* Flap is elevated, revealing sinus in the bone. Calculus revealed by elevating the flap is removed. *D,* Continuity between the alveolar crest, the abscess on the root and the external surface of the facial plate. *E,* Root surface scaled and smoothed. *F,* Flap replaced.

Determining the operation approach

The first requirement is to determine the relative facial or lingual location of the purulent focus of the abscess. Lingual abscesses may produce swelling on the facial surface and vice versa. To locate the abscess area, probe around the gingival margin following tortuous pockets to their termination. If a sinus is present, the abscess may be probed through it.

Because it offers better accessibility and visibility, the facial approach is preferred,

and is the one that is used unless the abscess is close to the lingual surface.

The incisions

After the approach is decided upon, the superficial calculus is removed and two vertical incisions are made from the gingival margin to the mucobuccal fold, outlining the field of operation (Fig. 48–3, A). If the lingual approach is used, the incisions are made from the gingival margin to the level

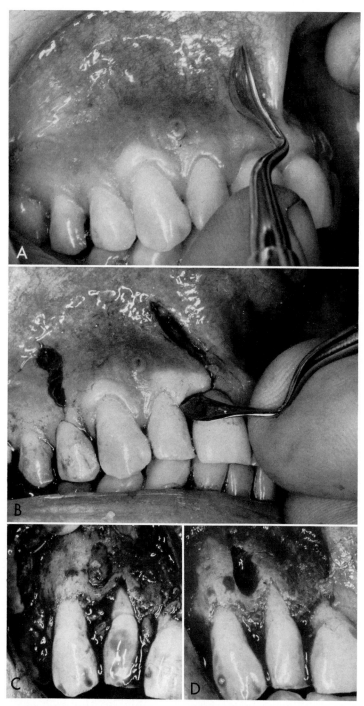

Figure 48–3 Simple Full Thickness Flap Operation for Periodontal Abscess. *A,* Chronic periodontal abscess with sinus between the maxillary canine and lateral. #20G periodontal knife in position for vertical incision. *B,* Operative field is outlined with two vertical incisions. Horizontal incision being made across the interdental papilla with a periodontal knife preparatory to elevating a full thickness flap. Note how the knife is stabilized by the finger rest. *C,* Full thickness flap is elevated, showing granulation tissue at the gingival margin and sinus opening filled with spongy purulent tissue. *D,* Sinus curetted. Note the narrow marginal bridge of bone which is usually infected and removed to facilitate healing.

of the root apices. The operative field should be large enough to allow unhampered visibility and accessibility. A flap that is too narrow or too short jeopardizes the outcome of treatment.

Elevating the flap

After the vertical incisions are made, a mesiodistal incision is made across the interdental papilla with a periodontal knife to facilitate detachment of the flap (Fig. 48–3, B). A full thickness flap is raised with a periodontal knife or periosteal elevator and held in position with a retractor. A flap on either the facial or lingual surface usually suffices. In the case of an abscess which was initially acute, the edges of the incision, made the previous day, are usually united so that the flap may be raised in one piece. An aspirator is essential to maintain a clean field and provide the necessary visibility.

Elevation of the flap reveals some or all of the following conditions (Fig. 48–3, C):

1. Granulation tissue at the gingival margin.
2. Calculus on the root surface.
3. Bony surfaces with multiple pinpoint bleeding areas.
4. A sinus opening on the external bone, which can be probed inwardly to the tooth.
5. Purulent spongy tissue in the orifice of the sinus.

Removal of the granulation tissue and calculus, and smoothing the root

After the field is carefully surveyed, the granulation tissue is removed with curettes to provide a clear view of the root. All deposits are scaled from the teeth, and the root surfaces are planed with hoe scalers and smoothed with curets. If a sinus is present, it is explored and curetted (Fig. 48–3, D).

The location of the sinus determines the manner in which the bone is managed. The bone is not disturbed except in cases in which only a thin rim of bone separates the sinus from the crest of the alveolar bone (Fig. 48–4). Thin marginal bridges of bone are removed, because they are usually pathologically involved and act as foreign bodies which impair healing.

Replacing the flap

The area is cleansed with warm water preparatory to replacing the flap. The margin of the flap usually contains a periodontal pocket lined by epithelium which prevents the flap from reattaching to the tooth. To remove the pocket epithelium the margin of the flap is everted and an internal bevel is cut along the margin with a scissors (Fig. 48–5).

The facial and lingual surfaces are covered with a piece of gauze shaped into a "U," which is held in position until bleeding stops. The gauze is removed and the flap is sutured and covered with periodontal pack.

The patient is instructed not to rinse until the next day, when a pleasant-tasting mouthwash diluted one to three in warm water is used every two hours. The area should be cleansed gently with a soft toothbrush and water irrigation under medium pressure. The patient is to return in one week, at which time the pack and sutures are removed and the patient is instructed in

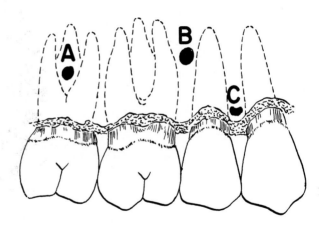

Figure 48–4 Various Levels at Which the Sinus from a Periodontal Abscess May be Located. In the case of C, the narrow marginal bridge of bone is removed during treatment.

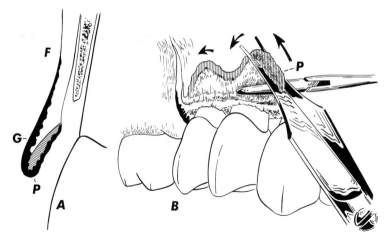

Figure 48–5   Simple Flap for the Treatment of Periodontal Abscess. *A,* Flap (F) elevated from the bone. The marginal gingiva is shown at G. P is the inner surface of the periodontal pocket (*shaded area*). *B,* Flap everted with hemostat. Inner pocket wall (P) (*shaded area*) removed with scissors.

plaque control. Repacking is usually not necessary.

The normal appearance of the gingiva is attained within six to eight weeks; repair of the bone requires approximately nine months. The prospects for bone repair and fill are better for osseous defects produced by rapidly destructive periodontal disease[1] (Fig. 48–6).

THE GINGIVECTOMY OPERATION FOR THE PERIODONTAL ABSCESS IN THE WALL OF A PERIODONTAL POCKET

Day one

If the abscess is acute, preliminary measures are instituted as described on page 783.

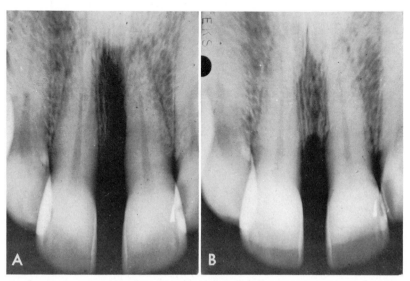

Figure 48–6   Repair of Osseous Defect Following Treatment of Periodontal Abscess. *A,* Bone destruction and osseous defect produced by periodontal abscess. *B,* Bone repair one year after treatment by flap operation without osseous surgery.

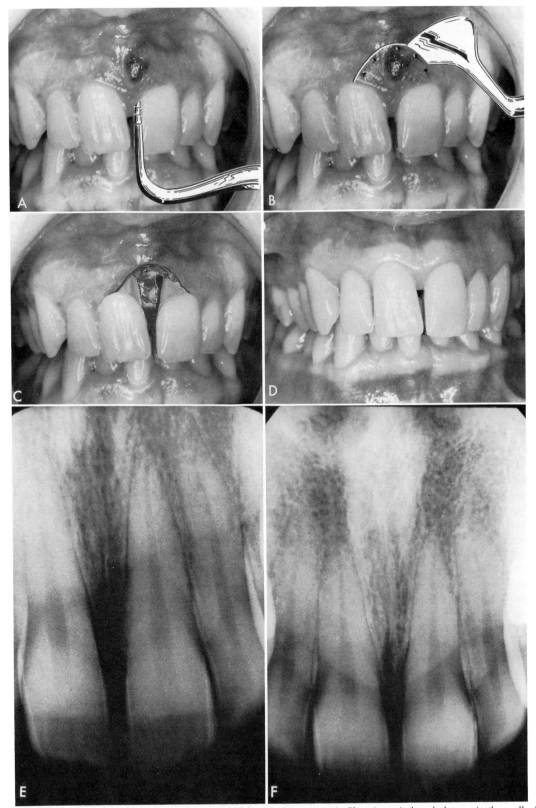

Figure 48–7 Chronic Periodontal Abscess Treated by Gingivectomy. *A,* Chronic periodontal abscess in the wall of a deep pocket is explored with Glickman periodontal probe #26G. *B,* Semilunar incision approximately 2 mm. apical to bleeding points made by pocket marker (composite illustration). *C,* Removal of pocket wall reveals abscess tract along incisor root (composite illustration). *D,* Appearance of healed gingiva after one year. *E,* Radiograph before treatment. *F,* Bone repair one year after treatment.

Day two

After the acute symptoms have subsided, the treatment is the same as that employed if the patient presented initially with a chronic abscess.

The area is isolated, dried and painted with an antiseptic solution and injected to ensure adequate anesthesia. The abscess is probed to determine the extent of involvement, and the pocket is marked with a pocket marker (Fig. 48–7, A).

The Incision

The supragingival calculus is removed and a semilunar incision is made approximately 2 mm. peripheral to the pinpoint markings with the periodontal knives #20G and #21G (Fig. 48–7, B). The incised gingiva is removed with a surgical hoe #19G, exposing the following: granulation tissue, calculus, and a tract of bone destruction along the root (Fig. 48–7, C).

The granulation tissue and calculus are removed and the roots are smoothed. The bone is not disturbed.

The area is cleansed with warm water and covered with a gauze pad until bleeding stops, after which a periodontal pack is applied. Both the lingual and facial surfaces should be packed to provide better retention of the pack. The patient is dismissed with a list of instructions usually provided after gingivectomy (see page 656), and instructed to return in one week, when the pack is removed. It is not necessary to replace the pack for another week, unless the area is particularly sensitive. The patient is instructed in plaque control (see page 467). Gingival health is restored within six to eight weeks (Fig. 48–7, D), and bone repair is observed radiographically after nine months (Fig. 48–7, E and F).

REFERENCE

1. Nabers, J. M., Meador, H. L., and Nabers, C. L.: Chronology, An Important Factor in the Repair of Osseous Defects. Periodontics, 2:304, 1964.

Chapter 49

TREATMENT OF GINGIVAL ENLARGEMENT

Treatment of gingival enlargement is based upon an understanding of the etiology and underlying pathologic changes (see Chap. 7). Enlargements caused by inflammation alone can be treated effectively by local procedures. When systemic or unknown conditions are partly or entirely responsible, local treatment will only reduce the enlargement by the extent to which inflammation contributes to it. Because gingival enlargements differ in etiology, their treatment is best considered under separate headings.

TREATMENT OF CHRONIC INFLAMMATORY GINGIVAL ENLARGEMENT

Scaling and curettage

Chronic inflammatory enlargements, which are soft and discolored and are caused principally by edema and cellular infiltration, are treated by scaling and curettage, provided the size of the enlargement does not interfere with complete removal of deposits from the involved tooth surfaces (Fig. 49–1).

Gingivectomy

Since most chronic inflammatory gingival enlargements consist of a significant fibrotic component that will not undergo shrinkage following scaling and curettage, or are of such size that they obscure deposits on the tooth surfaces and interfere with access to them, gingivectomy (Chap. 43) is the treatment of choice. (See Fig. 49–2, *A* and *B*, opposite page 792.) **The location and bevel of the incision are particularly critical.** The following procedure is used:

After the area is anesthetized, the junction of the enlarged gingiva with the adjacent mucosa is probed and outlined with pinpoint markings (Fig. 49–3, *A*). The incision is made **apical to the markings and sufficiently close to the bone to assure**

791

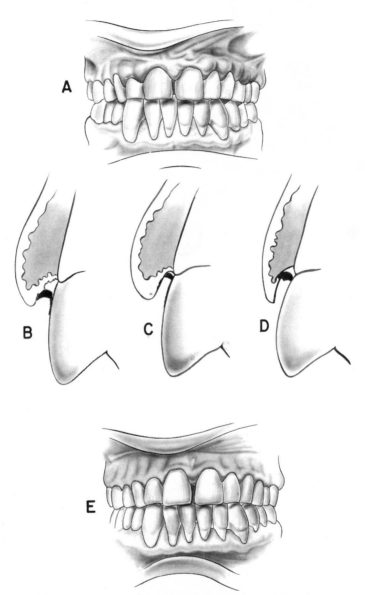

Figure 49–1   Treatment of Chronic Inflammatory Gingival Enlargement by Scaling and Curettage. *A,* Chronic inflammatory gingival enlargement in the maxilla. *B,* Removal of the calculus with a superficial scaler, shown in cross section. *C,* Removal of subgingival calculus using a deep scaler. *D,* Smoothing the tooth surface and removing inner lining of the pocket formed by the enlarged gingiva with a curet. *E,* Appearance of the healed gingiva.

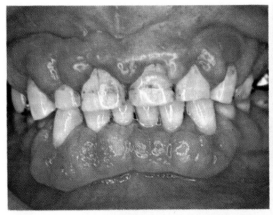

A. Chronic inflammatory gingival enlargement.

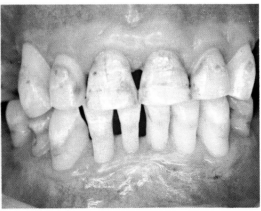

B. After treatment.

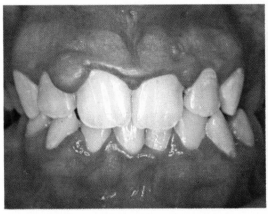

C. Chronic inflammatory enlargement associated with mouth breathing.

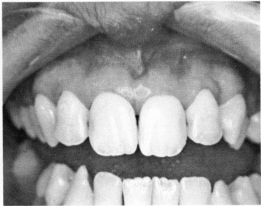

D. After treatment.

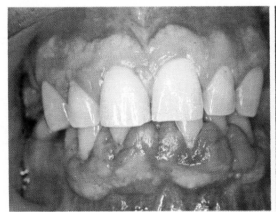

E. Gingival enlargement associated with Dilantin therapy.

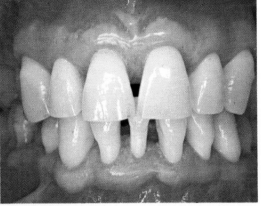

F. After treatment.

Figure 49–2

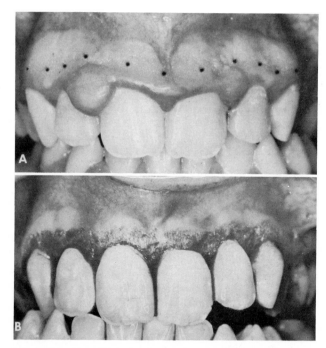

Figure 49–3 Gingivectomy Incision for Gingival Enlargement. *A,* Chronic inflammatory gingival enlargement with tumor-like area. Pin-point markings outline extent of the enlargement. *B,* Enlarged gingiva removed. Note the bevelled incision. (For the pre- and post-treatment appearance see Figure 49–2, *C* and *D.*)

complete removal of the enlarged tissue and complete exposure of all root deposits. No extraneous fibrous tissue should be left on the bone, because it interferes with the attainment of normal gingival contour. The mucosa adjacent to the enlargement should be tapered by beveling the incision (Fig. 49–3, *B*). The teeth are scaled and planed, and a periodontal pack is inserted for one week.

Tumor-like inflammatory enlargement

Tumor-like inflammatory enlargements are treated by gingivectomy as follows:

Under local anesthesia the tooth surfaces beneath the mass are scaled to remove calculus and other debris (Fig. 49–4). The lesion is separated from the mucosa at its base with a Bard-Parker blade #12 (Fig. 49–4). If the lesion extends interproximally, the interdental gingiva is included in the incision to ensure exposure of irritating root deposits. After the lesion is removed, the involved root surfaces are scaled and smoothed, and the area cleansed with warm water. A periodontal pack is applied and removed in a week, at which time the patient is instructed in plaque control.

TREATMENT OF THE GINGIVAL ABSCESS

In contrast with a periodontal abscess which involves the supporting periodontal tissues, the *gingival abscess is a lesion of the marginal or interdental gingiva, usually produced by an impacted foreign object.* It is treated as follows:

Under topical anesthesia, the fluctuant area of the lesion is incised with a Bard-Parker blade, and the incision gently widened to permit drainage. The area is cleansed with warm water and covered with a gauze pad. After bleeding stops, the patient is dismissed for 24 hours and instructed to rinse every two hours with a glass of warm water.

When the patient returns, the lesion is generally reduced in size and symptom-free. Topical anesthetic is applied and the area is scaled and curetted. If the residual size of the lesion is too great, it is removed surgically.

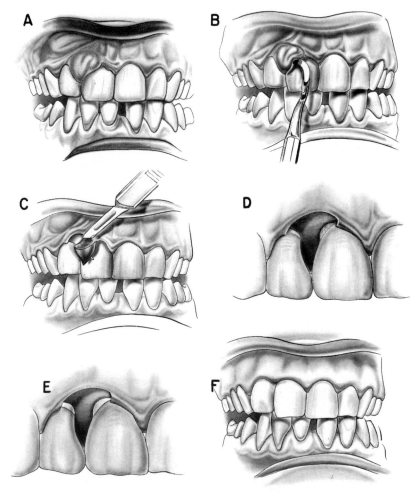

Figure 49–4   Treatment of Tumor-like Inflammatory Gingival Enlargement. *A,* Appearance of the lesion between the maxillary central and lateral incisors. *B,* The nature of attachment of the lesion is explored and the superficial calculus removed with a scaler. *C,* The lesion is excised with a #12 Bard-Parker blade. *D,* After the lesion is removed, calculus deposits are noted on the root surfaces. *E,* The tooth surfaces are scaled and smoothed. *F,* Appearance of the area one month after treatment. (Compare with *A*.)

TREATMENT OF GINGIVAL HYPERPLASIA ASSOCIATED WITH DILANTIN THERAPY

Gingival enlargement does not occur in all patients receiving Dilantin; when it does occur, it may be of three types:

Type I. **Noninflammatory hyperplasia caused by the Dilantin (Fig. 49–5, *A*).** Discontinuing the Dilantin is the only method of eliminating it. Ths is usually not feasible, but if it is done, the enlargement disappears after one or two months.

Type II. **Chronic inflammatory enlargement entirely unrelated to the Dilantin (Fig. 49–5, *B*).** The enlargement is caused entirely by local irritants, similar to the inflammatory enlargement in patients not receiving Dilantin, and can be treated successfully by gingivectomy and fastidious plaque control, without recurrence.

Type III. **Combined enlargement is a combination of hyperplasia caused by Dilantin plus inflammation caused by local irritation (Fig. 49–5, *C*). This is the most common type of enlargement in Dilantin patients.** It is treated by gingivectomy and elimination of all sources of local irritation, plus fastidious plaque control by the patient. The enlarged gingiva is removed with periodontal knives, scalpels or electrosurgery; more recently, cryosurgery[8] has been used for this purpose.

The initial treatment of combined enlargement presents no difficulty; the prob-

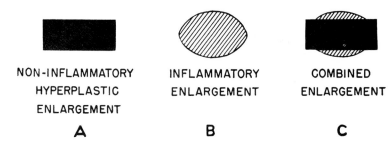

NON-INFLAMMATORY
HYPERPLASTIC
ENLARGEMENT

INFLAMMATORY
ENLARGEMENT

COMBINED
ENLARGEMENT

A   B   C

Figure 49–5 Types of Gingival Enlargement in Patients Under Dilantin Therapy. *A,* Non-inflammatory hyperplastic enlargement caused by the Dilantin alone. *B,* Inflammatory enlargement caused by local irritation without Dilantin-induced hyperplasia. *C,* Combined enlargement which results from inflammation superimposed upon Dilantin-induced hyperplasia.

lem is with recurrence. Recurrence can be kept to a minimum by periodic scaling and diligent plaque control by the patient (see Fig. 49–2, *E* and *F,* opposite page 792).[6] A hard natural rubber fitted bite guard worn at night sometimes assists in the control of recurrence.[1, 2]

Local treatment is very effective; it keeps patients comfortable and without disfigurement for years,[3, 5, 7] but it does not keep them entirely free of enlargement. It prevents the return of that part of the enlargement caused by inflammation (Fig. 49–6); it does not usually prevent the recurrence of the hyperplastic component of the enlargement caused by the Dilantin, although it

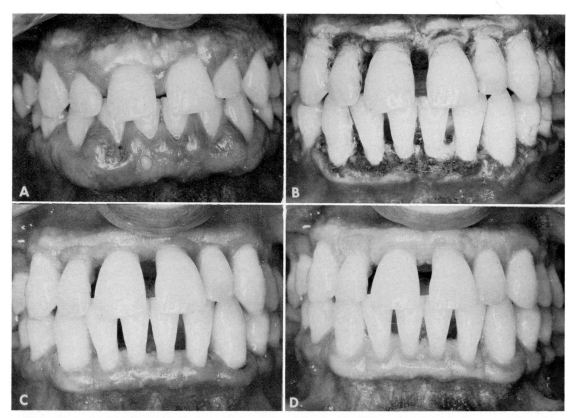

Figure 49–6 Combined Type of Gingival Enlargement Associated with Dilantin Therapy. *A,* Enlargement caused by Dilantin combined with superimposed inflammation. *B,* Appearance at time of pack removal, one week after complete mouth gingivectomy. *C,* After four months. *D,* After five years. There is some hyperplasia caused by the Dilantin, but its size has been kept to a minimum by periodic scalings and diligent plaque control which prevent inflammation from recurring.

has been reported to do so in some cases.[4, 6] In Dilantin patients with gingival enlargement caused by local irritation alone, with no drug-induced hyperplasia, recurrence is totally preventable by local measures.

TREATMENT OF LEUKEMIC ENLARGEMENT

Leukemic enlargement occurs in acute or subacute leukemia and is uncommon in the chronic leukemic state. The medical care of leukemic patients is often complicated by gingival enlargement with superimposed painful acute necrotizing ulcerative gingivitis which interferes with eating and creates toxic systemic reactions. The bleeding and clotting times and platelet count of the patient are checked and the hematologist consulted before periodontal treatment is instituted.

Treatment of the acute gingival involvement is described in Chapter 50. After the acute symptoms subside, attention is directed to correction of the gingival enlargement. The rationale is to remove the local factors responsible for the inflammation, because leukemic enlargement does not occur in the absence of local irritants.

The enlargement is treated by scaling and curettage carried out in stages under topical anesthesia. The first visit consists of gently removing all loose accumulations with cotton pellets, superficial scaling and instruction in oral hygiene procedures for plaque control. Oral hygiene is extremely important in these cases and should be performed by the nurse, if necessary.

Progressively deeper scalings are carried out at subsequent visits. Treatments are confined to a small area to facilitate control of bleeding. Antibiotics are administered systemically the evening before and for 48 hours after each treatment to reduce the risk of infection.

TREATMENT OF GINGIVAL ENLARGEMENT IN PREGNANCY

Treatment requires elimination of all local irritants which are responsible for precipitating the gingival changes in pregnancy. **Elimination of local irritants early in pregnancy is a preventive measure against gingival disease which is preferable to treatment of gingival enlargement after it occurs.**

Marginal and interdental gingival inflammation and enlargement are treated by scaling and curettage (see Chap. 58). Treatment of **tumor-like gingival enlargements** consists of surgical excision plus scaling and smoothing of the tooth surface. **The enlargement will recur unless all irritants are removed.** Food impaction is second only to dental plaque as a cause of tumor-like gingival enlargement in pregnancy.

When to treat

The lesion should be treated as soon as it is detected. It should not be permitted to remain until the pregnancy terminates, on the assumption that it will disappear spontaneously. This invites the possibility of increased growth of the lesion during pregnancy, with added patient discomfort. It also misleads the patient into thinking that parturition will solve her gingival problem. **Gingival enlargements do shrink after pregnancy, but they do not disappear.** There is a residual area of local irritation and inflammation which, if untreated, may cause progressive destruction of the periodontal tissues.

TREATMENT OF GINGIVAL ENLARGEMENT IN PUBERTY

Gingival enlargement in puberty is treated by scaling and curettage and the removal of all sources of irritation and plaque control. Gingivectomy may be required in severe cases. The problem in these patients is recurrence because of poor oral hygiene.

DRUGS IN THE TREATMENT OF GINGIVAL ENLARGEMENT

Gingival enlargement can be reduced by escharotic drugs, but this is not a recommended form of treatment. The destructive action of the drugs is difficult to control; injury to healthy tissue and root surfaces, delayed healing and excessive postoperative pain are complications which can be avoided when the gingiva is removed with periodontal knives, scalpels or electrosurgery.

Removal of the enlarged gingiva by any method must be accompanied by elimination of local irritants.

RECURRENCE OF GINGIVAL ENLARGEMENT

Recurrence following treatment is the most common problem in the management of gingival enlargement. Residual local irritation and systemic or hereditary conditions that cause noninflammatory gingival hyperplasia are the responsible factors.

If chronic inflammatory enlargement recurs immediately after treatment, it indicates that all irritants have not been removed. Contributory local conditions, such as food impaction and overhanging margins of restorations, are factors which are commonly overlooked. If the enlargement recurs after healing is complete and normal contour is attained, inadequate plaque control by the patient is the most common cause.

Recurrence during the healing period appears as red, bead-like granulomatous masses which bleed upon slight provocation. This is a proliferative vascular inflammatory response to local irritation, usually a fragment of calculus on the root. The condition is corrected by removing the granulation tissue and smoothing the root surface.

Familial, hereditary or *idiopathic* gingival enlargement recurs after surgical removal even if all local irritants have been removed. The enlargement can be maintained at minimal size by preventing secondary inflammatory involvement.

REFERENCES

1. Aiman, R.: The Use of Positive Pressure Mouthpiece as a New Therapy for Dilantin Gingival Hyperplasia. Chron. Omaha D. Soc., *131*:244, 1968.
2. Babcock, J. R.: The Successful Use of a New Therapy for Dilantin Gingival Hyperplasia. Periodontics, *3*:196, 1965.
3. Bergmann, C. L.: Dilantin: Its Effects on the Gingival Tissue, D. Dig., *73*:63, 1967.
4. Cianco, S. G., et al.: Gingival Hyperplasia and Diphenylhydantoin (Dilantin): A Longitudinal Study. I.A.D.R. Abst., #65, 1970, p. 65.
5. Ginwalla, T. M., et al.: Management of Gingival Hyperplasia in Patients Receiving Dilantin Therapy. J. Indian D. Assn., *39*:124, 1967.
6. Hall, W. B.: Dilantin Hyperplasia: A Preventable Lesion. J. Periodont. Res., *4*:36, 1969.
7. Miller, F. D.: Multipronged Attack Against Dilantin Gingival Hyperplasia. D. Survey, *42*:51, 1966.
8. Sanders, R. E.: Cryogenic Treatment of Dilantin Gingival Hyperplasia. Chron. Omaha D. Soc., *33*:48, 1969.

Chapter 50

THE TREATMENT OF ACUTE GINGIVAL DISEASE

The treatment of acute gingival disease entails the alleviation of the acute symptoms and the elimination of all other periodontal disease, chronic as well as acute, throughout the oral cavity. **Treatment is not complete so long as periodontal pathology** or factors capable of causing it are still present.

Acute necrotizing ulcerative gingivitis occurs in a mouth essentially free of any other gingival involvement, or superimposed upon underlying chronic gingival disease. **The simplest part of clinical treatment is the alleviation of the acute symptoms; correction of underlying chronic gingival disease requires more comprehensive procedures.**

The treatment of acute necrotizing ulcerative gingivitis consists of the following phases:

1. LOCAL. Alleviation of the acute inflammation plus treatment of chronic disease either underlying the acute involvement or elsewhere in the oral cavity.

2. SYSTEMIC. *A. Supportive Treatment.* Alleviation of generalized toxic symptoms such as fever and malaise.

B. Etiotropic Treatment. The correction of systemic conditions which contribute to the initiation or progress of the gingival changes.

Treatment should follow an orderly sequence, as described in the following paragraphs.

COMPREHENSIVE TREATMENT OF ACUTE NECROTIZING ULCERATIVE GINGIVITIS

At the **first visit** the dentist should obtain a general impression of the patient's background, including information regarding recent illness, living conditions, dietary background, type of employment, hours of rest and mental stress. Observe the general appearance, the apparent nutritional status, responsiveness or lassitude, and **take the patient's temperature.** Palpate the submaxillary and submental areas for enlarged lymph glands.

Examine the oral cavity for the "characteristic lesion" of acute necrotizing ulcerative gingivitis (Chap. 11), its distribution and possible involvement of the oropharyngeal region. Evaluate the oral hygiene; check for the presence of pericoronal flaps, periodontal pockets and local irritants. A bacterial smear may be made from the material in the involved areas, but this is merely corroboratory and is not to be relied upon for diagnosis.

Examine the occlusion and check for bruxism, clamping or clenching.

Question the patient regarding the history of the acute disease, its onset and duration. Is it recurrent? Are the recurrences associated with specific factors such as menstruation or foods, exhaustion or mental stress? Has there been any previous treatment? When, and for how long? Inquire as to the type of treatment and the patient's impression regarding its effect.

After the diagnosis is established, the patient is treated as either "nonambulatory" or "ambulatory," based upon the following criteria:

NONAMBULATORY PATIENTS. These are patients with symptoms of generalized toxicity, such as high fever, malaise and lassitude; bed rest is often necessary, and extensive office treatment should not be undertaken until the systemic symptoms subside.

AMBULATORY PATIENTS. In these patients, there may be localized adenopathy and a slightly elevated temperature, but no serious systemic complications.

Preliminary Treatment for Nonambulatory Patients

Day one

1. Local treatment is limited to gently removing the necrotic pseudomembrane with a pellet of cotton saturated with hydrogen peroxide.

2. The patient is advised to rest in bed and rinse the mouth every two hours with a glass of an equal mixture of warm water and 3 per cent hydrogen peroxide. For systemic antibiotic action, penicillin is administered either intramuscularly in a dose of 300,000 units or as 250 mg. tablets every four hours. For penicillin-sensitive patients, other antibiotics such as erythromycin (250 mg. every four hours) are prescribed. Keep a carbon copy of the prescription in the patient's file for future reference. The patient is to report to the dentist after 24 hours.

Always stipulate the period for which the instructions are intended, and check the condition of the patient the next day. It is poor practice to place the patient on a home regimen for a protracted period of time. There may be a severe reaction to the antibiotic, and the peroxide mouthwash may produce diffuse erythema and ulceration of the oral mucosa and swelling of the tongue.

Day two

If the patient's condition has improved, proceed to the treatment described below under Treatment for Ambulatory Patients. If there is no improvement at the end of 24 hours, a bedside visit should be made. **The instrumentarium required for this visit includes a mirror, explorer, cotton pliers, flashlight, thermometer, a container of cotton pellets, and a glass-stoppered bottle of peroxide.** At the bedside, the oral condition, the possibility of oropharyngeal involvement and the patient's temperature are checked. The involved gingiva is again gently swabbed with peroxide, and the instructions for the previous day are repeated. The patient is to communicate with the dentist after 24 hours.

Day three

In most instances, the patient is improved by this time and is started on the treatment for ambulatory patients described below.

Treatment for Ambulatory Patients

The following is the procedure for ambulatory patients and for initially nonambulatory patients after satisfactory response to preliminary treatment:

Day one

Instrumentarium: two dappen dishes, one containing topical anesthetic, the other 3 per cent hydrogen peroxide; cotton pellets and cotton rolls, mirror, explorer, cotton pliers, and superficial scalers.

Treatment is confined to the acutely involved areas, which are isolated with cotton rolls and dried. Topical anesthetic is applied, and after two or three minutes the areas are gently swabbed with a cotton pellet to remove the pseudomembrane and nonattached surface debris. Each cotton pellet is used in a small area and is then discarded; sweeping motions over large areas with a single pellet are not used. After cleansing with warm water, the superficial calculus is removed.

Deep scaling and curettage are contraindicated at this time because of the possibility of extending the infection into deeper tissues, and also of causing a bacteremia. Unless an emergency exists, surgical procedures such as extractions or gingivectomy are postponed until the patient has been symptom-free for a period of four weeks in order to minimize the likelihood of exacerbation of the acute symptoms.

The patient should be advised of the extent of the total treatment the condition requires and that treatment is not complete when the pain stops. He should be informed of the presence of chronic gingival and periodontal disease which must also be eliminated in order to prevent recurrence of acute symptoms. The patient is to return in 24 hours.

INSTRUCTIONS TO THE PATIENT. The patient is dismissed with the following instructions: **Avoid tobacco, alcohol and condiments.** Heat and the products of tobacco irritate the inflamed tissue and retard healing. If the patient is a heavy smoker, it is preferable to recommend less smoking, rather than complete abstinence. A heavy smoker who might disregard a drastic order to discontinue smoking entirely may be more cooperative if he is permitted to indulge in tobacco occasionally. The occasional use of tobacco is obviously better than total disregard of unacceptable instructions.

Rinse with a glassful of an equal mixture of 3 per cent hydrogen peroxide and warm water every two hours.

Pursue usual activities, but avoid excessive physical exertion or prolonged exposure to sun as required in golf, tennis, swimming or sunbathing.

Confine toothbrushing to the removal of surface debris with a bland dentifrice; overzealous brushing will be painful. Dental floss, interdental cleansers and water irrigation under medium pressure are recommended.

The patient need not be placed in isolation, but **use of a separate set of dishes is recommended and intimate contacts are discouraged.** The contagiousness of acute necrotizing ulcerative gingivitis has not been demonstrated; but until such time as it is conclusively ruled out, methods of transmitting organisms should be avoided as a precautionary measure.

Day two

The patient's condition is usually improved; the pain is diminished or no longer present. The gingival margins of the involved areas are erythematous, but without a superficial pseudomembrane.

Deep scalers and curets are added to the instrumentarium, and the procedures performed on Day One are repeated. Shrinkage of the gingiva may expose previously covered calculus, which is removed along with gentle curettage of the gingiva. Instructions to the patient are the same as the previous day. If there have been undesirable effects of the peroxide, warm water alone is used for rinsing.

Day three

The patient is essentially symptom-free. There is still some erythema in the involved areas, and the gingiva may be slightly painful to tactile stimulation (Fig. 50–1). Scaling and curettage are repeated. The patient is instructed in plaque control procedures (described on page 467) which are essential for the success of the treatment and maintenance of periodontal health. The peroxide rinses are discontinued.

Day four

Tooth surfaces in the involved areas are scaled and smoothed, and plaque control by the patient is checked and corrected if necessary.

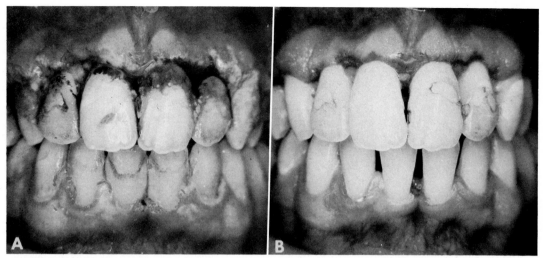

Figure 50–1 **Initial Response to Treatment of Acute Necrotizing Ulcerative Gingivitis.** *A,* Severe acute necrotizing ulcerative gingivitis. *B,* Third day. There is still some erythema but the condition is markedly improved.

Day five

Unfortunately, treatment is often stopped at this time because the acute condition has subsided, but this is when comprehensive treatment of the patient's chronic periodontal problem should start. Appointments are scheduled for the treatment of chronic gingivitis, periodontal pockets and pericoronal flaps, and the elimination of all forms of local irritation, plus occlusal adjustment if necessary.

Patients without gingival disease other than the treated acute involvement are dismissed for 1 week. If the condition is satisfactory at that time, the patient is dismissed for one month when the schedule for subsequent recall visits is determined according to the patient's needs.

Gingival Changes with Healing

The characteristic lesion of acute necrotizing ulcerative gingivitis undergoes the following changes in the course of healing in response to treatment:

Removal of the surface pseudomembrane exposes the underlying red hemorrhagic crater-like depression in the gingiva.

In the next stage the bulk and redness of the crater margins are reduced, but the surface remains shiny.

This is followed by the early signs of the restoration of normal gingival contour and color.

In the final stage the normal gingival color, consistency, surface texture and contour are restored. Portions of the root exposed by the acute disease are covered by healthy gingiva (Figs. 50–2 and 50–3).

CONTOURING THE GINGIVA AS AN ADJUNCTIVE TREATMENT PROCEDURE

Even in the cases of severe gingival necrosis, healing ordinarily leads to restoration of the normal gingival contour (Fig. 50–4). However, if the teeth are irregularly aligned, healing sometimes results in the formation of a shelf-like gingival margin which favors the retention of food and recurrence of gingival inflammation. This can be corrected by reshaping the gingiva with a periodontal knife or electrosurgery (Figs. 50–5, 50–6 and 50–7). Effective plaque control by the patient is particularly important to establish and maintain normal gingival contour in areas of tooth irregularity.

SURGICAL PROCEDURES AND ACUTE NECROTIZING ULCERATIVE GINGIVITIS

Tooth extraction or extensive gingival surgery should be postponed until four
(Text continued on page 806)

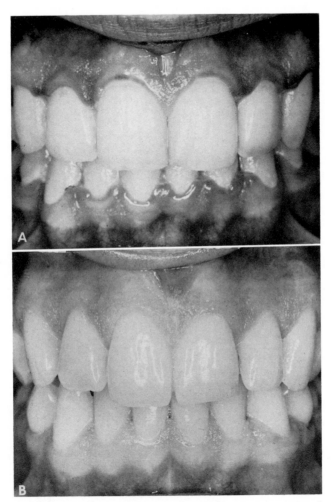

Figure 50–2 Treated Acute Necrotizing Ulcerative Gingivitis. *A,* Before treatment. Note the characteristic interdental lesions. *B,* After treatment, showing restoration of gingival health contour.

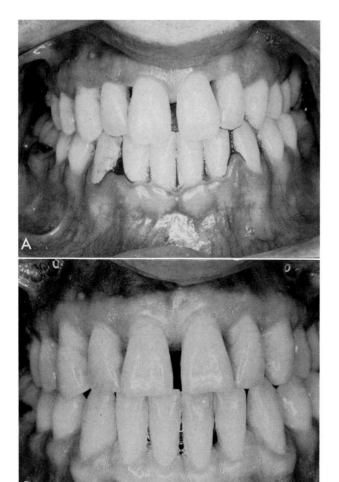

A

Figure 50-3 Physiologic Contour and Reattachment of Gingiva Following Treatment of Acute Necrotizing Ulcerative Gingivitis. A, Acute necrotizing ulcerative gingivitis showing the characteristic punched-out eroded gingival margin with surface pseudomembrane. B, After treatment. Note the restoration of physiologic gingival contour and reattachment of the gingiva to the surfaces of the mandibular teeth, which had been exposed by the disease.

Figure 50-4 Gingival Healing Following Treatment. A, Before treatment. Severe acute necrotizing ulcerative gingivitis with crater formation. B, After treatment. Note the restored gingival contour.

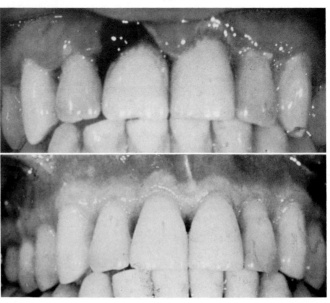

B

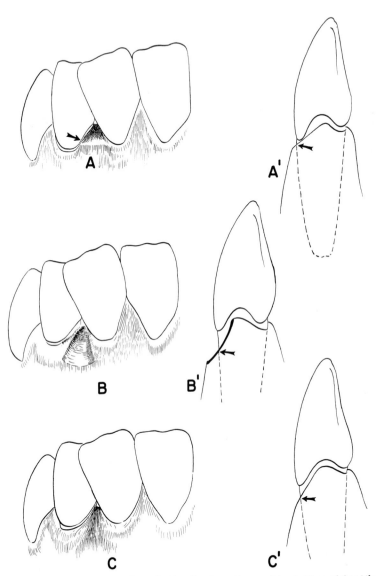

Figure 50–5   Contouring the Gingiva as an Adjunct in Treating Some Cases of Acute Necrotizing Ulcerative Gingivitis.
A, "Gingival shelf" (*arrow*) which remains in an area of tooth irregularity, after the acute symptoms are alleviated. *A',* Facio-lingual view showing outline of the gingival shelf. *B,* The gingiva is contoured to eliminate the shelf. *B',* Corrected contour of the gingiva. *C,* Physiologic gingival contour after healing. *C',* Faciolingual view of healed gingiva.

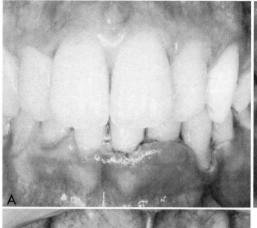
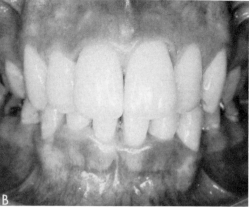
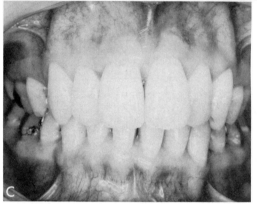

Figure 50–6   Reshaping the Gingiva in the Treatment of Acute Necrotizing Ulcerative Gingivitis. A, Before treatment, showing bulbous gingiva and interdental necrosis in the mandibular anterior area. B, After treatment, gingival contours still undesirable. C, Final result; physiologic contours obtained by reshaping the gingiva.

weeks after the acute signs and symptoms of necrotizing ulcerative gingivitis have subsided. If emergency surgical interference is required in the presence of acute symptoms, prophylactic chemotherapy with penicillin or other antibiotics is indicated to prevent worsening or spread of the acute disease. Penicillin is administered systemically either by intramuscular injection of phenoxymethyl penicillin, 300,000 units once daily for three days beginning the evening before the surgical procedure, or by oral administration of 250 mg. tablets, one every four hours, beginning the evening before the operation and continuing for 48 hours after it.

THE MENSTRUAL PERIOD AND THE TREATMENT OF ACUTE NECROTIZING ULCERATIVE GINGIVITIS

When the menstrual period occurs in the course of treatment, there is a tendency for exacerbation of the acute signs and symptoms, giving the appearance of a "relapse."

Patients should be informed of this possibility and spared unnecessary anxiety regarding their oral condition.

ROLE OF DRUGS IN THE TREATMENT OF ACUTE NECROTIZING ULCERATIVE GINGIVITIS

A large variety of drugs have been used topically in the treatment of acute necrotizing ulcerative gingivitis, some of which are listed in Table 50–1. **Topical drug therapy is only an adjunctive measure in the treatment of acute necrotizing ulcerative gingivitis;[3] no drug, when used alone, can be considered complete therapy.**

Escharotic drugs such as phenol, silver nitrate and chromic acid should not be used. They are necrotizing agents that alleviate the painful symptoms by destroying the nerve endings in the gingiva. They also destroy the young cells necessary for repair and delay healing. Their repeated use results in loss of gingival tissue which is not restored when the disease subsides.[4]

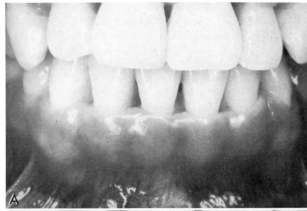

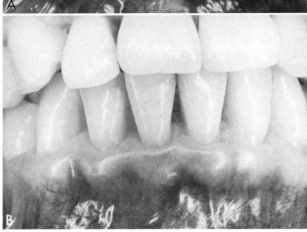

Figure 50-7 Craters Corrected by Reshaping the Gingiva. *A,* Gingival craters which remain after the treatment of acute necrotizing ulcerative gingivitis. *B,* Healed gingiva after recontouring with a periodontal knife.

TABLE 50-1 TOPICALLY APPLIED DRUGS USED IN TREATMENT OF ACUTE NECROTIZING ULCERATIVE GINGIVITIS

Oxygen-Liberating Agents
Zinc peroxide
Hydrogen peroxide
Sodium perborate
Potassium chlorate
Potassium permanganate
Sodium peroxyborate[27]

Mercurial Derivaties
Tinct. Metaphen 1:200 (untinted)
Mercuric cyanide 1%
Merthiolate 1:1,000
Mercuric chloride 1:2,000

Spirocheticides
Sodium carbonate 10% aqueous
Arsphenamine 10% aqueous
Mapharsen
Neoarsphenamine
Fuadin

Escharotics (Caustics)
Copper sulfate and zinc chloride
Chromic acid 8%
Negatan
Zinc chloride 8%
Phenol 95%
Trichloroacetic acid 50%
Iodine 16.5% and silver nitrate 35%

Aniline Dyes
Viogen (Berwick's solution)
Acriviolet 1%
Gentian violet 1%
Acriflavine 1%
Methylene blue 1%

Other Agents
Ascoxal[12]
Copper sulfate, phenol, glycerin and water
Metronidazole[9, 14]
Penicillin
Sulfonamide in paraffin—especially sulfadiazine
Surgical pack (zinc oxide–resin, eugenol)
Vancomycin[13, 21]

SYSTEMIC ANTIBIOTICS IN THE TREATMENT OF ACUTE NECROTIZING ULCERATIVE GINGIVITIS

Antibiotics are administered systemically in patients with toxic systemic complications or local adenopathy but are not recommended for topical use because of the risk of sensitization. Phenoxymethyl penicillin is the drug of choice. It may be administered as follows: (1) in table or capsule form, 400,000 units every three hours (V-Cillin K, Penn-Vee and other effective preparations); (2) intramuscular injection, 300,000 units, repeated at 24-hour intervals until the systemic symptoms subside. In penicillin-sensitive patients, other antibiotics such as erythromycin or lincomycin, 250 mg. four times daily, may be used.

Antibiotics are continued until the systemic complications or local lymphadenopathy subside. Systemic penicillin also effects some reduction in the oral bacterial flora and temporary alleviation of the oral symptoms,[26] but it is only an adjunct to the complete local treatment the disease requires. Patients treated by systemic antibiotics alone should be cautioned that the acute painful symptoms may recur after the drug is discontinued.

SUPPORTIVE SYSTEMIC TREATMENT

In addition to systemic antibiotics, supportive treatment consists of copious fluid consumption and analgesics for relief of pain. Bed rest is necessary for patients with toxic systemic complications such as high fever, malaise, anorexia and general debility.

ETIOTROPIC SYSTEMIC TREATMENT

Etiotropic treatment consists of measures for the correction of systemic conditions which contribute to the initiation or progress of acute necrotizing ulcerative gingivitis. Since the role of systemic etiologic factors has not been established, the indications for and value of systemic therapy are not clearly defined.

Nutritional supplements

The role of nutritional therapy in the treatment of gingival and periodontal disease in general is considered in Chapter 57. The rationale for nutritional supplements in the treatment of acute necrotizing ulcerative gingivitis is based upon the following: (1) Experimental evidence that lesions resembling acute necrotizing ulcerative gingivitis have been produced in animals in certain nutritional deficiencies (Chap. 11); (2) the possibility that difficulty in chewing raw fruits and vegetables in a painful condition such as acute necrotizing ulcerative gingivitis could lead to the selection of a diet inadequate in vitamins B and C. Because these are water-soluble vitamins which are not stored in the body and require continual replenishment, daily supplements may be needed to prevent a nutritional deficiency; (3) there are isolated clinical studies[5, 6] reporting fewer recurrences when local treatment of acute necrotizing ulcerative gingivitis is supplemented with vitamin B or vitamin C.

When the intake of water-soluble vitamins B and C has been severely curtailed because of pain in acute necrotizing ulcerative gingivitis, nutritional supplements may be indicated along with local treatment in order to ward off deficiencies in the aforementioned vitamins. Under such circumstances the patient may be started on a standard multivitamin preparation combined with a therapeutic dose of vitamin B and C such as the following:

Thiamine	10 mg.
Riboflavin	10 mg.
Niacinamide	100 mg.
Calcium pantothenate	20 mg.
Pyridoxine HCl	2 mg.
Folic acid	1.5 mg.
Ascorbic acid	300 mg.
Vitamin B_{12}	4 mmg.

The patient should be placed on a natural diet with the required detergent action and nutritional content as soon as the oral condition permits. Nutritional supplements may be discontinued after two months.

Local procedures are the keystone of the treatment of acute necrotizing ulcerative gingivitis. Inflammation is a local conditioning factor which impairs the nutrition of the gingiva regardless of the systemic nutritional status. Local irritants should be eliminated in order to foster normal metabolic and reparative processes in the gingiva. Persistent or recurrent acute necrotizing ulcerative gingivitis is more likely to be caused by failure to remove local irritants and inadequate plaque control than by nutritional deficiency.

SEQUELAE THAT MAY FOLLOW TREATMENT OF ACUTE NECROTIZING ULCERATIVE GINGIVITIS

Persistent or "nonresponsive" cases

If the dentist finds himself changing from drug to drug in an effort to relieve a "stubborn" case of acute necrotizing ulcerative gingivitis, something is wrong with the over-all treatment regimen which is not likely to be corrected by changing drugs. **When confronted with such a problem: (1) All local drug therapy should be discontinued so that the condition may be studied in an uncomplicated state.** (2) Careful differential diagnosis is undertaken to rule out diseases which resemble acute necrotizing ulcerative gingivitis. (See Chap. 11.) (3) A search is made for contributing local and systemic etiologic factors that may have been overlooked. (4) Special attention is given to instructing the patient in plaque control before undertaking comprehensive local treatment.

Recurrent acute necrotizing ulcerative gingivitis

The following factors should be explored in patients with recurrent acute necrotizing ulcerative gingivitis:

INADEQUATE LOCAL THERAPY. Too frequently, treatment is discontinued when the symptoms have subsided, without eliminating the chronic gingival disease and periodontal pockets which remain after the superficial acute condition is relieved. Persistent chronic inflammation causes degenerative changes which predispose the gingiva to recurrence of acute involvement.

PERICORONAL FLAP. **Recurrent acute involvement in the mandibular anterior area is often associated with persistent pericoronal inflammation arising from difficult eruption of third molars.**[2] The anterior involvement is less likely to recur after the third molar situation is corrected.

ANTERIOR OVERBITE. Marked overbite is often a contributing factor in the recurrence of disease in the anterior region. Where the incisal edges of the maxillary teeth impinge upon the labial gingival margin, or the mandibular teeth strike the palatal gingiva, the resultant tissue injury predisposes to recurrent acute disease. Less severe overbite produces food impaction and gingival trauma. Correction of the overbite is necessary for the complete treatment of acute necrotizing ulcerative gingivitis.

Inadequate plaque control and heavy use of tobacco are common causes of recurrent disease.

TREATMENT OF ACUTE PERICORONITIS

The treatment of pericoronitis depends upon the severity of the inflammation, the systemic complications and the advisibility of retaining the involved tooth. All pericoronal flaps should be viewed with suspicion. **Persistent symptom-free pericoronal flaps should be removed as a preventive measure against subsequent acute involvement.**

The following is the procedure for the treatment of acute pericoronitis:

Visit 1

1. Determination of the extent and severity of involvement of adjacent structures and toxic systemic complications (Fig. 50–8).

2. The area is gently flushed with warm water to remove superficial debris and surface exudate, and a topical anesthetic is applied.

3. The area is swabbed with antiseptic, and the flap is gently elevated from the tooth with a scaler. The underlying debris is removed, and the area is flushed with warm water (Fig. 50–8). Extensive curettage or surgical procedures are contraindicated at the initial visit. Instructions to the patient include hourly rinses with a solution of a teaspoonful of salt in a glass of warm water, rest, copious fluid intake and systemic antibiotics for fever. The patient is to return in 24 hours.

4. If the gingival flap is swollen and fluctuant, an anteroposterior incision is made with a #15 Bard-Parker blade to establish drainage, followed by insertion of a ¼″ gauze wick.

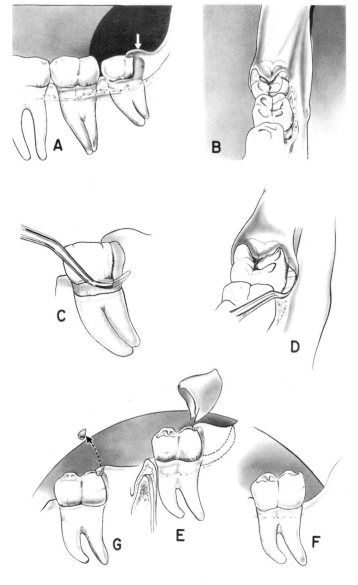

Figure 50–8 Treatment of Acute Pericoronitis. *A,* Inflamed pericoronal flap in relation to the mandibular third molar. *B,* Anterior view of third molar and flap. *C,* Lateral view with Younger-Good scaler in position to gently remove debris under flap. *D,* Anterior view of scaler in position. *E,* Removal of section of the gingiva distal to the third molar, after the acute symptoms subside. The line of incision is indicated by the dotted line. *F,* Appearance of the healed area. *G,* Incorrect removal of the tip of the flap, permitting deep pocket to remain distal to the molar.

Visit 2

After 24 hours, the condition is usually markedly improved. If a drain had been inserted, it is removed. The flap is gently separated from the tooth and the area flushed with warm water. The patient is to continue with the instructions of the previous day and return in 24 hours.

Visit 3

At this visit, a determination is made as to whether the tooth is to be retained or extracted. This decision is governed by the likelihood of further eruption into a good functional position. Bone loss on the distal surface of the second molars is a hazard following the extraction of partially or completely impacted third molars[8] which is significantly greater if the third molars are extracted after the roots are formed or in patients beyond their early twenties. **To reduce the risk of bone loss around second molars, partially or completely impacted third molars should be extracted as early as possible in their development.**

If it is decided to retain the tooth, the necessary surgical procedures are performed at this visit, provided there are no acute symptoms. Periodontal knives or electrosurgery are used for this purpose. Under anesthesia, an incision is begun just anterior to the border of the ramus and brought downward and forward to the distal surface of the crown, as close as possible to the level of the cemento-enamel junction. This will detach a wedge-shaped section of tissue that includes the gingival flap (Fig. 50–8).

It is necessary to remove the tissue distal to the tooth as well as the flap on the occlusal surface. Incising only the occlusal portion of the flap leaves a deep distal pocket which invites recurrence of acute pericoronal involvement.

After the tissue is removed, a periodontal pack is applied. The pack may be retained by bringing it forward along the facial and lingual surfaces into the interproximal space between the second and third molars. The pack is removed after one week.

Pericoronitis and acute necrotizing ulcerative gingivitis

Pericoronal flaps which are chronically inflamed may become the sites of acute necrotizing ulcerative gingivitis. The disease is treated in the same manner as elsewhere in the mouth and, after acute symptoms have subsided, the flap is removed. Pericoronal flaps are often referred to as "primary incubation zones" in acute necrotizing ulcerative gingivitis; their elimination is one of many measures required to minimize the likelihood of recurrent disease.

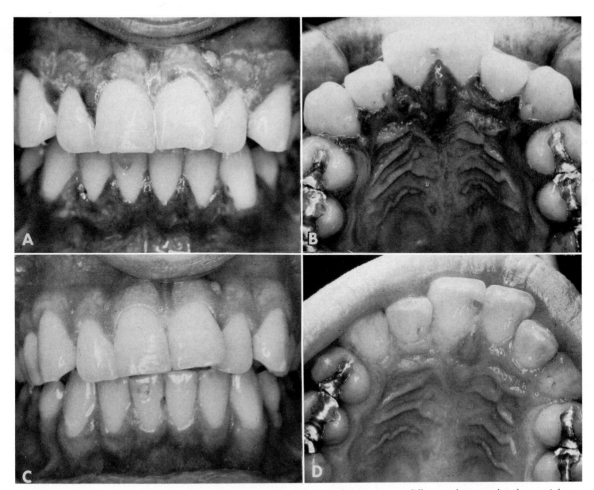

Figure 50–9   Treatment of Acute Herpetic Gingivostomatitis. *A,* Before treatment, diffuse erythema and surface vesicles. *B,* Before treatment, lingual view showing gingival edema and ruptured vesicle on palate. *C,* One month after treatment showing restoration of normal gingival contour and stippling. *D,* One month after treatment, lingual view.

TREATMENT OF ACUTE HERPETIC GINGIVOSTOMATITIS

Various medications have been used in the treatment of this condition, including local applications of 8 per cent zinc chloride, camphorated phenol, spirits of camphor. Talbot's iodine, phenol, sulfonamide solutions, moccasin snake venom,[17] systemically administered yeast,[19] riboflavin, vitamin B complex,[11] thiamine and radiation therapy. Aureomycin has been used successfully as a mouthwash,[10] applied topically in a 3 per cent ointment[16] or administered systemically in the form of 250 mg. capsules for a total dosage of 3 grams.[20] Vaccination with smallpox vaccine or a vaccine prepared from the contents of the vesicles has been described both as a therapeutic measure and also for the prevention of recurrence,[18,22] but the results are doubtful.

Treatment consists of palliative measures to make the patient comfortable until the disease runs its course (seven to ten days).

Plaque, food debris and superficial calculus are removed to reduce gingival inflammation which complicates the acute herpetic involvement. Extensive periodontal therapy should be postponed until the acute symptoms subside in order to avoid the possibility of exacerbation (Fig. 50–9). Painful, swollen herpetic infection of a dentist's finger after preparing a crown in a patient with herpetic lesions on the lower lip has been reported.[24]

Relief of pain to enable the patient to eat comfortably is obtained with Dyclone (dyclonic hydrochloride), a topical anesthetic mouthwash[28] which is available in 0.5 per cent solution which may be diluted 1 to 1 with water. It is held in the mouth for one or two minutes and swished around, to produce an anesthetic effect that lasts for 40 minutes. It is helpful when used before meals, but may be used more often without toxic effects.

Supportive treatment

Supportive measures include copious fluid intake and systemic antibiotic therapy (Aureomycin, 250 mg. four times daily) for the management of toxic systemic complications. For the relief of pain, systemically administered aspirin or Bufferin is usually sufficient. A dosage of 10 grains of the former or 2 tablets of the latter, every three hours, may be prescribed for adults, with smaller doses used for children.

REFERENCES

Acute Necrotizing Ulcerative Gingivitis

1. Burket, L. W.: Oral Medicine. 3rd ed. Philadelphia, J. B. Lippincott Co., 1946, p. 53.
2. Frankl, Z.: Dentitio Difficilis and Parodontosis. Paradentologie, 1:107, 1947.
3. Glickman, I.: The Use of Pencillin Lozenges in the Treatment of Vincent's Infection and Other Acute Gingival Inflammations. J.A.D.A., 34:406, 1947.
4. Glickman, I., and Johannessen, L. B.: The Effect of a Six per cent Solution of Chromic Acid on the Gingiva of the Albino Rat—A Correlated Gross, Biomicroscopic, and Histologic Study. J.A.D.A., 41:674, 1950.
5. King, J. D.: Nutritional and Other Factors in "Trench Mouth" with Special Reference to the Nicotinic Acid Component of the Vitamin B₂ Complex. Brit D. J., 74:113. 1943.
6. Linghorne, W. J., McIntosh, W. G., Tice, J. W., Tisdall, F. F., McCreary, J. F., Drake, T. G. H., Greaves, A. V., and Johnstone, W. M.: The Relation of Ascorbic Acid Intake to Gingivitis. J. Canad. D. A., 12:49, 1946.
7. Roth, H.: Vitamins as an Adjunct in the Treatment of Periodontal Disease. J.A.D.A., 32:60, 1945.

Acute Pericoronitis

8. Ash, M. M., Jr., Costich, E. R., and Hayward, J. R.: A Study of Periodontal Hazards of Third Molars. J. Periodont., 33:209, 1962.
9. Wade, A. B., Blake, G., and Mirza, K.: Effectiveness of Metronidazole in Treating the Acute Phase of Ulcerative Gingivitis. D. Practit. & D. Rec., 16:440, 1966.

Acute Herpetic Gingivostomatitis

10. Arnold, H. L., Domzalski, C. A., and Austin, E. R.: Aureomycin Mouthwash for Herpetic Stomatitis. Proc. Staff Meet. Honolulu, 15:85, 1949.
11. Burket, L. W., and Hickman, G. C.: Oral Herpes (Simplex) Manifestations: Treatment with Vitamin B Complex. J.A.D.A., 29:411, 1942.
12. Clausen, F. P.: Local Treatment of Acute Necrotizing Ulcerative Gingivitis with Ascoxal: Clinical Experiences from Treatment of Military Personnel. Tandlaegebladet, 70:1009, 1966.
13. Collins, J., and Hood, H. M.: Topical Antibiotic Treatment of Acute Necrotizing Ulcerative Gingivitis. J. Oral Med., 22:59, 1967.
14. Duckworth, R., Waterhouse, J. P., Britton, D. E. R., Nuki, K., Sheiham, A., Winter, R., and Blake, G. C.: Acute Ulcerative Gingivitis: A Double-Blind Con-

trolled Clinical Trial of Metronidazole. Brit. D. J., *120*:599, 1966.

15. Emslie, R.: Treatment of Acute Ulcerative Gingivitis. A Clinical Trial Using Chewing Gum Containing Metronidazole or Penicillin. Brit. D. J., *122*:307, 1967.

16. Everett, F. G.: Aureomycin in the Therapy of Herpes Simplex Labialis and Recurrent Oral Aphthae. J.A.D.A., *40*:555, 1950.

17. Fisher, A. A.: Treatment of Herpes Simplex with Moccasin Snake Venom. Arch. Derm. & Syph., *43*:444, 1941.

18. Frank, S. B.: Formalized Herpes Virus Therapy and the Neutralizing Substance in Herpes Simplex. J. Invest. Dermat., *1*:267, 1940.

19. Gerstenberger, H. J.: The Etiology and Treatment of Herpetic (Aphthous and Aphthoulcerative) Stomatitis and Herpes Labialis. Am. J. Dis. Child., *26*:309, 1923.

20. Jacobs, H. G., and Jacobs, M. H.: Aureomycin: Its Use in Infections of the Oral Cavity. Oral Surg., Oral Med. & Oral Path., *2*:1015, 1949.

21. Mitchell, D. F., and Baker, B. R.: Topical Antibiotic Control of Necrotizing Gingivitis. J. Periodont., *39*:81, 1968.

22. Savitt, L. E., and Ayres, S., Jr.: Persistent Multiple Herpes-like Eruption. Response to Repeated Intradermal Injections of Smallpox Vaccine. Arch. Derm. & Syph., *59*:653, 1949.

23. Shinn, D. L. S., Squires, S., and McFadzean, A.: The Treatment of Vincent's Disease with Metronidazole. D. Practit., *15*:275, 1965.

24. Synder, M. L., Church, D. H., and Rickles, N. H.: Primary Herpes Infection of Right Second Finger. Oral Surg., *27*:598, 1969.

25. Stephen, K. W., McLatchie, M. F., Mason, D. K., Noble, H. W., and Stevenson, D. M.: Treatment of Acute Ulcerative Gingivitis (Vincent's Type). Brit. D. J., *121*:313, 1966.

26. Wade, A. B., Blake, G. C., Manson, J. D., Berdon, J. K., Mathieson, F., and Bate, D. M.: Treatment of the Acute Phase of Ulcerative Gingivitis (Vincent's Type). Brit. D. J., *115*:372, 1963.

27. Wade, A. B., and Mirza, K. B.: The Relative Effectiveness of Sodium Peroxyborate and Hydrogen Peroxide in Treating Acute Ulcerative Gingivitis. D. Practit., *14*:185, 1964.

28. Weisberger, D.: Treatment of Some Diseases of the Soft Tissues of the Mouth. D. Clin. North America, March 1960, p. 215.

Chapter 51

DRUGS AND OTHER PERIODONTAL THERAPEUTIC AIDS

Most techniques for the treatment of gingival and periodontal disease do not rely on the use of drugs; however, there are many situations in which they serve a useful purpose. This chapter contains pertinent information regarding representative drugs used in the management of periodontal disorders.*

SYSTEMICALLY ADMINISTERED DRUGS

For systemic action drugs are administered parenterally (intramuscularly, subcutaneously, intravenously) and orally.

Parenteral

Parenteral use provides rapid drug absorption and effect; surgical asepsis is essential to prevent infection. Intravenous injection results in almost immediate action and is usually employed with relatively innocuous drugs and the vitamins.

Oral

Oral administration depends upon absorption of the drug from the gastrointestinal tract. Its advantages over parenteral injections are ease of administration, relative safety because of gradual absorption, and the absence of complications at the site of injection. However, the facts that many drugs are destroyed in the gastrointestinal tract and that the time lapse

---

*For more extensive coverage of useful drugs, see the current edition of Accepted Dental Therapeutics, published by the Council on Dental Therapeutics of the American Dental Association.[1]

between administration and action is relatively long, preclude oral administration in some instances.

CHEMOTHERAPEUTIC AGENTS

Chemotherapy is the treatment of disease by administrating chemicals which adversely affect the causative agents without injuring the patient. Chemotherapy is used in periodontics for the prevention and treatment of systemic complications of acute oral infections, and (2) as a preoperative prophylactic measure against infections or bacteremia following scaling and curettage or surgical periodontal procedures. This is imperative in patients with a history of rheumatic fever or congenital cardiac valve injury.

Bacteremia following periodontal treatment

Bacteremia may occur in as many as 88 per cent of patients following periodontal treatment,[67b] but lower incidences have been reported (16–46 per cent following prophylaxis;[76a] 8 per cent[67a] and 83.8 per cent[42a] following scaling; 26.3 per cent following scaling and curettage,[77a] and 24.56[76a] 38.18[33a] and 83.3[42a] per cent following gingivectomy). The size of the blood sample, the time at which it is taken, the ratio of sample to medium and the nature of the culture media may account for the differences in the findings in the various studies.[67b] Bacteremia has also been noted in patients with periodontal disease previous to treatment.[42a]

Post-treatment bacteremias are transient, with most of the bacteria eliminated within 10 minutes by the natural defense mechanisms. The bacteremia is likely to persist as long as surgical manipulation of the tissues is in progress. In some cases, bacteria are recovered from the blood stream more than two hours after gingivectomy.[76a] The incidence of bacteremia is related to the duration of the treatment, and may[21a, 77b] or may not[33a, 76b] be related to the severity of the disease or the mobility of the teeth.

Seventy different strains of organisms have been recovered at different times following scaling and curettage and gingivectomy,[67b] including strains of *Streptococcus, Diphtheroid, Vibrio, Spirillum,* *Tetracoccus, Bacteroides, Veillonella, Fusobacterium, Actinomyces, Micrococcus, Leptotrichia* and two nontypable anaerobes. Streptococci and diphtheroids were found most frequently.[33a, 76a]

The greatest interest is in *S. viridans*, the most common organism. Transient bacteremia is usually unattended by clinical sequelae, but in patients with a history of rheumatic fever or congenital heart valve injury, it constitutes a real menace. The circulating bacteria may lodge and vegetate on the injured valve and establish bacterial endocarditis. *S. viridans* is almost always the responsible organism. Two cases of subacute bacterial endocarditis associated with *Lactobacillus acidophilus* have been reported,[14a] and one with *S. mitis*.[23a]

The incidence of postgingivectomy bacteremia may be reduced by a preliminary root-planing one week earlier;[42a] however, the reduction is offset by the additional bacteremia caused by the root planing itself. Bacteremia may be reduced by flooding periodontal pockets with a mixture of phenol, aconite, iodine and glycerine for five minutes before scaling and curettage,[77b] but not by spraying with cetyl pyridinium chloride.[21b] Pretreatment with chemotherapy is the most effective way of reducing the incidence of bacteremia.

The effectiveness of chemotherapeutic agents results from retardation of the rate of multiplication of microorganisms (inhibitory), cessation of multiplication (bacteriostatic or fungistatic) and/or destruction of viable organisms (bactericidal or fungicidal). Antibiotics and sulfonamides are the commonly used chemotherapeutic agents.

Antibiotics

Antibiotics are substances produced by living organisms such as molds and bacteria that inhibit or destroy infective agents. There are numerous antibiotics, with new ones effective against different spectra of organisms constantly being developed. Selection should be based upon the specificity of the drug for the needs of the patient.

The following antibiotics are effective against the common gram-positive organisms and are of principal interest in periodontics:

Potassium penicillin G (Pentids), sodium penicillin G (Bicillin) and phenoxymethyl penicillin (V-Cillin, V-Cillin K, Pen Vee, Compocillin-V).

Erythromycin (Erythrocin stearate) and erythromycin estolate (Ilosone); the latter is contraindicated in patients with liver disease or dysfunction.

Lincomycin hydrochloride (Lincocin), and the cephalosporins, cephalothin and cephaloridine (also effective against gram-negative organisms).

There are many antibiotics which are effective against a **wide spectrum of organisms,** but they introduce the risk of disrupting the intestinal flora and producing resistant strains of organisms. It is preferable to select antibiotics based upon their specificity for the patient's needs.

The tetracyclines are a group of wide spectrum antibiotics which include tetracycline (Achromycin, Panmycin and Tetracyn), chlortetracycline hydrocloride (Aureomycin), oxytetracycline (Terramycin) and demeclocycline hydrochloride (Declomycin). Tetracyclines ingested when teeth are being formed may produce permanent discoloration and hypoplasia.

Streptomycin is not recommended for dental use because it may produce permanent vertigo and/or hearing loss and is also nephrotoxic; kanamycin, vancomycin, colistin and gentamicin may create similar results.[57]

Phenoxymethyl penicillin is the systemic antibiotic of choice for most periodontal needs; it is essentially nontoxic with no ill effects with blood levels 100 times the therapeutic level. It is an analogue of penicillin G which is absorbed more rapidly, is less susceptible to inactivation by acids and can be given with meals. The usual dosage for oral administration is one 250 mg. tablet or capsule (400,000 units) four times a day, or intramuscularly, 300,000 units, every 24 hours.

Allergic reactions caused by sensitization occur more frequently with penicillin than with other antibiotics; urticaria is the most common type. Other allergic reactions include exfoliative dermatitis, angioneurotic edema and a syndrome including fever, joint pains and lymph node enlargement.[39] The reactions generally occur one to two weeks after the initiation of therapy. They may be alleviated by discontinuing the drug and prescribing antihistamines such as Pyribenzamine or Benadryl. Continued use of penicillin may lead to the development of penicillin-resistant strains of bacteria and require the substitution of a different antibacterial agent. In patients with known sensitivity, alternate drugs such as erythromycin or lincomycin in 250 mg. tablets or capsules every four hours, which are effective against the same organisms, should be used. Other antibiotics are used for infections with penicillin-resistant organisms.

PROPHYLACTIC "ANTIBIOTIC UMBRELLA" IN PERIODONTAL TREATMENT. Antibiotics do not participate in healing, but may affect it favorably by preventing infection, or hinder it by disrupting protein synthesis. If antibiotics are administered as a protective "umbrella" to prevent infection, they should be started the evening before treatment and continued for 48 hours after the operative procedure. Longer postoperative periods invite the risk of superimposed infection from organisms which thrive when the susceptible flora is reduced.

Nystatin (Mycostatin) is a fungistatic antibiotic with some effectiveness in the treatment of oral moniliasis (thrush). It is administered systemically three times daily in a 500,000 unit tablet or as Mysteclin tablets (500,000 units of nystatin and 250 mg. of tetracycline), one every six hours. Nystatin cream, 100,000 units per gram, is helpful in the treatment of chronic angular cheilitis.[72] Amphotericin B is an antifungal antibiotic administered by slow intravenous infusion in a dosage of 0.25 mg. per kilogram of body weight.[35] Even under supervised hospital conditions, the use of this drug is limited because of its potential toxicity. Local irritation and allergic dermatitis may follow its topical use.

Oral change such as generalized stomatitis, "black tongue" and acute moniliasis may occur in patients under systemic antibiotic therapy. They result from the disruption of the normal microbial symbiosis and overgrowth of ordinarily inhibited pathogens. Many antibiotics (among them are penicillin, tetracycline, erythromycin, chloramphenicol and streptomycin) and sulfonamides are secreted in the oral cavity through the salivary glands.[2,9,10,18,32,65]

Sulfonamides

The sulfonamides are used as chemotherapeutic agents in patients sensitive to antibiotics. They are effective against coccal infections—streptococcal, diplococcal, and micrococcal. Sulfonamides have many toxic effects; they are insoluble and tend to precipitate in the kidneys. Sulfisoxazole (Gantrisin) may be used without danger of renal complications. An initial dose of four to six 0.5 gm. tablets is followed by one tablet every four or five hours.

Analgesics and narcotics

Analgesics and narcotics are drugs used for the relief of pain. Acetylsalicylic acid—aspirin—is effective in adults in dosages of two five grain tablets every three hours. Smaller doses are used for children.

Acetophenetidin (phenacetin) is an analgesic usually used in mixtures with acetylsalicylic acid and caffeine as follows:

Acetylsalicylic acid	3½ grains
Phenacetin	2½ grains
Caffeine	½ grain

Buffered acetylsalicylic acid (Bufferin) comes in tablets containing acetylsalicylic acid, 0.3 gm.; magnesium carbonate, 0.1 gm.; aluminum glycerate, 45 mg.; and excipients, 0.12 gm. Adult dosage is two tablets every three hours. It is effective and unattended by the gastric complaints sometimes reported with acetylsalicylic acid. Acetaminophen, 325 to 650 mg. daily, may be used as a substitute for aspirin.

Darvon Compound 65 is a non-narcotic analgesic for severe pain. Each capsule contains 65 mg. dextropropoxyphene hydrochloride, 227 mg. aspirin, 162 mg. acetophenetidin, and 32.4 mg. caffeine. Dosage is one capsule every three or four hours. Pentazocine hydrochloride (Talwin) is also an effective non-narcotic analgesic. The usual dosage is 50 mg. every four hours. There are reservations regarding its use in children under 12, and during pregnancy.

Codeine is a narcotic with analgesic, hypnotic and sedative effects. It is usually administered in tablet preparations together with acetylsalicylic acid, phenacetin and caffeine, as follows:

Acetylsalicylic acid	3½ grains
Phenacetin	2½ grains
Caffeine	½ grain
Codeine	¼ grain

Two tablets every three hours is an effective dose in cases of severe pain.

Demerol hydrochloride (meperidine hydrochloride) is a narcotic for severe pain, and for insomnia that may accompany pain. It may be administered orally in 50 mg. tablets every four hours, or intramuscularly.

Morphine surpasses all other analgesics in effectiveness, particularly for persistent pain. Habituation is readily established, and for this reason morphine should be used only when adequate relief from pain cannot be obtained from other drugs. Morphine is usually prescribed as morphine sulphate, 8 to 10 mg. every four to six hours—orally, subcutaneously or intramuscularly.

SEDATIVES AND HYPNOTICS

Barbiturates

The barbiturates are effective sedatives and hypnotics for preoperative sedation of apprehensive patients; they are not used for relief of pain. These drugs should not be administered in the office unless someone is available to accompany the patient home.

Pentobarbital (Nembutal) is a short-acting barbiturate; a 100 mg. capsule approximately 30 minutes before operative procedures is usually effective. Seconal (100 mg. capsule) is another barbiturate that may be used in this way.

Promethazine hydrochloride (Phenergan hydrochloride) is an effective sedative and antihistaminic. The preoperative dosage for adult patients is 25 to 50 mg. It should not be given to ambulatory patients who are going to drive after they leave the office.

Phenobarbital is a long-acting sedative and hypnotic. Large doses may cause severe circulatory depression. Patients with toxic goiter react with severe rashes. The average dosage is 50 mg.

Tranquilizers

These drugs are useful for the relief of anxiety, tension and fear. Among the commonly used tranquilizers are chlordiazepoxide (Librium), adult dosage 5 or 10 mg., three or four times daily; meprobamate (Miltown), a tranquilizer with muscle relaxant action, adult dosage 200 or 400 mg., three times a day; diazepam (Valium), adult dosage 2 to 10 mg., two to four times daily; and hydroxyzine hydrochloride (Vistaril), 25 to 100 mg., three or four times daily. Patients using tranquilizers often complain of having a dry mouth.

SKELETAL MUSCLE RELAXANTS

These drugs are useful in patients with painful temporomandibular joint disorders or painful muscle spasms. Mephenesin (Tolserol) or mephenesin carbamate (Tolseram), in a dosage of 2 to 3 gm. 20 minutes prior to the time the patient is seen, provides the muscle relaxation necessary for dental procedures. Relief of painful muscle spasms may also be obtained with methocarbamol (Robaxin),[43] 1.5 to 2 gm., four times daily for two or three days and 1 gm. daily thereafter, or chlorphenesin carbamate, 1.6 to 2.4 gm. daily in divided doses.[3]

DRUGS USED LOCALLY IN PERIODONTAL TREATMENT

Antibiotics

Transitory relief of the symptoms of acute oral infections may be obtained from antibiotics in lozenge or troche form. However, because of untoward effects, such as edema of the oral mucosa (with sloughing in extreme cases), painful glossitis, the occurrence of acute oral moniliasis and the possibility of sensitizing the patient and causing allergic side reactions in other areas of the body, **the topical use of antibiotics is discouraged.**

Corticosteroids

KENALOG IN ORABASE. Kenalog, triamcinolone acetonide 0.1 per cent (a derivative of triamcinolone), is a potent synthetic glucocorticoid used topically for the treatment of certain acute and chronic mucous membrane lesions. Orabase is a nontoxic vehicle which is adhesive and maintains drug contact with the oral mucosa. It is applied topically to the lesions four times daily, after meals and before retiring.[79] Sex hormones sometimes used in the treatment of gingival disorders may cause local vascular abnormalities.[44]

Local anti-infectives

These are substances which act as disinfectants, destroying bacteria at the site of application, or antiseptics, preventing the growth of bacteria at the site of application as long as the drug is present. The efficacy of an antiseptic or disinfectant is expressed in terms of its phenol coefficient; that is, the ratio of its germicidal power to that of phenol. An ideal antiseptic must have a high efficiency and low toxicity, must be active in the presence of purulent material, should be nonirritating and should act against a wide range of bacteria. Those commonly used in periodontal practice are peroxides, mercury preparations and dyes.

PEROXIDES. The oxygen liberated by unstable peroxides is responsible for their germicidal power. Hydrogen peroxide is decomposed by tissue catalase and bubbles of oxygen are formed. A 3 per cent hydrogen peroxide solution is a useful adjunct as a cleaning agent and antiseptic in scaling and curettage. Other forms of oxygen therapy such as insufflation into the gingival tissues, Superoxol (30 per cent hydrogen peroxide), zinc peroxide, carbamide peroxide in glycerin and sodium perborate serve no useful purpose.

Sodium perborate has been widely used in the care of the mouth, and specifically for acute necrotizing ulcerative gingivitis, despite reports from different clinical sources and animal experiments describing unfavorable sequelae following its use. Edema of the lips, necrosis of the oral mucosa[35] and mat-like brownish-black patches on the tongue,[15, 55, 77] which heal after the drug is discontinued, have been observed in patients using sodium perborate mouthwash. Under experimental conditions, when sodium perborate was applied in poultices in humans[70] and daily as a paste in animals,[28] inflammation, vesication, necrosis and sloughing of the oral mucosa resulted. The validity of the assumption that "neutralized" preparations of sodium perborate are less likely to produce undesirable tissue changes has not been established.[28]

MERCURY PREPARATIONS. Merthiolate,

Metaphen, Merbromin and Mercresin are relatively nonirritating mercurial antiseptics useful in pre- and postoperative cleansing of the field of operation.

DYES. Local antiseptic action is due to their bacteriostatic and bactericidal powers. Commonly employed dyes are:

Acriflavine	1% aqueous solution
Gentian violet	1% in 50% alcohol solution
Brilliant green	1% in 50% alcohol solution

The dyes are effective antiseptic agents that can be used as an adjunct in the treatment of periodontal disease without risk of tissue irritation. Gentian violet is used as a specific treatment for moniliasis. A word of caution is indicated regarding the indiscriminate use of dyes. *By staining the tissues, these agents obscure the clinical features of the disease and complicate diagnosis.*

ANESTHETICS

These are used by injection or topically to prevent pain during surgical procedures or subgingival scaling and curettage. Those commonly administered by injection are procaine hydrochloride, lidocaine hydrochloride, butethamine hydrochloride (Monocaine)[34] and mepivacaine hydrochloride (Carbocaine).

There are many topical anesthetics, in liquid, gel and aerosol forms (Topanol, Butyn, Cetacaine, Xylocaine); butacaine sulfite, benzyl alcohol and benzocaine are the usual components. Applied liberally to the field of operation these are helpful in scaling and curettage, incising acute periodontal abscesses or pericoronitis. Care must be exercised in the use of spray anesthetics to prevent inhalation, which may cause a toxic reaction.

Dyclone (0.5 per cent dyclonine hydrochloride) is used as a topical anesthetic mouthwash. A small amount; five minutes before eating, swished thoroughly around the mouth, provides sufficient anesthesia to enable patients with painful mucous membrane lesions to eat comfortably. It lasts for about 40 minutes and may be repeated to provide continuous relief from pain.

ASTRINGENTS

These are drugs that temporarily reduce or condense the surface area of moderately inflamed, engorged or edematous mucous membranes or other tissues, and thereby reduce the likelihood of bacterial invasion. Tannic acid, tincture of myrrh, ferric chloride and ferric subsulfate powder are commonly used astringents. The latter two drugs are also useful for the control of bleeding.

Hemostatics and vasoconstrictors

Hemostatics are drugs that stop bleeding from lacerated capillaries and arterioles by producing a rapid coagulation of the blood about the vessels. They are ineffective in cases of severe hemorrhage, where sutures or compression must be employed.

Ferric subsulfate powder is useful to arrest gingival bleeding. A cotton pellet dipped in the powder is applied to the bleeding area and kept there for about 20 minutes.

Thrombin is a drug capable of hastening the process of blood clotting. It is intended for topical application only and is applied as a liquid or a powder.

Oxidized cellulose (Novacell, Oxycel) and absorbable gelatin sponge (Gelfoam) are useful hemostatics in deep wounds, rather than for gingival surface bleeding. Epinephrine is sometimes used to control bleeding during scaling and curettage (1:25,000) and in gingival retraction (1:10,000). Because it increases the blood pressure and heart rate it must be used guardedly; allergic manifestations have also been reported.

PERIODONTAL PACKS (PERIODONTAL DRESSINGS)

These are used for postoperative care following surgical periodontal procedures. Two principal types are in use (with and without eugenol), and plastics are being investigated.

Eugenol packs

Most periodontal packs consist of zinc oxide and eugenol, with varied ingredients.

The Kirkland-Kaiser periodontal pack is in this group. The pack is prepared from a powder and liquid (Chap. 43).

The powder consists of zinc oxide, powdered rosin and tannic acid flakes. It is prepared as follows: Mix the zinc oxide and powdered rosin in equal proportion by weight. To four parts of this mixture add one part by weight of tannic acid flakes. Mix thoroughly. The liquid is a mixture of one part peanut oil and two parts eugenol. It is prepared as follows: Pour the eugenol into a test tube, add a lump of rosin about the size of the last joint of the thumb and warm over a burner flame until the rosin is liquefied. After this is cooled, add the peanut oil.

The pack is ready for use immediately after it is mixed. Wrapped in wax paper it retains its working qualities for an entire day. It may also be frozen and stored for longer periods and removed from the freezer prior to use.

Another pack in this group is the following:

	Powder
Zinc oxide	63 gm.
Rosin	30 gm.
Asbestos fiber	5 gm.
Zinc acetate	2 gm.
	Liquid
Eugenol	80 cc.
Olive oil	20 cc.

Non-eugenol packs

A typical non-eugenol, fat-containing pack consists of:

Powder
Zinc oxide
Rosin Powder
Zinc bacitracin

Ointment
Zinc oxide
Hydrogenated fat

Coe-Pack is a non-eugenol pack with demonstrated antimicrobial action (in vitro)[63] which is well accepted by patients. It is supplied in two tubes and must be used when it is mixed.

Tube 1
Metallic oxides
Lorothidol
Tube 2
Nonionizing carboxylic acids
Chlorothymol

Cyanoacrylate pack

N-butyl cyanoacrylate is a periodontal dressing which is applied in drops or as a spray and solidifies in five to ten seconds.[7, 13] Polymerization from liquid to solid state is catalyzed by moisture, heat and pressure. It adheres to smooth and irregular surfaces for periods of from two to seven days. N-butyl cyanoacrylate has been studied extensively in clinical trials, but has not as yet been released for general periodontal use.

Each of the above packs has its proponents, but the choice is often a matter of individual preference. Some claim that non-eugenol packs produce less inflammation when used on exposed bone,[6, 8] but others find no such differences.[26, 60] No differences have been observed in the tissue reaction around eugenol and non-eugenol implants.[33]

Degenerative changes occur in healing epithelium beneath eugenol and non-eugenol packs,[64] and they produce no difference in postoperative sequelae following scaling and curettage or gingivectomy.[61] Comparable healing has been reported following gingivectomy with or without a pack.[73] Comparison of the effects of eugenol, non-eugenol and N-butyl cyanoacrylate on denuded bone, partial thickness flaps and mucoperiosteal flaps reveals no microscopic differences in healing, but the cyanoacrylate-packed areas appear better clinically.[60] Cyanoacrylate is normally phagocytized by leukocytes, but some report that it may delay healing by producing foreign body granulomas.[78]

Antibiotics in packs

Improved healing and patient comfort,[5] with less odor and taste,[7] have been obtained by including zinc bacitracin (3000 units per gram) in the pack. Other antibiotics such as Terramycin[25] (125 mg. powdered drug in six drops of liquid), neomycin and nitrofurazone have also been tried, but all produce hypersensitivity reactions.[53]

An "intraoral adhesive bandage" (consisting of pectin, gelatin, sodium carboxymethyl cellulose and polyisobutylene, coated on the outside with a polyethylene film) has been tried to secure periodontal grafts without suturing.

Wax packs and periodontal varnish

At one time very popular, these are no longer widely used. A typical wax pack consists of a mixture of cocoa butter and paraffin, one to two parts by volume, cut into strips and applied following gingivectomy with slight pressure interproximally, facially or lingually.

Periodontal varnish serves as a protection following scaling and curettage.[15] The area is dried before it is applied; a typical varnish consists of:

Gum copal	
Gum mastic	āā16.0
Tr. myrrh	
Ether	āā20.0
Collodion	40.0

DRUGS IN POCKET ERADICATION

Through the years some clinicians have felt that escharotic drugs improve the effectiveness of scaling and curettage procedures for pocket elimination by destroying degenerated tissue in the pocket wall and facilitating healing. Silver nitrate, chromic acid and phenol are examples of such drugs. Although they are used in small quantities, there is no assurance that these drugs will not also destroy healthy tissue and inadvertently delay healing.

McCall's[52] *epithelial solvent* is a solution of sodium sulfide used in pocket eradication for the removal of the lateral epithelial wall; opinions differ regarding its effectiveness.[12,56] Sodium hypochlorite (Antiformin), advocated for its supposed selective action as an epithelial solvent, has been demonstrated[29,37] to have a nonspecific necrotizing effect upon both the epithelium and the connective tissue of the pocket wall.

PREPARATIONS FOR DESENSITIZING TEETH

There are many methods of desensitizing hypersensitive cervical areas of teeth in the dental office; our choice is sodium fluoride paste. It is prepared by mixing 10 gm. each of sodium fluoride and kaolin with sufficient glycerin to form a paste which is stored in a closed container, and is used as follows:

The tooth surface is dried and the paste burnished with a metal instrument and left in position for two minutes. The patient may report an initial sensation of cold. The paste is removed with warm water, and the mouth is thoroughly rinsed. Burnishing is important; comparable results are not obtained when the paste is applied with a rubber cup. It may be repeated after two weeks if necessary. Sodium fluoride paste is effective, and does not injure the gingiva or discolor the teeth; it should not be used on freshly cut tooth surfaces.

Other desensitizing agents for office use are zinc chloride, 8 per cent solution, liquid phenol, formaldahyde, ammoniacal silver nitrate; a mixture of sodium carbonate monohydrate, 2.5 gm., with potassium carbonate, 12.5 mg.; and sodium silico-fluoride.[36,51] Except for the last two, these chemicals are not to be used on freshly cut dentin to avoid injury to viable tissue.

Desensitizing preparations used by the patient

The following solution, which is applied by the patient, is helpful for generalized sensitivity:

R
2% aqueous solution sodium fluoride	8 oz.
Color and flavor	

Pour small amount into glass. Dip toothbrush in solution and use as dentifrice. *Caution:* Do not swallow.

Sensitivity is usually relieved by the time the 8 oz. is used. Sodium fluoride paste may be used for areas where sensitivity persists.

Reduction in sensitivity has also been reported with a stannous fluoride–containing gel used as a dentifrice[54] and with a sodium monofluorophosphate dentifrice.[38] Some patients report relief with dentifrices containing formalin (Thermodent)[24] and strontium chloride (Sensodyne).[16,68] Corticosteroid hormones are also being tried for desensitizing exposed root surfaces.[59]

DENTIFRICES

Dentifrices are aids for cleaning and polishing tooth surfaces and may be used in the form of paste, powder or liquid. Powders and pastes contain abrasives, such as calcium carbonate, calcium phosphate, calcium sulfate, sodium bicarbonate and sodium chloride, soaps or synthetic detergents and flavoring agents. In addition, the pastes contain humectants (glycerin, sorbitol), water, thickening agents (carboxymethyl cellulose, carrageen) and foaming agent.

There is considerable interest in improving dentifrices by adding chemicals with a potential for inhibiting plaque and calculus.* One such enzyme-containing dentifrice (Extar) prevents deposition of supragingival calculus on surfaces that are mechanically cleansed with the brush, but not in inaccessible areas. Substances such as penicillin, dibasic ammonium phosphate, vaccines[14] and chlorophyll in dentifrices are of no demonstrable value in the treatment of gingival disease.

Abrasivity of dentifrices

Dentifrices should be sufficiently abrasive for satisfactorily cleansing and polishing but should provide a margin of safety to protect the aggressive toothbrusher from wearing away tooth substance and soft restorative materials.[41, 67] The abrasive quality of dentifrices affects enamel, but it is more of a concern in patients with exposed, less resistant, cementum and dentin.[74] The Council on Dental Therapeutics of the American Dental Association has graded the abrasion of many popular dentifrices, based upon the removal of dentin by standardized brushing in an in vitro system.[66] Dentifrices which provide the cleansing effectiveness required for plaque control, with a minimum of abrasion, may be selected from this list for periodontal patients. Inasmuch as the formulations of dentifrices are occasionally changed, the most current information should be obtained from the Council.

MOUTHWASHES

Mouthwashes are usually pleasant-tasting, aromatic solutions which rinse away loose debris but are not substitutes for the cleansing attainable by toothbrushing and other oral hygiene aids. Many mouthwashes produce a temporary re-

duction of oral bacteria,[45, 48, 49] but there is no evidence that this is beneficial or desirable. Some popular mouthwashes decrease plaque accumulation;[40, 75] the effect may be slight.[11]

The flavoring and aromatic chemicals in mouthwashes make the mouth feel refreshed, and some produce a temporary reduction in mouth odors beyond the masking effect of the mouthwash.[21, 58] Mouth odors are caused by local and/or systemic factors.* Cleansing thoroughly to remove debris from around the teeth and from the surface of the tongue is a more meaningful approach to the reduction of locally caused mouth odors than rinsing away the debris and bacteria feeding on it.

When rinsing action is desired, the popular mouthwashes diluted one to three with warm water may be used. The following are representative prescriptions for mouthwashes:

1. Isotonic sodium chloride solution
2. Hypertonic sodium chloride solution (2% aqueous solution)
3. Sodium bicarbonate   2 gm.
   Water to make   100 cc.
4. Sodium chloride   2 gm.
   Sodium bicarbonate   1.9 gm.
   Amaranth solution   2 cc.
   Peppermint water
   to make   240 cc.

Mouthwashes are often used by the profession as vehicles for the topical use of chemicals in the oral cavity. Reduction in oral bacteria, plaque formation and gingivitis has been reported with chlorhexidine gluconate (Hibitane).[46, 69] Plaque reduction has also been reported with oxygenating agents,[71, 80] but prolonged use of hydrogen peroxide may result in acute inflammation[50] and increased mitotic rate[27] in the oral tissues. Daily use of 0.05 per cent sodium flurode dentifrices does not affect the gingiva, but a 0.5 per cent NaF rinse every other week may induce or aggravate gingival inflammation.[42]

DISCLOSING SOLUTIONS

The following are solutions and wafers used in the dental office to disclose plaque

---

*For potential plaque and calculus inhibitors, see page 467.

*Mouth odors are discussed on page 488.

prior to and after oral prophylaxis, and at home to check the effectiveness of patients' plaque control.

Solutions

1. Basic fuchsin   6 gm.
   Ethyl alcohol, 95%   100 cc.
   Add two drops to water
   in a dappen dish
2. Potassium iodide   1.6 gm.
   Iodine crystals   1.6 gm.
   Water   13.4 cc.
   Glycerin to make   30.0 cc.

Wafers

The wafer is crushed between the teeth, followed by water swished around the mouth for about 30 seconds. Two such wafers are Red-Cote (certified color, mannitol, sucaryl and artificial flavor) and an erythrosin wafer[4] which contains:

F.D.C. Red #3 (erythrosin) 15 mg.
Sodium chloride   .747%
Sodium sucaryl   .747%
Calcium stearate   .995%
Soluble saccharin   .186%
White oil   .124%
Flavoring (F.D.A.
approved)   2.239%
Sorbitol to make a 7 grain wafer

Disclosing solution which stains dental plaque without discoloring the mucosa or dental restorations is also available.

REFERENCES

1. Accepted Dental Therapeutics. 34th ed. Chicago, American Dental Association, 1971-1972, pp. 257–262.
2. Alder-Hradecky, C., and Kelentey, B.: Salivary Excretion and Inactivation of Some Penicillins. Nature, 198:792, 1963.
3. American Medical Association Council on Drugs: A New Skeletal Muscle Relaxant: Chlorphenesin Carbamate. J.A.M.A., 196:783, 1966.
4. Arnim, S. S.: The Use of Disclosing Agents for Measuring Tooth Cleanliness. J. Periodont., 34: 227, 1963.
5. Baer, P. N., Goldman, H. M., and Scigliano, J.: Studies on a Bacitracin Periodontal Dressing. Oral Surg., Oral Med. & Oral Path., 11:712, 1958.
6. Baer, P. N., Sumner, C. F., III, and Scigliano, J.: Studies on a Hydrogenated Fat-Zinc Bacitracin Periodontal Dressing. Oral Surg., Oral Med. & Oral Path., 13:494, 1960.
7. Baer, P. N., Sumner, C. F., III, and Miller, G.: Periodontal Dressings. Dent. Clin. North America, 13:181, 1969.
8. Baer, P. N., and Wertheimer, F. W.: A Histologic Study of the Effects of Several Periodontal Dressings on Periosteal-Covered and Denuded Bone. J. D. Res., 40:858, 1961.
9. Bartels, H. A., Cohen, G., and Scopp, I. W.: Alterations in the Oral Microbial Flora Accompanying Local and Systemic Drug Therapy. J. Periodont.–Periodontics, 40:421, 1969.
10. Bender, I. B., Pressman, R. S., and Tashman, S. G.: Studies on Excretion of Antibiotics in Human Saliva. I. Penicillin and Streptomycin. J.A.D.A., 46:164, 1953.
11. Bergenholtz, A., Hugoson, A., Lundgren, D., and Östgren, A.: The Plaque Inhibiting Activity of Some Mouthwashes. J. Periodont. Res., 2:246, 1967.
12. Beube, F. E.: An Experimental Study of the Use of Sodium Sulfid Solution in Treatment of Periodontal Pockets. J. Periodont., 10:49, 1939.
13. Bhaskar, S. N., Frisch, J., Margetis, P. M., and Leonard, F.: Oral Surgery–Oral Pathology Conference Number 18, Walter Reed Army Medical Center. Oral Surg., 22:526, 1966.
14. Bibby, B. G.: A Consideration of Vaccine Therapy in Periodontal Disease. J. Periodont., 28:300, 1957.
14a. Biocca, E., and Seppilli, A.: Human Infections Caused by Lactobacilli. J. Infect. Dis., 18:112, 1947.
15. Blass, J. L.: The Uses and Abuses of Drugs in Dentistry. New York. J. Den., 5:139, 1935.
16. Blitzer, B.: A Consideration of the Possible Causes of Dental Hypersensitivity: Treatment by a Strontium-Ion Dentifrice. Periodontics, 5:318, 1967.
17. Block, P. L., Dooley, C. L., and Howe, E. E.: The Retardation of Spontaneous Periodontal Disease and the Prevention of Caries in Hamsters with Dextranase. J. Periodont.–Periodontics, 40:105, 1969.
18. Borzelleca, J. F., and Cherrick, H. M.: The Excretion of Drugs in Saliva. Antibiotics. J. Oral Therap. & Pharm., 2:180, 1965.
19. Bressman, E., Kaslick, R. S., and Chasens, A.: Use of an Adhesive Bandage to Stabilize Free Gingival Grafts. J. Periodont., 42:40, 1971.
20. Campbell, J. B., Seguin, L., Kutscher, A. H., and Zegarelli, E. V.: Activity of Amphotericin B Against Candida Albicans–Disc Sensitivity Studies. Oral Surg., Oral Med. & Oral Path., 13: 1273, 1960.
21. Canadian Consumer, 5:163, 1968.
21a. Conner, H., Haberman, S., Collings, C., and Winford, T.: Bacteremias Following Periodontal Scaling in Patients with Healthy Appearing Gingiva. J. Periodont., 38:466, 1967.
21b. Cutcher, J. L., et al.: Control of Bacteremia Associated with Periodontal Procedures. IADR Abstr., 1971, p. 91, No. 154.
22. Department of Health, Education and Welfare, Food and Drug Administration (21 CFR, Part 3): Labeling of Mouthwash, Mouth Freshener, and Gargle Preparations – Statement of Policy.
23. Eisenbrand, G. F.: A Method for Making an Efficient and Adherent Periodontal Pack. D. Digest, 68:210, 1962.
23a. Eisenbud, L.: Subacute Bacterial Endocarditis Precipitated by Non-Surgical Dental Procedures. Oral Surg., Oral Med. & Oral Path., 15:624, 1962.
24. Forrest, J. O.: A Clinical Assessment of Three

Desensitizing Toothpastes Containing Formalin. Brit. D. J., *114*:103, 1963.

25. Fraleigh, C. M.: An Evaluation of Topical Terramycin in Postgingivectomy Pack. J. Periodont., *27*:201, 1956.

26. Frisch, J. E., and Bhasker, S. N.: Response of Rat Tissues to Eugenol-Containing and Eugenol-Free Periodontal Packs. I.A.D.R. Abstr., 507, 1967, p. 165.

27. Gargiulo, A. W.: Biologic Effect of Hydrogen Peroxide upon the Human Gingiva. Periodontics, *1*:199, 1963.

28. Glickman, I., and Bibby, B. G.: Effect of Sodium Perborate upon the Gingival Mucosa: A Controlled Experiment. J.A.D.A., *31*:1201, 1944.

29. Glickman, I., and Patur, B.: Histologic Study of the Effect of Antiformin on the Soft Tissue Wall of Periodontal Pockets in Human Beings. J.A.D.A., *51*:420, 1955.

30. Gottlieb, S. J., and Falliers, C. J.: Dental Anesthesia with Lidocaine Hydrochloride for Children with Intractable Asthma and Associated Allergies. J. Oral Therap., & Pharm., *3*:468, 1967.

31. Griffin, L. H., Wagner, M. J., and Collings, C. K.: Noninhibition of Bone Resorption by Topically Applied Fluoride During Periodontal Flap Surgery. J. Periodont.–Periodontics, *40*:427, 1969.

32. Gross, A., and Uotinen, K. G.: Elimination of Antibiotics in Submaxillary and Parotid Saliva of Unanaesthetized Dogs. Pharm. & Therapeutics in Dentistry, *1*:46, 1970.

33. Guglani, L. M., and Allen, E. F.: Connective Tissue Reaction to Implants of Periodontal Packs. J. Periodont., *36*:279, 1965.

33a. Gutverg, M., and Haberman, S.: Studies on Bacteremia Following Oral Surgery: Some Prophylactic Approaches to Bacteremia and the Results of Tissue Examination of Excised Gingiva. J. Periodont., *33*:105, 1962.

34. Hiatt, W.: Local Anesthesia: History; Potential Toxicity: Clinical Investigation of Mepivacaine. Dent. Clin. North America, July 1961, p. 243.

35. Hirschfeld, I.: Vincent's Infection of Mouth: Clinical Incidents in Its Diagnosis and Treatment. J.A.D.A., *21*:768, 1934.

36. Hunter, G. C., Jr., Barringer, M., and Spooner, G.: Analysis of Desensitization of Dentin by Sodium Silico-fluoride and Gottlieb's Solution by Use of Radioactive Silver Nitrate. J. Periodont., *32*:333, 1961.

37. Hunter, H. A.: A Study of Tissues Treated with Antiformin-Citric Acid. J. Canad. D. A., *21*:344, 1955.

38. Kanouse, M. C., and Ash, M. M., Jr.: The Effectiveness of a Sodium Monofluorophosphate Dentifrice on Dental Hypersensitivity. J. Periodont.–Periodontics, *40*:38, 1969.

39. Kaplan, S. I., and Hurwitz, G.: Reactions to Penicillin. Oral Surg., Oral Med. & Oral Path., *2*:21, 1949.

40. Kennedy, P. T., and Knewets, T. F.: Plaque Removal and the Use of an Antibacterial Mouthwash. U.S. Navy Medical Newsletter, *55*:39, 1970.

41. Kitchin, P. C., and Robinson, H. B. G.: How Abrasive Need a Dentifrice Be? J. D. Res., *27*:501, 1948.

42. Koch, G., and Lindhe, J.: The Effect of Supervised Oral Hygiene on the Gingivae of Children. The Effect of Sodium Fluoride. J. Periodont. Res., *2*:64, 1967.

42a. Korn, N. A., and Schaffer, E. M.: A Comparison of the Post-Operative Bacteremias Induced Following Different Periodontal Procedures. J. Periodont., *33*:226, 1962.

43. Kunin, I. J.: Methocarbamol in the Treatment of Temporomandibular Joint Syndrome. Oral Surg., Oral Med. & Oral Path., *14*:296, 1961.

44. Lindhe, J., and Brånemark, P.: Changes in Microcirculation after Local Application of Sex Hormones. J. Periodont. Res., *2*:185, 1967.

45. Litsky, B. Y., Mascis, J. D., and Litsky, W.: Mouthwash to Minimize Aerosol from High-Speed Drill. Oral Surg., *29*:25, 1970.

46. Löe, H., and Schiøtt, C. R.: The Effect of Mouthrinses and Topical Application of Chlorhexidine on the Development of Dental Plaque and Gingivitis in Man. J. Periodont. Res., *5*:79, 1970.

47. Lukomsky, E. H.: Fluorine Therapy for Exposed Dentin and Alveolar Atrophy. J. D. Res., *20*:649, 1941.

48. Manhold, J. H., Jr., and Manhold, B. S.: Further *in vivo* Study of Commercial Mouthwash Efficacy. New York J. Dent., *33*:383, 1963.

49. Manhold, J. H., Jr., Parker, L., and Manhold, B. S.: Efficacy of a Commercial Mouthwash: *In Vivo* Study. New York J. Dent., *32*:165, 1962.

50. Martin, J., Bishop, J., Guentherman, R., and Dorman, H.: Cellular Response of Gingiva to Prolonged Application of Dilute Hydrogen Peroxide. J. Periodont., *39*:208, 1968.

51. Massler, M.: Desensitization of Cervical Cementum and Dentin by Sodium Silicofluoride. J. D. Res., *34*:761, 1955.

52. McCall, J. O.: The Measure of Success in Periodontic Practice. J.A.D.A., *15*:279, 1928.

53. Meyler, L.: Side Effects of Drugs, Vol. 5. Amsterdam, Excerpta Medica Foundation, 1966.

54. Miller, J. T., Shannon, I. L., Kilgore, W. G., and Bookman, J. E.: Use of a Water-Free Stannous Fluoride–Containing Gel in the Control of Dental Hypersensitivity. J. Periodont.-Periodontics, *40*:490, 1969.

55. Miller, S. C. et al.: Hydrogen Peroxide and Sodium Perborate: Their Comparative Oral Irritant Action. J.A.D.A., *25*:1957, 1938.

56. Miller, S. C., and Sorrin, S.: The Action and Use of Sodium Sulfide Solution as Epithelial Solvent. D. Cosmos, *69*:1113, 1927.

57. Mopsik, E. R.: Infections and Antibiotics. Dent. Clin. North America, *15*:327, 1971.

58. Morris, P. P., and Read, R. R.: Halitosis: Variations in Mouth and Total Breath Odor Intensity Resulting from Prophylaxis and Antisepsis. J. D. Res., *28*:324, 1949.

59. Mosteller, J. H.: Use of Prednisolone in the Elimination of Postoperative Thermal Sensitivity. J. Pros. Dent., *12*:1176, 1962.

60. Ochstein, A. J., Hansen, N. M., and Swenson, H. M.: A Comparative Study of Cyanoacrylate and Other Periodontal Dressing on Gingival Surgical Wound Healing. J. Periodont.–Periodontics, *40*:515, 1969.

61. Oliver, W. M., and Heaney, T. G.: Sequelae Following the Use of Eugenol or Non-Eugenol Dressings after Gingivectomy and Subgingival Curettage. D. Pract. (Bristol), *21*:49, 1970.

62. Ostrolenk, M., and Weiss, W.: The Effect of Mouth-washes on the Oral Flora. D. Abst., 5:51, 1960.

63. Persson, G., and Thilander, H.: Experimental Studies of Surgical Packs. 1. *In Vivo* Experiments on Antimicrobial Effect. Odont. T., 76:147, 1968.

64. Persson, G., and Thilander, H.: Experimental Studies of Surgical Packs. 2. Tissue Reaction to Various Packs. Odont. T., 76:157, 1968.

65. Rammelkamp, C. H., and Keefer, C. S.: The Absorption, Excretion, and Distribution of Peni-cillin. J. Clin. Invest., 22:425, 1943.

66. Report of the Council on Dental Therapeutics of the American Dental Association: Abrasivity of Current Dentifrices. J.A.D.A., 81:1177, 1970.

67. Robinson, H. B. G.: Individualizing Dentifrices: The Dentist's Responsibility. J.A.D.A., 79:633, 1969.

67a. Robinson, L., et al.: Bacteremias of Dental Origin. Oral Surg., Oral Med. & Oral Path., 3:519, 923, 1950.

67b. Rogosa, M., Hampp, E. G., Nevin, T. A., Wagner, H. N., Jr., Driscoll, E. J., and Baer, P. N.: Blood Sampling and Cultural Studies in the Detection of Post-Operative Bacteremias. J.A.D.A., 60:71, 1960.

68. Ross, M. R.: Hypersensitive Teeth; Effect of Strontium Chloride in a Compatible Dentifrice. J. Periodont., 32:49, 1961.

68a. Royer, R. G., Gaines, R., and Kruger, G.: Bacter-emia Following Exodontia, Prophylaxis, and Gingivectomy. J. D. Res., 43:877, 1964.

69. Schiøtt, C. R., Löe, H., Jensen, S. B., Kilian, B., Davies, R. M., and Glavind, K.: The Effect of Chlorhexidine Mouthrinses on Human Oral Flora, J. Periodont. Res., 5:84, 1970.

70. Schroff, J.: The Effect of Sodium Perborate on Oral Tissues—A New Method for Determining Chemical Irritability on Oral Mucous Membrane. D. Items Int., 60:203, 1938.

71. Shipman, B., Cohen, E., and Kaslick, R. S.: The Effect of a Urea Peroxide Gel on Plaque Deposits and Gingival Status. J. Periodont., 42:283, 1971.

72. Shuttleworth, C. W., and Gibbs, F. J.: Aetio-logical Significance of Candida Albicans in Chronic Angular Cheilitis and Its Treatment with Nystatin. Brit. D. J., 108:354, 1960.

73. Stahl, S. S., et al.: Gingival Healing. III. The Effects of Periodontal Dressings on Gingivectomy Repair. J. Periodont.–Periodontics, 40:34, 1969.

74. Stookey, G. K., and Muhler, J. C.: Laboratory Studies Concerning the Enamel and Dentin Abrasion Properties of Common Dentifrice Polishing Agents. J. D. Res., 47:524, 1968.

75. Sturzenberger, O. P., and Leonard, G. J.: The Effect of a Mouthwash as Adjunct in Tooth Clean-ing. J. Periodont.–Periodontics, 40:299, 1969.

76. Thomas, B. O. A.: The Limitations of a Calculus Preventing Agent. J. Periodont., 27:314, 1956.

76a. Vargas, B., Collings, C. K., Polter, L., and Haber-man, S.: Effects of Certain Factors on Bacteremias Resulting from Gingival Resection. J. Periodont., 30:196, 1959.

76b. Wada, K., Tomizawa, M. and Sasaki, I.: Study on Bacteremia in Patients with Pyorrhea Alveolaris Caused by Surgical Operations. Periodont. Abstr., 18:27, 1970.

77. Williams, C. H. M.: Harmful Effects of Sodium Perborate Preparations. J. Canad. D. A., 1:267, 1935.

77a. Winslow, M. B. and Kobernick, S. D.: Bacteremia After Prophylaxis. J.A.D.A., 61:69, 1960.

77b. Winslow, M. B., and Millstone, S. H.: Bacteremia After Prophylaxis. Part II. J. Periodont., 36:371, 1965.

78. Woodward, S. C., et al.: Histotoxicity of Cyano-acrylate Tissue Adhesive in the Rat. Ann. Surg., 162:113, 1965.

79. Zegarelli, E. V., Kutscher, A. H., and Silvers, H. F.: Triamcinolone Acetonide in the Treatment of Recurrent Ulcerative Stomatitis. Preliminary Report. J. Periodont., 30:63, 1959.

80. Zinner, D. D., Duany, L. F., and Chilton, N. W.: Controlled Study of the Clinical Effectiveness of a New Oxygen Gel on Plaque, Oral Debris and Gin-gival Inflammation. Pharm. & Therapeutics in Dentistry, 1:7, 1970.

Part III • Functional Phase of Periodontal Treatment

Chapter 52

PRINCIPLES OF OCCLUSION

The recognition and correction of occlusal relationships that are injurious to the periodontium and may give rise to disorders of the masticatory musculature and temporomandibular joint require an understanding of the principles of occlusion. Fundamentals of occlusion are presented here; their clinical application is described in subsequent chapters.

DEFINITION OF OCCLUSION

The term occlusion refers to the contact relationships of the teeth resulting from neuromuscular control of the masticatory system (musculature, temporomandibular joint, mandible and periodontium).[108] Occlusion is more than just the static relationship of the teeth when the jaws are closed;[15] it consists of all contacts during chewing and swallowing. These are referred to as the *functional contacts of the dentition. Contacts during bruxing, clamping and clenching are called parafunctional contacts.* The normality or abnormality of an individual occlusion is determined by the manner in which it functions and by its effect upon the periodontium, musculature and temporomandibular joint rather than by the alignment of the teeth in each arch and the static relationship of the arches to each other.

THE FORCES OF OCCLUSION

The forces of occlusion are created by the musculature in chewing, swallowing and speech, and are transmitted through the teeth to the periodontium. These forces function in synchronized balance and guide the alignment of the teeth as they erupt, and participate in maintaining the position of the teeth in the arches. Tooth position and arch form are not static; they are maintained by the balance among the various forces of occlusion. Disturbance of this balance may lead to altered tooth positions and changes in functional environment that may be injurious to the periodontium.

The following factors are involved in the creation and distribution of the forces of occlusion: (a) **muscular activity,** (b) **inclined planes of the teeth and the anterior component of force,** (c) **proximal contacts,** (d) **design and inclination of the teeth** and (e) **atmospheric balance.**

Muscular activity

The forces of occlusion are created by two groups of muscles: the muscles of mastication, and the counteracting oral musculature. The forces created by the muscles of mastication are distributed in several directions by the inclined planes of the teeth. This occurs in chewing, either directly through tooth contact or indirectly through a resistant bolus of food, and in swallowing.[14] The resultant forces tend to displace the maxillary teeth facially and the mandibular teeth lingually, and tend to move all the teeth mesially.

Counteracting forces exerted by the tongue, the lips and the cheek

These forces balance the tendency toward displacement of the teeth created by the muscles of mastication. The orbicularis oris counteracts the labially directed force exerted by the mandibular teeth and the tongue against the maxillary anterior teeth. The tongue is a versatile muscle which exerts pressure in various directions, balancing the inward pressure of lips and buccinator muscles, and balancing the tendency of inclined planes to force the mandibular premolars and molars lingually. The buccinator balances the tendency of inclined planes to force the maxillary molars buccally.

The balance between the antagonistic forces of occlusion has been summarized by Breitner[11] as shown in Table 52–1.

The inclined planes of the teeth and the anterior component of force

As noted above, the forces exerted by the muscles on closure of the mandible are distributed in several directions by the inclined planes of the teeth. *The resultant of the occlusal forces gives rise to an anterior force, which tends to move the teeth mesially and is termed the anterior component of force* (Fig. 52–1). The anterior component of force on one side of the arch is transmitted from the molars through the contact points of the teeth to the midline, where it is neutralized by the force from the other side of the arch.

The anterior component of force pushes the teeth mesially in their sockets. When the force is released, the teeth move back

TABLE 52–1 BALANCE BETWEEN ANTAGONISTIC OCCLUSAL FORCES

Lips ⟶	⟵Tongue
Cheeks⟶	⟵Tongue
Eruption (growth of teeth)⟶	⟵Masticatory muscles (masseter, temporalis, internal pterygoid)
Air pressure on skin and nasal cavity⟶	⟵Tongue in closed mouth, air pressure in open mouth
Masseter⟶	⟵Elasticity of periodontal ligament, particularly of molars, and suprahyoid muscles
Internal pterygoid	
in vertical movement ⟶	⟵Same as masseter
in lateral movement⟶	⟵Internal pterygoid of other side
External pterygoid	
in anterior movement⟶	⟵Posterior third of temporalis, suprahyoid group, diagastricus, muscles of the neck
in lateral movement⟶	⟵External pterygoid of other side

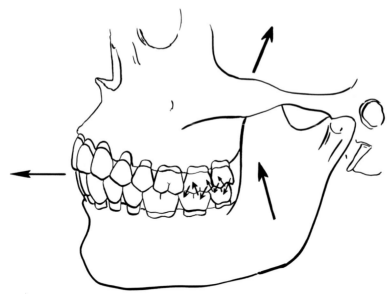

Figure 52–1 Anterior Component of Force. Masticatory muscle forces are indicated by the large arrows on the right. Forces induced by intercuspation of the teeth are represented by the small arrows. The anterior component of force that is the resultant of all the forces of occlusion is indicated by the horizontal arrow (*left*).

to their previous position because of the resilience of the periodontal ligament. With time, the areas of proximal contact are flattened by wear, permitting mesial movement of the teeth, referred to as physiologic mesial migration. The overall effect is a reduction of 0.5 cm. in the length of the dental arch from the third molars to the midline by the age of 40 years.

Proximal contacts

Proximal contact relationships are important in maintaining the stability of the dental arch. The anterior component of force is transmitted through intact proximal contacts. Contacts malpositioned in a cervicoincisal or faciolingual direction deflect the forces of occlusion and may cause displacement of the teeth (Fig. 52–2) and create abnormal forces on the periodontium.

Tooth design and inclination

Certain features of tooth design affect the transmission of occlusal forces.[15] For example, the maxillary central incisor is shaped so that it is inclined mesially to

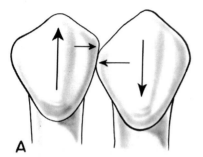
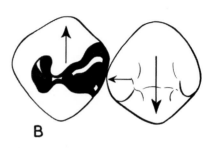

Figure 52–2 *A,* **Improper Proximal Contact Relationship** (*horizontal arrows*). This relationship is a potential source of excessive force in the directions indicated by the vertical arrows. *B,* Improper contact relationship in the faciolingual plane (*horizontal arrows*). This relationship is a potential cause of displacement of the teeth facially and lingually as indicated by the vertical arrows. (After R. A. Jentsch.)

provide maximum efficiency of its cutting edge. In function, the maxillary incisors tend to be driven mesially and buttress each other. The root of the maxillary incisors is shaped so that there is greater area of attachment of periodontal fibers on the palatal and distal sides, which counteract the tendency toward facial and mesial displacement during function. The molars are inclined mesially so as to transmit a component of the vertical occlusal forces to the premolars and canines.[74]

Atmospheric balance

Breathing is an important factor in maintaining normal atmospheric balance in the nasal and oral cavity. After swallowing with the lips together, a vacuum is created between the tongue and the palate, which is a factor in the development of the palate and the shape of the maxillary dental arch.

THE POSTURAL POSITION OF THE MANDIBLE (PHYSIOLOGIC REST POSITION) AND THE FREE WAY SPACE

When the teeth are not in contact in mastication, swallowing or speech, the lips are at rest and the jaws are apart. This is termed the *postural position of the mandible.* It is often referred to as the *"physiologic rest position,"*[103] but *"postural position" is more appropriate.*[69] **This position is no more "physiologic" than other positions of the mandible and the musculature is not really "at rest." In order to maintain the mandible in this position it is necessary to support it against the force of gravity; the muscles are in a mild state of contraction.** The postural position is not constant; it varies with the position of the head and body, and proprioceptive stimuli from the dentition and emotional factors also affect it.[77]

The space between the mandibular and maxillary teeth when the mandible is in the postural position is called the free way space. The average normal space is 1.7 mm.[26,65] It ranges between 0.9 and 2.5 mm. in 90 per cent of individuals.

The postural position and free way space are ordinarily stable and reproducible but are not necessarily constant throughout life. Aging, malocclusion, tooth mobility and periodontal disease, unreplaced posterior teeth, improperly constructed dental restorations, excessive occlusal wear or unilateral chewing, which change the teeth and their functional relationships, may also change the muscle tonus, which in turn may alter the postural position and the free way space.[22,99]

VERTICAL DIMENSION

The term *vertical dimension designates the distance between the maxilla and mandible when the teeth are in occlusion.* The vertical dimension is maintained by a balance between the rate of occlusal wear and continuous tooth eruption. If occlusal wear is more rapid than tooth eruption, loss of vertical dimension results, accompanied by an increased free way space. Insufficient function, on the other hand, may be followed by extrusion of the teeth.

THE PHYSIOLOGY OF MASTICATION

Mastication consists of the coordinated function of various parts of the oral cavity to prepare food for swallowing and digestion. Although the teeth are the most essential unit in mastication, there are other important related factors, such as the lubricating and enzymatic action of the saliva, the lips, cheeks, tongue, the hard palate and the gingiva, the muscles of mastication and the temporomandibular articulation.

Incision

Incision reduces the food to sizes suitable for mastication. It involves coordinated action of the hand, arm, head, neck and shoulders as well as the teeth and masticatory musculature.[39] To engage the food the mouth is opened and the mandible is protruded. Shearing strokes of the anterior teeth penetrate the food until it is thinned. The food is not "cut apart" by tooth to tooth contact. The hand and head move in opposite directions to separate the food so that part of it remains in the oral cavity. The tongue and cheek direct the bolus of food to the occlusal table of the posterior teeth for mastication.

The masticatory cycle

The pathway of the mandible in chewing is referred to as the chewing cycle or the masticatory cycle. It is usually represented as being of teardrop shape when viewed in the frontal or lateral planes (Fig. 52–3, A). The average jaw opening during mastication of most foods[64] is 18.2 mm. The duration of the average chewing cycle is 1.046 seconds.[71] The pattern of the masticatory cycle varies considerably, depending upon the consistency and shape of the food bolus, the nature of the occlusion and individual chewing habits[93, 96] (Fig. 52–3, B).

In the early stages of chewing a resistant bolus of food, the closing strokes terminate far short of occlusal contact. As the food softens and is reduced in size, the strokes approach occlusal contact more closely and often reach it.[4] The duration of the average chewing contact is 0.1 to 0.15 second.

The end of the closing stroke, when the mandibular cusps enter the confines of the fossae of the maxillary teeth in intercuspation, is the critical phase of the chewing cycle. It is sometimes referred to as the *terminal functional orbit*[62] (Fig. 52–3). In the transition from the end of the closing stroke to the beginning of the opening stroke, the mandibular cusps most often enter the maxillary fossae directly, but they may also rub against the fossa walls, laterally and anteroposteriorly.[1, 93] Although supposedly guided by the inclined planes of the cusps (cusp guidance),[71] the rubbing

contacts are sporadic and do not conform to an orderly pattern.[7]

Deglutition

Swallowing occurs approximately 600 times in a 24-hour period.[51] It occurs most frequently during eating and drinking, at a lesser rate during the usual indoor activities and least frequently when asleep. The total time of tooth contact in chewing and swallowing in a 24-hour period has been estimated to be 17.5 minutes[31] (Table 52–2).

In swallowing, the palatal muscles seal off the oropharynx from the nasopharynx, the suprahyoid muscles raise and tilt the hyoid bone and larynx, and the tongue forcibly propels the food bolus or liquid posteriorly over the epiglottis into the esophagus. To provide firm anchorage for the action of the tongue, and to oppose the depressing action of the suprahyoid muscles, the mandible is braced against the maxilla and cranium by the masseter, temporal and internal pterygoid muscles.[39]

Muscles of mastication*

The **lateral (external) pterygoid muscle**, especially the inferior belly, is the main trigger muscle in opening the jaw;[45] it is

---

*For a comprehensive electromyographic study of the action of the muscles of mastication in chewing and swallowing, see Møller.[67]

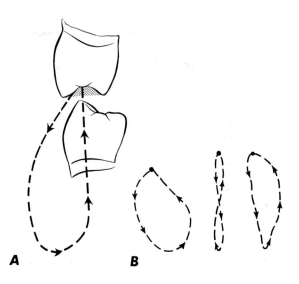

Figure 52–3 The Chewing Cycle and Terminal Functional Orbit. *A*, Frontal view of teardrop shaped chewing cycle which starts with the jaws slightly apart. The **Terminal Functional Orbit** is represented by the dotted area between the maxillary cusps. *B*, Variations in chewing cycle patterns including a "cross-over" near the center.

A   **B**

TABLE 52–2 TOTAL DURATION OF TOOTH CONTACTS IN A 24-HOUR PERIOD*

Chewing:		
Actual chewing time per meal	450 sec.	
4 meals a day	1800 sec.	
Each second 1 chewing stroke	1800 strokes	
Duration of each stroke	0.3 sec.	
Total chewing forces per day	540 sec. = 9.0 min.	
Swallowing:		
1. Meals		
Duration of 1 deglutition movement	1 sec.	
During chewing 3 × per minute		
⅓ of movements with occlusal force only	30 sec.	0.5 min.
2. Between meals		
Daytime 25 per hour (16 hrs.)	400 sec.	6.6 min.
Sleep 10 per hour (8 hrs.)	80 sec.	1.3 min.
TOTAL	1050 sec. ca. 17.5 min.	

*From Graf, H.[31]

coordinated with the activities of the **supra-hyoid muscles** (the **diagastric**, the **mylohyoid**, and the **geniohyoid**), which assist in retracting and depressing the mandible and also in fixing and elevating the hyoid bone. The **masseter, medial (internal) pterygoid**, and **temporal muscles** are the principal muscles involved in closing the jaw, and in the regulation of the position of the mandible in space.

Protrusion of the jaw is accomplished by simultaneous bilateral contraction of the **lateral pterygoid muscles;** the jaw-closing muscle groups may also participate. Retrusion of the jaw is produced by simultaneous contraction of the **middle and lateral portions of the temporal muscles,** assisted by **masseter, digastric,** and **geniohyoid muscles.** Lateral movements are achieved by the contraction of the **lateral and medial pterygoid muscle** on one side and the contralateral **temporal muscle.**

NEUROMUSCULAR CONTROL OF MANDIBULAR MOVEMENTS*

The motor area for the stomatognathic structures which controls movement of the jaw, tongue and face is located in the frontotemporal part of the cortex of the brain.[43] Opening of the jaw is initiated in

*For detailed presentations of this subject, see Kawamura, Y.,[42] and Jerge, C.[41]

the cortical jaw motor area, closing movements in the amygdaloid-hypothalamic area.[43, 86]

A proprioceptive neuromuscular reflex system regulates the muscular activity responsible for mandibular movements. By feeding back information to the central nervous system,[79] it provides a constant awareness of the movements of the mandible and the muscular contractions producing them. Sensory impulses transmitted through fibers located within the muscles, in the periosteum of the bone, the oral mucosa, periodontal ligament and the ligaments and capsule of the temporomandibular joint participate in controlling jaw movements.[46]

The cells of the sensory fibers synapse with motor neurons of the trigeminal nerve, forming a reflex arc. This in turn regulates the motor stimulations to the muscles, which then modify the movement of the mandible. In addition to regulating mandibular movements, neuromuscular reflexes are involved in the establishment of centric and habitual occlusion, and in maintaining the mandible in the postural position.

Neuromuscular reflexes that protect the tissues from painful or injurious stimuli are called nociceptive reflexes. When a hard object is unexpectedly encountered in chewing, the impact upon the periodontal ligament initiates a nociceptive reflex, which stimulates the muscular action required for immediate opening of the mandible.

According to Kawamura,[44] chewing starts as a conscious act and becomes a cyclic subconscious motion controlled by three reciprocal reflexes: (1) the jaw-opening reflex, which is initiated by stimuli applied to the teeth (periodontal ligament) and oral tissues; (2) the jaw-closing reflex, which occurs in swallowing in response to weak mechanical stimulation on the dorsum of the tongue; and (3) the jaw-jerk reflex, in response to forceful stretching of the closing muscles when the jaw is opened. The jaw then begins to close, and the jaw-closing muscles produce electromyographic discharges which inhibit the jaw-opening muscles.

Jerge[41] feels that the reflexes responsible for jaw opening and closing are separate and dissimilar, rather than interrelated. Opening is initiated by intraoral pressure receptors, and stretch of the opening muscles initiates reflex jaw closing.[41]

Electromyography

Each time a muscle contracts, electrical energy is liberated, which can be recorded by electromyography. Normal muscle contractions produce synchronous patterns of electrical activity, without necessarily distinguishing between closure in centric or habitual occlusion.[17] Occlusal disharmonies cause asynchronous and hypertonic muscular activity (Fig. 52-4) that returns to normal after the occlusion is corrected.[80] By recording alterations in muscular activity, electromyography reveals the presence of subtle occlusal disharmonies that may escape detection by clinical examination.

Occlusion should not be thought of in terms of the oral structures alone. The bodily posture and position of the patient's head affect the muscular closure of the mandible and the pattern of tooth contacts[12] (Fig. 52-5).

The field of occlusion has a vocabulary of its own; some of the most frequently used terms are explained below.

CENTRIC RELATION, CENTRIC AND HABITUAL OCCLUSION

Centric relation refers to the position of the mandible. It is the most posterior relation of the mandible to the maxillae at the established vertical dimension.[30] In this position the condyles are located as far posteriorly in the glenoid fossa as the ligaments[6] and musculature[30] of the temporomandibular joint permit.

The term centric occlusion refers to the position of the teeth. It is the position in which the teeth are intercuspated, with the mandible in centric relation.[*] Other terms for it are retruded contact position, centric relation occlusion, terminal hinge position and ligamentous position.

The term habitual occlusion also refers to the position of the teeth. It is the position in which the teeth are intercuspated with the mandible not in centric relation.[53,61] Other terms for it are functional[†] occlusion, acquired occlusion, convenience occlusion, intercuspal position and pseudocentric occlusion. In habitual occlusion the mandible is usually anterior to or anterolateral to centric relation.

Tooth contacts in chewing and swallowing

The subject of occlusion presents something of a paradox: there is more information regarding how to correct and reconstruct the occlusion than there is regarding how the dentition functions. There are many detailed systems for occlusal adjustment and carving tooth cusps in order to attain "proper" occlusion. But there are relatively few facts regarding jaw relationships and tooth contacts during function, which supposedly would be the basis for dentistry's corrective and restorative efforts.

It has been difficult to capture and record jaw movements and tooth contacts in the functioning dentition, despite the imaginative techniques used for this purpose. Hesse[34] traced the masticatory movements of the mandible with a lead point in the space of a missing tooth which marked the opposing tooth surface. Hildebrand[35] followed jaw movements and tooth contacts by roentgen kymography and kinematography (photography with x-ray of a metal

---

[*]The term centric occlusion is sometimes applied to intercuspation of the teeth regardless of whether the mandible is in centric relation. This usage is not followed here.

[†]Because it is the position in which most functional contacts occur, this term is preferred by the author.

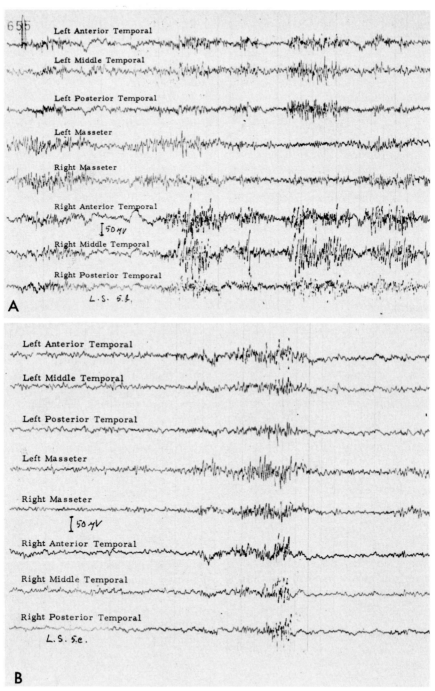

Figure 52–4 Electromyogram of Patient with Bruxism. *A,* Spastic disharmonious muscle contractions in swallowing associated with central prematurity. *B,* Same patient. Harmonious muscle activity in swallowing after elimination of centric prematurity by occlusal adjustment. (Courtesy of Dr. Sigurd P. Ramfjord, Ann Arbor, Michigan.)

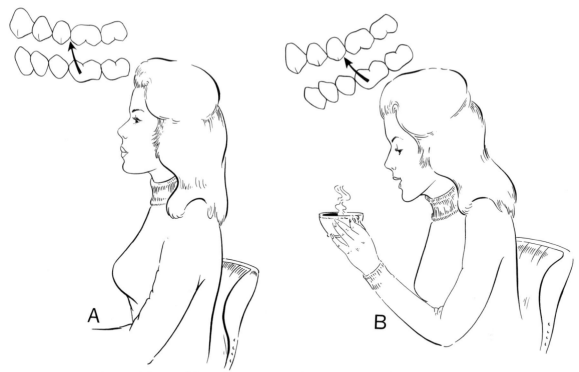

Figure 52–5 Closure of the Mandible and Pattern of Tooth Contacts Affected by Bodily Posture and Head Position.
A, Patient sitting with head erect. Arrow shows pathway of mandibular closure. B, Patient eating, head tilted forward. Arrow shows mandibular pathway shifted anteriorly.

indicator ligated to the lower teeth). Jankelson and co-workers[39] studied tooth contacts with orthodontic bands on gold crowns connected to a power supply and a recorder. Yurkstas and Emerson[111] used electrical contacts in full dentures. Anderson and Picton[4] studied tooth contacts in opposing teeth by means of fine insulated wires embedded in amalgams. Messerman, Reswick and Gibbs[63] developed a gnathic replicator for registering and reproducing jaw motion during function.

Part of the difficulty in obtaining information regarding the function of the natural dentition has been the fact that instruments used for this purpose often introduce the risk of inciting artificial muscle activity which distorts the individual's natural functional patterns. In 1961 Brewer and Hudson[13] overcame this problem by using miniaturized radio transmitters fitted into artificial dentures which registered tooth contacts without artificial encumbrance. Their work introduced a technique for studying occlusion which has become known as **intraoral telemetry** and has been applied to the natural dentition by numerous investigators.[2, 16, 19, 27, 29, 32, 76, 84, 87-90, 94]

Intraoral telemetry is in its early stages; because of the small number of cases studied thus far, the findings must be considered as suggestive rather than conclusive. However, whereas in the past most concepts regarding occlusion were based on speculation, monitoring the occlusion with intraoral telemetry provides accurate documentation of tooth contacts and jaw movements while food is being chewed and swallowed (Figs. 52–6, 52–7 and 52–8).

There is some variation in the findings in different telemetric studies, but the preponderance of evidence indicates that (1) **tooth contacts do occur in chewing and swallowing;** (2) **almost all chewing contacts and most swallowing contacts occur in habitual occlusion;** and (3) **centric occlusion is rarely used in chewing and is only occasionally used in swallowing.**[29] Chewing contacts in habitual occlusion are brief (0.1 to 0.15 sec.), compared with the duration of swallowing contacts (0.298 to 0.300 sec.).

Habitual occlusion, formerly considered an acquired or second-best occlusion, is really the functional working occlusion of the human dentition. It is not a detour

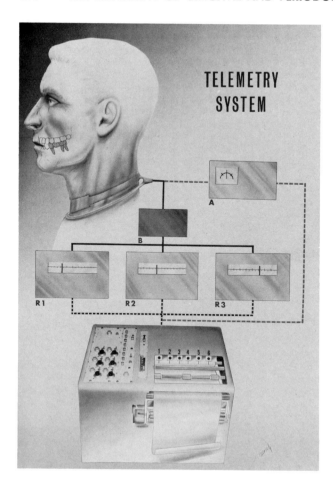

Figure 52–6 Intraoral Telemetry System.
Miniaturized radio in fixed bridge emits signals upon tooth contact. A, Amplifier for swallowing sensor. B, Antenna coupler. R_1, R_2, R_3, Radio receivers which lead into six-channel oscillograph recorder.

Figure 52–7 Assembly of Miniaturized Telemetry Unit in Mandibular Molar Pontic. *Left,* Battery. *Top center,* Multilayered switch. *Right,* Oscillator.

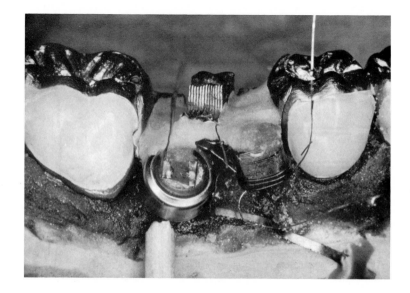

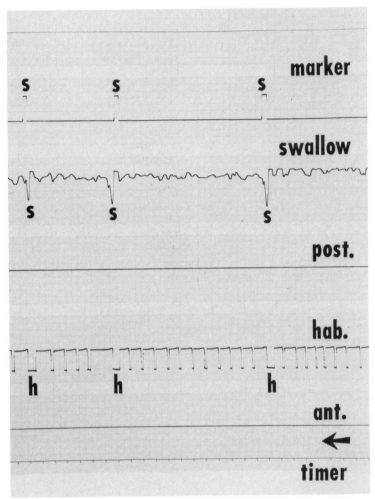

Figure 52–8 Intraoral Telemetry Recording of Tooth Contacts Made by Patient While Eating. Six channels are shown along the right margin as follows: **Marker channel,** Individual swallowing (s), recorded manually with telegrapher's key. **Swallow channel,** Individual swallows (s), recorded by sensor. **Post. channel,** Tooth contacts in centric occlusion. (There are none on this recording.) **Hab. channel,** Tooth contacts in habitual occlusion. Note that the tooth contacts (h) made in habitual occlusion during swallowing are of longer duration than the adjacent contacts made during chewing. **Ant. channel,** Position anterior to habitual occlusion. No contacts are shown in this position. **Timer channel,** Calibrated to time the duration of each contact.

position into which the jaw is deflected by premature contacts which prevent the teeth from reaching centric occlusion; the teeth ordinarily go directly into habitual occlusion (Fig. 52–9). Elimination of centric pathway prematurities does not necessarily result in increased use of centric occlusion.[73] The mandible may follow many paths in opening and closing, but they are all anterior to centric relation.[75] The postural position of the mandible is also anterior to centric relation.

Centric relation is the posterior border position of the mandible which is repro-

ducible and therefore may be a useful reference position in the diagnosis and correction of occlusal problems. **Centric relation is not a physiologic functional position of the dentition (Fig. 52–9).** After the entire dentition is reconstructed with maximum intercuspation in centric relation, a patient may persist in using habitual occlusion.[28] Occlusion, like other physiologic body processes, changes with age. **The therapist should consider the needs of the individual occlusion at the patient's age, rather than attempt a standard occlusion for all ages.**

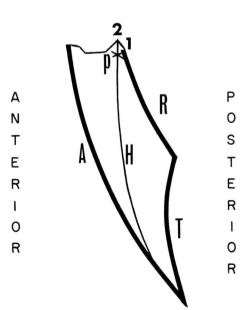

Figure 52–9 Rhomboid Figure Represents Sagittal View of the Border Pathways of Mandibular Movement (Posselt).[75] 1, Centric occlusion, 2, Habitual occlusion. R, The most retruded (centric) pathway of the mandible with the condylar movement, predominantly rotary around a hinge axis (the terminal hinge axis). T, Most retruded pathway of the mandible with the condylar movement predominantly translatory. A, Anterior border pathway of the mandible. H, Habitual (functional) opening and closing pathway of the mandible. P, The postural position of the mandible is located on the habitual pathway. O, The occlusal plane.

Lateral excursions

Movements of the mandible with the teeth in contact are termed excursions, and may be lateral, protrusive, lateral-protrusive or retrusive. Side-to-side contacts of the mandibular posterior teeth along the buccal cusps, central fossae and lingual cusps of the maxillary teeth (lateral excursions) do not regularly occur in chewing and swallowing; **they occur most often in bruxism.** Protrusive excursions are also uncommon in the normal function of the dentition. **In chewing and swallowing more of the contacts are single thrusts rather than glides.**

OTHER CONCEPTS OF OCCLUSION

Balanced occlusion

The term balanced occlusion refers to simultaneous contact between the right and left posterior segments of the arch in lateral excursions of the mandible, and simultaneous contact between the posterior and anterior segments of the arch in protrusive excursion. At one time considered to be an ideal type of functional relationship, balanced occlusion is rarely encountered in the natural dentition.[12] Balancing tooth contacts introduce a risk of damage to the periodontium which outweighs the ostensible benefits of attempting to create bilateral balance by occlusal adjustment or prosthetic restorations.[91, 101] In patients with periodontal disease, molars with nonworking side contact (more than 50 per cent of the teeth examined) showed significantly greater mobility, bone loss and pocket depth than teeth which did not contact on the nonworking side.[109]

Cuspid-protected occlusion

According to the concept of a cuspid-protected occlusion,[23] the interlocking relation of the maxillary canines between the mandibular canines and first premolars is the most important articulation in the natural dentition. In closure of the jaws in mastication the maxillary canines act as protective stress breakers that bear the brunt of the muscular forces and guide the mandible so that the posterior teeth come into closure with a minimum of horizontal forces. In lateral and protrusive excursions, the mandibular canines and first premolars engage the palatal surface of the maxillary canines so as to disocclude the incisors, premolars and molars and protect them from undesirable horizontal forces. This concept hypothesizes that the maxillary canines are especially equipped to absorb lateral forces because of the size of the root and radicular bone and because of an especially sensitive proprioceptive mechanism which reflexly reduces muscle forces when the canines make occlusal contact.

Cuspid-guided occlusion

According to this concept, the canines "guide" rather than "protect" the occlusion. The lingual inclines of the maxillary canines (cuspal guidance) is similar to that of the lingual surface of the maxillary incisors (incisal guidance). In functional movement of the mandible, the lingual surface of the maxillary canines and the cusps of the posterior teeth on one side are engaged simultaneously by the mandibular teeth so that the occlusal forces are distributed throughout the segment of the arch. In protrusive excursion the forces are shared by the incisors and canines.

Group function

Beyron[9] describes "group function," the simultaneous gliding contact of teeth on the working side, as an important feature of optimal occlusion, along with the following: (1) Bilateral contact of most teeth in the habitual position, and between posterior teeth in centric relation. The distance between the two positions should be about 1 mm. or less. (2) Axial loading of the posterior teeth in the retrusive range. (3) Acceptable interocclusal distance.

Hinge axis occlusion

This concept (gnathology) is based upon centric relation and the centric pathway as the functional aspects of occlusion. It hypothesizes that functional mandibular movements start with the condyles in centric relation; that excursive movements are functional; and that the factors that govern mandibular movements dictate the occlusal morphology of the teeth.[33]

Functionally generated occlusion

According to this concept, the excursive movements of the mandible are the functional pathways of occlusion.[59] The occlusal surfaces of the maxillary posterior teeth are reconstructed in conformity with the individual excursive movements, and in optimal occlusion there is maximum tooth contact on the "working side," with no "balancing side" contact. The occlusion is characterized by a "long centric," in which the mandible can move between centric occlusion and habitual occlusion with the dentition in contact.

Masticatory efficiency

The size of the food platform area, or the total available functional contact surface, is a major factor in determining the chewing efficiency of the dentition.[37, 110] The food platform area is diminished by such factors as missing teeth,[58] cuspal interferences,

incomplete eruption, tilting and other forms of malocclusion, and may be increased by attrition. In mouths with no missing teeth, the first molar provides 36.7 per cent of the total effective chewing area.[57] The second molar, third molar, second premolar, and first premolar follow in order of decreasing relative contribution to the total chewing area, with percentages of 27.9, 15.4, 12.9 and 8.1 respectively.

Loss of the first molar is often compensated for by mesial drifting of the second and third molars, and the dentition performs as if only the third molars were absent. Consideration of the effect of tooth loss on masticatory performance is complicated by the fact that mastication is usually performed on only one side of the dentition at a time. When both sides of the dentition are about equal in performance, there is a tendency for right side chewing.

Pain from caries or periodontal involvement influences the choice of the mastication side, and reduces the masticatory performance as well as the occlusal force that can be exerted on the affected side. Severe bone loss in periodontal disease also appears to reduce the maximum occlusal force.

OCCLUSAL DISHARMONY (OCCLUSAL DYSTROPHY)

Occlusal disharmonies are tooth relationships capable of injuring the supporting periodontal tissues. The most common type is premature tooth contacts which interfere with mandibular movement, referred to as occlusal prematurities. Tooth contacts which interfere with closure in centric occlusion are termed centric prematurities (centric pathway prematurities); those which interfere with closure in habitual occlusion are called habitual prematurities (habitual pathways prematurities).

The significance of occlusal prematurities*

There are several possible results of premature tooth contacts in centric or habitual occlusion or in both. They may incite muscle activity in an effort to wear away the obstructing tooth surfaces, which become

*For the detection and correction of occlusal prematurities, see Chapter 53.

repetitive and develop into bruxism, clamping or clenching habits.[80] They may cause destruction of the periodontal tissues, loosening of the teeth (trauma from occlusion) and deflection of the pathway of the mandible[102] (Fig. 52–10). They may produce instability of the dentition in closure and disturbed muscle patterns in an effort to overcome instability.[79] This, in turn, may lead to muscle spasm and temporomandibular joint disorders. The fact that most people have occlusal prematurities without necessarily suffering their harmful effects is indicative of the adaptability of the oral tissues.

ATTRITION

The term *attrition* refers to *the wearing away of teeth in the course of functional and parafunctional mandibular movement.*

A certain amount of tooth wear is physiologic. It normally occurs on the occlusal surface of the posterior teeth, the incisal edges of the anterior teeth, the lingual surfaces of the maxillary anterior teeth, the facial surfaces of the mandibular anterior teeth, and at the proximal contact points associated with physiologic migration of the dentition. Wear increases with age and is characterized by a reduction in cusp height and inclination, and the formation of facets. Tooth surfaces worn by attrition are hard, smooth and shiny, and frequently present yellowish brown discoloration (Fig. 52–11).

Excessive wear may result in obliteration of the cusps and the formation of either a flat or cupped-out occlusal surface and reversal of the occlusal plane of the premolars and first and second molars, referred to as the "curve of Pleasure" or the "anti-Monson" curve (Fig. 52–12).

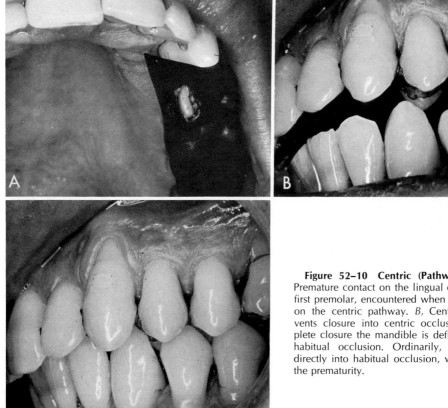

Figure 52–10 Centric (Pathway) Prematurity. *A,* Premature contact on the lingual cusp of the maxillary first premolar, encountered when the mandible moves on the centric pathway. *B,* Centric prematurity prevents closure into centric occlusion. *C,* Upon complete closure the mandible is deflected anteriorly into habitual occlusion. Ordinarily, the mandible goes directly into habitual occlusion, without encountering the prematurity.

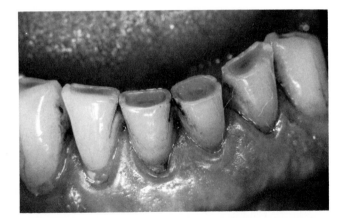

Figure 52–11 Occlusal Wear. Flat shiny discolored surfaces produced by occlusal wear.

Parafunctional movements of the mandible such as bruxism and clenching are the most common causes of excessive occlusal wear. Abrasive foods[20] and the presence of abrasive particles in the atmosphere encountered in some industries, intensify tooth wear. Malocclusion often results in excessive and abnormally located wear.

Facets are isolated flat or concave planes worn on tooth surfaces (Fig. 52–13). They

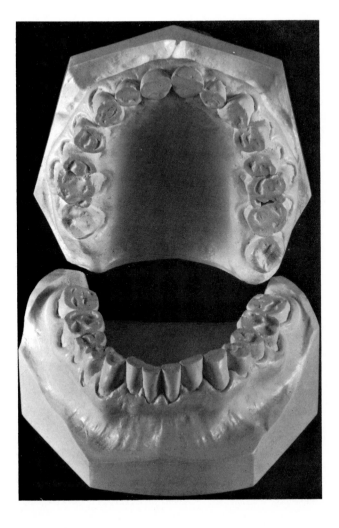

Figure 52–12 Reversed Faciolingual Occlusal Plane (Curve of Pleasure). The normal occlusal plane is sometimes reversed by excessive wear so that in the mandible the occlusal surfaces slope facially instead of lingually, and in the maxilla they are inclined lingually. The third molars are not usually affected.

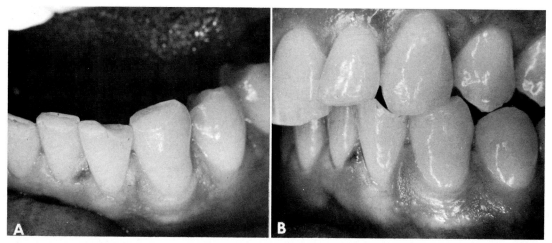

Figure 52–13 Wear Facets. *A,* Flat facets worn on incisal edges of anterior teeth. Note the notch on lateral incisor also produced by wear. *B,* Maxillary canine fits into notch on lateral incisor produced by parafunctional mandibular movements.

are generally caused by abnormal occlusal wear from parafunctional tooth contacts such as bruxism, and by premature tooth contacts, but may also be produced by physiologic wear. Facets vary in size and location, depending upon whether they are produced by physiologic or abnormal wear.[6, 8, 105] They have been reported in 98 per cent of adults and 83 per cent of all teeth examined.[106] Facets are usually not sensitive to thermal and tactile stimulation. Unworn teeth in a mouth with generalized cuspal wear are often sites of premature occlusal contact.

The angle of the facet upon the tooth surface is of potential significance to the periodontium. Horizontal facets tend to direct forces in the vertical axis of the teeth to which the periodontium can adapt most effectively. **Angular facets direct occlusal forces laterally and increase the risk of periodontal injury.**

THE TEMPOROMANDIBULAR JOINT

Temporomandibular joint function is a critical component of the physiology of occlusion. Within certain border limits imposed by its structure, the temporomandibular joint permits complete freedom for three types of mandibular movement: (1) opening and closing, (2) protrusion and retrusion and (3) lateral movements. In addition, the temporomandibular joint assists in stabilizing the mandible against the maxilla and cranium during the complex interaction of muscular forces exerted in chewing and swallowing.

Anatomic features[21, 52]

The temporomandibular joint is a ginglymoarthrodial type of articulation. The parts entering into it are (Fig. 52–14) the **condyle of the mandible,** the **mandibular fossa** and the **articular eminence of the squamous portion of the temporal bone,** the **articular disc,** the **capsule and the ligaments.** The anterosuperior surface of the condyle articulates with the lower third of the posterior surface of the articular eminence, from which it is separated by the articular disc. The space between the posterior surface of the condyle and the anterior wall of the external auditory meatus is occupied by loose, highly vascular connective tissue (Fig. 52–14). The articulating surfaces of the condyle, the mandibular fossa and the eminence are covered with fibrous connective tissue, which sometimes contains cartilage cells.

The inclination of the posterior surface of the articular eminence is correlated with that of the lingual surface of the maxillary anterior teeth (incisal guidance) but not necessarily with the cuspal inclines of the posterior teeth[48] (Fig. 52–15).

The **articular disc** is a plate of fibrocartilage situated between the condyle and the articular eminence. Its upper surface is saddle-shaped, concave anteroposteriorly, and slightly convex mediolaterally to permit gliding movement. Its lower surface is con-

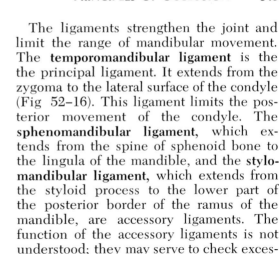

Figure 52–14 Diagrammatic Representation of the Temporomandibular Joint. A, Articular disc. C, Condyle. E, Articular eminence. T, Vascular connective tissue posterior to the condyle. S, Upper joint space. SS, Lower joint space. M, Upper and lower heads of the lateral pterygoid muscle.

cave to receive the head of the condyle and permit hinge or rotary movement.

The **capsule** covers the joint and unites its parts. It is composed of (1) an outer dense fibrous layer attached around the periphery of the articular disc and (2) a loose inner vascularized synovial layer.

The ligaments strengthen the joint and limit the range of mandibular movement. The **temporomandibular ligament** is the the principal ligament. It extends from the zygoma to the lateral surface of the condyle (Fig 52–16). This ligament limits the posterior movement of the condyle. The **sphenomandibular ligament,** which extends from the spine of sphenoid bone to the lingula of the mandible, and the **stylomandibular ligament,** which extends from the styloid process to the lower part of the posterior border of the ramus of the mandible, are accessory ligaments. The function of the accessory ligaments is not understood; they may serve to check excessive mandibular movement.

The joint is richly supplied with **pain receptors** and **proprioceptors.** Reflex mechanisms in the joint affect the opening and closing movements of the jaws.[72, 83] Afferent neurons in the capsule participate with the intraoral muscle receptors in the reflex control of cyclic jaw movements.[83]

Adaptive remodeling of the temporomandibular joint

Throughout life mechanical forces produce a slow remodeling of the articular

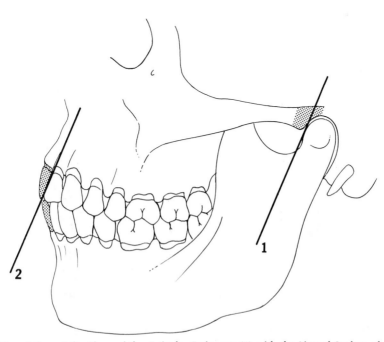

Figure 52–15   Correlation of the Plane of the Articular Eminence (1) with the Lingual Surface of the Maxillary Incisors (2).

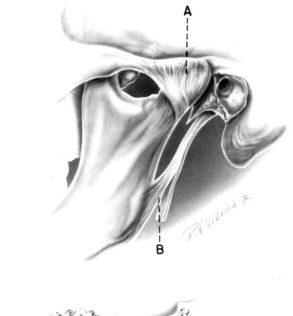

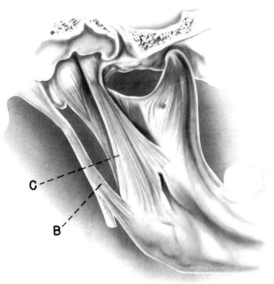

Figure 52–16 The Ligaments of the Temporomandibular Joint. *Above,* Lateral view. *Below,* Medial view. *A,* Temporomandibular ligament. *B,* Stylomandibular ligament. *C,* Sphenomandibular ligament.

surfaces of the joint to enable it to adapt to changing occlusal forces.[10, 66] The result is continuous physiologic change in the condyle and temporal bone to preserve the congruity of opposing surfaces.

Remodeling occurs in three ways:

Regressive remodeling occurs on the articular eminence of the temporal bone and the posterior aspect of the articular surface of the condyle. This leads to a loss of convexity or flattening of the joint, not necessarily associated with degenerative or osteoarthritic changes.

Progressive remodeling involves the addition of bone to the articular surface of the condyle, which brings it closer to the joint cavity.

Peripheral remodeling is similar to the progressive type, except that bone formation may also take place at the neck of the condyle. It occurs most often on the anterior condylar margin, and if excessive may produce lipping of the joint margins.

Remodeling of the temporomandibular joint has also been produced in experimental animals by altering occlusal forces. Continuous retraction of the mandible with a chin strap device resulted in resorption of the posterior border of the condyle and the opposing glenoid fossa, as well as bone formation on the anterior surface of the condyle with a slight reduction in fossa depth, without inflammation or degenerative changes.[40] **Anterior[36] and posterior[81] displacement of the mandible with dental restorations created traumatic changes in the periodontium and tooth movement which were more severe than the changes in the joint.** The condyle was initially displaced but tended to return to its original position. Experimental distal displacement of the mandible also stimulated growth activity in the embryonic condylar cartilage, but the fossa and disc remained unaltered.[24]

Functional movements

The mandible is activated by the masticatory musculature, but the extent to which condylar movements are influenced by neuromuscular stimulation,[104] the contour of the articulating surfaces in the joint and the inclined surfaces of occluding teeth has not been established.[95] Function of the joint is best understood by correlating condylar activity with various positions and movements of the mandible as follows:

When the mandible is in centric relation and the teeth are in centric occlusion, the condyles are behind the posterior surface of the articular eminence, at the level of the lower third and separated from it by the articular disc. This is the most posterior position to which the condyle can be brought by the musculature. **It is limited from further posterior movement by the musculature[30] and temporomandibular ligament.[6, 75]**

When the teeth are in habitual occlusion the mandible is anterior or anterolateral to centric relation and the condyles are slightly anterior to and inferior to their most retruded position. When the mandible is in the postural position, the condyles are usually inferior to their position in habitual occlusion.[56]

In opening and closing the jaw, the condyles are capable of two types of movement: Rotation and translation.

Rotation consists of a hinge-like movement of the condyles about an axis without change in their position. The axis about which the condyles rotate is termed the **hinge axis,** which is an imaginary horizontal line through the center of rotation of both condyles.[55]

Translation consists of forward and downward movement of the condyles. The condyles and articular discs glide along the posterior slope of the articular eminence and in some instances beyond the eminence. The discs move with the condyles and adapt themselves to the changing condylar positions, and fill the changing space between the two bone surfaces. In maximum opening the condyle may move anterior to the articular eminence in a normally functioning joint.[107] With the jaw opened wide there

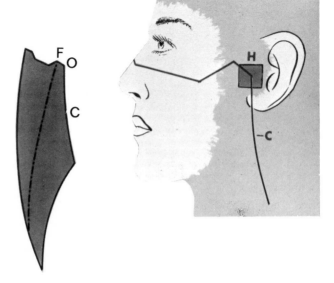

Figure 52–17 Terminal Hinge Axis. The terminal hinge axis (H) of the condyles (*right side*) corresponds to the centric relation of the mandible and centric occlusion of the dentition (O) in Posselt's rhomboid representation of the border movements of the mandible (*left side*). The centric pathway of the mandible is shown at C, the habitual occlusion is at F and the dotted line extending beneath it is the habitual pathway.

may be a slight reduction (approximately 0.09 mm.) in the width of the mandible in the molar area.[82]

The jaws ordinarily open and close into habitual occlusion, not in centric relation.[98] Opening consists of simultaneous rotation and downward and forward translation of the condyle; the reverse occurs in closure. Pure condylar rotation may occur in some instances of habitual opening and closing but only for the short distance between the closed position and the postural position. Closure is usually a simple vertical (elevator) motion.[98] In centric relation the condyles undergo pure rotation for opening up to approximately 2 cm. at the incisors. The axis of this rotation is called the *terminal hinge axis* (Fig. 52–17).

In lateral movements of the mandible from the closed position, the condyle on the side toward which the mandible is moving either rotates about a vertical axis or combines lateral movement with rotation (Fig. 52–18). *The lateral shift of the condyle on this side is called the Bennett movement.*[78] The condyle on the other side moves downward and forward, and inward.

TEMPOROMANDIBULAR JOINT DISORDERS

Developmental abnormalities, disease processes and trauma which do not originate in dental structures or the masticatory musculature may impair movement of the temporomandibular joint and disturb occlusal function.[60, 85] Most often, however, temporomandibular joint disorders are caused by **dysfunction of the dentition and the masticatory musculature.**

Clinical features

Temporomandibular joint disorders are characterized by impaired function and pain. Impairment in function varies from slight to complete limitation of movement with inability to open the jaws (trismus). The pain may be localized to the joint or radiate to the masticatory muscles, particularly the temporal; it may be referred to other areas of the face, the occipital region, the tongue or the ear. Vertigo occurs in some cases.[47]

The pain may be constant or recurrent. It may be precipitated by movement of the mandible, or it may occur without provocation. It may be elicited only by digital pressure on a muscle or the joint. Painless limitation of joint movement does occur, but infrequently. Temporomandibular disorders are more common in females than in males (3 to 1).[25]

Symptoms of temporomandibular joint disorders may be precipitated by a variety of circumstances, such as opening the mouth at a long dental appointment, sudden opening such as yawning, the insertion of exten-

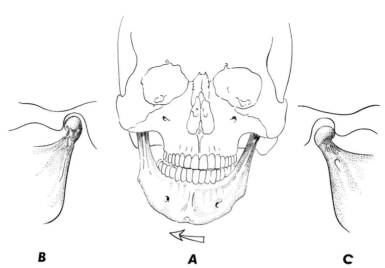

Figure 52–18   Bennett Movement of the Condyle. *A,* Lateral movement of the mandible in the direction of the arrow. *B,* Condyle on the side to which the mandible is moving either rotates about a vertical axis or combines a lateral shift with rotation. The lateral shift is called the Bennett movement. *C,* Condyle on the other side moves downward, forward and inward.

sive dental restorations which modify occlusal relationships, improper occlusal adjustment, and insertion of removable orthodontic appliances. Patients who brux often complain of temporomandibular joint symptoms in the morning upon arising.

"Grating," "clicking" or "snapping" noises upon opening and closing the jaws may accompany a joint disorder or may precede it asymptomatically for months or years.[38] The presence of such noises without symptoms is not always followed by joint disorders, nor do they necessarily occur more frequently in such patients.

Etiology

ABNORMAL OCCLUSAL FUNCTION. **Abnormal occlusal function is the principal cause of temporomandibular joint disorders. Occlusal abnormalities create joint disorders indirectly by causing excessive tension upon the masticatory musculature, which in turn disrupts joint function.** Spasm (myospasm) occurs in severe cases. It is characterized by abrupt involuntary painful contraction of a muscle or group of muscles, which seriously limits joint movement and may aggravate existing occlusal abnormalities and worsen the dysfunction of the joint. Direct injury to the joint by abnormal occlusal forces such as condylar displacement is usually repaired by adaptive changes without lasting effects.

MUSCLE SPASM. In the opinion of some,[92] muscle spasm rather than occlusal abnormality is the primary cause of temporomandibular joint disturbances. According to this concept, muscle spasm is caused primarily by emotional tension[50, 68] and individual temperament and constitution. These may increase the susceptibility of muscle to spasm induced by occlusal forces which act as secondary or precipitating factors. It has been demonstrated that emotional stress alters the stroke, volume and rate of the heart beat and also produces intermittent tooth contacts in functional occlusion.[18]

From a clinical viewpoint it is generally more difficult to find predisposing constitutional and emotional factors than it is to locate occlusal abnormalities. This does not mean that occlusion is the sole etiologic factor; occlusal dysfunction is extremely common, but only a small percentage of the patients who have it suffer from joint disorders.[54] Nevertheless, abnormal muscle contraction and joint disorders usually respond to occlusal correction.[80] Emotional disorders should be treated regardless of whether the patient's temporomandibular symptoms are corrected by occlusal adjustment.

Occlusal abnormalities that may lead to temporomandibular joint disorders are premature tooth contacts in centric or habitual occlusion, (2) overclosure from loss of posterior tooth support or from excessive tooth wear uncompensated by continuous eruption and (3) parafunctional habits such as bruxing and clenching.

YOUR OWN JAW MOVEMENTS

It will help to understand occlusion if you think in terms of your own jaw and the movements it can make:

The border movements

The border movements are the limits to which the mandible can move in any direction. Posselt, in a classic study,[75] developed a rhomboid figure which represents a sagittal view of the border movements of the mandible (Fig. 52–19). Look at Figure 52–19, and, as you read this, do the following:

1. Close your jaw and retrude the mandible as far as you can, keeping your teeth together. If you succeed, you will reach position 1 in Figure 52–19. This is the centric relation of the mandible; the condyles are in their most retruded position in the temporomandibular joints. Your dentition is in maximum intercuspation, with **the mandible in centric relation. This is centric occlusion.** (You may not be able to reach centric occlusion because one or more teeth are in the way.)

Habitual or functional occlusion

2. Keep your teeth together and move your jaw slightly forward to the next comfortable position. This is your **habitual** or **functional occlusion;** most of your teeth will be in contact in this position. It is represented by position 2 in the rhomboid diagram.

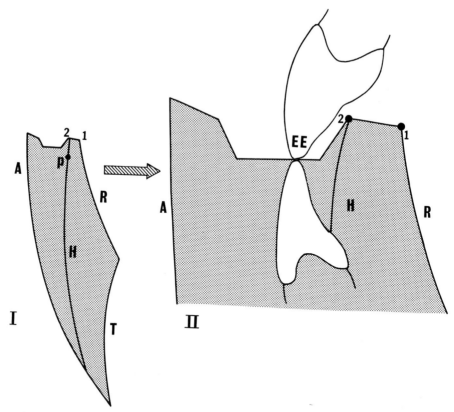

Figure 52–19 Comparison of the Border Movements and Habitual (Functional) Movements of the Mandible I. Rhomboid figure of the border mandibular movements in the sagittal plane (Posselt), showing the following: 1, Centric occlusion. 2, Habitual occlusion (functional occlusion). R, Centric (retruded) pathway of opening and closing with the condyles rotating around a hinge axis (terminal hinge axis). T, Retruded pathway of mandibular opening and closing. The action of the condyles is mainly sliding or translatory. A, Anterior border of mandibular movement. H, Habitual (functional) pathway of the mandible. p, The postural position of the mandible.

II. Enlarged view of the rhomboid, showing the relationship of the edge-to-edge position (EE) of the mandibular and maxillary incisors to habitual occlusion (2).

3. Now, slide your teeth back to position 1. Hold them there a few seconds and, still trying to retrude your mandible as far as you can, slowly open your mouth. Your mandible is now moving along the line R in Figure 52–19, which is the **most retruded** or **centric pathway of the mandible.** As you open, the condyles may remain in position and rotate in a simple hinge movement around the imaginary axis—the hinge axis. Since centric relation is the most retruded position of the condyles, the axis around which the condyles move at this stage is called the **terminal hinge axis.** As you continue to open your jaw, more **translation** or sliding creeps into the condylar movement, and the mandibular path changes from R to T in Figure 52–19. Continue to open along line T to the bottom of the rhomboid. As

your mandible moves along line T, the principal motion of the condyle is a sliding one, combined with slight axial rotation. The condyles in the temporomandibular joints are now down and forward behind the articular eminences, or below or in front of them.

4. From the bottom of the rhomboid, start to close, protruding your jaw as far as possible. You are now moving along the A. Continue to the top of line A; your mandibular incisors will now be in front of, and higher than, the incisal edges of the maxillary incisors.

5. Bring your jaw back until your incisors are edge to edge, and look at Figure 52–19. You are now at EE. Slide back a little more and your teeth will come into occlusion. **This is position 2,** your **habitual occlusion.**

Your jaw has traveled the **perimeter of the border movements of the mandible.** To reach back to position 1, it would be necessary to make a special effort to retrude your jaw.

The habitual pathway of opening and closure

6. Now, open your jaw and rest. Then open and close loosely several times. You are now opening and closing on the **habitual pathway, line H in Figure 52–19. The habitual pathway is the working pathway of the mandible, where it usually functions.** You will notice that it is anterior to the centric pathway. This means that the centric pathway is a border movement of the mandible; the habitual pathway is not.

If you wanted to open your jaw along the centric pathway (line R), the way you initially did, it would be necessary to make a special effort to retrude your mandible into centric relation and keep it back as you opened. When we want our patients to open and close along the centric pathway, we often put a little pressure on the chin to help them retrude the jaw. Tooth contacts which obstruct your mandible as it tries to reach centric occlusion are called "**centric pathway prematurities**" or "**centric prematurities**"; interfering contacts in the habitual path are called "**habitual prematurities.**"

7. Now rest. Wet your lips with your tongue, swallow and just sit there for a minute. The chances are that, when you swallowed, your teeth closed into habitual occlusion. While you are resting, your teeth are apart; your mandible is in the **postural or rest position** and, if you look at Figure 52–19 you will notice that this **position (P) is on the habitual pathway, H.**

REFERENCES

1. Adams, S.: Tooth Contact in Lateral Excursions During Mastication. J. Am. Soc. Periodont. *1*:160, 1963 (Abst.).
2. Adams, S. H., and Zander, H. A.: Functional Tooth Contacts in Lateral and in Centric Occlusion. J.A.D.A., *69*:465, 1964.
3. Anderson, D. J.: The Physiology of Mastication. D. Practit. & D. Record, 5:389, 1955.
4. Anderson, S. J., and Picton, D. C. A.: Tooth Contact During Chewing. J. D. Res., *36*:21, 1957.
5. Anderson, J. R., Jr., and Myers, G. E.: Nature of Contacts in Centric Occlusion in 32 Adults. J. D. Res., *50*:7, 1971.
6. Arstad, T.: The Capsular Ligaments of the Temporomandibular Joint and Retrusion Facets of the Dentition in Relationship to Mandibular Movements. Oslo, Academisk Forlag, 1954.
7. Atkinson, H., and Shepherd, R.: Masticatory Movements and the Resulting Force. Arch. Oral Biol., *12*:195, 1967.
8. Beyron, H. L.: Occlusal Changes in the Adult Dentition. J.A.D.A., *48*:674, 1954.
9. Beyron, H. L.: Optimal Occlusion. Dent. Clin. North America, *13*:537, 1969.
10. Blackwood, H. J. J.: Adaptive Changes in the Mandibular Joints with Function. Dent. Clin. North America, *10*:559, 1966.
11. Breitner, C.: The Tooth-Supporting Apparatus under Occlusal Changes. J. Periodont., *13*:72, 1942.
12. Brenman, H. S., and Amsterdam, M.: Postural Effects on Occlusion. D. Progress, *4*:43, 1963.
13. Brewer, A. A., and Hudson, D. C.: Application of Miniaturized Electronic Devices to the Study of Tooth Contact in Complete Dentures. J. Pros. Dent., *11*:62, 1961.
14. Brill, N., Lammie, G. A., Osborne, J., and Perry, H. T.: Mandibular Positions and Mandibular Movements: A Review. Brit. D. J., *106*:391, 1959.
15. Brodie, A. G.: Orthodontics. *In* Lippincott's Handbook of Dental Practice. Philadelphia, J. B. Lippincott Co., 1948, p. 65.
16. Butler, J. H.: Recent Research on Physiology of Occlusion. Dent. Clin. North America, *13*:555, 1969.
17. Butler, J. H., and Stallard, R. E.: Effect of Occlusal Relationships on Neurophysiological Pathways. J. Periodont. Res., *4*:141, 1969.
18. Butler, J. H., and Stallard, R. E.: Physiologic Stress and Tooth Contact. J. Periodont. Res., *4*: 152, 1969.
19. Butler, J. H., and Zander, H. A.: Evaluation of Two Occlusal Concepts. Periodont. Acad. Rev., *2*:5, 1968.
20. Carlsson, G. E., Hugoson, A., and Persson, G.: Dental Abrasion and Alveolar Bone Loss in the White Rat. IV. The Importance of the Consistency of the Diet and its Abrasive Components. Odont. Revy, *18*:263, 1967.
21. Choukas, N. C., and Sicher, H.: The Structure of the Temporomandibular Joint. Oral Surg., Oral Med. & Oral Path., *13*:1203, 1960.
22. Cohn, L. A.: Factors of Dental Occlusion Pertinent to the Restorative and Prosthetic Problem. J. Pros. Dent., *9*:256, 1959.
23. D'Amico, A.: The Canine Teeth: Normal Functional Relation of the Natural Teeth of Man. J. South. Calif. D. A., *26*:6, 49, 127, 175, 194, 239, 1958.
24. Folke, L., and Stallard, R.: Condylar Adaptation to a Change in Intermaxillary Relationship. J. Periodont. Res., *1*:79, 1966.
25. Franks, A. S.: The Social Character of Temporomandibular Joint Dysfunction. D. Practit. & D. Rec., *15*:94, 1964.
26. Garnick, J., and Ramfjord, S. P.: Rest Position. An Electromyographic and Clinical Investigation. J. Pros. Dent., *12*:895, 1962.
27. Gillings, B. R. D., Kohl, J. T., and Zander, H. A.: Contact Patterns Using Miniature Radio Transmitters. J. D. Res., *42*:177, 1963.

28. Glickman, I., Martignoni, M., Haddad, A., and Roeber, F. W.: Further Observations on Human Occlusion Monitored by Intraoral Telemetry. I.A.D.R. Abstracts, #612, 1970, p. 201.

29. Glickman, I., Pameijer, J. H. N., Roeber, F. W., and Brion, M. A. M.: Functional Occlusion as Revealed by Miniaturized Radio Transmitters. Dent. Clin. North America, 13:667, 1969.

30. Glossary of Prosthodontic Terms. J. Pros. Dent., 20:443, 1968.

31. Graf, H.: Bruxism. Dent. Clin. North America, 13:659, 1969.

32. Graf, H.: Occlusal Tooth Contact Patterns in Mastication. Thesis, University of Rochester, 1963.

33. Guichet, N. F.: Applied Gnathology: Why and How. Dent. Clin. North America, 13:687, 1969.

34. Hesse, F.: Zur Mechanik der Kaubewegung des menschlichen Kiefers. Deutsch. Mo. f. Zahnh., 15:517, 1897; D. Cosmos, 42:1004, 1900.

35. Hildebrand, G. Y.: Studies in the Masticatory Movements of the Lower Jaw. Scand. Arch. Physiol., Suppl., 61, 1931. Berlon & Leipzig, Walter De Gruyter & Co., 1931.

36. Hiniker, J. J., and Ramfjord, S. P.: Anterior Displacement of the Mandible in Adult Rhesus Monkeys. J. D. Res., 43:811, 1966.

37. Howell, A. H., and Manly, R. S.: An Electronic Strain Gauge for Measuring Oral Forces. J. D. Res., 27:705, 1948.

38. Ireland, V. E.: Problem of "the Clicking Jaw." D. Digest, 57:549, 1951.

39. Jankelson, B., Hoffman, G. M., and Hendron, J. A.: The Physiology of the Stomatognathic System. J.A.D.A., 46:375, 1953.

40. Janzen, E. K., and Bluher, J. A.: The Cephalometric, Anatomic, and Histologic Changes in *Macaca mulatta* After Application of a Continuous-Acting Retraction Force on the Mandible. Am. J. Ortho., 51:823, 1965.

41. Jerge, C. R.: The Neurologic Mechanism Underlying Cyclic Jaw Movements. J. Pros. Dent., 14:667, 1964.

42. Kawamura, Y.: Neurophysiologic Background of Occlusion. Advances in Oral Physiology, Osaka Univ., 1968.

43 Kawamura, Y.: Neurophysiologic Background of Occlusion. Periodontics, 5:175, 1967.

44. Kawamura, Y., and Fujimoto, J.: Study on the Jaw Opening Reflex, Med. J. Osaka Univ., 9:377, 1958.

45. Kawamura, Y., Kato, I., and Miyoshi, K.: Functional Anatomy of the Lateral Pterygoid Muscle in the Cat. J. D. Res., 47:1142, 1968.

46. Kawamura, Y., and Majima, T.: Temporomandibular-Joint's Sensory Mechanisms Controlling Activities of the Jaw Muscles. J. D. Res., 43:150, 1964.

47. Kelly, H. T., and Goodfriend, D. J.: Vertigo Attributable to Dental and Temporomandibular Joint Causes. J. Pros. Dent., 14:159, 1964.

48. Koyoumdjisky, E.: The Correlation of the Inclined Planes of the Articular Surface of the Glenoid Fossa with the Cuspal and Palatal Slopes of the Teeth. J. D. Res., 35:890, 1956.

49. Kydd, W. L., and Sander, A.: A Study of Posterior Mandibular Movements from Intercuspal Occlusal Position. J. D. Res., 40:419, 1961.

50 Laskin, D. M.: Etiology of the Pain-Dysfunction Syndrome. J.A.D.A., 79:147, 1969.

51. Lear, C. S. C., Flanagan, J. B., Jr., and Moorees, C. F. A.: The Frequency of Deglutition in Man. Arch. Oral Biol., 10:83, 1965.

52. Lindblom, G.: On the Anatomy and Function of the Temporomandibular Joint. Acta Odont. Scandinav., 17:7, Suppl. 28, 1960.

53. Lindblom, G.: The Term, "Balanced Articulation," Its Origin, Development and Present Significance in Modern Odontology. D. Record, 69:304, 1949.

54. Loiselle, R.: Relation of Occlusion to Temporomandibular Joint Dysfunction: The Prosthodontic Viewpoint. J.A.D.A., 79:145, 1969.

55. Lucia, V. O.: The Fundamentals of Oral Physiology and Their Practical Application in the Securing and Reproducing of Records to Be Used in Restorative Dentistry. J. Pros. Dent., 3:213, 1953.

56. Lundberg, M.: Free Movements in the Temporomandibular Joint. A Cineradiographic Study. Acta Radiol., Suppl. 220, 1963.

57. Manly, R. S.: Practical Application of Research on Mastication. Monthly Report of Office of Naval Research, Feb. 1, 1950.

58. Manly, R. S., and Shiere, F. R.: The Effect of Dental Deficiency on Mastication and Food Preference. Oral Surg., Oral Med. & Oral Path., 3:674, 1950.

59. Mann, A. W., and Pankey, L. D.: Concepts of Occlusion—The Pankey-Mann Philosophy of Occlusal Rehabilitation, Dent. Clin North America, 7:621, 1963.

60. Mayne, J., and Hatch, G.: Arthritis of the Temporomandibular Joint. J.A.D.A., 79:125, 1969.

61. McLean, D. W.: Physiologic vs. Pathologic Occlusion. J.A.D.A., 25:1583, 1938.

62. Messerman, T.: A Concept of Jaw Function with a Related Clinical Application. J. Pros. Dent., 13:130, 1963.

63. Messerman, T., Reswick, J. B., and Gibbs, C.: Investigation of Functional Mandibular Movements. Dent. Clin. North America, 13:629, 1969.

64. Mitani, H., and Kawamura, S.: Frontal Plane Movement of Incision Inferius During Mastication. *In* Functional Movement of the Jaw. Med. J. Osaka Univ., 1971, p. 37.

65. Mitani, H., and Kawazoe, T.: Kinesiological Studies on the Rest Position of the Mandible. *In* Functional Movement of the Jaw. Med. J. Osaka Univ., 1971, p. 39.

66. Moffett, B. C., Johnson, L. C., McCabe, J. B., and Askew, H. C.: Articular Remodeling in the Adult Human Temporomandibular Joint. Am. J. Anat., 115:119, 1964.

67. Møller, E.: The Chewing Apparatus, Acta Physiologica Scandinav., 69: Suppl. 280, 1966.

68. Moulton, R. E.: Psychiatric Considerations in Maxillofacial Pain. J.A.D.A., 51:408, 1955.

69. Moyers, R. E.: Some Physiologic Considerations of Centric and Other Jaw Relations. J. Pros. Dent., 6:183, 1956.

70. Murphy, T. R.: The Movement of Translation at the Temporomandibular Joint as it Occurs in Mastication. Brit. D. J., 118:163, 1965.

71. Murphy, T. R.: The Timing and Mechanism of the Human Masticatory Stroke. Arch. Oral Biol., 10:981, 1965.

72. Olsson, A.: Temporomandibular Joint Function and Functional Disturbances. Dent. Clin. North America, 13:643, 1969.

73. Pameijer, J. H. N., Brion, M. A. M., Glickman, I., and Roeber, F. W.: Intraoral Occlusal Telemetry., V. Effect of Occlusal Adjustment upon Tooth Contacts During Chewing and Swallowing. J. Pros. Dent., 24:492, 1970.

74. Picton, D. C. A.: Tilting Movements of Teeth During Biting. Arch. Oral Biol., 7:151, 1962.

75. Posselt, V.: Studies in the Mobility of the Human Mandible. Acta Odont. Scandinav., 10(Suppl. 10), 1952.

76. Powell, R. N.: Tooth Contact During Sleep. Thesis, University of Rochester, 1963.

77. Preiskel, H. W.: Some Observations on the Postural Position of the Mandible. J. Pros. Dent., 15:625, 1965.

78. Prothero, J. H.: Prosthetic Dentistry. 4th ed. Chicago, Medico Dental Publishing Co., 1928, pp. 21, 27, 30, 46.

79. Pruzansky, S.: Applicability of Electromyographic Procedures as a Clinical Aid in the Detection of Occlusal Disharmony. Dent. Clin. North America, March 1960, p. 117.

80. Ramfjord, S. P.: Bruxism, a Clinical and Electromyographic Study. J.A.D.A., 62:21, 1961.

81. Ramfjord, S. P., and Hiniker, J. J.: Distal Displacement of the Mandible in Adult Rhesus Monkeys. J. Pros. Dent., 16:491, 1966.

82. Regli, C. P., and Kelly, E. K.: The Phenomenon of Decreased Mandibular Arch Width in Opening Movements. J. Pros. Dent., 17:49, 1967.

83. Richter, J. L., Daugherty, W. F., and Beaudreau, D. E.: Responses in the Mesencephalic Nucleus to Temporomandibular Joint Stimulation. I.A.D.R. Abst., #636, 1970, p. 207.

84. Roeber, F. W., Pameijer, J. H. N., and Glickman, I.: An Intraoral Electronic System for the Study of Dental Occlusion. Med. & Biol. Engng., 6:677, 1968.

85. Sarnat, B.: Developmental Facial Abnormalities and the Temporomandibular Joint. J.A.D.A., 79:108, 1969.

86. Schärer, P. Kasahara, Y., and Kawamura, Y.: Tooth Contact Patterns during Stimulation of the Rabbit Brain. Arch. Oral Biol., 12:1041, 1967.

87. Schärer, P., LeGault, J. V., and Zander, H. A.: Mastication Under Anesthesia. Helv. Odont. Acta, 10:130, 1966.

88. Schärer, P., and Stallard, R. E.: The Effect of an Occlusal Interference on the Tooth Contact Occurrence During Mastication. Helv. Odont. Acta, 10:49, 1966.

89. Schärer, P., and Stallard, R. E.: The Use of Multiple Radio Transmitters in Studies of Tooth Contact Patterns. Periodontics, 3:5, 1965.

90. Schärer, P., Stallard, R. E., and Zander, H. A.: Occlusal Interferences and Mastication: An Electromyographic Study. J. Pros. Dent., 17:438, 1967.

91. Schuyler, C. H.: Factors Contributing to Traumatic Occlusion. J. Pros. Dent., 11:708, 1961.

92. Schwartz, L. L.: Temporomandibular Joint Syndromes. J. Pros. Dent., 7:489, 1957.

93. Schweitzer, J. M.: Masticatory Function in Man. J. Pros. Dent., 11:625, 1961.

94. Scott, I., and Ash, M. M.: A Six-Channel Intraoral Transmitter for Measuring Occlusal Forces. J. Pros. Dent., 16:56, 1966.

95. Shanahan, T. E. J., and Leff, A.: Mandibular and Articulator Movements. Part VII: Concepts of Lateral Movements and Condyle Paths. J. Pros. Dent., 14:279, 1964.

96. Shepherd, R. W.: A Further Report on Mandibular Movement. Aust. D. J., 5:337, 1960.

97. Sheppard, I., Sheppard, S., and Rakoff, S.: The Mandibular Sideshift and Lateral Excursions. J. Oral Med., 22:115, 1967.

98. Silverman, M. M.: Character of Mandibular Movement During Closure. J. Pros. Dent., 15:634, 1965.

99. Sloane, R. B.: Kinesiology and Vertical Dimension. J. Pros. Dent., 2:12, 1952.

100. Stallard, H.: The Anterior Component of the Force of Mastication and Its Significance to the Dental Apparatus. D. Cosmos, 65:457, 1923.

101. Stallard, H. and Stuart, C. E.: Eliminating Tooth Guidance in Natural Dentitions. J. Pros. Dent., 11:474, 1961.

102. Thielemann, K.: Biomechanik der Paradentose ins besondere Artikulationsausgleich durch Einschleifen. 2nd ed. München, Barth, 1956.

103. Thompson, J. R.: The Rest Position of the Mandible and Its Significance to Dental Science. J.A.D.A., 33:151, 1946.

104. Von Puff, A. and Krause, G.: Röntgenkinematographische Untersuchungen am Kiefergelenk unter funklioneller Belastung. Deutsche Zahn. Zeit., 20:189, 1965.

105. Weinberg, L. A.: Diagnosis of Facets in Occlusal Equilibration. J.A.D.A., 52:26, 1956.

106. Weinberg, L. A.: The Prevalence of Tooth Contact in Eccentric Movements of the Jaw: Its Clinical Implications. J.A.D.A., 62:402, 1961.

107. Wooten, J. H.: Physiology of the Temporomandibular Joint. Oral Surg., 21:543, 1966.

108. World Workshop in Periodontics, Edited by Ramfjord, S., Kerr, A., and Ash, M. Ann Arbor, Michigan, University of Michigan, 1966, p. 265.

109. Yuodelis, R. A., and Mann, W. V., Jr.: The Prevalence and Possible Role of Nonworking Contacts in Periodontal Disease. Periodontics, 3:219, 1965.

110. Yurkstas, A. A.: The Masticatory Act. J. Pros. Dent., 15:248, 1965.

111. Yurkstas, A. A., and Emerson, W. H.: A Study of Tooth Contacts During Mastication with Artificial Dentures. J. Pros. Dent., 4:168, 1954.

Chapter 53

OCCLUSAL ADJUSTMENT

Occlusal adjustment is the establishment of functional relationships favorable to the periodontium by one or more of the following procedures: reshaping the teeth by grinding, dental restorations and tooth movement. **There is a tendency to identify occlusal adjustment solely in a negative sense—namely, as a method of eliminating injurious occlusal forces, which indeed it**

should do. But its equally important purpose is to provide the functional stimulation necessary for the preservation of periodontal health, a positive dimension which occlusal adjustment adds to the practice of all phases of dentistry.

ENVIRONMENTAL CONTROL AND THE PERIODONTIUM

The local environment of the periodontium and periodontal health

The local environment of the periodontium consists of two principal factors: (1) the saliva with its microbial population, and (2) the occlusion. Two environmental pollutants adversely affect the periodontium; they are (1) dental plaque formed by oral bacteria, which leads to destructive periodontal inflammation; and (2) injurious occlusal forces which damage the supporting periodontal tissues.

The establishment of a satisfactory local environment is essential in the treatment of periodontal disease and in the preservation of periodontal health. The urgency of controlling plaque is well recognized; occlusal adjustment to eliminate injurious forces and create forces favorable to the periodontium is equally important in the control of the total local environment.

THE RATIONALE OF OCCLUSAL ADJUSTMENT

Occlusal adjustment is based upon the premises that tissue damage and excessive tooth mobility[22] caused by unfavorable occlusal forces undergo repair when the injurious forces are corrected; and that realignment of occlusal forces by creating unobstructed functional contacts provides trophic stimulation beneficial to the periodontium.

For which patients is the occlusion adjusted?

The occlusion is adjusted for patients with evidence of trauma from occlusion, manifested in one or more of the following ways: (1) **periodontal injury** (excessive tooth mobility, angular thickening of the periodontal ligament, angular (vertical) bone destruction, infrabony pockets, some instances of furcation involvement and migration of maxillary anterior teeth); (2) **muscle dysfunction**; and (3) **temporomandibular disorders**. These patients are represented diagrammatically in Fig. 53–1.

Most of the population has centric prematurities in the permanent[2,5,12] (approximately 90 per cent)[24] and deciduous dentitions,[13] and prematurities in habitual occlusion are also extremely common (Fig. 53–1, Group 1). All patients with occlusal prematuries do not have trauma from occlusion. It is assumed that trauma from occlusion is caused by repetitive parafunctional forces (bruxism, clamping and clenching) rather than by chewing and swallowing. This is because it has been estimated that teeth are in functional contact for approximately 17.5 minutes[10] in a 24-hour period, which leaves ample time for the periodontium to recover if it were injured by functional occlusal forces.

Occlusal prematurities are inciting causes of bruxism. Of the many people with occlusal prematurities, only some (the percentage has not been determined) develop parafunctional habits (Fig. 53–1, Group 2). Bruxism* is common, but only some patients who brux develop trauma from occlusion (Fig. 53–1, Group 3).

The occlusion is adjusted for patients with occlusal prematurities who brux and present evidence of trauma from occlusion (the vertical crosshatched column in Fig. 53–1).

---

*Used throughout the chapter to include clamping and clenching habits.

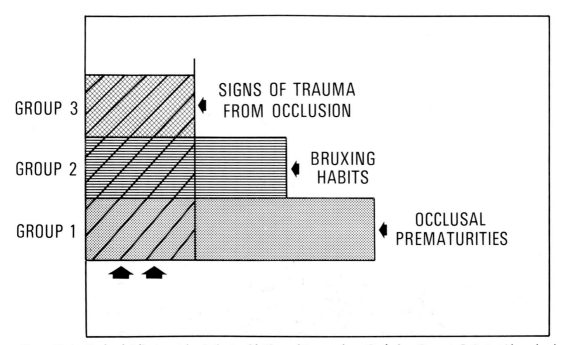

Figure 53–1 Occlusal Adjustment for Patients with Signs of Trauma from Occlusion. Group 1, Patients with occlusal prematurities. Group 2, Patients with prematurities who develop bruxing habits. Group 3, Patients with bruxing habits who develop trauma from occlusion. Occlusal adjustment is for patients in the cross-hatched vertical column *(double arrow)*.

Preventive occlusal adjustment

We do not recommend preventive occlusal adjustment—the correction of what appear to be abnormal occlusal relationships in patients without signs of trauma from occlusion, for the ostensible purpose of preventing future damage. It is the tissue response in the periodontium, masticatory musculature and temporomandibular joints which determines whether an occlusion is traumatic; the determination is not made by the alignment of the teeth and the presence or absence of occlusal prematurities. The absence of tissue injury means that the occlusal forces are acceptable to the tissues despite the fact that the alignment and relationship of the teeth may appear abnormal. Changing the occlusion in anticipation of future injury without any indication that it will necessarily occur, may upset the present satisfactory balance between the occlusion and the tissues. **The occlusion must satisfy the needs of the periodontium, the musculature and the temporomandibular joints, not the desires of the therapist.**

When to adjust the occlusion in the sequence of periodontal treatment

We are often confronted with patients suffering from both inflammation and trauma from occlusion; it would be best to eliminate both at the same time. This is not always feasible, and when a choice must be made **the occlusion is usually adjusted after gingival inflammation and periodontal pockets have been eliminated,** for the following reasons:

1. Inflammation in the periodontal tissues interferes with repair and diminishes the benefits from occlusal adjustment.

2. Teeth with periodontal disease often migrate. After the inflammation is eliminated, the teeth shift again, often in the direction of their original position (Fig. 53–2). If the occlusion is adjusted before the inflammation is alleviated, it will have to be repeated after gingival health is restored.

The usual sequence of treatment is modified under the following conditions: **In infrabony pockets, excessive occlusal forces are important in determining the pattern of the osseous defects.** To provide optimal conditions for repair of the bony defect with or without the use of osseous and marrow implants, the occlusion is adjusted before or along with the pocket elimination procedures.[30]

In mucogingival surgery, because occlusal forces affect the post-treatment contour of the facial bony plate;[9] and in cases of excessive tooth mobility in which trauma from occlusion is a major causative factor, the occlusion is adjusted before or along with the treatment of the inflammation.

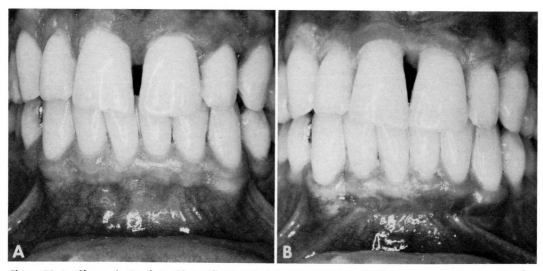

Figure 53–2 Change in Tooth Position Following Periodontal Treatment. *A,* Before treatment. Note the diastema between the maxillary central incisors. *B,* In the course of treatment the teeth return to their normal position following resolution of inflammation.

Explaining occlusal adjustment to the patient

Patients may be concerned that grinding their teeth will change their appearance, and cause tooth decay and increased sensitivity. It should be explained that their teeth are not going to be "ground down," but that they will be reshaped so that they will function better. The reshaping is done in areas where tooth decay rarely occurs. It should also be made clear that adjusting the occlusion is a necessary part of the total periodontal treatment, which benefits the periodontal tissues and prolongs the life of their teeth. The appearance of the teeth will not be spoiled; if anything, they will look better and feel more comfortable. Above all, the patient should understand that occlusal adjustment is not permanent, that the teeth and the occlusion change with time, and that their occlusion will be checked at their periodic recall visits and minor adjustments will be made, if necessary.

TECHNIQUES OF OCCLUSAL ADJUSTMENT

All methods of occlusal adjustment are empirical; they correct occlusal abnormalities, without necessarily affecting the factors which cause them. Occlusal adjustment techniques are flexible and subject to refinement as new information regarding the genesis of occlusal aberrations becomes available. There are many methods of occlusal adjustment; two are presented here: (1) the functional technique, and (2) the Schuyler technique.

I. The Functional Technique of Occlusal Adjustment

This technique includes procedures previously described in the literature (James,[15] Grove,[11] Jankelson[16]), but it represents a departure from previous occlusal adjustment techniques in that **most of the correction is done in habitual, rather than centric occlusion.** It is based upon the recently demonstrated principle that **habitual occlusion is the most commonly used functional occlusion of the dentition.**[8] It includes elimination of centric pathway prematurities,[26] as well as habitual occlusal

prematurities,[31] because both types may incite parafunctional habits (bruxing, clamping and clenching), which in turn produce trauma from occlusion.

Lateral and protrusive excursions of the mandible are not corrected because they are nonphysiologic parafunctional movements rather than regular features of chewing and swallowing.[8,17] Instead of reshaping teeth to accommodate potentially injurious parafunctional habits, this technique attempts to correct the prematurities which cause the habits. However, testing for premature contacts in lateral and protrusive excursions after the occlusion is adjusted usually reveals that most have been eliminated by the corrective procedures in this technique.

OBJECTIVES

The objectives of the functional technique are as follows:

1. To establish functional occlusal relationships beneficial to the periodontium.

2. To eliminate premature tooth contacts in centric and habitual occlusion capable of inciting parafunctional habits.

3. To restore teeth to their unworn contours and preserve the vertical dimension.

SCHEDULE OF OCCLUSAL ADJUSTMENT

The occlusion is adjusted systematically according to the schedule in Table 53–1. The usual interval between visits is one week, to permit patients to become accustomed to the altered occlusion; however, patients may be seen as frequently as every 24 hours. The procedures scheduled for each visit are outlined in Table 53–1; they sometimes require additional sessions, but the sequence of the adjustment should not be changed.

CASTS

Casts should be made before the teeth are altered by occlusal adjustment, and after occlusal adjustment is complete. They are permanent records for pre- and post-treatment comparisons and for reference at check-up visits. Casts also provide a lingual view of the dentition, which is useful in locating gross occlusal disharmonies. Mounting the casts on an articulator

TABLE 53–1 THE FUNCTIONAL METHOD OF OCCLUSAL ADJUSTMENT—SCHEDULE OF VISITS

Visit 1*	Eliminate Class III prematurities in centric occlusion	
Visit 2	Recheck Class III prematurities in centric occlusion	Eliminate Class I prematurities in habitual occlusion
Visit 3	Recheck Class I prematurities in habitual occlusion	Eliminate Class II prematurities in habitual occlusion
Visit 4	Recheck Class I and II prematurities in habitual occlusion	Eliminate Class III prematurities in habitual occlusion
Visit 5	Recheck all classes of prematurities	Polish all tooth surfaces and obtain wax registration of the adjusted occlusion

*Supplemental sessions may be required to complete the purposes of each visit.

is helpful but not necessary for occlusal adjustment.

ARMAMENTARIUM

Use 30 gauge adhesive wax strips, a grease marking pencil, articulating paper, medium grit carborundum stones or diamond points, sandpaper disks and rubber polishing wheels (Fig. 53–3). High-speed handpieces may be used for maximum efficiency, but conventional handpieces are recommended for initial experience in occlusal adjustment.

CLASSIFICATION OF OCCLUSAL PREMATURITIES

To accomplish the objectives of this technique, occlusal prematurities in centric and habitual occlusion are classified into Class I, Class II and Class III, as follows:

Class I Prematurity: The buccal surfaces of the buccal cusps of the mandibular molars and premolars, against the lingual inclines of the buccal cusps of the maxillary molars and premolars (Fig. 53–4); and the facial surfaces of the mandibular anterior teeth, against the lingual surfaces of their maxillary antagonists.

Class II Prematurity: The lingual surfaces of the lingual cusps of the maxillary molars and premolars, against the buccal inclines of the lingual cusps of the mandibular molars and premolars (Fig. 53–4).

Class III Prematurity: The buccal inclines of the lingual cusps of maxillary molars and premolars, against the lingual inclines of the buccal cusps of the mandibular molars and premolars (Fig. 53–4).

How to Correct Occlusal Prematurities. **The correction of occlusal prematurities after they have been located and marked on the teeth is a technique in itself. Its aim is to reduce the prematurities so as to create unobstructed closure of cusps into fossae, while restoring and preserving original tooth anatomy.** It is not simply a matter of grinding down premature contacts. This is incorrect because it creates flattened planes which will further disrupt the occlusion. The correction of occlusal prematurities consists of the following three procedures: (1) **grooving**, (2) **spheroiding** and (3) **pointing**.

Grooving consists of restoring the depth of developmental grooves made shallow by occlusal wear. It is done with a tapered diamond point, which is slowly rotated in the groove until the desired depth is attained (Fig. 53–5).

Spheroiding consists of reducing the prematurity and restoring the original tooth contour. Starting 2 or 3 mm. mesial or distal to the prematurity, the tooth is recontoured from the occlusal margin to a distance 2 or 3 mm. apical to the marking (Figs. 53–5 and 53–6). It is done with a light "paintbrush" stroke, gradually blending the area of prematurity with the adjacent tooth surface. A special effort is made to preserve the occlusal height of the cusps (Figs. 53–7 and 53–8).

The purpose of spheroiding is not simply
(Text continued on page 860.)

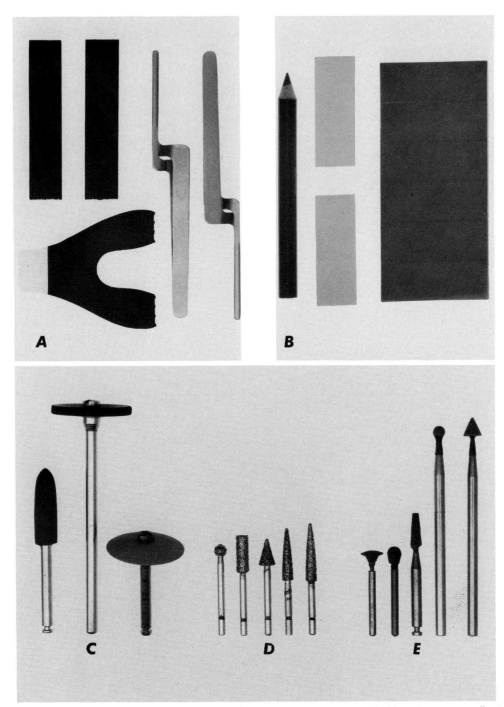

Figure 53–3 Armamentarium for Occlusal Adjustment. *A,* Articulating paper and holders. *B,* 30 gauge adhesive wax and grease marking pencil. *C,* Polishing wheels. *D,* Diamond points. *E,* Carborundum stones.

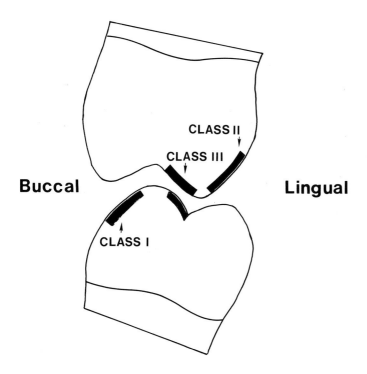

CLASS II

CLASS III

Buccal

Lingual

CLASS I

Figure 53–4 Class I, Class II, and Class III Prematurities.

Figure 53–5 Grooving to Restore the Depth of Developmental Grooves on Worn Tooth Surfaces. A tapered diamond stone (1) is rotated slowly in the groove as indicated. After the desired depth is attained, the stone is moved (2 and 3) to spheroid the adjacent tooth surface.

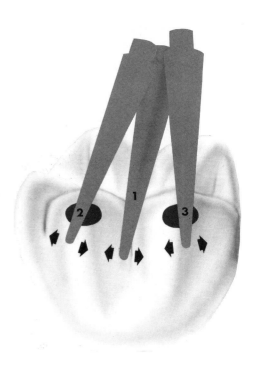

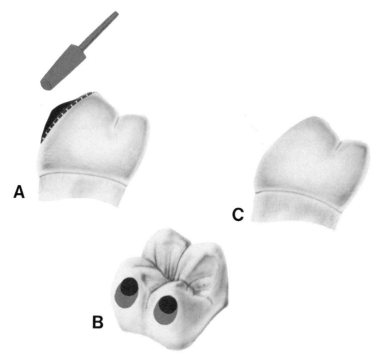

Figure 53–6   Spheroiding to Restore the Original Tooth Contour. *A,* Recontouring prematurity. *B,* Recontouring extends several millimeters below the black marking. *C,* Corrected contour.

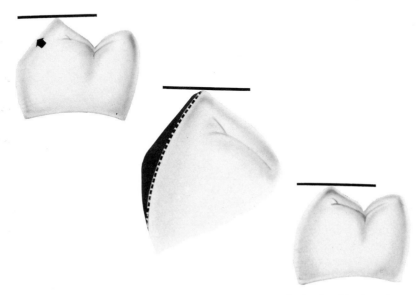

Figure 53–7   Correct Method of Spheroiding *(Broken line)* and preserving the height of the buccal cusp *(horizontal line).* The arrow points to the prematurity.

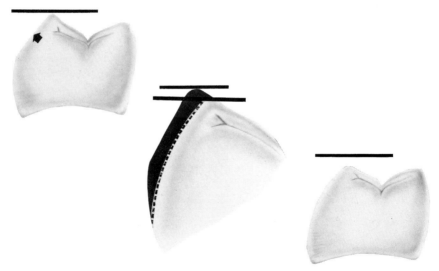

Figure 53–8 Incorrect Method of Spheroiding *(broken line)* results in excessive reduction in buccal cusp height *(horizontal line).* The arrow points to the prematurity.

to narrow occlusal surfaces. When teeth are flattened by wear, the buccolingual diameter of the occlusal surface is increased. Spheroiding restores the buccolingual width of the occlusal surface to what it was before wear occurred (Fig. 53–9).

Pointing consists of restoring cusp point contours (Fig. 53–10). It is done by reshaping the tooth with rotating diamond points.

As a general rule Class I prematurities are corrected on mandibular teeth and Class II and Class III prematurities on the maxilla. However, if doing all the correction on one jaw would entail mutilation of tooth anatomy, the opposing teeth are included in the correction process. The emphasis is always upon restoring and preserving unworn tooth anatomy. When adjustment is completed, the appearance and the function of the dentition are both improved.

Visit 1. Eliminate Class III prematurities in centric occlusion (Fig. 53–11)

HOW TO LOCATE CENTRIC PREMATURITIES. To locate centric prematurities it is necessary to have the patient open and close with the mandible in centric relation. There are many methods of doing this; the following is effective:

The patient is seated in an upright position with the headrest adjusted to a comfortable, unstrained erect position of the

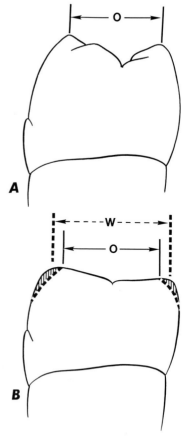

Figure 53–9 Flattened Occlusal Surface Restored to Unworn Width. *A,* Occlusal diameter (O) of unworn mandibular molar. *B,* Widened occlusal diameter (W) of worn molar restored to diameter of unworn surface (O) by recontouring *(shaded areas).*

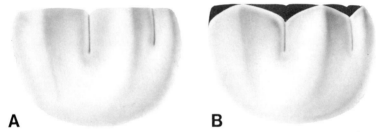

Figure 53–10 Pointing. *A,* Buccal margin of mandibular molar flattened by wear. *B,* Tooth recontoured to restore cusp points.

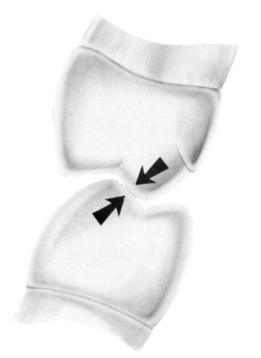

Figure 53–11 Class III Prematurity. The buccal surface of the lingual cusp of the maxillary molars and premolars, with the lingual aspect of the buccal cusps of the mandibular teeth.

head. The operator first demonstrates retrusion of his own chin and then requests the patient to bring his jaw back as far as he can, with the teeth slightly apart. The patient is then instructed to open and close repeatedly; as he does, the operator places his thumb and forefinger on the chin and exerts a gentle pressure on it. This retrudes the mandible, and is repeated until the patient opens and closes in the retruded pathway without assistance.

To detect Class III prematurities, the wax is first placed on the maxillary molars and premolars. The teeth are dried, and strips of 30 gauge wax, adhesive on one side, are placed over the occlusal surface and pressed firmly into position with the adhesive side on the teeth (Fig. 53–12). The patient moistens the exposed wax surface to prevent adherence to the mandibular teeth and is instructed to open and close rapidly with the jaw retruded, assisted by the operator if necessary, to ensure closure in centric relation. Mobile teeth are stabilized with the fingers so that prematurities will register in the wax and not be pushed aside.

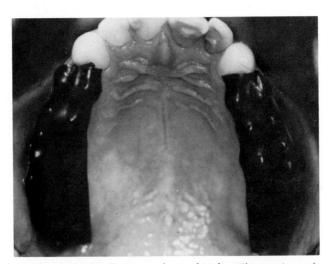

Figure 53–12 Wax Strips on the Maxillary Premolars and Molars. The anterior teeth are not covered.

If there are no obstructing tooth surfaces in centric closure of the jaw, the wax will be uniformly transparent in areas where the cusps and fossae contact the opposing teeth.

If there are Class III prematurities, they appear on the buccal inclines of the lingual cusps, as localized thinned areas with wax piled up at the periphery (Fig. 53–13, A). The wax need not necessarily be perforated. The prematurities are marked on the teeth through the wax with a pencil, and the wax strips are removed (Fig. 53–13, B).

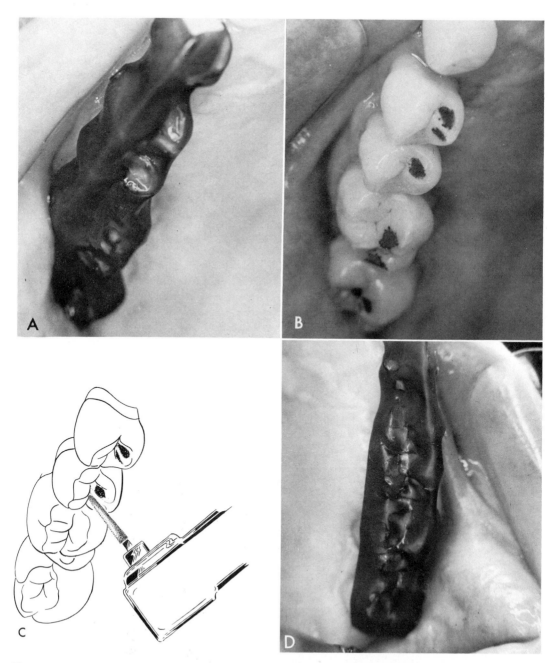

Figure 53–13 Correction of Class III Prematurities. A, Indentations in wax show Class III prematurities on the buccal aspect of maxillary lingual cusps. B, Prematurities marked on the teeth. C, Prematurities corrected with tapered diamond point. Note the position of the diamond in the groove. D, After correction, wax shows contact on cusp tips and fossae.

CORRECTION OF CLASS III PREMATUR-
ITIES IN CENTRIC OCCLUSION. The tapered diamond point is placed in the groove
mesial or distal to the premature marking,
and, after groove depth is restored, the
stone is carried over the triangular ridge,
reducing the prematurity and restoring the
pointed contour of the cusp (Figs. 53–13, C,
and 53–14). The correction procedure is
repeated with new wax strips until only
cusp tips and the bottom of the fossae register transparencies in the wax. To avoid
excessive grinding of the maxillary teeth it
is frequently necessary to do part of the
correction on the mandible. Wax strips are
placed on the opposing mandibular teeth;
the remaining Class III prematurities in
centric occlusion are registered on the
lingual aspect of the mandibular buccal
cusps and are corrected (Fig. 53–15).

**Visit 2. Recheck Class III
prematurities in centric
occlusion and eliminate Class I
prematurities in habitual
occlusion** (Fig. 53–16)

Residual Class III prematurities in centric occlusion are located and corrected. The
remainder of the occlusal adjustment is
done in habitual occlusion, which is the
functional position of the dentition.

HOW TO LOCATE CLASS I PREMATUR-
ITIES IN HABITUAL OCCLUSION. Ask the
patient to moisten his lips, swallow and
close his teeth together in their most comfortable position. Have him repeat this
process several times; the teeth will meet
in the same position. This is the habitual
occlusion.

Wax is placed on the occlusal and incisal
surfaces of the mandibular teeth (Fig. 53–
17), and the patient is asked to open and
close again as he did before. This will produce many transparencies in the wax, but
only those on the facial surface of the teeth
are dealt with at this time (Fig. 53–18).
The transparent areas are marked on the
mandibular teeth with a pencil, and the wax
is removed (Fig. 53–19, A and B).

Correction is started on the posterior
teeth with grooving on the facial surface of
of the molars (Fig. 53–19, C), followed by
spheroiding and pointing of the molars and
premolars (Fig. 53–20).

After the posterior segments are corrected,
attention is directed to the anterior teeth
(Fig. 53–21). The facial surfaces are sphe-
roided mesiodistally to relieve the prematurities and at the same time to reduce
the width of the worn incisal edges. Extruded teeth are reduced in the adjustment
procedure (Fig. 53–22). Wax strips are
placed on the teeth again, and correction is
repeated until transparencies appear only
(Text continued on page 868.)

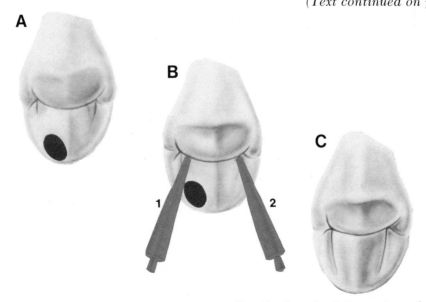

Figure 53–14 Correction of Class III Prematurity on a Maxillary First Premolar. *A,* Prematurity on the mesiobuccal
aspect of the lingual cusp. *B,* Diamond point (1) carried from the mesial groove, over the prematurity and triangular ridge
into the buccal groove (2). *C,* Prematurity corrected. The original occlusal anatomy is restored.

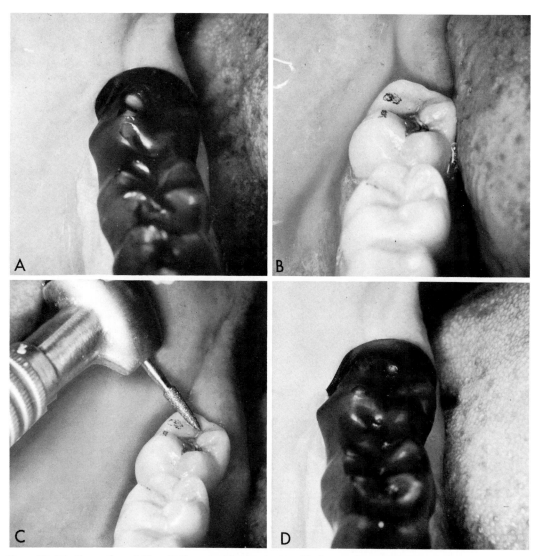

Figure 53–15 Correction of Class III Prematurities on the Mandibular Teeth. *A,* Class III prematurities on the lingual aspect of the mandibular buccal cusps. *B,* Class III prematurities marked on the tooth. *C,* Correction of the prematurities, starting with grooving the occlusal surface. *D,* Prematurities eliminated — wax registrations on cusp tip and fossa.

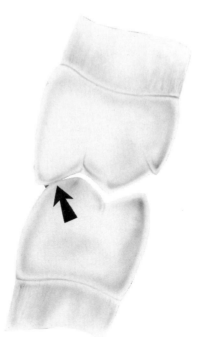
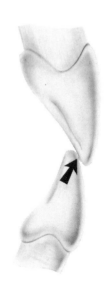

Figure 53–16   Class I Prematurities in Habitual Occlusion. Class I prematurities on the facial surface of the mandibular anterior and posterior teeth indicated by arrows.

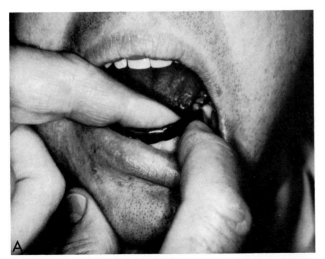

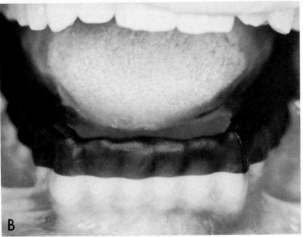

Figure 53–17   Correcting Class I Prematurities in habitual occlusion. *A,* Placing the wax on the mandibular teeth. *B,* Wax in position.

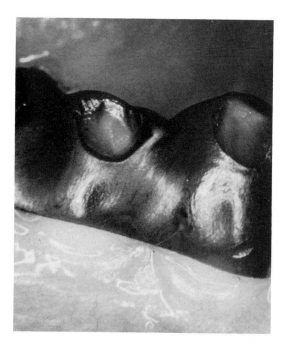

Figure 53–18 Class I Prematurities in Habitual Occlusion on the Premolars. Note the piling up of the wax around the translucent areas.

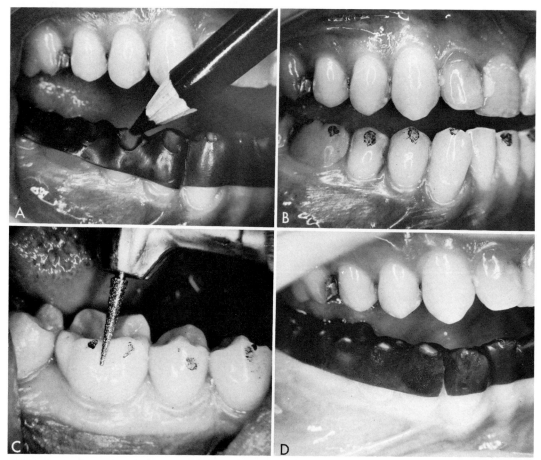

Figure 53–19 Correction of Class I Prematurities in Habitual Occlusion. *A,* Prematurities are marked through the wax onto the teeth. *B,* Prematurities marked on the teeth. *C,* Grooving the buccal surface with a tapered diamond. *D,* After correction, contact is shown on the cusp tips.

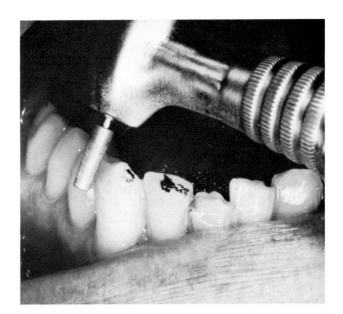

Figure 53–20 Spheroiding the Facial Surface of a Mandibular Premolar to Correct a Class I Prematurity.

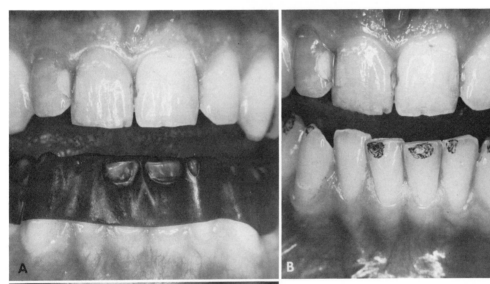

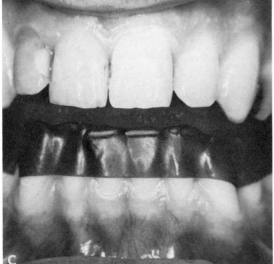

Figure 53–21 Correction of Class I Prematurities in Habitual Occlusion on the Mandibular Anterior Teeth. A, Class I prematurities on the facial surface registered in the wax. B, Prematurities marked on the teeth. C, After the prematurities are corrected, only the incisal edges contact the maxillary teeth.

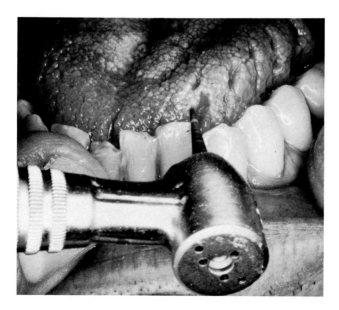

Figure 53–22   Reduction of Extruded Mandibular Incisors.

on the cusp tips and incisal edges (Fig. 53–21, *C*). This usually requires several applications of wax strips. It may be necessary to complete the correction on the opposing maxillary surfaces in order to avoid excessive reduction of the mandibular teeth. After the prematurities are eliminated, the teeth are smoothed and the patient is dismissed.

Teeth tend to upright themselves and to erupt into the spaces created by the correction of Class I prematurities (Fig. 53–23). This reduces lateral stresses and redirects occlusal forces in the long axis of the teeth, but often creates new Class I prematurities which are corrected at the next visit.

Visit 3. Recheck Class I prematurities in habitual occlusion and eliminate Class II prematurities in habitual occlusion (Fig. 53–24)

Class I prematurities in habitual occlusion which may have developed because of the uprighting of the teeth since the previous visit are corrected.

HOW TO LOCATE CLASS II PREMATURITIES IN HABITUAL OCCLUSION.   To locate

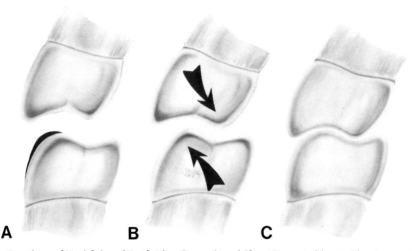

A   B   C

Figure 53–23   Eruption and Uprighting of Teeth After Correction of Class I Prematurities. *A,* Class I prematurity indicated in black. *B,* Direction of tooth movement after correction of prematurity. *C,* Teeth in adjusted position.

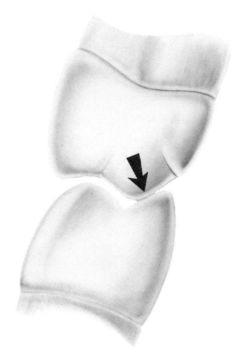

Figure 53-24 Class II Prematurity in Habitual Occlusion on the Lingual Surface of Maxillary Molar indicated by arrow.

Class II prematurities in habitual occlusion, the wax is applied to the maxillary posterior teeth. The patient again closes in habitual occlusion, and Class II prematurities are registered on the lingual surface of the lingual cusps (Fig. 53–25, A, B and C). Prematurities are corrected by grooving and spheroiding (Fig. 53–25, D), which are repeated until only the tips of the lingual cusps register in the wax (Fig. 53–25, E). The teeth are smoothed, and the patient is dismissed.

Visit 4. Recheck Class I and II prematurities in habitual occlusion and eliminate Class III prematurities in habitual occlusion

Class I and Class II prematurities in habitual occlusion which may have appeared because of the uprighting of the teeth since the previous visits are corrected. To locate Class III prematurities in habitual occlusion, wax is placed on the maxillary posterior teeth. The patient closes in habitual occlusion, and the Class III prematurities are registered in the wax on the buccal surface of the lingual cusps. The Class III prematurities in habitual oc-

clusion are corrected by grooving and pointing procedures described for correcting Class III prematurities in centric relation. Class III prematurities in habitual occlusion are not common at this stage, because the uprighting of the teeth after the relieving of the Class I and Class II prematurities tends to reduce excessive contact between the buccal inclines of the maxillary lingual cusps and the lingual inclines of the mandibular buccal cusps (Fig. 53–23).

Visit 5. Recheck all classes of prematurities, polish all tooth surfaces and make a wax registration in habitual occlusion

At this visit, Class III prematurities in centric occlusion and Class I, II, and III prematurities in habitual occlusion are checked and corrected, and all tooth surfaces are smoothed and polished. Registrations are taken in habitual occlusion with the wax on the maxilla and then with the wax on the mandible. At this stage the occlusal adjustment is completed; the wax should show transparent areas on the tips of the occluding cusps, at the base of the fossae into which they occlude and on the incisal edges of the anterior teeth. The wax registrations are filed for reference.

MAINTENANCE OF THE OCCLUSION

Teeth and dental restorations wear with use, and as a result the occlusion changes. No method of occlusal adjustment creates a permanent occlusal relationship. The occlusion must be checked periodically for minor adjustments, and the patient should be advised accordingly.

II. Schuyler Technique for Occlusal Adjustment

This technique is based upon centric occlusion and the principle that lateral and protrusive excursions are functional movements of the mandible. It initially included bilateral balance in lateral excursion,[34] but balancing side contacts were eliminated from the procedure because of their potential for creating occlusal trauma.[33] The technique is presented here with minor variations.[21]

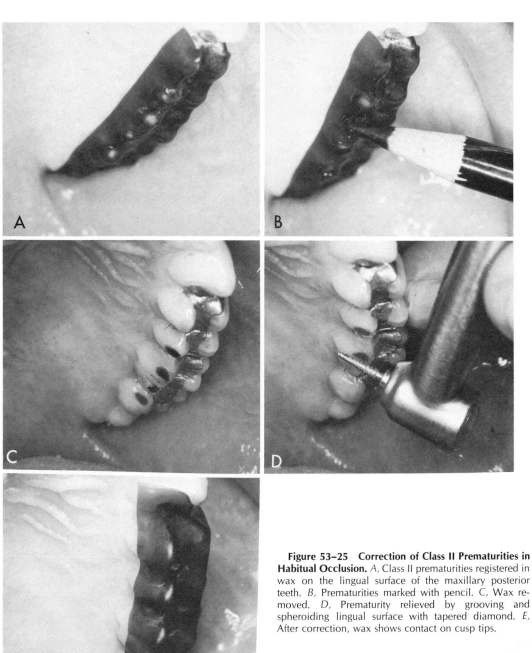

Figure 53–25 Correction of Class II Prematurities in Habitual Occlusion. *A,* Class II prematurities registered in wax on the lingual surface of the maxillary posterior teeth. *B,* Prematurities marked with pencil. *C,* Wax removed. *D,* Prematurity relieved by grooving and spheroiding lingual surface with tapered diamond. *E,* After correction, wax shows contact on cusp tips.

STEP 1. ELIMINATE GROSS OCCLUSAL DISHARMONIES

1. EXTRUDED TEETH. Extruded teeth are reduced to the level of the occlusal plane by grinding and reshaping within the limits permitted by the position of the pulp. If large areas are exposed by grinding, a dental restoration in conformity with the corrected occlusal relationship is indicated.

Extruded unopposed third molars may irritate the mucosa of the opposing jaw, interfere with closure in centric occlusion and deflect the mandible. Food impaction is also common between extruded third molars and the second molar. Extruded molars should be extracted or reduced to the occlusal plane and splinted to the second molar.

When an unopposed maxillary third molar is removed, the interdental space be-

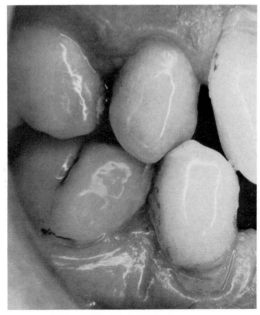

Figure 53–27 Plunger Cusp on the Maxilla. The premolar forces food between the mandibular teeth, causing gingival inflammation.

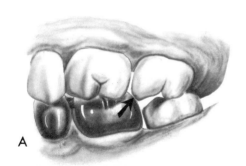

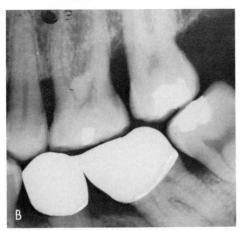

Figure 53–26 Displacement of Maxillary Second Molar in the Absence of Distal Support. *A,* Impact of mandibular first molar *(arrow)* leads to displacement of maxillary second molar and creates area of food impaction. Note absence of contact between the mandibular molars. *B,* Radiograph showing accentuated bone loss in area of food impaction on mesial surface of maxillary second molar.

tween the first and second molars should be watched for evidence of food impaction. Distal thrusts produced on occlusal contact may momentarily break the contact between the maxillary first and second molars and permit impaction of food (Fig. 53–26). At the first sign of such impaction the first and second maxillary molars should be splinted together.

2. PLUNGER CUSPS. Plunger cusps are cusp points that wedge into the interproximal spaces between opposing teeth and cause food impaction (Fig. 53–27). The cusp points should be rounded and shortened and, if this does not suffice, the opposing interproximal space can be protected by splinting the teeth adjacent to it.

3. UNEVEN ADJACENT MARGINAL RIDGES. Differences in the height of adjacent marginal ridges may cause food impaction and should be corrected by either reducing the height of the relatively high marginal ridge or increasing the height of the low one with a restoration (Fig. 53–28). Extreme differences are overcome by using both procedures. In grinding the marginal ridges the natural tooth contour should be preserved. The marginal ridge should not be reduced if it entails sacrifice of occlusal contact.

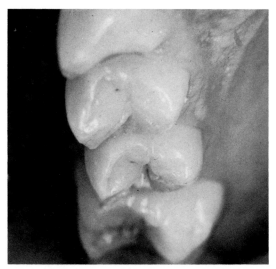

Figure 53–28 Uneven marginal ridges.

4. ROTATED, MALPOSED AND TILTED TEETH. Teeth that are rotated or in a facial or lingual version may interfere with functional movement of the mandible and cause food accumulation and impaction. Depending upon their severity, such conditions can be corrected by orthodontic procedures (Chap. 56), reshaped by grinding, or restorations which conform to the corrected occlusal and proximal relationship of the dentition (Fig. 53–29).

Tilted teeth create abnormal occlusal forces which may lead to periodontal injury. They should be realigned orthodontically to direct the functional forces within the confines of the root. However, it is sometimes expedient to accomplish the desired correction by reshaping the crown with a restoration.

5. *Facets and Flat Occlusal Wear.* Facets are flattened planes produced by wear on a convex tooth surface[42] (Fig. 53–30), which vary in size and outline. They are detected by examination after the teeth have been dried. Study casts are also helpful. Occlusal contact at the periphery of broad facets may create lateral or tipping forces potentially injurious to the periodontium.

Correction of Facets. To correct a facet, the periphery is progressively reduced by grinding until normal convexity of the tooth is restored, and only a small area remains in occlusal contact (Fig. 53–31).

6. FLAT OCCLUSAL WEAR. When excessive wear produces broad flat or cupped-out occlusal surfaces, forces applied at the periphery are directed outside the confines of the root and may create tipping forces injurious to the periodontium. The occlusal surface is modified by grinding to restore the normal faciolingual and mesiodistal diameters, cuspal anatomy, grooves and marginal ridges (Fig. 53–32). Proximal contact relationships must be maintained. If the desired correction is not attainable by grinding, the use of a restoration is indicated (Fig. 53–32). Incisal edges flattened by excessive occlusal wear are also reshaped by grinding (Fig. 53–33).

STEP II. ELIMINATE CENTRIC PREMATURITIES

The purpose of this step is to eliminate prematurities that interfere with final closure of the mandible in centric occlusion and to establish simultaneous contact when the teeth are intercuspated. The normal areas of contact in centric occlusion are

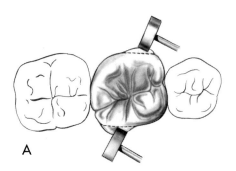
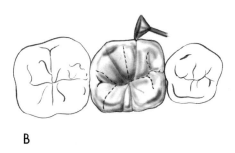

A   **B**

Figure 53–29 Reshaping Slightly Rotated Tooth by Grinding. A, Slightly rotated molar. Areas removed by grinding indicated by dotted lines. B, Occlusal surface recontoured (*dotted lines*) and buccal grooves relocated.

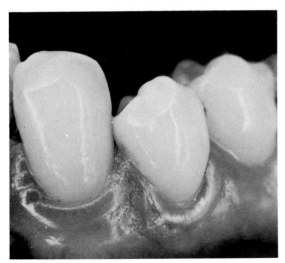

Figure 53–30 Prominent facets on the premolars.

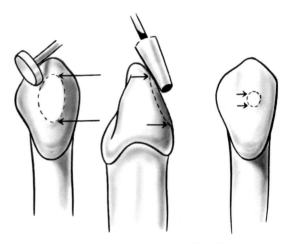

Figure 53–31 Reduction of Facet by Grinding. The dimensions of the facet before and after reduction are indicated by the arrows.

referred to as areas of centric maintenance (Fig. 53–34).

How to detect centric prematurities

The following is one of several methods available for this purpose.[4,5,16,17,20,22,23]

Seat the patient in a relaxed, erect posi-tion with the head unsupported by the head rest. Explain the purpose of the pro-cedure to follow, especially what is ex-pected of the patient. Gently hold the patient's chin with the thumb and index finger of the right hand (Fig. 53–35). Request the patient to relax the jaw.

Instruct the patient to tap the teeth to-

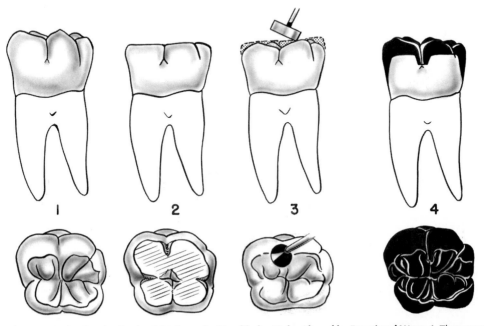

Figure 53–32 Reshaping the Occlusal Surface of a Mandibular Molar Altered by Functional Wear. *1,* The unworn molar crown. *2,* The molar crown altered by wear. *3,* Reshaping the molar crown to reduce the area of the occlusal surface and restore cuspal inclines and marginal ridges. (The outlined stippled area is the portion of the tooth surface removed.) *4,* The use of a restoration to reshape a worn molar crown where correction by grinding is not feasible. (After S. C. Miller.)

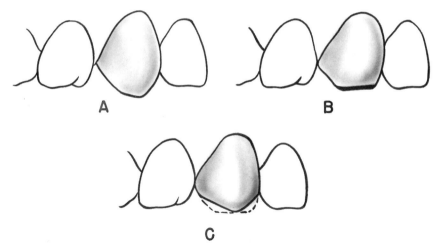

Figure 53–33 Recontouring Canine Altered by Incisal Wear. *A,* Contour of unworn maxillary canine. *B,* Facet frequently seen at incisal edge of canine. *C,* Correction of facet. Areas of tooth removed are indicated by the broken line.

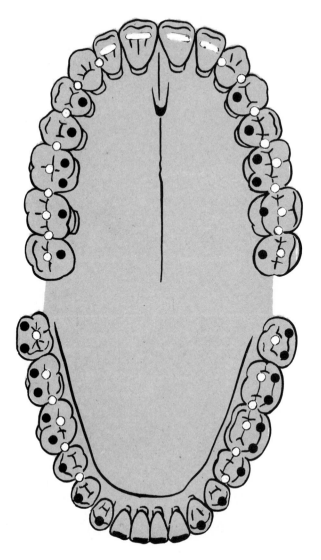

Figure 53–34 Areas of Centric Maintenance in the Mandible and Maxilla. In centric occlusion, the buccal cusps of the mandibular teeth *(black dots)* occlude into the central areas of the maxillary posterior teeth *(white dots).* The lingual cusps of the maxillary teeth *(black dots)* occlude into the central areas of the mandibular posterior teeth *(white dots).* The incisal edges of the mandibular anterior teeth *(black markings)* contact the lingual surface of the maxillary anterior teeth *(white markings).*

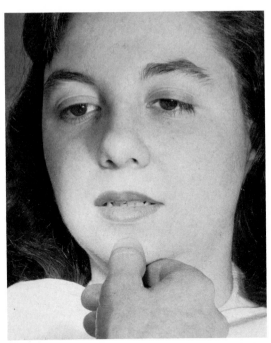

Figure 53–35 Determination of Centric Occlusion. Gentle guidance of the mandible aids in determining the pathway of centric closure.

gether lightly and rapidly while you guide the mandible along its most retruded path of closure with your right hand on the chin. Be careful not to deflect the mandible to the left or right. It is sometimes difficult to obtain complete patient relaxation. Premedication with mephenesin (Tolserol), 1 to 3 gm., or meprobomate (Equanil), 0.4 gm., is helpful.

The above procedure is repeated until you can feel that the mandibular closure is unstrained and it can be repeated by the patient without guidance by your hand. This mandibular movement represents terminal hinge rotation of the condyles in their most retruded position in the glenoid fossa, or the pathway of centric closure.[1]

Determine whether there are any pre-mature tooth contacts preventing the teeth from closing in centric occlusion. Question the patient as to the teeth which seem to "hit first" as the jaws close. The patient's impression is often useful in locating the areas of the mouth, if not the exact tooth surfaces, where prematurities occur.

Common sites of prematurities are the mesial inclines of the lingual cusps and marginal ridges of the maxillary molars and premolars and their opposing tooth surfaces. **The mesial incline of the lingual cusp of the maxillary first premolars is the most common initial prematurity.**

THE ACENTRIC GLIDE. When *initial tooth contact* is made in centric relation, centric prematurities cause the mandible to glide into habitual occlusion *on complete closure* (Fig. 53–36). This is termed the *acentric glide,* and is a common occurrence.[2] Occlusal adjustment eliminates the prematurities and provides for unobstructed closure into centric occlusion and also eliminates the acentric glide.

To locate the prematurities, soften a double thickness of base plate wax or aluwax cut to proper size, using the study casts as a pattern. Insert the wax and adapt it to the occlusal surfaces of the maxillary teeth. Hold the wax in position with the thumb and index finger of the left hand (Fig. 53–37). Request the patient to repeat the previously exercised opening and closing movement, gently guiding the mandible with the right hand for the first few closures. Explain to the patient that he is to close into the wax, but not "bite through it."

After the patient has repeatedly tapped the teeth together without assistance, remove the wax and examine it against a strong light. It will be very thin or perforated where there is a prematurity (Fig. 53–38). If there is generalized perforation or thinning of the wax, it indicates

Figure 53–36 Acentric Glide. Premature contact on the mesial surface of the distobuccal cusp of the maxillary first molar *(small arrow)* leads to anterior deflection of the mandible *(large arrow).*

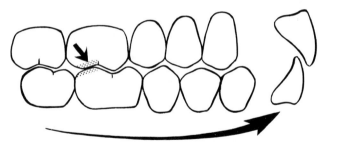

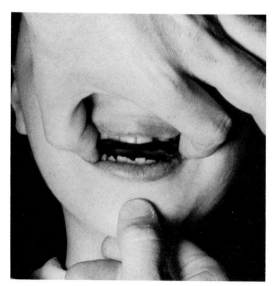

Figure 53–37 Use of Wax Template to Locate Prematurities. Wax template adapted to the functional surfaces of the teeth held in position on the maxilla as the mandible moves in the centric pathway.

either that the teeth meet uniformly in centric occlusion or that the patient slid into habitual occlusion after encountering a prematurity. To clarify this situation the procedure is repeated with a new wax template until the operator is satisfied that the imprint is valid.

When a prematurity is registered, the wax template is replaced on the maxillary teeth and the offending surface is marked with a pencil. The wax template is then placed on the mandibular teeth and the contacting mandibular surface is marked.

After the initial prematurity is adjusted by grinding, other prematurities may become apparent. A new wax template is made to reveal whether the initial prematurity is eliminated and also whether there are other prematurities. When the wax template shows uniform contact throughout the dentition, centric occlusion is established (Fig. 53–39).

How to determine whether to grind the cusp or fossa to eliminate a centric prematurity

When a prematurity is detected, the operator must decide whether to relieve the offending cusp or the tooth surface with which it occludes. This requires examina-

tion of the relationship of the cusp in other positions and excursions of the mandible, such as protrusive and lateral (described below). If the cusp will also interfere with the protrusive or lateral movements, then it should be adjusted to eliminate the premature contact in centric occlusion. If the offending cusp is in proper contact or not in occlusion in the excursions, it should not be disturbed in centric occlusion; the opposing tooth surface is reduced to correct the centric prematurity.

STEP III. PROTRUSIVE POSITION AND EXCURSION

Protrusive excursion refers to *the path of the mandible as it moves anteriorly or posteriorly between the centric occlusion and the edge-to-edge relationship of the*

Fig. 53–38

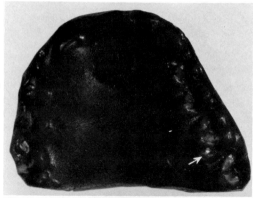

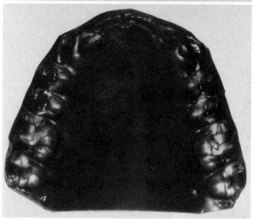

Fig. 53–39

Figure 53–38 Prematurity on Distolingual Cusp of Maxillary First Molar Indicated by Perforation of Wax Template.

Figure 53–39 Wax Template Showing Uniform Contact Throughout the Dentition in Centric Occlusion.

anterior teeth. The latter is called the *protrusive position.* Protrusive position and excursion are corrected separately and in the following order.

1. Correction of protrusive position

Protrusive position correction is directed at attaining maximum contact of incisal edges of the maxillary and mandibular anterior teeth. This is done as follows: The patient is instructed to open and close on the incisal edges with articulating paper between the teeth. Progressively relieving the marked areas permits the unmarked incisal edges to come into contact (Fig. 53–40). Wherever possible, adjustment is confined to the maxillary teeth. The mandibular teeth are ground (a) when because of pain, proximity to the pulp or esthetic reasons, the limit of grinding of the maxillary teeth has been reached, and (b) when individual mandibular teeth protrude either incisally or facially. It is important not to grind the mandibular teeth so that they would be out of contact in the

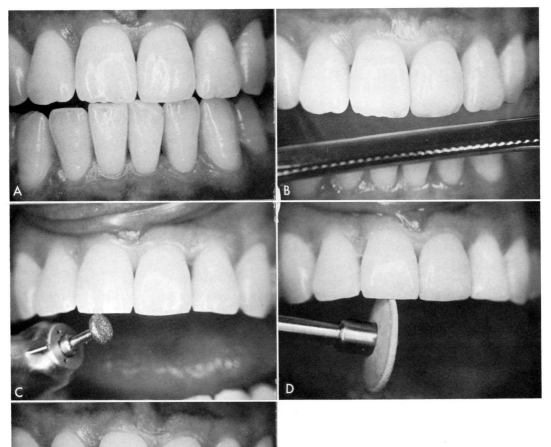

Figure 53–40 Correction of the Anterior Teeth in Protrusive Position. *A,* Before correction. *B,* Articulating paper in place to detect areas of contact. *C,* Marked areas on maxillary teeth reduced. *D,* Smoothing the ground surfaces with rubber wheel. *E,* Uniform contact of anterior teeth in protrusive position.

various mandibular excursions. If such contact is not maintained, the mandibular teeth will extrude and recreate prematurities.

The production of flat broad incisal surfaces by grinding should be avoided. After the maximum number of anterior teeth are in contact, the width of the incisal edges is reduced by grinding the facial margin of the maxillary teeth and the lingual margin on the mandible. The anterior teeth are also reshaped to improve esthetics. The ideal result of correction of protrusive position is contact between the twelve anterior teeth. This may not be attainable in cases of tooth irregularity.

To stabilize the mandible and avoid overloading the anterior teeth, it is desirable to have as many of the posterior teeth as possible in contact when the anterior teeth are in the protrusive position. Uniform contact of all posterior teeth in protrusive position is not generally attainable, but it is often possible to adjust the anterior teeth so that there are some areas of posterior contact. **The anterior teeth should not be mutilated in an effort to bring the posterior segments into contact.**

2. Correction of protrusive excursion

Protrusive excursion is corrected to provide freedom of movement and equalized contact between the mandibular and maxillary teeth as the mandible moves back and forth between centric occlusion and protrusive position. The lingual surfaces of the maxillary anterior teeth serve as the "incisal guidance" for the movement of the mandible in protrusive excursion. Under ideal conditions, the movement of the mandibular anterior teeth in protrusive excursion is matched by the sliding contact of the cusps of the posterior teeth so that the jaws remain in contact anteriorly and posteriorly throughout the protrusive excursion. This ideal (balanced occlusion) is rarely encountered. Usually protrusive excursion consists of (a) an initial phase in which there is contact in the anterior and posterior segments (Fig. 53–41) and (b) a terminal phase supported solely by the anterior teeth. PROCEDURE FOR CORRECTING PROTRUSIVE EXCURSION. Insert articulating paper and instruct the patient to move the

jaw forward and back with the teeth in contact. Mobile teeth should be stabilized by the operator's fingers to prevent them from moving away from the articulating paper. Areas in excessive contact will be most prominently marked.

Reduce the prominently marked areas. In the posterior part of the mouth this entails grinding cuspal inclines. Do not disturb the cusp tips and contacting surfaces required for maintenance of centric occlusion. In the anterior region grinding is confined to the lingual surfaces of the maxillary teeth, except when extensive adjustment is required. In such cases the marked areas on the mandibular teeth are also adjusted. The above procedure is repeated until simultaneous contact of the anterior and posterior segments throughout the protrusive excursion is either attained or approached.

The lingual surface of the maxillary teeth is adjusted as follows: The gingival portion of the area marked by the articulating paper represents the initial phase of the excursive movement during which there is contact in both anterior and posterior segments (Fig. 53–42). The incisal portion marked by the articulating paper represents the terminal phase when contacts may be limited to the anterior teeth. Grinding is confined to the incisal portion of the marked surfaces unless the gingival portion is prominent and interferes with protrusive excursion. The area of centric contact on the lingual surface is not disturbed.

There are several types of problems that require correction in protrusive excursion. Disharmony between the cuspal planes of the posterior teeth and the lingual surfaces of the anterior teeth may deflect the mandible laterally from the median line and/or vertically, taking the anterior teeth out of contact. In cases of pronounced overbite with little overjet, the maxillary and mandibular anterior teeth extend beyond the occlusal planes of the posterior teeth. Posterior tooth contact is lost shortly after protrusive excursion begins. The brunt of the mandibular movement is borne by the anterior teeth. Grinding of the anterior teeth to reduce the overbite is indicated in this type of case (Fig. 53–43). If this is not feasible, the anterior overbite is reduced by orthodontic and prosthetic measures.

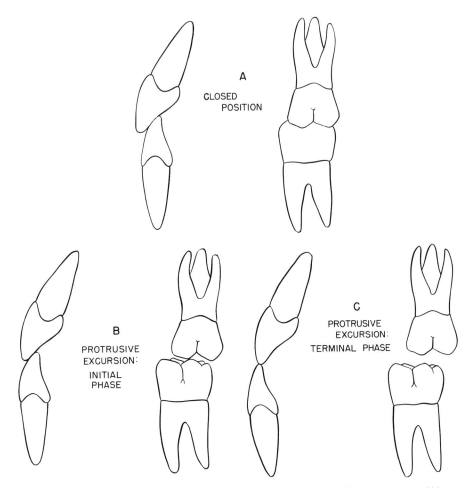

Figure 53–41 Two Phases of Protrusive Excursion. *A,* Closed position. *B,* Initial phase. As the mandible moves forward contact is maintained in both the anterior and posterior regions. *C,* Terminal phase. Only the anterior teeth are in contact.

Figure 53–42 Protrusive Excursion Adjustment. Lingual surface of maxillary incisor showing articulating paper markings in protrusive excursion. *A,* The area of centric maintenance, which should not be disturbed. *B,* The area of combined contact of the posterior and anterior teeth. This should not be disturbed. *C,* The area when only the anterior teeth are in contact, which should be reduced.

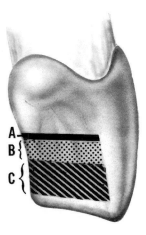

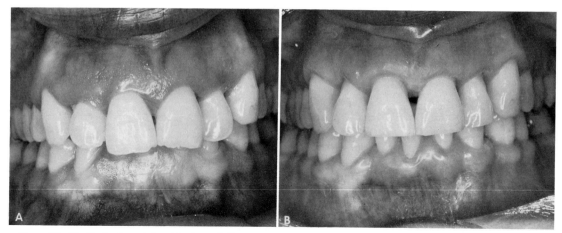

Figure 53–43 Reduction of Overbite by Grinding. A, Before treatment. Pronounced anterior overbite. B, After occlusal correction, overbite reduced.

STEP IV. LATERAL EXCURSION

Lateral excursion is the sideward and return movement of the mandible from centric occlusion to a position in which the buccal cusps of the mandibular and maxillary molars, premolars and canines are in edge-to-edge contact (lateral position). The combination of sideward and forward movement of the mandible is referred to as *lateral protrusive excursion*. The side to which the mandible moves is called the *working side;* the other side is customarily referred to as the *balancing side*, although bilateral balance is no longer sought in occlusal adjustment because it is commonly a cause of periodontal injury. When the mandible moves in lateral excursion (Fig. 53–44), the mandibular buccal cusps move along the lingual planes of the maxillary buccal cusps and the lingual cusps of the maxillary teeth are in contact with the buccal planes of the mandibular lingual cusps. There should be no contact on the balancing side.[33]

Procedure for correcting lateral excursion

In lateral excursion correction of one working side and its corresponding balancing side are completed before the other working side is treated.

LEFT WORKING AND BALANCING SIDE. Using bilateral articulating paper, have the patient move the mandible with the teeth in contact from centric occlusion to the left side until the buccal surfaces of the left mandibular and maxillary molars, premolars and canines are in alignment.

Remove the articulating paper and examine the markings on the working and balancing sides. The prominent inclined planes will be most heavily marked. Correction of the working side is concerned primarily with the *lingual planes of the buccal cusps of the maxillary teeth* and *the buccal planes of the lingual cusps of the mandibular teeth* (Fig. 53–45). After the most heavily marked surfaces are relieved, repeat the excursion procedure, progressively adjusting the heavily marked surfaces until there is uniform contact of the teeth on the working side (Figs. 53–45 and 53–46) without contact on the balancing side.

Balancing side

Prematurities on the balancing side can interfere with correction of the working side and even prevent working side contact (Fig. 53–47). The *buccal inclines* of the *maxillary lingual cusps* and the *lingual inclines* of the *mandibular buccal cusps* are common sites of balancing side prematurity (Fig 53–48). In relieving these cuspal inclines, the teeth are taken out of contact in lateral excursion, but the areas of centric occlusal maintenance should not be disturbed (Fig. 53–47).

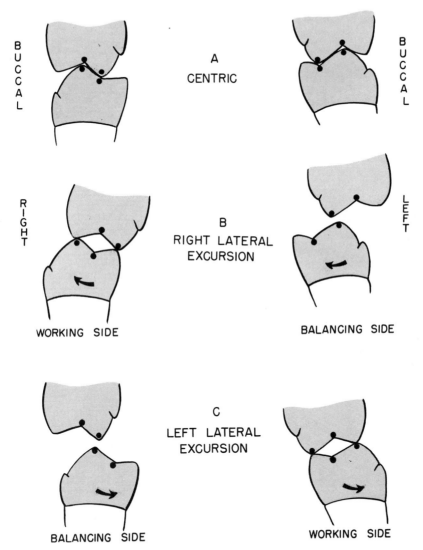

Figure 53–44 Right and Left Lateral Excursions. *A,* Centric occlusion. The areas of centric maintenance are indicated by the black dots. *B* and *C,* Right and left lateral excursions. In each instance only the working side is in contact.

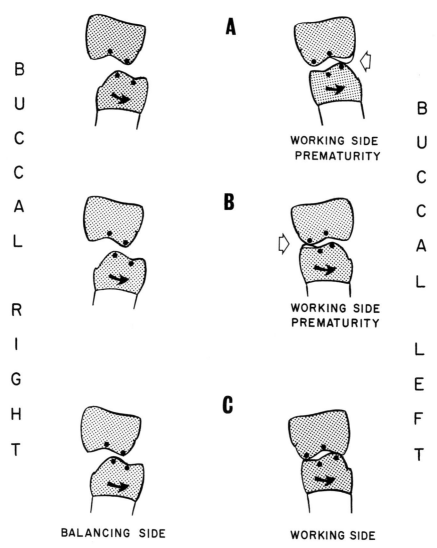

Figure 53–45 Correction of Working Side Prematurity in Lateral Excursion *(indicated by dark arrows).* A, Working side prematurity on the buccal cusps *(white arrow).* B, Working side prematurity on lingual cusps *(white arrow).* C, Proper working side contact established after correction of prematurities. The areas of centric maintenance *(black dots)* are not disturbed. Note the absence of contact on the balancing side.

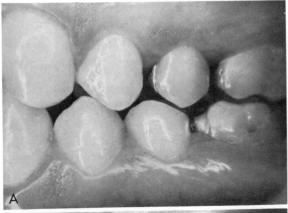

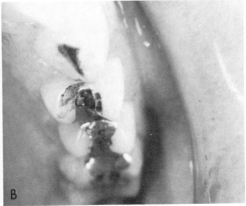

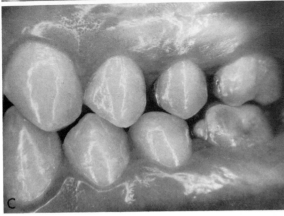

Figure 53–46 Correction of Lateral Excursion.
A, Lateral excursion with contact only on the canines and first premolars. *B,* Articulating paper markings on the prominent canine and first premolar. *C,* Uniform contact of buccal cusps in lateral excursion.

RIGHT WORKING AND BALANCING SIDES. After the left working and balancing sides are corrected, the procedures are repeated with the mandible moving to the right.

Correction of lateral protrusive excursion

Adjustment of lateral protrusive excursion is often required in the canine area after protrusive and lateral excursions have been corrected (Fig. 53–49).

CROSSBITE. This is a reversal of the normal buccolingual relationship of the maxillary and mandibular teeth. When only a few teeth are involved, orthodontic corrective measures should be employed. When a large segment of the arch is in crossbite relationship, special principles must be employed in adjusting the occlusion. The areas of centric maintenance in crossbite are the tips of the buccal cusps of the maxillary teeth and the tips of the lingual cusps of the mandibular teeth, and the areas into which they occlude (Fig.

53–50). The cusp surfaces relieved in adjusting the occlusion in crossbite are the reverse of those in patients with a normal buccolingual relationship.

STEP V. REFINEMENT OF THE ADJUSTED OCCLUSION

Rechecking tooth relationships

The tooth relationships are rechecked in all functional positions and movements, and the tooth surfaces are smoothed and polished.

OCCLUSAL ADJUSTMENT IN THE TREATMENT OF BRUXISM

Bruxism* is common, but all patients with the habit are not necessarily injured by it.

---

*Includes clamping and clenching habits.

(Text continued on page 886.)

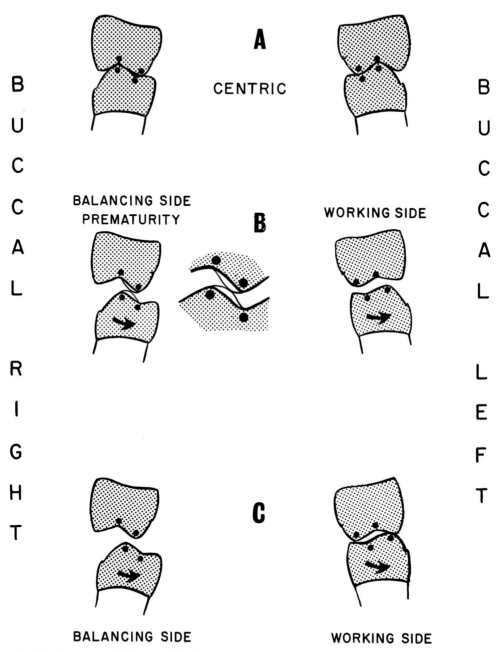

Figure 53–47 Correction of Balancing Side Prematurity. *A,* Centric occlusion. Black dots indicate areas of centric maintenance. *B,* Balancing side prematurity prevents contact on the working side. Movement of mandible indicated by arrows. *C,* Balancing side prematurity eliminated bringing working side into proper contact. Note absence of contact on the corrected balancing side.

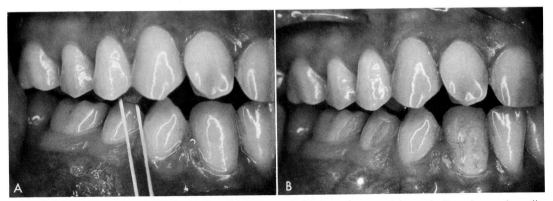

Figure 53–48 Correction of Balancing Side Prematurity. *A,* Balancing side prematurity on the lingual cusp of maxillary first premolar. Tooth contact obstructs passage of dental floss. *B,* Balancing side prematurity eliminated.

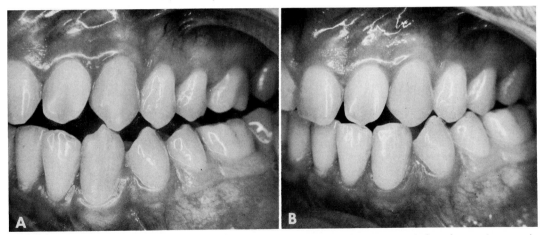

Figure 53–49 Correction of Lateral Protrusive Excursion. *A,* Premature contact on canine in lateral protrusive excursion. *B,* After correction.

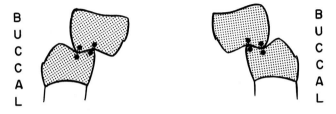

CROSSBITE

Figure 53–50 Crossbite showing reversal of normal buccolingual cuspal relationships. Black dots indicate the areas of centric maintenance.

Those who are, suffer from trauma from occlusion in the periodontium, musculature[23] and temporomandibular joint. Occlusal prematurities, excessive muscle tension and emotional factors singly or together are the accepted causes of bruxism, but opinions differ as to which is the primary or most critical factor. (For a discussion of bruxism, see Chapter 25).

The keystone of the treatment of bruxism is occlusal adjustment to correct occlusal prematurities, habitual and centric, which are usually responsible for triggering the bruxing habit. How severe a prematurity must be to incite bruxing depends upon the individual's emotional status, which also influences the aggressiveness of the muscular response. This means that psychological guidance may be necessary for some patients,[4, 23, 36, 39] but the treatment of bruxism starts with adjusting the occlusion.

Occlusal adjustment, even when combined with psychologic therapy may not be effective in all patients. Bite guards are used as a palliative measure in resistant cases.[25] Bite guards are removable acrylic appliances which cover the occlusal and incisal surfaces and extend to the maximum prominence facially and lingually (Fig. 53–51). They provide a hard, smooth surface to protect the periodontium and musculature from the impact of lateral tripping forces ordinarily created by bruxing mandibular movements. They are worn at night on the maxilla and mandible, but a single splint may be used by patients who cannot tolerate both. The occlusal surface of the splints must be flat and smooth; single splints should be checked regularly to eliminate indentations made by the opposing teeth.

OCCLUSAL ADJUSTMENT IN THE TREATMENT OF TEMPOROMANDIBULAR JOINT DISORDERS

Except for conditions caused by joint disease,[29] injury or developmental anomalies, temporomandibular joint disorders can usually be treated effectively by elimination of the etiologic occlusal disharmonies and the establishment of physiologic occlusal relationships. Treatment is sometimes initiated on a psychologic basis.[19] The occlusal approach is more fruitful,[35] but emotional considerations should not be disregarded.

Diagnosis

Diagnosis involves correlation of the patient's history, clinical examinations and radiographs.

Clinical examination

Gently palpate the external surface in the area of the joint. A painful response suggests the possibility of periarticular inflammation.[3] Also check for pain on opening and closing the jaw. If myospasm is present, pain may be localized in a muscle or radiate to other areas: the masseter myospasm radiates to the ear, the joint and the mandibular teeth; spasm in the temporalis radiates to the maxillary teeth, the temple area and the orbit; spasm in the medial pterygoid radiates to the postmandibular and infraauricular area; spasm in the lateral pterygoid radiates to the temporomandibular joint.

Pain may be elicited by palpating individual malfunctioning muscles, which may or may not be in spasm. Opening and closing the jaw should be studied for restriction and deviation of mandibular movement.

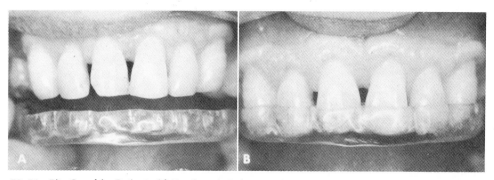

Figure 53–51 Bite Guard for Patient with Bruxism. *A,* Preliminary to insertion on maxillary teeth. *B,* Bite guard inserted.

The limits of maximum opening decrease with age. Thirty-five to 40 mm. is considered the minimal normal interincisal distance.[37]

If the mandible deviates to the side of the painful joint, malfunction of the masseter or the temporalis on that side may be responsible. If the mandible deviates to the side opposite the painful joint, malfunction of the medial pterygoid may be the cause. Simultaneous shortening of the masseter and medial pterygoid on the same side restricts mandibular movement without deflection. Auscultation of the joints with a stethoscope provides additional information about the condylar movement before, during and after treatment.[7, 28]

Radiographs

X-rays of the joint are useful but not conclusive; negative radiographic findings do not rule out the existence of a functional joint disorder. There are many special techniques for joint radiographs,[6, 20, 27] of which tomographs are the most reliable.[18, 43]

Occlusal adjustment

Centric and habitual pathway prematurities which disrupt occlusal function should be located and corrected; this procedure often results in dramatic relief of acute symptoms (Fig. 53–52), after which the

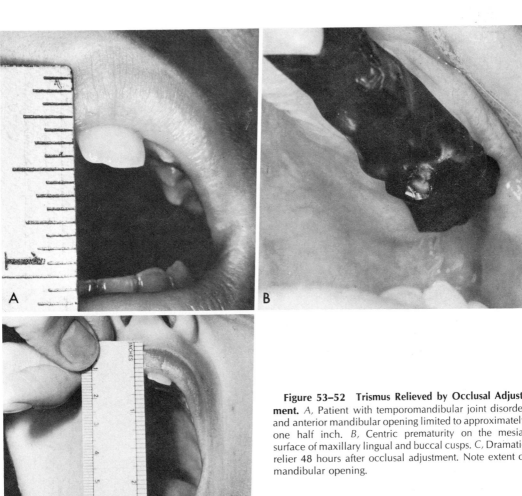

Figure 53–52 Trismus Relieved by Occlusal Adjustment. *A,* Patient with temporomandibular joint disorder and anterior mandibular opening limited to approximately one half inch. *B,* Centric prematurity on the mesial surface of maxillary lingual and buccal cusps. *C,* Dramatic relief 48 hours after occlusal adjustment. Note extent of mandibular opening.

occlusion of the entire dentition should be adjusted.

If pain or limitation of movement interferes with locating premature tooth contact, impressions are taken and a therapeutic bite guard is constructed with a thin smooth occlusal surface for the maxilla or mandible. Its purpose is to relieve muscle dysfunction by eliminating abnormal cuspal contacts. The bite guard is worn throughout the day and night, including at meal-times.

After 24 to 48 hours of use of the bite guard, joint and muscle pain is usually relieved sufficiently to permit opening and closure of the jaws with the bite plane in position. Articulating paper is used to detect premature contacts on the bite guard, which are relieved by grinding. The procedure is repeated daily until unimpaired closure in habitual and centric occlusion is attained. The bite guard is discontinued and final occlusal adjustment is made in the natural dentition.

Joint pain or muscle spasm which prevents opening of the mouth sufficiently to obtain impressions may be relieved temporarily with ethyl chloride. It is sprayed on the skin in the painful areas at an acute angle from a distance of 24 inches, with a slow sweeping motion to prevent frosting of the tissues[35] and with the patient's eyes and nose shielded. This will relax the musculature so that impressions can be taken for the construction of a therapeutic bite-plane.

Continuous joint and muscle pains are relieved by the application of heat with a towel soaked in hot water for 15 minutes hourly. Sedation with phenobarbital, 30 mg. three times a day, or tranquilizers such as meprobamate, 400 mg., or reserpine, 0.25 mg., three times a day, is also helpful.

Subluxation of the temporomandibular joint

It is within the range of normal for the condyle to move anterior to the articular eminance. However, if the condyle becomes temporarily locked in this position with pain and clicking during mastication, the condition is referred to as subluxation. Subluxation of the mandible is a self-reducing incomplete dislocation of the temporomandibular articulation. It may be caused by chronic degenerative changes in the joint. Acute trauma, previous dislocation of

the mandible or excess manipulation of the jaw during a dental procedure may cause abnormal looseness of the capsule and recurrent subluxation.[28] Chronic cases may be relieved by intra-articular injection of sclerosing solutions to restrain jaw movement.

REFERENCES

1. Arstad, T.: The Capsular Ligaments of the Temporomandibular Joint and Retrusion Facets of the Dentition in Relationship to Mandibular Movements. Akademisk Forlag (Oslo), 1954.
2. Bell, D. H., Jr.: Sagittal Balance of the Mandible. J.A.M.A., 64:486, 1962.
3. Bell, W. H., and Ware, W. H.: Management of Temporomandibular Joint Pain Dysfunction Syndrome. Dent. Clin. North America, 15:487, 1971.
4. Clark, T. D., Perachio, A., and Mahan, P.: A Neurophysiological Study of Bruxism in the Rhesus Monkey. I.A.D.R. Abstr., p. 190, #566, 1970.
5. Cohen, W. E.: A Study of Occlusal Interferences in Orthodontically Treated Occlusions and Untreated Normal Occlusions. Am. J. Ortho., 51:647, 1965.
6. Cross, W. G.: Selective Grinding as a Means of Prevention and Treatment of Periodontal Disease. D. Practit., 2:300, 1952.
7. Freese, A. S., and Scheman, P.: Management of Temporomandibular Joint Problems. Postgraduate Dental Lecture Series. St. Louis, C. V. Mosby, 1962.
8. Glickman, I., Pameijer, J. H., Roeber, F. W., and Brion, M. A. M.: Functional Occlusion as Revealed by Miniaturized Radio Transmitters. Dent. Clin. North America, 13:667, 1969.
9. Glickman, I., Smulow, J. B., Vogel, G., and Passamonti, G.: The Effect of Occlusal Forces on Healing Following Mucogingival Surgery. J. Periodont., 37:319, 1966.
10. Graf, H.: Bruxism. Dent. Clin. North America, 13:659, 1969.
11. Grove, C. J.: Trauma Produced by Occlusion, Due to Horizontal Stress. J.A.D.A., 11:813, 1924.
12. Ingervall, B.: Retruded Contact Position of Mandible. A Comparison Between Children and Adults. Odont. Revy, 15:130, 1964.
13. Ingervall, B.: Retruded Contact Position of Mandible in the Deciduous Detition. Odont. Revy, 15:414, 1964.
14. Ingle, J. I.: Determination of Occlusal Discrepancies. J.A.D.A., 54:6, 1957.
15. James, A. F.: A discussion by Correspondence. D. Items Int., 45:584, 1923.
16. Jankelson, B.: A Technique for Obtaining Optimum Functional Relationship for the Natural Dentition. Dent. Clin. North America, March 1960, p. 131.
17. Jankelson, B.: Physiology of Human Dental Occlusion. J.A.D.A., 50:664, 1955.
18. Klein, I. E., Blatterfein, L., and Miglino, J. C.: Comparison of the Fidelity of Radiographs of

Mandibular Condyles Made by Different Techniques. J. Prosth. Dent., 24:419, 1970.

19. Lupton, D.: Psychological Aspects of Temporomandibular Joint Dysfunction. J.A.D.A., 79:131, 1969.

20. Markowitz, H. A., and Gerry, R. G.: Temporomandibular Joint Disease (A Collective Review). Oral Surg., Oral Med. & Oral Path., 3:75, 1950.

21. Miller, S. C.: Textbook of Periodontia. 3rd ed. Philadelphia, The Blakiston Co., 1950, p. 343.

22. Mühlemann, H. R., Herzog, H., and Rateitschak, K. H.: Quantitative Evaluation of the Therapeutic Effect of Selective Grinding. J. Periodont., 28:11, 1957.

23. Nadler, S.: The Importance of Bruxism. J. Oral Med., 23:142, 1968.

24. Olsson, A.: Temporomandibular Joint Function and Functional Disturbances. Dent. Clin. North America, 13:643, 1969.

25. Posselt, V., and Wolff, I. B.: Treatment of Bruxism by Bite Guards and Bite Plates. J. Canad. D. Assn., 29:773, 1963.

26. Ramjford, S. P.: Bruxism, a Clinical and Electromyographic Study. J.A.D.A., 62:21, 1961.

27. Ricketts, R. M.: Laminagraphy in the Diagnosis of Temporomandibular Joint Disorders. J.A.D.A., 46:620, 1953.

28. Sarnat, B. G.: The Temporomandibular Joint. 2nd ed. Springfield, Ill., Charles C Thomas, Publisher, 1964.

29. Sarnat, B. G., and Laskin, D. M.: Diagnosis and Surgical Management of Diseases of the Temporomandibular Joint. Springfield, Ill., Charles C Thomas, 1962.

30. Schärer, P., Butler, J., and Zander, H.: Die heilung parodontaler Knochentaschen bei okklusalar

Dysfunktion. Schweiz. Mschr. Zahnheilk., 79:244, 1969.

31. Schmidt, J. R., and Harrison, J. D.: A Method for Simultaneous Electromyographic and Tooth-Contact Recording. J. Pros. Dent., 24:387, 1970.

32. Schreiber, H. R.: Occlusal Equilibration in Abnormal Occlusions. J. Periodont., 27:47, 1956.

33. Schuyler, C. H.: Factors Contributing to Traumatic Occlusion. J. Pros. Dent., 11:708, 1961.

34. Schuyler, C. H.: Fundamental Principles in the Correction of Occlusal Disharmony. Natural and Artificial. J.A.D.A., 22:1193, 1935.

35. Schwartz, L.: Disorders of the Temporomandibular Joint. Philadelphia, W. B. Saunders Co., 1959.

36. Shapiro, S., and Shannon, J.: Bruxism—as an Emotional Reactive Disturbance. Psychosomatics, 6:427, 1965.

37. Sheppard, I. M., and Sheppard, S. M.: Range of Condylar Movement During Mandibular Opening. J. Pros. Dent., 15:263, 1965.

38. Shore, N. A.: Equilibration of the Occlusion of Natural Dentition. J.A.D.A., 44:414, 1952.

39. Thaller, J. L., Rosen, G., and Saltzman, S.: Study of the Relationship of Frustration and Anxiety to Bruxism. J. Periodont., 38:193, 1967.

40. Thomas, B. O. A., and Gallagher, J. W.: Practical Management of Occlusal Dysfunctions in Periodontal Therapy. J.A.D.A., 46:18, 1953.

41. Vauthier, U.: Functional Equilibration and Analysis of Occlusal—Articular Relationship by Waxbites. Paradontologie, 10:54, 1956.

42. Weinberg, L. A.: Diagnosis of Facets in Occlusal Equilibration. J.A.D.A., 52:26, 1956.

43. Yale, S. H.: Radiographic Evaluation of the Temporomandibular Joint. J.A.D.A., 79:102, 1969.

Chapter 54

RESTORATIVE-PERIODONTAL INTERRELATIONSHIPS

Dental restorations and periodontal health are inseparably interrelated; periodontal

health is necessary for the proper function of all restorations, and the functional stimulation provided by dental restorations is essential for the preservation of the periodontium. Technical excellence is important in restorative dentistry. The adaptation of the margins, the contours of the restoration, the proximal relationships and the surface smoothness fulfill critical biologic requirements of the gingiva and supporting periodontal tissues. But in the final analysis, we restore cusps and fossae, entire teeth and groups of teeth for the purpose of restoring function. The word "restorative" in restorative dentistry refers primarily to the restoration of occlusion, not only of the teeth being restored and their antagonists, but of the remainder of the dentition as well. Dental restorations are therefore as much a part of the treatment of periodontal disease as are scaling and curettage and surgical procedures.

PERIODONTAL HEALTH ESSENTIAL FOR PROPER FUNCTION OF PROSTHESIS

Gingival and periodontal disease must be eliminated before restorative procedures are begun, for the following reasons:

Tooth mobility and pain from food impaction in periodontal pockets interfere with mastication and function of the prosthesis.

Inflammation and degeneration of the periodontium impair the capacity of abutment teeth to meet the functional demands of the prosthesis. Restorations constructed so as to provide beneficial functional stimulation to a healthy periodontium become a destructive influence when superimposed upon existing periodontal disease, **and shorten the life span of the teeth and the prosthesis.**

The position of teeth is frequently altered in periodontal disease. Resolution of inflammation and regeneration of periodontal ligament fibers following periodontal treatment cause the teeth to move again, often in the direction of their original position. Prosthesis designed for teeth before the periodontium is treated may produce injurious tensions and pressures upon the treated periodontium.

Partial prosthesis constructed on casts made from impressions of diseased gingiva and edentulous mucosa will not fit properly when periodontal health is restored. When the inflammation is eliminated, the contour of the gingiva and adjacent mucosa is altered (Fig. 54–1). Shrinkage creates spaces beneath the pontics of fixed bridges and the saddle areas of removable prosthesis. Resultant food accumulation leads to inflammation of the mucosa and gingiva of the abutment teeth.

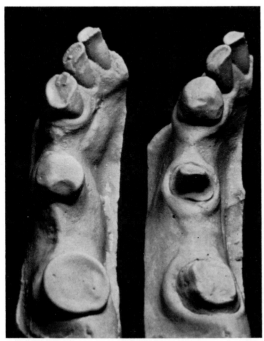

Figure 54–1 Change in Contour of Edentulous Mucosa Following Resolution of Inflammation. *Left,* Before treatment. Note the pyramidal contour of the edentulous mucosa. *Right,* The contour of the edentulous mucosa changes after resolution of inflammation. The teeth are in process of preparation.

To properly locate the gingival margin of restorations, the position of the healthy gingival sulcus must be established before the tooth is prepared. Margins of restorations hidden behind diseased gingiva will be exposed when the inflamed gingiva shrinks following periodontal treatment.

Modified preparation technique

In patients with mutilated dentitions and extensive periodontal disease, the usual sequence is changed and a temporary prosthesis is constructed before the periodontal pockets are eliminated. The teeth are prepared with provisional margins which are relocated after the gingivae heal. This provides improved occlusal relationships and splinting during the healing period. Approximately two months after periodontal treatment, when gingival health is restored and the location of the gingival sulcus is established, the **preparations are modified to relocate the margins in proper relation to the healthy gingival sulcus,** and a final restoration is constructed.

PREPARATION OF THE MOUTH FOR PROSTHESIS

The aims of periodontal treatment are not limited to the elimination of periodontal pockets and the restoration of gingival health. **It should also create the gingival-mucosal environment necessary for the proper function of fixed and removable partial prosthesis.** Preparation of the mouth for prosthesis consists of soft tissue corrective measures performed as part of surgical periodontal treatment or as an adjunct to scaling and curettage.

Periodontal pockets and adjacent edentulous mucosa

Periodontal pockets on teeth adjacent to edentulous spaces, and deformed edentulous mucosa are conditions that require correction before prosthesis is constructed. Periodontally involved teeth adjacent to edentulous spaces present two problems, which must be treated together: (1) elimination of the pockets and (2) management of the edentulous mucosa. Inflammation from the periodontal pockets extends for varying

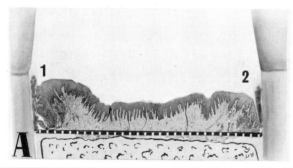

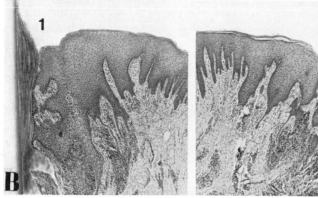

Figure 54–2 Preparation of the Mouth for Prosthesis. *A,* Edentulous mucosa with periodontal pockets (1 and 2) on the adjacent teeth. The location of the necessary incision is indicated by the dotted line. *B,* Inflammation from the periodontal pockets (1 and 2) extends into the edentulous mucosa.

distances into the adjacent edentulous mucosa (Fig. 54–2) and alters its color, consistency and shape. The edentulous mucosa affected by inflammation may present various degrees of discoloration and edema with a smooth glistening surface, depending upon the relative predominance of cellular and fluid exudate or fibrosis. If principally fibrotic, it is pink, firm and enlarged with a lobulated surface.

The contour of the edentulous mucosa and gingiva is affected by mechanical factors as well as inflammation from adjacent pockets. The edentulous mucosa may conform to the shape of the underlying bone or it may be swollen and rounded faciolingually, or lateral pressure from the tongue and cheek and food excursion may cause a pyramiding of the mucosa to form an elongated triangular ridge (Fig. 54–3). Because of the absence of the normal protective action of the embrasure, the gingiva is often similarly deformed.

The deformed edentulous mucosa re-

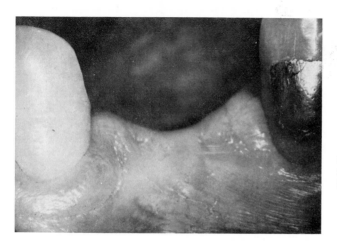

Figure 54–3 "Pyramiding" of Edentulous Mucosa and Adjacent Gingiva. The gingiva and mucosa are contoured by pressure from the tongue and food excursion.

duces the vertical height available for prosthetic replacements. It does not provide a reliable base for the support of saddle areas or the proper design of pontics. The triangular-shaped mucosa is unsatisfactory for the placement of pontics. In an effort to overcome the problem, short pontics with a deep V-shaped base, which straddles the ridge, are used. These are unsatisfactory because food wedges between the mucosa and pontics and causes inflammation which jeopardizes retention of the bridge (Fig. 54–4).

Management of pockets and edentulous mucosa

The area is prepared for prosthesis with the following objectives:

1. To establish a healthy gingival sulcus so that the pontics adjacent to the natural teeth can be designed to create the gingival embrasure necessary for preservation of gingival health.

2. To eliminate extraneous mucosal tissue to permit adequate vertical space for the replacements.

3. To provide a firm healthy mucosal base for placement of saddles or pontics.

The periodontal pockets and mucosa are resected together by an incision made across the edentulous area from tooth to tooth below the level of the base of the pockets and close to the crest of the edentulous ridge (Fig. 54–5). Periodontal knives or

Bard-Parker blades may be used. The tissue is removed and the tooth surfaces are scaled and planed. The flat plane created by the incision is tapered facially and lingually so that the tissue conforms to the shape of the ridge. Periodontal pack is placed around the teeth and across the ridge for a period of a week and repeated if necessary. A dental floss loop across the edentulous area will assist in retention of the pack (Chap. 43). A month is usually required for complete healing.

Treatment of the periodontal pockets as separate entities does not produce the desired results. It leaves a trough adjacent to the tooth surfaces, which retains debris after the pontics or saddles are constructed, causing recurrence of periodontal disease.

It should be noted that uninflamed gingiva and adjacent edentulous mucosa may be deformed by mechanical factors and require correction before inserting prosthesis.

PERIODONTAL ASPECTS OF PROSTHESIS

In addition to esthetics, the purposes of fixed and removable prosthesis include the improvement of masticatory efficiency and the prevention of tilting and extrusion of teeth and the resultant disruption of the occlusion and food impaction. **However, the most critical purpose of prosthesis is to provide the functional stimulation essential for the preservation of the periodontium of the remaining natural dentition.**

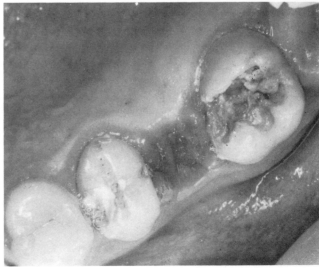

Figure 54–4 Chronic Inflammation of Edentulous Mucosa under bridge with ridge-lap type of pontic.

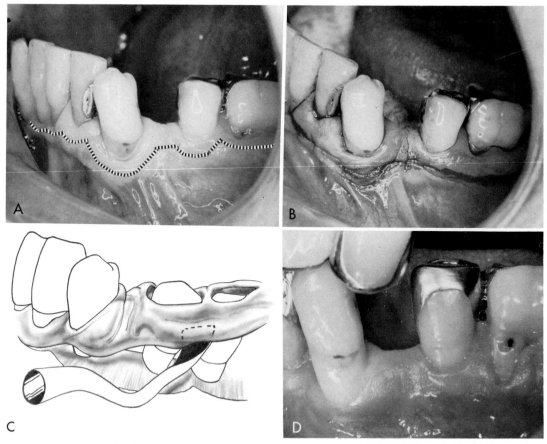

Figure 54–5 Preparation for Prosthesis. *A,* Deformed edentulous mucosa and adjacent periodontal pockets. The incision is indicated by the dotted line. *B,* The incision. *C,* Inflamed gingiva and edentulous mucosa removed. *D,* Mucosa and gingiva healed with deformity corrected.

Occlusal adjustment before prosthesis

Traumatic occlusal relationships should be eliminated before restorative procedures are begun, and restorations should be constructed in conformity with the newly established occlusal patterns. If this is not done, the prosthesis perpetuates occlusal relationships injurious to the periodontium.

The harmful effects of occlusal trauma are not confined to the teeth involved in the restoration and their antagonists. Other areas of the dentition are secondarily affected by an occlusal disharmony created or perpetuated by an inlay or bridge. Delaying occlusal adjustment until the restorations are inserted often necessitates grinding through the occlusal surface of the newly constructed restorations.

The occlusion must be checked at regular intervals after prosthesis is inserted. Oc-clusal relationships change with time as the result of wear of restorative materials and settling of saddle areas of removable prosthesis, especially those without distal support.

Tooth preparation in relation to the gingival margin

The first requirement for proper location of the gingival margin of a crown or other restoration close to the gingiva is a healthy gingival sulcus. Preparation should not be finalized until the gingiva is healthy and its position on the root has been established. Periodontal pockets should not be permitted to remain undisturbed for the ostensible purpose of "keeping the root covered," or "hiding the margins of the restoration." When the gingiva is treated, as it eventually must be, the denuded root and margins of the restoration that were "hidden" by the inflamed gingiva become visible. In the interim, the patient has suffered unnecessary destruction of the periodontium, and the longevity of the tooth and restoration has been jeopardized.

Treatment of the gingiva, final tooth preparation and impression taking should not be attempted in one operation. This does not allow time for the gingiva to heal, and the location of the margin of the restoration in relation to the healed gingival sulcus can only be estimated. The margin of the restoration and adjacent root surface are often exposed after healing occurs.

Location of the margin of restorations in relation to the gingiva

Crown margins should be located at the base of the gingival sulcus[10, 14, 34, 52] (Figs. 54–6 and 54–7, A, B and C). **This is the level reached when a blunt probe is inserted without pressure into the sulcus.** In this position, the gingival fibers brace the gingiva against the tooth and margin of the completed restoration (Fig. 54–8).

The margin of the preparation should not terminate at the crest of the marginal gingiva (Fig. 54–7, D). **Regardless of how perfect**

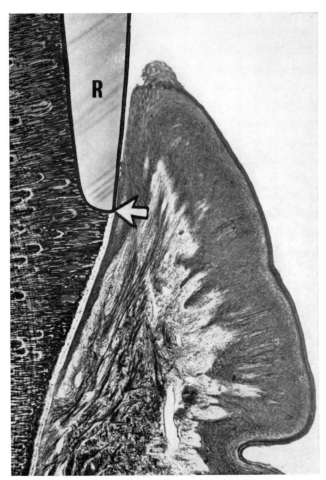

Figure 54–6 Correct Location of Restoration in the Gingival Sulcus. Margin of restoration (R) is located at the base of the gingival sulcus (*arrow*) at the coronal level of the epithelial attachment. Note the gingival fibers which brace the marginal gingiva against the tooth.

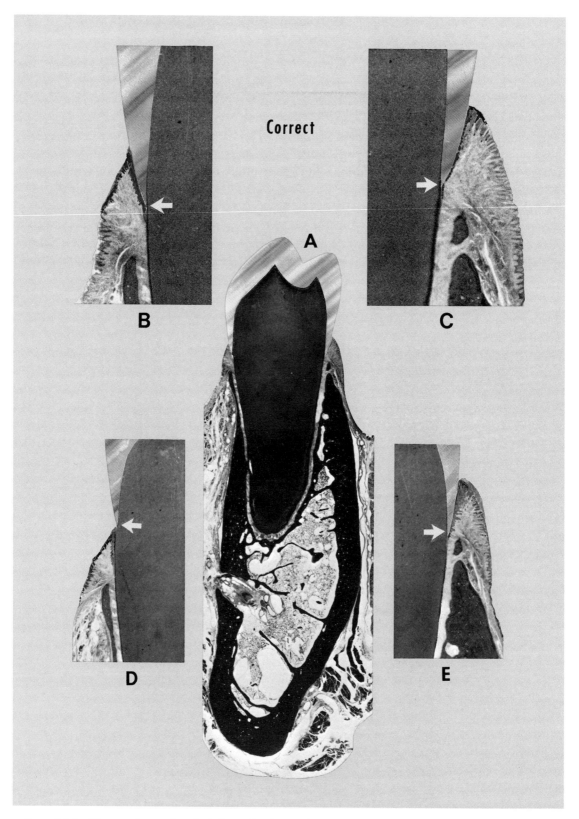

Figure 54–7   Where to Locate the Gingival Margin of Dental Restorations (a Composite Illustration). *A,* Faciolingual section through a crown on a mandibular premolar. *B* and *C,* Correct location of the margin of the restoration at the base of the gingival sulcus (*arrow*). *D,* Less desirable location at the tip of the gingival margin (*arrow*). *E,* Incorrect location—the restoration extends into the connective tissue beyond the base of the sulcus (*arrow*), forcing the epithelium to proliferate along the root and the gingival margin to bulge away from the tooth.

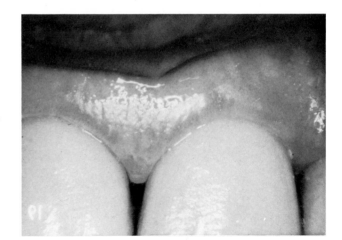

Figure 54–8 Marginal Gingiva Around Porcelain Crowns prepared to the base of the gingival sulcus. (Dr. Mario Martignoni, Rome, Italy.)

the margin of the cemented restoration appears by clinical standards, it is a broad rough area when viewed microscopically. Plaque-forming bacteria cling and grow there and cause gingivitis and caries of the narrow band of tooth structure apical to the margin of the restoration, which is a non-self-cleansing area. In some animal experiments, crown margins at the crest of the gingiva resulted in less gingivitis than restorations above or below it.[29]

Restorations should not be forced into the gingival connective tissue beyond the epithelial attachment (Fig. 54–7, *E*). Preparations beyond the base of the sulcus detach the epithelial attachment and the gingival fibers which cannot reattach when tooth structure is replaced by the crown. The epithelial attachment proliferates along the restoration and the gingiva bulges away from the tooth, leading to pocket formation.

"AVOID THE GINGIVAL THIRD." The full crown is extremely useful because it fulfills requirements that can be met by no other type of restoration (Fig. 54–9). However, even when ideally constructed in relation to the gingival sulcus, the full crown introduces the risk of gingival inflammation. Crowns substitute a foreign substance such as gold, acrylic or porcelain for the natural tooth wall of the gingival sulcus. The materials are not irritating, but they favor the accumulation of plaque which irritates the gingiva and, if not removed within 24 to 48 hours, may undergo calcification and develop into calculus. The junction of the crown and the tooth also presents a problem. Even with perfect

marginal fit, an extremely thin cement line, which attracts plaque,[50] in unavoidable.

The risk of irritation to the gingiva is reduced by restorations which terminate coronal to the gingival margin,[41] preferably **without encroaching upon the gingival third of the tooth**[47] (Fig. 54–10). Wherever possible, inlays,[40] pinledges and three-quarter crowns should be used as individual restorations and retainers for fixed prosthesis. This is not a matter of substituting

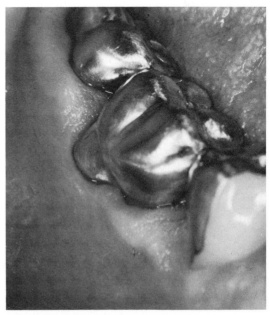

Figure 54–9 Tooth Contour Restored by Crown. Note the excellent condition of the gingiva in the bifurcation area.

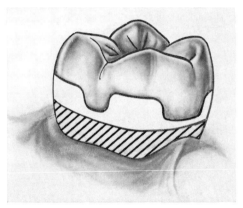

Figure 54–10 "Avoid the Gingival Third." Inlay constructed without involving the gingival third of the crown.

other restorations for purposes that can only be fulfilled by crowns. However, when there is a choice and high caries incidence is not a problem, the gingival third of the tooth should not be involved in the restoration.

Gingival retraction for taking impressions

When using elastic impression materials it is often necessary to retract the gingiva to gain access to the gingival margin of the preparation. Several methods of accomplishing this are described below. **These are methods for retracting healthy gingiva. They are not for the removal, displacement or shrinkage of inflamed, swollen gingival tissue. The gingiva must be healthy and its position on the tooth established before the impression is taken.**
METHODS OF RETRACTING THE GINGIVA. *Surgery.* Surgical resection of the gingiva is the preferred method for providing access to the margin of the preparation. Under local anesthesia the gingiva is excised **apical to the margin of the preparation** with periodontal knives or Bard-Parker blade, #11 or #12 (Fig. 54–11). Bleeding is controlled with a cotton pellet under pressure, moistened with epinephrine if necessary. **The gingiva will regenerate and be restored to its normal position, provided it was healthy when the preparation was started.** If the gingiva is diseased when the tooth is prepared, resection of the gingiva or inadvertent removal of plaque and calculus during tooth preparation would affect

shrinkage in the pocket wall and exposure of tooth surface beyond the margin of the preparation (Fig. 54–12). The recession is sometimes erroneously attributed to the surgery.
Electrosurgery. The gingiva may also be retracted by electrosurgery without the problem of bleeding. However, if it is used close to bone, it may cause painful injury and irreparable destruction of supporting tissues (see Chap. 37 for a discussion of Electrosurgery).
Mechanical. With the *mechanical method*[23] of gingival retraction an aluminum shell is trimmed so that it rests on the occlusal surface of the prepared tooth without touching the gingival margin, but is shaped to conform with it. The shell is filled with softened temporary stopping and replaced on the tooth so that the stopping is extruded and displaces the gingiva. The shell is then removed and the margin of the temporary stopping is trimmed so that when the shell is replaced the gingival tissue is retracted without blanching.
Retraction Strings. Strings impregnated with chemicals are used for gingival retraction. Among the types of chemicals for this purpose are[13] **vasocontrictors** (8 per cent recemic epinephrine). These cause rapid transient elevation in blood pressure and blood sugar and are contraindicated in patients with coronary disease, hyperthyroidism or diabetes. They also produce local ischemia which may be injurious to the gingiva. Also used are **corrosives** (zinc chloride 8 per cent, tannic acid 20 per cent and trichloracetic acid 10 per cent); and **astringents** (aluminum sulfate 14 per cent).
Impregnated strings will cause the gingiva to wilt away from the tooth and expose the margin of the preparation. The gingiva will ordinarily return to its proper position, provided it was healthy at the outset and the string is not permitted to keep the gingiva separated long enough to permit disease-producing plaque and food debris to accumulate in the sulcus. Impregnated strings should not be used on diseased gingiva; pocket walls temporarily retracted from the root will return and jeopardize the tooth and restoration (Fig. 54–13). Because the effects of the chemicals cannot be controlled, pressure retraction of the gingiva with chemical-free strings or other methods of retraction are preferred.

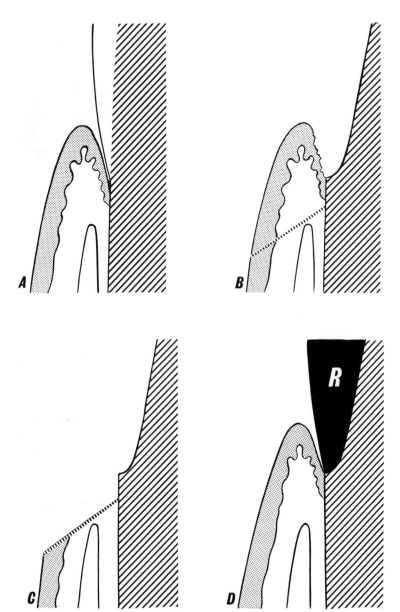

Figure 54–11 Marginal Gingiva Removed to Provide Access for Taking Impressions. *A,* Normal dentogingival relationship before preparing tooth. *B,* Champfer-type tooth preparation. The gingival margin is slightly lacerated during preparation. Gingiva incised at dotted line. *C,* Gingival margin removed using periodontal knife or electrosurgery. *D,* Restoration (*R*) in position at the base of the healed gingival sulcus.

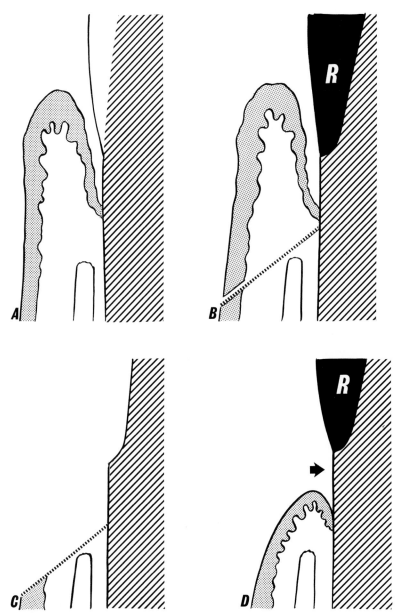

Figure 54–12 Recession Following the Restoration of Teeth with Untreated Periodontal Disease. *A,* Periodontal pocket present before tooth preparation. *B,* Restoration (*R*) erroneously inserted in tooth with untreated periodontal pocket. The dotted line shows incision required for elimination of pocket. *C,* Diseased gingiva removed. *D,* Gingiva heals revealing the root surface (*arrow*) which had been denuded by periodontal disease before restoration was inserted.

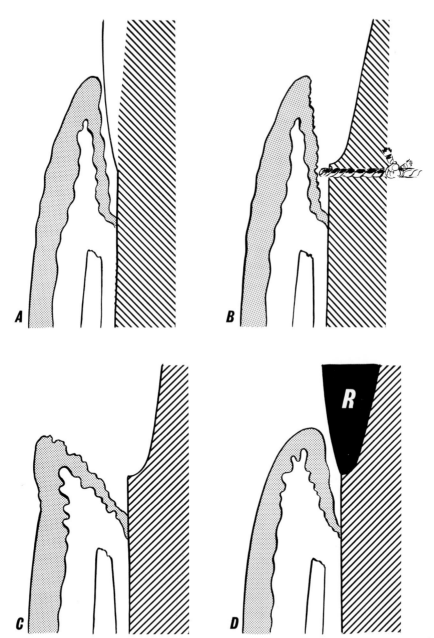

Figure 54–13   Periodontal Pocket Persists After Retraction. *A,* Periodontal pocket present before tooth is prepared. *B,* Tooth prepared, retraction string placed to retract diseased gingiva. *C,* Diseased gingiva temporarily retracted to provide access to tooth for impression. *D,* Restoration (*R*) inserted, the periodontal pocket has returned.

When impressions are taken with copper bands the gingiva may be temporarily detached from the root without permanent injury. This detachment is followed by healing and restoration of the gingival margin,[48] provided no particles of impression material remain in the sulcus.

Even with extreme care the gingiva is often lacerated in the course of tooth preparation. If the gingiva is healthy before the restoration is started, it will regenerate and return to its previous position on the tooth,[17, 18] provided the area to which it was attached is not cut away and included in the preparation.

Temporary coverage

The interim of temporary coverage between the time of the impression and cementation of the completed restoration is a critical one. Proper occlusal relationships, proximal contour and contact and smooth margins are essential. The entire preparation should be covered so that there is no exposed space at the gingival margin. Granulation tissue and exudate from the gingiva tend to fill such spaces and create problems unless removed prior to cementation of the restoration.[51] The granulation tissue may interfere with proper seating of the restoration and cause a marginal defect and ultimate loss of the restoration (Fig. 54–14). Finishing temporary restorations 1 mm. short of the gingiva and covering the area with periodontal pack may help prevent gingival problems.[20]

Overextended temporary crowns create problems. Detachment of the gingival fibers for a short period is unlikely to produce permanent damage, but after one month such crowns introduce the risk of permanent gingival recession.[16] The best gingival response is obtained if temporary coverage is given the same careful attention as the completed restoration.

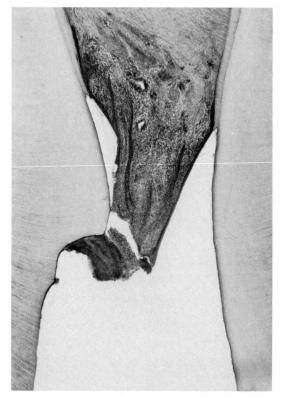

Figure 54–14 Calculus in Space Under Improperly Seated Restoration. Tooth in experimental animal showing calculus formed in space created when granulation tissue prevented proper seating of crown. The gingival margin of the preparation is shown here; the restoration has been removed. There is suppurative inflammation of the gingiva adjacent to the calculus.

The embrasures

When teeth are in proximal contact, *the spaces that widen out from the contact are known as embrasures.* The interdental space is divisible into a facial and lingual embrasure (Fig. 54–15), an occlusal or incisal embrasure that is coronal to the contact area (Fig. 54–16, A), and a gingival embrasure, which is the space between the contact area and the alveolar bone.[4, 55] The gingival embrasure is filled with soft tissue,

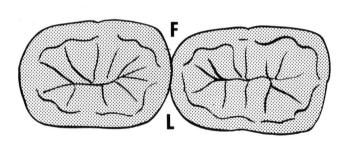

Figure 54–15 Occlusal View of Mandibular Molars Showing Facial (F) and Lingual (L) Embrasures.

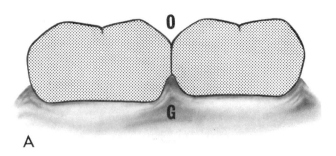

Figure 54–16   Occlusal (O) and Gingival (G) Embrasures. A, Interdental gingiva fills gingival embrasure (G). B, Open gingival embrasure (G) in patient with periodontal disease.

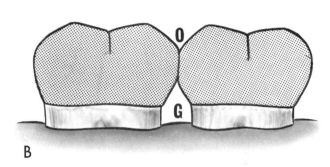

but with age and in periodontal disease (Fig. 54–16, B) spaces are created in the gingival embrasure. Embrasures protect the gingiva from food impaction and deflect food so as to massage the gingival surface. They provide spillways for food during mastication and relieve occlusal forces when chewing resistant foods.

THE GINGIVAL EMBRASURE.   Embrasures are critical considerations in restorative dentistry. Proximal surfaces of dental restorations are important because they create the embrasures essential for gingival health (Fig. 54–17). From the periodontal viewpoint, the gingival embrasure is the most significant. Periodontal disease causes tissue destruction which reduces the level of the alveolar bone, increases the size of the gingival embrasure and creates open interdental spaces. Restorations may be constructed so as to preserve the morphology of the crown and root and retain the enlarged embrasure and the open interdental space (Fig. 54–18, A and B); or the teeth may be reshaped by the restorations so as to *relocate the gingival embrasure* close to the new level of the gingiva. This is accomplished by changing the contour of the proximal surfaces and locating the contact areas further apically (Fig. 54–18, C). The interdental gingiva will assume its normal shape by filling the new embrasure

provided for it, which must be adequate in all dimensions.

The following dimensions of the gingival embrasure are important to the preservation of gingival health:

A. *Height.* The distance between the contact area and the bone margin (Fig. 54–19, A). When the contact area is too close to the cervical line of the tooth, the embrasure is shortened.

B. *Width.* The distance mesiodistally between the proximal surfaces (Fig. 54–19, B).

C. *Depth.* The distance faciolingually from the contact area to a line joining the proximofacial or proximolingual angles (Fig. 54–19, C).

The proximal surfaces of crowns should taper away from the contact area—facially, lingually and apically. Excessively broad proximal contact areas and inadequate contour in the cervical region crowd out the facial and lingual gingival papillae. The prominent papillae entrap food debris, which leads to gingival inflammation and pocket formation (Fig. 54–20).

Proximal contacts that are too narrow faciolingually create enlarged facial and lingual embrasures that do not provide sufficient protection against interdental food impaction.

The facial and lingual contours of res-

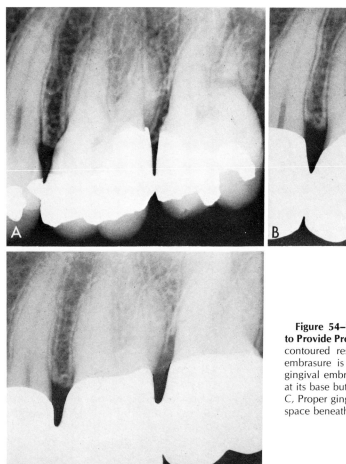

Figure 54–17 Contour of Restoration Corrected to Provide Proper Gingival Embrasures. *A,* Improperly contoured restorations on the molars; the gingival embrasure is too narrow. *B,* New restorations, the gingival embrasure between the molars is now wider at its base but is too narrow beneath the contact area. *C,* Proper gingival embrasure created by widening the space beneath the molar contact area.

torations are also important in the preservation of gingival health. Undercontoured facial and lingual surfaces may disturb normal food deflection and cause food impaction and accumulation in the gingival sulcus (Fig. 54–21). Overcontouring the facial surfaces creates a ledge which deflects food beyond the gingival margin onto the attached gingiva (Fig. 54–21). This deprives the gingival margin of the mechan-

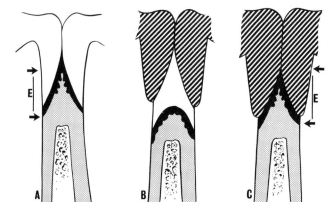

Figure 54–18 Relocation of the Gingival Embrasure. *A,* Normal gingival embrasure (E) filled with gingival tissue. *B,* Space created in gingival embrasure by periodontal disease and restorations constructed to retain the space. *C,* Restorations constructed so as to relocate the gingival embrasure (E) close to the gingiva by recontouring the proximal surfaces and locating the contact area further apically.

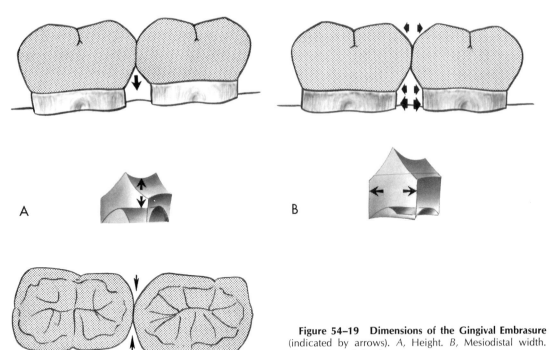

A

B

C

Figure 54–19 Dimensions of the Gingival Embrasure (indicated by arrows). *A*, Height. *B*, Mesiodistal width. *C*, Faciolingual depth.

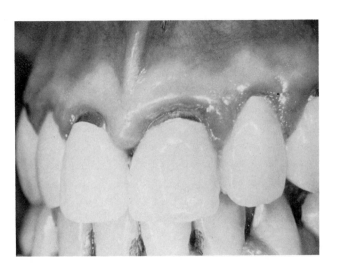

Figure 54–20 Inadequate Gingival Embrasures Lead to Gingival Disease.

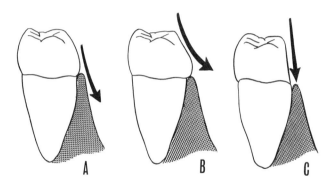

Figure 54–21 Improperly Contoured Restorations Result in Gingival Disease on the Facial Surface. *A,* Normal gingivodental relationship. *B,* Overcontour creates undesirable ledge which deflects food away from the gingival margin. *C,* Undercontour results in food impaction.

ical cleansing action of the food, which may stagnate in the overprotected gingival sulcus. Overcontouring of the facial surface may also interfere with mechanical cleansing action of the cheek against the tooth surface.[30]

The occlusal surface

Occlusal surfaces should be designed so as to direct forces in the long axis of the teeth. They should restore occlusal dimensions and cuspal contours in harmony with the remainder of the natural dentition—after occlusal abnormalities have been eliminated by occlusal adjustment. **The occlusal surfaces of the teeth should not be arbitrarily narrowed.** Proper occlusal relationships are more important than the width of the occlusal table in the attainment of physiologic occlusal forces. The anatomy of the occlusal surface should provide well-formed marginal ridges and occlusal sluiceways to prevent interproximal food impaction.

Restoration materials and surface finish

The surface of restorations should be as smooth as possible, because roughness results in plaque accumulation,[25, 50] followed by calculus formation. Less plaque forms on porcelain than on polished or unpolished gold.[24] Self-curing acrylic accumulates plaque and should not be used near the gingiva.[53]

Pontics

A pontic should meet the following requirements: it should (a) be esthetically acceptable; (b) provide occlusal relationships that are favorable to the abutment teeth and opposing teeth and the remainder of the dentition; (c) restore the masticatory ef-

fectiveness of the tooth it replaces; (d) be designed to minimize accumulation of irritating dental plaque and food debris, and to permit maximum access for cleansing by the patient; and (e) provide embrasures for passage of food.

Plaque which causes inflammation of the mucosa under pontics and the gingiva around abutment teeth tends to accumulate around fixed prostheses because it requires a special effort to keep them clean. **The health of the tissues around fixed prostheses depends primarily upon the patient's oral hygiene; the materials of which pontics are constructed appear to make little difference, and pontic design is important only to the extent that it enables the patient to keep the area clean.** Plaque accumulates to an equal degree upon pontics made of glazed and unglazed porcelain,[15] polished gold and polished acrylic resin,[36, 46] despite the finding that the surfaces of the latter two are smoother.[5]

The bullet-shaped spheroidal pontic is the most hygienic (Fig. 54–22) (next to the sanitary type, Fig. 54–28). The proximal sur-

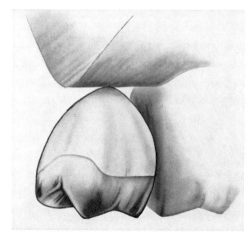

Figure 54–22 Bullet-Shaped Spheroidal Type Pontic.

faces are tapered to create spaces between adjoining pontics for self-cleansing passage of food, stimulation of the edentulous mucosa by food excursion, and for cleansing with toothbrush and dental floss. It should also re-create spaces adjacent to the abutment teeth that approach the shape and dimension of the natural embrasure to protect the marginal gingiva (Fig. 54–23). A pontic no larger than a premolar may be cantilevered off the end of a multiunit bridge to prevent extrusion of opposing teeth. Proper contour of such terminal pontics is especially important (Fig. 54–23, E) because the absence of protection from a proximal tooth increases the risk of food accumulation under the pontic.

Anteriorly, where esthetics is a greater consideration, a modified ridge-lap design is used (Fig. 54–24). The pontic follows the facial contour of the ridge to the crest where it joins the lingual surface. The lingual surface of the pontic should follow the normal tooth form for a distance of approximately half of its occlusogingival length, then taper in a convex line to meet the facial portion at the crest of the ridge.[56]

The natural teeth should guide the design of the occlusal surface of pontics. The width of the occlusal surface should not be narrowed beyond that of the tooth being replaced. The assumption that reduced occlusal width provides occlusal forces more favorable to the periodontium of the abutment teeth has not been proved.

Narrowing the proximal contact areas of posterior teeth causes recession and inflammation of the interdental gingiva. Restoring the width of the contact area leads to resolution of the inflammation and

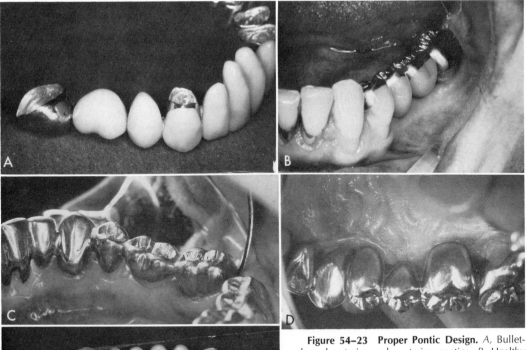

Figure 54–23 Proper Pontic Design. A, Bullet-shaped anterior and posterior pontics. B, Healthy gingiva and edentulous mucosa with bullet-shaped pontics. C, Lingual view showing spaces required between the pontics and the natural teeth. Note anatomical reconstruction of the occlusal surface of the pontics. D, Healthy gingiva and mucosa in relation to bullet-shaped second premolar pontic. Note the inflammation between the first premolar and canine caused by inadequate gingival embrasure. E, Pontics with properly constructed modified ridge-lap design. Note the cantilevered pontic (arrow).

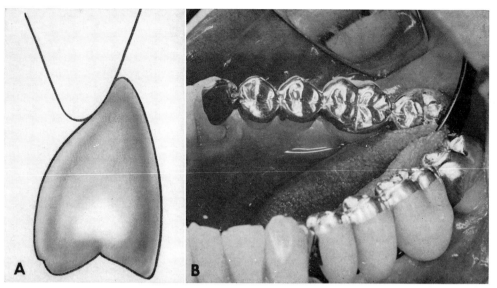

Figure 54–24 Modified Ridge-lap Pontic for Esthetics. *A,* Bullet-shaped pontic extended onto the facial aspects of the edentulous ridge. *B,* Modified ridge-lap type of pontic replacing the first molar. The premolars are bullet-shaped. Note the excellent condition of the mucosa made possible by adequate spaces for food passage.

keratinization of the interdental gingiva. Abnormally shaped spaces between narrowed pontics and broad proximal surfaces of adjacent natural teeth create food impaction problems (Fig. 54–25). Occlusal width is also necessary to shunt the food laterally so that it is not forced into the tissue around the base of the pontic; the gingiva of abutment teeth is especially vulnerable to inflammation and pocket formation.[10]

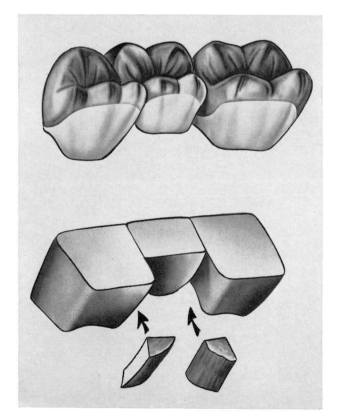

Figure 54–25 *Above,* Pontic with narrow occlusal width creates food impaction problems. *Below,* Occlusal width required to provide proper proximal relations between pontic and adjacent teeth.

The functional relationships of the cusps are the most critical consideration in the design of the occlusal surface of pontics. The cusps should be in harmony with the functional pattern of the entire dentition. Abnormal occlusal relationships jeopardize the opposing teeth and the remainder of the dentition as well as the periodontium of the abutment teeth.

The tip of the pontic should just barely contact the edentulous mucosa (Fig. 54–22). The casts should not be scraped or scored in an attempt to seat the pontic into the mucosa. This creates a pseudo-sulcus around the pontic where food debris accumulates. Inflammation and swelling of the mucosa and further food retention are sometimes followed by abscess formation, which jeopardizes the bridge. Small spaces between the base of the pontic and the edentulous mucosa also tend to trap irritating food debris. Saddle-type pontics, which straddle the ridge, retain macerated food debris beneath their base, leading to inflammation of the periodontium of the adjacent natural teeth and the edentulous mucosa (Figs. 54–26 and 54–27).

The "sanitary-type" fixed bridge, which consists of a cast occlusal surface connecting the abutment teeth (Fig. 54–28), reduces the risk of periodontal problems. Esthetics permitting, this is the bridge of choice from the periodontal viewpoint. Food passes under the occlusal connection

and cleanses the surface of the mucosa and gingiva. The undersurface of the connector should be rounded faciolingually.

Cementation

Retained cement particles irritate the gingiva and should be removed. Removal of cement from interproximal joints of pontics and abutments can be facilitated by coating the exterior surfaces of the prosthesis with mineral oil prior to cementation.

Occasionally it may be necessary to delay permanent cementation until functional and phonetic evaluations can be made. This is especially true with large multiple units, which involve full coverage. The period of temporary cementation should not exceed 30 days. Long term "temporary" cementation and repeated removal and recementation are discouraged.

The dentition should be evaluated periodontally, and the teeth to be included in the prosthesis should be determined before the prosthesis is designed. Permanent cementation should not be postponed indefinitely for the ostensible purpose of "testing" questionable teeth.

Failure to finalize cementation of prosthesis is contraindicated for several reasons:

1. It interferes with adaptation of the gingiva to the margin of the restorations.

2. Seepage under temporarily cemented restorations may lead to caries and pulp

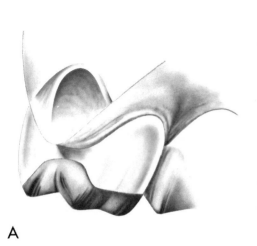

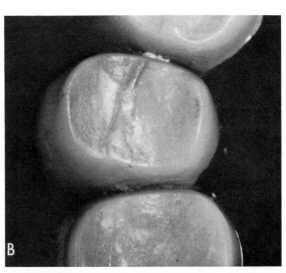

Figure 54–26 Saddle-Type Pontics. *A,* Diagrammatic view of saddle-type pontic in position. *B,* Under surface of saddle-type pontic. Note the irregularities which conform to surface of the underlying mucosa and trap food debris.

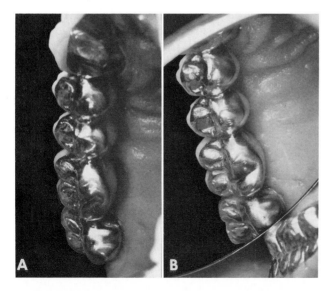

Figure 54–27 Replacement of Saddle-Type Pontics by Bullet-Shaped Pontics Leads to Resolution of Mucosal Inflammation. *A,* Bullet-shaped pontics inserted in area previously covered by saddle-type pontics. Note the inflammation where the saddle-type pontics had been. *B,* After several months note the excellent condition of the mucosa under the bullet-shaped pontics.

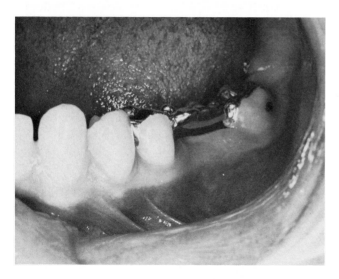

Figure 54–28 Sanitary-Type Fixed Bridge with Healthy Gingiva and Edentulous Mucosa.

involvement that escape detection, particularly if patients do not adhere to the schedule of periodic removal and recementation.

3. It encourages diagnostic indecision.

4. It is an unnecessary burden to the patient who is never finished with treatment, while the dentist is repeatedly confronted with a problem case.

5. The technical excellence required for a permanent restoration is often unwittingly compromised by the thought that required corrections can be made "the next time."

Removable partial denture prosthesis

From the periodontal viewpoint, fixed prosthesis is the restoration of choice, but removable partial prosthesis is also extremely effective. Its usefulness in the total treatment of periodontal problems should not be minimized.[11] The periodontal implications of removable partial prosthesis must be understood so that it will benefit the periodontium and not cause periodontal destruction and tooth mobility.[7, 27, 32, 38]

DESIGN. To provide maximum stability for removable partial prosthesis, every effort should be made to retain posterior teeth for the distal support of the saddle areas.

Finger-like projections between the teeth (Fig. 54–29) irritate the interdental and marginal gingiva and lead to food impaction, periodontal pockets[38] and gingival enlargement. These problems can be avoided by using a wide major connector on the palate

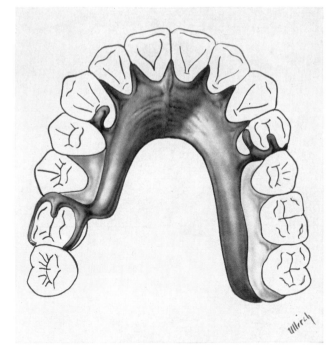

Figure 54–29 Incorrect Design—Interdental Projections on Partial Prosthesis are Periodontally Undesirable.

(Fig. 54–30) rather than a horseshoe-type design which encroaches upon the gingiva.

The margins of facial and lingual flanges adjacent to abutment teeth should be thinned and rounded with a wide taper from the crest of the ridge (Fig. 54–31). The design provides for self-cleansing action of unobstructed food passage. Blunt borders close to the abutment teeth form narrow troughs which trap irritating food debris.

Insufficient saddle coverage is responsible for torsional and lateral stresses[8] upon abutment teeth, which lead to periodontal destruction and premature tooth loss. With lingual bars without distal support, this is a particular problem. To provide maximum

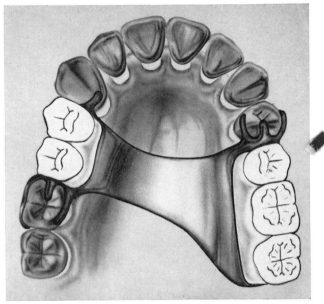

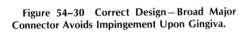

Figure 54–30 Correct Design—Broad Major Connector Avoids Impingement Upon Gingiva.

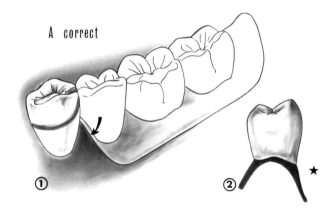

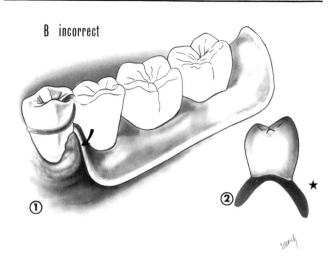

Figure 54–31 Junction of Partial Prosthesis and Abutment Teeth. *A,* Correct. (*1*) The margin of the saddle area is thinned and flared distally (*arrow*) to permit unobstructed food passage over the gingival margin. (*2*) Cross section of saddle area showing properly thinned margin of the facial flange (*asterisk*). *B,* Incorrect. (*1*) Thick margin of partial denture adjacent to abutment tooth forms trough (*arrow*) which traps debris and causes gingival inflammation and periodontal pocket. (*2*) Cross section of saddle area showing thick blunt margin of facial flange (*asterisk*).

stability, saddles should be extended on the facial and lingual surfaces as far as the patients' tissues permit.

Tissue-borne areas of removable partial dentures should not be relied upon to restore vertical dimension, particularly saddle areas without distal support. Such attempts are followed by rapid bone resorption under the saddles, settling of the dentures, distal tilting of the abutment teeth, food impaction, periodontal pocket formation, tooth mobility and a return to the pre-existent reduced vertical dimension. To prevent such sequelae the vertical dimension should be established in the natural dentition before the partial denture is constructed.

CLASPS. Clasps should be designed so that they are passive; that is, exert no pressure or tension upon the abutment teeth when the denture is at rest.[45] Torque and tension on clasped teeth can be kept to a minimum by using a wrought wire on the facial surface, by increasing the length of the clasp arms and by reducing the cross section.

Stress breakers, which connect the retainer and saddle areas by flexible and movable joints, are sometimes used to prevent excessive occlusal forces on abutment teeth. However, comparisons have revealed no advantage of stress breakers over rigid connectors in this respect.[2] With rigid connectors between clasps and saddle areas, the resilience of the mucosa acts as a stress breaker. It permits controlled movement of the prosthesis so that the tissue-borne sections take the initial occlusal stress and prevent sudden impact on the periodontium of the natural teeth.

OCCLUSAL RESTS. Occlusal rests should be designed *to direct the forces along the vertical axis of the tooth.* To accomplish this, the rest is seated in a spoon-shaped preparation in the abutment tooth with the floor inclined so that the deepest point is toward the vertical axis of the tooth (Fig. 54–32).[22] This purpose is also accomplished by extending occlusal rests beyond the central zone of the occlusal surface of premolars or covering the occlusal surface overlying one of the roots of the molars.[35]

Lug rests on inclined lingual surfaces of anterior teeth tend to be spread by occlusal forces so that settling of the denture results. This is followed by impingement of the facial and lingual arms of the clasp upon the gingiva, and digging of the connecting bar into the lingual mucosa with pocket formation and denudation of the roots (Fig. 54–33).

Spreading of lug rests on anterior teeth can be prevented by constructing a restoration on the abutment teeth with a horizontal ledge on the lingual surface into which the clasp fits (Fig. 54–34). The floor of the ledge should be sloped so as to direct the forces axially. An incisal stop will also prevent settling of clasps (Fig. 54–35). The notch is cut for a slight distance into the tooth substance, at a point approximately one third from the distoincisal angle. The incisal rest fits into the notch and is tapered to terminate in a point on the facial surface.

Removable partial prosthesis should always be constructed with occlusal rests. They are sometimes omitted for the ostensible purpose of reducing axial load on teeth with weakened periodontal support. Such dentures jeopardize the teeth because they settle and cause gingival and periodontal disturbances.

PRECISION ATTACHMENTS. Precision attachments are used for esthetic reasons and to direct occlusal forces axially rather than laterally. There are many types of precision attachments, and advantages have been demonstrated for some.[21] They cause greater stress and displacement on the abutment teeth of free-end saddle prostheses than is produced by conventional back-action clasps.[39] More evidence is required to establish the relative merits of precision attachments and clasps in terms of their effects upon the periodontium.

Multiple abutments

Multiple abutments reduce injurious lateral and tortional stresses on abutment teeth and should be standard procedure in patients with reduced periodontal support. Multiple abutments are made by connecting inlays or crowns or clasping abutment and adjacent teeth in sequence. **When the terminal tooth is periodontally weak, more than one adjacent tooth should be used for added support. Joining a weakened tooth to a strong one is just as likely to weaken the strong tooth as it is to strengthen the weakened one (Fig. 54–36). It is always advisable to consider whether the long-term interest of the patient would be better served by extracting the prospective weak abutment tooth and making a multiple abutment of two adjacent, relatively well-**

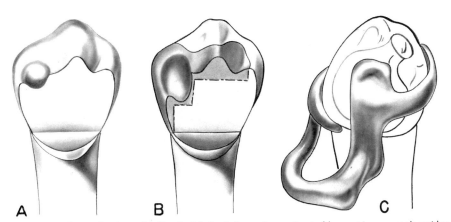

Figure 54–32 Occlusal Rests in Line With Vertical Axis. *A,* Properly constructed lug rest in a premolar without a restoration. *B,* Properly constructed lug rest in a restoration in a premolar. *C,* Clasp in position on a premolar with a lug rest in a restoration. (After Dr. Irving R. Hardy, Boston.)

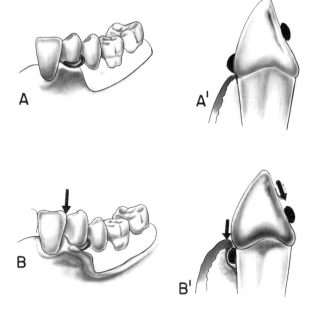

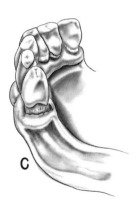

Figure 54–33   "Settling" of a Lingual Bar With an Inadequate Lug Rest on the Canine. *A,* Lingual bar in position. *A',* Labiolingual view showing cross section of labial and lingual arms of the clasp. *B,* Lingual bar settles in direction indicated by the arrow. *B',* The labial arm digs into the gingiva, the lingual arm slides down along the inclined plane of the lingual surface. *C,* View of the distal surface of the canine showing recession of the gingiva and marginal gingival disease resulting from settling of the partial denture.

Figure 54–34   A Method of Preventing "Settling" of a Clasp on the Mandibular Canine. *A,* A restoration is made for the canine including a ledge on the lingual surface. *B,* The lingual arm of the clasp fits into the ledge on the lingual surface.

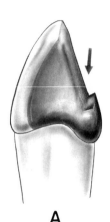

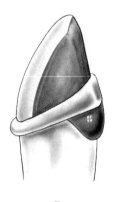

A   B

supported teeth. In patients who have had generalized periodontal involvement, all teeth should be joined together by the partial denture, either by clasping or inclusion in continuous clasps.

Combined fixed and removable partial prosthesis

Isolated teeth with reduced periodontal support are particularly vulnerable to periodontal injury and loosening when used as abutments in removable partial prosthesis. They lack mesial and distal buttressing action to assist in withstanding forces transmitted by the denture. In such cases, fixed and removable prosthesis should be combined. The isolated teeth should be joined to their nearest neighbors by a fixed bridge (Fig. 54–37) and can then be used as abutments for removable prosthesis.

Periodontal injury from operative procedures

Forceful wedging of teeth to facilitate restoration of proximal contour and overzealous malleting of restorations are potential sources of trauma to the peri-

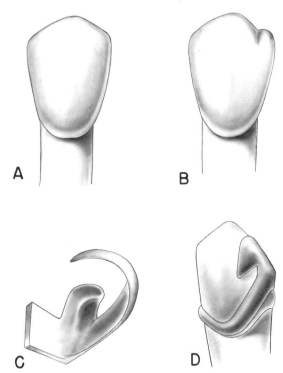

Figure 54–35 Incisal Stop on Anterior Tooth. *A,* Mandibular canine. *B,* A notch is cut in the incisal edge. *C,* View of clasp with incisal rest. *D,* Clasp in position on the tooth. (After Dr. Irvin R. Hardy, Boston.)

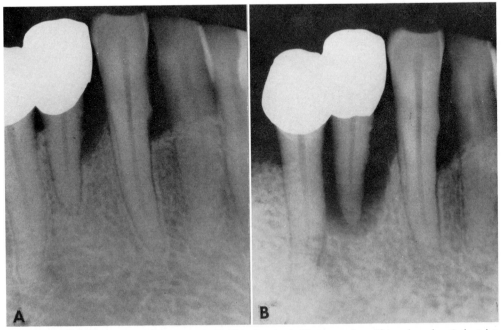

Figure 54–36 Weakened Tooth Splinted to Single Firm Tooth. *A,* First premolar with weakened periodontal support splinted to firm second premolar. *B,* After three years the periodontal condition is worse, the second premolar is also denuded of bone, and both premolars are mobile.

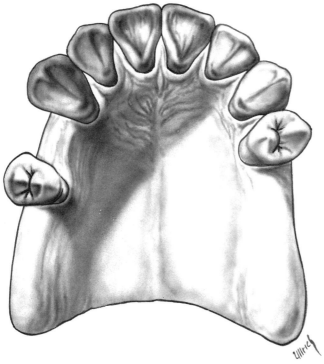

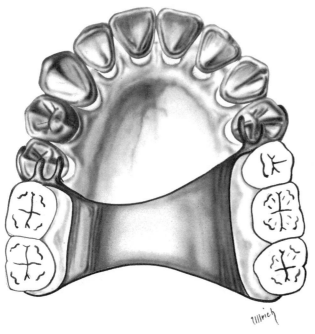

Figure 54–37 Combined Fixed and Removable Partial Prosthesis. *Above,* prosthesis required for mouth with isolated second premolar. *Below,* isolated second premolar included in fixed prosthesis before the palatal bar is constructed. The first premolar is replaced by a pontic.

odontium. Failure to "tailor" matrix bands and abusive use of the rubber dam may cause painful laceration of the gingiva, which may become infected. Retained fragments of rubber dam may cause a periodontal abscess. Abrupt removal of cotton rolls may denude the mucosa of surface epithelium and lead to herpetic viral infection with vesicle formation in such areas. Escharotic drugs sometimes used in cavity sterilization may seep onto the gingiva and produce a chemical burn.

PERIODONTAL SPLINTS

A splint is an appliance for the immobilization or stabilization of injured or diseased parts. They are useful adjuncts in periodontal therapy and serve the following purposes:

1. Protect loose teeth from periodontal injury by stabilizing them in a favorable occlusal relationship.

2. Distribute occlusal forces so that teeth weakened by loss of periodontal support do not become loose.

3. Retain teeth in positions to which they have been moved by orthodontic procedures.

4. Prevent pathologic migration.

DISTRIBUTION OF OCCLUSAL FORCES IN SPLINTS. Splints are primarily functional catalysts and not simply devices for holding loose teeth tightly. By stabilizing weakened teeth, they maintain satisfactory relationships between occlusal forces and the periodontium.

Loose teeth tilt into positions in which occlusal relationships are altered and axial forces are converted into potentially injurious lateral forces. Splinting prevents such movement and reduces the likelihood of injurious occlusal forces.

Occlusal forces applied to a splint are shared by all the teeth within it, even if the force is applied to only one section of the splint. Because of this, teeth weakened by periodontal disease may benefit from support provided by teeth with an intact periodontium. On the other hand, including a weakened tooth in a splint does not completely relieve it of the burden of occlusal forces, nor does it immunize it against injury from excessive occlusal forces. If only one tooth in a splint is in a traumatic occlusal relationship, the periodontal tissues of the remaining teeth may also be injured[12] (Fig. 54–38).

GUIDELINES FOR CONSTRUCTING PERIODONTAL SPLINTS. **The occlusion of the entire dentition should be adjusted before the splint is prepared, and the splint must be in harmony with the corrected occlusion.** A rigid splint in occlusal disharmony accelerates the destruction of the periodontium of all the splinted teeth, not simply the tooth that is being traumatized.

Include a sufficient number of firm teeth in the splint. The functioning surface of the firm teeth should be at least one and a half to two times that of the mobile teeth. If the functioning surface of the weak teeth is the same as or greater than that of the firm teeth, the firm teeth will become loose.

Splint around the arch. Avoid straight line splints confined to a segment of the arch. For example, in splinting the anterior teeth include a tooth distal to each canine. This prevents faciolingual and anterior-posterior tipping movements and prevents excessive lateral forces[54] (Fig. 54–39). When splinting the posterior segment, extend the splint anteriorly beyond the canine as a precautionary measure against faciolingual movement of the splint (Fig. 54–40).

The splint should not irritate the gingiva, cheeks, lips or tongue. It should not trap food and should provide adequate embrasures and also protect the gingiva from food impaction.

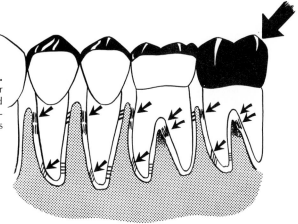

Figure 54–38 Transmission of Forces in a Splint. Excessive occlusal force applied only to the second molar (*large arrow*) injures the periodontium of all the splinted teeth, and in comparable locations. The small arrows indicate the areas of injury. The location of injury depends upon the direction of the occlusal force.

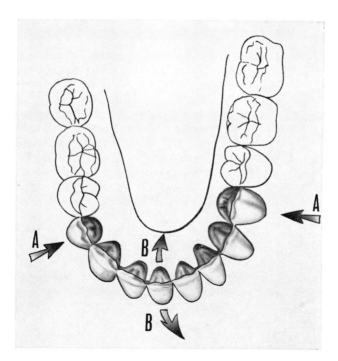

Figure 54–39 Premolars Included in Anterior Splint (*arrows A*) to Minimize Labiolingual Tipping Action (*arrows B*).

Figure 54–40 Splint Extended Beyond Canine to Minimize Faciolingual Movement. *A,* Splint from canine to molars susceptible to faciolingual movement (*arrows*). *B,* Lateral incisor (*asterisk*) included in splint.

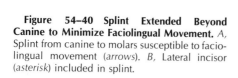

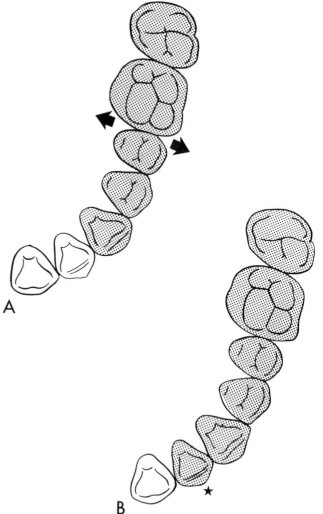

Impress the patient with the importance of keeping the splint meticulously clean. Dental plaque and food debris cause inflammation, which jeopardizes the periodontal tissues and defeats the purpose of the splint.

Splints are valuable adjuncts in periodontal therapy, provided they are used intelligently. They are no better than the judgment which selects the teeth for which they are employed.[31] Splints are not devices for retaining teeth the patient would be better off without. It is well to bear in mind that **the period of usefulness of the most carefully constructed splint is measured by the lifespan of the poorest tooth contained within it.**

CLASSIFICATION OF SPLINTS. Periodontal splints may be temporary (provisional) or permanent. Temporary splints are employed for a limited period of time to aid healing by limiting the mobility of the healing tissues, and to assist in determining the prognosis of questionable teeth. Permanent splints serve as constant adjuncts to the maintenance of periodontal health. Splints may be *fixed* or *removable* and are classified according to type of construction as *external splints*, which engage the external surfaces of the teeth, or *internal splints*, which replace part of the tooth structure.

Temporary (Provisional) Splints

Treatment splints are employed to assist healing of mobile teeth following scaling and curettage or surgical periodontal treatment procedures. The teeth may be splinted previous to or along with the other treatment. Excessive tooth mobility causes movement of periodontal tissues and disrupts and retards healing. The tissues ultimately heal, but the periodontal ligament is abnormally wide and the teeth remain mobile. The temporary splint aids healing by stabilizing the teeth. It should remain in position for periods of up to two months. If there is marked improvement when the splint is removed, the teeth are retained and usually splinted permanently to prevent recurrence of mobility.

Temporary splints are also used to assist in determining whether teeth with a borderline prognosis should be retained or extracted. The temporary splint aids in reaching decisions, but it should not become an excuse for indecision. There are instances in which the operator desires to know more about the behavior of a questionable tooth before embarking on an extensive restorative program. Two months under a temporary splint will provide the answer whether such teeth should be retained or extracted. If stability is not restored within two months, no further improvement is obtained from continued temporary splinting.

Making a practice of indecision by prolonged temporary splinting is contrary to the basic principle that treatment should not be undertaken until the diagnosis and prognosis of every tooth and the treatment plan have been established. It bears emphasis that the clinical concept of periodontal therapy is predicated upon the welfare of the dentition as a whole. Prolonged provisional treatment of isolated teeth postpones definitive treatment of the entire mouth. In an effort to favor the questionable teeth, the patient may develop abnormal functional patterns injurious to the remainder of the dentition.

The following are among the types of appliances used for temporary splinting.[1, 9, 42, 49]

Metal Wire Ligature. This is the most common form of temporary splint and its use is essentially limited to anterior teeth (Fig. 54–41). It is constructed as follows: A 0.002 stainless steel wire is doubled and formed into a horizontal loop enclosing the teeth from canine to canine. If first premolars are present, they should be included in the splint for added stability. The ends of the loop are twisted just enough to hold it in position incisal to the cingula (Fig. 54–41, A). Interproximal loops are positioned which engage the facial and lingual sections of the horizontal loop. The horizontal loop is tightened and then the interproximal loops are tightened in sequence. After all the loops are tight, the ends are bent in and tucked interproximally to prevent irritation to the gingiva or the tongue and cheek (Fig. 54–41, E). Acrylic is then brushed onto the wire to further limit tooth movement and prevent slipping of the wire, minimize food accumulation and protect the lips and tongue from irritation.

Gaps between the teeth are bridged by twisting the horizontal loop. The horizontal wire can be secured against slipping

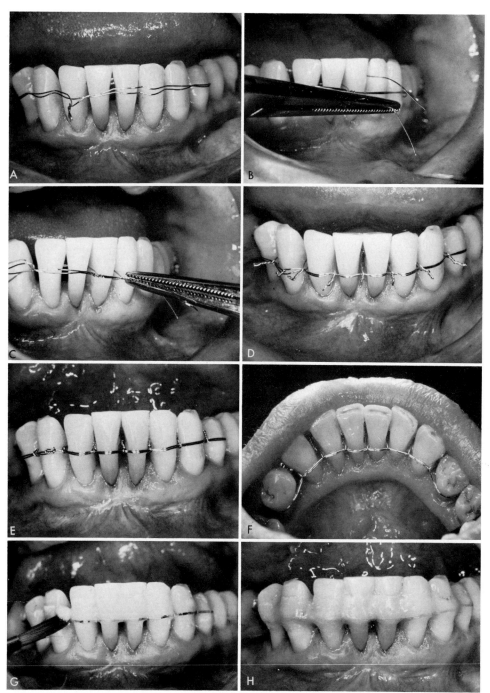

Figure 54–41   Construction of Temporary Wire Ligature Splint. *A,* Horizontal loop loosely aligned in position incisal to the cingula. *B,* Interdental loops are inserted. *C,* Interdental loops tightened. *D,* All the interdental loops and the horizontal loops are tightened. *E,* Splint in position with interdental loops bent inward to avoid tissue irritation.

F, Lingual view showing position of splint in relation to cingula. *G,* Acrylic is brushed onto the wire to stabilize splint, to minimize food accumulation and protect the tissues from irritation. *H,* Acrylic polished. **Notice that the acrylic tapers toward the incisal edges and does not encroach upon the gingival embrasure.**

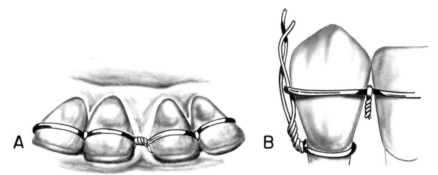

Figure 54–42 A, Space between splinted teeth maintained by twisting the arch wire. B, Wire from cervical line prevents splint from slipping. (After L. Hirschfeld.)

on conical teeth by joining it to a secondary loop at the neck of the tooth (Fig. 54–42).[19]

Orthodontic Band Splint. An effective temporary splint can be made by uniting a series of orthodontic bands.[3] This type of splint is used more often on posterior teeth (Fig. 54–43). The bands (0.005 stainless steel) may be fastened directly on the teeth and then welded into one unit, or the entire splint may be constructed on a cast. The bands should be properly contoured and be free of the gingiva.

A Fixed External Acrylic Splint (Sorrin).[43] This is a clear acrylic splint that fits onto the teeth like a multiple clasp; it is rigid, esthetically acceptable, and does not irritate the lips, tongue or cheek. The splint is cemented in place and may be left for a period up to two months (Fig. 54–44). Similar splints made of metal are more durable but less satisfactory esthetically.

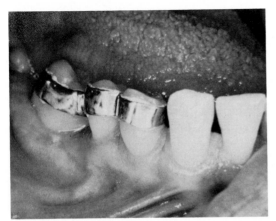

Figure 54–43 Orthodontic Band Splint to Stabilize Weak Second Premolar.

A Fixed Internal Temporary Acrylic Splint.[31] This type of splint consists of acrylic restorations reinforced with an embedded horizontal wire and joined together (Fig. 54–45). It is usually used on anterior teeth; posteriorly, amalgam is substituted for acrylic.

The splint is prepared as follows: The mobile teeth are stabilized with a ligature, and a compound or plaster impression is taken to be used as a matrix when the plastic filling material is inserted. The teeth are prepared so as to provide retention for the acrylic, which is placed in the cavity, covered with cellophane, and held under pressure with the matrix. The reinforcing stainless steel wire is embedded in the soft acrylic. After setting, the acrylic is polished and the ligature placed at the outset to stabilize the teeth is removed.

A Removable-Fixed Periodontal Splint. This is a rigid cast appliance that can be used to splint an entire arch.[1] It is constructed so that it fits both above and below the heights of contour of the teeth in order to provide maximum stability. The splint is constructed with two free ends to permit insertion. It consists of bilateral continuous clasps posteriorly, connected by an anterior lingual segment (Fig. 54–46). Interproximal wiring through holes in the splint secure it to the teeth.

Permanent Splints

The question is sometimes raised regarding the possible detrimental effects of restricting tooth movement by splinting. The reduction of physiologic movement of teeth

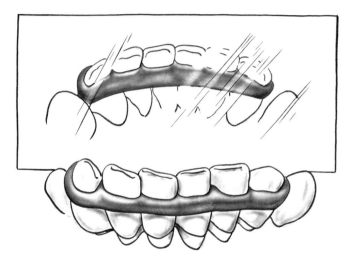

Figure 54–44 Removable External-Type Splint.

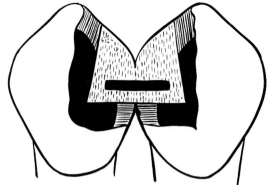

Figure 54–45 Temporary Internal Splint of Self-Curing Acrylic (*dotted lines*) containing a wire reinforcement. (After J. N. Obin and A. N. Arvins, New York.)

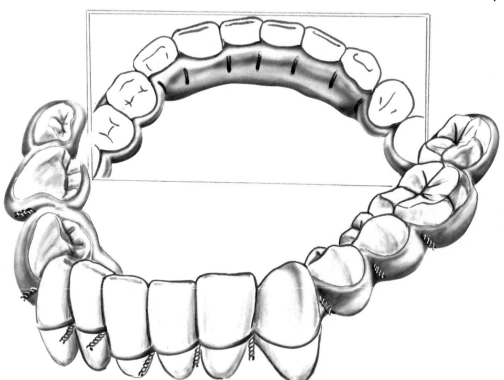

Figure 54–46 Removable Fixed Periodontal Splint. Bilateral continuous clasps ligated into position stabilize the posterior teeth. The anterior teeth are ligated individually to the lingual segment of the casting (shown in mirror view). After they have been tightened, the wire ligatures are bent inward to avoid tissue irritation. (After Baer, P. N., Malone, F. J., and Boyd, C. R.)

with a healthy periodontium could result in atrophy. However, permanent splints are employed when the periodontal support has been lost so that ordinarily physiologic forces may become injurious. The weakened teeth are assisted in withstanding occlusal forces by support from adjacent firm teeth.

Permanent splints may be (a) the removable external type or (b) the fixed internal type.

REMOVABLE EXTERNAL SPLINTS. Removable partial prosthesis may serve as a satisfactory permanent splint. Although this is not as desirable as the fixed type of splint, it offers the advantage of convenience. To obtain maximum stability with the removable type of splint, the continuous clasp construction is used and all the natural dentition should be included.

REMOVABLE SPLINTS AND PATHOLOGIC MIGRATION. Special types of removable appliances may be constructed for the specific purpose of splinting rather than replacing teeth (Fig. 54–47). However, removable splints should not be used if there is a tendency for the teeth to migrate,

particularly if the splints are worn only at night. The teeth move during the day, and when the appliance is inserted at night it feels tight and fits into position with difficulty. By morning the teeth have been moved back into position, and the splint is easily removed. Daily back-and-forth movement of the teeth injures the periodontium and increases tooth mobility, defeating the purpose for which the splint was constructed. To prevent this situation the teeth should be brought into proper position, the occlusion should be adjusted, and the teeth should be joined with a fixed internal type splint (Fig. 54–47, C).

The Overby Splint. The Overby[33] splint consists of a lingual or occlusal metal bar attached to the teeth by screws fitted into gold-threaded sleeves. The sleeves are cemented into bur holes at the cingula of anterior teeth or on the occlusal or lingual surfaces of posterior teeth (Fig. 54–48). The splint is screwed into place, but it may be removed and added to, should it become necessary to extract teeth and replace them.

The Fixed Internal Splint. The fixed

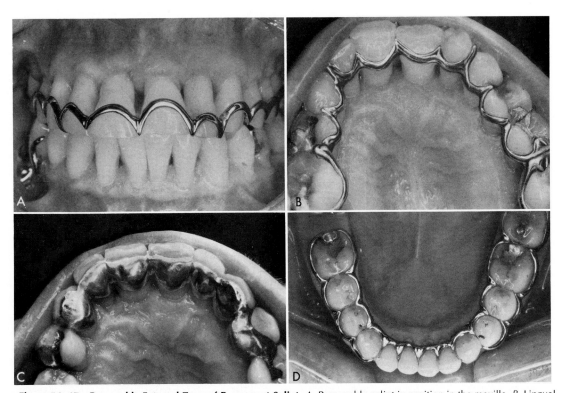

Figure 54–47   Removable External Type of Permanent Splint. *A,* Removable splint in position in the maxilla. *B,* Lingual view. *C,* Removable maxillary splint replaced by fixed internal splint from first premolar to first premolar. *D,* Removable splint in the mandible.

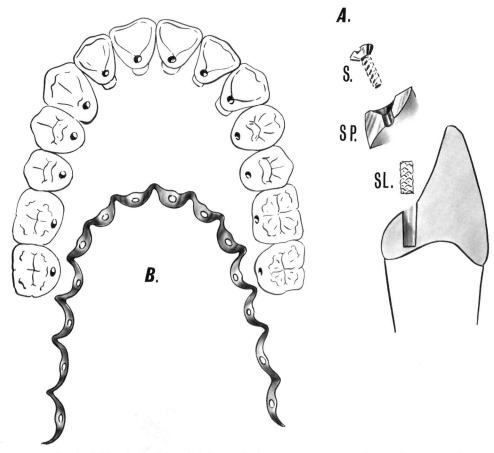

Figure 54–48 Overby Splint. *A,* Gold threaded sleeve (SL) fits into groove prepared in tooth. Screw (S) fits into sleeve and fastens splint (SP) to tooth. *B,* Splint ready for insertion with holes which correspond with sleeves cemented in teeth.

internal splint is the most efficient and durable type of permanent splint. It entails the construction of various types of prosthetic restorations for each of the teeth participating in the splint. The restorations are joined together to form a rigid unit and cemented in position. Fixed splinting with crowns is described in detail in Chapter 55. However, inlays and three quarter crowns can also be used effectively for this purpose (Fig. 54–49).

ENDOSSEOUS IMPLANTS IN RESTORATIVE DENTISTRY

Recent years have brought a revival of interest in endosseous implants as abutments for dental restorations. Their use has spread more rapidly then information regarding their merits and limitations has been developed. The different types of implants and techniques for using them are described in detail in a book edited by A. N. Cranin.[6] The superiority of stable fixed prostheses over free-end removable appliances had led to clinical experimentation with the use of a variety of endosseous implants as distal abutments. The thin blade types, vented to increase their retentive qualities, are commonly used.[28] Their insertion entails a demanding technique which consists of exposing the edentulous section of bone with a mucoperiosteal flap, drilling a slit the length of the blade through the cortical bone at the crest of the edentulous ridge, tapping the implant into the bone and suturing the flaps back in position. Good results are obtained in many patients but not always on a predictable basis (Fig. 54–50).

The use of endodontic endosseous implants as an adjunct to periodontal therapy is described in Chapter 45.

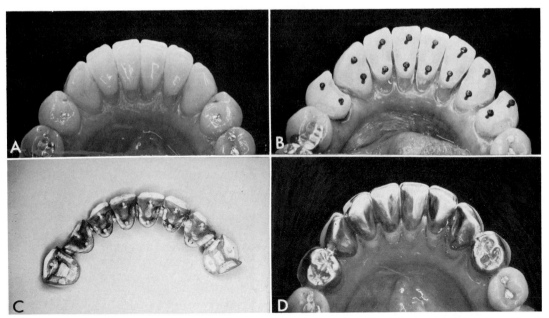

Figure 54–49 Fixed Internal Splinting With Inlays. *A,* Anterior teeth to be splinted. *B,* Anterior teeth prepared for pinledge inlays. *C,* Splint constructed, showing pins. *D,* Splint in place. Note that it includes the mandibular premolars to prevent faciolingual tipping.

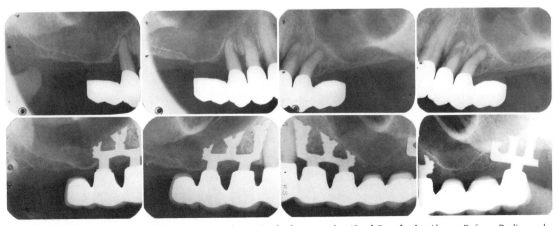

Figure 54–50 Endosseous Blade Implant Used as Distal Abutment for Fixed Prosthesis. *Above,* Before. Radiographs showing periodontal and periapical involvement of maxillary premolars with cantilevered distal pontics. *Below,* Endosseous blade implants, replacing two premolars (*left*), and replacing two premolars and providing a distal abutment for the fixed prosthesis (*right*). The entire restoration is a single unit.

CARE OF THE MOUTH WITH EXTENSIVE DENTAL RESTORATIONS

It makes little sense for the dentist to spend time designing, preparing and perfecting dental restorations without making a comparable effort to provide for their care after insertion in the patient's mouth. **Dental restorations function only** as long and as satisfactorily as the condition of the periodontium permits. **Instruction in plaque control is just as much a part of the restorative service rendered a patient as are the fit of the margins, the contour of the proximal surfaces and the occlusion. Failure to provide instruction in plaque control is an omission—a "short cut"— which jeopardizes the outcome of restorative procedures.**

When restorations are inserted the dentist and patient should join in a plaque control program to prevent the onset of periodontal disease. (For Patient Motivation and Instruction in Plaque Control, see page 467). The patient should be persuaded to take care of his mouth for his own sake. He should understand that by doing what he is being taught to do he will prolong the usefulness of his natural teeth as well as the restorations.

Plaque control procedures are the same for mouths with and without extensive reconstruction, but certain aspects warrant special mention:

The Bass method of tooth brushing is recommended (see page 449), with a soft or medium bristle brush. The patient may use a manual or electric brush, depending upon his ability to use them effectively.

Abusive brushing, long horizontal strokes with a hard brush, will abrade the gingiva and wear away tooth structure and some restorative materials, but proper brushing, even when vigorously performed, will not wear away plastic crowns or facings. Patients should not be instructed to "go easy" with their toothbrush to protect their restorations; this will initiate periodontal disease and premature loss of the restorations and the restored teeth.

Interproximal cleansing is critical, because most gingival disease starts there. Dental floss is most effective for this purpose, but when teeth are splinted greater reliance must be placed upon rubber tips and wooden and plastic interdental cleansers. Pontic surfaces may be cleaned with dental floss, pipe cleansers or the Zon Dental Bridge Cleaners. Toothbrushing and interdental cleansing should be followed by water irrigation under pressure, which is especially useful for cleansing around dental restorations.

THE FALLACY OF EARLY TOOTH EXTRACTION TO PRESERVE THE ALVEOLAR RIDGE

Teeth are sometimes unnecessarily extracted early in periodontal disease in an ill-advised attempt to retain the bone support for artificial dentures. Such extraction is contraindicated for the following reasons:

1. It condemns teeth which, with proper treatment, could be retained, and prematurely deprives the patient of his natural dentition.

2. Artificial forces produced by dentures are not physiologic for the bone; they accelerate normal postextraction atrophy. Forces created by complete dentures are not comparable to the occlusal forces of the natural dentition. The former produce a foreign external force on a remnant of the jaws which is not designed to support it; the latter provide functional stimulation for alveolar bone created for the purpose of supporting it.

3. **If a patient with early periodontal disease has enough bony support to provide a well-formed ridge for a denture, the best way to preserve the bone is to treat the periodontal disease.**

4. In young patients with rapid bone destruction ("periodontosis") not completely controllable by periodontal treatment, the rate of bone loss is accelerated by complete dentures. Wearing dentures is a problem because of rapid changes in the bone. Periodontal therapy, which postpones the need for complete dentures, is better for the patient than early extraction of the teeth.

REFERENCES

1. Baer, P. N., Malone, F. J., and Boyd, C. R.: A Removable-Fixed Periodontal Splint. Oral Surg., Oral Med. & Oral Path., 9:1057, 1956.
2. Barkann, L.: The Case for Metal Ligatures in Periodontia. J. Sec. District D. Soc. (N.Y.), 31:341, 1945.
3. Block, P.: A Wire-Band Splint for Immobilizing Loose Posterior Teeth. J. Periodont., 39:17, 1968.
4. Bryan, A. W.: Some Common Defects in Operative Restorations Contributing to the Injury of the Supporting Structures. J.A.D.A., 14:1486, 1927.
5. Clayton, J. A., and Green, E.: Roughness of Pontic Materials and Dental Plaque. J. Pros. Dent., 23:407, 1970.
6. Cranin, A. N. (Ed.): Oral Implantology. Springfield, Ill., Charles C Thomas, 1970.
7. Fenner, W., Gerber, A., and Mühlemann, H. R.: Tooth Mobility Changes During Treatment with Partial Denture Prosthesis. J. Pros. Dent., 6:520, 1956.
8. Frechette, A. R.: The Influence of Partial Denture Design on Distribution of Force to Abutment Teeth. J. Pros. Dent., 6:195, 1956.
9. Friedman, N.: Temporary Splinting—an Adjunct in Periodontal Therapy. J. Periodont., 24:229, 1953.
10. Fröhlich, Von E.: Zahnfleischrand und künstliche Krone in pathologisch-anatomischer Sicht. Dtsch. Zahn. Ztschr., 22:1252, 1967.
11. Glickman, I.: The Periodontal Structures and Re-

movable Partial Denture Prosthesis. J.A.D.A., 37:311, 1948.

12. Glickman, I.: Stein, R. S., and Smulow, J. B.: The Effect of Increased Functional Forces upon the Periodontium of Splinted and Non-Splinted Teeth. J. Periodont., 32:290, 1961.

13. Goransson, P., and Nyman, L.: Review of Methods for Exposing the Gingival Margin. Scientific and Educational Bulletin (International College of Dentists), 2:24, 1969.

14. Gottlieb, B.: Die Prinzipien der Stumpfpräparation. Ztschr. f. Stomat., 22:473, 1924.

15. Henry, P. J., Johnston, J. F., and Mitchell, D. F.: Tissue Changes Beneath Fixed Partial Dentures. J. Pros. Dent., 16:937, 1966.

16. Hildebrand, G. Y.: Studies in Dental Prosthetics. Stockholm, Aktiebolaget Fahlcrantz' Boktryckeri, 1937, p. 256.

17. Hildebrand, G. Y.: The Problem of the Cervical Preparation. Proc. Swedish Dental Soc., 1927, S.T.T. p. 14.

18. Hildebrand, G. Y.: Studies in Dental Prosthetics. Stockholm, Aktiebolaget Fahlcrantz' Boktryckeri, 1937, p. 226.

19. Hirschfeld, L.: The Use of Wire and Silk Ligatures. J.A.D.A., 41:647, 1950.

20. Hirshberg, S. M.: Compatible Temporary Tooth Health and Gingival Protection. J. Pros. Dent., 18:151, 1967.

21. Homma, S., Homma, M., and Nakamura, Y.: Dynamic Study of Attachments (Abst.). J. D. Res., 40:228, 1961.

22. Ito, H., Inoue, Y., and Yamada, M.: Three Dimensional Photoelastic Studies on the Clasp-Rest and Tooth Extraction (Abst.). J. D. Res., 38:203, 1959.

23. Johnston, J. F., Phillips, R. W., and Dykema, R. W.: Modern Practice in Crown and Bridge Prosthodontics. Philadelphia, W. B. Saunders Company, 1960, p. 189.

24. Kaqueler, J. C., and Weiss, M. B.: Plaque Accumulation on Dental Restorative Materials. IADR Abst., 1970, p. 202, Abst. 615.

25. Knowles, J. W., and Snyder, D. T.: The Effect of Roughness on Supragingival and Subgingival Plaque Formation. IADR Abst., 1970, p. 135, Abst. 345.

26. Koivumaa, K. K., and Wennström, A.: A Histological Investigation of the Changes in Gingival Margins Adjacent to Gold Crowns. A pilot study. Odont. Tskr., 68:373, 1960.

27. Krogh-Poulsen, W.: Partial Denture Design in Relation to Occlusal Trauma and Periodontal Breakdown. Internat. D. J., 4:847, 1954.

28. Linkow, L. I.: Endosseous Blade-vent Implants: A Two-Year Report. J. Pros. Dent., 23:441, 1970.

29. Marcum, J. S.: The Effect of Crown Marginal Depth Upon Gingival Tissue. J. Pros. Dent., 17:479, 1967.

30. Morris, M. L.: Artificial Contours and Gingival Health. J. Pros. Dent., 12:1146, 1962.

31. Obin, J. N., and Arvins, A. N.: The Use of Self-Curing Resin Splints for the Temporary Stabilization of Mobile Teeth Due to Periodontal Involvement. J.A.D.A., 42:320, 1951.

32. Osborne, J., Brills, N., and Lammie, G. A.: Partial Dentures. Internat. D. J., 7:26, 1957.

33. Overby, G. E.: Intracoronal Splinting of Mobile Teeth by Use of Screws and Sleeves. J. Periodont., 33:270, 1962.

34. Pichler, H.: Das Herrichten von Zahnstümpfen für Kronenringe. Ztschr. f. Stomat., 18:299, 1920.

Der Schutz des freien Zahnfleischrandes bei Kronen-und Brückenarbeiten. Ztschr. f. Stomat., 22:483, 1924.

35. Plitzner, J.: Role of Occlusal Rest Lug as Transmitter of Masticating Stress. Dentist. Reform., 42:77, 1938.

36. Podshadley, A. G.: Gingival Response to Pontics. J. Pros. Dent., 19:51, 1968.

37. Posselt, U., and Wolff, I. B.: Treatment of Bruxism by Bite Guards and Bite Plates. J. Canad. D. A., 29:773, 1963.

38. Seemann, S. K.: A Study of the Relationship Between Periodontal Disease and the Wearing of Partial Dentures. Australian D. J., 8:206, 1963.

39. Shohet, H.: Relative Magnitudes of Stress on Abutment Teeth with Different Retainers. J. Pros. Dent., 21:267, 1969.

40. Shooshan, E. D.: A Pin-ledge Casting Technique – Its Application in Periodontal Splinting. Dent. Clin. North America, March 1960, p. 189.

41. Silness, J.: Periodontal Conditions in Patients Treated with Dental Bridges. III. The Relationship Between the Location of the Crown Margin and the Periodontal Condition. J. Periodont. Res., 5:225, 1970.

42. Simring, M., and Thaller, J. L.: Temporary Splinting for Multiple Mobile Teeth. J.A.D.A., 53:429, 1956.

43. Sorrin, S.: The Use of Fixed and Removable Splints in the Practice of Periodontia. Am. J. Ortho. & Oral Surg., 31:354, 1945.

44. Stafne, E. E., and Schaffer, E. M.: The Changes in Morphology of the Periodontal Col of Rhesus Monkeys with Alterations in Tooth Contact Relations. IADR Abst., 1965, p. 55, Abst. 76.

45. Steffel, V. L.: Clasp Partial Dentures, J.A.D.A., 66:803, 1963.

46. Stein, R. S.: Pontic-Residual Ridge Relationship: A Research Report. J. Pros. Dent., 16:251, 1966.

47. Stein, R. S., and Glickman, I.: Prosthetic Considerations Essential for Gingival Health. Dent. Clin. North America, March, 1960, p. 177.

48. Swenson, H. M.: Experimental Periodontal Pockets in Dogs. J. D. Res., 26:273, 1947.

49. Talkov, L.: Temporary Acrylic Fixed Bridgework and Splints. J. Pros. Dent., 2:693, 1952.

50. Waerhaug, J.: Effect of Rough Surfaces Upon Gingival Tissue. J. D. Res., 35:323, 1956.

51. Waerhaug, J.: Histologic Considerations Which Govern Where the Margin of Restorations Should Be Located in Relation to the Gingiva. Dent. Clin. North America, March 1960, p. 161.

52. Waerhaug, J.: Tissue Reactions Around Artificial Crowns. J. Periodont., 24:172, 1953.

53. Waerhaug, J., and Zander, H. A.: Reaction of Gingival Tissues to Self-Curing Acrylic Restorations. J.A.D.A., 54:760, 1957.

54. Weinberg, L. A.: Force Distribution in Splinted Anterior Teeth. Oral Surg., Oral Med. & Oral Path., 10:484, 1957.

55. Wheeler, R. C.: A Textbook of Dental Anatomy and Physiology. 3rd ed. Philadelphia. W. B. Saunders Co., 1958, pp. 64–65.

56. Wing, G.: Pontic Design and Construction in Fixed Bridgework, D. Practit. & D. Rec., 12:390, 1962.

57. Wust, B. P. Von, Rateitschak, K. H., and Mühlemann, H. R.: The Effect of Local Periodontal Treatment on Mobility and Gingival Inflammation. Helv. Odont. Acta. 6:58, 1960.

Chapter 55

OCCLUSO-REHABILITATION AND THE PERIODONTAL PROBLEM*

DEFINITION

The term "occluso-rehabilitation" desig-nates the procedures employed to restore

the dentition for the purpose of establish-ing an optimal functional relationship, ac-ceptable phonetics and desirable esthetics. Other terms such as "bite raising," "bite revision" and "mouth rehabilitation" are also used in referring to these procedures. Occluso-rehabilitation entails the applica-tion of the various phases of dentistry, such as selective grinding, orthodontic tooth movement, and the restoration of parts of teeth, individual teeth or groups of teeth. All these procedures must be coordinated so as to establish a functional environment conducive to the health of the periodontium. In this manner, restorative efforts serve along with other forms of local treatment as therapeutic aids in the management of periodontal disease (Figs. 55–1 and 55–2).

INDICATIONS FOR OCCLUSO-REHABILITATION

In the total management of periodontal disease there are circumstances in which the establishment of an optimal functional relationship requires the integration of a variety of corrective procedures attainable only by occluso-rehabilitation. Such condi-tions include:

1. Loss or absence of tooth substance because of caries, abrasion, erosion and congenital or developmental defects.

2. Multilation of the dentition because of failure to replace missing teeth. Such failure

---

*Original draft submitted by Louis Alexander Cohn, D.D.S., F.A.C.D.

928

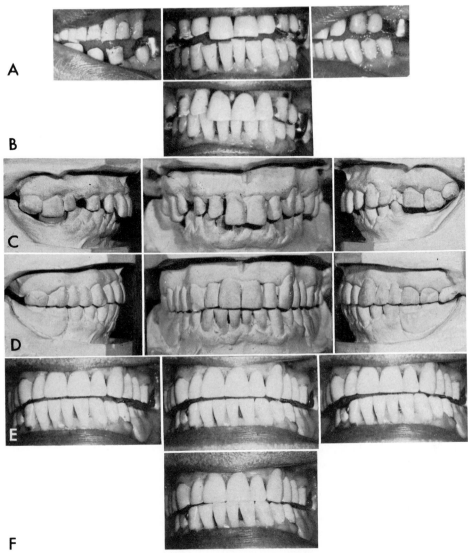

Figure 55–1   A Case of Periodontal Disease in Which There is Loss of Posterior Tooth Support with Resultant Excessive Anterior Overbite and Extrusion of Teeth. *A,* Before treatment—centric relation, left, front, and right views. There is premature contact on the mandibular second premolars and maxillary first molars. Note marked attrition of maxillary canine (*left*), mandibular anterior teeth, as well as spreading of the mandibular anterior teeth. *B,* Before treatment—from the premature contact the mandible slides forward into habitual occlusion. *C,* Before treatment—casts, left, front, and right views. Note extruded maxillary molars and maxillary central incisors. *D,* After treatment—casts, left, front, and right views in centric occlusion. Note reduced occlusogingival length of maxillary molars. Also note maxillary central incisors. The clinical crowns have been shortened into line with the maxillary lateral incisors which were not restored, but selectively ground. *E,* After treatment—right lateral excursion, centric occlusion, and left lateral excursion. Note harmony of the line of occlusion, closing of mandibular incisal contacts, and reduction of overbite. Compare this position with that at *A.* Note disocclusion of anterior teeth in centric occlusion. *F,* After treatment—protrusive position. Note harmony of functional contact of the incisors. The mandibular incisors were treated by selective grinding without orthodontic measures.

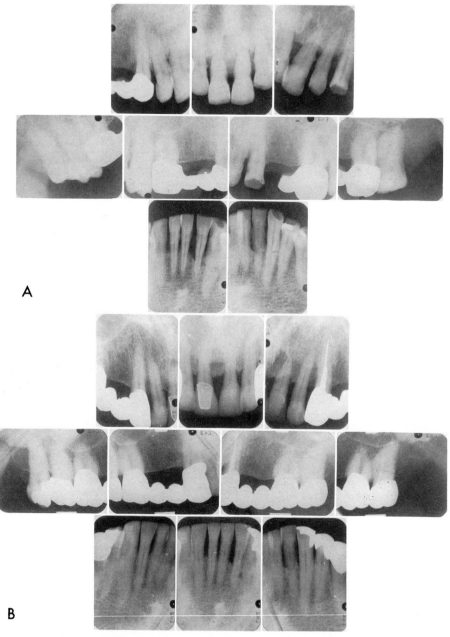

Figure 55–2   Roentgenograms Before and After Treatment of Patient Shown in Figure 55–1. *A,* Before treatment. Note generalized loss of bone and pathologic migration of mandibular anterior teeth. *B,* Twelve years after treatment. Note improved appearance of the bone in the maxillary and mandibular anterior regions. Also note that the proximal contact of the mandibular anterior teeth has been restored following occluso-rehabilitation.

usually leads to a series of changes in the position of the remaining teeth such as tipping, rotation or extrusion with loss of proximal contact followed by food impaction. **When many posterior teeth are lost, collapse of the dental arch may occur with increase in the overbite relationship of the anterior teeth and loss of vertical dimension.**[6] Such collapse not only impairs the functioning of the dentition and alters the esthetics, but of greater importance, it adversely affects the leverage on the periodontal tissues. Lateral, tipping or torsional stresses are induced, and destruction of the periodontal tissues and tooth mobility may result (Figs. 55–1 and 55–2).

3. **Tooth habits such as tapping or clamping the teeth, are hyperfunctional states which can adversely influence the periodontal tissues,** particularly if the teeth are incorrectly related in occlusion. The harmful effects of such habits can be ameliorated by occluso-rehabilitation.

4. **In teeth with markedly reduced periodontal support,** disproportion in the clinical crown-root ratio leads to traumatic occlusal forces which are correctable by occluso-rehabilitation. In such cases occluso-rehabilitation entails corrective measures to eliminate the traumatic effects of the occlusal forces.

5. **Excessive mobility is also a factor which is dealt with by occluso-rehabilitation.** Excessive mobility is detrimental to the healing processes. In the treatment of periodontal disease where such mobility exists, occluso-rehabilitation can serve a vital role by stabilizing the teeth and creating a favorable environment for healing.

SPECIFIC OCCLUSO-REHABILITATION PROCEDURES

The basic goal in occluso-rehabilitation is to construct an occlusion which is beneficial to the periodontium. Recent evidence that habitual occlusion* rather than centric occlusion† is the most frequently used functional relationship of the dentition,[3]

---

*Habitual occlusion: The position of the dentition in which the teeth are intercuspated with the mandible not in centric relation.

†Centric occlusion: The position of the dentition in which the teeth are intercuspated with the mandible in centric relation.

and that patients may continue to function in habitual occlusion after the dentition is reconstructed in centric occlusion,[4] has not as yet had significant impact upon the field of occluso-rehabilitation. Most techniques of occluso-rehabilitation are based upon centric relation* and centric occlusion, and in varying degrees are concerned with lateral and protrusive excursions and balanced occlusion.

The technique described here embodies these principles; the following are its procedures and the specific manner in which each contributes toward the attainment of the overall purpose:

I. Determination of Centric Relation

With the exception of temporomandibular joint dysfunctions, the position of centric relation can be determined by restrained guided positioning of the mandible to the maxilla and controlled manipulation about its hinge axis. The patient is asked to let the jaw relax, or "let it hang loosely," swallowing and moistening the lips several times. The chin is then held lightly between the index finger and thumb and the patient is asked to protrude, retrude and move into the lateral positions until the operator is assured that the relaxed unstrained retruded position of the mandible has been obtained, without pressure. Once certain of the latter position, again without exerting pressure in a posterior direction, the operator oscillates the mandible vertically as a simple hinge, without benefit of the patient's muscular effort, permitting the teeth to tap several times and come slowly into resting contact. Thereupon the patient should press the teeth forcibly together and the path of closure should be noted. Ideally, all of the mandibular and maxillary teeth should contact simultaneously.

Detection of centric prematurities

Gross areas of premature contact will be disclosed by visual examination. Minor prematurities are located by the following methods: (1) questioning the patient re-

---

*Centric relation: The most posterior relation of the mandible to the maxilla at the established vertical dimension.

garding his sensations of tooth contact, and (2) testing by drawing dental floss posteroanteriorly between the maxillary and mandibular teeth. Interference in the passage of the dental floss indicates the location of the area of premature contact.

For more definitive location of prematurities wax is used as follows: Depending on the degree of separation of the jaws caused by the prematurities, one or more well-warmed sheets of base plate wax are wrapped over the maxillary teeth on the side of the jaw opposite the premature contact. The mandible is then eased into its most retruded position and moved upward until the premature contact is attained as described above. Chilling the wax will create a key whereby the prematurity can be relocated. If the premature contact is on both sides, the wax is placed on both sides, either anterior to or posterior to the premature contact region. The wax key can also be used in studying the occlusion because it serves as a means of orienting the casts at the centric relationship on an articulator. There are other recordings which may be required for more thorough study of the occlusion, such as the hinge axis determination,[2, 10] face-bow registrations and protrusive and lateral tracings or positional wax check bites of the mandibular glides.

II. Determination of the Postural Position (Rest Position) and Free Way Space

Although the postural position is sometimes difficult to appraise, it can be disclosed by careful study or by use of suitable techniques.[14, 23, 24] The following is a recommended method:

The patient is either seated upright in the dental chair with the head off the head rest or in a standing position. He is instructed to alternately swallow and moisten the lips several times, then to let the jaw and lips hang loosely, and start humming the sound "mmm" without effort, continuing the sound but permitting it to fade out. The patient is told that during the interval when the sound is fading the lips will be parted by the operator but that he is to **continue the humming.** Separation of the lips will disclose the free way space. It is of paramount importance to stress to the patient **that the lips should be relaxed while the humming sound is made.**

The free way space is the distance between the jaws when the postural position of the mandible is established. The maintenance of the free way space is of paramount significance in the diagnosis and treatment planning involved in occlusorehabilitation. The extent of the free way space should be determined at the time of examination. It it is excessive, it may be reduced in occluso-rehabilitation, but it should never be obliterated.

In patients with pronounced overbite, altered muscle activity patterns complicate determination of centric relation and the free way space. In such cases relaxing drugs such as mephenesin (Tolserol), 1 to 3 gm., or meprobamate (Equanil, Miltown), 0.4 gm., are helpful.

III. Correction of Tooth Position and Cuspal Relationships in Centric Occlusion

Ideally, the proximal contacts in centric occlusion should be aligned anteroposteriorly and faciolingually so that the arch shape is not deformed (Fig. 55-3). The maxillary teeth overjet the mandibular teeth; the maxillary canine and all maxillary posterior teeth engage their antagonists at one half cusp distal to the corresponding mandibular teeth. The incisal edges of the mandibular anterior teeth engage the lingual surfaces of the maxillary teeth anywhere from a point incisal to the cingulum. The buccal cusps of the posterior mandibular teeth are related to the middle* of the occlusal surfaces of the maxillary teeth (Fig. 55-4), and conversely the lingual cusps of the maxillary teeth are related to the middle of the occlusal surfaces of the mandibular teeth. This results in a facial overjet of all the maxillary teeth and a lingual overjet of the mandibular teeth. It is also important that the maxillary posterior teeth be inclined in a facioaxial direction, with the mandibular posterior teeth in a linguoaxial inclination (Fig. 55-5). This effects a reciprocal axial relationship of the posterior teeth most satisfactory to the reception of forces by the periodontium.

If the teeth are not correctly intercuspated at the centric relation of the mandible in

---

*Middle: This term designates a linear area which lies midway between the buccal and lingual marginal ridges on the occlusal surface.

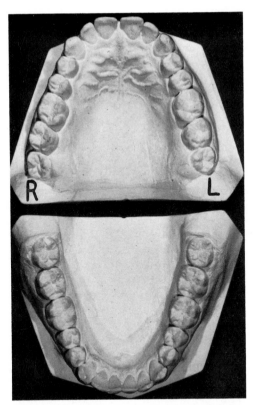

Figure 55–3 Excellent Arch Form and Tooth Relationship With a Small Diastema Between the Maxillary Central Incisors. Note the difference between the left and right sides of the maxillary arch. On the left side, (L), there is a perfect relationship of all the contact points. On the right side, (R), there is an incorrect contact relationship between the second and third molars. The mandibular arch is perfectly formed and the contact relationships of the mandibular left side up to and including the lateral incisor are ideal. On the right side, there are small variations in the contact point relationships.

the course of function, an individual tooth or group of teeth momentarily carries the burden of the entire occlusal force upon closure. This initial contact is commonly referred to as "centric premature contact," "centric prematurity" or "centric interference." In the presence of centric premature contact, the mandible may continue to close to centric relation after the initial tooth contact is made, or may be deflected to a habitual occlusion.[8–11]

IV. Proximal Contact and Stability of Arch Form

Stability of the arch form depends on the correct location of the proximal contact point relationships of the teeth. In drifted, tipped or extruded teeth, the convex proximal surface of one tooth contacts with the inclined surface of the adjacent tooth in an abnormal location. Forces applied against such teeth tend to displace them, further accentuating the abnormal tooth positions.

The correct proximal contact point relationships of the canine, first premolar and lateral incisor teeth are of particular importance to arch stability. It is in this area of the arch that the anterior component of force[22] meets the force from the lips. Depending on the relative location of the proximal contact point of these teeth, slow but continuous change in the position of any one of the aforementioned teeth can occur. Unless resisted by an equal and opposite force, the forces are resolved at right angles

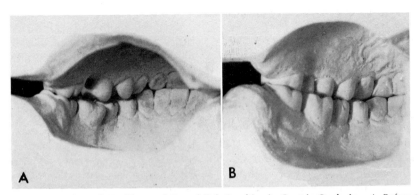

Figure 55–4 Correction of Tooth Position and Cuspal Relationships in Centric Occlusion. A, Before treatment. Note incorrect relationship of maxillary lingual cusps to the middle areas of the mandibular teeth. The terminal molars present an end to end relationship. B, After treatment. Note the changed relationship accomplished by occluso-rehabilitation. The maxillary lingual cusps are now contacting the middle areas of the opposing teeth in centric occlusion.

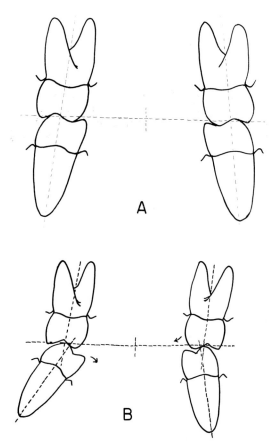

Figure 55–5 *A,* **Ideal Situation in Which the Maxillary Lingual Cusps Meet the Middle Areas of the Mandibular Teeth and Conversely the Mandibular Buccal Cusps Meet the Middle areas of the Maxillary Teeth.** Note the facial overjet of the maxillary tooth and the lingual overjet of the mandibular tooth and the faciolingual axial inclination of the teeth. *B,* Incorrect axial-inclination of the teeth coupled with incorrect cuspal relationships.

tion of the teeth in the arch. If the proximal contact points of the anterior teeth are not in proper position, these teeth may overlap, or existing irregularities may be accentuated. Malposition of a posterior tooth may also be aggravated by growth pressure associated with eruption of the third molar.

The integrity of the proximal contact areas is important to the stabilization of the arch and the maintenance of a stable occlusion (Fig. 55–8). Of paramount importance is the perfection of the proximal contacts and the functional occlusal relationships of the posterior teeth and the canines. **The canine acts as the keystone between the incisor teeth and the posterior teeth.** If the posterior arch segments are in perfect proximal and occlusal relationships, the anterior teeth, though irregular, may be maintained with minimal change over a long period of time (Fig. 55–8).

V. Modification of Tooth Form and Crown-Root Ratio

The tooth is an individual functioning unit which is subject to various biomechanical influences. **There are two basic considerations regarding the crown of the tooth which are particularly pertinent in occluso-rehabilitation: one is the relationship of the crown form to the gingiva, and the other is the relationship of the crown to the root insofar as it affects the leverage on the periodontium.**

The relationship of the crown form to the gingiva

The crown form is one of the controlling influences in the maintenance of the health of the gingivae.[25] By the anatomic relationship of the crown to the gingiva, food is shunted away from the gingival sulcus and irritation from food retention is prevented (Fig. 55–9). This is particularly true of the mandibular facial, maxillary lingual and interproximal gingival areas. Loss of periodontal tissue exposes the root and alters the normally protective gingiva-tooth relationship (Fig. 55–9). Such loss readily permits the retention of food, and if the teeth are not thoroughly cleansed, mechanical as well as bacterial irritation results. Despite instruction in plaque con-

to the surface against which they are applied (Fig. 55–6).

When the mandibular anterior teeth are lingually inclined or are irregular, and the overbite is deep, further lingual inclination and extrusion of these teeth are apt to occur. This is most evident if the first premolar proximal contact meets the canine below the normal contact area of the canine. During mastication, the bolus of food and the pressure of the lip applied through the maxillary anterior teeth cause lingual tipping forces to the mandibular incisors, which are not counteracted by the anterior component of force (Fig. 55–7).

The growth force associated with erupting third molars also may disturb the posi-

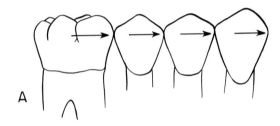

A

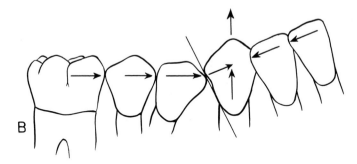

B

Figure 55–6 *A,* **Normal Direction of Anterior Component of Force Through the Posterior Teeth.** *B* and *C,* Instability of teeth and arch collapse which result when the premolar contact with the canine is gingival to its normal position. The various directions in which the teeth tend to move are indicated by the arrows.

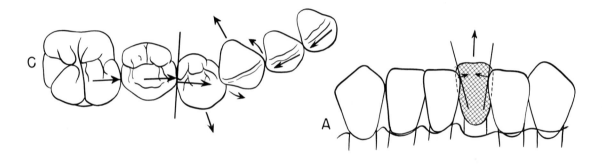

C

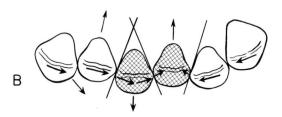

A

B

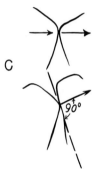

C

Figure 55–7 If the Anterior Component of Force Is Not Correctly Neutralized in the Midline, Changes in the Position of Any Tooth in the Arch May Occur. The direction of the anterior component of force, and the forces which result from malposition of the teeth are indicated by arrows. *A,* Facial view. Mandibular incisor in lingual version may be forced incisally and lingually as indicated by the arrows. *B,* Incisal view. Progressive crowding of irregularly aligned mandibular teeth as the result of deflection of the anterior component of force. *C,* Diagrammatic representation of the resolution of forces at the contact point in a normal (*above*) and abnormal proximal relationship (*below*).

935

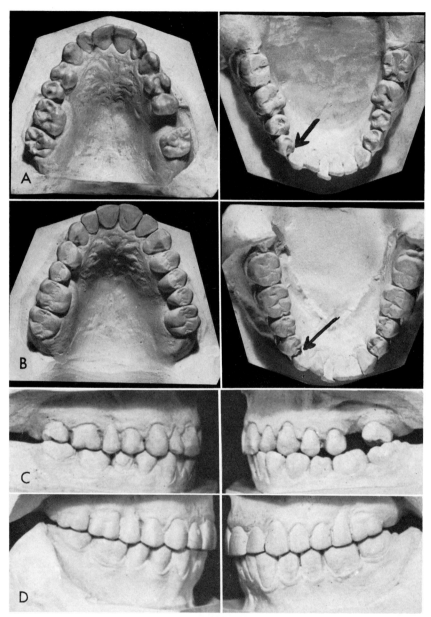

Figure 55–8   Correction of Proximal Contact Relationships and Establishment of Proper Arch Form by Occluso-Rehabilitation. *A,* Before treatment. Note crowded mandibular anterior teeth, and irregular arch form with incorrect proximal contact relationships. The arrow indicates abnormal premolar-canine relationship. The mandibular first premolar contacts the mandibular canine at a point gingival to the usual position. *B,* After treatment. Note correction of arch form and proximal contact. Particularly note the correction of the contact relationship indicated by the arrow. *C,* Before treatment. Lateral view. *D,* After treatment. Lateral view.

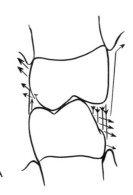
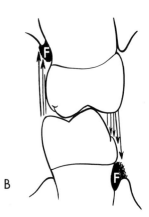

Figure 55–9 *A,* **Normal Relationship of the Crown to the Gingiva.** Note the pathways of food excursion (indicated by the arrows) which tend to shunt the food laterally over and onto the gingiva. *B,* **Abnormal Relationship of the Gingiva to the Tooth in Periodontal Disease.** Note the food retention areas (*F*) which result because the normal protective relationship of the crown to the gingiva is distorted.

trol, removal of such debris by the patient may be difficult, and at times, incomplete.

The relationship of the crown to the root

There are three basic considerations in the development of leverage upon the periodontium: **(1) the crown-root ratio, (2) the width of the crown and (3) the position and form of the cusps.**

THE CROWN-ROOT RATIO.   Tooth stability is influenced by the leverage exerted upon the periodontium. The nature of this leverage depends on the amount of tooth that is retained in bone (clinical root) in relation to the tooth portion not so retained (clinical crown). Increase in the length of the clinical crown creates an unfavorable leverage upon the periodontium. The clinical root may be short because of morphologic variation in the anatomy of the root, or as a result of alveolar bone loss or a combination of both factors (Fig. 55–10).

THE WIDTH OF THE CROWN AND FORM OF THE CUSPS.   Lateral and tipping stresses arise during function when the cuspal inclines are steep or the morsal platform is

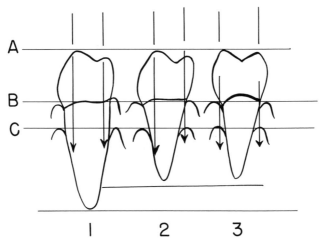

Figure 55–10   The Unfavorable Distribution of Functional Forces Associated With Variations in Crown-Root Relationship Is Accentuated in Cases of Reduced Periodontal Support. *1,* Normal premolar. Vertical forces of occlusion fall within the confines of the root when the periodontium is at the cemento-enamel line (*B*), and also when the height of the periodontium is reduced (*C*). In the first instance the clinical crown is (*A-B*) and in the second instance (*A-C*). *2,* Premolar with normal crown and short root. Vertical forces of occlusion just barely fall within the confines of the root when periodontium is at cemento-enamel line (*A*). However, when periodontium is reduced (*C*) the vertical forces of occlusion fall outside the root. *3,* Premolar with abnormally wide crown and short root. The vertical forces of occlusion are directed beyond the periphery of the root when the periodontium is at the cemento-enamel line (*B*) and also when the level of the periodontium is reduced (*C*).

wide in relation to the root (Fig. 55–10). Ideally, forces applied to the teeth should fall within the peripheral contours of the root structure retained in alveolar bone. In the mandible, this force should be transmitted to the root by way of the buccal cusps, and in the maxillary teeth it should be transmitted to the root by way of the lingual cusps. The location of the cusp in relation to the root in the faciolingual direction influences the direction of the transmitted force upon the periodontium (Fig. 55–10). If the direction of the functional forces falls within the lateral border of the clinical root, stress is directed vertically upon the periodontium. If, on the other hand, the force is directed beyond the confines of the root, lateral or tipping stresses are induced.

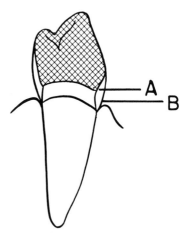

Figure 55–11 Change in Crown Form in Order to Reestablish the Normal Tooth-Gingiva Relationship in a Case of Treated Periodontal Disease. The original crown form is shown in cross-hatching (A). The corrected form is shown at (B).

How to modify tooth form and crown-root ratio

There are two methods of modifying the crown surfaces to eliminate unfavorable forces upon the periodontium. **One is the construction of a new crown form in gold, percelain fused to gold, porcelain or gold with an acrylic facing. The other is the use of inlays to change the morsal surface anatomy.** The choice depends on the condition of the tooth, caries susceptibility, the position of the tooth in the arch, the prosthetic demands upon the tooth as an abutment and the esthetics.

Protection of exposed sensitive surfaces and the elimination of irritation from food to the gingiva can be accomplished by changing the contour of the entire crown.[13] The new form changes the relationship to the gingiva by re-establishing the protective anatomic contour of the teeth and promoting a more normal function (Figs. 55–11 and 55–12). With change in crown from, the proximal tooth contact areas can be restored at locations which **prevent mesiodistal shifting or food impaction.[1]**

In all instances, reduction of the length of the clinical crown, change of the cuspal positions and modification of the cusp inclines can be accomplished simultaneously when reconstructing the crown surface artificially (Fig. 55–13).

Narrowing the faciolingual width of the morsal tooth surface of the reconstructed crown attains the correct location of the mandibular buccal and maxillary lingual

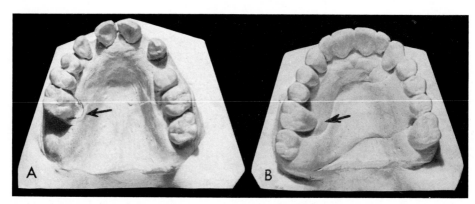

Figure 55–12 *A,* **Recession in Relation to the Lingual Root of the Maxillary Molar** (*arrow*) *B,* The same tooth treated with a full cast crown. The previously exposed tooth surface is covered by the crown (*arrow*). Note the improvement in the appearance of the gingiva in relation to the tooth. The other teeth have also been crowned. Note that the design of the partial denture avoids impingement upon the gingiva.

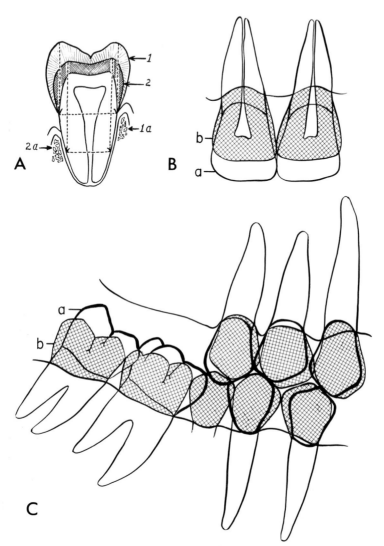

Figure 55–13 Schematic Drawing Showing the Need for Altering the Tooth Form in Cases of Chronic Destructive Periodontal Disease. *A,* The original tooth form and periodontium at the cemento-enamel junction are shown at *1* and *1a*. The vertical functional forces upon the crown (*vertical lines*) fall within the root. The altered bone level in destructive periodontal disease is shown at *2a*. The manner in which the tooth is modified so as to conform with the altered bone level is shown at *2*. Note that by altering the tooth form the vertical forces upon the newly contoured crown are kept within the root (*vertical lines*). Note the alteration in cusp inclination. *B,* Shortening and recontouring the clinical crown using restorations. (a) Original clinical crown; (*b*) corrected clinical crown. *C,* Correction of improper functional relationships by occluso-rehabilitation. The pre-existent condition which requires correction is indicated by the heavy outline (a). The corrected relationships are shown in cross-hatching (*b*). Note establishment of line of occlusion to permit replacement of maxillary molars. Also note restoration of proper proximal contact relationships.

cusps in relation to the root (Fig. 55–13, A). The facial cusps of the mandibular teeth and the lingual cusps of the maxillary teeth should be in such a position that centric occlusion tooth contact is made in the middle position of the occlusal surfaces of their antagonists. After the location of these cusps is determined, the lingual cusps of the mandibular teeth and the buccal cusps of the maxillary teeth are built to the minimum width of the morsal platform required for contact in all functional positions of the mandible.

VI. The Attainment of Balanced Occlusion

In order to understand the meaning of balanced occlusion, it is necessary to analyze its various components. **Balanced occlusion entails simultaneous contact between the right and left posterior segments of the arch in the lateral excursions of the mandible, and simultaneous contact between the posterior segments of the arch and the anterior segment in protrusive excursion (Fig. 55–14).** In occluso-rehabilitation, an effort should be made to create balanced occlusion, but this is not always possible, and in the opinion of some, may not be desirable. Many deformities of the tooth relationships with which we deal are mutilations of a previous malocclusion, rather than a previous normal relationship of the teeth and jaws. In the former type of case, attainment of bilateral balance by occluso-rehabilitation is difficult.

VII. Modification of Crown Morphology and Crown-Root Ratio to Attain Balanced Occlusion

In attempting to attain balanced occlusion, it is generally necessary to alter the crown morphology or the crown-root ratio. These procedures should be instituted without creating leverage relationships which will adversely affect the periodontium. It would defeat the purpose of occluso-rehabilitation if the health of the periodontium of the individual teeth is jeopardized in order to attain the mechanical ideal of balanced occlusion. In isolated instances, it may be preferable to remove a tooth which is so incongruous with proper functional patterns that modifying it would create a weak link in the dentition. In order to safeguard teeth against adverse leverage, it is necessary to avoid excessive increase in the crown-root ratio, excessive

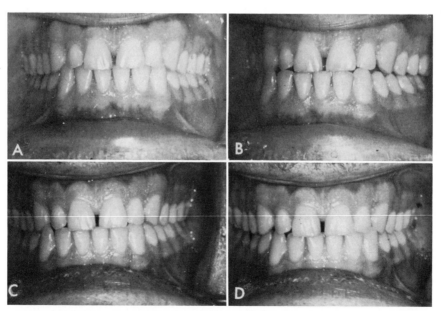

Figure 55–14   An Ideal Occlusion in Which the Centric Occlusion and Centric Relationship are Identical Which has Never Been Treated by Selective Grinding. (Casts shown in Figure 55–3.) *A,* Centric occlusion. *B,* Protrusive position. All the posterior teeth and the incisal edges of the anterior teeth make simultaneous contact. *C* and *D,* Left and right lateral positions with ideal cuspal relationships and bilateral balance.

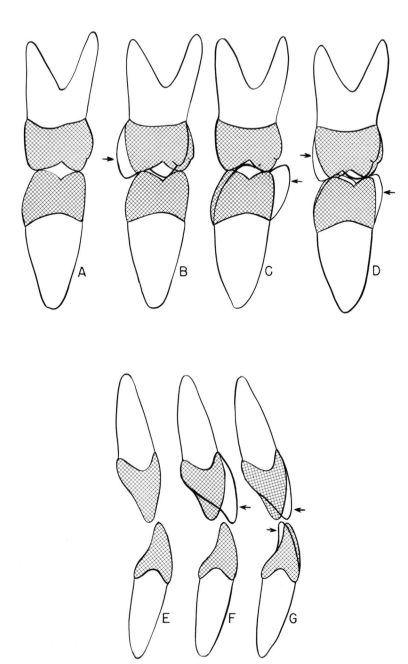

Figure 55–15 **Diagrammatic Representation of Incorrect Tooth Relationships in Centric and a Method of Correcting Them.** *A,* Incorrect molar relationship *(faciolingual view) B* and *C,* Incorrect treatment. The Incorrect relationship is shown in cross hatching and the alterations in crown form are indicated by the arrows. In both *B* and *C* the alteration has been limited to one tooth. This necessitates distortion of the crown form in relation to the root. *D,* Correct treatment indicated by the arrows. Both the maxillary and mandibular crowns are altered without distortion of the crown-root relationship. *E,* Diagrammatic representation of incorrect relationship of the incisors in centric. *F,* Incorrect treatment attempting to remedy the condition by changing only the maxillary tooth *(arrow).* Distortion of the crown-root relationship results. *G,* Correct treatment: a restoration is used on both the maxillary and mandibular teeth *(arrows).*

faciolingual width of the morsal platform or distorted cuspal positions in relation to the periphery of the clinical root (Fig. 55–15).

In isolated instances, because of the tooth positions at centric relation, it would be necessary to distort the crown forms faciolingually to obtain ideal functional contacts. This cannot be condoned if it would result in a situation in which the force applied to the crown will not be properly translated to the root. In such circumstances, as a first choice, corrective treatment requires orthodontic movement of the tooth. When the tooth has been moved to a favorable position, the crown can be restored without excessive distortion of the crown-root relationship and the root will receive the correct force.

When dealing with shifted tooth positions, the mesiodistal cuspal anatomy may have to be modified to avoid cuspal interference. To meet the needs of lateral balance and function, unorthodox location of a cusp form may be required in planning morsal anatomy (Fig. 55–16). It is well to

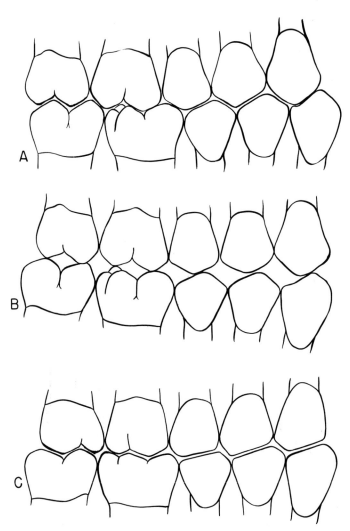

Figure 55–16 *A,* **Ideal Cuspal Relationships in Lateral Excursion,** showing intercuspation. *B,* A condition in which cuspal intercuspation is lacking in lateral excursion. *C,* The condition shown in *B* is corrected by occluso-rehabilitation. The mesial slopes of the maxillary canine and premolars and the distal slopes of the mandibular canine and premolars are modified so as to attain intercuspation. Particular note should be made of the *changed anatomy of the maxillary molars* which includes relocating the facial grooves and changing the size and location of the cusps. Such modifications vary with the individual needs according to the malposition of the teeth.

bear in mind that the typical cusp location is not always most satisfactory from a functional viewpoint.

In order to reduce lateral stresses, the inclinations of proposed cusp restorations should be modified (Fig. 55–13, A). Such modification should not be so severe as to produce flat, horizontal cusps. A flat, horizontal occlusal surface would neither function in harmony with the excursive movements of the mandible, nor would the force be applied in the long axis of the root.

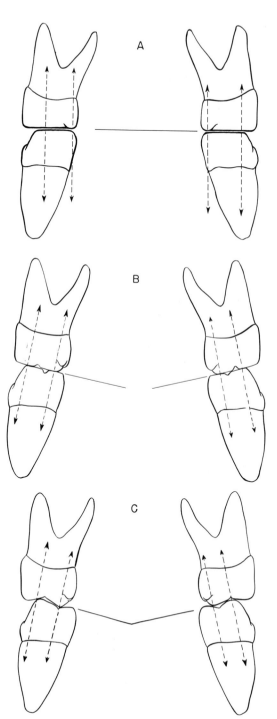

Figure 55–17 Cuspal Inclination and Modified Cusp Anatomy Necessary for Optimal Function. *A,* Flat occlusal surfaces on a horizontal plane are contraindicated. They are incompatible with the excursive movements of the mandible. The functional forces are not in line with the vertical axis of teeth. *B,* Flat occlusal surfaces, but the plane of the occlusal surface is such that the functional forces are in line with the vertical tooth axis. Note the occlusal surface sluiceways and reduced area of occlusal contact. *C,* Example of modified cusp anatomy. The functional forces are in line with the vertical tooth axis. Note the reduced area of occlusal contact.

Therefore, to accomplish the functional needs of occlusion, cusps must have suitable lateral inclinations synchronized with the lateral and protrusive movements of the mandible (Fig. 55–17). **There is a minimum cusp inclination that is required in all cases in order to assure function in all excursions of the mandible, and at the same time provide optimal forces to the periodontium.**

Modification of the cuspal anatomy referred to above is not to be construed as synonymous with establishment of arbitrary mechanical forms of the morsal surfaces. **Teeth designed with cuspal modification should be essentially anatomic in form.** In modifying the cusp, the main change is in the cusp ridge which may be markedly reduced or completely eliminated. All other details of the anatomic tooth form should be faithfully reproduced, and particular emphasis placed on correctly locating the sluiceways, spillways and accessory grooves on tooth surfaces which are contacted by the opposing cusps. This will permit the escape of food between the tooth surfaces in function. Insufficient attention to natural anatomic details leads to difficulty in mastication with possible attendant injurious stresses upon the periodontium. When teeth come into final functional positions only minimal areas of the occlusal surfaces should contact (Fig. 55–17).

VIII. Correction of Excessive Overbite

As a background for consideration of the function of the anterior teeth, it is helpful to differentiate between the process of "incision" which is carried out by the anterior teeth and chewing of food which is performed by the posterior teeth. Ideally, when food is chewed in the posterior part of the mouth, the anterior teeth are in "balanced functional relationship" (Fig. 55–14). However, if the ideal relationship between the posterior and anterior teeth in function is not attainable, it is imperative that the anterior teeth should be *free of trauma while the posterior teeth are functioning.* In all instances, as many of the anterior teeth as possible should function as a unit or group, and isolated incisal tooth contacts should be avoided.

The deep overbite case involves the consideration of the interrelationship of the anterior and posterior teeth more pointedly than any other functional problem. **A deep overbite may exist as a result of abnormal development, or be acquired from tooth loss and arch collapse (Fig. 55–18).** In both instances, the anterior teeth "lock the occlusion" so that eccentric function of the posterior teeth cannot be achieved. The anterior teeth interfere in the mandibular functional movements and are constantly being traumatized.

Orthodontic treatment is the method of choice for the reduction of excessive overbite. The qualifying limitation in the use of restorative measures for reduction of excessive overbite is the free way space and excessive increase in the crown-root ratio of the teeth. If the free way space is normal, and this is often the case in the overbite which results from abnormal development, then there is no room for increase in the height of the posterior teeth by occlusal restorations. The latter would encroach upon the free way space and would result in trauma to the periodontium, with ultimate re-establishment of the free way space and return of the excessive overbite.[14] When periodontal involvement exists, attempts to increase the posterior height and steepen the cusp inclines to harmonize with a severe anterior overbite are contraindicated. Where the periodontal involvement is not severe, the combined treatments of orthodontics, selective grinding and some restorative dentistry are helpful in selected cases of excessive overbite.

Restoring vertical dimension

In the acquired deep overbite, orthodontic treatment alone is not always feasible.[7] Acceptable compromise treatment consists of combining a minimum amount of orthodontic treatment, selective grinding, and reduction of the overbite by restorative measures, with or without increase in the vertical dimension, depending upon the individual case (Figs. 55–19 and 55–20).

When increase in the vertical dimension is indicated it is essential that this should not be accomplished at the expense of the free way space.[5, 21] If the vertical dimension is increased to such a degree that the normal free way space is reduced or obliterated,

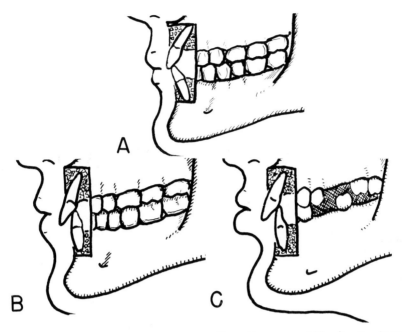

Figure 55–18 *A,* **Normal Anterior Overbite.** *B,* **Deep overbite** without appreciable alteration in vertical dimension or free way space. Occluso-rehabilitation is not feasible. Orthodontic measures are indicated. *C,* **An Acquired Deep Overbite** resulting from loss of posterior tooth support. The free way space is increased and is sufficient to permit treatment by occluso-rehabilitation, with or without supplemental orthodontic measures.

several unfavorable sequelae may result. Unless rapid wear of the occluding surfaces occurs, patient discomfort is experienced when masticating and speaking, the teeth clicking or loosening. Abnormal tooth clamping habits are induced. Subsequently, depression of teeth takes place until the normal free way space is established.[12, 20, 23] Trauma to the periodontium or temporo-mandibular joint[16] may be incurred during this process. Failure to maintain the free way space in occluso-rehabilitation is an even greater menace in patients with treated periodontal disease. The expected benefits from occluso-rehabilitation do not material-ize, but, instead, destruction of the peri-odontium is aggravated by trauma induced because of insufficient free way space.

In reduction of the overbite by restorative measures, it may not be necessary to involve the anterior teeth. Selective grinding of the anterior teeth may be sufficient. When the anterior teeth must be involved restor-atively, operative procedures are limited by the position of the pulp. It should be borne in mind that regardless of the type of treatment used in the reduction of excessive overbite, the ideal of a balanced functional relationship between the anterior and poste-rior segments of the dentition is not always attainable.

IX. Parafunctional Habits (Bruxism) and Occluso-Rehabilitation

When planning for occluso-rehabilita-tion, unless the habit of tooth grinding can be arrested or materially reduced, increase of the vertical dimension to the total amount permissible by the free way space may be contraindicated. **Continued grinding by the patient will rapidly wear restored tooth surfaces back to their former level.** In these instances, planning for the restoration of the proper tooth relationships should in-corporate minimal change in the vertical dimension wherever possible. On the other hand, when the teeth are not being used sufficiently, it is important to instruct the patient regarding the need for adequate use of the teeth to help prevent unfavorable changes in the tooth relationships following occluso-rehabilitation. **The use of similar materials on rebuilt occluding surfaces is of prime importance to maintain even wear.**

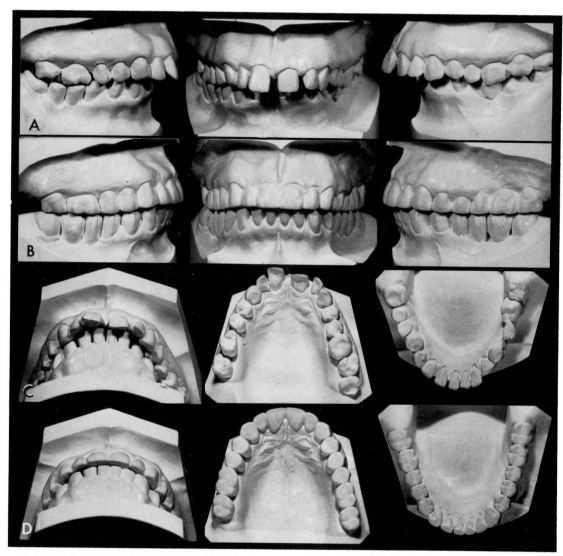

Figure 55–19 Deep Overbite and Overjet Corrected by Occluso-Rehabilitation. *A,* Before treatment. Front and side views in centric occlusion showing deep overbite and overjet. *B,* After treatment. Overbite and overjet corrected by the following procedures: (1) Orthodontic correction of maxillary anterior segment. (2) Restoration of all the maxillary teeth and the mandibular posterior teeth with acrylic faced gold crowns. (3) Increase in vertical dimension. Note change in the line of occlusion by comparing the side views in *A* and *B. C,* Before treatment. Note extent of overbite (*left*). Note missing maxillary first molar and mandibular molars which accentuated the overbite. *D,* After treatment. Note reduction in the overbite. Anterior teeth are out of contact in centric occlusion. However, contact is made in functional excursions. Excellent maxillary and mandibular arch form, modified cuspal contours and realignment of the mandibular anteriors established by occluso-rehabilitation. Stability of non-splinted mandibular anterior teeth attained by corrected proximal and functional relationships.

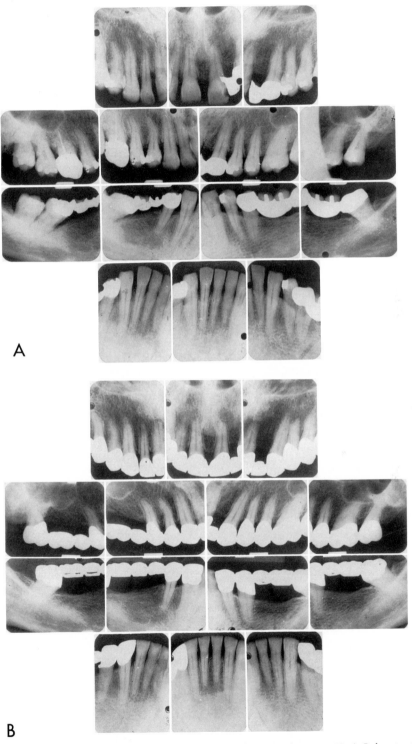

Figure 55–20   Before and After Correction of Overbite. Patient Shown in Figure 55–19. *A,* Before treatment. *B,* Seven years after treatment. Compare with *A* and note improvement in the appearance of the bone in the following areas: maxillary anterior, mandibular and maxillary third molars (*left*). Also note fixed splinting by multiple restorations.

X. The Use of Removable Prosthesis in Occluso-Rehabilitation

Wherever possible, a fixed prosthesis should be employed to supply missing teeth in occluso-rehabilitation because it is the best means of stabilizing teeth. When a removable prosthesis is used, several qualifying limitations should be borne in mind (Chap. 54).

Removable prosthetic replacements are supported by the abutment teeth as well as by the tissues overlying the edentulous areas. The abutment teeth are subjected to increased functional demands. To reduce the load on the abutments, a balance should be effected between the tissues under the saddle area of the appliance and the abutment teeth.[18] A precise prosthetic technique is needed to assure this result. The form of the edentulous areas should be procured by a separate impression which registers the tissues in their relaxed state without displacement or compression.[17] This type of impression, ("mucostatic") is obtained by using an individually fitted tray adjusted in the mouth to be free of all muscular interferences. Any zinc oxide-eugenol paste that will flow freely and set rigidly may be used. From a model secured from this impression a metallic base is accurately constructed. The base is positioned in the mouth and an impression taken to establish its proper relationship to the abutment teeth. This technique fosters equalized distribution of functional stresses between the tissues in the edentulous areas and the periodontium of the abutment teeth.

Precision attachments or a suitably designed clasp with a vertical rest which fits into a restoration on the abutment tooth, such as the Gillette or Neurohr types, serve as satisfactory retainers.

The functional relationships of the teeth on removable partial dentures as well as the natural teeth must be harmoniously articulated to the individual mandibular movements.

XI. The Use of Fixed Prosthesis in Occluso-Rehabilitation

Fixed bridges serve both to replace missing teeth and to establish proper occlusal relationships in the dentition. **When con-** structing extensive fixed bridge replacements, multiple abutments are indicated to prevent mobility or to reduce it.[15]

Splinting with fixed prosthesis

Splinting with fixed prosthesis is employed for three purposes:

1. To stabilize mobile natural teeth where no teeth are missing.

2. To supply missing teeth and simultaneously stabilize mobile natural teeth.

3. To prevent firm natural abutment teeth from becoming loose.

The number of teeth required to stabilize a loose tooth depends upon the degree and direction of mobility, the amount of remaining bone, the location of the mobile tooth in the arch and whether or not it is to be used as an abutment. As a general rule, the mesiodistal component of tooth mobility is reduced, with greater facility than mobility in other directions. This is so because the approximating teeth in the arch aid in the tooth support. For the stabilization of faciolingual movement, sole reliance is of necessity placed upon the firm teeth included in the splint. In general, it is safer to use more than one firm tooth to support a mobile tooth. **If more than one mobile tooth is to be splinted, then the number of firm teeth required for stable splinting increases.** The exact number of firm teeth which must be included in such a splint varies, depending upon the individual conditions (Fig. 55–21).

When a fixed bridge is used to both supply missing teeth and stabilize natural teeth, attention should be directed to the following considerations; **If the distal abutment tooth of the bridge is the terminal tooth in the arch, and is mobile, multiple firm anterior abutments are required to stabilize the restoration.** In some instances, the degree of the terminal tooth mobility precludes satisfactory splinting with fixed prosthesis, and it is necessary to resort to a bilateral removable partial denture. Splinting with fixed prosthesis entails the use of mesio-occluso-distal inlays, three-quarter crowns or full crowns. All restorations used in splinting must be particularly well constructed to resist displacement forces. **The individual units of the splint should be soldered together; semi-fixed attachments should not be used (Fig. 55–22).**

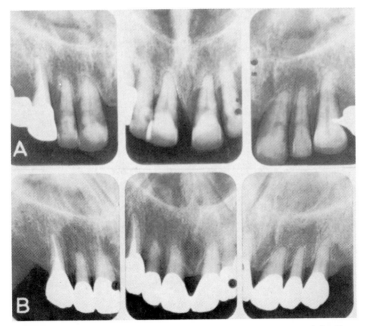

Figure 55–21 **Pathologic Migration With Advanced Periodontal Disease Corrected by Treatment of the Tissues, Orthodontic Measures, Fixed Splinting, and Modification of the Crown-Root Ratio.** *A,* Radiographs before treatment. *B,* After two years, marked improvement in the qualitative appearance of the bone and also in the bone height. Note that the overall length of teeth has been reduced in the treatment procedure. This is not the result of technical variations in obtaining the radiographs.

The physical support gained by splinting is also of value in preventing injury from **tooth-clamping habits.** If the hyperfunctional state cannot be aided by other therapy, a fixed splint should be used. Clamping habits vary, so that different areas of the dentition may be subjected to trauma. The splint should include uninvolved teeth as well as those in the involved area. This will reduce mobility of the involved teeth.

In cases in which some question exists regarding the number of teeth to be in-

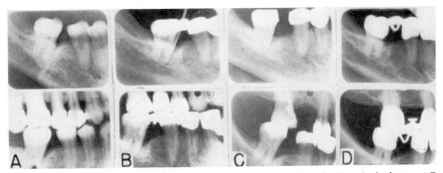

Figure 55–22 **Example Depicting the Need for Rigid Fixation When a Posterior Terminal Abutment Tooth is Periodonally Involved.** *A,* Original condition: Note the bone loss in relation to the mandibular molar. Following periodontal treatment, a fixed bridge was inserted to restore the missing tooth. It was anchored rigidly to the posterior tooth but was attached anteriorly by means of a precision rest. Despite the corrected occlusion and accuracy of the fit of the rest, faciolingual movement in function was not adequately restricted. *B,* Three years later: The periodontal condition was aggravated as a result of the improperly connected bridge. *C,* The bridge was removed. Periodontal treatment for the mandibular terminal molar was reinstituted and a new fixed bridge was inserted, rigidly connected to both the anterior and posterior abutment teeth. (The maxillary premolar was removed because of a root fracture.) *D,* After six years. Note improvement in the bone height.

cluded in a fixed splint, a temporary acrylic splint should be inserted on the prepared teeth for a short period of time* to test whether or not the mobility is reduced. Such a trial will indicate the need for including additional firm teeth in the splint.

Splinting is the added mechanical factor used to prevent, reduce or eliminate tooth movement. Alone, it is not always sufficient to accomplish the desired goal. To obtain

*The time interval of a test varies. At most, two months may be needed to evaluate the benefits of the temporary splinting. If stability is to be attained it will occur during that period. It is important that the temporary splint be constructed in conformity with correct functional relationships and not violate any of the fundamentals of occluso-rehabilitation. Splinted units should be watched carefully and the teeth under question observed frequently for change in mobility status.

maximum benefits, splinting should be combined with redesign of the crown surface, and the teeth should be in functional harmony with the mandibular movements of the patient (Figs. 55–23 to 55–25).

GENERAL CONSIDERATIONS REGARDING OCCLUSO-REHABILITATION

A properly functioning occlusion cannot always be established by the transfer of a "bite" from the mouth to the articulator, followed by building the occlusion on the articulator and then transferring it back to the mouth without change or adjustment. There are a number of considerations which influence mechanical constructions in transfer between the articulator and the

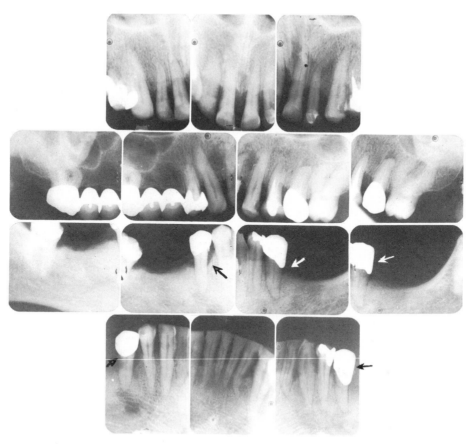

Figure 55–23 Radiographs of a Case of Periodontal Disease in a Forty-Four Year Old Patient With a Tooth-Clamping and Grinding Habit. There is generalized bone loss. Note particularly the mandibular left and right second premolars (*arrows*) which are serving as abutment teeth for a partial denture.

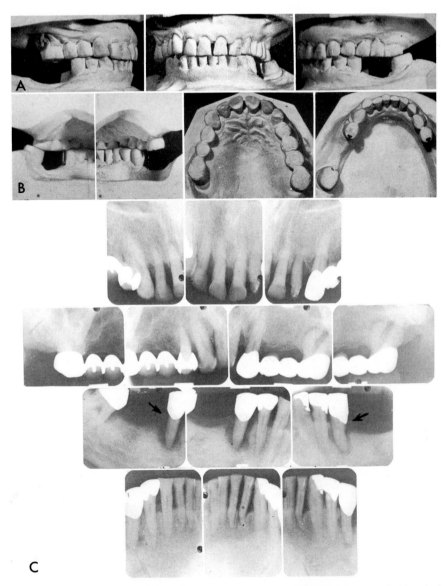

Figure 55–24   Casts and Radiographs of Case Shown in Figure 55–23 After Seven Years. *A,* Note lack of harmony between the occlusal line of the posterior teeth in relation to the anterior teeth. *B,* Note that the maxillary lingual cusps are not in the middle areas of the mandibular teeth. Also note incorrect arch form and incongruity in cuspal contours in various parts of the mouth. *C,* The mandibular premolars had been splinted to the first premolars for a period of seven years. Despite this fact, the periodontal condition had become progressively worse (compare with Fig. 55–23). Sufficient attention had not been given to establishing satisfactory functional relationships.

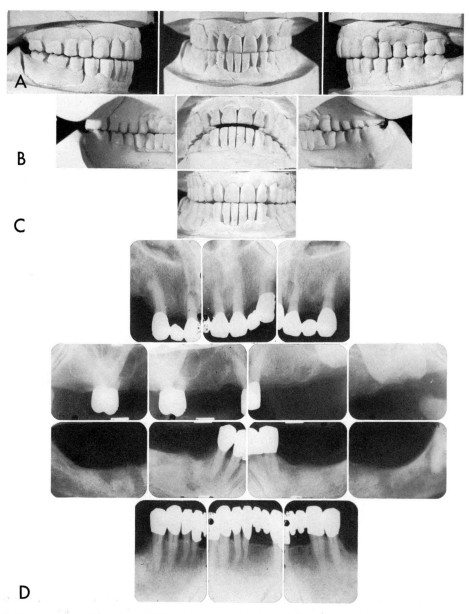

Figure 55–25 Four Years After the Institution of Occluso-Rehabilitation to Correct the Conditions Shown in Figure 55–24. *A,* Casts in centric occlusion. Compare with Figure 55–24. *B,* Note proper position of the lingual cusps of the maxillary posterior teeth in the middle areas of the mandibular teeth. Also note dis-occlusion of the anterior teeth. *C,* The anterior teeth are in contact in the protrusive position. There is simultaneous contact of the posterior teeth. *D,* Radiograph showing fixed splinting. Note improvement in the bone picture as compared with Figure 55–24. Note that the anterior missing teeth are replaced as part of a fixed splint and not by the removable denture which supplies the posterior teeth.

mouth.[19] These depend on the method of transfer, the skill of the operator and the biological adaptability of the involved structures.

While a discussion of technique is not part of the context of this chapter, whatever method is used in occluso-rehabilitation, the new tooth relationships should be tested by the following wax bite method before and after final cementation, and at periodic intervals thereafter. Wax check bites are taken in all functional positions. These should always show an even distribution of forces as evidenced by the thinning out of a standard thickness of a base plate wax which has been thoroughly softened and placed between the opposing arches. Uneven perforations are an indication of imbalance in the occlusion and should be rectified by selectively grinding the teeth concerned. Any new relationship of the crown surfaces of the teeth requires an equilibrium between the periodontium, the muscles of mastication, the temporomandibular joint and the mucosal base support of the partial denture, if used.

In the final analysis, the value of occluso-rehabilitation can only be proved by response of the tissues. Any concept of occluso-rehabilitation, if it is to serve a useful purpose in oral health, must demonstrate clinical and radiographic evidence of its value as an adjunct in the treatment of periodontal disease. Mobile teeth should return to firmness, and the healthy color, tone and texture of the gingivae attained by periodontal therapy should be maintained. Radiographically, the periodontal space, lamina dura and the density of the bone should be restored to normal. In some instances, the height of bone in relation to the teeth may be increased. **It should be borne in mind that dental restorations are subject to wear and change; therefore periodic supervision is necessary for all cases of occluso-rehabilitation, particularly those in patients with treated periodontal disease.**

REFERENCES

1. Burch, J. G.: Ten Rules for Developing Crown Contours in Restorations. Dent. Clin. North America., 15:611, 1971.
2. Clayton, J. A., Kotowicz, W. E., and Myers, G. E.: Graphic Recordings of Mandibular Movements: Research Criteria. J. Prosth. Dent., 25:287, 1971.
3. Glickman, I.: Role of Occlusion in the Etiology and Treatment of Periodontal disease. J. D. Res., 50:199, 1971.
4. Glickman, I., Martignoni, M., Haddad, A., and Roeber, F. W.: Further Observations on Human Occlusion Monitored by Intraoral Telemetry. I.A.D.R. Abstracts, #612, 1970, p. 201.
5. Harris, H. L.: Effect of Loss of Vertical Dimension on Anatomic Structures of the Head and Neck. J.A.D.A., 25:175, 1938.
6. Hirschfeld, I.: The Individual Missing Tooth, A Factor in Dental and Periodontal Disease. J.A.D.A., 24:67, 1937.
7. Lee, R. L., and Gregory, G. G.: Gaining Vertical Dimension for the Deep Bite Restorative Patient. Dent. Clin. North America, 15:743, 1971.
8. Lindblom, G.: The Importance of Balanced Occlusion. D. Record, 59:1, 1939.
9. Lindblom, G.: The Term "Balanced Articulation," Its Origin, Development and Present Significance in Modern Odontology. D. Record, 69:304, 1949.
10. McCollum, B. B.: Fundamentals Involved in Prescribing Restorative Dental Remedies. D. Items Int., 61:522, 1939.
11. McLean, D. W.: Physiologic vs. Pathologic Occlusion. J.A.D.A., 25:1593, 1938.
12. Mershon, J. V.: Possibilities and Limitations in the Treatment of Closed Bites. Internat. J. Orthodont., 23:581, 1937.
13. Morris, M. L.: Artificial Crown Contour and Gingival Health. J. Prosth. Dent., 12:1146, 1962.
14. Niswonger, M. E.: The Rest Position of the Mandible and the Centric Relation. J.A.D.A., 21:1572, 1934.
15. Pugh, C. E., and Smerke, J. W.: Rationale for Fixed Prostheses in the Management of Advanced Periodontal Disease. Dent. Clin. North America, 13:243, 1969.
16. Riesner, S. E.: Temporomandibular Reaction to Occlusal Anomalies. J.A.D.A., 25:1938, 1938.
17. Rudd, K. D., and Dunn, B. W.: Accurate Removable Partial Dentures. J. Prosth. Dent., 18:559, 1967.
18. Rudd, K. D., and O'Leary, T. J.: Stabilizing Periodontally Weakened Teeth by Using Guide Plane Removable Partial Dentures: A Preliminary Report. J. Prosth. Dent., 16:721, 1966.
19. Schuyler, C. H.: Intra-Oral Method of Establishing Maxillo-Mandibular Relation. J.A.D.A., 19:1012, 1932.
20. Schuyler, C. H.: Problems Associated with Opening the Bite Which Would Contraindicate It as a Common Procedure. J.A.D.A., 26:734, 1939.
21. Sloane, R. B.: Kinesiology and Vertical Dimension. J. Pros. Den., 2:12, 1952.
22. Stallard, H.: The Anterior Component of the Force of Mastication and Its Significance to the Dental Apparatus. D. Cosmos, 65:457, 1923.
23. Thompson, J. R.: The Rest Position of the Mandible and Its Significance to Dental Science. J.A.D.A., 33:151, 1946.
24. Thompson, J. R., and Brodie, A. G.: Factors in the Position of the Mandible. J.A.D.A., 29:925, 1942.
25. Wheeler, R. C.: Complete Crown Form and the Periodontium. J. Prosth. Dent., 11:722, 1961.

Chapter 56

PERIODONTAL-ORTHODONTIC INTERRELATIONSHIPS

ORTHODONTIC PROCEDURES IN PERIODONTAL TREATMENT

Orthodontic procedures to restore satisfactory functional relationships[1, 8, 14, 15] are often required in periodontal therapy. The advisability of undertaking orthodontic correction depends upon the following factors: (1) the severity of the occlusal problem and its correctability by orthodontics, (2) the level of the remaining bone and (3) the possibility of the periodontal and occlusal conditions worsening without orthodontic correction. Reduced bony support as the result of periodontal disease does not contraindicate orthodontic treatment unless the remaining bone is insufficient to withstand ordinary functional requirements. **Reposi-**tioning teeth in the bone so as to direct occlusal forces in the vertical axis increases the longevity of teeth with reduced bony support.

Gingival and periodontal disease interfere with the effectiveness of orthodontic appliances and should be eliminated before orthodontic treatment is begun. Inflammation causes degeneration of periodontal ligament fibers and impairs their ability to transmit external forces to the bone. This dissipates the orthodontic forces and delays the desired bone response and tooth movement.

Teeth can often be repositioned in relatively uncomplicated mechanotherapy with the Hawley appliance, grassline or wire ligatures or rubber dam elastics, either singly or in combination. **No tooth movement should be undertaken before the patient's problem has been thoroughly analyzed.** Supposedly "minor tooth movement" may lead to unexpected complications unless it is planned in conformity with the overall pattern of forces involved in the maintenance of tooth-to-tooth and arch-to-arch relationships.

Correction of Pathologic Migration

The following factors should be considered when orthodontic correction of migrated teeth is contemplated:

1. The availability of space for the teeth to be repositioned.

2. The absence of interference from teeth in the opposing arch.

3. The extent to which loss of posterior tooth support, reduced vertical dimension and accentuated anterior overbite complicate tooth movement.

4. The availability of sufficient anchorage from which forces can be applied.

5. Habits which may interfere with the desired tooth movement.

Hawley appliance for the correction of pathologic migration

The Hawley appliance is a removable, tissue-borne appliance with an anterior wire frame extension or labial bow. It may be modified in a variety of ways for moving individual teeth (Fig. 56–1) and is most often used on the maxilla. The tissue-borne portion covers the palate, is usually con-structed of acrylic, and may have clasps on the posterior teeth for added retention. To prevent irritation to the gingiva it should cover approximately one third the length of the crowns. The margin is cut away when necessary to create space for the desired tooth movement.

The labial bow is embedded in the acrylic and extends through the interproximal spaces between the canines and premolars onto the facial surfaces of the anterior teeth (Fig. 56–1). When used on the mandible, the tissue-borne portion is horseshoe shaped, and may be made of acrylic or metal, depending upon the strength required.

To correct pathologic migration of maxil-lary anterior teeth, the wire labial bow or rubber dam elastics attached to hooks em-

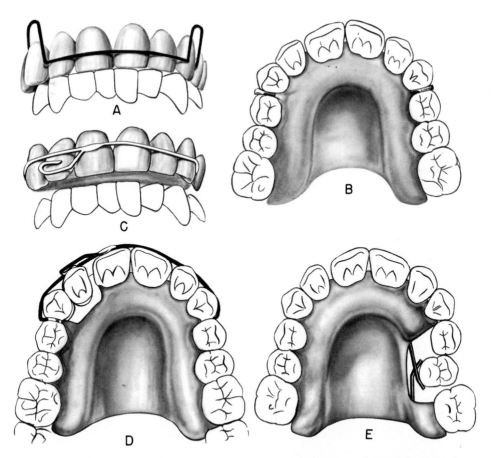

Figure 56–1 The Hawley Appliance. *A,* Hawley appliance with labial bow. *B,* Acrylic tissue-borne portion covers ap-proximately one third of the length of the crowns. *C,* Wire soldered to labial bow to move lateral incisor. The palatal acrylic is used as an anterior bite palate. *D,* Palatal view showing acrylic cut away to provide space for the lateral incisor. *E,* Wire spring embedded in acrylic to move the second premolar buccally. If necessary the proximal tooth surfaces are stripped to provide space.

bedded in the acrylic at the distal surface of each canine are used. The appliance should be worn at all times until the desired tooth movements are affected (Fig. 56–2).

When excessive overbite interferes with the movement of the anterior teeth, the acrylic may be brought onto the occlusal surfaces of the posterior teeth to create enough space anteriorly to permit the lingual movement of the maxillary anterior teeth (Fig. 56–3). After the desired anterior tooth movement is attained, the Hawley appliance is replaced by prosthesis on the posterior teeth to retain the vertical dimension.

When the mandibular anterior teeth are procumbent so that there is insufficient overjet to permit lingual movement of the maxillary teeth, the mandibular teeth are retracted to provide the necessary space.

Stabilization of migrated anterior teeth

After the migration has been corrected, an effort is made to create an environment in which the teeth will be stable, without artificial retention. The entire occlusion is adjusted to eliminate prematurities that would tend to displace the teeth. Grinding the anterior teeth alone may leave the patient with posterior prematurities that deflect the mandible anteriorly against the maxillary teeth and cause them to migrate again. Tongue-thrusting habits, grinding and clenching also tend to displace the teeth, particularly those with weakened periodontal support.

If the teeth tend to separate after the occlusion is adjusted, they should be stabilized with fixed internal retention. The teeth are brought back into position and splinted from first premolar to first premolar with inlays which require a minimal loss of tooth structure.

Correction of Malposed Teeth

Grassline ligatures and rubber dam elastics[9] are useful for the correction of malposed individual teeth. With grassline ligatures, tooth movement is effected by contraction of the ligature after it absorbs moisture from the mouth. The dry ligature is applied in such a manner that the force created by contraction is in the direction of

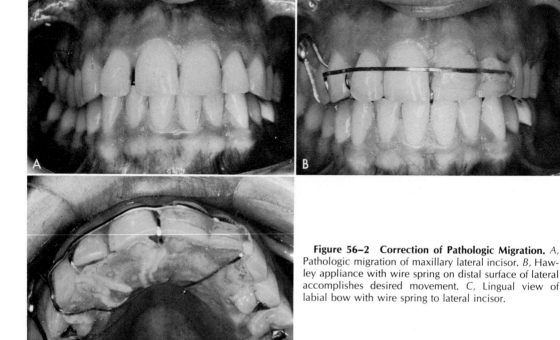

Figure 56–2 Correction of Pathologic Migration. *A,* Pathologic migration of maxillary lateral incisor. *B,* Hawley appliance with wire spring on distal surface of lateral accomplishes desired movement. *C,* Lingual view of labial bow with wire spring to lateral incisor.

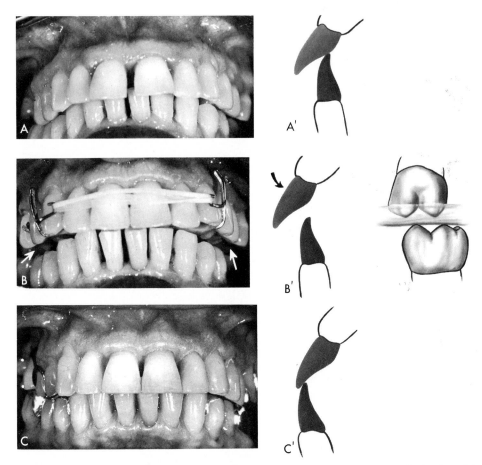

Figure 56–3 Correction of Excessive Overbite and Pathologic Migration by Combining Orthodontic and Prosthetic Procedures. *A,* Excessive anterior overbite and spacing of anterior teeth in patient with periodontal disease. *A',* diagrammatic representation of anterior overbite. *B,* Hawley appliance used to correct migration of anterior teeth using elastics. The acrylic portion of the appliance is extended over the occlusal surfaces of the posterior teeth (*arrows*) to increase the vertical dimension and permit lingual movement of maxillary anterior teeth. The appliance is constructed of clear acrylic which is not visible on the photograph. *B',* Space created between anterior teeth by using posterior acrylic bite plane. *C,* Prosthesis constructed to retain newly established vertical dimension. *C',* Newly established relationships of anterior teeth.

desired tooth movement. Particular care must be taken to include a sufficient number of teeth for anchorage (Figs. 56–4 and 56–5). **The ligature should be placed close to the contact points, incisal to the cingulum, to prevent slipping and irritation of the gingiva.** Ligatures are usually replaced weekly until the desired tooth movement is attained.

Teeth can be moved more rapidly with rubber dam elastics, with a greater risk of damage to the supporting tissues. Rootward sliding of the band with injury to the periodontium and extrusion of teeth are infrequent complications of the use of rubber dam elastics.

Crowded mandibular anterior teeth

Crowded and malposed teeth frequently present a problem from both the periodontal and orthodontic viewpoints (Fig. 56–6). The gingiva around teeth in labial version is often attached apical to the level on the adjacent teeth. On teeth in lingual version, the labial gingiva is often enlarged and attracts irritating plaque and debris. Orthodontic correction of malposed teeth creates gingival contours more conductive to periodontal health (Fig. 53–6, *C*).

A tooth may be extracted to correct crowding (Fig. 56–7), provided it creates sufficent space for proper alignment of the

(Text continued on page 961)

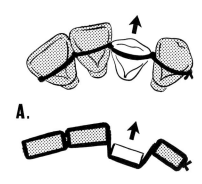

A.

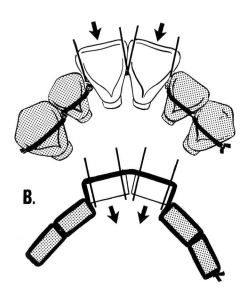

B.

Figure 56–4 Grassline Ligature to Correct Malposition. *A,* Repositioning of lingually placed lateral incisor. *B,* Two labially placed central incisors are brought into proper alignment. The proximal surfaces of the incisors may be trimmed (*vertical lines*) to fit into available space.

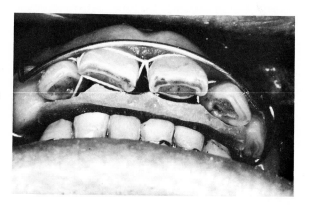

Figure 56–5 Grassline Ligature used in conjunction with bite plate to correct rotated teeth.

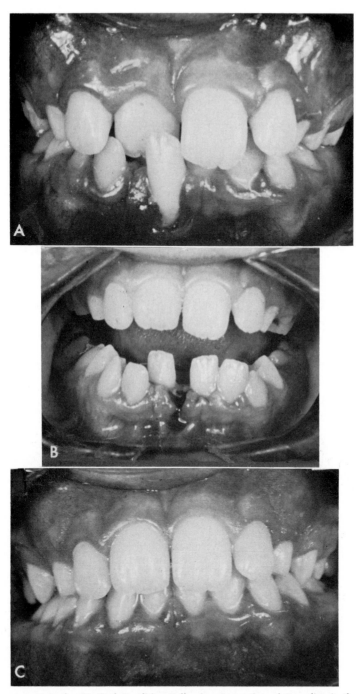

Figure 56–6 Improvement in the Gingival Condition Following Correction of Crowding in the Mandibular Anterior Region. *A,* Marked gingival disease associated with malocclusion. *B,* Central incisor removed. *C,* Improved condition of the gingiva associated with improvement in the tooth relationship after orthodontic treatment. (Courtesy Dr. Coenraad F. A. Moorrees, Forsyth Dental Center.)

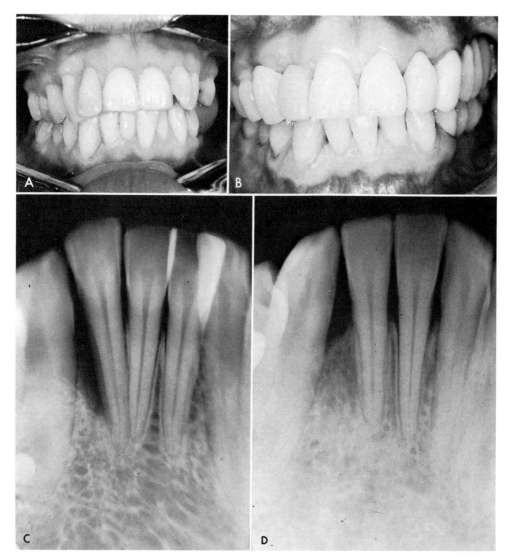

Figure 56–7 Improvement in the Condition of the Bone Following Correction of Anterior Irregularity. *A,* Crowding of mandibular teeth with left central incisor in labial version. *B,* After treatment which included extraction of the right lateral incisor, alignment of the anterior teeth and prosthesis. *C,* Before treatment. Note the angular bone defect. *D,* Three years after treatment. Note improvement in the bone. (Restorations by Dr. Philip Williams, Lynn, Mass.)

teeth which remain. Another consideration when tooth extraction is being considered is the degree of overbite. Normally the mandibular teeth are "contained within" the maxillary arch. Extraction of a mandibular incisor may result in "closing in" of the arch with increase in the overbite and the possibility of undersirable periodontal sequelae.

Another consideration when tooth extraction is contemplated is the mechanics required to realign the remaining teeth without proximal tipping. Improper proximal contacts create areas of potential food impaction. Where possible it is preferable to avoid tooth extraction by judicious grinding of the proximal surfaces to create space for the crowded teeth (Fig. 56–8).

Crossbite relationship

Crossbite relationships often result in food impaction and trauma from occlusion. A comparatively simple procedure may be used effectively to correct single teeth in labial, buccal or lingual version if space in the arch permits. The malposed tooth on each arch is banded with a hook on the facial surface of the tooth in buccal version and the lingual surface of its antagonist. A "cross" elastic attached to the hooks

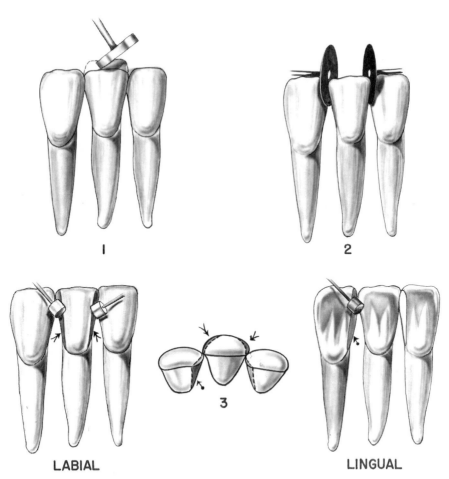

LABIAL   LINGUAL

Figure 56–8 Grinding as an Adjunct to the Treatment of Malposed and Extruded Anterior Teeth. *1,* Reduction of the incisal edge of a prominent mandibular anterior tooth. *2,* Grinding of the proximal surfaces of a mandibular tooth in labial version as well as the proximal surfaces of the adjacent teeth to provide space for proper alignment. *3,* Where space cannot be provided by grinding the proximal surfaces as illustrated in (2), the mesial and distal aspects of the labial surface of the malposed tooth are reduced along with the marginal ridges on the lingual surfaces of the adjacent teeth.

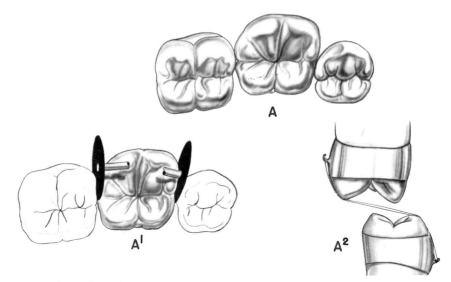

Figure 56–9 Crossbite Relationship of First Molars Corrected by Intermaxillary Elastics. *A,* Mandibular first molar in buccal version. *A¹,* Reduction of the mesiodistal diameter to permit the molar to fit into the available space. *A²,* Orthodontic bands and intermaxillary elastic in position.

results in the restoration of proper alignment (Fig. 56–9). The occlusion should then be adjusted.

Occasionally an anterior crossbite occurs in patients with a pseudoprognathic mandibular relationship. The maxillary teeth are in lingual version, but the anterior teeth are edge-to-edge when the mandible is retruded (Fig. 56–10, *A* and *B*). The condition may sometimes be corrected with a Hawley appliance by temporarily opening the bite and pushing the maxillary anterior teeth forward, but comprehensive mechanotherapy on both jaws is often required (Fig. 56–10, *C*).

Correction of Anterior Open Bite

An anterior open bite may impair periodontal health if attended by inadequate functional stimulation to the gingiva and the supporting tissues. Some of the undesirable sequelae include accumulation of plaque and food debris with resultant chronic gingivitis, atrophy of the alveolar bone around the anterior teeth and trauma to the periodontium of the posterior teeth. Bites which are slightly open anteriorly may be reduced by judiciously grinding the posterior teeth; but if this is not feasible, orthodontic therapy is indicated.

OCCLUSAL ADJUSTMENT IN ORTHODONTIC THERAPY

Occlusal forces created by orthodontically corrected dentitions affect the condition of the periodontium upon which the stability of the renovated occlusion depends. The anatomic and esthetic goals of orthodontics have been expanded to include the attainment of satisfactory occlusal relationships, and occlusal adjustment has become an integral part of orthodontic therapy.

Occlusion During Active Orthodontic Treatment

The periodontal tissues cannot differentiate between the forces of occlusion and those created by orthodontic appliances. Both types of forces are transmitted to the periodontium together, and tooth movement results from their combined effect rather than from the appliances alone. Injurious occlusal forces in the course of tooth movement detract from the efficiency of orthodontic appliances. Unfavorable occlusal forces may be unavoidable during tooth movement, but the damage they produce should be minimized by checking the occlusion each time appliances are adjusted and correcting gross prematurities in centric

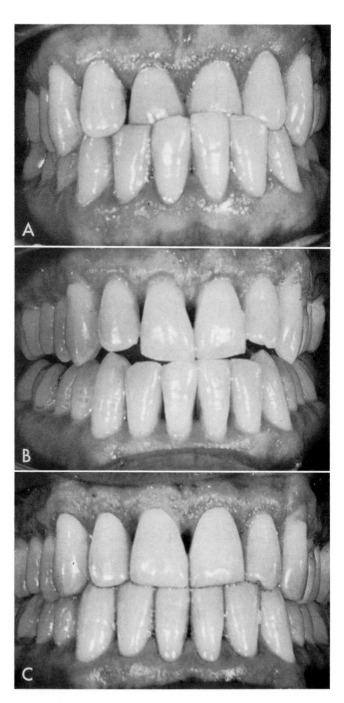

Figure 56–10 Anterior Crossbite Relationship. *A,* Patient with anterior crossbite and associated periodontal disease. *B,* Determination of centric indices that the crossbite is a "habitual" occlusion and that the anterior teeth are edge to edge when the mandible is in centric. *C,* After periodontal treatment which includes orthodontic correction (compare with *A*).

and habitual occlusion (for occlusal adjustment, see Chap. 53).

Occlusion During and After the Retention Period

Orthodontic therapy is incomplete so long as the dentition functions so as to injure the periodontium. The occlusion should be adjusted before and during the retention period for several reasons: injurious occlusal forces during the retention period interfere with the maturation of bone and the stabilization of tooth position, and may defeat the purpose of the retaining device. Teeth held firmly in a retaining device are more vulnerable to trauma from occlusion because they cannot move away from injurious forces.

After retainers are removed, uncontrolled drifting of the teeth ("settling in") cannot be relied upon to provide satisfactorily functioning occlusion. Teeth may "settle into" positions which are esthetically acceptable and meet the requirements of static jaw relationships, but the dentition must be checked in function. "Settling in" should be accompanied by occlusal adjustment to avoid trauma which injures the periodontium and increases the risk of collapse of the newly created occlusion.

Hawley appliances should not be used as permanent retainers in orthodontically treated patients; they are periodontally contraindicated. The appliances are usually worn at night with the result that the periodontium is injured and the teeth become loosened from the interplay between daytime pressures in one direction and nighttime pressures in the other. Young adults who do not wear their appliance until spaces reappear between their teeth create greater periodontal damage when they try to force the teeth back into the retainer.

For teeth with a persistent tendency toward migration after orthodontic therapy, the interest of the periodontium is best served by adjusting the entire occlusion and splinting the offending teeth into the adjusted occlusion.

PERIODONTAL PROBLEMS ASSOCIATED WITH ORTHODONTIC THERAPY

RETENTION OF PLAQUE. Orthodontic appliances tend to retain irritating plaque and food debris, which cause gingivitis (Fig. 56–11). Patients should be taught proper oral hygiene methods when applances are inserted, and their importance should be stressed. The condition of the periodontium should be checked regularly during orthodontic treatment and periodontal care instituted at the earliest sign of gingival disease. Water irrigation under pressure is a helpful oral hygiene aid for these patients.

IRRITATION FROM ORTHODONTIC BANDS. Orthodontic treatment is often started at a stage of tooth eruption when the epithelial attachment is still on the enamel. The bands should not extend into the gingival tissues beyond the level of attachment. Forceful detachment of the gingiva from the tooth followed by apical proliferation of the epithelial attachment results in increased gingival recession sometimes seen in orthodontically treated patients.[11] If gingival inflammation is present, the gingival margin is prevented from following the migrating epithelium and pocket formation results.

TISSUE RESPONSE TO ORTHODONTIC FORCES. Orthodontic tooth movement is possible because the periodontal tissues are responsive to externally applied forces.[12, 14] The bone is remodeled by an increase in osteoclasts and bone resorption in areas of pressure, and by increased osteoblastic activity and bone formation in areas of tension. Orthodontic forces also produce vascular changes in the periodontal ligament which may influence the bone resorptive and bone formative patterns.[4, 7]

Radioautographic and histochemical studies indicate that cellular proliferation in the periodontal ligament may be related to the magnitude of orthodontic forces;[17] that alkaline phosphatase in periodontal ligament cells is decreased in areas of pressure;[16] and that oxidative enzyme activity is intensified in the periodontium in areas of orthodontically induced bone resorption and formation.[5]

TISSUE INJURY FROM ORTHODONTIC FORCES. From the periodontal viewpoint, it is important to avoid excessive forces and too rapid tooth movement in orthodontic treatment. Excessive force may produce necrosis of the periodontal ligament and adjacent alveolar bone, which ordinarily undergo repair. However, destruction of the periodontal ligament at the crest of the alveolar bone may lead to

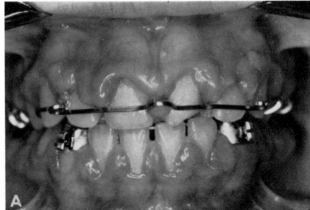
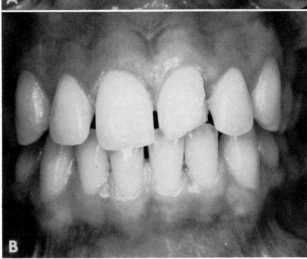

Figure 56–11 Gingival Inflammation and Enlargement Associated with Orthodontic Appliance and Poor Oral Hygiene. *A,* Gingival disease with orthodontic appliance in place. *B,* After removal of the appliance and periodontal treatment.

irreparable damage. If the periodontal fibers beneath the epithelial attachment are destroyed by excessive force and the epithelium is stimulated to proliferate along the root by local irritants, **the epithelium will cover the root and prevent re-embedding of the periodontal fibers in the course of repair. Absence of functional stimulation from the periodontal fibers may result in atrophy of the crest of the alveolar bone.** Excessive orthodontic forces also increase the risk of apical root resorption.[18]

It has been reported that the marginal and attached gingiva are "pulled" when teeth are orthodontically rotated,[6] and that relapse of the occlusion after orthodontic treatment can be reduced by surgical resection or removal of free gingival fibers, combined with a brief retention period.[3, 10] Temporary separation of the reduced enamel epithelium on the tension side of orthodontically moved teeth and displace-

ment and folding of the interdental papillae on the pressure side have also been noted.[2]

REFERENCES

1. Alexander, P. C.: Orthodontic Procedures in Periodontal Therapy. J. Periodont., *28*:46, 1957.
2. Atherton, J. D., and Kerr, N. W.: Effect of Orthodontic Tooth Movement upon the Gingivae. Brit. D. J., *124*:555, 1968.
3. Brain, W. E.: The Effect of Surgical Transsection of Free Gingival Fibers on the Regression of Orthodontically Rotated Teeth in the Dog. Am. J. Orthodont., *55*:50, 1969.
4. Castelli, W. A., and Dempster, W. T.: The Periodontal Vasculature and Its Responses to Experimental Pressures. J.A.D.A., *70*:891, 1965.
5. Deguchi, T., and Mori, M.: Histochemical Observations on Oxidative Enzymes in Periodontal Tissues During Experimental Tooth Movement in the Rat. Arch. Oral Biol., *13*:49, 1968.
6. Edwards, J. G., A Study of the Periodontium During Orthodontic Rotation of Teeth. Am. J. Orthodont., *54*:441, 1968.

7. Gianelly, A. A.: Force-Induced Changes in the Vascularity of the Periodontal Ligament. Am. J. Orthodont., 55:5, 1969.
8. Granerus, R.: Some Orthodontic-Therapeutic Aspects of the Treatment of Periodontal Diseases. Sveriges Tandlak. Forb. Tidn., 47:455, 1955.
9. Hirschfeld, L., and Geiger, A.: Minor Tooth Movement in General Practice. St. Louis, C. V. Mosby Co., 1966.
10. Moffett, B. C.: Remodeling Changes of the Facial Sutures, Periodontal and Temporomandibular Joints Produced by Orthodontic Forces in Rhesus Monkeys. Bull. Pacif. Coast Soc. Orthodont., 44:46, 1969.
11. Pearson, L. E.: Gingival Height of Lower Central Incisors, Orthodontically Treated and Untreated. Angle Orthodont., 38:337, 1968.
12. Reitan, K.: Tissue Changes Following Experimental Tooth Movement as Related to the Time Factor. D. Record, 73:559, 1953.
13. Rothenberg, S., and Shapiro, E.: The Orthodontic Management of Functional Problems in Periodontal Therapy. Dent. Clin. North America, March, 1960, p. 143.
14. Schwartz, A. M.: Tissue Changes Incidental to Orthodontic Tooth Movement. Ortho., Oral Surg. and Rad., Int. J., 18:331, 1932.
15. Shapiro, M.: Orthodontic Procedures in the Care of the Periodontal Patient. J. Periodont., 27:7, 1956.
16. Takimoto, K., Deguchi, T., and Mori, M.: Histochemical Detection of Acid and Alkaline Phosphatases in Periodontal Tissues After Experimental Tooth Movement. J. D. Res., 47:340, 1968.
17. Tayer, B. H., Gianelly, A. A., and Ruben, M. P.: Visualization of Cellular Dynamics Associated with Orthodontic Tooth Movement. Am. J. Orthodont., 54:515, 1968.
18. Tirk, T. M., Guzman, C. A., and Nalchajian, R.: Periodontal Tissue Response to Orthodontic Treatment Studied by Panoramix. Angle Orthodont., 37:94, 1967.

Part IV • *The Systemic Phase of Periodontal Treatment*

Nutritional Therapy in Periodontal Treatment; and Systemic Conditions Which Require Special Considerations

Treatment of Chronic Desquamative Gingivitis (Gingivosis) and Menopausal Gingivostomatitis, and Gingival Disease in Puberty, Pregnancy and Menstruation

Chapter 57

NUTRITIONAL THERAPY IN PERIODONTAL TREATMENT; AND SYSTEMIC CONDITIONS WHICH REQUIRE SPECIAL PRECAUTIONS

The treatment of gingival and periodontal disease consists for the most part of local procedures. This is understandable because the local factors so important in the etiology are accessible for correction; whereas in many cases in which systemic causative factors are suspected, it is frequently difficult to establish their nature.

The following are conditions requiring systemic therapy as part of their overall management: (1) **oral manifestations of certain dermatologic diseases (Chap. 13)**, (2) **gingival disturbances attributed to hormonal imbalance (Chap. 58)**, (3) **systemic toxicity in patients with acute gingival disease (Chap. 50)**, (4) **nutritional deficiencies** and (5) **systemic conditions requiring special precautions in patient management.** Of these, the latter two are presented in this chapter.

NUTRITIONAL THERAPY IN THE TREATMENT OF GINGIVAL AND PERIODONTAL DISEASE

Nutritional therapy may be required as an adjunct in the treatment of the following: chronic gingivitis, chronic periodontal disease, acute necrotizing ulcerative gingivitis and other acute conditions of the oral mucous membrane. When indicated, nutritional therapy serves two basic functions in regard to the periodontium: (1) it satisfies the chemical requirements of the tissues by supplying the necessary nutriments, and (2) provides mechanical stimulation to the tissues in the course of mastication.

Nutritional therapy in chronic periodontal disease

Nutritional therapy[16,37] **in the treatment of gingival and periodontal problems should be based upon a demonstrated need,** which is determined as follows:

If when examining a patient it is the operator's impression that the response of the periodontium to existing local factors varies from what he would ordinarily expect, then he may suspect the existence of contributing systemic factors, one of which may be nutritional.

This suspicion must be corroborated by evaluation of the patient's nutritional status (Chap. 33). This entails the medical and dietary history and a physical examination for signs of nutritional disturbances in areas other than the oral cavity. In some instances biochemical tests are indicated.

When existence of a nutritional disturbance has been established, nutritional therapy should be provided as follows:

1. Modify the patient's diet so as to include the necessary nutriments and also satisfy caloric requirements. Standard texts are useful aids in diet analysis and construction.[30] It is preferable to use a protective natural diet rather than to continue a poor diet and attempt to supplement it.

2. Consideration should be given to the **physical character of foodstuffs;** the mechanical stimulation from hard and detergent foods such as raw fruits and vegetables, as well as chewy foods, such as meat, aids in the maintenance of periodontal health.

Nutritional supplements may improve the effectiveness of local periodontal treatment, provided the patient has a nutritional deficiency. The evidence that nutritional supplements (protein,[8,24,39] fats,[38] multivitamins,[14] trace minerals,[40,41] and water-soluble bioflavonoids[6]) prevent gingival or periodontal disease in man or improve the response to local treatment is not conclusive.[15] Some clinical studies[11] indicate that scaling and polishing reduce the severity of gingivitis by 30 per cent, whereas 45 per cent reduction is obtained by the

systemic administration of **synthetic vitamin C alone,** and 67 per cent reduction follows the combination of scaling and polishing with systemic **synthetic vitamin C.** Others[32] note that **increasing the plasma ascorbic acid levels** by dietary supplements in patients with gingival disease and below average plasma ascorbic levels does not improve the condition of the gingiva, and find no significant relationship between either whole blood or urine **ascorbic acid** levels and the periodontal status.[42] It has also been reported that elevating the **ascorbic acid** level of the blood by dietary supplements does not decrease **tooth mobility** or affect the ascorbic acid level of inflamed gingiva or influence the outcome of local treatment.[17,31]

It has been suggested that gingivitis is more severe and the response to oral prophylaxis is poor in individuals with inadequate **carbohydrate metabolism** as reflected in **nonfasting blood glucose levels,**[9] whereas other investigators find no significant relationship between the periodontal status and either **fasting or postprandial serum glucose levels.**[43]

Some investigators have suggested beneficial effects from **fluoride in the treatment of osteoporosis and other human metabolic bone disease,**[4,10] and fluoride concentrations from 4 to 5.8 p.p.m. in water have been shown to reduce the prevalence and severity of osteoporosis.[3] Others[21] have found that the addition of **fluoride** to the diet has no effect on osteoporosis induced in dogs by feeding low calcium–high phosphorus diets. Periodontal disease has been reported to be less severe in individuals using drinking water with 1.2 p.p.m. **fluoride,** compared with those using water containing 0.1 p.p.m.[12] X-ray diffraction studies of human bone indicate that a rise in fluoride content is accompanied by an increase in apatite crystal size, which produces a more stable bone apatite.[35] In tissue cultures, low concentrations of **fluoride** inhibit bone resorption without any apparent effect on bone formation, but high concentrations of fluoride inhibit both bone formation and resorption.[18] Systemic **fluoride** has been recommended for the treatment of alveolar atrophy,[26] but there are conflicting reports regarding the effectiveness of high doses of fluoride in preventing alveolar bone loss in rats.[22,49]

Oral mucosal lesions caused by nutritional deficiency respond to nutritional therapy alone (Fig. 57–1). However, in nutritionally deficient patients with periodontal disease nutritional therapy is only an adjunct to local treatment. **The eradication of gingivitis and periodontal pockets requires removal of all forms of local irritation and the maintenance of effective oral hygiene.**[32, 34]

Removal of local irritants is essential for other reasons. **The chronic inflammation and circulatory congestion they produce interferes with the transport of nutrients.** This may create a local conditioned nutritional deficiency in the periodontium of individuals with a satisfactory nutritional status—and prevent the periodontium from benefiting from nutritional therapy where nutritional deficiencies exist. In addition, the degeneration that often accompanies inflammation or is caused by injurious occlusal forces impairs the capacity of the periodontal tissues to utilize nutrients.

Patients on special diets for medical reasons

Patients on low residue, nondetergent diets often develop gingivitis because the foods lack cleansing action and the tendency for plaque and food debris to accumulate on the teeth is increased. Because fibrous foods are contraindicated, special effort is made to compensate for the soft diet by emphasizing the patient's oral hygiene procedures. Patients on salt-free diets should not be given saline mouthwashes, nor should they be treated with saline preparations without consulting the patient's physician. Diabetes, gallbladder disease and hypertension are examples of conditions in which particular care should be taken to avoid the prescription of contraindicated foodstuffs.

Supportive nutritional therapy in acute necrotizing ulcerative gingivitis and other acute conditions of the oral mucous membrane

Nutritional considerations in the treatment of acute necrotizing ulcerative gingivitis in nutritionally deficient patients were presented in Chapter 50. Severe cases of acute necrotizing ulcerative gingivitis or other painful conditions, such as acute herpetic gingivostomatitis, aphthous stomatitis, desquamative gingivitis, erythema multiforme, bullous lichen planus or pemphigus, are often accompanied by poor appetite, inability to chew or swallow food and excessive loss of fluids, nitrogen and water-

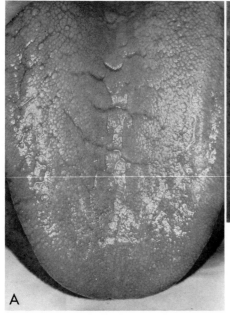

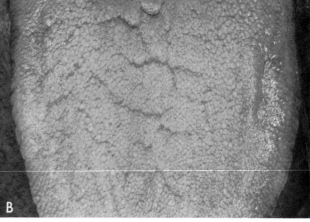

Figure 57–1 Tongue Changes Following Nutritional Therapy. *A,* Atrophy of the papillae in patient with vitamin B complex deficiency. *B,* Regeneration of papillae after nutritional therapy.

soluble vitamins (vitamin B complex and vitamin C). In such patients nutritional therapy may be indicated as a supportive measure to restore a chemically adequate nutrition in order to obtain maximum benefits from local treatment.

SYSTEMIC THERAPY FOR CHRONIC PERIODONTAL DISEASE

There are two aspects of systemic therapy to supplement local procedures in the treatment of chronic periodontal disease. The first deals with **patients with a known systemic disease, such as hyperthyroidism, osteoporosis or diabetes, in which the effectiveness of local treatment in attaining cessation of bone destruction depends upon treatment of the systemic disturbance.** The desired results are obtained by a close working relationship with the patient's physician.

The second aspect of systemic therapy for chronic periodontal disease is still in its experimental stage. It consists of the systemic use of drugs or tissue extracts (Herosteon L3532, Vaduril, Alveoactive, Ebosone and Siccacel)[5, 20] for the purpose of stimulating cellular activity in the periodontium in an effort to improve the response to local treatment.

SYSTEMIC CONDITIONS WHICH REQUIRE SPECIAL PRECAUTIONS

Acute and subacute leukemia

Patients with acute and subacute leukemia often present periodontal problems which, in addition to being painful, jeopardize the systemic management of the patient. **Gingival enlargement that interferes with mastication, persistent gingival bleeding, and acute gingival and periodontal infection that cause severe systemic complications,** are examples of conditions requiring immediate periodontal care.

Periodontal treatment in acute and subacute leukemia introduces risks of troublesome **hemorrhage** and severe **infection** and should be approached with proper precautions.[36] **The hematologic findings should be checked with particular reference to bleeding and clotting time, platelet count and prothrombin time.**

One of the most common problems in these patients is **gingival enlargement** (Chap. 28), which produces deepened gingival crevices in which plaque, food debris and bacteria accumulate. The resulting gingival inflammation is usually aggravated by the fact that the patients have stopped toothbrushing, either because they were frightened by gingival bleeding or preoccupied with concern regarding their "blood condition," or because of physical weakness.

In most cases, the first thing to do is remove the accumulated plaque and debris, and carefully cleanse around the necks of the teeth with a pellet of cotton saturated with 3 per cent hydrogen peroxide. Place the patient on a plaque control regimen, preparing the patient to expect some gingival bleeding during the cleansing procedures. After 24 to 48 hours the gingival condition is usually improved. Superficial scaling is carried out to further reduce the the inflammation and the enlargement (Fig. 57–2).

In patients with persistent gingival bleeding the source is usually deep in a periodontal pocket. Surface hemostatics alone are not effective in controlling such bleeding. The following procedure is recommended: Carefully cleanse the area with a pellet of cotton saturated with 3 per cent hydrogen peroxide to remove partially clotted debris. Locate the bleeding point in the periodontal pocket. Carefully explore along the tooth surface adjacent to the bleeding point to locate calculus and other deposits and remove them, making every effort to avoid injury to the gingiva. Clean the area again with hydrogen peroxide. Place a cotton pellet saturated with thrombin or dipped in ferric subsulfate (Monsel's Salt) against the bleeding point. Cover the area with a gauze sponge and maintain it in position under pressure for at least 20 minutes. Remove the gauze; if there are still signs of oozing; a periodontal pack should be applied for at least 24 hours.

Acute necrotizing ulcerative gingivitis often complicates the oral picture in acute and subacute leukemia. The regular treatment (Chap. 50) is followed; its primary purpose is to make the patient comfortable and eliminate a source of systemic toxicity. Systemic antibiotics are essential to prevent complications.

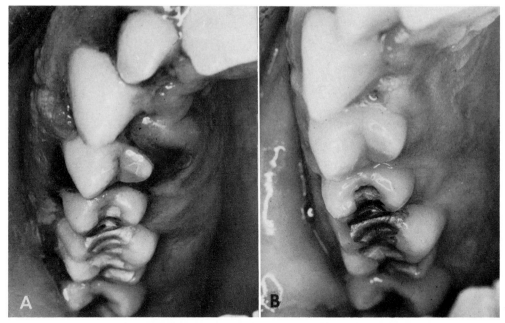

Figure 57–2 Acute Monocytic Leukemia. *A,* Gingival enlargement and bleeding in leukemic patient. *B,* After careful scaling and curettage and improved oral hygiene.

Acute gingival or periodontal abscesses are common sources of pain in these patients, with regional adenopathy and systemic complications. The latter are controlled by systemic antibiotics. Under topical anesthesia—using a Bard-Parker #11 or #12 blade—the abscess is incised to provide drainage, and cleaned with cotton pellets saturated with 3 per cent peroxide. Bleeding is stopped with a gauze sponge held under pressure for 20 minutes. The acute symptoms generally subside after 24 hours.

In **chronic leukemia** gingival and periodontal disorders may be treated by scaling and curettage without complications; but an effort should be made to avoid periodontal surgery. Adherent superficial deposits not dislodged with cotton pellets are removed with the scalers, making every effort to avoid injuring the gingiva, and the patient is instructed in plaque control.

Hemorrhagic disorders

HEMOPHILIA. Scaling and curettage and periodontal surgery can be performed on patients with hemophilia provided sufficient precautions are taken;[25] it is preferable to avoid surgery. The precautions include hospitalization before treatment, trans-fusions with fresh whole blood, fresh human plasma or intravenous Factor VIII (2.5 ml./kg./hour) for 10 hours to achieve a 30 per cent blood level of Factor VIII. Factor VIII may be given postoperatively (1 ml./kg./hour) until bleeding has stopped.[14]

After scaling and curettage or surgery, dried thrombin and oxidized cellulose are packed around the area previous to insertion of the periodontal pack. Other local measures for the control of bleeding include electrocautery and Monsel's solution.

Christmas Disease (Hemophilia B). **Periodontal therapy should present no problems, since the clotting defect responds to administration of blood or plasma.**[28] Surgery should be confined to small areas. Before the periodontal pack is inserted, bleeding points should be controlled by cotton pellets saturated with Monsel's solution applied under pressure or electrocautery.

PROTHROMBIN DEFICIENCY. **Bleeding tendencies caused by prothrombin deficiency**[29] **can be remedied by the systemic administration of vitamin K, except in patients with advanced liver disease.** Vitamin K, 50 mg., or menadione sodium bisulfite, a synthetic vitamin K analogue, 72 mg., is administered intravenously immediately preceding treatment, and may be repeated daily if necessary. In patients with advanced liver disease, daily intravenous doses of vitamin K, 150 mg., may be tried, but administration of fresh whole blood or plasma may also be required.

It should be emphasized that difficulties in patients with bleeding tendencies can be reduced by operating with extreme care with a minimum of tissue laceration.

Diabetes

Special precautions are indicated in the periodontal care of diabetic patients.[19] Treatment should not be undertaken until the diabetes is under control. Dental visits should not interfere with the patients' eating schedule so as to minimize the likelihood of diabetic acidosis, coma or insulin reaction. **Elderly chronic diabetics are prone to arteriosclerosis, hypertension and coronary artery disease.** In such pa-

tients the need for periodontal surgery should be weighed against the risk involved. It is preferable to perform the surgery in a hospital where cardiovascular complications can be handled properly.

In diabetics, resistance to infection is reduced. The causes are not understood, but the decreased resistance has been attributed to impaired antibody formation, reduced phagocytic activity, and a lowered state of cellular nutrition.[27] Therefore antibiotics should be prescribed before and after extensive scaling and curettage or surgical procedures (penicillin, 250 mg. every four hours, beginning the evening before treatment and continuing for 48 hours postoperatively).

Controlled diabetics should respond well to periodontal therapy (Fig. 57–3). All local etiologic factors must be eliminated, and the patient must provide fastidious oral hygiene. In young adult

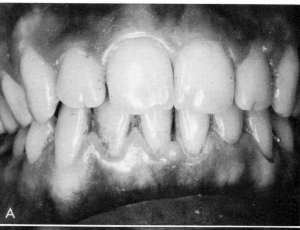

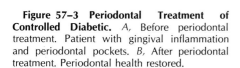

Figure 57–3 Periodontal Treatment of Controlled Diabetic. *A,* Before periodontal treatment. Patient with gingival inflammation and periodontal pockets. *B,* After periodontal treatment. Periodontal health restored.

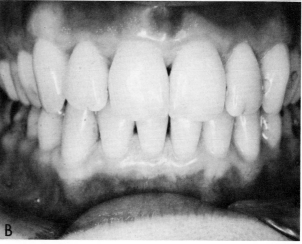

diabetics elimination of gingival and periodontal disease may reduce the insulin required to control the diabetes.[47]

Cardiac disorders

Patients with a history of **coronary insufficiency** or **hypertensive heart disease**, which may be accompanied by symptoms of **angina pectoris**, are ordinarily under medical care and required to avoid exertion and excitement, or excessive activity. **The patient's physician should be consulted before undertaking periodontal treatment.** The patient should be sedated at home before leaving for the office or sedated at the office 30 minutes before beginning treatment. If barbiturates are used, someone should accompany the patient; if this is not feasible, the patient should be hospitalized. Treatment done at each visit should be limited. Local anesthetics should be used without vasoconstrictor drugs,[1] or with a minimal adequate amount (epinephrine, 1:100,000).[7]

In patients with a history of **congenital cardiac defects, plastic valve replacements or rheumatic heart disease, premedication with antibiotics or chemotherapeutic agents is indicated before scaling and curettage or surgical periodontal procedures.** There are several premedication procedures; the following is recommended.[13] Procaine penicillin, 600,000 units, supplemented by crystalline penicillin G, 600,000 units, intramuscularly one to two hours before the dental procedure, and 600,000 units of procaine penicillin intramuscularly daily for two days postoperatively. If oral penicillin is used, the dosage is 250 mg. of phenoxymethyl penicillin one to two hours before the dental procedure, and every four hours after for two days. In penicillin-sensitive patients other antibiotics (see page 816) or chemotherapeutic agents may be used.

Patients on anticoagulant therapy

Anticoagulants are used as continuous therapy in patients with coronary artery disease for the purpose of preventing intravascular clotting. Drugs used for this purpose are heparin, bishydroxycoumarin (Dicumarol), warfarin sodium (Coumadin), phenindione derivatives (Hedulin and Danilone), cyclocumarol (Cumopyran) and ethyl biscoumacetate (Tromexan ethyl acetate).[23, 44]

Heparin inactivates thrombin and has an almost immediate anticoagulant effect; the other drugs depress prothrombin synthesis in the liver, and require a longer period to develop their anticoagulant effect.[2] Dosage is generally adjusted so that the patient's normal prothrombin time (Quick test) is increased one-and-a-half to two-and-a-half times. Vitamin K, or a synthetic analogue, is used to reduce the prothrombin time if it becomes excessive.

An increasing number of patients are being placed on anticoagulant therapy, and appropriate inquiry should be included in every case history. **The patients are on a scheduled recall program for check of prothrombin time and physical examination by their physician, who should be consulted before periodontal treatment is begun.** The danger of clotting if the anticoagulant is stopped is greater than the problem of bleeding under drug therapy, provided proper precautions are taken.[45] **The range within which moderate scaling procedures can be safely performed is one and one half to two times the average normal prothrombin time (12 to 14 seconds).**[13] Aspirin should not be prescribed for these patients, because when combined with anticoagulants it may lead to excessive bleeding.

Scaling and curettage can usually be performed without difficulty, but patients should not be dismissed until bleeding has stopped. A gauze sponge is applied under moderate pressure to hasten the clotting. Periodontal surgery may be performed in such patients, but factors other than the risk of hemorrhage should be considered. Because of the cardiac condition for which the anticoagulants are being used, elective surgery may be contraindicated. In older patients scaling and curettage is often an advisable compromise.

It is preferable to perform periodontal surgery in a hospital, where emergency care is available, but it may also be performed in small segments in the dental office. Resection of the gingiva with electrosurgery reduces the bleeding. Local anesthesia with epinephrine or other vasoconstrictors 1:100,000 is preferred to general anesthesia. Before the periodontal pack is applied, bleeding is stopped by packing cotton pellets interproximally and applying pressure facially and lingually with a gauze sponge. The periodontal pack is inserted over the cotton pellets.

Patients on corticosteroid therapy

Corticosteroid hormones are used widely for the long-term treatment of a variety of conditions such as rheumatoid arthritis, lupus erythematosus, periarteritis nodosa, dermatomyositis, scleroderma, bronchial asthma, allergic vasomotor rhinitis, pulmonary fibrosis, sarcoidosis, ulcerative colitis, regional ileitis, pemphigus, psoriasis, atopic dermatitis, acute gouty arthritis, and certain renal diseases and hematologic disorders.

The prolonged administration of potent corticosteroids may lead to inactivity and atrophy of the adrenals, resulting in hypoadrenalism. Sustained hormonal therapy with cortisone or ACTH results in a variety of side effects, many of which resemble naturally occurring Cushing's syndrome,[48] are characterized by fever, hypertension and anoxia, and may be fatal. In addition, these patients cannot tolerate the stress of an operative procedure[33] and are less capable of coping with infection. Topically applied corticoids in the form of ointments or eyedrops may not have this depressant effect upon the adrenals.[46]

Patients on prolonged corticosteroid therapy should be given an additional 100 mg. of cortisone acetate or 20 mg. of Prednisone administered orally two hours before periodontal surgery to prevent acute adrenal crisis. As a precautionary measure Solu-Cortef should be available for intravenous administration. Prophylactic antibiotic therapy (250 mg. of penicillin orally three times a day, or other antibiotics) should begin 24 hours before each periodontal treatment and continue for 48 hours postoperatively.

ADDISON'S DISEASE. Patients with Addison's disease ordinarily receive a daily oral dose of 25 to 37.5 mg. of cortisone, which is equivalent to 5 to 7.5 mg. of prednisolone. For periodontal surgery, these patients should receive 100 to 200 mg. of cortisone intramuscularly, 18 to 24 hours before operation. The regular oral dose is omitted. On the day of surgery, the patients receive 100 mg. of cortisone intramuscularly. The next day they return to their regular daily oral dose.

Hyperthyroidism

In hyperthyroidism the patient's condition should be under control before extensive periodontal treatment is undertaken. Periodontal surgery may be performed in an uncontrolled or unsuspected hyperthyroid without complication but thyrotoxic episodes characterized by angina, tachycardia or other cardiac arrhythmias may occur.

Apprehensive and neurotic patients

Apprehensive and neurotic patients require special management. The former are premedicated with Nembutal or Seconal, 100 mg. 30 minutes before operating, or are treated with tranquilizing drugs. Neurotic patients with deep-seated anxieties are more complicated problems. The success of treatment may be jeopardized by a peculiar reaction of such patients to some aspect of the case management.

REFERENCES

1. American Dental Association and American Heart Association: Management of Dental Problems in Patients with Cardiovascular Disease. J.A.M.A., 187:848, 1964, Summary.
2. Behrman, S. J., and Wright, I. S.: Dental Surgery During Continuous Anticoagulant Therapy. J.A.D.A., 62:172, 1961.
3. Bernstein, D. S., et al.: Prevalence of Osteoporosis in High- and Low-Fluoride Areas in North Dakota. J.A.M.A., 198:499, 1966.
4. Bernstein, D. S., et al.: The Use of Sodium Fluoride in Metabolic Bone Disease. In Proceedings of the American Society for Clinical Investigation. J. Clin. Invest., 42:916, 1963.
5. Bertolini, A. G.: Behandlung parodontaler Kollagenopathien mit lebenden Liophilzellen Siccacel. Parodontol., 16:66, 1962.
6. Carvel, R. I., and Halperin, V.: Therapeutic Effect of Water-Soluble Bioflavonoids in Gingival Inflammatory Conditions. Oral Surg., Oral Med. & Oral Path., 14:847, 1961.
7. Chamberlain, F. L.: Management of Medical-Dental Problems in Patients with Cardiovascular Diseases. Mod. Concepts Cardiovasc. Disease, 30:697, 1961.
8. Cheraskin, E., and Ringsdorf, W. M., Jr.: Perio-

dontal Pathosis in Man. X. Effect of Combined Versus Animal Protein Supplementation upon Sulcus Depth. J. Oral Ther., 1:497, 1965.

9. Cheraskin, E., and Ringsdorf, W. M., Jr.: Resistance and Susceptibility to Oral Disease. I. A study in Gingivitis and Carbohydrate Metabolism. J. D. Res., 44:374, 1965.

10. Cohen, P., and Gardner, F. H.: Induction of Subacute Skeletal Fluorosis in a Case of Multiple Myeloma. New England J. Med., 271:1129, 1964.

11. El-Ashiry, G. M., Ringsdorf, W. M., Jr., and Cheraskin, E.: Local and Systemic Influences in Periodontal Disease: II. Effect of Prophylaxis and Natural Versus Synthetic Vitamin C upon Gingivitis. J. Periodont., 35:250, 1964.

12. Englander, H. R., Kesel, R. G., and Gupta, O. P.: The Aurora-Rockford, Illinois, Study. II. Effect of Natural Fluoride on the Periodontal Health of Adults. Am. J. Pub. Health, 53:1233, 1963.

13. Fay, J. T.: Dental Procedures for the Patient with Cardiovascular Disease. J.A.D.A., 78:105, 1969.

14. Febbraro, E. E.: New Experiences with Vitamin E in Periodontis. Rev. Gaucha Odont., 7:25, 1959.

15. Glickman, I.: Nutrition in the Prevention and Treatment of Gingival and Periodontal Disease. J. D. Med., 19:179, 1964.

16. Glickman, I.: The Role of Nutritional Therapy in the Management of Periodontal Disease. J.A.D.A., 52:275, 1956.

17. Glickman, I., and Dines, M. M.: Effect of Increased Ascorbic Acid Blood Levels on the Ascorbic Acid Level in Treated and Non-treated Gingiva. J. D. Res., 42:1152, 1963.

18. Goldhaber, P.: The Inhibition of Bone Resorption in Tissue Culture by Nontoxic Concentrations of Sodium Fluoride. Israel J. Med. Sci., 3:617, 1967.

19. Gottsegen, R.: Dental and Oral Considerations in Diabetes. In Ellenberg, M., and Rifkin, H. (eds.): Clinical Diabetes Mellitus. New York, McGraw-Hill, 1962.

20. Held, A. J.: Endogenous Therapy in Parodontolysis. Paradentologie, 3:7, 1949.

21. Henrikson, P., et al.: Fluoride and Nutritional Osteoporosis: Physicochemical Data on Bones from an Experimental Study in Dogs. J. Nutr., 100:631, 1970.

22. Kristoffersen, T., Bang, G., and Meyer, K.: Lack of Effect of High Doses of Fluoride in Prevention of Alveolar Bone Loss in Rats. J. Periodont. Res., 5:127, 1970.

23. Kwapis, B. W.: Anticoagulant Therapy and Dental Practice, J.A.D.A., 66:172, 1963.

24. Lederman, N. J., and Hazen, S. P.: Relationship Between Supplementary Dietary Protein and Periodontal Health. I.A.D.R. Abst., 1965, p. 53, #66.

25. Leonard, M. E.: Hemophilia. In Conn, H. F. (ed.): Current Therapy. Philadelphia, W. B. Saunders Co., 1957, p. 183.

26. Lukomsky, E. H.: Fluorine Therapy for Exposed Dentin and Alveolar Atrophy. J. D. Res., 20:649, 1941.

27. Marble, A., White, H. J., and Fernald, A. T.: The Nature of the Lowered Resistance to Infection in Diabetes Mellitus. J. Clin. Invest., 17:423, 1938.

28. McIntyre, H., Nour-Eldin, F., Israels, M. C. G., and Wilkinson, J. F.: Dental Extractions in Patients with Haemophilia and Christmas Disease. Lancet, 2:642, 1959.

29. Meyers, M. C.: Hemorrhagic Disorders. In Conn, H. F. (ed.): Current Therapy. Philadelphia, W. B. Saunders Co., 1957, p. 184.

30. Nizel, A. E.: The Science of Nutrition and Its Application in Clinical Dentistry, 2nd ed. Philadelphia, W. B. Saunders Co., 1966, p. 185.

31. O'Leary, T. J., Rudd, K. D., Crump, P. P., and Krause, R. E.: The Effect of Ascorbic Acid Supplementation on Tooth Mobility. J. Periodont.–Periodontics, 40:284, 1969.

32. Parfitt, G. J., and Hand, C. D.: Reduced Plasma Ascorbic Acid Levels and Gingival Health. J. Periodont., 34:347, 1963.

33. Parnell, A. G.: Adrenal Crisis and the Dental Surgeon. Brit. D. J., 116:294, 1964.

34. Pierce, H. B., Newhall, C. A., Merrow, S. B., Lamden, M. P., Schweiker, C., and Laughlin, A.: Ascorbic Acid Supplementation: I. Response of Gum Tissue. Am. J. Clin. Nut., 8:353, 1960.

35. Posner, A. S., et al.: X-Ray Diffraction Analysis of the Effect of Fluoride on Human Bone Apatite. Arch. Oral Biol., 8:549, 1963.

36. Prichard, J. F.: Periodontal Case Management in Hemorrhagic Disease. J. Periodont., 26:247, 1955.

37. Radusch, D. F.: The Periodontal Benefits of Well-Planned Diets. J.A.D.A., 47:14, 1953.

38. Rao, S. S., Shourie, K. L., and Shankwalker, G. B.: Effect of Dietary Fat Variations on the Periodontium. An Experimental Study on Rats. Periodontics, 3:66, 1965.

39. Ringsdorf, W. M., Jr., and Cheraskin, E.: Periodontal Pathosis in Man: IV. Effect of Protein Versus Placebo Supplementation upon Gingivitis. J. D. Med., 18:92, 1963.

40. Ringsdorf, W. M., Jr., and Cheraskin, E.: Periodontal Pathosis in Man. VI. Effect of Multivitamin-Trace Minerals Versus Placebo Supplementation on Gingivitis. J. West. Soc. Periodont., 11:85, 1963.

41. Ringsdorf, W. M., Jr., and Cheraskin, E.: Periodontal Pathosis in Man. VII. Effect of Multivitamin-Trace Mineral Versus Placebo Supplementation on Sulcus Depth. J.A.D.A., 68:1, 1964.

42. Shannon, I. L., and Gibson, W. A.: Intravenous Ascorbic Loading in Subjects Classified as to Periodontal Status. J. D. Res., 44:355, 1965.

43. Shannon, I. L., and Gibson, W. A.: Relationship of Oral Health to Fasting and Postprandial Serum Glucose Levels. J. D. Med., 20:3, 1965.

44. Shira, R. B., Hall, R. J., and Guernsey, L. H.: Minor Oral Surgery During Prolonged Anticoagulant Therapy. J. Oral Surg., Anesth. Hosp. & D. Serv., 20:93, 1962.

45. Waldrep, A. C., Jr., and McKelvey, L. E.: Oral Surgery for Patients on Anticoagulant Therapy. J. Oral Surg., 26:374, 1968.

46. Williams, L. F., Jr., and Wynne, G. F.: Fundamental Approach to Surgical Problems. Springfield, Ill., Charles C Thomas, 1962, p. 127.

47. Williams, R. C., Jr., and Mahan, C. J.: Periodontal Disease and Diabetes in Young Adults. J.A.M.A., 172:776, 1960.

48. Zimmerman, B.: The Endocrine Glands. In Textbook of Surgery. 8th ed. New York, Appleton-Century-Crofts, 1963, Chap. 39.

49. Zipkin, I., Larson, R. H., and Bernick, S.: Blocking of the Nutritionally Induced Periodontal Disease Syndrome with Fluoride. I.A.D.R. Abst., 1970, p. 134.

Chapter 58

TREATMENT OF CHRONIC DESQUAMATIVE GINGIVITIS (GINGIVOSIS), MENOPAUSAL GINGIVOSTOMATITIS AND GINGIVAL DISEASE IN PUBERTY, PREGNANCY AND MENSTRUATION

TREATMENT OF CHRONIC DESQUAMATIVE GINGIVITIS (GINGIVOSIS)

Chronic desquamative gingivitis is more likely a clinical syndrome produced by a variety of diseases than a separate and specific disease entity. It may be an oral manifestation common to bullous derma-

tologic disease, such as benign mucous membrane pemphigoid, lichen planus and pemphigus. The etiology of chronic desquamative gingivitis is not known, although it has long been suspected as being caused by gonadal hormone insufficiency. From the viewpoint of treatment it is more realistic to consider the clinical features without inferring that they are unique to a single disease.

Chronic desquamative gingivitis is treated in two phases:[3]

Phase I. Local treatment of the marginal gingivitis

This consists of scaling and curettage and the elimination of all forms of local irritants. The patient is instructed in plaque control procedures but cautioned not to scuff the gingiva with the toothbrush.

Elimination of the marginal inflammation

also improves the condition of the attached gingiva. Discoloration and edema of the attached gingiva, often a striking clinical finding, is caused by extension of inflammation from the gingival margin. The lingual surface, which is cleansed by the mechanical action of the tongue and by food excursion, is usually less severely involved than the facial surface where local irritants accumulate.

Phase II. Systemic treatment

Systemic corticosteroids are used to supplement the local treatment. Celestone, 0.6 mg. tablets, is prescribed in a dosage of four tablets daily for the first week, decreasing by one-half tablet daily until a symptom-free maintenance dose is attained. Prednisone or prednisolone (5 mg. tablets in an initial dosage of four tablets daily, which is subsequently reduced to meet individual requirements) may also be used. Corticoid

therapy relieves the pain and improves the gingival response to local treatment (Figs. 58–1 and 58–2), but the results are not predictable. Corticosteroids are usually withdrawn gradually after one month, but some patients require continued therapy. Systemic corticoid therapy should not be employed indiscriminately, as side effects of prolonged therapy may be more distressing than the oral symptoms (Chap. 57).

When the desquamative gingival changes result from benign mucous membrane pemphigoid, there may be accompanying ocular and vaginal lesions. Systemic corticoids are effective treatment for this condition and may be combined with the topical use of Kenalog applied three times daily if the oral lesions are severe. Therapy is continued until it can be withdrawn without recurrence of symptoms. The condition of the gingiva improves considerably, but complete restoration of gingival health may not be attained.

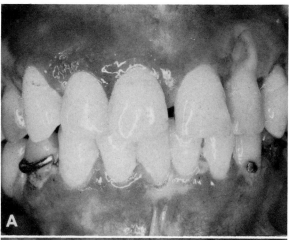
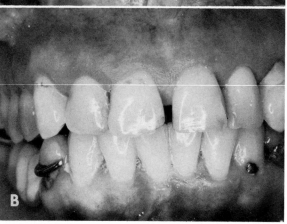

Figure 58–1 Chronic Desquamative Gingivitis. *A,* Before treatment. Diffuse desquamation and surface erosion. *B,* After one month. Condition improved by systemic corticosteroid therapy plus scaling and curettage.

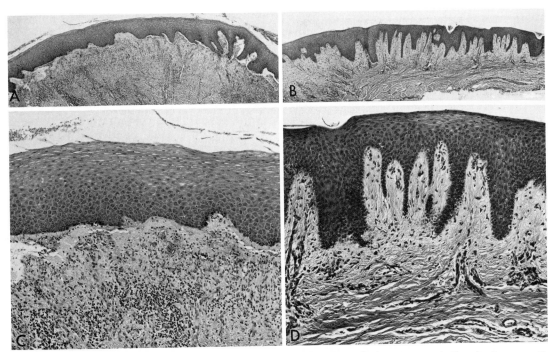

Figure 58–2 Restoration of Normal Microscopic Features Following the Treatment of Chronic Desquamative Gingivitis. *A,* Before treatment. Chronic desquamative gingivitis showing blunting of rete pegs with subepithelial vesicle formation. Compare with *B* which shows same patient after treatment. *B,* Sixteen months after treatment, showing normal histologic features. *C,* Before treatment. Detailed study of area in *A* showing subepithelial vesicle and replacement of connective tissue by edema fibrin and inflammatory cells. Note the blunting of the epithelial rete pegs. *D,* After treatment. Detailed study of area in *B* showing well-formed epithelial rete pegs and papillary connective tissue layer.

Imbalance of gonadal hormones is uncommon in patients with desquamative gingivitis. If it exists, relief of symptoms and improvement in the gingival condition may be obtained by systemic administration of estrogens in females (ethinyl estradiol, 0.05 to 0.15 mg. daily) and androgens in males (methyl testosterone, 5 mg. daily).[2, 7, 12-15] The hormones are administered to stimulate hyperplasia of the atrophic oral epithelium.[10] The symptoms are relieved promptly by this therapy, but improvement in the condition of the gingiva requires at least six months and in many instances it does not occur even after prolonged therapy.

Topical hormones (for female patients Premarin cream, 1.25 mg. of conjugated estrogen per gram; for male patients methyltestosterone ointment, 2 mg./gm. of ointment [Oreton-M]) may be used as a supplement to local therapy in severe cases of desquamative gingivitis. Prolonged topical or systemic estrogen therapy should not be used in patients with a history of suspected malignancy or endometriosis, or with a familial disposition to cancer.[9] In all patients the estrogens are used on alternate months rather than continuously. Successful results with desquamative gingivitis have been reported by supplementing scaling and curettage with topical Kenalog in Orabase (triamcinolone).[13]

In most patients with desquamative gingivitis the etiology cannot be determined. Treatment consists of eliminating the local irritants supplemented with systemic corticosteroid therapy for a limited period. Recurrence is prevented by regular dental visits combined with plaque control by the patient.

Gingival desquamation caused by local factors

Irritation from mouthwashes or hot foods may cause diffuse erythema and desquamation of the gingiva, which may be distinguishable from chronic desquamative gingivitis. **The history and biopsy provide** the basis for differential diagnosis. Discontinuing the offending agent is usually followed by uneventful recovery.

TREATMENT OF MENOPAUSAL GINGIVOSTOMATITIS

The principal problems in these patients are oral pain, dryness, burning and sensitivity to temperature changes; in addition, some patients present painful fissures, erosions or vesicles. Treatment consists of estrogen administered systemically for the pain, either orally, 1 mg. of stilbestrol daily, or parenterally as estradiol dipropinate, 10,000 R.U. in 1 cc. of sesame oil daily. The symptoms usually subside within ten days, when treatment is stopped. It may be continued, if necessary, in smaller doses. Patients should be advised that menstruation may start again under estrogen therapy.

Topical corticosteroid (Kenalog in Orabase) is applied to surface erosions and fissures three times a day after meals for relief of pain. Marginal gingival inflammation is treated by scaling and curettage.

Patients with removable partial prosthesis or complete dentures may complain of soreness under the saddle area or denture. The prosthesis should be checked for sources of irritation, occlusion, peripheral extension and adaptation to the mucosa. If all of these are ruled out as sources of difficulty, the saddle area or denture is then lined with Premarin cream, 1.25 mg. of conjugated estrogen per gram, three times a day after meals.

The cushioning effect of the ointment produces relief lasting about 30 minutes even in the initial stage of treatment. The long-term purpose of the estrogen is to stimulate epithelial hyperplasia so that the mucosa can withstand the pressure of the prosthesis. This usually takes several months. Topical estrogens should be used with caution because they are absorbed and have systemic effects.[6] Absorption may be reduced by using dosages below the threshold of effective systemic action.[1]

Menopausal gingivostomatitis has been treated successfully with injections of estradiol dipropionate under the mucobuccal fold (1 mg. in sesame oil once or twice a week, diminished to once every two or three weeks).[8] This treatment also produced microscopic evidence of hyperplasia of the prickle cell layer of the epithelium with increased activity of the basal cells, and in some instances surface keratinization.

In some cases symptoms may be relieved by intensive systemic vitamin B complex therapy or estrogen therapy singly or in combination,[5] and with daily topical estrogen therapy over a long period. Hormonal therapy is not effective in all cases of menopausal gingivostomatitis. Other possible causative factors for the symptoms, such as vitamin deficiency, diabetes, anemia and psychic disorders, should be explored.[11] **Local irritation from irregularly aligned teeth, sharp incisal edges, rough margins of restorations or calculous deposits should be ruled out before seeking remote causes of the tongue symptoms.**

TREATMENT OF THE GINGIVA IN PUBERTY

Gingivitis in puberty is caused by an exaggerated response to local irritation. Removal of all local irritants combined with plaque control is essential for establishing and maintaining periodontal health. The initial elimination of the gingivitis by scaling and curettage presents no problem; the difficulty lies in preventing recurrence. Slight local irritation causes severe gingival inflammation and edema so that frequent recall visits and repeated instruction in plaque control are necessary to prevent gingival disease during puberty. The problem usually subsides by the age of 17 or 18 when the difference in the response of the gingiva is striking. Areas that were persistent sources of difficulty during puberty are easily brought under control by local treatment and patient care.

TREATMENT OF THE GINGIVA IN PREGNANCY

In pregnancy the emphasis should be upon (1) preventing gingival disease before it occurs, and (2) treating existing gingival disease before it becomes worse. All patients should be seen as early as possible in pregnancy. Those without gingival disease should be checked for potential sources of local irritation, and should be

instructed in plaque control procedures (see page 467). Those with gingival disease should be treated promptly, before the conditioning effect of pregnancy upon the gingiva becomes manifest.

Every pregnant patient should be scheduled for periodic dental visits, and their importance as a preventive against serious periodontal disturbances should be stressed.

The treatment of tumorlike enlargement in pregnancy is described in Chapter 49; other periodontal disorders are treated by scaling and curettage. Periodontal surgery is contraindicated, except for painful conditions which cannot be treated any other way. Other periodontal conditions requiring surgery should be treated palliatively during pregnancy, but definite arrangements should be made for their treatment after parturition.

It is misleading to advise pregnant patients that their periodontal condition is transitory and will disappear after delivery. The severity of gingival disease diminishes after parturition, but the tissues do not return to normal. Those which are untreated or treated palliatively during pregnancy will persist in a less severe form after delivery (Fig. 58–3). Failure to provide the necessary treatment and eliminate the responsible local factors invites worsening of the disease.

TREATMENT OF GINGIVAL CHANGES ASSOCIATED WITH THE MENSTRUAL CYCLE

The menstrual cycle is not usually accompanied by notable gingival changes, but minor disorders such as "periodic bleeding gums" or a bloated congested feeling in the gingiva in the days preceding the menstrual period are occasionally encountered. These occur in areas of chronic inflammation

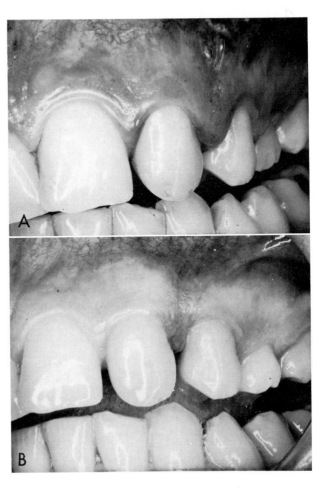

Figure 58–3 Gingiva in Pregnancy, Before and After Parturition. A, Inflamed edematous gingiva treated palliatively in the third trimester of pregnancy. B, One month post-parturition. The gingival condition is markedly improved, but there is residual inflammation which must be treated.

where the circulatory congestion is aggravated by vascular engorgement just previous to the menstrual period. **The removal of local irritants and improved oral hygiene before the next menstrual period usually suffice to correct these problems.**

Recurrence of acute necrotizing ulcerative gingivitis may occasionally be correlated with the onset of the menstrual period. Thorough treatment of the initial episode, which is not confined to relieving acute symptoms but includes complete restoration of periodontal health, reduces the likelihood of such recurrences. Patients under active treatment for acute necrotizing gingivitis may suffer a relapse at the onset of menstruation. The patient is treated palliatively until the menstrual period is over, when the regular course of treatment is continued.

Extensive periodontal curettage and surgery may be followed by excessive gingival bleeding and should be avoided during the menstrual period or in the days just preceding it. Patients with gingival problems during the menstrual period ordinarily require no hormonal therapy; elimination of local irritants and improved oral hygiene usually resolve their problems. **However, patients with persistent cyclical bleeding despite local therapy, or recurrent ulceration or aphthous lesions associated with the menstrual cycle, should be studied medically.**

REFERENCES

1. Chamberlin, T. L., Gardner, W. U., and Allen, E.: Local Responses of the 'Sexual Skin' and Mammary Glands of Monkeys to Cutaneous Applications of Estrogen. Endocrinology, 28:753, 1941.
2. Dreizen, S., Stone, R. E., and Spies, T. D.: A Note on the Use of Pituitary Adrenocorticotropic Hormone (ACTH) and Estradiol Benzoate (Progynon B) in the Treatment of Gingivitis Associated with Endocrine Imbalance. Surg., Gynec. & Obstet., 90:580, 1950.
3. Glickman, I., and Smulow, J. B.: Chronic Desquamative Gingivitis — Its Nature and Treatment. J. Periodont., 35:397, 1964.
4. Goldman, H. M., and Ruben, M. P.: Desquamative Gingivitis and Its Response to Topical Triamcinolone Therapy. Oral Surg., 21:579, 1966.
5. Massler, M., and Henry, J.: Oral Manifestations During the Female Climacteric. The Post-menopausal Syndrome. Alpha Omegan, 44:105, 1950.
6. Moore, C., Lamar, J. K., and Beck, N.: Cutaneous Absorption of Sex Hormones. J.A.M.A., 111:11, 1938.
7. Perl, P.: Testicular Hormone (Methyltestosterone) Used for the Treatment of an Acute Inflammatory Gingival Condition. S. African D. J., 19:339, 1945.
8. Richman, M. J., and Abarbanel, A. R.: Effects of Estradiol, Testosterone, Di-ethylstilbestrol and Several of Their Derivatives upon the Human Oral Mucous Membrane. J.A.D.A., 30:913, 1943.
9. Speert, H.: Local Action of Sex Hormones. Physiol. Review, 28:23, 1948.
10. Ziskin, D. E.: Hormonal Therapy for Some Gingival Conditions. J. D. Res., 18:329, 1939.
11. Ziskin, D. E., and Moulton, R.: Glossodynia: A Study of Idiopathic Orolingual Pain. J.A.D.A., 33:1422, 1946.
12. Ziskin, D. E., and Silvers, H. F.: Two Cases of Subgingival Proliferative Lesions of Probable Hormonal Origin. J. Periodont., 14:89, 1943.
13. Ziskin, D. E., and Silvers, H. F.: Report of a Case of Desquamative Gingivitis and Lichen Planus. J. Periodont., 16:7, 1945.
14. Ziskin, D. E., Silvers, H. F., Stein, G., Kutscher, A. H., and Karshan, M.: Treatment of Some Chronic Lesions of the Oral Mucous Membranes. Oral Surg., Oral Med. & Oral Path., 4:422, 1951.
15. Ziskin, D. E., and Zegarelli, E. V.: Chronic Desquamative Gingivitis. Am. J. Orthodont. & Oral Surg., 31:1, 1945.

Part V • *THE MAINTENANCE PHASE OF PERIODONTAL TREATMENT*

Chapter 59

MAINTENANCE CARE

Preservation of the periodontal health of the treated patient requires as positive a program as the elimination of periodontal disease. After treatment is completed, patients are placed on a program of periodic recall visits for maintenance care to prevent recurrence of the disease.

Transfer of the patient from active treatment status to a maintenance program is a definitive step in total patient care which requires time and effort on the part of the dentist and his staff. Patients must be made to understand the purpose of the maintenance program, with emphasis on the fact that preservation of the teeth is dependent upon it. It is meaningless to simply inform patients that they are to return for periodic recall visits without pinpointing their significance and without describing what is expected of the parents between visits.

THE MAINTENANCE PROGRAM

Periodic recall visits form the foundation of a meaningful long-term prevention program. The interval between visits is set initially at three months, but may be varied according to the patient's needs.

In addition to periodontal considerations, recall visits include examination for dental caries and lesions of the oral mucosa. A complete series of intraoral radiographs is taken every two years and compared with previous radiographs for the preservation of bone height,[5] the repair of osseous defects, signs of trauma from occlusion, periapical pathology and caries.

Periodontal care at each recall visit consists of two phases: one is concerned with gingival health, the other with occlusion.

984

Phase 1. Gingival health

Plaque control should be checked, in the patient's mouth, with disclosing tablets (for plaque control procedures, see page 467). It is helpful to store patients' toothbrushes and rubber interdental cleansers in the dental office in individual plastic boxes for use at recall visits (other plaque control equipment such as dental floss and plastic interdental cleansers, tips for water irrigation devices and mirrors should be provided). **Plaque control must be reviewed and corrected until the patient demonstrates the necessary proficiency, even if it requires additional instruction sessions. Patients' needs in this respect cannot be compromised.**

Plaque control, which is essential for the prevention of gingival disease and as an adjunct to active treatment, is a critical factor in the post-treatment preservation of periodontal health.[5] Patients instructed in plaque control have less plaque and gingivitis than uninstructed patients.[1-3,6]

Review of plaque control is followed by examination for gingival disease and periodontal pockets, plus the required scaling and curettage. Plaque, gingivitis and periodontal pockets tend to recur following all forms of periodontal treatment; periodic scaling and curettage combined with plaque control is the most effective means of minimizing recurrence.

Phase II. The occlusion

The occlusion changes as the natural dentition and dental restorations wear with use. Patients must be checked for the earliest signs of trauma from occlusion (see Chap. 24), and the occlusion should be adjusted when necessary. Periodic evaluation of the occlusion is especially important in patients whose periodontal treatment included correction of the occlusion with extensive dental restorations, or occlusal adjustment.

REFERENCES

1. Lindhe, J., and Koch, G.: The Effect of Supervised Oral Hygiene on the Gingiva of Children. J. Periodont. Res., 1:260, 1966.
2. Lindhe, J., and Koch, G.: The Effect of Supervised Oral Hygiene on the Gingivae of Children. J. Periodont. Res., 2:215, 1967.
3. Rateitschak, K. H.: The Therapeutic Effect of Local Treatment on Periodontal Disease Assessed upon Evaluation of Different Diagnostic Criteria. 2. Changes in Gingival Inflammation. J. Periodont., 35:155, 1964.
4. Rateitschak, K. H., Engelberger, A., and Marthaler, T. M.: The Therapeutic Effect of Local Treatment on Periodontal Disease Assessed upon Evaluation of Different Diagnostic Criteria. 3. Radiographic Changes in Appearance of Bone. J. Periodont., 35:263, 1964.
5. Simaan, C., and Skach, M.: Clinical and Histological Evaluation of Gingival Massage in the Treatment of Chronic Gingivitis. J. Periodont., 37:383, 1966.
6. Stahl, S. S., et al.: Gingival Healing. IV. The Effects of Home Care on Gingivectomy Repair. J. Periodont. – Periodontics, 40:264, 1969.

Index

Page numbers in *italic* type refer to illustrations. Page numbers in **boldface** type refer to tables.